Scientific Foundations of
Trauma

This volume is dedicated to
Major General Robert Scott 1929–1991

Quiet but persistent in his pursuit of scientific answers to military injury he contributed greatly to the protection of service personnel against injury. Dedicated to peace, he yet served the machine of defence and was foremost in the idea for this volume. Regrettably one of his main interests – sailing – led to his death before its completion so we regard it as both a duty and an honour that he should be remembered through this dedication.

Scientific Foundations of
Trauma

Editors

Graham J. Cooper OBE, PhD

Technical Manager/Trauma and Surgery, Chemical and Biological Defence Establishment, Defence Evaluation and Research Agency, Porton Down, Salisbury, UK

Hugh A. F. Dudley CBE, MCh, FRCS

Emeritus Professor, Strathdon, Aberdeenshire, UK

Donald S. Gann MD

Professor of Surgery and Physiology, Executive Vice-chairman, Department of Surgery, University of Maryland, Baltimore, USA

Roderick A. Little PhD, FRCPath, FFAEM

Professor of Surgical Sciences, Director, North Western Injury Research Centre and Head, MRC Trauma Group, Manchester, UK

Robert L. Maynard BSc, MB, BCh, MRCPath, MRCP

Senior Medical Officer, Department of Health, London, UK

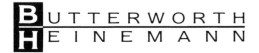

Butterworth-Heinemann
Linacre House, Jordan Hill, Oxford OX2 8DP
A division of Reed Educational and Professional Publishing Ltd

 A member of the Reed Elsevier plc group

OXFORD BOSTON JOHANNESBURG
MELBOURNE NEW DELHI SINGAPORE

First published 1997

British Library Cataloguing in Publication Data
A catalogue record for this book is available from the British Library

Library of Congress Cataloguing in Publication Data
A catalogue record for this book is available from the Library of Congress

ISBN 0 7506 1585 0

Coventry University

Composition by Genesis Typesetting, Laser Quay, Rochester, Kent
Printed and bound in Great Britain by The Bath Press plc, Bath

Contents

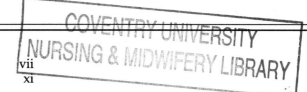

Part 1: Mechanisms of Injury

Part 2: Pathophysiology of Injury

Contributors

T. A. Abbott BSc
Formerly Head of Ballistic Protection Section,
Stores and Clothing – Research and Development
Establishment, Colchester, UK

I. V. Allen MD, DSc, FRCPath
Professor, Department of Neuropathology, The
Queen's University of Belfast, Institute of
Pathology, Belfast, UK

D. J. Anton MSc(OccMed), MB, BS, FFOMD, Av
Med, MAE
Honorary Consultant Occupational Physician,
Frenchay NHS Healthcare Trust, Bristol, UK

S. Bahrami PhD
Docent, Ludwig Boltzmann Institute for
Experimental and Clinical Traumatology, Vienna,
Austria

Y. S. Bakhle MA, DPhil, DSc
Reader in Biological Pharmacology, Department
of Applied Pharmacology, National Heart and
Lung Institute, London, UK

R. N. Barton PhD
MRC Scientific Staff, North Western Injury
Research Centre, University of Manchester,
Manchester, UK

J. Björk MD, PhD
Research Scientist, Pharmacia and Upjohn, Lund
Research Center, Lund, Sweden

G. W. Bowyer MA(Camb), FRCS(Orth)
Major, formerly Lecturer in Military Surgery,
Royal Army Medical College, London, UK

T. G. Buchman PhD, MD
Professor of Surgery, Director of Burn, Trauma
and Critical Care, Department of Surgery,
Washington University School of Medicine,
St Louis, Missouri, USA

G. B. Bulkley MD
Mark M. Ranitch Professor of Surgery, Johns
Hopkins Hospital, Baltimore, Maryland, USA

R. Bullock MD, PhD, FRCS(SN)
Lind Lawrence Associate Professor, Neurological
Surgery, MCV Neurosciences Center, Virginia
Commonwealth University, West Hospital,
Virginia, USA

†S. Burzstein MD
Formerly Professor of Technion, Faculty of
Medicine and Director of Department of Intensive
Care, Rambam Medical Centre, Haifa, Israel

G. Carlson BSc, FRCS
Clinical Scientist, MRC Trauma Group, North
Western Injury Research Centre and Honorary
Surgeon, Department of Surgery, Hope Hospital,
Salford, UK

F. B. Cerra MD, FACS, FCCM
Professor of Surgery, Department of Surgery,
Medical School, University Hospital and Clinic,
University of Minnesota, USA

W. G. Cioffi, Jr MD, FACS
Associate Professor of Surgery, Chief, Division of
Trauma and Burns, Rhode Island Hospital, Brown
University, USA

G. Cliff MSc(Cape Town)
Executive Officer: Research, Natal Sharks Board,
Durban, Republic of South Africa

G. J. Cooper OBE, PhD
Technical Manager/Trauma and Surgery,
Chemical and Biological Defence Establishment,
Defence Evaluation and Research Agency, Porton
Down, Salisbury, UK

D. L. Coppel FFARCS
Consultant in Anaesthesia/Intensive Care
Medicine, Regional Intensive Care Unit, Royal
Victoria Hospital, Belfast, UK

J. W. L. Davies BSc, PhD
Honorary Scientist, Laing Laboratories, Salisbury
District Hospital, UK

E. A. Deitch MD
Professor of Surgery, Department of Surgery,
Louisiana State University Medical Centre, USA

H. A. F. Dudley CBE, MCh, FRCS
Emeritus Professor, Strathdon, Aberdeenshire, UK

R. G. Evans BSc, PhD
Professor, Department of Physiology, Monash
University, Clayton, Victoria, Australia

J. Flor PhD
Department of Physiology and Cell Biology,
Albany Medical College, New York, USA

B. L. Furman BPharm, PhD, FRPharmS
Senior Lecturer in Pharmacology and Head,
Department of Physiology and Pharmacology,
University of Strathclyde, Glasgow, UK

R. R. Gandhi MD, PhD
Surgical Resident, Department of Surgery, New
York Medical College, Vahalla, USA

D. S. Gann MD
Professor of Surgery and Physiology, Executive
Vice Chairman, Department of Surgery, University
of Maryland, School of Medicine, Baltimore, USA

P. J. Garlick BA, PhD
Professor of Surgery, Department of Surgery,
Health Sciences Center, SUNY at Stony Brook,
New York, USA

R. J. N. Garth FRCS
Consultant Otolaryngologist, Department of
Otolaryngology, Head and Neck Surgery, Royal
Devon and Exeter Hospital, Exeter, UK

D. Glaister OstJ, PhD, MBBS, FFOM, RAF(Ret^d)
Group Captain, Head Biodynamics Division,
Consultant in Aviation Medicine, Whittingham
Professor in Aviation Medicine, Deputy Director,
Royal Air Force, Institute of Aviation Medicine,
Farnborough, UK

R. D. Goldfarb PhD, FAPS
Professor of Physiology and Medicine, Sections of
Cardiology and Critical Care Medicine,
Department of Medicine, Rush-Presbyterian-
St Luke's Medical Centre Chicago, Illinois, USA

D. I. Graham MB, BCH, PhD, FRCP(Glasg),
FRCPath, FRSE
Professor, Department of Neuropathology,
Institute of Neurological Sciences, The Southern
General Hospital, Glasgow, UK

U. Haglund MD
Chairman, Department of Surgery, University
Hospital, Uppsala, Sweden

H. W. Hopf MD
Assistant Professor of Anaesthesia and Surgery,
Department of Anaesthesia, University of
California, San Francisco, USA

J. B. Hull MD, FRCS(Orth)
Consultant Orthopaedic Surgeon, Ministry of
Defence Hospital Unit, Frimley Park Hospital,
Camberley, UK

T. K. Hunt MD
Professor and Vice Chairman for Research,
Wound Healing Research Laboratory, Department
of Surgery, School of Medicine, University of
California, San Francisco, USA

M. J. Iremonger BSc(Eng), PhD
Senior Lecturer, School of Engineering and
Applied Science, Royal Military College of
Science, Cranfield University, Swindon, UK

B. Janzon MSc(EngPhys), PhD(MedSci)
Director, Department of Weapons and Protection,
FOA – National Defence Research Establishment,
Tumba, Sweden

A. Jönsson PhD(MedSci)
Assistant Director of Research, Solna, Sweden
(formerly, FOA – National Defence Research
Establishment, Tumba, Sweden)

E. Kirkman PhD
MRC Non-clinical Scientific Staff, Honorary
Lecturer in Physiology, North Western Injury
Research Centre, University of Manchester, UK

B. Lawton BSc, PhD, CEng, MIMechE
Reader in Thermal Power, School of Engineering
and Applied Science, Royal Military College of
Science, Cranfield University, Swindon, UK

G. Leichtfried BSc
Technician, Ludwig Boltzmann Institute for
Experimental and Clinical Traumatology, Vienna,
Austria

A. K. C. Li MA, MD(Cantab), FRCS(Eng and
Edin), FRACS, FACS, Hon FPCS,
Hon FRCS(Glasg)
Vice Chancellor and Professor of Surgery, The
Chinese University of Hong Kong, Shatin, Hong
Kong

R. A. Little PhD, FRCPath, FFAEM
Professor of Surgical Sciences, Director, North
Western Injury Research Centre and Head, MRC
Trauma Group, Manchester, UK

K. G. Lowry MBCh, MMedSc, FFARCSI
Intensive Care Consultant, Royal Victoria
Hospital, Belfast, UK

J. Ludbrook MD, DSc, ChM, FRCS, FRACS
National Health and Medical Research Council of
Australia Senior Principal Research Fellow,
Cardiovascular Research Laboratory, University of
Melbourne, Department of Surgery, Royal
Melbourne Hospital, Parkville, Victoria, Australia

C. Lundberg MD, PhD
Assistant Professor and Head, Division of
Biotechnology, Medical Products Agency, Uppsala,
Sweden

M. Mars MBChB
Associate Professor, Department of Physiology,
University of Natal, Durban, South Africa

R. L. Maynard BSc, MB, BCh, MRCPath, MRCP
Senior Medical Officer, Department of Health,
London, UK

W. F. McManus MD, FACS
Formerly Director of the Clinical Division of the
US Army Institute for Surgical Research, Fort Sam
Houston, Texas, USA

S. G. Mellor MS, FRCS, RAMC
Lt Colonel and Clinical Director of Surgery, The
Department of Surgery, Royal Naval Hospital,
Portsmouth, UK

T. R. Mokoena MB, ChB(Natal), DPhil(Oxon),
FRCS
Professor and Chief Surgeon, University of
Pretoria, Kalafong Hospital, Pretoria, Republic of
South Africa

G. M. Moss MSc, FRAeS, CEng
Senior Lecturer, Royal Military College of Science,
Cranfield University, Swindon, UK

R. V. Mueller MD
Fellow, Department of Plastic Surgery, University
of California, San Francisco, USA

M. S. Mulligan MD
Resident in Thoracic Surgery, Department of
Pathology, The University of Michigan Medical
School, Ann Arbor, USA

J. R. Parratt PhD, DSc, MDhc, FRCPath, FESC,
FRSE
Professor, Department of Physiology and
Pharmacology, University of Strathclyde, Glasgow,
UK

S. Paterson-Brown FRCS
Consultant Surgeon, University of Edinburgh,
Royal Infirmary, Edinburgh, UK

L. D. Payne BDS, LDS
Honorary Archivist, Ballistic Injury Archives,
Department of Military Surgery, Royal Defence
Medical College, London, UK
e-mail to lpayne@easynet.co.uk

Y. Phillips MD, COL, MC
Colonel, Medical Corps, Department of Medicine,
Walter Reed Army Medical Centre, Washington
DC, USA

B. A. Pruitt, Jr MD, FACS
Colonel, MC, Commander and Director,
Department of the Army, US Army Institute of
Surgical Research, Fort Sam Houston, Texas, USA

H. Redl PhD
Professor, Ludwig Boltzmann Institute for
Experimental and Clinical Traumatology, Vienna,
Austria

P. M. Reilly MD
Trauma Fellow, Department of Surgery – Division
of Trauma and Critical Care, Hospital of the
University of Pennsylvania, Philadelphia, USA

P. Rice BM, MRCPath
Head of Pathology and Clinical Toxicology,
Chemical and Biological Defence Establishment,
Porton Down, Salisbury, UK

G. R. Ripple MD, FCCP, LTC, MC
Staff, Pulmonary and Critical Care Medicine
Centre, Walter Reed Army Medical Centre,
Washington, USA

J. V. Robbs ChM, FRCS, FRCP(G)
Professor and Head, Division of Surgery, Chief
Metropolitan Vascular Service, Department of
Surgery, University of Natal Medical School,
South Africa

N. J. Rothwell BSc, PhD, DSc
Professor, School of Biological Sciences,
Manchester University, Manchester, UK

L. W. Rue III MD, FACS
Associate Professor of Surgery, Chief, Section of
Trauma, Burns and Surgical Critical Care,
Department of Surgery, University of Alabama
School of Medicine, Birmingham, USA

J. M. Ryan MCh, FRCS
Visiting Professor and Senior Lecturer in Trauma
Care, The University College London Hospitals,
Accident and Emergency Directorate, University
College Hospital, London, UK

H. J. Schiller MD
Assistant Professor of Surgery, SUNY Health
Service Center, Department of Surgery, Syracuse,
New York, USA

G. Schlag MD
Professor, Director of the Ludwig Boltzmann
Institute for Experimental and Clinical
Traumatology, Vienna, Austria

R. G. Shephard MA, PhD, CPhys, MInstP
Head Energetic Materials Department, Defence
Research Agency, Fort Halstead, Kent, UK

G. Smedegård PhD
Head, Department of Inflammation Research,
Pharmacia and Upjohn, Uppsala, Sweden

R. F. Spencer MD, FRCS, FCS(SA) Orth
Consultant Orthopaedic Surgeon, Weston General
Hospital, Weston-super-Mare, Honorary
Consultant, Avon Orthopaedic Centre, Bristol and
Honorary Senior Lecturer, University of Bristol,
UK

H. B. Stoner MD, FRCPath, FRCS
Professor, c/o North Western Injury Centre,
University of Manchester, UK

Z. Török MBChB, MSc(Biological Engineering),
MFOM(Lond)
Technical Manager (Medicine), Chemical and
Biological Defence Establishment, Ministry of
Defence, Porton Down, Salisbury, UK

D. D. Trunkey MD, FACS
Professor of Surgery, Chairman, Department of
Surgery, Oregon Health Sciences University,
Portland, Oregon, USA

D. C. Viano PhD
Principal Research Scientist, Research and
Development Center, General Motors
Corporation, Warren, Michigan, USA

A. A. Vlessis MD, PhD
Senior Cardiothoracic Surgery Resident,
University of Michigan Medical Center, Ann
Arbor, USA

P. A. Ward MD
Chairman, Department of Pathology, The
University of Michigan Medical School, Ann
Arbor, USA

M. Waters FRCS
Senior Registrar in Accident and Emergency
Medicine, Westbrook, Rhuddlan, UK

J. Wernerman MD, PhD
Associate Professor at the Karolinska Institute,
Department of Anaesthesiology and Intensive
Care, Huddinge University Hospital, Sweden

D. W. Wilmore MD
Frank Sawyer Professor of Surgery, Department of
Surgery, Harvard Medical School, Brigham and
Women's Hospital, Boston, Massachusetts, USA

R. R. Wolfe PhD
Professor, University of Texas Medical Branch at
Galveston and Chief of Metabolism, Shriners
Burns Institute, Galveston, Texas, USA

D. W. Yates MD, MCh, FRCS
Professor of Accident and Emergency Medicine,
University of Manchester, Manchester, UK

J. T. Yelverton MS
Principal Investigator, EG & G Management
Systems Inc., Albuquerque, New Mexico, USA

Preface

Scientific knowledge potentially applicable to the understanding and management of trauma has increased markedly during this current injury-ridden century. However, we have seen two obstacles to its availability. First, the professional team at the sharp end dealing with the victims in both peace and war is often unaware of the advances in understanding that have taken place at the bench or in the laboratory. This is especially true in relation to military causes and effects as much relevant research is not reported in the general scientific literature. Second, and in spite of the growing interest by the clinician in the scientific underpinning of management, there is still not a complete interlock between the methods of going about obtaining scientific understanding and the putting of the results obtained into action. Vocabularies and attitudes often differ.

This volume arose from an appreciation of the above problems and is an attempt to make some of the scientific foundations of trauma more readily available. It has been somewhat long in gestation which attests to the complexity of the task and the difficulty of knowing exactly what to include from across a very wide range. We are especially grateful to our contributors who have endured long hold-ups with grace and patience. We can only hope that they and our readers will be pleased with the result.

We also owe a considerable debt to Susan Devlin at Butterworth-Heinemann and her team, whose enthusiasm has kept the project alive.

Graham Cooper
Donald Gann
Roderick A. Little
Robert Maynard
Hugh Dudley

PART 1
MECHANISMS OF INJURY

SECTION 1
PENETRATING INJURY BY PROJECTILES

1. Wound Ballistics Research Before 1945

L. D. Payne

The bizarre effects of missiles on tissues are very puzzling. (Wilson, 1921)

INTRODUCTION

No historical review of traumatic injury research can omit to mention the work of Ambrose Paré; a man both skilled and confident enough to use the evidence of his own eyes in the development of new treatment methods not based on inaccurate, orthodox folklore, but on the application of accurate observation of the effects of various procedures.

Paré maintained that gunshot wounds were not poisonous in the sense previously held and would in fact respond to gentle salves and innocuous wound drainage. That the latter may have initially been the result of necessity does not detract either from Paré's ability to learn immediately from the careful observations, experience, or the importance of his contribution to military surgery.

Advances of the kind achieved by Paré and by surgeons during war, based entirely on clinical observation and experiment made in this way, have been of great significance in wound ballistics. Studies undertaken by laboratory workers have often been designed to confirm, extend and explain advances made in the field.

John Hunter in 1792 described wounds caused by musket ball during his service on Belle Isle in 1761, and his observations on the optimal treatment of these wounds reflect the nature of his meticulous investigation. Hunter took great pains to note the relationship between the velocity of the ball and the nature of the wound: 'Velocity in the ball makes parts less capable of healing, than when it moves with a small velocity' (Hunter, 1812).

However, Hunter's detailed recommendations for treatment are less satisfactory and Guthrie in 1815 commented on this in his textbook of gunshot injuries. He based his recommendations on his experience in the Peninsular War, added to and revised after the battle of Waterloo (Guthrie, 1815). Billroth and Bircher considered Guthrie's contribution and that of Hennen (Hennen, 1818) to be among the most important made by the earlier workers. Billroth also pointed out that Guillaume

Dupuytren, the leading French surgeon of his generation, 'contributed more exact studies of the effects of projectiles, as modified by their speed and the resistance encountered. Dupuytren attempted to support his claim that the greater the distance from which the shot is fired, the larger the wound of exit as compared to the wound of entrance. He states that the wounds of exit in soft parts more closely resemble torn than crushed injuries' (Billroth, 1859; Bircher, 1986).

EARLY STUDIES ON THE MECHANISM OF INJURY BY HIGH-VELOCITY PROJECTILES

Huguier, after assisting in the case of the wounded during the 'February Revolution' in Paris of 1848, came to the conclusion that the mechanism of destruction of tissues by projectiles involved a sudden catastrophic rise in pressure. The effect of the tissue being flung aside or bursting from within had led to the assertion that explosive bullets were being used (Huguier, 1848).

Huguier fired into cadaver material (liver and muscle) and convinced himself that the energy of the moving projectile being imparted to the 'water' in the tissues caused the dispersion of these parts in a hydrodynamic fashion. This conclusion was later supported as the cause of the extensive tissue disruption produced by projectiles (Horsley, 1894; Kramer and Horsley, 1897). The importance of these observations appears to have been ignored by contemporary writers, including Billroth.

Sarazin provided evidence of the increasing power of the military rifle (Sarazin, 1867). He fired the 11-mm-bore Chassepot rifle at a suspended human cadaver and drew attention to the remarkable amount of internal damage produced. He also commented on the size of the exit wounds and recommended a detailed review of all aspects of military surgery.

Kocher, in 1875, published the first results of a series of experiments on wounds caused by relatively high-velocity missiles, using the Vetterli rifle, methodically investigating all the physical variables he felt might have a bearing on the nature of wounds produced. He examined such variables as size of projectile, velocity, relative hardness and the possibility of fragmentation within the tissues. He supported this work with experimental data and included in the text the methods of calculation used to evaluate it (Kocher, 1875).

Kocher confirmed Huguier's theory that it was not the bullet, *per se*, but the motion of the tissues that gave the impression of an explosion. It is interesting to note that the bullet velocities studied (1800–2000 ft/s, 591–656 m/s) were similar to those of the American rifles in use in the American war between the States. Kocher continued his interest in terminal effects into the early twentieth century and a photograph in his biography shows him probably in 1904 demonstrating a military rifle fixed in a modified 'Mann Rest' to an interested audience of English surgeons (Bonjour, 1952). Dougherty *et al.* (1987) credits Kocher with disproval of the current theory that tissue disruption was due to the high-speed rotation of a projectile fired from a rifle barrel, by demonstrating that equally destructive wounds could be caused by conoidal bullets from smooth-bore weapons (Kocher, 1879, 1880).

Kocher also showed the pseudo-explosive effect of high-speed rifle bullets by firing them into cans filled with water. Bellamy (Bellamy and Zajtchuk, 1991) have pointed out that Kocher emphasized the importance of maintaining projectile integrity and limiting projectile deformation if the extent of injury was to be limited. Sadly, Kocher's recommendations communicated in 1894 to an International Medical Conference, that to reduce tissue damage a tapered point should be employed (Kocher, 1895), may well have contributed to the introduction of the 'spitzer bullet' which in effect enhanced wounding by ensuring its instability in dense media as described by Pilcher (1911, 1915) and Kirschener (1915).

Wilson in his paper of 1921 gives credit to Kocher as the pioneer in accurate observations on the wounding effects of high-velocity bullets.

Sir Thomas Longmore (Surgeon-General) encapsulated almost the whole of accepted thinking on the mechanisms of wound production in his major work *Gunshot Injuries* published in 1877, pirated editions of which were widely used by the US Army surgeons of the time. He gave a detailed account of the weaponry and ammunition available, as well as extensive statistics of battle casualties. The mid nineteenth century was a period of great change, especially in small-arms development, and he charted this in detail. He commented on the wounds likely to have been produced by muskets of the seventeenth and eighteenth century and he clearly described wounds produced during the nineteenth century when British troops fought against 'uncivilized enemies who were still using weapons whose effects were very similar to early arms'. He continued, 'Out of 211 wounds inflicted on British troops in the Ashanti War of 1873/74 only 18 entailed fatal consequences, either on the field of battle or subsequently'. Those received at close range, however, were very severe with a high mortality. Longmore's experimental work on conoidal bullets had been published earlier in 1863 (Longmore, 1863), and he continued to comment and update his work up to and beyond the second edition of his textbook published in 1897 (Longmore, 1863, 1877, 1881).

The effect of the 'new' Rumanian 6.5-mm Mannlicher rifle bullet was described by Demosthen in experiments which involved 'wartime cartridges with the full charge, fired at metal plates, wooden boards and cubes, tree trunks, sawdust, powder, paraffin, sulphur, clothed corpses, and live horses' (Demosthen, 1894).

These tests were conducted at a comprehensive set of ranges which increased by 10 increments from 5 to 1400 m. In all, some 30 whole corpses and eight live horses were used and 70 photographic figures produced. The wounds in the horses and the corpses were dissected at the end of each session. Demosthen commented on the extravasation of blood in all the perforated organs and on the tendency of the bullet hole in contracted muscle tissue to split along the direction of the muscle fibres. He vigorously disputed the practical use of the findings of Habert and Von Bruns that clean perforations without fracture would be produced in wounds of the skull sustained at long range (600 paces according to Habert and 800 m according to Von Bruns), and attributed these erroneous assertions to the use of reduced charges to simulate the effect of long-range shots (Demosthen, 1894). He also took issue with the statements made by Von Bruns, Habart and Seydel (Seydel, 1893) that at long ranges (1000 paces or 1200 m) clean perforations of long bones could be expected, again attributing this to their use of reduced charges to simulate impact at long range. His experience was that in tests ranging from 100 to 1400 m, wounds of the diaphysis of long bones led to extensive fracture and comminution of the bone. He also emphasized the extent to which the metal-jacketed, higher-velocity rounds were prone to deformation and fragmentation on entering the body, especially after hitting bone. This observation that metal jacketing does not always prevent fragmentation of high-velocity projectiles is important and was confirmed during the Vietnam War when 5.56-mm-calibre bullets were found to be liable to considerable fragmentation (Fackler *et al.*, 1984; Stevens and Ezell, 1987).

Military surgeons Delorme and Chavasse undertook a number of studies on the effects of French military rifles during the late nineteenth century (Delorme and Chavasse, 1891). Stevenson quotes their work frequently as evidence of the devastating short-range wounding effect of the large-bore rifle bullet (Stevenson, 1897). Delorme's textbook on war surgery produced in 1915 contains interesting observations on the terminal effects of the unusual solid bronze 'Balle D' French service round (Delorme, 1915).

Sir Victor Horsley, considered by many to be the doyen of wound ballistics researchers, brought a considerable intellect to bear on the interpretation of the effects of missiles on the head, especially the brain. Horsley's major ballistic investigations began in 1893 and, working with Dr S. P. Kramer, a dentist from Cincinnati, a long series of experiments were undertaken (Paget, 1919).

Horsley described the mechanism by which the effects of missile injury were caused and at the same time dispelled a number of myths concerning the transfer of energy from the projectile to the target. He demolished the old idea that the 'wind of the shot' had any destructive power by demonstrating that the air movements of the projectile could not even rotate a delicate paper vane. Horsley also attempted to investigate the laws of dispersion of energy by firing directly into blocks of soap and clay and studying the track of the missile so recorded. In his laboratory behind University College Hospital Medical School he mounted on a bench a specially constructed 0.22-inch-calibre rifle, provided by Sir Andrew Noble and modified to allow a 40-grain bullet to be fired at velocities ranging from a few hundred to 3500 ft/s, (1150 m/s) (Horsley, 1894; Horsley, 1894/95; Kramer and Horsley, 1897; Horsley, 1915).

Small-calibre bullets were also being studied by others. Von Bruns produced a comprehensive monograph on the wounding capabilities of the then 'state of the art' self-loading pistol – the Mauser of 1897. Using X-ray, he demonstrated extensive comminuted fractures of limb bones in human cadavers. He also produced photographs of the reconstructed bones after dissection and reassembly of the fragments (Von Bruns, 1897).

Writing for a continental surgical audience, Von Bruns also produced extensive information on the effects of soft-nosed bullets on tissue. Much of the work was intended as a direct attack on the use by the British in colonial encounters of the Mark IV Dum-dum round. The motivation behind his work did not reduce its impact and he returned to the theme of excessive wounding on numerous occasions over the next few years. Von Bruns' work had great influence in Europe and a considerable body of opinion opposed to British ammunition was established (Von Bruns, 1889, 1898, 1900).

The writings of Sir Alexander Ogston should be read to balance those views so strongly advocated by Von Bruns in which he refuted Von Bruns' allegations regarding the Mark IV round, by demonstrating similar effects produced by regular rifle bullets. He also took issue with the use of soft-nosed sporting bullets or over-modified service ammunition to mimic the wounds supposedly caused by the official British Mark IV Dum-dum round (Ogston, 1898, 1899a,b).

The paper produced by Keith and Rigby in 1899 also sought to provide more detailed models of the volume of tissue damaged by bullets of contentious designs. These authors used plaster-of-Paris approaching its setting point as a means of modelling and permanently recording the extent of the temporary wound tract in living tissues of the same texture, and it was used to fill in bandage-wrapped skulls as a model for brain tissue. Ordinary yellow soap and paraffin wax were also used as model fillers and to investigate the possible damaging effect of rapid spinning of a bullet within a wound.

A cadaver specially preserved to retain tissue elasticity but firm enough to enable clean sectioning was used to compare the effects of the 0.303-inch-calibre Dum-dum, the Mark II, and Mark IV, service rounds as well as the 0.275-inch Mauser bullet which was used by the Boers in the South African War. They also compared the 0.45-inch Webley service revolver round (often known as a 'man stopper') and the Mauser hollow-nose pistol bullet and illustrated the wound tracts with drawings of sagittal sections of the wounds (Keith and Rigby, 1899).

Marine engineers studying the interaction between propeller blades and water had coined the term 'cavitation' (Barnaby and Thornecroft, 1897) to describe the formation of vapour-filled voids which could then give rise to pitting on moving surfaces. C.E. Woodruff (1898) was the first to adopt this to describe the behaviour of tissue through which the missile had passed.

Woodruff's diagram of the path of a round, with its oscillating cavity outlined in a simple line drawing, illustrates the concept clearly.

The actual process of cavitation could not be recorded visually until the advent of high-speed photography and radiography used by Black, Zuckerman, Burns, Krohn and the Americans under Newton Harvey during the Second World War (see below). Although Woodruff had suggested the possible use of the cinematograph as a technique to record the predicted ballooning of a fluid-filled target, he also predicted the possibility of tissue damage resulting from the violent collapse of a cavity (Woodruff, 1898).

H.G. Beyer in 1898 investigated the effects of bullets fired from the recently introduced Lee straight-pull rifle and demonstrated the ability of a small-calibre, high-velocity round to cause effective incapacitation. The more general acceptance of such small-calibre rounds was thwarted by the failings of the propellent rather than the design concept – a problem which was still causing trouble in the early M-16 rifles in the Vietnam War 65 years later (Stevens, 1987).

Surgeon-Colonel William Flack Stevenson, the second professor of military surgery at the Royal Army Medical College, London, reinforced the need for surgeons to have a practical knowledge of weapons and their effects if they were to appreciate the nature of the injuries they were to treat. Surgeon-Colonel W.F. Stevenson's career spans the period of transition between that of his predecessor, Longmore, and the large-bore single-shot weapons, and that of Spencer, his successor, with magazine rifles and machine guns. In his textbook *Wounds in War* published in 1897, he reviewed, recorded and reported, in great detail, contemporary views and works on terminal ballistics. He confirmed the view of Von Coler and Schjerning (1894) that energy transfer to the tissues was not simply due to hydraulic pressure, as open water-filled lead cans were just as extensively damaged as water-filled closed cans when struck by rifle bullets (Stevenson, 1897, 1898b, 1910).

Stevenson reinforced his position as the leading British authority on terminal effects as a result of taking part in the extensive investigations into the effects of various shapes of bullets at the firing ranges of the Woolwich Arsenal (Stevenson, 1898a). This involvement by professors of surgery of The Royal Army Medical College has become a tradition and continues up to the present.

In 1910 Reverdin produced a comprehensive text entitled 'Lessons in War Surgery', directed mainly towards descriptions of contemporary ballistics and terminal effects. Among the illustrations is a set of high-speed 'Cinematographie' stills demonstrating the effect of a perforating wound of the intact head. The photographs clearly demonstrate the ejection of material from both entry and exit wounds as well as the gross plastic deformation of the skull (Reverdin, 1910). These details were not fully appreciated or further investigated until the work of Zuckerman and Harvey in the Second World War (see below).

Louis A. Lagarde figures prominently in the American literature on wound ballistics as a result of his extensive account in the 'Report of the Surgeon General of the Army for 1893' (Lagarde, 1893) of the effects to be anticipated with the use of the new high-velocity small-calibre rounds, compared to the 0.45-calibre Springfield rifle, and his extensive lecturing on wound ballistics (Lagarde, 1894, 1900).

Lagarde's work on poisoned wounds also demonstrated the failure of the heat generated in firing to sterilize bullets by firing anthrax-contaminated bullets into animals and observing them until they developed the disease (Lagarde, 1903).

The demand to examine the requirements needed to produce adequate 'stopping power' in the US Army's side-arm, after the failure of the 'long 38 round' to incapacitate Moro Guerillas in the Phillipines, led to the classic study by Thompson and Lagarde reporting the effects of pistol rounds on steers (Thompson and Lagarde, 1904). However, the work seems to have been little studied since it has recently been summarized by Leone Day (Day, 1983). Lagarde's experience led him to revise the interpretation of some of the earlier conclusions of others, and his comprehensive work, first published in 1914 and revised in 1916, provides an extensive account of experimental studies and should be consulted by all interested in the history of wound ballistics (Lagarde, 1914).

EARLY TWENTIETH-CENTURY STUDIES

Journée, a young French artillery officer, carried out a wide-ranging review of actual bullet wounds in corpses examined on the battlefield, as well as comprehensive and more controlled experiments on horses. His purpose was to determine the relationship between the kinetic energy of a bullet and the gravity of the wounds inflicted (Journée, 1907). His experiments compared the injuries produced by a soft lead ball, cylindro-conoidal lead bullets and jacketed round-nosed bullets. However, he also compared the effect of an 'elephant gun' of 21.2 mm calibre with what appears to a very modern round of 4.5 mm calibre and a muzzle velocity of 1000 m/s. From these comparisons he concluded that the force required to fracture a human femur was 16 kg/cm^2, and for that of a horse 35 kg/cm^2. The minimum force needed to cause perforating wounds in man was about 2 kg/cm^2 and 10 kg/cm^2 in horses.

In 1908 a naval surgeon published his views based on an extensive reading of contemporary small-arms literature and a description of his own research work (Beadnell, 1908). He reported an unusual experiment designed to investigate the transmitted effects of shock waves and, though he did not identify it as such, temporary cavitation. Some 50 frogs were attached, at varying distances from the centre, to a circular board some 4.5 ft in diameter. The board was submerged and a rifle bullet fired through a hole in the centre of the board. The apparatus was recovered and the effects on the frogs noted. The first four rows died immediately, with many of the smaller bones broken. The damage decreased until those placed 15 in from the centre were unaffected by the 'hydrodynamic effect'. He commented also on the vacuum behind any high-speed projectile and how debris is sucked into the wound tract by it.

Wilson, in 1921, briefly outlined the history of the experimental approach to wound ballistics and summarized the gross effects so far described: 'The comminution of bone, the blasting out of soft tissue at the point of exit, the pulping of soft tissues around the track of the missile and injuries to distant parts by energy transmitted through fluid'. The major remaining question was at what distance from the missile path might energy transfer still be expected to produce tissue damage. This question led him to suggest the use of gelatine blocks of various densities as a substitute for tissue. He stated that, in general terms, 'the energy of a high velocity missile passing through gelatine masses of different percentage densities is dispersed in an explosive degree to distances approximately inversely as the square of the percentage densities'. Wilson also modified the blocks by inserting threads to demonstrate the distortion caused by the rotation of the tissue induced by the spin of the projectile (Wilson, 1921).

Wilson had already produced two works of direct interest to the research before he was asked to serve on the major investigation into wounding effects

(US Chief of Ordnance, 1928). One study related to the use of gelatine to simulate tissue and the other was a major chapter on 'Firearms and projectiles: their bearing on wound production' (US Surgeon General, 1927, A History of the United States Medical Services).

'Stopping Power', an article by Calvin Goddard published in 1935, investigated those factors believed to result in enhanced energy transfer of pistol bullet energy. He examined the theories of Lagarde, Hatcher and Medinger who had devised a formula using muzzle velocity, a form factor for bullet shape, gravity and the sectional area of the bullet to calculate the stopping power. He reached the conclusion that the most important factors in pistol bullets are sectional area and velocity (Goddard, 1935).

STUDIES UNDERTAKEN BETWEEN THE FIRST AND SECOND WORLD WARS

In the late 1920s there had been increasing official interest in the possibility of using smaller calibre rounds as replacements for the existing 0.303-in. and 0.30-in. bullets. Greener in the ninth edition of his book *The Gun* had reported on the work of Heubler in Switzerland, who had already proposed calibres as small as 0.22 (5.5 mm) in the late nineteenth century (Greener, 1910). The British War Office had investigated and seriously considered this concept prior to 1914, and only the problems of availability and supply during the early part of the First World War prevented the introduction of the 0.274-inch calibre P13 rifle into service.

In the summer of 1928 an extensive study was begun at the Aberdeen Proving Ground (US, Chief of Ordnance, 1928). This work, which went on well into 1934, brought together under Colonel Louis B. Wilson, then Medical Director of the Mayo Foundation, a team, the members of which would later become some of the best-known researchers in the field of wound ballistics, small-arms technology and casualty incapacitation in the first half of the twentieth century. The scope of the work was 'from the Ordnance standpoint to ascertain the effects of the caliber .30 bullets on body tissues, and to determine whether or not calibers as small as the .256 (6.5 mm) would have the necessary shocking and debilitating effects at the maximum battle ranges (1200 yards)' (Hatcher, 1948). In addition, extensive medical studies of the wounds were to be carried out in order to identify those factors which would be of value in the future treatment of gunshot wounds, and would enable the subject to be better presented for teaching purposes and for future study.

One simple and interesting innovation was the use of a bag made of two sheets of target cloth with a small amount of charcoal dust between the layers and placed over the entry point, in an effort to ascertain to what distance foreign bodies would be carried into the tissues.

This work is well described in the papers of Callender and French (Callender and French, 1935; Callender, 1943; French and Callender, 1962). A further and more unusual personal insight is that of Chamberlin, one of the surgeons involved. The accuracy of his account will be recognized by all who have undertaken similar studies (Chamberlin, 1978).

The results of the tests are also summarized by Julian Hatcher in *The Book Of The Garand* which also details the prolonged development of a military rifle from the concept stage to combat reports and beyond. Hatcher developed an empirical method of assessing the effectiveness of pistol ammunition, known as the 'Relative Incapacitation Index' (RII) which related bullet geometry to predicted performance with a high degree of correlation with actual results (Hatcher, 1935).

Kent, a physicist at the Aberdeen Proving Grounds in the 1930s, laid down important principles in research in this field and in its application to bullet design (Kent, 1930). He was also instrumental in encouraging the National Research Council to convene the Conference on Wound Ballistics in 1943, and the granting of contracts leading to the extensive work reported by Newton Harvey (Beyer, 1962).

WOUND BALLISTICS RESEARCH IN THE SECOND WORLD WAR

Zuckerman and the Oxford Extra-mural Unit

In 1939 Zuckerman began the study of the effects of shock waves generated by detonation of high explosives on people sheltering in underground shelters. Monkeys were secured to shelter walls and then a bomb, buried nearby, was detonated. Post-explosion examination of the monkeys demonstrated that the likely injurious effect was negligible (Zuckerman, 1939; Zuckerman and Black, 1940). Zuckerman also carried out a comprehensive review of the published works on the effects of explosives on the human body: this confirmed his suspicion that little of actual value was known and many of the collected reports were seriously misleading. When he began work on the problem of blast injury, he made the chance but important observation of the asymmetrical distribution of parenchymal lung injury, more severe on the side closer to the explosion in guinea-pigs exposed to low-pressure shock waves from exploding gas balloons (Zuckermann, 1978). This discredited the idea that injury was 'due to a wave of pressure passing through the nose and into the lungs' as was currently thought, though this idea promulgated at least until 1945 (Young, 1945; see also Barcroft, 1939 and HMSO, 1953). Krohn and Zuckerman later confirmed the hypothesis that blast injury was due to the direct effect of the pressure pulse on the body, by subjecting rabbits protected by steel boxes with only their heads exposed to very high blast pressures. The animals suffered no internal injury, nor did they lose consciousness, the only physical injuries found being ruptured eardrums (Fisher *et al.*, 1941; Krohn, Whitteridge and Zuckerman, 1942). This success enabled him to recruit researchers into the Oxford Extra-mural Unit (OEMU) with a brief to study all aspects of ballistic injury. Zuckerman had been greatly impressed by the wounding power of small splinters from exploding bombs or shells or grenades. In a review of the injuries of battle casualties he commented on the effect of a minute piece of metal weighing no more than one-fiftieth of an ounce (about half a gramme) which had fractured both radius and ulna in a young soldier (Zuckerman, 1942, 1978). This observation called into question the standard procedure for assessing the relative wounding power of fragmenting weapons where fragments of less than a twenty-fifth of an ounce (about a gramme) were ignored.

Zuckerman set about investigating his hypothesis (based on the work of the German ballisticians, Crantz and Becker, 1921, 1925) that small fragments were dangerous because of the momentum they donated to the tissues through which they passed. Zuckerman's 'guns' consisted of steel blocks, bored out to take a detonator to which a small ball bearing had been attached. The ball bearing was ejected at very high velocity when the detonator exploded, so simulating the effect of an individual fragment.

Using the technique of spark photography, a series of studies was undertaken to assess the effects of the energy transferred to an elastic target. These progressed from blocks of meat to rabbits' legs and gelatine blocks, and demonstrated for the first time the existence of the temporary cavity and that the series of rapid pulsations which followed was the likely cause of the damage produced by small fast moving fragments. The mechanism of bone fracture without actual contact was also elucidated (Black *et al.*, 1941).

Having confirmed that minute fragments could cause wounds out of all proportion to their size, the problem of how much of the wounding effect of fragmenting weapons was actually caused by splinters was then investigated. This required the integration of information on vulnerability and mean presented target area, which was obtained by photographing nude models and measuring the presented area in various postures. A figure of $0.4\,m^2$ was adopted, with 10–15% of this area representing the exposed body surface area of highly vulnerable organs such as the heart. Using fragments as small as 11 mg, taken from bomb casings, or 52 mg, in preformed weapons, threshold incapacitation velocities were established. A 52 mg fragment at 2300 ft/s was deemed to have a 37.9% chance of causing incapacitation with a random strike, while at 4920 ft/s it was 92.8% (Zuckerman, 1952). A fragment as small as 2.3 mg was observed to have penetrated up to an inch into muscle (Burns and Zuckerman, 1942).

An interesting phenomena was that tissue destruction did not necessarily increase with an increase of impact velocity. As expected, the amount of destruction rose with velocity up to the perforation velocity and then decreased up to the highest nominal velocities tested (1200 m/s). This confirmed that the length of the wound track in the tissue must be taken into account in estimating the potential for damage. The degree of internal destruction in a normal limb seemed to be approximately proportional to the momentum lost by the projectile in the tissues (Burns and Zuckerman, 1941).

Incapacitation appeared to be unaffected by the sum of the mass of the multiple fragments, and only when a critical mass of 1.3 g was reached was the effect enhanced. These comments discounted special areas including the eyeball (Zuckerman 1942).

This work was extended by Gruneberg in his analysis of the Ministry of Home Security Casualty Survey and the Army Training Accidents Survey (Gruneberg *et al.*, 1943).

The work of American investigators in the Second World War

Callender and French continued their active investigation into wound ballistics of both small-arms ammunition and fragments. They used a series of witness screens as described by Mann (1909) to demonstrate the extent of yaw. Steel cylinders filled with clay and fitted with internal pressure gauges connected to oscillographs recorded the extent and history of the pressure waves generated during the passage of a missile. Their revised conclusions published in 1943 took account of Zuckerman's work in demonstrating the extent of the temporary cavity (Callender, 1943), but still tried to use the 'laws of hydraulics' to explain the effects. In summary, they concluded that the measure of severity of a wound is related to the rate of energy transmission or the power expended in creating the wound. In simple terms, the likely severity was related to the cube of the velocity of the missile.

The National Research Council Conference on Wound Ballistics in 1943 led on to extensive basic work on wound ballistics, ultimately reviewed in *Advances in Military Medicine* (Harvey, 1948).

The access to spark photography, velocity measurement by rotating paper disks or rotary impact recorder, high-speed cameras and X-ray equipment with exposure times of only one-millionth of a second enabled the further analysis of the actual mechanisms involved (Harvey *et al.*, 1944). Piezo-electric crystal gauges inserted into the target material gave insight into the pressures involved in wound formation. Most of the early work was concerned with the explanation of the explosive effect of high-velocity projectiles (Harvey *et al.*, 1945); shots were fired into various standard materials such as gelatine blocks, gelatine in rubber tubes, water or dough as recommended by Wilson (Wilson, 1921) and Zuckerman (Black *et al.*, 1941). The use of a water tank with Plexiglas sides was especially useful in allowing high-speed photography to be used to record the events (McMillen and Harvey, 1946). Scaling down of the contemporary military rifle bullet of 9.6 g and its 70 kg target to a 0.4-g steel sphere striking a 3-kg target, enabled quantitative studies on temporary cavitation volume to be conducted. The effects of the shock wave produced during cavity formation and the possibility of damage at a distance was intensively investigated (Harvey *et al.*, 1947). The possibility of injury to peripheral nerves from the indirect effects of passage of a missile, or the fracture of bone during the formation of the temporary cavity, was explored. Early studies showed an incidence of 45% of fracture of the femur where the velocity of the sphere had a velocity of 4432 ft/s (1400 m/s) (Butler and Puckett, 1944; Harvey, 1948).

German research in the Second World War

The Crantz Laboratory was a centre of terminal ballistic work during this period. The development of the Crantz–Schardin camera which could take pictures at a rate of five million per second enabled detailed study of terminal ballistic and detonation phenomena (Simon, 1945). The influence of Carl Crantz was felt throughout the whole range of applied ballistics investigations, and of the research community involved in this area (Schardin, 1959). Zornig, regarded as the 'father' of the Ballistics Research Laboratories (BRL) in Maryland, had studied with Crantz, and Kent the most distinguished civilian member on the staff at BRL has called Crantz its 'Grandfather' (Poor, 1959). A spin off from the early work of Crantz and Becker had led to Zuckerman's further investigations and a later text of Crantz, quoted in Thoresby's review of the mechanism of 'Cavitation' in 1966, indicated the importance of the former's work in the whole field of terminal ballistics (Thoresby, 1966).

Detailed examination of the effects of fragment patterns and perforation characteristics was conducted at the 'Ballistischen Institut der Lufttechnischen Akademie at Berlin-Gatow' under the direction of Schardin (Benzinger, 1950; Desaga, 1950; Schardin, 1950).

Research into the effects of bullets and other projectiles upon tissue has continued since 1945 and the advances made are examined in detail in the specialist chapters which follow.

REFERENCES

Barcroft J. (1939). *Sectional Steel Shelters; Report on the Investigation of the Standard of Protection Afforded.* Office of the Lord Privy Seal. London: HMSO, Command Paper 6055, July.

Barnaby S.W. and Thornecroft J.I. (1897). *Trans. Inst. Naval Architects*, **39**, 139–44.

Beadnell C.M. (1908). On some functions of the projectile from a surgical aspect. *J.R. United Serv. Inst.*, **52**, 1235–47, 1360–74, 1518–31.

Bellamy R.F., Zajtchuk R. (1991). The evolution of wound ballistics: A brief history. In *Textbook of Military Medicine*, Part 1, vol. 5 (Bellamy R.F. and Zajtchuk R., eds) *Conventional Warfare; Ballistic, Blast and Burn injuries.* Washington: Office of the Surgeon General, Department of the Army.

Benzinger T. (1950) German aviation medicine in World War II. US Government Printing Office, Washington.

Beyer H.G. (1898–99). Observations on the effects produced by the 6mm Rifle and projectile. An experimental study. *J. Bost. Soc. Med. Sci.*, **iii**, 117–36.

Beyer J.C. (1962). *Wound Ballistics* (Coates and Beyer, eds). Washington, DC: Office of the Surgeon General, Department of the Army, pp. xi–xix.

Billroth T. (1859). Historical studies on the nature and treatment of gunshot wounds from the fifteenth century to the present time, 1859. *Yale J. Biol. Med.* Vol. **4**, (1, 2, 3), 16–36, 119–48, 225–57.

Black A.N., Burns B.D., Zuckerman S. (1941). An experimental study of the wounding mechanisms of high velocity missiles. *Br. Med. J.*, **2**, 872–4.

Bonjour E. (1950). *Theodor Kocher*: Bern: Paul Haupt (in German).

Burns B.D., Zuckerman S. (1941). *The Relationship between striking-velocity and the Damage Caused to Materials by a 3/32 in. Steel Ball.* Ministry of Home Security, RC 232.

Burns B.D., Zuckerman S. (1942). *The Wounding Power of Small Bomb and Shell Fragments.* Ministry of Home Security, RC. 350.

Butler E.G., Puckett W.O. (1944). Damage to bone produced by steel spheres. In *The Mechanism of Wounding by High Velocity Missiles. 1. Quantitative Data* (Harvey E.N., Butler E.G., McMillen J.H., Puckett W.O., eds). National Research Council, Division of Medical Sciences, Office of Scientific Research and Development, Missiles Casualties Report No. 2 (Interim Report) 15th December Section E, pp. 58–9.

Callender G.R., French, R.W. (1935). Wound ballistics – studies in the mechanism of wound production by rifle bullets. *Milit. Surg.*, **77**, 177–201.

Callender G.R. (1943). Wound ballistics; mechanism of production of wounds by small arms bullets and shell fragments. *War Med. Chicago*, **3**, 337–50.

Chamberlin F.T. (1978). Gun shot wounds. In *Handbook for Shooters and Reloaders*, vol. 2 (Ackley P.O., eds) UT: Plaza Publishing, pp. 48–64.

Crantz C., Becker K. (1921). *Handbook of Ballistics*, vol. 1, London: HMSO (trans. of 2nd German edition).

Crantz C., Becker K. (1925). *Aussere Ballistik*, vol. 1, 5th edn. Berlin: Julius Springer.

Day L. (1983). The holes in stopping power theory. In *Gun Digest*, 37th edn. pp. 24–8.

Dean B. (1920). Helmets and Body Armour in Modern Warfare, PhD Yale University Press.

Delorme E., Chavasse (1891). Etude comparative des effects produit par les balles du fusil gras de 11 mm, et du fusil lebel de 8 mm. *Arch. Med. Pharm. Mil.*, **xvii**, 8–112.

Delorme E. (1915). *War surgery.* London: H.K. Lewis (trans De Meric).

Demosthen A. (1894). Experiences sur les effets du projectile du fusil Mannlicher. *Trans. 11th Int. Med. Con. Rome*, 4, 254–60.

Desaga H. (1950). Blast injuries. In *German Aviation Medicine; World War II*, vol. 2. The Surgeon General, US Air Force, Department of the Air Force, pp. 1274–93.

Dougherty P.J. (1987). Theodor Kocher and the foundation of scientific wound ballistics. Paper presented at the Surgical Associates Day, Uniformed Services University of the Health Sciences, Bethesda, Maryland.

Fackler M.L., Surinchak J.S., Malinowski J.A., Bowen R.E. (1984). Bullet fragmentation: a major cause of tissue disruption. *J. Trauma*, **24**, 35–9.

Fisher E.B., Krohn P.L., Zuckerman S. (1941). *The Relationship Between Body Size and the Lethal Effects of Blast.* Ministry of Home Security, RC 284, December.

French R.W., Callender G.R. (1962) Ballistic characteristics of wounding agents. In *Wound Ballistics* (Beyer J.C. ed.). Washington DC: Office of the Surgeon General, Department of the Army.

Goddard C. (1935). Stopping Power. *Milit. Sur.*, **76**, (2), 57–71.

Greener W.W. (1910). *The Gun and its Development*, 9th edn. (Republished by Arms and Armour Press, SBN 85368–073–6, Undated.)

Gruneberg H., Powell R., Spicer C.C. (1943). *The Relationship Between Anti-Personnel Effect and Size of Projectile.* Ministry of Home Security RC. 406.

Guthrie G.S. (1815). *Treatise on Gunshot Wounds of the Extremities Requiring Amputation.* London: Longman.

Harvey E.N., Butler E.G., McMillen J.H., Puckett W.O. (1944). *The Mechanism of Wounding by High Velocity Missiles, 1, Quantitative Data.* National Research Council, Division of Medical Sciences, Office of Scientific Research and Development, Missiles Casualties Report No. 2 (Interim Report) 15th Dec.

Harvey E.N., Butler E.G., McMillen J.H., Puckett W.O. (1945). Mechanisms of wounding. *War Med.*, **8**, 91.

Harvey E.N., Korr I.M., Oster G., McMillen J.H. (1947). Secondary damage in wounding due to pressure changes accompanying the passage of high velocity missiles. *Surgery*, **V21**, 218.

Harvey E.N. (1948). Studies on wound ballistics. In *Advances in Military Medicine*, vol. 1, part 2 (Andrus E.C. et al., eds). Boston: Little, Brown & Co., chap. 18.

Hatcher J.S. (1935). *Textbook of Pistols and Revolvers.*

Hatcher J.S. (1948). *The Book of the Garand.* Washington: Infantry Journal Press.

Hennen J. (1818). *Remarks Concerning Several Important Subjects in Military Surgery.* Edinburgh: Constable.

HMSO Medical Research (1953). (Green F.H.K. and Corell Sir G., eds). London: HMSO, chap. 11

Horsley V. (1894). The destructive effects of small projectiles. *Nature*, **50**, (1283), 104–8.

Horsley V. (1894–5). The destructive effects of projectiles. *Proc. Roy. Inst. Great Britain*, **xiv**, 228–38.

Horsley V. (1915). Remarks on gunshot wounds of the head. *Br. Med. J.*, 20 Feb.; *Proc. Med. Soc. Lond.*, 8 Feb.

Huguier (1848). Plaies D'Armes A Feu. *Bull. Acad. Nat. Med.*, tome 14, 7–112.

Hunter J. (1812). *A Treatise on the Blood, Inflammation and Gun-shot Wounds*, 2 vols. London.

Journée Col. (1907) Rapport entre la force vive des balles et la gravite des blessures qu'elles peuvent causer. *Rev. Artillerie*, **70**, 81–120.

Keith A., Rigby H.M. (1899). Modern military bullets; a study of their destructive effects. *Lancet*, 1499–507.

Kent R.H. (1930). The theory of the motion of a bullet about its center of gravity in dense media with applications to bullet design, Aberdeen proving ground. *B.R.L Report*, X–65.

Kirschener M. (1915). Remarks on the action of the regular infantry bullet and of the dum-dum bullet on the human body. *JRAMC*, **24**, (6), 605–11.

Kocher T. (1875). Uber die sprengwirkung der modernen kleingewehr-geschosse. *Cor. Blat. f. Schweiz Aerzte*, **v**, 3–7, 29–33, 69.

Kocher T. (1879). Neue beitrage zur kenntniss der wirkung der mordernen kleingewehr-geschosse. *Cor. Blat. f. Schweiz Aerzte*, **IX**, 65–71.

Kocher T. (1880). *Uber Schusswunden. Experimentelle Untersuchungen uber die Wirkungsweise der Modernen Kleine-Gewehr-Geschosse.* Leipzig: Vogel.

Kocher, T. (1895). *Zur Lehre von den Schusswunden Durch Kleinkalibergeschosse*, Kassel: Fischer.

Kramer S.P., Horsley V. (1897). On the effects produced on the circulation and respiration by gunshot injuries of the cerebral hemispheres. *Phil. Trans. Roy. Soc., series B*, **188**.

Krohn P.L., Whitteridge D., Zuckerman S. (1942). Physiological effects of blast. *Lancet*, **i**, 252.

Lagarde L.A. (1893). Report on effects of small-arms firing with new calibres and velocities. *Rep. Surgeon-General Army*, June, 73–95.

Lagarde L.A. (1894/5). The difference between certain wounds inflicted by the projectiles of large and small calibre hand weapons. *Int. Med. Magazine Philadelphia*, **3**, 87–97.

Lagarde L.A. (1900). Gunshot injuries by weapons of reduced calibre. *Johns Hopkins Hosp. Bull.* (106), 20–4.

Lagarde L.A. (1903) Poisoned wounds by the implements of warfare. *JAMA Mutter Lecture*, **40**, 984–9, 1062–9.

Lagarde L.A. (1914). *Gunshot Injuries, How They Are Inflicted, Their Complications and Treatment.* New York: William Wood & Co., pp. 1–457.

Longmore T. (1863). On the probable surgical effects in battle in the case of the employment of projectiles of a more elongated form such as the Whitworth projectiles. *Army Med. Rep.*

Longmore T. (1877). *Gunshot Injuries.* London: Longman Green & Co.

Longmore T. (1881). Some observations on the wounds inflicted by the bullets of the Martini-Henry Rifle. *Trans. 7th Int. Med. Cong. London*, **2**, 583–6.

Mann F.W. (1909). *The Bullet's Flight*: New York: Munn & Co.

McMillen J.H., Gregg J.R. (1945). The Energy, Mass and velocity which is required of small missiles in order to produce a casualty. National Research Council,

Division of Medical Sciences, Office of Scientific Research and Development. *Missiles Casualties Rep.*, **12**, 6 Nov.

Ogston A. Sir (1898). The wounds produced by modern small bore bullets. *Br. Med. J.*, **2**, 813–15.

Ogston A. Sir (1899a). Continental criticism of English rifle bullets. *Br. Med. J.*, **1**, 752–7.

Ogston A. Sir (1899b). The peace conference and the dumdum bullet. *Br. Med. J.*, **2**, 278–81.

Paget S. (1919). *Sir Victor Horsley; A Study of His Life and Work*. London: Constable and Co.

Pilcher E.M. (1911). The pointed bullet. *J. R. Army Med. Corps*, **17**, 607–18.

Pilcher E.M. (1915). Notes on the terminal effects of the 0.303 Mark VII service round. *J. R. Army Med. Corps*, **24**, (6), 611–14.

Poor C.L. (1959). Exterior Ballistics developments in the United States since the time of Crantz. In *Selected Topics in Ballistics* (Nelson W.C., ed.), Agardograph No. 32. Oxford: Pergamon Press.

Reverdin J.-L. (1910). *Lecons de Chirurgie de Guerre, Des Blessure Faites Par Les Balles De Fusils*. Paris: Felix Alcan, Editure.

Sarazin (1867). Des effets produits par le projectile du fusil chassepot sur le cadavre. *Gazette Medicale de Strasbourg*, (18), 223–4, 25 Sept. 1867.

Schardin H. (1950). The physical principles of the effects of a detonation. In *German Aviation Medicine; World War II*, vol. 2. The Surgeon General, US. Air Force, Department of the Air Force, pp. 1207–24.

Schardin H. (1959). La vie et l'oeuvre de C. Cranz. In *Selected Topics in Ballistics* (Nelson W.O. ed.). Agardograph No. 32. Oxford: Pergamon Press.

Seydal K. (1893). *Lehrbuch der Kriegschirurgie*. Stuttgart.

Simon L.E. (1945). *Report on German Scientific Establishments*, Office of Technical Services, United States Department of Commerce.

Stevens R.B., Ezell E.C. (1987). *The Black Rifle; M16 Retrospective*. Toronto: Collector Grade Publications.

Stevenson W.F. (1897). *Wounds in War*, 1st edn. London: Longman Green & Co.

Stevenson W.F. (1898a). *Further Trial of Dum Dum Bullets, and of Bullets to R.L. Designs Nos 9063B and 9063B**. London: Departmental Committee, Small Arms Report 17. War Office.

Stevenson W.F. (1898b). The effects of the dum-dum bullet from a surgical point of view. *Br. Med. J.*, 1324–5.

Stevenson W.F. (1910). *Wounds in War*, 3rd edn. London: Longman Green & Co.

Thompson J.T., Lagarde L.A. (1904). Untitled. *Series of Reports of the Board Designated to Investigate Short Range Stopping and Shocking Power*. Record of the Ordnance Department, United States Army, File no. 38449–48–1. Washington DC: National Archives.

Thoresby F.P. (1966). 'Cavitation'; The wounding process of the high velocity missile, a review. *JRAMC*, **112**, (2), 89–99.

US Chief of Ordnance (1928). *Report of Experimental Gunshot Wounds in Live Animals*. Aberdeen Proving Ground. June–July.

US Surgeon General (1927). The Medical Department of the United States Army in the World War. *Surgery*, **XI**, (One).

Von Bruns P. (1889). *Die Geschosseinwirkung der Neuen Kleinkalibergewehre, ein Beitrag zur Beurteilung der Schusswunden in Kunftigen Kriegen*. Tubingen: Verlag Der H. Laupp' schen Buchhandlung.

Von Bruns P. (1897). *Ueber die Wirkung und Kriegschirurgische Bedeutung der Selbstladepistole System Mauser*. Tubingen.

Von Bruns P. (1898). Ueber die wirkung der bleispitzengeschosse, (dum-dum-geschosse) (The effect of lead-nosed (dum-dum-bullets) *Tubingen Surg. Clin, Tubingen*, **21**. (In Translation see Dric-T-7713, June 1986.)

Von Bruns P. (1898). Inhumane Kriegsgeschosse. *Arch. Klin. Chir.*, **V57**, 602 et seq.

Von Bruns P. (1900). Die neuesten kriegserfahrungen uber die gewehrschusswunden. *Munchener Medicinische Wochenschrift*, **15**, 485–6.

Von Coler and Schjerning (1894). *Ueber die Wirkung und die Kriegschirurgische Bedeutung der Neuen Handfeuerwaffen*. Berlin: Koniglich Preussichen Kriegsministeriums. 1894

Wilson L.B. (1921). Dispersion of bullet energy in relation to wound effects, *T Mil. Surg.*, **xlix**, 241–51.

Woodruff C.E. (1898). The cause of the explosive effect of modern small-caliber bullets. *New York Med. J.*, **xvii**, 593–601.

Young M.W. (1945). Mechanics of blast injury. *War Med.*, **8**, n(2), 73–8.

Zuckerman S. (1939). *The Effects of Direct Concussion on Monkeys in Underground Shelters*. Ministry of Home Security, A.R.P.D., Research and experimental branch, R.C. 65, December 1939.

Zuckerman S. (1942). *Sizes of Shell, Mortar and Bomb Fragments Causing Wounds, (Dieppe Series)*. Advisory Council on Scientific Research and Technical Development. AC 3142.

Zuckerman S. (1952). Vulnerability of human targets to fragmenting and blast weapons. In *A Textbook of Air Armament*. Ministry of Supply. Ref. TAA/2/12/52, part 2, chap. 10.

Zuckerman S., Black, A.N. (1940). *The effects of impact on the head and back of monkeys*. Ministry of Home Security, Research and Experiments Department, R.C. 124, August.

Zuckerman S. (1978). *From Apes to Warlords*. London: Hamish Hamilton.

2. Projectiles: Types and Aerodynamics

G. M. Moss

TYPES OF PROJECTILE

There are many objects which, acting as projectiles, can cause physical injury. However, because this section is concerned mainly with ballistics, the objects considered are those designed to cause penetrating injury when fired from a tube either individually or as components of a 'round' of ammunition. This condition excludes:

1. Explosively formed projectiles or EFPs: slugs of material, usually metallic, which are generated by means of careful explosive shaping. There is usually one per warhead, although they may be used in tandem to attack explosively reacting armour (ERA). They travel at high speed and are also known by the acronym PFF (preformed fragments).
2. Shaped charges: metallic jets formed in a similar way to EFPs and are also designed to attack the same type of target. The tip of the jet is normally travelling at 8 or 9 km/s and is followed by a larger slug of metal moving at a much lower speed, typically between 300 and 900 m/s.
3. Anti-riot projectiles (baton rounds; rubber bullets): designed specifically not to penetrate. They observe the general principles of flight outlined below.

Injuries from projectiles in categories 1 and 2 can be substantial, however they are unlikely to be targeted specifically at personnel. Therefore we discuss antipersonnel projectiles only.

Bullets are projectiles which are stabilized by the use of axial spin or by means of afterbody flaring. *Darts* are stabilized by the use of rear-mounted fins. The general principles which apply to bullets can also be extended to artillery shells because they share the same external shape and method of stabilization. Similarly, the principles which apply to the flight of darts can be applied to other fin-stabilized projectiles (e.g. flechettes and long rod penetrators used to attack armour).

Fragments are any pieces of material which are given additional velocity by means of an explosive charge near the end of the trajectory of a projectile. These may include the products of a fragmentation warhead in which score marks in the case of a projectile that contains an explosive charge generate large numbers of fairly regularly shaped high-velocity elements.

There are a whole range of possible projectile shapes which could be considered, many of them based on perceptions of supposed mechanisms for wounding. The designer may seek to maximize projectile momentum, or kinetic energy, or the rate of deposition of kinetic energy, or cavity size, or propensity to tumble, or ability to fragment or lose velocity at impact.

In choosing a design, he/she must be aware of article 23e of the Hague Convention of 1899, as specified in the accompanying Declaration of 29 July 1899: 'The contracting Parties agree to abstain from the use of bullets which expand or flatten easily in the human body, such as bullets with a hard envelope which does not entirely cover the core or is pierced with incisions.' Also he should be aware of the unanimous UN resolution of 29 July 1979 which 'Appeals to all governments to exercise utmost care in the development of small-calibre weapon systems so as to avoid an unnecessary escalation of the injurious effects of such systems.'

The rounds dealt with here have axial symmetry or near symmetry, and are assumed to exhibit, at least for the external ballistic part of their flight, some degree of directional stability and to remain intact and essentially undeformed. The latter requirement is often violated by bullets in common use, but again the general principles of ballistics and aerodynamics can be applied to any ensuing fragments equally as well as to the complete round.

Projectiles which travel through a medium (usually air) at a velocity greater than that of sound in the same medium are supersonic; below that velocity they are subsonic. The classification is based on the Mach number (M) for the medium:

$$M = \frac{\text{speed of projectile}}{\text{speed of sound}}$$

The denominator varies with the compressibility and mass density of the medium. For example, in air at sea level on an average day in continental Europe, it is about 340 m/s and is dependent on the square root of the temperature. In fresh water, the corresponding speed is about 1450 m/s.

A flight Mach number less than unity typifies a subsonic projectile and above about Mach 1.2 a supersonic one. The range Mach 0.8–1.2 is known as the transonic region. Above Mach 5, the projectile is defined as hypersonic, though the prefix hyper- is now somewhat uncritically applied to projectiles with speeds of about 1000 m/s and more.

Any given projectile may be supersonic, transonic or subsonic at different parts of its flight depending on the Mach number at the time. For example, even a projectile which was highly supersonic in air would become subsonic on entering water (or body muscle tissue in which the speed of sound is very similar to that in water).

AERODYNAMICS OF PROJECTILES

Aerodynamic drag

In a vacuum the only force acting on a projectile in flight is that of gravitational acceleration – its weight. Consequently, it may be shown that the *in vacuo* trajectory for a flat earth is parabolic and is symmetrical about the vertex, i.e. the angle of descent is equal to the angle of launch. The projectile speed at impact is equal to the speed at launch and the maximum range is achieved at a launch angle of 45° to the horizontal (Moss *et al.*, 1995). In a fluid medium, there is an additional force opposing forward motion caused by the resistance of the medium and known as *drag*. In general terms, for speeds up to about Mach 0.8, this force varies approximately as the square of the forward speed. For projectiles which fly above Mach 2, it varies approximately linearly with forward speed and it is the dominant force on the projectile. It then substantially modifies the trajectory in the way shown in Figure 2.1 to reduce range and steepen the angle of descent and impact.

A 155-mm artillery shell fired at its maximum muzzle velocity has aerodynamic drag about five times the weight of the shell at launch. The drag is produced by the stresses generated in the air as it flows over the projectile. Force is equal to stress times the area over which the stress acts and so the drag force is proportional to the area of the projectile. However, the weight of a projectile is equal to the density of the projectile multiplied by its volume. Area is proportional to length squared for a given shape, and volume to length cubed. It follows that as the projectile reduces in size, i.e. in linear dimension, its volume decreases more rapidly than its area.

Hence, for small projectiles, such as those fired from small arms, the importance of aerodynamic drag becomes more pronounced. Considering a NATO standard 7.62-mm bullet, at its design muzzle velocity of 837 m/s (Mach 2.46 at sea level on a standard day), the aerodynamic drag at launch is just over 60 times the weight of the round. This profoundly modifies the *in vacuo* trajectory, to reduce the theoretical range by a factor of about 20. At any speed above about 160 m/s, the drag force is greater than the weight of the round.

Though a projectile passes through a (usually) static medium, it is sometimes analytically convenient to consider the object as stationary and the fluid

moving. In most cases, these different reference frames can be used interchangeably and this will be done here; where the distinction is significant it will be commented upon.

Types of drag

Essentially, there are three separate contributions to the drag force on an object moving through a fluid medium. These may be summarized as:

● skin friction
● pressure drag
● yaw-dependent drag.

Skin friction Skin friction is produced directly by the viscosity of the fluid, which in turn is a measure of resistance to shear. The molecules immediately adjacent to the surface of a moving object stick firmly to the surface. Those a little further away move parallel to it. There is then a thin layer of fluid close to the surface of the body in which shearing is taking place, known as the *boundary layer*.

The resolution in the direction of flight of the force generated by these shear stresses is skin friction. For objects of reasonable size travelling at typical projectile speeds, it varies approximately as the square of the forward speed.

The shear forces acting on the projectile that are slowing it down are exactly equal to the shear forces acting on the fluid medium which carry the medium along with the projectile. These tangential forces may be of consequence in penetrating injury.

Pressure drag The viscosity of air is small. Nevertheless, it can still make a substantial contribution to the drag of a projectile because of its effect on the pressure drag.

Any motion through a fluid medium causes the static pressure in the medium to change (static pressure is the kind of pressure measured by a barometer). In a reference frame fixed with respect to the object, there is a basic relationship between the static pressure in the fluid (p) and the speed of the flow (V). This states that, for steady flow in which the effects of viscosity are not large,

$$\frac{\gamma}{\gamma - 1} \frac{p}{\rho} + \frac{1}{2} V^2 = \text{a constant}$$

in which γ is the ratio of specific heats for the fluid (taken as 1.4 for air).

At very low speeds, the air density ρ remains constant and the equation can be written:

$$p + \frac{1}{2} \rho V^2 = \text{a constant}$$

This is Bernoulli's equation. It shows that if the fluid speed rises, the static pressure will fall (and

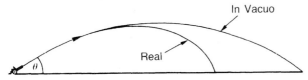

Figure 2.1 Trajectories in a vacuum and in air.

vice versa). It is useful in gaining a qualitative idea of the consequences of fluid flow.

In general, as a consequence of the motion, the average static pressure at the front of the moving body is greater than that at the rear. This imbalance produces a force acting towards the rear of the body against the motion of the body, which is known as *pressure drag*.

If pressure drag is to be minimized at subsonic speeds, smooth shapes with rounded noses and gently tapering rear sections with sharp trailing edges are required. If sharp corners are present elsewhere on the object or if cross-sectional shape changes too sharply, the boundary layer may separate from the surface to cause the formation of a region of fluid (the wake) behind, which moves with it. In the wake, the static pressure is lower than it would otherwise be and therefore drag is increased. By application of Bernoulli's equation, it might be supposed that in the wake, where the

velocity is low, the static pressure would be high. However, to reach the wake from the free stream it is necessary to cross the separated boundary layer in which viscous forces are important. This changes the constant in the equation so that low velocities and low pressures exist together. To a first order, the average pressure in the wake is the same as at the separation point. This is normally quite close to the point of minimum pressure on the body and so the wake pressure is usually quite low.

Objects are streamlined to reduce the pressure drag caused by boundary layer separation. Examples of the flow around high drag and low drag objects are given in Figure 2.2. In this, Figure 2.2 (a) is a flat plate at right angles to its direction of motion. In this case, flow separates at the sharp corners to produce a large wake and hence large drag. Even if the edges are significantly rounded (Figure 2.2 (b)), flow separation and hence high drag forces still occur. It is necessary to use

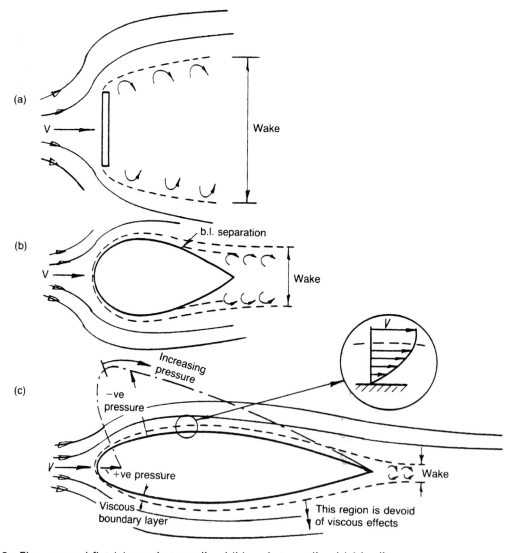

Figure 2.2 Flow around flat (a), semi-streamlined (b) and streamlined (c) bodies.

highly streamlined bodies before flow separation is averted. Figure 2.2(c) is a well-streamlined shape for which most of the drag is skin friction. For the same frontal area at the same speed, this fully streamlined body could have a drag two orders of magnitude less than the drag of the flat plate.

At low subsonic speeds, pressure drag for most bodies varies almost exactly as the square of the speed.

Cavitation In a gas, the minimum pressure that can be reached is theoretically zero – a complete vacuum. In practice, pressures less than about 30% of the ambient static pressure are not observed in the vicinity of bodies in motion. In a liquid medium, however, a reduction of local static pressure below the vapour pressure of the liquid will cause the liquid to change to its vapour phase. The consequent massive reduction in density causes vapour-filled voids to appear in the liquid. If the local static pressure rises above the vapour pressure, these voids collapse. The impact of the previously separated fluid surfaces can itself produce very large and destructive pressure pulses within the fluid medium.

Liquids usually contain dissolved air, and air bubbles will begin to form at pressures well above the vapour pressure of the liquid itself, leading to similar phenomena to that described above but which occur at considerably lower speeds.

Wake flow Another consequence of the slow-moving wake behind a body with a blunt base is that, relative to the fluid itself, the wake flow is moving in the same direction as the projectile and at nearly the same speed – the projectile motion is accompanied by the fluid in its wake.

Figure 2.3(a) shows the flow pattern about a circular cylinder drawn with it as the reference frame – the flow pattern which would be seen by an observer moving with the cylinder. Figure 2.3(b) is the same flow pattern drawn with respect to a reference frame fixed in the fluid. The 'sink effect' of the wake can be clearly seen. This can lead to contamination of penetrating wounds made by high-speed projectiles as the wake moves material into the cavity.

Shock waves An inevitable accompaniment of movement at supersonic speeds is a system of shock waves. The way in which these are produced is illustrated in Figure 2.4. Imagine a very slender object moving through otherwise stationary air at speed V. At each instant, the object is pushing aside some of the air. Each of these 'little pushes' is a small pressure wave which travels radially away from its point of generation at the speed of sound, a, and triggers the adjustment of the air ahead to flow smoothly around the projectile.

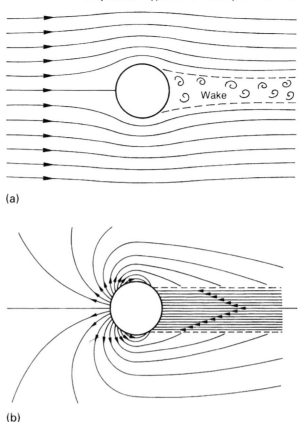

Figure 2.3 (a), (b) Flow around a circular cylinder.

Figure 2.4(a) shows what happens when the object is moving at Mach 0.5. The circles represent the positions that the pressure waves, generated at various past times, have reached at the present (on the diagrams, t is the time from the present, reckoned backwards). For example, the circle labelled *1* is the present position of the pressure wave which was generated when the object was at point *1*. It can be seen that, although the waves travelling ahead of the object are closer together than those travelling behind it, the fluid still receives warning of the approach of the object.

The instantaneous situation for Mach 2 is represented in Figure 2.4(b). Here the pressure waves which are attempting to travel ahead of the object coalesce into a straight line, which intersects the line of flight at the object itself. This Mach line, or in three dimensions, Mach cone, is a very weak pressure pulse. It is clear that any air to the left of this line/cone remains undisturbed. Because the individual pressure waves propagate outwards at the local speed of sound, it follows that the included angle between the Mach line/cone and the line of flight can be found as in terms of the Mach number, and is known as the Mach angle.

With a real object, the individual pressure waves are stronger and travel correspondingly

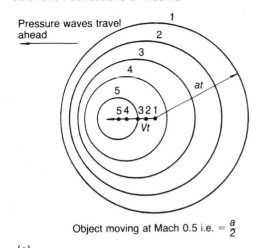

Object moving at Mach 0.5 i.e. $= \frac{a}{2}$

(a)

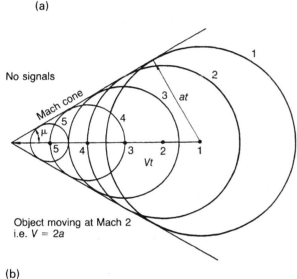

Object moving at Mach 2
i.e. $V = 2a$

(b)

Figure 2.4 (a), (b) The generation of shock waves. *a* is the ambient speed of sound.

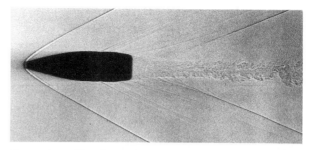

Figure 2.5 The flow about a supersonic projectile.

faster. The included angle of the common tangent to the pressure pulses now produced is larger than the Mach angle and the coalescence of the pulses produces a pressure wave travelling at rather more than the ambient speed of sound – the wave is known as a *shock wave*. It is physically very thin, typically less than 10^{-5}m in air at sea level, and is the first indication which the air receives of the approach of an object travelling at supersonic speeds. It can represent a pressure increase of several atmospheres and the heating which takes place as the fluid is compressed requires a constant supply of energy. This appears as an additional drag force on the body, known as wave drag.

As the air passes through the shock wave, it changes direction to pass around the nose of the body. As the air moves further back over the projectile, it encounters changes in geometry. If the local slope of the body surface increases, another shock wave will be formed. If reductions in surface slope are met, the air changes direction through a broader region known as an expansion fan. A typical supersonic flow field is shown in Figure 2.5. This picture of a bullet in flight was taken at a flight Mach number of 2.5, with a special optical technique being used to make the shock waves and expansion fans visible.

The larger the change in local slope of the surface, the stronger is the shock wave and the larger is the drag produced. For bluff-nosed bodies, the wave is at right angles to the flow and generates large amounts of drag. If drag is to be kept small for supersonic projectiles, it is important that they have slender nose shapes. The implications for stability are discussed below.

Yaw-dependent drag In general, a projectile will not fly with its body axis aligned with the direction of flight. The angle between the two is called the *yaw angle*. It may arise from a variety of causes, but its presence usually generates a sideforce normal to the body axis and therefore with a component in the drag direction.

For small angles of yaw, the sideforce is proportional to the yaw angle and the drag is equal to the sideforce multiplied by the yaw angle. Therefore, the drag due to sideforce varies with the square of the yaw angle.

Drag coefficient
The total drag of the projectile is the sum of the three components described above. In each case, the individual drag force is produced by a stress acting on an area, either normal stresses (pressures), or tangential (shear) stresses. Additionally, the forces generated depend on the density of the fluid in which motion is occurring. It is therefore logical to divide the drag force on the projectile by the product of air density, the square of the forward speed and a reference area. The denominator has the units of force and therefore the quantity formed by this division has no units or dimensions – a *drag coefficient* written C_D. In practice, for theoretical reasons, a 2 is introduced into the numerator and,

for projectiles, the reference area used is the frontal area of the round. In analytical form:

$$C_D = \frac{8 \cdot \text{Drag force}}{\rho V^2 \pi d^2}$$

in which ρ is the fluid density, V is flight speed and d is projectile maximum diameter (calibre).

The use of drag coefficient as a measure of the efficiency of a projectile is universal. By measuring drag in terms of this coefficient, the first-order effects of air density, flight speed and projectile size are removed. In consequence, drag coefficient becomes a function of Mach number only. This dramatically reduces the problem of data presentation since the drag characteristics of a given shape can now be presented by a single curve. This curve is illustrated in Figure 2.6(a), in which the drag coefficient for the typical bullet shape shown is plotted against Mach number. Note that there are no effects of fluid density, flight speed or projectile size on this curve. Shown in Figure 2.6(b) is the actual drag force in Newtons for a 7.62 mm round at sea level on a standard day. Also given on this plot is the drag curve which would result if the drag coefficient were truly constant, i.e. independent of Mach number.

For hand guns which are meant for shooting at close ranges, the ammunition is not always designed to have low drag. Some virtue may be perceived in designing the bullet to move extremely fast while giving it a non-aerodynamic shape. This may produce more damage on arrival than a more conventional bullet. The French THV (Très Haute Vitesse) bullet is an example of this kind of thinking (for a description of this round see Knudsen, 1990).

It should be mentioned that if the viscosity of the fluid in which motion occurs is significantly raised, this can also cause changes in the value of the drag coefficient for a given shape.

The estimation of drag coefficient

The basic drag coefficient versus Mach number relationship can either be estimated from scratch or it can be deduced from range measurements. Knowledge of this enables trajectories for the round to be predicted.

If an analytical approach is adopted, it is usual to consider the drag of the projectile to be made up of individual contributions from the nose or forebody, from the base, with boat-tail if present and from skin friction and excrescence drag.

At low subsonic speeds, the drag of the nose is almost independent of shape. Figure 2.7 shows the variation for four different noses; the main

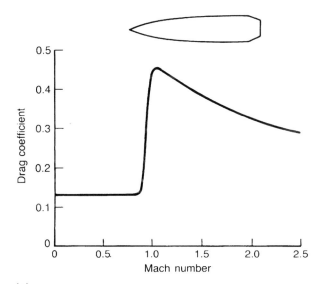

(a)

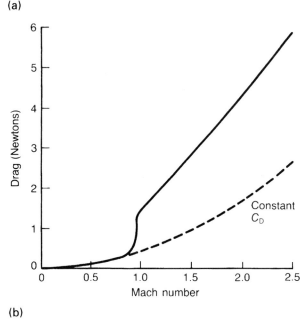

(b)

Figure 2.6 (a), (b) The variation of drag coefficient and drag force with Mach number for a typical projectile shape.

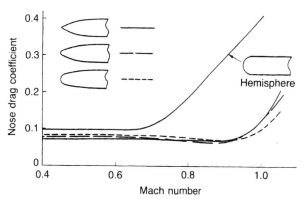

Figure 2.7 The variation of drag coefficient with Mach number for different forebody shapes at subsonic speeds.

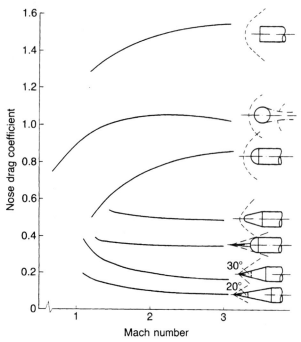

Figure 2.8 The variation of drag coefficient with Mach number for different forebody shapes at supersonic speeds.

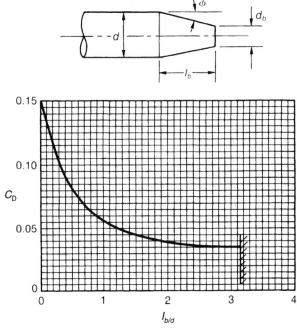

Figure 2.9 The variation of base drag with boat-tail length at subsonic speeds.

difference is in the Mach number at which the drag coefficient starts to rise – the more rounded the nose, the sooner the drag rise occurs. This is the outcome of the presence of small shock waves in the flow, which are themselves a consequence of local supersonic regions. These exist because the air is speeded up as it passes around the projectile. Therefore there are regions in which the speed of the air is greater than the speed of the object. Hence there will be regions in the flow for which the local Mach number is greater than unity, even when the flight Mach number for the projectile is still less than 1. The bluffer the projectile, the greater the increase in speed, therefore the lower the Mach number at which these supersonic regions occur.

At supersonic speeds, nose shape is much more critical. Figure 2.8 shows the variation of drag coefficient with Mach number for various simple shapes at supersonic speeds. The drag force is proportional to drag coefficient multiplied by the square of the speed (or multiplied by M^2). It is clear that noses need to be fairly slender if very large drag is to be avoided.

Base drag is essentially due to the change in pressure on the base of the projectile caused by boundary layer separation. It may be minimized by using a tapered base – a technique known as boat-tailing. Figure 2.9 gives the variation in base drag for a tapered afterbody of various length at low subsonic speeds. The taper angle (ϕ) is 9° which is about optimum, and brings the body to

a point when the afterbody is 3.15 diameters in length. It is noteworthy that a boat-tail of only 0.5 body diameters in length reduces the base drag by a factor of 2.

Similar considerations apply at supersonic speeds. Figure 2.10 shows the variation of base drag coefficient against Mach number for a plain base and a boat-tailed base. This time the taper angle is 6.5° which is about optimum at supersonic speeds.

Skin friction is normally estimated by 'unrolling' the surface of the projectile to produce a flat plate and using semi-empirical skin friction formulae for flat plates to give the coefficient. Excrescences are also usually tackled empirically, the main contribution being from the driving band, if present.

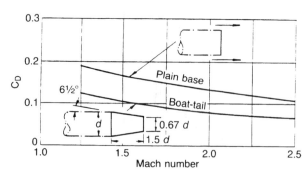

Figure 2.10 The effect of boat-tailing on base drag at supersonic speeds.

TABLE 2.1

DRAG BREAKDOWN FOR A TYPICAL BULLET SHAPE

Drag component	Mach number				
	0.5	0.8	1.0	1.2	2.0
Forebody	0.007	0.007	0.048	0.106	0.074
Skin friction	0.053	0.047	0.044	0.041	0.032
Driving band	0.005	0.005	0.010	0.015	0.011
Base with boat-tail	0.051	0.058	0.142	0.172	0.144
Base no boat-tail	0.128	0.176	0.214	0.270	0.212
Total with boat-tail	0.116	0.117	0.244	0.334	0.261
Total no boat-tail	0.193	0.235	0.316	0.432	0.329

Table 2.1 gives the drag breakdown for a typical artillery shell over a range of Mach numbers, both for a shell with a boat-tail and for the same shell with a plain base. It is noteworthy that the drag expressed in coefficient form is very similar to that for the 7.62-mm round given in Figure 2.2, in spite of the fact that one is 20 times the linear size of the other. This illustrates the value of the use of drag coefficients because the same shape at the same Mach number has the same drag coefficient (though not the same drag), regardless of speed, size and air density.

An alternative approach to the estimation of drag is to measure the decay in speed of a round in flight at a ballistic range. Since the deceleration of the round is produced by the drag force, it follows that:

$$\frac{\Delta V}{V} = - \frac{\rho \pi d^2}{8 \cdot \text{mass}} \cdot \Delta \text{ range} \cdot C_D$$

in which ΔV is the velocity drop over the distance Δ *range*.

This equation can also be expressed as:

$$\frac{\Delta V}{V} = - \frac{\rho \pi d^2 C_D V}{8 \cdot \text{mass}} \cdot \Delta t$$

At high supersonic speeds, the product $C_D \cdot V$ is approximately constant and so the rate of speed loss is a fixed proportion of the speed. For example, the 7.62-mm round initially loses 7% of its speed every one-tenth of a second.

The rate at which velocity decays is a potential measure of penetration and is often referred to by the term ballistic coefficient. This is derived from an obsolete technique for trajectory estimation. It is a measure of the mass per unit frontal area of a projectile (often still expressed in lb/in^2). The deceleration of the projectile is inversely proportional to the coefficient.

Fragments Fragments are usually characterized by bluff and irregular shapes and have drag coefficients which are virtually constant over the whole supersonic Mach range. Given that M > 1, the drag force varies as the square of the speed and consequently the velocity decays exponentially:

$$\frac{V}{V_o} = \exp \left(- \frac{\rho \cdot S \, C_D}{2m} \cdot r \right)$$

in which V_o is the initial velocity, S is the reference area of the fragment (the area upon which C_D is based), m is the mass of the fragment and r is the radial distance travelled.

In view of the variation of the individual terms for real fragments, this is often expressed in the general form:

$$\frac{V}{V_o} = \exp \left(- \frac{r}{c \cdot m^{1/3}} \right)$$

in which c is a constant. A typical variation of fragment velocity with radial flight distance is given in Figure 2.11.

Aerodynamic moments

A tube-launched projectile in ballistic flight will normally experience yaw disturbances. The cause may be: disturbances as it leaves the tube because of tube motion; the effects of the propellant gases which overtake it as it first leaves the tube; crosswinds or gusts; or simply the effect of gravity in curving the trajectory downwards (Figure 2.1).

The presence of yaw generates a sideforce on the projectile. Theoretically, the local sideforce is proportional both to the yaw angle and locally to the rate of change of cross-sectional area of the projectile. For the slender projectile shape which is

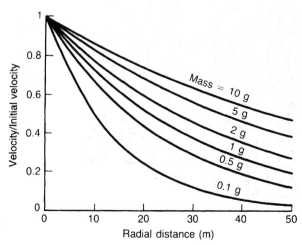

Figure 2.11 The reduction of flight speed with distance from launch for typical fragments.

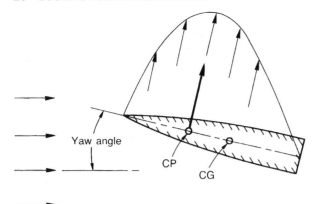

Figure 2.12 Sideforce distribution on a yawed projectile of typical shape.

needed to minimize drag (especially at supersonic speeds), this produces a sideforce distribution similar to that outlined in Figure 2.12.

This sideforce exerts a total moment about the centre of gravity (CG) of the projectile which is found by multiplying the local sideforce by its distance from the CG. This moment can be represented by the total sideforce acting at a single point known as the centre of pressure (CP). If nose-up moments are reckoned to be positive, the relationship is:

Moment = Sideforce × distance of CP forward of CG

Theoretically, the centre of pressure position can be calculated from the formula:

$$\frac{\text{CP position aft}}{\text{of nose apex}} = \frac{\text{projectile length} -}{(\text{volume/base area})}$$

(in practice both this and the previous theoretical result for sideforce give reasonable approximations to measured values, except at very high speeds).

For a normal low drag shape, the centre of pressure is forward of the centre of gravity and nose-up yaw generates a corresponding nose-up moment.

For the same reasons advanced earlier for drag, the aerodynamic moments on a projectile are expressed in dimensionless form as a coefficient. The same normalizing parameters are used, except that, because a moment is involved, an extra length is required to make the ratio non-dimensional. The length used is the projectile maximum diameter or calibre. The expression for the yawing moment coefficient C_m therefore becomes:

$$C_m = \frac{8 \cdot \text{Yawing moment}}{\rho V^2 \pi d^3}$$

This coefficient, at least for small yaw angles, varies linearly with yaw angle. Because the rate at which the moment increases with increase in yaw angle is critical for stability, the derivative of this

coefficient with respect to yaw angle is the usual form in which this quantity appears in stability assessment is $dC_m/d\alpha$ which is written $C_{m\alpha}$. It is further deduced that $C_{m\alpha}$ is positive for a directionally unstable projectile, zero for a neutrally stable projectile and negative for a directionally stable projectile. These terms are defined in the next section. For all normal shapes of projectile body $C_{m\alpha}$ is positive.

Stability

The stability of a projectile is concerned with its motion following a disturbance from an equilibrium condition. A distinction is made between the initial tendency of the projectile to return to its starting position after a disturbance and any subsequent motion. Because the first can be analysed without any reference to the resulting motion, it is termed static stability. Examination of the motion itself is referred to dynamic stability analysis.

There are three possible classes of static stability:

1. Stable – the projectile tends to return to its starting condition.
2. Neutrally stable – the projectile remains in its disturbed condition.
3. Unstable – the projectile tends to move further away from its starting condition in the same direction as that of the disturbance.

These three classes can be illustrated by considering a cone on a horizontal surface as shown in Figure 2.13. In Figure 2.13(a), the cone is standing on its base. If the apex is displaced sideways and

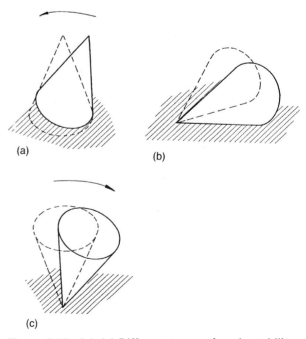

Figure 2.13 (a)–(c) Different types of static stability.

then released, the cone will return to its original, equilibrium position. It is therefore statically stable. When placed on its side as in Figure 2.13(b), a sideways displacement simply produces a change in the rest position. The cone is then neutrally stable. Finally, if the cone is balanced on its apex (Figure 2.13(c)), any sideways displacement will cause it to tip further away from the initial condition in the direction of the disturbance. The cone is now statically unstable.

This idea can now be applied to a projectile in flight. If it is subjected to a yaw disturbance then the sign of the resulting yawing moment generated will also define the static stability. In the low drag shape described above for which the centre of pressure is forward of the centre of gravity, the yawing moment generated by a yaw disturbance is in the same direction as the yaw disturbance and hence will tend to make the projectile tumble – the projectile is statically unstable. If the centre of pressure and centre of gravity coincide, there is no moment generated by a yaw disturbance and so the projectile is neutrally stable. Finally, if the centre of pressure is aft of the centre of gravity, a yaw disturbance generates a yawing moment which tends to remove the disturbance and so the projectile is then statically stable.

There is clearly an important correspondence in the distance between the centre of pressure, the centre of gravity and the static stability of the round. This distance is called the static margin. It is positive for positive static stability (when the centre of pressure is behind the centre of gravity), zero for neutral stability and negative for negative stability (static instability).

To minimize the longitudinal deceleration of the projectile in flight, it is necessary to fly nose forwards. Figure 2.14 shows the drag coefficient as a function of yaw angle for the 7.62-mm round. If the round tumbles, the average drag would rise by a factor of about 10. Additionally, the flight would become more variable and dispersion would increase. It is clear, therefore, that some means must be found for stabilizing the round so as to ensure that the nose points essentially along the trajectory.

The nature of the sideforce generated by yaw suggests one possibility: the local sideforce is proportional to the rate of change of cross-sectional area. Therefore, if boat-tailing is used to reduce drag, it will make instability worse. This is because the static margin can be written:

Static margin = – (Moment about CG/Total sideforce)

and the boat-tail, since its area is reducing will generate a negative sideforce. Hence, as shown in Figure 2.15(a), the moment is increased while the total sideforce is reduced, giving a more negative static margin and hence a further forward centre of pressure and a greater instability. The remedy for this is to increase the body cross-section towards the rear, which has exactly the reverse effect and so can be used to stabilize the projectile.

The increase in area towards the base is known as a flare and so this is flare stabilization. It suffers from increased drag compared with a normal round but may be used in special cases, such as at very high speeds when fins would become too hot to be sustainable. A flared skirt is also used in air

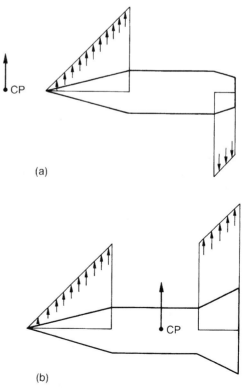

(a)

(b)

Figure 2.15 (a), (b) The effect of afterbody shape on centre of pressure position.

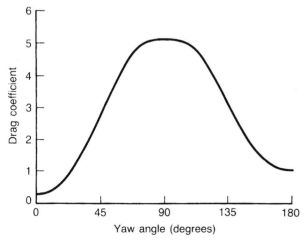

Figure 2.14 The variation of drag coefficient with yaw angle for the M80 round at a Mach number of 2.5.

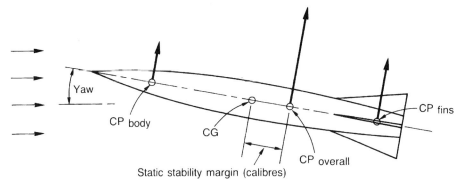

Figure 2.16 The way in which rear-mounted fins confer directional stability.

gun pellets, which otherwise do not have sufficient spin to be directionally stable.

Apart from the use of a flare, which is not common, there are two standard techniques of generating directional stability:

1. By the use of fins.
2. By the use of spin.

Fin stabilization
As described earlier, it is only necessary to move the centre of pressure aft of the centre of gravity to confer static directional stability on a projectile. This may be done by providing a lifting surface aft of the centre of gravity of the round.

In Figure 2.16, the body lift is well ahead of the centre of gravity but is, as explained below, rather small. The lift generated by the stabilizing fins is behind the centre of gravity and is relatively large. Taking moments about, for example, the body nose apex, produces the position for the resultant of both

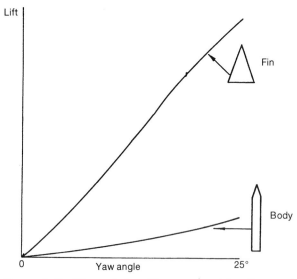

Figure 2.17 The relative lift generated by fins and bodies.

lift forces. This is the overall centre of pressure for a projectile with fins and if this is aft of the centre of gravity, the projectile will be directionally statically stable.

Two-dimensional flat surfaces are far more efficient at generating lift than are three-dimensional bodies. This is indicated in Figure 2.17, in which the lift from a flat plate of triangular form (a delta fin) is compared with that from a circular body with a conical nose, both of which have the same plan area. The fin gives much more lift per unit plan area at the same yaw angle than does the body. Therefore, relatively small fins at the rear of projectiles are effective. Fin-stabilized projectiles will normally have a static margin of between one and four calibres, depending mainly on the type of target to be attacked.

The main disadvantages of fin stabilization are that room must be found for the fins inside the barrel (the body of the round must be sub-calibre and be sabot launched) or they must deploy after launch. The fins also increase drag, typically by between 25% and 40%. However, the very low frontal area does give the dart configuration good penetration.

Because fins provide stability by using the same mechanism (aerodynamic forces) as that which produces instability in the body, a dart remains stable if it enters a dense medium, as long as it stays intact. This is in contrast to the behaviour of spin-stabilized rounds.

Spin stabilization
Spin stabilization is based on the properties of a gyroscope.

The gyroscope A gyroscope which is spinning very fast has a large angular momentum with respect to its spin axis. If it is assumed that the gyroscope has a moment of inertia of A about the spin axis and a rotation rate of p, angular momentum will be $A \cdot p$. If an impulsive moment of $m\delta t$ is now applied at right angle to the spin axis, then the resulting position of the net angular momentum vector will have rotated

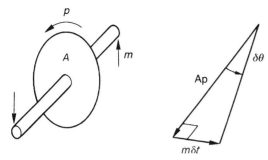

Figure 2.18 The action of a gyroscope.

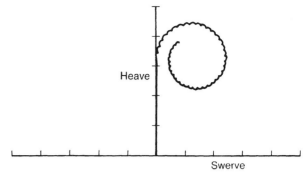

Figure 2.20 The motion of the nose of a spin-stabilized projectile following a yaw disturbance.

by the angle $\delta\theta$ from its original position (Figure 2.18).

For small angles, $\delta\theta = m\delta t / Ap$, that is

$$\frac{d\theta}{dt} = \frac{m}{A_p}$$

Thus a gyroscope subjected to a moment acting at right angles to its spin axis actually rotates about an axis delayed by 90° in the direction of the spin. This motion is *precession*. The rate at which it precesses is determined by the ratio of the applied moment to the angular momentum of the gyroscope.

The use of spin to stabilize projectiles It has already been indicated that most projectile body shapes are aerodynamically directionally unstable. They can be made directionally stable by the use of axial spin.

Consider a spin-stabilized projectile which is spinning clockwise as viewed from the rear (the common mode) and is aerodynamically statically unstable, and suppose that it is subjected to a nose-up yaw disturbance in (say) the vertical plane. Because $C_{m\alpha}$ is positive, the projectile will experience a nose-up moment attempting to increase the yaw angle. However, if it is spinning fast enough,

this moment, by the argument advanced above, causes the nose of the projectile to move to the right (Figure 2.19).

The projectile yaw angle is now the resultant of the original yaw in the vertical plane, and the consequent yaw in the horizontal plane. The net yaw has now therefore moved in a clockwise direction when viewed from the front of the projectile. The argument can now be repeated and the consequence of the original yaw disturbance is that the nose of the projectile describes a spiral of declining amplitude (Figure 2.20). Note that in this figure 'heave' refers to movement in the vertical plane and 'swerve' to movement in the horizontal plane.

The main motion here is precession but it may be noticed that there is a small higher frequency motion superimposed. This is normally present in gyroscopic motion and is known as nutation. The amplitude and frequency of the motion, in the case of a projectile in flight, are determined by the dynamic stability of the projectile. This motion is not usually of great importance in the design of ammunition for small arms and so will not be discussed further here.

The gyroscopic stability coefficient In the discussion above, it has only been stated that the projectile is spinning 'fast enough'. There are, in fact, both upper and lower bounds to the amount of spin which can be employed in the stabilization of projectiles. It has already been shown that the angular momentum of the projectile and its yawing moment curve slope are important quantities for achieving stability. In fact it may be shown that (see for example Moss, 1995) the spin rate for neutral stability p_o is given by:

$$p_o = \frac{1}{A} \sqrt{4BM_\alpha}$$

in which B is the transverse moment of inertia of the projectile about an axis through its centre of gravity, M_α is the yawing moment curve slope and

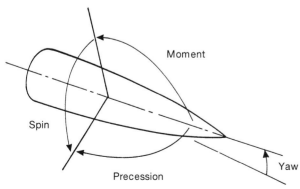

Figure 2.19 The basic mechanism of spin stabilization.

A is the axial moment of inertia. This may be viewed as the lower bound of spin rate for stability of the round.

Any increase in the spin rate above this value will increase the stability of the round, i.e. it will increase its resistance to a yaw disturbance. This criterion is usually expressed in terms of a gyroscopic stability coefficient s_g defined as:

$$s_g = \frac{A^2 p^2}{4BM_\alpha}$$

This will have a value of unity for a neutrally stable spin stabilized projectile and a larger value for a stable projectile. It is usual to consider $s_g = 1.2$ as the lower bound for stability in practice. If s_g is less than this value, the round is likely to tumble in flight leading to shorter ranges and lower accuracy. However, it is possible to deliberately produce rounds with s_g less than 1 in order to improve their 'stopping' capability (e.g. see Long, 1985).

The upper bound to spin rate is also related to stability. If the round is spun much too fast, it will strongly resist any attempts to perturb it and the consequence is that it will fly like the lower diagram of Figure 2.21. This again produces a round flying at larger yaw angles than necessary and reduces range.

For most conventional small arm ammunition, the design value of s_g is taken to be around 2. This value for small-diameter rounds can produce remarkably high spin rates. Once again this is a consequence of the square-cube law referred to earlier. Stability is being conferred by the inertial properties of the round – these vary as the mass, i.e. as length cubed. The disturbances are aerodynamic

TABLE 2.2
SPIN RATES FOR STABILITY FOR DIFFERENT CALIBRE PROJECTILES

Projectile	Calibre (mm)	Spin rate (rev/min)
L15	155	16 500
M1	105	25 600
M80	7.62	167 000
CB10	5.56	334 000

in origin – they come from air pressure and vary with area, i.e. as length squared. Therefore, as the calibre reduces the spin rate has to increase to maintain stability. Table 2.2 gives the spin rates required for a variety of spin-stabilized projectiles at a constant speed corresponding to launch at sea level at a Mach number of 2.5. It can be seen that spin rate times calibre is approximately constant as argued above.

The spin of the round is produced by rifling the barrel, that is by machining spiral grooves into the barrel. If the helix angle of the rifling twist is expressed as θ then the spin rate of the round at the muzzle (p) for a given muzzle velocity (V) is given by:

$$p = \frac{2 \cdot V \tan(\theta)}{d}$$

Since we require V/d to be almost constant, it follows therefore that θ is also almost constant, regardless of the calibre of the gun. It is usually in the range 5–10°.

Still more can be learned from the expression for the gyroscopic stability coefficient by expressing it in a different way. Using the definition of $C_{m\alpha}$ used earlier, the stability coefficient may be written:

$$s_g = \frac{8A^2 p^2}{B\rho V^2 \pi d^2 C_{m\alpha}}$$

A further point emerges from this re-arrangement. If during flight, the round enters a medium for which the density is significantly higher than for air (such as human tissue), the round will theoretically become very unstable and should tumble very rapidly. This motion is not normally observed. For a discussion of a proposed resolution of this problem, see Kneubuehl and Sellier (1992), where it is argued that with high-speed bullets in high-density media, the presence of cavities around the bullet profoundly modify the forces and moments generated and hence the consequent path of the projectile.

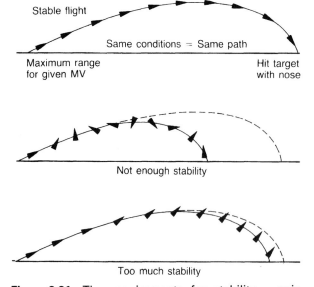

Figure 2.21 The requirements for stability – spin stabilization.

REFERENCES

Kneubuehl B.P., Sellier K. (1992). Wound ballistics: a new understanding of the behaviour of a bullet in a dense medium. In *Proceedings of the 13th International Symposium on Ballistics Stockholm, Sweden*.

Knudsen P.J.T. (1990). The ballistician's dilemma. Internal Security & Co. *Int. Defense Rev.*, *23*, (suppl), 5.

Long D. (1985). *The AR-15/M16 A Practical Guide*. Paladin Press.

Moss G.M., Leeming D.W., Farrar C.L. (1995). *Military Ballistics – A Basic Manual, vol 1*. Brassey's New Battlefield Weapon Systems and Technology Series into the 21st Century. London/Washington.

3. Projectile–Material Interactions: Simulants

B. Janzon

Tissue simulants are used in experimental wound ballistic and related research for many purposes. In order to appreciate their different properties and how well they represent the tissues they are intended to simulate, brief overviews of the properties of bullets and their behaviour during trajectory and/or penetrating media of the same density as tissues, as well as the responses of the target to penetration, are required.

Different kinds of projectiles

Many different kinds of projectiles can be involved in wounding processes, from automobiles, very large pieces of machinery thrown or falling at low velocity in industrial accidents, rocks and debris scattered by an explosion, fragments from artillery and mortar shells, bombs and grenades, bullets from machine guns, assault rifles, submachine guns and hand guns. Obviously there are many different mechanisms involved in their effects on living tissues.

The discussion in this chapter concentrates merely on fragments and bullets. Low-velocity impacts of heavy objects may sometimes give injuries similar to air blast, and are dealt with elsewhere.

The term bullet denotes a non-explosive, ballistically stable projectile, fired from a barrel of a calibre usually below 14.5 mm. The bullet can contain a pyrotechnic tracer, or an incendiary charge.

The armed forces of countries which used to comprise the Soviet Union possess large quantities of 14.5-mm heavy machine guns; the US and NATO counterpart is of calibre 0.50 in (12.7 mm). Military assault rifles are commonly of calibre 7.62, 5.56 or 5.45 mm, although some older calibres are still in use. Some newer smaller calibres are appearing, down to about 4.5 mm.

A 7.62-mm NATO assault rifle bullet typically has a muzzle velocity of just over 800 m/s and an energy of about 3000 J. The 5.56-mm NATO assault rifle, with a bullet of less than half the weight of the earlier model, has almost 2000 J of muzzle energy, reached by increasing the muzzle velocity of the bullet to about 900 m/s or more.

Submachine guns and hand guns may have larger calibres – such as 9-mm parabellum, 10-mm or 0.45-in ACP – and relatively heavy bullets. Muzzle velocities are, however, much lower, and seldom exceed 400 or 450 m/s. Some modern submachine guns have the calibre 5.56 mm and fire standard assault rifle ammunition; their shorter barrel gives rise to a somewhat lower velocity than the 900 m/s mentioned.

A shell, bomb or grenade fragment may have any shape, size and weight. The most usual material is steel. The most common shape derived from the usual modern shells and grenades is relatively 'chunky', in contrast to older artillery ordnance made of less brittle steels and with a long cylindrical, central part, which gave rise predominantly to elongated 'splinters'. The launch velocity of a fragment may be up to 2000 m/s or more. In modern and prefragmented munitions the majority of fragments are, however, relatively small. Nevertheless a fragment much less than 1 g in weight may still cause serious injury. Such small fragments will be retarded very rapidly during their air trajectory, and quickly lose their velocity and capacity to injure. In order to extend the radius of efficacy, fragments of heavy materials, such as tungsten, are used in some prefragmented munitions.

A spherical steel ball, for example a ball bearing, constitutes a very suitable projectile for wound ballistic research, especially preferable for a laboratory study using animal models (see, among others, Berlin *et al.*, 1979; Janzon and Seeman, 1985). One of the most important reasons for this is the reproducibility of its energy transfer in the wound, this being dependent only on the wound channel length in soft tissue, impact velocity and projectile diameter. Such 'bullets' may be easily fired from smooth-bore barrels, with or without a sabot.

THE PHYSICAL MECHANISMS OF WOUNDING

Projectile flight in air

Whereas a fragment usually tumbles in its air trajectory, causing high drag and rapid retardation, a bullet is designed to be ballistically stable. If a small disturbance, such as may occur on exit from the muzzle, or from side winds, causes destabilization, the ensuing oscillatory motion is attenuated and the bullet will return to a stable position in its trajectory.

Most bullets are spin-stabilized, the spin being imparted by a low-angle thread ('rifling') in the barrel, which engraves itself into the bullet and forces it to rotate as it accelerates down the barrel. To give the bullet optimum stability, the rate of spin must be neither too small nor too great.

During air trajectory, bullet velocity will usually decline faster than does its spin. A small bullet may thus become over-stable at longer ranges, meaning that it will fly at increasing angles of yaw relative to its downward-curving trajectory. (Yaw is the angle between the trajectory and the bullet axis, see

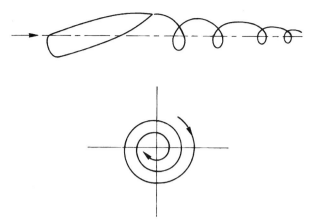

Figure 3.1 Principle sketch of attenuated precession motion of a spin-stabilized bullet.

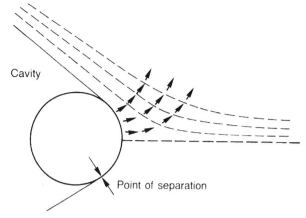

Figure 3.2 Cavitating flow around sphere (May, 1975).

Sebourn, 1996.) The bullet does not, as one might expect, fly like a gyroscope with a constant angle in space, but it displays a conical, rotating motion pattern called precession, occurring at a much lower rate than its spin. A disturbance in the bullet's path will also, after an initial period of more complex motion, create a precession motion (Figure 3.1), which will, however, be attenuated if the bullet has good stability.

Even a ballistically stable bullet usually flies at small angles of yaw because of errors in the position of its centre of mass, surface imperfections and asymmetries in its shape, often caused during passage down the barrel. Large angles of yaw may be caused by hitting obstacles close to the target. Even very small angles of yaw on impact, of the order of one or a few degrees, have been shown to be decisive for the bullet's subsequent tumbling in the target (Janzon, 1982a).

Cavitation

One very important physical phenomenon characterizing the wounding process of fast projectiles is cavitation (Woodruff, 1898; Janzon, 1983). When a projectile moves through a liquid or a medium with similar properties, such as muscle tissue, the material is accelerated away from the path of the projectile by high pressures created around its path (Figure 3.2). This causes a temporary cavity behind the bullet, filled with air or vapour at sub-atmospheric pressure. Matter is sucked into this

low-pressure cavity at both the points of entry to and exit from the penetrated medium (Dziemian and Herget, 1950; Thoresby and Darlow, 1967).

At the moment of maximum expansion of the cavity, energy transfer from the bullet is distributed as follows: rupture and laceration of the tissue as it retards the projectile's passage; propagation as pressure moves to the rest of the target; and stored (potential) energy in the surrounding tissues as a result of elastic deformity. Collapse of the cavity occurs as a result of the last. Very high pressures, of the same order as those created during the passage of the projectile, of up to tens or hundreds of Megapascals [MPa], may arise in the tissues during the collapse. There may be one or more oscillatory re-expansions of the cavity (Figure 3.3).

The effect of cavitation may vary depending on the strength of the material affected and its other properties and will generally cause star-like lacerations around the wound path (Janzon, 1983). Boundary effects and the inflow of air through the entrance and exit apertures normally make the temporary cavity there smaller than elsewhere (Janzon, 1983; Janzon and Persson, 1990).

Bullet tumbling and energy transfer

All small-calibre ammunition currently issued to armed forces is spin-stabilized. The spin rate, bullet design and mass must be suitably matched to allow stability in air, in order to achieve sufficient accuracy and effective ranges. In human muscle,

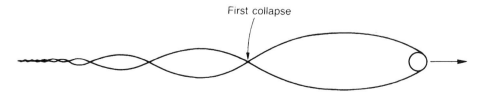

Figure 3.3 'Cavity train' behind fast-moving sphere in an infinite medium.

with a density about 800 times that of air, the angular momentum of the bullet and the consequent stabilizing moment arising as the response to a disturbance, are insufficient to retain stabilization and tumbling commences as soon as penetration begins. The shape of the projectile and its behaviour, relative to the cavity it creates, determines the outcome.

When penetration has begun, the tumbling moment on the projectile will increase with the yaw, causing a cumulative increase of the yaw angle, soon resulting in overturning by 90 degrees or more (Figure 3.4) (Janzon, 1983). For very small yaws the growth rate of the tumbling is low, and the bullet may thus penetrate deeply before finally tumbling. The growth rate increases with increasing yaw, and even a few degrees of yaw angle, of the bullet on impact, may be enough to cause early tumbling.

Bullets of the same type, fired from the same weapon under the same conditions, seem to follow exactly the same tumbling sequence in the target, but with different points of onset, determined by stochastical variations of impact conditions. As a consequence, the records of different shots may be superimposed, using yaw angle as a function of penetration depth to determine the 'tumbling point' for each shot as a common point of reference (Janzon et al., 1979; Kokinakis et al., 1979; Janzon, 1982a, see Flash X-ray registration below). Tumbling is dependent largely on the angle of yaw on impact, to a certain extent on the obliquity of the impact, and on the structure of target material close behind the point of impact, but not on the rate of the yaw on impact.

The variation of the retardation force with the bullet's penetration depth (Figure 3.4) is denoted as the 'energy transfer characteristics'. Integrating that force over penetrated distance will yield the energy transferred to the target. Considerable variation may occur between shots, especially due to the variation of the bullet's small angle of yaw upon impact.

Factors influencing tumbling

As indicated, the bullet's angle of yaw upon impact is a very important determining factor for its motion in the target. Figure 3.5 shows some of the factors influencing the tendency of the bullet to tumble in dense materials. A blunt tip gives rise to a cavity which detaches from the leading edge of the projectile at some angle of yaw. A cylindrical base (Figure 3.5) may cause a stabilizing lift force when the projectile meets the wall of the cavity (May, 1975). A boat-tail base (which is usual) is likely to result in an absence of any stabilizing force, or there may even be a destabilizing lift force, sucking the projectile base further into the wall of the cavity (May, 1975). The more pointed the tip, the less are the chances that any stabilizing force would affect the rear, as the cavity would be attached along the entire length of the leading edge of the projectile (Figure 3.5).

A finned, or similarly aerodynamically stabilized projectile is characterized by its centre of pressure (the effective site of a turning force) being located behind its centre of mass, independent of yaw angle, and it is consequently always stable, even after a severe disturbance, and regardless of the density of the target material (Janzon, 1983). In this case, other factors such as deformation of the projectile upon impact, determine whether the projectile remains stable or not in a material much denser than air. The deformation mechanism is usually bending of the projectile body, which may well be sufficient to cause instability. The fins may also be torn away following impact, or the rear part of the projectile may break loose, with the same effects.

If a stabilizing effect is not imparted by the shape of the base, the factors which determine how fast the bullet tumbles are: the degree of lift, affected by the shape of the bullet, and by the current yaw; the distance between centre of mass and centre of pressure, which may also change with the yaw (Peters et al., 1996a); and the bullet's longitudinal

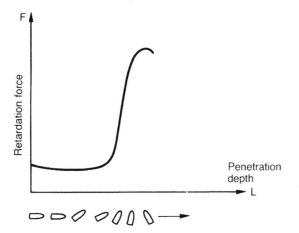

Figure 3.4 Tumbling sequence of bullet, and consequence for the retardation force affecting it.

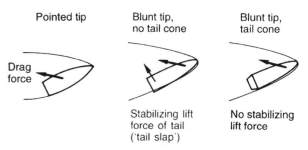

Figure 3.5 Cavitation by yawing projectiles of different shape.

moment of inertia. Thus a long bullet will usually tumble relatively more slowly than a short one.

The tumbling of the projectile is far more central to the bullet's capacity to transfer energy than is any other factor, including velocity. The retardant force on a projectile at 90 degrees of yaw may be more than ten times that in its head-on position (Janzon, 1983).

Bullet break-up

When tumbling, or when hitting a hard object, even a fully jacketed bullet may break up. If the bullet is soft-nosed – and consequently not legal for use in armed conflict according to the 'Dum-Dum' ban contained in the 1899 Hague Declaration – it will expand when it strikes tissue, provided that the velocity is sufficient to generate high enough pressures to deform the tip. Such deformable hand gun ammunition is, however, commonly used for law enforcement purposes, especially in the USA. Deformable rifle ammunition is used throughout the World for hunting. For an interesting background to the Dum-Dum bullet ban the reader is referred to Von Bruns (1898).

Most non-military bullets have some kind of jacket, designed to reduce wear of and deposits in the gun barrel, but some have no jacket, and consist merely of a slug, usually made of hardened lead. In a bullet with a full jacket, factors, such as jacket design, core material strength, bullet-tip design and impact velocity, are important determinants of whether deformation and break-up occur, and to what extent. A lead projectile with an uncovered nose will usually deform quite easily and this usually occurs very soon after the bullet has struck the target (Berlin et al., 1988b).

There are, primarily for law-enforcement purposes, designs involving other, stronger, core materials, such as steel, copper or bronze, which may resist deformation better, or which may give only limited and well-controlled deformation. Their main purpose is often to provide a good penetration of hard targets, while retaining desirable wound ballistic properties. An excellent survey of the deformation properties of primarily hand-gun bullets can be found in Sellier et al. (1977).

The full metal jacket of a military bullet is also intended to prevent deformation and break-up, in addition to complying with internal and exterior ballistic considerations. If, however, a military rifle projectile tumbles very rapidly in the wound, it has been shown (Nordstrand et al., 1979) that the centrifugal forces affecting the alloy lead core are sufficient to allow break-up. Whether or not the bullet will fragment then depends upon the design of the jacket, especially at the rear (Berlin et al., 1976, 1977), at the crimping cannelure of the jacket (Herget, 1953) and at the interface between different parts of an inhomogeneous core (Berlin et al.,

1988a). Blunt-nosed bullets appear to have a tendency to break at the tip, because the entire drag force is concentrated on a much smaller area at the tip than in a pointed bullet (Callender and French, 1935).

Scaling

Scaling allows predictions to be made of the behaviour of different shapes and sizes of projectiles in materials of different sizes and properties, using both experimental and behaviour data acquired under defined geometric conditions. A scaling analysis of the wounding process was made by Janzon (1983). Many scaling laws are possible (Birkhoff, 1960; Baker et al., 1973); the simplest one obviously being linear (replica) scaling, where all lengths are scaled, and consequently areas and retardation forces scale as $(\text{length})^2$, and volume and mass as $(\text{length})^3$.

All densities and other bulk properties, shapes, velocities and pressures remain the same.

Another possible scaling law is that of Reynolds, that is the dimensionless number, Re, expressed as the product:

$$Re = (\text{density}) \cdot (\text{velocity}) \cdot (\text{length})/(\text{viscosity})$$

must be kept constant. This scaling law, widely used in aero- and hydrodynamics, is relevant if only the hydrodynamic portion of the retardation process is considered.

If flow in the trans- and supersonic ranges is to be considered, Mach scaling should be used, that is the ratio

$$(\text{velocity})/(\text{sonic velocity})$$

should be maintained constant. The sonic velocity of muscle tissue is about 1450 m/s (Berlin et al., 1979). For a blunt fragment or a tumbling bullet, transonic flow may begin to occur at 700–800 m/s.

If flow is strongly affected by the presence of a free surface, such as in the case of cavitation flow, a relevant approach is to keep the property

$$Fr = (\text{velocity})/\sqrt{(\text{length})}$$

constant, that is Froude scaling.

It is obvious that no model can simultaneously comply with all these scaling laws, unless it involves exactly the same bullet, target and sizes as the event it is intended to simulate. Choice of models becomes, then, a matter of deciding which important properties of the event are to be considered, and which ones may be disregarded without biasing the outcome. This usually requires a profound knowledge of the physics involved, and mistakes are easily made. In doubtful cases, experiments to calibrate the model should always be used.

Projectile retardation

The law governing the retardation of a projectile in tissue or simulant may be written (Peters, 1990, 1996a):

$$F = C_{Dv} \cdot A \cdot \rho \cdot v^2/2 + C_{Dv} \cdot A \cdot R \qquad (1)$$

where A is the projectile's displayed cross-section area, ρ is target density and v projectile velocity. The first term describes the hydrodynamic (inertial) component required to accelerate the target material from the projectile, the second is dependent on the strength of the target, that is the force required to damage and displace the material in the projectile's path. C_{Dv} is not a true constant, but depends on velocity and cavitation conditions.

The 'rupture modulus', R, which is contained in equation (1), seems to be dependent on the strain rate of the target material – how rapidly it is deformed. Thus, more energy is required to damage a certain volume of tissue as the strain rate increases, or the same energy deposited in a larger volume of tissue causes a greater injury (Janzon et al., 1988; Peters, 1990, 1996a). A proportionality was found:

$$R = c \cdot (v/d)^{1/2} \qquad (2)$$

where c is a constant and d is a relevant, characteristic size of the target (Peters, 1990). Typically, the velocity at which the hydrodynamic drag force equals the rupture force is from 50 to about 200 m/s in soft tissue, gelatin and certain soft soap (Peters, 1990). The demonstrated importance of strain rate affects the validity of scaled experiments and their value in estimating tissue damage.

SIMULATING BULLET INTERACTION WITH LIVE TISSUE

There are many reasons for using simulant materials to study bullet interaction with a live target. Obviously the best simulant for tissue is live tissue. Another possibility is to use cadavers, human or animal, either in their entirety or to take out selected organs for further study.

Skin is very strong compared with muscle tissue, and very resistant to damage. Several animal species have a loose skin of much greater strength and resistance to that of man. In such cases, the removal of the skin over the area to be used should be considered.

In order to study bullet behaviour, a considerable number of other materials have been used over the years. Among the most common are a 20% cured gelatin-water solution and soft soap.

Animal models

Dogs, cats, horses, cattle, goats, sheep and pigs have been much used for the purpose of simulating human tissue. In ethically satisfactory studies animals are deeply anaesthetized and remain so for the duration of the experiment. Using an animal model enables the study of physiological parameters and other tissue responses to the trauma. In choosing a species, the purpose for which it is to be used is important: e.g. for simulating ballistic injury for the training of medical personnel, or as part of a standardized and well-controlled laboratory model. The legal status of studies involving the use of deeply anaesthetized animals for training medicine personnel varies from country to country. Such studies are not permitted, for example, in the UK.

If extrapolations are to be made from animal models to wounding in man there must be a close resemblance between the organ system to be studied, and that of man (Schantz, 1979). The species chosen must enable a sufficient and representative wound channel length to be obtained so as to reproduce the tumbling behaviour of the bullet in a wound in man. It is also important that the anaesthetic, or other drugs used, should not interfere with or affect the system response studied.

Smaller mammal species

Little can be learned regarding wound ballistics from studies undertaken in laboratory rodents; scaling problems become almost insuperable, unless small spherical steel balls are used as projectiles. They enable accurate determination of the energy to be transferred. Dogs are easy to handle, tolerant to prolonged and deep anaesthesia, and their peripheral veins and arteries are readily accessible. They may be considered appropriate for the study of haemodynamic responses (Rybeck, 1974); however, it may be impossible to obtain adequate missile trajectory lengths through muscle. Dog muscle is relatively stronger than many other species (Peters, 1990) and thus the effect of cavitation will be relatively small. Dogs have loose skin which is both strong and furry.

Cats have an additional drawback of being rather small, though effective scaled studies have been undertaken in this species (Harvey et al., 1962). Like dogs they have loose, strong skin and a furry coat. Their muscle tissue is, like the dog's, stronger than most other species.

Horses, cattle, goats and sheep

Horses and cattle were used in some of the earliest experiments on wound ballistics. Their use began on the battlefields of the 1870–1 Franco–Prussian War, with carcasses of horses – and of humans also (Journée, 1907). Horses and cattle are characterized by large muscle masses, making it possible to obtain long wound paths. Due to their size, live animals are, however, difficult to handle, and it is not easy to sustain prolonged anaesthesia (Schantz, 1979).

Goats and sheep have been extensively used. Like cattle they are ruminants, and thus their intestinal organs are quite different from those of humans. They may be anaesthetized using the same methods as for humans, and are much easier to handle than cattle (Schantz, 1979). Their skin is fairly thin and supple, but is usually covered with a thick woolly coat. Their limb muscles are long and slender, necessitating the use of relatively large animals and carefully selected wound paths to obtain sufficient channel lengths.

Pigs

Pigs seem to be selected with increasing frequency as the animal of choice for biomedical research relevant to man (Mount and Ingram, 1971; Schantz, 1979), and their characteristics are well known. They appear similar to man in many respects – their skin (although there are some differences), intestinal system (except for the colon) (Schantz, 1979) and muscle tissue. Their size can be chosen widely, and even in smaller specimens, adequate wound channel lengths in muscle can easily be achieved. Pigs are easy to handle and anaesthetize, and endure long anaesthesia well. The shape of their limbs, however, makes it difficult to apply wound dressings designed for use in man.

Another problem is that animals of 25–30 kg, as are commonly used, are still juvenile, and full-grown animals may reach prohibitive weights. There is thus a demand for smaller species – so-called miniature pigs – which are, however, costly, difficult to obtain, and are also said to be ill-tempered compared with the common domestic species (Schantz, 1979). Pigs are an obvious choice, both to simulate man for training medical personnel, and for use in a laboratory model.

Human bodies and organs

Information on wounds in man stems mainly from analyses of battle casualties in armed conflicts (Coates, 1962; Dimond and Rich, 1967; Rich, 1968; Rich et al., 1968, 1969; Carey, 1988, 1996).

The data collected during wars has a number of general shortcomings: they are incomplete; selection may be biased by the evacuation procedures used; and the source and properties of the wounding agent are seldom exactly known. Valuable additional sources of information are forensic investigations, where the possibilities of ascertaining the exact circumstances of wounding are better (Sellier et al., 1992). Experiments have been performed on cadavers (MacCormack, 1895; Von Bruns, 1898; Journée, 1907). Human skulls filled with gelatin, in order to simulate brain, have been used to simulate the effects of bullet impacts in the head (Watkins et al., 1988; see Chapter 4).

Simulant materials

As seen from the discussion of 'scaling', a good simulant material must have many properties in common with the tissue penetrated. At high velocities, undoubtedly the most important property is the material's density, for example soft tissue has a common density around 1050 kg/m^3 and a velocity of sound of about 1450 m/s (Berlin et al., 1979). Other properties of simulants are defined by the purposes of the study.

Gelatin Gelatin, dissolved in water to various concentrations, is undoubtedly the most commonly used simulant in wound ballistic research. Twenty per cent gelatin at 24°C has been shown to give similar retardation to steel spheres as dog muscle (Harvey et al., 1962), though penetration depths were found to be greater in gelatin than in tissue (Harvey et al., 1962; Peters, 1990). Better simulation can be obtained by using the gelatin at 10°C, at which temperature an approximately correct 'rupture modulus' occurs (Watkins et al., 1982; Peters, 1990). It also yields the same drag coefficient for spherical bullets as does pig muscle (Berlin et al., 1979).

Gelatin, standardized during the manufacturing procedure and prepared in this way, is widely used throughout the US and by other NATO countries for munitions testing. The size of the block used is of importance to the results: commonly 150 × 150 mm blocks will accommodate most military-type bullets without disintegrating. Such blocks may, however, be too small to study expanding bullets including hunting ammunition.

Ten per cent gelatin at 4°C has been used by Fackler and Malinowski (1985). It has a somewhat lower density, about 1030 kg/m^3, and allows greater projectile penetration than tissue (Peters, 1990). The sonic velocity is, for both concentrations, similar to that of tissue.

Gelatin behaves in a manner similar to muscle, in that the passage of a high-velocity bullet causes a violent pulsating temporary cavity which then collapses, leaving only a permanent 'wound' cavity (of similar dimensions to the projectile) surrounded by longitudinal ruptures, appearing very similar to a wound in muscle. If a bullet fragments it is easily seen in the gelatin block which is more or less transparent. The rupture profile gives a good idea of the pattern of energy transfer in the target, and the transparency of the block makes it possible to use optical methods, such as high-speed still cine photography, to record penetration processes.

The drawbacks of gelatin are that it is relatively expensive, cannot be re-used, and is difficult and rather sensitive to manufacture as regards the quality of gelatin and water used and the manufacturing process. It cannot be stored without refrigeration except for a very short time, and it cannot be preserved to provide a permanent record

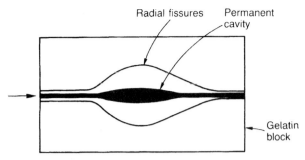

Figure 3.6 Wound profile in gelatin from typical 7.62-mm-calibre bullet.

of the experiment. An interesting way of providing a permanent record of the 'wound' is to use the gelatin block as a mould for a low-viscosity epoxy (Ragsdale *et al.*, 1990) or silicone rubber casting (E. Brown, 1988, personal communication). The liquid is poured into one end of the wound cavity, and will then penetrate all spaces inside it, including the star-like rifts around the wound track. After curing, the gelatin may be carefully removed from the cast, by spraying it with warm water.

A method to estimate the energy transfer characteristics of bullets using gelatin blocks as the muscle simulant was proposed by Harvey *et al.* (1945) and others, and revived by Fackler *et al.* (Fackler and Malinowski, 1985; Fackler *et al.*, 1988). This method gives reasonable qualitative data, and allows ready visualization of the result (Figure 3.6), but it does not yield good quantitative information unless very sophisticated measuring equipment is used. The result is also very sensitive to the quality of the gelatin, the manufacturing process, storage and temperature at the time of the experiment. Inaccuracies occur such as in trying to evaluate the energy transfer characteristics, or even the temporary cavity size, by measurement of the total length of fissures (Ragsdale and Josselson, 1988).

Soap Soap is another material which is widely used as a tissue simulant in wound ballistic research. In contrast to muscle and gelatin, which are highly elastic media, soft glycerin soap is a plastic (visco-plastic) medium with little elasticity. It has been shown (Janzon, 1982b; Scépanovic and Albreht, 1982) that there is no significant difference between the behaviour of tumbling bullets in soap and in pig muscle. The drag coefficient of spherical steel balls in soap is also the same as in pig muscle (Berlin *et al.*, 1979; Scépanovic, 1979). However, the target responds in a quite different way than does soft tissue. Instead of creating a cavity which will subsequently collapse, the approximate, maximum temporary cavity is permanently displayed in the soap. This cavity is almost circular in cross-section, and allows easy measurement of its shape and size. Soap-blocks of 200 × 200 mm cross-section are

suitable for all military bullets, as well as most types of hunting ammunition.

The density of the soap, about $1060 \, \text{kg/m}^3$, closely resembles that of tissue, as does the sonic velocity. The rupture modulus may also be kept approximately similar to that of tissue (Peters, 1990).

The advantages of soap are that it is readily available commercially, its properties may be varied to suit the strength requirements and it may be stored at room temperature for long periods without any other precautions than wrapping in plastic foil. It may also be used at room temperature, and provides a permanent record of the event. Used blocks may be kept for long periods of time. It is easy to handle, and not messy like gelatin. Soap-blocks may be re-cast and re-used, although temperature control of the melt is critical: too high temperatures may destroy the consistency and physical properties by formation of small bubbles of ethanol vapour. Finally soap makes it possible to estimate the energy transfer characteristics of the bullet without access to sophisticated measuring equipment (Janzon, 1982a).

A simple method of measurement of energy transfer from a tumbling bullet was achieved with soft soap-blocks, having a square cross-section of about 200 × 200 mm, and a length of about 270 mm (Berlin *et al.*, 1982; Janzon, 1982 a,b), as simulants. They were placed at the desired range, and fired at. As soap is a very plastic material, a permanent cavity was formed which could be cut open and its size and shape determined. The energy transfer from the bullet may be calculated with good precision from the data (Figure 3.7). The volume of the cavity may be determined by filling with water from a graduated cylinder.

The disadvantages of soap are that it does not give a true image of the appearance of the wound in

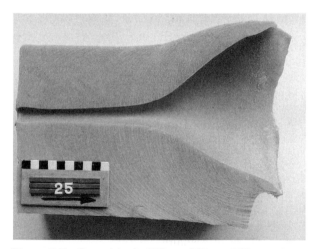

Figure 3.7 Soap-block 200 × 200 × 270 mm traversed by a 7.62-mm-calibre NATO bullet from the AK 4, range 100 m.

tissue, nor does it demonstrate the distribution of bullet fragments in the same way as does tissue. Although some soap may be translucent, soap-blocks are usually not entirely transparent.

Water and water-soaked materials As a high proportion of tissue contents is composed of water, water is an obvious choice as a simulant. Being completely transparent it is well suited for high-speed filming or photography. Its density is $1000\,kg/m^3$, though its strength is much lower than that of tissue, and the size of the cavity is determined by the ambient pressure and water temperature. However, in a solid container the walls of the vessel can strongly influence and suppress cavitation. If the bullet's energy release is high, a stiff vessel may also easily be damaged or destroyed. If water is loosely contained, such as in a plastic bag, the bag may be ruptured and the cavity will not collapse again after its maximal expansion. The drag coefficient for spherical bullets in water is lower than in pig muscle (Berlin *et al.*, 1979). Penetration of the bullet is greater than in tissue. One of the simplest demonstrations of the properties of a bullet is to fire at a water melon or a water-filled can; if the projectile causes high energy transfer, the entire target may disintegrate in a spectacular manner.

Water-soaked paper has been used as a simulant, and may be useful, although its density is low. Like soap, it may give a permanent record of the shot, which may be dried out and preserved.

Clay and similar materials Clay has been used, but should be avoided (Fackler and Kneubuehl, 1990). It may give a rough simulation of a very strong, non-deforming bullet's behaviour but, as its density is much higher than that of the tissue, the bullet is subject to much higher retardation loads, will thus be more prone to deform, tumble much faster, and its total penetration depth will be much less.

Other similar media to clay are plasticine or plastellina. They share the disadvantages of clay of too high density, however they are much easier and less smeary to handle and may be re-used. Both these have found use as a tissue simulant, especially in studies of blunt injury produced by a bullet striking body armour. There are also some types of silicon rubbers, used to make moulds, which may be useful as tissue simulants.

Wood Wood has been used as a tissue simulant. It is somewhat low in density, and has much higher strength than tissue, but it may be useful for some purposes. Practically no temporary cavity is formed when a bullet passes through wood. Among the early criteria of casualty creation – the amount of trauma caused by a fragment or splinter, required to put a soldier out of action – was the ability to penetrate 40 mm of poplar wood (Journée, 1907).

WOUND BALLISTIC MEASUREMENTS

Flash X-ray registration

In order to estimate accurately the performance of a bullet in live targets, multiple flash X-ray units, usually with flash durations of less than 100 ns, and equipped so as to allow delay in individual triggering of the flash X-rays, are the method of choice (Figure 3.8, Kokinakis *et al.*, 1979; Berlin *et al.*, 1982; Watkins *et al.*, 1988). At least 8–12 units are required, which may be of a type of between 100 and 300 kV. They may, preferably, be used with targets of simulant material (Figure 3.8), but may also be combined with live animals, such as pigs (Figure 3.9). Such equipment gives, in addition to an objective method of determining the actual retardation of the bullet, the possibility of observing and measuring bullet tumbling, deformation and break-up as well as the motion of the temporary cavity. The appearance of flash X-ray recordings are shown in Figures 3.10 and 3.11.

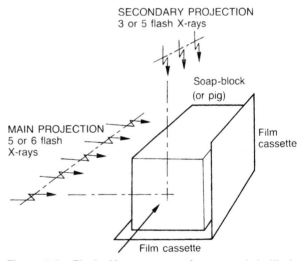

Figure 3.8 Flash X-ray set-up for wound ballistic studies.

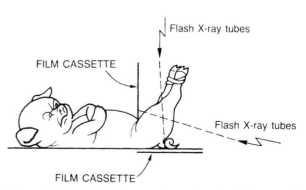

Figure 3.9 Flash X-ray set-up for bullet wound trauma studies on animals.

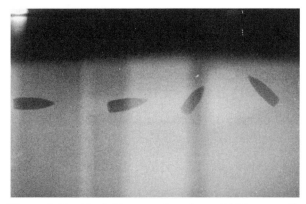

Figure 3.10 Flash X-ray registration of 7.62-mm-calibre NATO bullet penetrating a soap target. Note the cavity formation behind the bullet, which is much larger at the location of complete tumbling. The cavity will continue to expand long after the bullet has left, and the final result will appear similar to Figure 3.7.

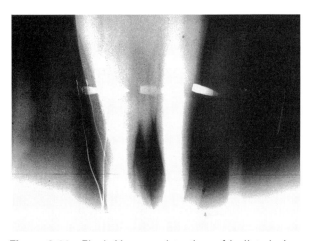

Figure 3.11 Flash X-ray registration of bullet during passage through both hind legs of pig.

Because of the strong dependence of bullet energy transfer on wound channel length, this quantity must always be accurately measured, especially in animal experiments where there may be considerable variation. It is preferable to do this immediately after the shot, before the animal has been moved.

By pooling the results of many shots registered by flash X-rays, using superimposition methods (Kokinakis *et al.*, 1979; Janzon *et al.*, 1979; Janzon, 1982a), measurement scatter may be diminished and a very good estimate of the projectile behaviour can be established. However, flash X-rays are available in only a few centres, are costly and require special skills in handling.

Also available are special stroboscopic flash X-rays, but the number of exposures tends to be limited and the frame rate relatively low. By combining a multiple flash X-ray source with a modern high-speed image converter camera, higher performance stroboscopic pictures can be taken.

High-speed photography and filming

When transparent targets are used, such as water or gelatin, high-speed filming with 500–25 000 frames per second, flash or stroboscopic photography may be used (Harvey *et al.*, 1962; Watkins *et al.*, 1982). Modern high-speed cameras – image converter cameras – can easily be applied to such use, and have high framing rates and good resolution. A drawback of this method is that, often, the bullet itself may not be visualized, as it is obscured inside the temporary cavity. Bullet position must be estimated from the motion of the tip of the cavity. As the cavity expands, so will the target block, giving rise to distortion, easily causing an overestimate of the cavity size. Yaw angle is also difficult to determine due to poor visualization of the bullet.

Velocity measurement

Experiments are often performed where the target has limited thickness, and the total energy deposited in the target is the quantity sought. It is then sufficient to measure entrance and exit velocities. For entrance velocity, photocells or laser barrier measurements are usually preferred, in order to avoid disturbing the bullet before it hits the target and thus possibly biasing the results. Velocity coils may also be used, either 'passive' ones where the bullet has to be magnetic, or 'active' ones, with an exciter coil and pick-up coils. For exit velocity, photocells or short-circuiting foil or laminate screens (break-screens) may be used. One particular problem is that, as the targets become longer, the existing bullet often tends to deviate from its original path, causing a need for a very large area break-screen.

After penetration, soft wall-board packs, sawdust or cotton wad, are suitable for collecting the remainder of the projectile. It will be easier to find if thin cardboard sheets are inserted at intervals in the packs.

If spherical steel balls are used as projectiles, simple short-circuiting wire or laminate screens or gauges, and a reliable electronic counter/chronograph, are sufficient to determine entrance and exit velocities. In water, gelatin and muscle tissue, a simple impact velocity measurement and an accurate measurement of the wound channel length should, together with drag coefficients (Berlin *et al.*, 1979), make it possible to determine energy transfers with enough precision for most purposes.

If photocells or similar devices are used, one must ensure that the triggering is actually caused by the bullet, since the bullet is preceded by a shock wave in air, and since parts of the target may be ejected at higher speed than the exiting bullet, and thus reach the exit velocity measurement devices before the bullet or its fragments. Flash X-ray or high-speed optical photography may also be used for both entrance and exit velocity measurements, and will diminish the risk of such error. Normally, the possibility of deviation of the bullet necessitates that the measurements station behind the target consists of a stereo pair and such a pair is often also required in front of the target, especially to determine bullet yaw.

Measurement of energy transfer characteristics

Measurement of energy transfer characteristics can be undertaken with good accuracy, without sophisticated measurements, using the simple method of firing through soap, described above under 'Soap' (and also by Berlin *et al.*, 1982). If the main objective is to get only a good qualitative view of the bullet's effects, the method described above under 'Gelatin' (and also Fackler and Malinowski, 1985; Fackler *et al.*, 1988) is well suited.

Yaw measurement

The bullet's yaw on impact is a very important property, and may best be measured using one, or preferably two stereo pairs, of optical high-speed photos immediately in front of the target, or, with somewhat less accuracy, using the same set-up equipped with flash X-ray units. A simpler way of estimating yaw is by means of a very thin piece of paper (Japan paper) mounted just before the target but without touching it. Examination of the shape of the hole produced in the paper allows an estimate of yaw angle to be made. This can be done to ensure that the bullet does not have a yaw exceeding, say, 5 degrees, but will not be sufficiently exact to determine angles of yaw of less than this. If the paper is thin, and close to the target, it should not upset the motion of the bullet enough to affect the results.

The need for testing

Nations and military forces must do experimental tests to determine the effects of small-calibre weapons ammunitions they intend to procure, to ensure that the ammunition meets the criteria laid down in the 1899 Hague Declaration (the Dum-Dum bullet ban), as well as possibly to put limits on the extent of local destruction.

The bullet designer may avoid surprises by testing his product extensively also from the wound ballistic aspect, during the entire development process, as well as during series production. Even small changes in ammunition or weapons tolerances may cause considerable differences in termi-

nal ballistics, which can only be detected by testing. The measurement methods reported here present solutions to this problem, without the investigators having to resort to complicated, extensive and costly testing. The involvement of military surgeons in the study of the ballistic properties of bullets is desirable and has provided insights of value in the management of bullet wounds.

REFERENCES

Baker W.E., Westine P.S., Dodge F.T. (1973). *Similarity Methods in Engineering dynamics*. Rochelle Park, NJ: Hayden.

Berlin R., Gelin L.E., Janzon B. et al. (1976). Local effects of assault rifle bullets in live tissues. *Acta Chir. Scand.*, (suppl. 459), 1–84.

Berlin R., Janzon B., Rybeck B. et al. (1977). Local effects of assault rifle bullets in live tissues. Part 2. Further studies in live tissues and relations to some simulant media. *Acta Chir. Scand.*, (suppl. 477), 5–48.

Berlin R.H., Janzon B., Rybeck B. et al. (1979). Retardation of spherical missiles in live tissue. *Acta Chir. Scand.*, (suppl. 489), 91.

Berlin R.H., Janzon B., Rybeck B. et al. (1982). A proposed standard methodology for estimating the wounding capacity of small calibre projectiles or other missiles. *Acta Chir. Scand. Suppl.*, **508**, 11–28 (FOA report B 20037-D4 (M3)).

Berlin R., Janzon B., Lidén E. et al. (1988a). Wound ballistics of Swedish 5.56 mm assault rifle AK 5. *J. Trauma*, **28**, (suppl.) S75–82.

Berlin R., Janzon B., Lidén E. et al. (1988b). Terminal behaviour of deforming bullets. *J. Trauma*, **28**, (suppl.), S58–62.

Birkhoff G. (1960). *Hydrodynamics*. Princeton, NJ: Princeton University Press.

Callender G.R., French R.W. (1935). Wound ballistics. Studies in the mechanism of wound production by rifle bullets. *Milit. Surg.*, **77**, 177–2011.

Carey M. (1988). An analysis of US Army combat mortality and morbidity data. *J. Trauma*, **28**, (suppl.), S183–8.

Coates J.B., ed. (1962). *Wound Ballistics*. Washington, DC: US Army Surgeon General.

Dimond F.C., Rich N.M. (1967). M-16 rifle wounds in Vietnam. *J. Trauma*, **7**, 619–25.

Dziemian A.J., Herget C.M. (1950). Physical aspects of the primary contamination of bullet wounds. *Milit. Surg.*, **106**, 294–9.

Fackler M.L., Malinowski J.A. (1985). The wound profile: a visual method for quantifying gunshot wound components. *J. Trauma*, **25**, 522–9.

Fackler M.L., Kneubuehl B. (1990). Applied wound ballistics: what's new and what's true. *J. Trauma (China)*, **6**(2), (suppl.), 32–7.

Fackler M.L., Bellamy R.F., Malinowski J.A. (1988). The wound profile: illustration of the missile–tissue interaction. *J. Trauma*, **28**, (suppl.), S21–9.

Harvey E.N., Butler E.G., McMillen J.H. et al. (1945). Mechanism of wounding. *War Med.*, **8**, 91–104.

Harvey E.N., McMillen J.H., Butler E.G. et al. (1962). Mechanism of wounding. In *Wound Ballistics* (Coates J.B., ed.): Washington DC: US Army Surgeon General, pp. 143–235.

Herget C.M. (1953). In *Surgery of Trauma* (Bowers W.F., ed.) Philadelphia, PA: Lippincott, pp. 494–510.

Janzon B., Berlin R., Nordstrand I., et al. (1979). Drag and tumbling behaviour of small calibre projectiles in tissue simulant. *Acta Chir Scand, Suppl.*, **489**, 57–70.

Janzon B. (1982a). Soft soap as a tissue simulant medium for wound ballistic studies, investigated by comparative firings with assault rifles Ak 4 and M16A1 into live, anesthetised animals. *Acta Chir. Scand. Suppl.*, **508**, 79–88 (FOA report B 20038-D4 (M3)).

Janzon B. (1982b). Edge, size and temperature effects in soft soap block tissue simulant targets used for wound ballistic studies. *Acta Chir. Scand. Suppl.*, **508**, 105–22 (FOA report B 20039-D4 (M3)).

Janzon B. (1983). *High Energy Missile Trauma. A Study of the Mechanisms of Wounding of Muscle Tissue.* Gothenburg, published by author (Engalls Väg 10, S-147 63 Uttran, Sweden).

Janzon B., Persson Å. (1990). Simulation and visualization of wound ballistic phenomena. *J. Trauma (China)*, **6**(2), (suppl.), 3–12.

Janzon B., Seeman T. (1985). Muscle devitalization in high-energy missile wounds, and its dependence on energy transfer. *J. Trauma*, **25**, 138–44.

Janzon B., Schantz B., Seeman T. (1988). Scale effects in ballistic wounding. *J. Trauma*, **28**, (suppl.), S29–32.

Journée (1907). Relations between the living force of bullets and the gravity of wounds that may be caused by them. *Rev. d'Artillerie*, May (in French).

Kokinakis W., Neades D., Piddington M. et al. (1979). A gelatin methodology for estimating vulnerability of personnel to military rifle systems. *Acta Chir. Scand. Suppl.*, **489**, 35–55.

MacCormack W. (1895). Some points of interest in connexion with the surgery of war. *Lancet*, **ii**, 290–2.

May A.W. (1975). *Water Entry and the Cavity-running Behaviour of Missiles TR 75-2.* Silver Spring, MD: NAVSEA Hydroballistics Advisory Committee (AD-A 020429).

Mount L.E., Ingram D.L. (1971). *The Pig as a Laboratory Animal.* London: Academic Press.

Nordstrand I., Janzon B., Rybeck B. (1979). Break-up behaviour of some small calibre projectiles when penetrating a dense medium. *Acta Chir. Scand. Suppl.*, **489**, 81–90.

Peters C.E. (1990). A mathematical model of wound ballistics. *Journal of Trauma (China)*, **6**(2), (suppl.) 303–18.

Peters C.E., Sebourn C.L., Crowder H.L. (1996a). Wound Ballistics of unstable projectiles. Part I: Projectile yaw growth and retardation. *J. Trauma*, **40**(3), (suppl.), S10–15.

Peters C.E., Sebourn, C.L. (1996b). Wound Ballistics of unstable projectiles. Part II: Temporary cavity formation and tissue damage. *J. Trauma*, **40**(3), (suppl.), S16–21.

Ragsdale B.D., Josselsson A. (1988). Predicting temporary cavity size from radial fissure measurements in ordnance gelatin. *J. Trauma*, **28**, (suppl.), S5–8.

Ragsdale B.D., Sohn S.S. (1990). The shape factor: terminal ballistics of dissimilar .38 cal. projectiles of uniform weight and velocity in ordnance gelatin. *Journal of Trauma (China)*, **6**(2), (Suppl.), 56–70.

Rich N.M. (1968). Vietnam missile wounds evaluated in 750 patients. *Milit. Med.*, **133**, 9–22.

Rich N.M., Johnson E.V., Dimond F.C (1968). Wounding power of missiles used in the Republic of Vietnam. *JAMA*, **199**, 157–68.

Rich N.M., Manion W.C., Hughes C.W. (1969). Surgical and pathological evaluation of vascular injury in Vietnam. *J. Trauma*, **9**, 279–91.

Rybeck B. (1974). Missile wounding and hemodynamic effects of energy absorption. *Acta Chir Scand. Suppl.*, 450.

Scépanovic D. (1979). Steel ball effect – investigation of shooting at blocks of soap. *Acta Chir. Scand. Suppl.*, **489**, 71–80.

Scépanovic D., Albreht M. (1982). Effects of small calibre arms projectiles in soap. *Acta Chir. Scand. Suppl.*, **508**, 49–60.

Schantz B. (1979). Aspects on the choice of experimental animals when reproducing missile trauma. *Acta Chir. Scand. Suppl.*, **489**, 121–30.

Sebourn C.L., Peters C.E. (1996). Flight dynamics of spin-stabilized projectiles and the relationship to wound ballistics. *J.Trauma*, **40**(3), (suppl.), S22–6.

Sellier K., Kneubühl B. (1992). *Wundballistik und ihren ballistichen Grundlagen.* Springer-Verlag, Berlin, ISBN 3-540-54855-6.

Thoresby F.P., Darlow H.M. (1967). The mechanisms of primary infection of bullet wounds. *Br. J. Surg.*, **54**, 359–61.

Von Bruns P. (1898). *On the Effects of Lead-tipped Bullets.* (In German: *Uber die Wirkung der Bleispitzengeschosse ['Dum-Dum Geschosse']*). From: Beiträge zur klinischen chirurgie, Band XXI. Tübingen: H Laupp'sche Buchhandlung.

Watkins F.P., Pearce B.P., Stainer M.C. (1982). Assessment of terminal effects of high velocity projectiles using tissue simulant. *Acta Chir. Scand. Suppl.*, **508**, 39–47.

Watkins F.P., Pearce B.P., Stainer M.C. (1988). Physical effects of the penetration of head simulants by steel spheres. *J. Trauma*, **28**, (suppl.), S40–53.

Woodruff C.E. (1898). The causes of the explosive effect of modern small calibre bullets. *N.Y. Med. J.*, **67**, 593–601.

4. Projectile–Material Interactions: Soft Tissue and Bone

B. Janzon, J. B. Hull and J. M. Ryan

TERMINOLOGY

The term 'high-energy missile wound' denotes, here, an injury from a typical assault rifle or machine-gun bullet, of velocities between about 600 and 1000 m/s, depending on weapon and range. The energy transferred to the tissues will typically be from one hundred to a few hundred Joules, in exceptional cases up to thousands. High-energy transfer wounds are characterized by injury peripheral to the tissue track. A 'low-energy missile wound' would be described as a typical one from a fully jacketed bullet from a hand gun. The length-to-calibre ratio of such bullets is relatively low, velocities are typically 200–400 m/s and the tissue destruction away from the track of the bullet is usually low.

A deforming or disintegrating bullet from a powerful hand gun may give similar 'high-energy' effects as the much faster assault rifle bullet.

The term 'high velocity', which became popular to describe the new 5.56-mm generation of light assault rifles emerging in the 1960s and 1970s, will not be used here. It clearly appears from Chapter 3 that it is not velocity, *per se*, but rather the ability of the projectile to transfer energy to the tissues ('energy-transfer characteristics') due to tumbling, deformation and fracture of the bullet, which is the cause of the dramatic effects sometimes found in injuries from bullets of 'high-impact' energy.

LOCATION OF THE ENTRY WOUND

The most important factor in determining the outcome of a bullet injury is not the energy of the bullet, nor its energy-transfer characteristics. Many efforts were made over the years to determine a bullet's 'stopping power' or its 'relative incapacitation index' (Kokinakis *et al.*, 1979). Whereas both concepts may be of some interest to the weapons and ammunition designers, or to the procurer, the most important characteristic of the injury for the surgeon, and certainly for the victim, is the location of the injury. If a vital organ is injured, even very small energy transfer can cause death.

'Immediate (or instant) incapacitation' is a concept sometimes discussed, especially in law-enforcement circles. This term is used to describe the objective of preventing a violent and desperate, armed criminal injuring somebody. There is, however, no bullet of the calibres and designs treated here, which is likely to have this property unless it hits, not only a vital organ, but in principle only the central nervous system (CNS). Serious damage to the CNS will cause immediate, uncoordinated motion or collapse and the cessation of voluntary action. Any other hit, lethal though it may be, may still enable the wounded person to pull the trigger he/she was squeezing, even bring up his/her weapon, aim and shoot, or throw the hand-grenade he/she was holding. If projected on the body surface, the CNS would be shown to constitute only about 15% of the frontal body area.

SOFT TISSUE

Entrance and exit wounds

The exit wound is usually larger than the entrance wound produced by an elongated, fully jacketed bullet, because of tumbling within the body and yaw at exit. If the bullet has not had time to tumble in the wound, the exit aperture will be small. The star-like appearance of the torn skin in large exit wounds (Figure 4.1) is caused by the expansion of a temporary cavity in contact with the skin (Harvey *et al.*, 1962; Berlin *et al.*, 1976, 1977). As the boundary effects are rather strong, both at the entrance and the exit, leading to a decrease in the size of the temporary cavity there (Janzon and Seeman, 1985), considerable tissue destruction can occur within the wound even when both apertures seem small. On the other hand, a large and jagged exit wound

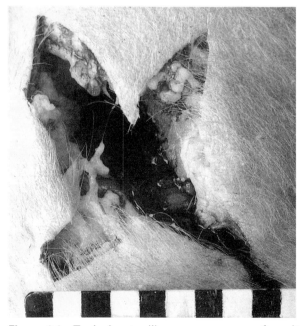

Figure 4.1 Typical star-like appearance of exit wound.

aperture is always a sign of very high energy transfers, associated with the expansion of a large temporary cavity or disruption of bone. It should be considered a warning sign, indicating that massive tissue destruction may be present in the wound, although this is not always so.

In fragment wounds, the entrance is almost always larger than the exit (Janzon and Seeman, 1985) – fragment wounds are often non-perforating (i.e. no exit). With fragments, tumbling and break-up do not usually affect the outcome to the same extent as with bullets. It is then only the velocity and shape which determine the energy transfer to the tissue and the corresponding injury.

If the wound channel is so long that a bullet may have turned 180 degrees inside the target, and may be exiting with the base first, or if the bullet has spent nearly all of its energy before exiting, a small exit wound could occur, notwithstanding tumbling and severe energy transfer within the wound (Figure 4.2). Severe bullet deformation and break-up are always associated with high-energy transfers and ensuing large injuries. It follows that bullet fragments – from jacket or core – found in a wound (e.g. by radiography), are indications of an extensive injury. The same is true for fragments of bone, shattered by a high-energy missile.

Debridement and excision

Wounds caused by high-energy missiles, in which there is significant tissue destruction, or contamination by foreign matter, must be debrided and excised (Heaton *et al.*, 1966). Debridement means laying the wound open; excision is the removal of all foreign objects and contaminants, especially all organic matter, from the wound. Debridement also means removing all non-viable tissue, leaving a live and healthy muscle surface in the wound.

Debridement should take place through wide incisions in skin and fasciae (Heaton *et al.*, 1966; Berlin, 1977; Owen-Smith, 1981; Dufour *et al.*, 1988). Thereby the location of foreign objects and non-viable tissue is facilitated, at the same time as decompression of the muscle bundles involved

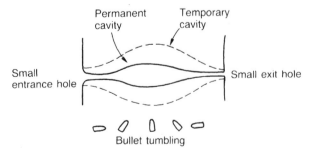

Figure 4.2 Wound where bullet has tumbled completely before exiting. Small entrance and exit holes may hide massive tissue destruction.

occurs. A through-and-through wound should be explored and debrided from both openings, usually starting with the exit wound (Owen-Smith, 1981).

To find the borderline between viable and non-viable tissue is an important task for the surgeon. It can be done with the aid of the classical 'four Cs' below (Whelan *et al.*, 1968; Berlin, 1977), where several of the criteria should be fulfilled to allow the judgement of muscle as non-viable.

The classical macroscopic criteria for non-viable muscular tissue are:

- Colour: A dark-red appearance indicates a lack of oxyhaemoglobin in the tissue, due to poor or absent circulation.
- Contractility: Healthy muscle contracts when touched or pinched.
- Consistency: A mushy appearance indicates damaged tissue.
- Capillary bleeding: When cut, blood from capillaries seeps out from healthy muscle.

Colour and the lack of capillary bleeding are essentially signs of impaired or lacking circulation. Lack of contractility indicates damage to either or both the nerve supply to and the metabolism of the tissue. Change in consistency is often a sign of mechanical disruption, combined with intramuscular bleeding.

Dependence of the injury in muscle on energy transfer

Several studies of the debridement and excision techniques (Haljamäe *et al.*, 1979; Röckert *et al.*, 1979; Almskog *et al.*, 1982; Dahlgren *et al.*, 1979, 1982; Hagelin, 1989) have compared surgeons' judgements, according to the criteria mentioned above, with objective data from histological, membrane potential and objective optical evaluations of the extent of the injury.

Most of these studies have employed the firing of spherical steel ball-bearing balls, launched from a smooth-bore barrel, at velocities typically between 500 and 1500 m/s. The ball diameter has, in most cases, been 6 mm. This model was characterized by very reproducible energy transfer. Measurement of impact and exit velocity was usually undertaken, yielding the energy transferred to the tissues. In addition, the wound channel length was always measured immediately after the shot, before the animal moved, giving another opportunity of estimating the energy deposited (Berlin *et al.*, 1979) in case of failure to measure the exit-velocity of the projectile.

A relationship can be demonstrated between the amount of tissue excised according to the accepted macroscopic criteria and the energy transferred by the bullet, in each separate experimental series (Figures 4.3, 4.4) (Janzon, 1983). Between the series considerable differences were found.

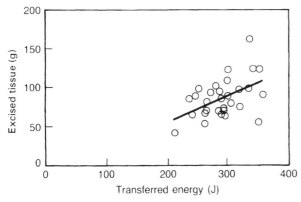

Figure 4.3 Regression of excised pig muscle on transferred energy (6-mm steel spheres, about 1000 m/s) (Berlin *et al.*, 1979).

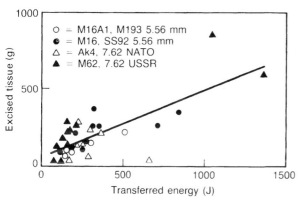

Figure 4.4 Regression of excised pig muscle on transferred energy (5.56- and 7.62-mm assault rifles) (Berlin *et al.*, 1976).

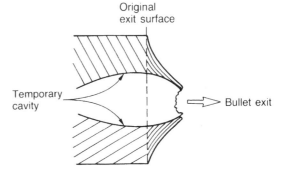

Figure 4.5 Exit wound creation and boundary effect.

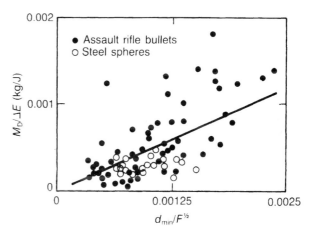

Figure 4.6 Amount of tissue destruction per unit of energy transfer vs: 'scaling parameter' $d_{min}/F^{1/2}$ (Janzon *et al.*, 1988).

The amount of tissue excised per Joule of energy transfer is generally much lower at the entrance and exit openings. Also superficial shots gave lower excision per unit of energy transferred (Janzon, 1983). The reason for this is found in the special character of the deformations near free boundaries (Figure 4.5), where the expansion of the temporary cavity will tend to occur in the direction of least resistance (Harvey *et al.*, 1947), thereby minimizing the radial expansion of the cavity, and limiting the extent of the injury (Berlin *et al.*, 1977). Also the amount of tissue excised per Joule of energy transfer seemed to be smaller in limbs of smaller size (Janzon, 1983; Janzon and Seeman, 1985; Janzon *et al.*, 1988).

Scale dependence – strain-rate sensitivity

This scale dependence was studied by analysing all available experimental results in Sweden (Janzon and Seeman, 1985). They are plotted in Figure 4.6, where each point represents a single firing. The abscissa variable is the 'scaling parameter' $d_{min}/$

$F^{1/2}$, where d_{min} is a measure characterizing the depth of the wound beneath the exterior surface and F is the average retardation force acting between bullet and tissue. The ordinate axis is relative tissue destruction – amount of tissue damaged per Joule of energy transfer. A linear regression could be computed by the least-squares method, yielding a correlation coefficient of 0.89.

The reasons for the scale effect are not obvious. According to Janzon (1983), the damage mechanism can be divided into four distinct processes (Figure 4.7):

1. Damage by direct contact with and static disruption of tissue (such as occurs in stab wound). This is clearly scale independent.
2. Damage caused by high overpressures in the immediate vicinity of a projectile, penetrating at a high velocity. These pressures are caused by the flow of tissue around the projectile (see Chapter 3, Figure 3.2). The mechanism causes a contusion- and a concussion-type injury (Wang *et al.*, 1982), and is independent of scale, except

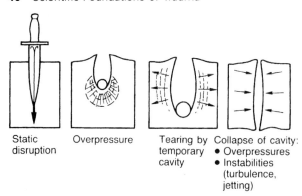

Static disruption | Overpressure | Tearing by temporary cavity | Collapse of cavity:
- Overpressures
- Instabilities (turbulence, jetting)

Figure 4.7 Wounding mechanisms active in high-energy missile trauma.

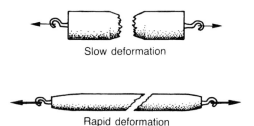

Slow deformation

Rapid deformation

Figure 4.8 Strain-rate dependence of mechanical properties and fracture behaviour of muscle.

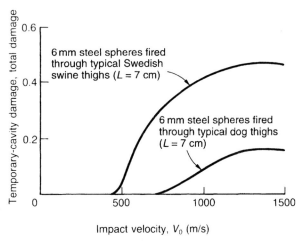

6 mm steel spheres fired through typical Swedish swine thighs ($L = 7$ cm)

6 mm steel spheres fired through typical dog thighs ($L = 7$ cm)

Impact velocity, V_0 (m/s)

Figure 4.9 Fraction of total tissue destruction attributable to temporary-cavity formation (Peters, 1990b).

where the boundaries are very close, such as close to the points of impact and exit.

3. Damage caused by expansion of a temporary cavity, reaching its maximum dimensions long after (milliseconds) the passage of the bullet. The injury is by tear damage, caused by stretching beyond the elastic limit of the tissues. Such damage does, however, often seem to follow fascial planes and the direction of the muscle fibres. It causes capillary bleeding, but often seems to be of less consequence to the total damage than might be expected (Harvey *et al.*, 1962; Berlin *et al.*, 1977; Janzon, 1983).

Mechanism 3 is clearly dependent on the size of the wounded part of the body. As shown by Janzon and Seeman (1985), the tissue damage diminished if expansion of the temporary cavity was suppressed (entirely or in part) by enclosing the injured zone in a solid plaster-of-Paris cast. This is reasonable since the temporary cavity's expansion will, primarily, cause damage by circumferential tearing of the tissues. Consequently, a greater mass surrounding the wound, such as a larger-sized limb, will diminish the maximum expansion of the cavity, and less tear damage will be expected to occur as the limb size increases, a scale dependence opposite to the one found.

4. Damage caused by the collapse of the temporary cavity. The injury could be of a contusion/ concussion type, as in 2 above, caused by the pressures being brought about by the violent collapse of the cavity (implosion). It could also be of a tear/disruption type, caused by instabilities of the interior cavity surface during collapse, with subsequent severe turbulence and jetting occurring (Birkhoff, 1960), cf. Figure 4.11. This may contribute to explain the scale dependence.

Notwithstanding the special character of mechanism 4, it seems very difficult to explain the scale

effect found by factors included in the dynamic term of Chapter 3, eq 1.

It may be explained by a strain-rate dependence of the strength of the muscle material – that it appears stronger, and elongates more before fracturing, when it is more rapidly stretched (Figure 4.8). Polymeric materials (i.e. plastics) are well known to show this behaviour (Bueche, 1962), as well as many others, and muscle is in reality a polymer. This is a very probable explanation of the size dependence found, as shown by Peters (1990 a,b). In fact it can be demonstrated that different types of muscle tissue seem to display a different strain-rate dependence, such as shown in Figure 4.9 (Peters, 1990b).

Appearance of the wound

Going from the bullet path outwards, different injury zones can be discerned in muscle. In Figure 4.10 zone 1 denotes the permanent wound channel, which is the cavity remaining after the pulsations of the temporary cavity have come to an end. Usually, part of the permanent cavity is caused by the pushing aside of tissues, rather than the expulsion

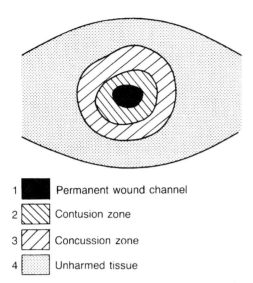

1 ⬛	Permanent wound channel
2 ▨	Contusion zone
3 ▨	Concussion zone
4 ▦	Unharmed tissue

Figure 4.10 Zones of injury in a bullet wound.

of material from the wound through the exit or entrance aperture. The amount of material ejected from the tissue is mostly small (Berlin *et al.*, 1976), the possible exception being wounds with extreme energy transfers close to the point of exit.

The size of the permanent wound channel may be an indication of the extent of energy transfer at that point (Fackler and Malinowski, 1985).

Next comes a zone (2) consisting of definitely non-viable tissue. The thickness of this zone is dependent on the amount of energy transferred at that point in the bullet's passage (for non-deforming and non-fragmenting bullets) and the other factors mentioned above. The muscle fibres will have lost their normal structure, are swollen or broken in pieces. Interstitial bleeding is seen throughout the tissue (Wang *et al.*, 1988; Zhang *et al.*, 1988). This zone is also denoted the 'contusion zone'.

If left in the wound, tissue from zone 2 will constitute an excellent growth medium for pyogenic bacteria which normally enter the wound during its formation, by the suction produced by cavitation (Dziemian and Herget, 1950) or colonize the wound later from the skin edges. Dahlgren *et al.*, (1979) found that in experimental wounds left without care, in reasonably clean pigs, there was a very high rate of serious anaerobic bacterial infection, including many cases of gas gangrene.

Zone 3 consists of tissue showing signs of damage (Wang *et al.*, 1988), such as swollen myofibres and obscure cross-striations. Nuclei are lightly stained or shrunk. Membrane dysfunction occurs. Some necrotic fibres may be found. Capillaries are congested and petechial bleeding and interstitial exudation are found. This zone may be called the 'concussion zone'. In this zone part of the tissue may survive, part may succumb. The tissue

closest to the wound track is normally the most seriously damaged. The border-line between zone 2 and zone 3 is not very clear.

Zone 4 is tissue which on macroscopical examination may appear normal. There may, however, be changes such as microthromboses present. The tissue affected in this way by the injury may be called 'shocked' tissue.

By scanning electron microscope studies of gunshot wounds (Lui *et al.*, 1990a), it was found that when muscle fibres intersected the projective trajectory at right or oblique angles, the projectile cut the myofibres by direct contact. Shearing forces ahead of the projectile also produced fibre damage. The temporary cavity seemed to have little effect in damaging these transverse myofibres. If the projectile's path was parallel to the muscle, the temporary cavity seemed to tear and stretch the fibres surrounding the path, causing an irregular shape of the wound channel.

Skin injury

Human skin is very resistant to damage (Heaton *et al.*, 1966), and has remarkable powers of recovery. The injury visible on the skin surface is usually much smaller than the underlying muscle injury. A large exit wound in the skin, with torn skin-flaps and star-like rifts, is always a sign of high energy transfer to tissue, and consequently a warning sign indicating massive destruction. The skin injury should always be treated conservatively (Whelan *et al.*, 1968; Owen-Smith, 1981). Only skin that is grossly pulped should be removed – usually less than 1–2 mm of the skin edge at the entry or exit wounds.

Heart and vascular injury

Direct high-energy impacts to the heart obviously carry a high mortality. Even if the heart is not directly struck by the missile, but is involved in the temporary cavitation, it may be displaced and cardiac arrest may occur. Also remote high-energy injuries may affect the heart, see 'Secondary damage' and 'Remote effects of pressure waves' below.

Blood vessels may be affected by the temporary cavitation. Arteries, however, seem to be resistant to stretching. Damage to all layers of the vessel wall may occur up to a distance of 20 mm or more from the area of visible gross damage (Rich, 1978; Chen *et al.*, 1990). This, however, seems to be of little importance to the outcome (Rich *et al.*, 1969; Amato *et al.*, 1970; Rich, 1978). Excision of the damaged part of an artery should usually be conservative (Owen-Smith, 1981).

Thromboses may be caused without a direct hit of a vessel (Chen *et al.*, 1990). They are probably caused by stretching or pressure waves which damage the cells of the endothelium.

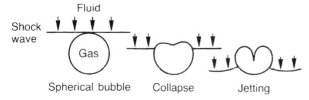

Figure 4.11 Collapse of gas-filled spherical bubble under the action of a shock wave in a dense medium.

Pulmonary injury

DeMuth (1968) and Harvey *et al.* (1962) found that in pulmonary tissue there is little or no evidence of temporary cavitation. Amato *et al.* (1974) documented the appearance of a small temporary cavity. This is due partly to the low-energy transfer, even from a very high velocity projectile, because of the low average density of the lung tissue, with great amounts of air interspersed, and partly to the damping properties of the air content, which prevent pressure waves from propagating very far from the wound track in the porous medium.

On the other hand, air-filled cavities are very vulnerable to shock waves reaching them. They may collapse, and severe disturbances of the inner surface may be caused, including jetting as shown in Figure 4.11. The jet may reach high velocities, up to hundreds of metres per second, and may cause tissue damage when it impacts and penetrates the other side of the cavity.

Liver, kidney, spleen, colon and intestine injury

Eason *et al.* (1975) found that in liver, the permanent cavity almost equalled the temporary one, because of the low strength of the tissue, which resulted in extensive star-patterned lacerations around the wound path in response to missile penetration. The temporary cavity is also larger in liver than in muscle (Amato *et al.*, 1974). Due to the abundance of blood vessels these lacerations constitute a much more serious injury than in muscle. At high-energy transfers, the entire liver may disintegrate.

Other encapsulated organs such as spleen or kidneys are also very vulnerable to high-energy projectile impact. However, the remarkable survival of kidney cells can be demonstrated *in vitro* (Tikka, 1989).

The colon seems to be very vulnerable to missile impact, and microscopical damage may extend up to 20 cm from the wound channel (Tikka, 1989). The intestines may contain gas pockets which may, by the action of pressure waves and the collapse mechanism described earlier, cause haematomas at distance from the site of wounding, which may later give rise to a risk of perforation.

Head injury

This is considered in detail in Chapters 5 and 9, and only a brief account is given here.

In head wounds (Butler *et al.*, 1945; Clemedson *et al.*, 1973; Watkins *et al.*, 1988) the retardation properties of the brain seem to be similar to those of muscle. The strength of brain tissue is, however, certainly much lower than muscle. The occurrence of temporary cavitation as a result of missile injury of the head will be diminished by the strong, non-deforming skull. Over a certain limit of energy release from the bullet, the cranium may be broken or shattered. Tangential wounds to the skull may cause serious brain damage without penetrating, through the action of shock and the pressure waves created, and cavitation caused in the brain closest to the location of the impact (Watkins *et al.*, 1988).

Because the brain is surrounded by the strong cranium, bullets hitting it may be induced to tumble, deform or fracture, which may aggravate the energy transfer compared to that of muscle tissue.

Missile injury to the brain, when cavitation or pressure waves are sufficient, causes many systemic responses which are especially severe in the respiratory and circulatory system (Lei *et al.*, 1990). Among these are apnoea immediately after the injury, bradycardia, hypotension, increased vascular resistance and reduction in cerebral blood flow. This will lead to anoxaemia of the brain, in turn aggravating the injury, and leading to a vicious circle of events.

Carey (1988) studied head injuries occurring in Vietnam, and concluded that bullet injuries to the brain caused a higher rate of fatalities than did fragment injuries. There was a very low incidence of clinically significant intracranial blood clots. He also concluded that men sustaining brain wounds, either fatal or non-fatal, became immediately militarily non-effective, only few being able to even aid themselves after the injury. About 85% of the injured survived, and about 30% could later return to some form of army duty (Carey, 1988).

Haemodynamic and metabolic effects

Rybeck (1974) found that the release of energy in muscle tissue of the hind leg of anaesthetized dogs, caused by the passage of a high-speed missile, had remarkable effects on the regional blood flow. There was pronounced vasodilatation in the wounded area. Thus, an increase of up to 100% or more of the flow in the injured leg occurred immediately after wounding, and then slowly declined. After more than 1 hour, there was still a pronounced increase in the blood flow. In the uninjured leg there was a corresponding decrease in the blood flow. No increase in cardiac output could be found, on the contrary there was a slight reduction with time.

Almskog *et al.* (1979) found that if both legs were injured, one immediately after the other, the flow increase still occurred, although there was no pronounced peak flow in the second injured leg. The flow was found to be diverted from the splanchnic area, and there was still no increase in cardiac output.

Missile trauma triggers a powerful sequence of events and responses in the circulatory and metabolical systems (Lewis, 1990). Some of the responses are characterized by release of mediators from damaged cells, loss of vascular control via the sympathoadrenal system, injury to endothelial cells, resulting in changes in capillary blood flow, transport and blood viscosity. Mediator release involves the activation of many systems (Lewis, 1990): coagulation system, fibrinolytic system, kallikrein – kinin system, arachidonic acid cascades and release of platelet activating factor.

The mechanisms in this complex interaction have not yet been clarified. The blood flow increase may serve the practical purpose of mobilizing the body's defences against the damaged tissues of the injury, and to combat the bacterial invasion in the wound, thereby limiting the amount of injury resulting. Some of these mechanisms may be adequate responses, others may not. It may, in future, be possible to modify these responses, with the intent of saving tissue which may otherwise be lost (Lewis, 1990).

Pronounced changes in cell metabolism in the area affected by missile trauma occur. In the concussion zone (zone 3), that is bruised tissue, and 'shocked' tissue (of zone 4), an experimental investigation of dogs (Fu *et al.*, 1990) showed a marked decrease in activity of SDH (succinate dehydrogenase) and H^+-ATP enzymes at 6 hours after wounding, a recovery of 12 hours, but still a marked loss of activity up to 24 hours after the injury. The conclusion was that without debridement, the condition of bruised and shocked tissue neither improved nor deteriorated. Recovery of tissue function might be expected in some areas between 6 and 12 hours after wounding, though in some areas a continued decline in function might be expected. It was shown that early debridement largely enabled the surrounding damaged tissue to recover its function.

It was also found by Dahlgren *et al.* (1979) that the apparent borderline between viable and non-viable tissue (the 'concussion' and the 'contusion' zone) seemed to change with time. Dahlgren *et al.* (1979) noted that the amount of tissue that was judged as non-viable increased with time after the wounding. The border between the discoloured contusion zone and the concussion zone appeared sharper after 12 hours (Dahlgren *et al.*, 1979; Hagelin, 1989).

The exact mechanisms causing a missile injury and affecting its development are still far from being completely known, and are difficult to resolve due to the difficulty of creating reproducible experimental methods and to the scatter always inherent in events involving biological material.

Secondary damage

Fragments, from a fractured bullet, or from a high-energy bone impact, are an obvious cause of secondary damage. In injuries involving high-energy femoral fracture, where bone fragments have been formed, abdominal injury may occur.

Organs close to the bullet trajectory may be damaged by pressure waves and by stretching and displacement caused by the temporary cavity. In high-energy injury, such secondary injury is frequent (Wang *et al.*, 1990). In maxillofacial injury, damage to the brain, sinuses or the skull may be expected.

In subcutaneous tissue injury to the thorax, damage to the lungs, heart, liver and brain are possible. If the subcutaneous tissue of the abdomen is affected, damage may be suspected to the liver, spleen, intestines, stomach, lungs or heart. In the investigation made by Liu *et al.* (1990b), the incidence of secondary damage was very high. The energy transfer of the projectiles was intermediate or high, and well representative of modern assault rifle bullets or high-velocity fragments.

In spinal injury (Ma, 1990), it was found that adjacent organs could easily be damaged, such as kidneys, liver, intestines and heart, when the spine was penetrated. Impacts in the spinous process, or soft tissue wounds of the back, were accompanied by very little secondary damage.

Remote effects of pressure waves

In studies of head injury by 7.62-mm assault rifle bullets in dogs, in 87% of all cases injury to the heart ensued, to lung (75%), liver (50%), spleen (62%) and kidney (25%) (Liu *et al.*, 1990b).

In studies of abdominal trauma in dogs and pigs using 7.62-mm and 5.56-mm bullets, and high-velocity fragments (1 g), injury to the spinal cord ensued only with the 5.56-mm projectiles (44%), to the heart, with all types of projectiles (45–60%) and likewise to the lungs (75%) (Liu *et al.*, 1990b).

In hind leg injury in dogs by 7.62-mm assault rifle bullets, 60–70% displayed injury to the heart, lungs (30–40%) and liver (20–30%) (Liu *et al.*, 1990b).

A pressure wave, especially a shock wave with a steep front passing through tissue, may cause secondary damage at large distances from its origin. This has been studied by extensive experimentation by Harvey *et al.* (1947), who introduced small gas-filled bubbles in gelatin and studied their behaviour when reached by a shock wave. It was shown that they may collapse violently (Figure 4.11). This phenomenon may be associated with jetting, and may cause serious injury. Harvey *et al.* found that rupture and severe damage to gas-filled viscera could ensue. A high-energy wound in the upper part of a leg may thus be suspected to cause damage to abdominal, gas-filled organs, although there may be no evidence of secondary fragments.

After thigh injury in anaesthetized pigs, blood extravasation and haemorrhage could be observed in small vessels and capillaries of the brain, heart, lung, liver, spleen, kidney and other organs (Liu *et al.*, 1990b). After injury to the thorax, in addition to lung injury there was usually myocardial haemorrhage. In the abdominal cavity some animals displayed haemorrhage of the intestines and/or stomach. In abdominal wounds, indirect injuries to thoracic organs also occurred (Liu *et al*, 1990b).

Local and remote nervous injury

Although nerve seems to be more resistant than muscle, function may be damaged without rupture (Harvey *et al.*, 1962; Suneson, 1989).

Suneson (1989) measured the pressure pulses transferred to the brain through the rather long distance of various tissues from the site of injury in the hind legs of pigs, and found them to be the order of parts of bars (1 bar = 760 mmHg = 14 psi) up to bars when the energy release was similar to that caused by the penetration of a typical assault rifle bullet. A typical apnoea lasting from approximately 6 to 40 seconds, immediately followed the shot. A second respiratory arrest often occurred within 1 minute. Disturbed breathing prevailed for longer or shorter periods after the injury. Most animals showed an increased breathing frequency up to 1 hour after the injury. A few animals had relatively normal breathing but took single deep breaths with intervals of 1–2 minutes.

BONE

Bone has much greater density and strength than its surrounding soft tissue and considerably less elasticity. These factors combine to not only ensure a greater degree of energy transfer from the missile to the wound, and therefore more severe injury, but also the stresses on the projectile itself are more pronounced, making missile deformation and break-up much more likely.

The energy required to disrupt bone integrity is greater than that needed to breach the skin or muscle tissue, and has been calculated to be of the order of 10 J (Amato *et al.*, 1974; Loh and Lee, 1990). The lack of elasticity in bone prevents true collapse of the temporary cavity; apparent collapse is seen due to the elasticity of the soft tissues enveloping the bone.

Understanding of how missiles react with bone has come from clinical experience gained both in war and peace, together with experimental studies using bone/gelatin models and animals. Experimental work over the past 20 years has been concerned with the indirect damage to bone that occurs as a result of adjacent soft tissue cavitation as well as direct bone injury. The interaction of high- and low-velocity missiles has been studied, as has the varied effects of different shaped fragments and those of different mass. In simple terms, the greater the energy transfer from missile to bone, the greater the damage incurred.

Bone injury is almost always accompanied by damage to the surrounding soft tissues and this may be of much greater clinical and pathological significance, especially when considering the skull or pelvis. Indirect bone injury is also partially dependent on the nature of the soft tissues surrounding the bone, as these will determine the extent of energy transfer from the missile to the wound track, and therefore the characteristics of the temporary cavity.

Low-energy transfer wounds

Experimental studies have shown that the minimum impact velocity required to penetrate bone is in the order of 65 m/s (Amato *et al.*, 1989; Loh and Lee, 1990). This is an approximation and is largely independent of the mass of the projectile. At impact velocities greater than this, but well below those causing true temporary cavity formation, drilling of cancellous bone occurs with the formation of a permanent wound track little wider than the calibre of the missile. Where there is little cancellous bone however, such as in the shafts of long bones, missile strike causes comminution even at low velocities, often with a large butterfly fragment (Huelke and Darling, 1964). Huelke *et al.* (1968) found that an impact velocity of 200 m/s was needed for complete perforation of the metaphyses of fresh human femora by 0.25-in. steel spheres, although osteoporotic bones could be perforated by missiles with lower striking velocities. The permanent cavities at these velocities were only slightly wider than the missile calibre. As striking velocity increased, the cylindrical permanent cavity was enlarged, and at 300 m/s there was chipping of the cortical bone around the exit hole. Further increase led to production of a large permanent cavity, and at impact velocities above 500 m/s there was shattering of the bone with separation of the condyles.

The mechanism of cavitation in bone appears similar to that in soft tissue. After penetrating the cortex, the projectile imparts radial energy to the cancellous spongy bone which disrupts the multiple thin plates of bone for a considerable distance from the wound tract. Expansion of the soft bone and medullary tissue creates an explosive exit hole in the opposite cortex, via which marrow and bony spicules are ejected.

Experimental work by Ragsdale and Josselson (1988) looked at the effects of various hand-gun and rifle bullets on human long bones suspended in 20% gelatin. At the lower velocity range of the spectrum, there was similar drilling of the bone with little or no fragmentation around the exit holes. Impact velocities in excess of 250 m/s resulted in increasing numbers of bone fragments and the development of a temporary cavity. The authors stress that although impact velocity and mass of the projectile is of great importance, the design and nature of the ammunition for various 'low velocity' hand guns influences energy transfer significantly.

High-energy transfer wounds

Comprehensive experimental work performed by Harvey *et al.* and reported in *Wound Ballistics* (Harvey *et al.*, 1962) defined much that is known today about the effects of high-energy missile injury to bone. Their work included direct observation of the involvement of bone in the temporary cavity caused by a high-velocity missile, and they showed that bone 'explodes' in a similar manner to the surrounding soft tissues. The question of whether bone fragments act as secondary missiles was addressed and the authors concluded that although bone fragments do fly out into the temporary cavity during its formation, once the cavity collapses the fragments usually return to the general area of their parent bone, possibly due to intact periosteal attachments. Dissection of wounds where bone disruption had been extensive rarely revealed the presence of fragments at any distance from the bone, suggesting that the fragments do not act as significant secondary missiles.

Indirect fracture

Indirect bone fracture was regularly observed. The passage of a high-velocity missile through the soft tissues adjacent to a bone causes a less severe fracture and is due to involvement of the bone in the temporary cavity. Harvey described the process 'as if the bone had received a heavy blow from the direction of the cavity'. He also related the likelihood of indirect fracture to the striking energy of the missile, finding that with striking velocities of 1500 m/s, there was an incidence of 45% of indirect fracture with 0.125-in. steel spheres fired close to femurs of a living cat. Finally, it was found that the femur appeared much more vulnerable to indirect fractures than did the humerus, possibly due to less effective soft tissue support of the former. More recent work by Janzon (1983) and Sun *et al.* (1990) has confirmed indirect fracture of bone by shock-wave propagation beyond the temporary cavity created by high-energy transfer wounds.

Extensive experimental work by Huelke, Harger *et al.* (1968) provided considerable information on the effects of mass and size of projectiles as well as impact velocity on bony damage. Using human cadaveric femurs, these workers demonstrated that drilling of cancellous bone in the metaphyseal region of long bones differed substantially from the shattering of the shaft cortical bone, even at low-impact velocities. This can be explained by the dissipation of the temporary cavity pressures within the multiple honeycomb spaces of cancellous bone; the brittle cortical bone of the diaphysis tends to explode due to cavitation.

Projectile size

In addition, Huelke *et al.* showed that the relative size of the projectile has a much greater influence on bone damage than does the mass of the missile. By comparing the effects of high-velocity steel spheres on the distal femoral metaphysis, they showed that doubling the density of 0.25-in. projectiles made no significant difference to observed damage; doubling the diameter to 0.406-in., however, considerably increased bony disruption. This can be explained by appreciating that increasing the surface area of the projectile in contact with bone must increase energy transfer, and hence lead to a greater degree of cavitation. Figure 4.12 relates energy transfer to impact velocity for different diameter steel spheres.

Secondary missiles

DeMuth and Smith (1966) reiterated many of the observations of Harvey *et al.*, including the conclusion that bone fragments did not appear to act as secondary missiles. This was challenged by Amato *et al.* (1974), who reported that during subsequent undulations of the temporary cavity, bone fragments tended to migrate along the path of the missile, possibly causing soft tissue damage, especially to skin around the exit wound. More recent work by Amato *et al.* (1989) using fresh calf femurs embedded in gelatin to simulate the soft tissues, and observation with high-speed photography and microsecond X-rays, confirmed temporary cavity formation in bone. It was also demonstrated that migration of secondary bone fragments occurred and that some were expelled from the exit hole in the gelatin block.

A recent observation by Ragsdale and Josselson (1989) was that there appears to be explosive decompression of the temporary cavity by dissection along the anterior gelatin–bone interface. This resembles a blow-hole through the line of least resistance and possibly mirrors what would occur *in vivo*, with stripping of the soft tissues from around a bone for some distance proximally and distally from the site of the missile wound (Figure 4.13). The effect of this would be to devascularize the bone cortex externally and could have a bearing

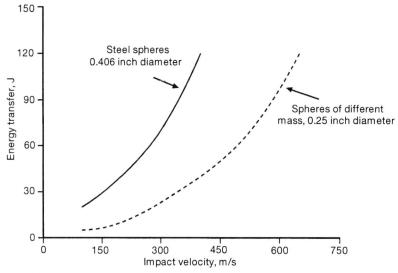

Figure 4.12 Relationship between energy transfer and impact velocity during penetration of distal femoral metaphysis by steel spheres of different diameters. (Reproduced from Harger and Huelke, 1970.)

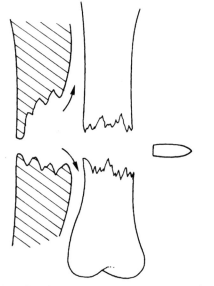

Figure 4.13 Diagramatic representation of 'blow hole' decompression of temporary cavity as described by Ragsdale and Josselson (1988).

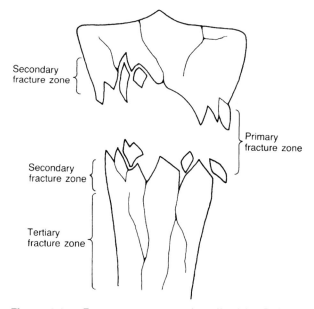

Figure 4.14 Fracture zones as described by Robens and Kusswetter (1983).

on the ability of subsequent healing. This phenomenon was only observed when energy transfer from projectile to wound was high, and has not been confirmed by live animal studies.

Classification

Little attempt has been made to classify bony injury by missiles, but experimental work by Robens and Küsswetter (1982) describes zones of bony injury around direct high-energy transfer wounds. They described three zones of damage around experimental wounding of cadaveric tibias using high-velocity 5.56-mm rifle bullets (Figure 4.14). The primary defect zone is the usually large area of cortical and cancellous bone loss surrounding the missile track. Outside this there is a secondary disorganized zone of comminuted bony fragments held in continuity by their soft tissue attachments, which may extend proximally and distally for up to 3 cm. Further still from the missile track, there exists a tertiary zone of linear cracks and spiral fractures which may extend for some 9 cm above and below the area of primary damage. The overlying soft tissues in the tertiary zone are intact and undamaged and this tertiary zone of damage does not cross adjacent joint lines.

Classification of the morphological appearances of bone fracture caused by high-energy missiles has been described by Loh and Lee (1990). They describe simple monofissure cortical fractures with low-energy impacts and progress through bifissure, trifissure and tetrafissure fractures through to complicated X and M shaped fracture patterns with high-energy transfer wounds to bone.

The effects of small fragments

When consideration is given to the effects on wounding of fragments from exploding munitions as opposed to bullets, there is little to be found in the literature specifically related to bone injury. The majority of wounds in war are attributable to fragments, and there is an increasing tendency for weapons manufacturers to develop ever more efficient preformed projectiles for mortars, bomblets and grenades which are designed primarily to incapacitate rather than kill.

Two recent experimental studies from China concentrate on the wounding effects of different shaped small projectiles and both remark on the incidence of direct and indirect fracture associated with penetrating soft tissue wounds. Liu *et al.* (1988) fired 0.44-g projectiles at dog hind limbs and observed the varying effects of triangular, square, cylindrical and spherical fragments. They found that with higher velocities of impact, fractures in the limbs were common and that indirect fractures tended to be oblique or transverse. Direct hits on the bone produced comminuted fractures as described above, but there appeared to be no correlation between shape of fragment and incidence of fracture.

Ma *et al.* (1988) used a similar model and also observed that projectile shape did not influence the rate of indirect fracture. They stressed, however, that velocity of impact was the main determinant of fracture and found that with a striking velocity of 1450 m/s, there was a 29% incidence of femoral fracture, regardless of projectile shape, even when the wound tract was as much as 15–20 mm from the bone. Their conclusion that energy transfer was related to projectile shape and a decreasing function of its mass, possibly explains this finding in that triangular- and square-shaped fragments give up energy rapidly and thus penetrate less, creating wide shallow wounds. Wide shallow wounds are obviously less likely to involve deep structures such as bone.

Spinal injuries

Spinal injuries constitute a special case. It has been shown by Ma (1990) that in spinal canal penetrating wounds from assault rifle bullets, spinal cord fracture and complete and irrecoverable paraplegia was normally immediately caused. In tangential wounds not penetrating the spinal canal, permanent paraplegia could result, but incomplete, recoverable paraplegia was also possible, depending on the energy transferred and pressures sustained by the spinal cord. With a direct impact on the spine there is usually damage to vertebral laminae and there may be fracture of the vertebra affected, as well as of the spinous process. Penetrations of the spinous process usually cause less damage. However, even extensive soft tissue damage close to the spinal cord, without directly involving the spine, caused no damage to spinal cord function (Ma, 1990).

MANAGEMENT PRINCIPLES – SOFT TISSUE

Injury to tissue caused by penetrating projectiles is usually obvious. An entry wound, and possibly an exit wound, will be present. What is rarely obvious, at first sight at least, is the degree and extent of tissue devitalization. This emphasizes that there should be no presumptions concerning injury severity when faced with a penetrating wound caused by a projectile. Lindsey's aphorism, 'treat the wound, not the weapon', is particularly appropriate. Knowledge of the wounding weapon or munition and presumed knowledge of projectile velocity are imprecise indicators of potential for injury, and should not be used to classify wounds or threats from weapons and munitions.

Contemporary literature reveals widespread disagreement on penetrating projectile wound management and this is not surprising. The conventional military approach to penetrating projectile wounds is: generous wound incision, fasciotomy or decompression for limb wounds, excision of devitalized or heavily contaminated soft tissue and careful dressing of the open wound. In an ideal civilian clinical setting it is now commonplace to rely on antibiotics alone or antibiotics with minimal surgical intervention for carefully selected projectile wounds, for example, low-energy-transfer wounds caused by low-velocity hand-gun bullets and modern, preformed military fragments. In wounds of this character, soft tissue injury is confined to a short wound track, is typically modest and foreign-body contamination is minimal. An important caveat concerns delay which must be minimal (<1 hour) if this approach is to be relied upon. These circumstances are exemplified in large urban centres in the USA where clinical conditions are ideal and the staff widely experienced.

Surgical debridement, wound excision and primary closure is a further approach practised widely in the USA. It is safe where wound contamination is minimal, as indicated by preoperative wound quantitative microbiology studies. Bacterial counts of less than 10^5 are widely accepted as indicative of a very low risk of wound infection; primary closure may be performed. Adjuvant antibiotic therapy is normally used additionally.

There is a re-awakening of interest in the technique of simple wound incision (no excision of tissue) and drainage followed by delayed primary closure – this was widely practised during the Second World War by experienced military surgeons for particular classes of wound. These were uncomplicated soft tissue extremity wounds caused by military rifle bullets; recent military research in the USA and the UK supports the validity of this approach.

It is clear from the literature that each of the management doctrines outlined above may be satisfactory for carefully selected wounds. The problem is to identify wounds and treat them appropriately. Because of factors unique to either battle or peacetime, and the wide variety of wounding profiles that may present in either situation, it is impossible to formulate a precise, single management doctrine that will meet all needs. Nevertheless, certain accepted treatment principles do exist and form the basis of widely adopted military doctrine for the management of projectile wounds. The doctrine makes a number of important assumptions. First, all penetrating projectile wounds are contaminated to a greater or lesser extent with bacteria from skin, soil and clothing; contamination may not be obvious during wound exploration. Second, antibiotics have an important role in the control of contamination and prevention of early wound infection but are of secondary importance to adequate surgery; they are never a substitute for surgery. Third, the majority of wounded patients will present to surgeons who will be experienced in the general sense but are unlikely to be familiar with projectile injury (at least in practice in the UK). Finally, postoperative patients may not remain under the care of the surgeon performing primary surgery and may require evacuation to other centres; this is a particular feature of battlefield management.

Assessment of early priorities

A full history and physical examination are vital in planning appropriate management. The history must include an estimate of delay from wounding to arrival in hospital; this will indicate the likelihood of wound infection or its imminence. Experience has shown that delay beyond 6 hours before the institution of antibiotics and surgery will result in infection rates approaching 100%. Knowledge of the wounding agent while allowing no assumptions on wound nature or severity is helpful. Fragments, for example, result in a more severe pattern of contamination. Police and hunting bullets are more likely to deform or fragment and usually result in more severe injury. Physical

examination of the undressed patient, including the back, may give an assessment of missile track and structures in its path, particularly if an exit wound is present.

Antibiotics and control of infection

Antibiotics are not a substitute for surgery. They have an important role in delaying the onset of systemic infection prior to surgical intervention. The overriding considerations are the prevention of gas gangrene, tetanus and haemolytic streptococcal septicaemia. Historically these are the organisms implicated in morbidity and mortality following projectile injury in war. Benzyl penicillin or an agent with an equivalent spectrum must be administered as quickly as possible, ideally within 1 hour of wounding. Dosage schedules must be designed to attain circulating and serum levels, three to four times the minimum inhibitory concentration for the expected bacterial species; the levels must be maintained over each 24-hour period.

Surgery

The surgical treatment of a penetrating wound caused by a projectile is at least a two-stage operation. The first operation is concerned with saving life and limb and the prevention of primary wound infection. The second is carried out 4–5 days later and comprises wound reappraisal and skin closure if appropriate. Subsequent procedures are frequently necessary (e.g. vascular or orthopaedic).

Skin incision

Adequate access to the recesses of many projectile wounds requires generous skin incisions and counter incisions may be carried out to relieve tension. Skin is remarkably resistant to projectile injury and may be safely conserved in most instances; where excision is necessary it should be kept to a minimum. Contaminated or damaged subcutaneous fat should be widely excised.

Fasciotomy and decompression

Deep fascia must be widely incised along the length of a wound. The aim is to unbridle injured muscle groups, relieve tension and permit a full evaluation of the extent of muscle injury. This is the UK understanding of the term debridement – a term derived from the French, *debrider*, meaning to slit up or unbridle. Failure to perform this manoeuvre will result in an underassessment of the extent of muscle injury – postoperative wound infection and compartment syndromes may result.

Assessment of extent of soft tissue injury

This step is central to successful management. Failure to exercise proper care during this stage is the commonest cause of morbidity and mortality. The two principle errors observed are overestimate and underestimate of the extent on non-viable muscle, both leading to inappropriate excision of muscle.

A full assessment of the extent of muscle and other soft tissue injury should be conducted in a rational way and requires a sound knowledge of standard surgical principles and the pathophysiology of projectile injury. Needless controversy surrounds this assessment. Clearly, wide variation in injury exists and the reasons have been outlined in an earlier chapter. Many wounds where low energy transfer has been a feature will have minimal muscle injury and there should be no problem in deciding on the extent, if any, of muscle excision. Difficulty may arise with more severe wounds. There is recent evidence that the immediate appearance of injured muscle is a poor indicator of devitalization. This is particularly true for uncomplicated wounds to soft tissue of limbs caused by modern assault rifle bullets. Many of these wounds present with large stellate exit wounds. It may appear that much muscle was ejected through the exit wound, however usually little is lost (Berlin *et al.*, 1976); the rest will just be displaced by the violent cavitation to which it was subjected. Stretching alone may not irreversibly damage the tissue, and especially if bullet tumbling occurred only close to the exit, little remaining non-viable tissue may be found at surgery, although extensive bruising and stretching may be evident. Under these circumstances minimal excision is appropriate provided widespread foreign-body contamination has not occurred. This may be difficult to determine, as high-energy transfer results in the contaminants being carried or drawn in and widely spread throughout the area of the temporary cavity which forms during wounding.

Recent military research has shown that this form of contamination is not visible at first surgery. In war, it is often necessary to embark on wound excision to excise some viable muscle where the value judgement of the surgeon suggests widespread contamination has taken place. This is a contentious view but one held by military and trauma surgeons. Muscle is remarkably resistant to injury during uncomplicated cavitation – the principal consequence is muscle stretch. Petechial haemorrhages and small radial lacerations are usually evident and, although the appearances may be dramatic, the majority of muscle fibres remain viable and will heal provided wound infection does not supervene. Cavitation associated with projectile fragmentation is quite different. The disruption of a bullet into small pieces produces irregular fragments which result in high retardation forces and the transfer of larger quantities of energy. The resulting large temporary cavity will be associated with multiple, diverging wound tracks causing multiple lacerations to muscle and other tissues. In this situation exploration will reveal very large quantities of lacerated, non-viable muscle caused not only by the cavitation process, but by rapidly moving pieces of metal.

The four traditional guidelines for wound excision – colour, contractility, consistency and capillary bleeding – must be assessed in the light of the observations outlined above. In practice, little difficulty will arise for most wounds and the advice from Lindsey: 'treat the wound, not the weapon' is most apt and helpful. This should prevent surgeons from carrying out an over-radical excision based on presumed injury derived from knowledge of the weapon or projectile. This is not academic nitpicking, as such practice is widespread.

Delayed primary closure

With notable exceptions, projectile wounds should be left open and dressed. The recent literature reveals a growing departure from this approach, but a general policy of leaving wounds open is still recommended and will cause no harm. Leaving wounds open improves drainage and reduces postoperative pain. Invasive infection in an open wound is rarely severe and is usually easy to manage, a feature recognized over a century ago by Friedrich (1898).

Correct dressing is by application of fine, fluffed, dry gauze over the wound surface, sufficient to fill the cavity. The wound must not be packed. Dressing is completed by overlaying multiple layers of gauze and cotton wool held in place with wide crepe bandages applied firmly but avoiding constriction.

Partial or complete primary closure

Partial or complete primary closure is appropriate under certain circumstances:

- *Head wounds*: scalp wounds should be closed and this becomes mandatory where the meninges are breached.
- *Face and neck*: an excellent blood supply permits primary closure, giving improved cosmetic results.
- *Hands and feet*: exposed tendons and neurovascular bundles should be covered by partial primary skin closure.
- *Joints*: joint capsules should be repaired if possible. Clean skin and soft tissue may be used to cover exposed synovium.
- *Laparotomy and thoracotomy incisions*: these should be closed using the surgeon's usual technique.

Surgery in war

Military surgeons have developed somewhat more didactic protocols for penetrating wound management in war. The general approach is based on the recommendations of the Inter-Allied Conference in 1917. It is very similar to the approach already outlined, but an important difference is the lack of flexibility and a leaning towards more radical excision of soft tissue. Many military and civilian surgeons find the approach unacceptable. It is seen as didactic and over radical, particularly in view of the reported success of early antibiotics and minimal surgical intervention in managing large numbers of projectile wounds. These critics either ignore or minimize two key features of projectile wounds in war: delay before surgical intervention, and heavy wound contamination associated with military fragment and bullet injury. Fragments are the most common wounding agents in war, accounting for between 44% and 92% of all surgical cases during recent campaigns. Two fragment families exist, one old, the other modern. Older fragments vary widely in size and shape and result from natural fragmentation of the casing of artillery shell and older mortars. Antipersonnel fragments from more modern military munitions are preformed and tend to be small and numerous, giving a high probability of multiple hits, and to be fairly regular in size and shape to ensure adequate range and consistent performance. Resulting casualties will present with multiple ragged wounds of varying severity; all will have wounds heavily contaminated with foreign bodies such as soil, dirty field clothing and fragments of skin. The principal threat to surviving casualties is potentially lethal wound infection. Delay before the institution of primary surgery is the norm and may exceed 12 hours. Primary surgery will take place under arduous field conditions and will be performed by youthful and relatively inexperienced teams. Reliance on antibiotics and surgical conservancy under these conditions is likely to herald disaster. It is obvious that this situation demands a somewhat didactic, straightforward and readily taught treatment approach that will be suitable for the majority.

Conclusion

Management for penetrating wounds caused by projectiles remains contentious. This need not unduly worry surgeons faced with their management. There is widespread agreement concerning the need to excise muscle that is obviously non-viable. A decision concerning the extent of excision for viable but heavily contaminated soft tissue is more contentious. Nevertheless, if these wounds are approached individually using surgical judgement and common sense, the surgeon will do no harm. The conditions on a battlefield will impose severe limitations and these must be recognized – here, the nature and extent of surgery must be influenced by factors such as delay, poor conditions, relative inexperience and large numbers. It is under these testing conditions that a tendency towards more radical excision of wounds is often appropriate. The corollary equally holds; in an ideal clinical setting where delay is minimal, it is increasingly appropriate to lean towards a more surgically conservative approach.

REFERENCES

Almskog B.A., Hasselgren P.O., Nordström G. et al. (1979). Circulatory changes following multiple wounds to soft tissue. *Acta Chir. Scand. Suppl.*, **489**, 261–70.

Almskog B.A., Haljamäe H., Hasselgren P-O. et al. (1982). Local metabolic changes in skeletal muscle following high energy missile injury. *J. Trauma*, **22**, 382–7.

Amato J.J., Billy L.J., Gruber L.P. et al. (1970). Vascular injuries. An experimental study of high and low velocity missile wounds. *Arch. Surg.*, **101**, 167–74.

Amato J.J., Billy L.J., Lawson N.S., Rich N.M. (1974). High velocity missile injury. An experimental study of the retentive forces of tissue. *Am. J. Surg.*, **127**, 454–9.

Amato J. J., Syracuse D., Seaver P. R., Rich N. (1989). Bone as a secondary missile: an experimental study in the fragmenting of bone by high velocity missiles. *J. Trauma*, **29**, 609–12.

Berlin R.H. (1977). Missile injury to live muscle tissue. *Acta Chir. Scand. Suppl.*, 480.

Berlin R., Gelin L.E., Janzon B. et al. (1976). Local effects of assault rifle bullets in live tissues. *Acta Chir. Scand. Suppl.*, **459**, 1–84.

Berlin R., Janzon B., Rybeck B. et al. (1977). Local effects of assault rifle bullets in live tissues. Part 2. Further studies in live tissues and relations to some simulant media. *Acta Chir. Scand. Suppl.*, **477**, 5–48.

Berlin R.H., Janzon B., Rybeck B. et al. (1979). Retardation of spherical missiles in live tissue. *Acta Chir. Scand. Suppl.*, **489**, 91.

Birkhoff G. (1960). *Hydrodynamics*. Princeton, NJ: Princeton University Press.

Bueche F. (1962). *Physical Properties of Polymers*. New York: Interscience, Wiley.

Butler E.G., Puckett W.C., Harvey E.N. et al. (1945). Experiments on head wounding by high velocity missiles. *J. Neurosurg.*, **2**, 358–83.

Carey M. (1988). An analysis of US Army combat mortality and morbidity data. *J. Trauma*, **28**, (suppl.), S183–8.

Carey M.E. (1996). Analysis of wounds incurred by US Army Seventh Corps personnel treated in corps hospitals during Operation Desert Storm Feb 20 to March 10, 1991. *J. Trauma*, **40** (3) suppl. S165–9.

Chen D.Y., Gu R.F., Li J.S. et al. (1990). The effect of high velocity missiles on adjacent blood vessels. *J. Trauma (China)*, **6**, (suppl.), 76–8.

Clemedson C.J., Falconer B., Frankenberg L. et al. (1973). Head injuries caused by small-calibre, high velocity bullets. An experimental study. *Z. Rechtsmedizin.* **73**, 103–14.

Dahlgren B., Berlin R., Janzon B. et al. (1979). The extent of muscle tissue damage following missile trauma one, six and twelve hours after the infliction of trauma, studied by the current method of debridement. *Acta Chir. Scand. Suppl.*, **489**, 137–44.

Dahlgren B., Almskog B., Berlin R. et al. (1982). Local effects of antibacterial therapy (benzyl-penicillin) on missile wound infection rate and tissue devitalization when debridement is delayed for twelve hours. *Acta Chir. Scand. Suppl.*, **508**, 271–9.

DeMuth W.E. Jr. (1966). Bullet velocity and design as determinants of wounding capability: an experimental study. *J. Trauma*, **6**, 222–32.

DeMuth W.E. Jr. (1968). High velocity bullet wounds of the thorax. *Am. J. Surg.*, **115**, 616–25.

DeMuth W.E., Smith J.M. (1966). High-velocity bullet wounds of muscle and bone: the basis of rational early treatment. *J. Trauma*, **6**, 744–55.

Dufour D. (ed.), Kroman Jensen S., Owen-Smith M. et al. (1988). *Surgery for Victims of War*. Geneva: International Committee of the Red Cross.

Dziemian A.J., Herget C.M. (1950). Physical aspects of the primary contamination of bullet wounds. *Milit. Surg.*, **106**, 294–9.

Eason R.L., Pryor W.H., Adams J.F. (1975). *Wound Studies in Porcine Skin, Muscle and Liver as Related to Variation of Velocities of Spherical Missiles*. NFMRL vol. XXV, no. 3., Camp Lejeune, NC: Naval Medical Field Research Laboratory.

Fackler M.L., Malinowski J.A. (1985). The wound profile: a visual method for quantifying gunshot wound components. *J. Trauma*, **25**, 522–9.

Friedrich P.L. (1898). The aseptic treatment of fresh wounds considering animal experiments on the development time of infection events. *Arch. Klin. Chir.*, **57**, 188 (in German).

Fu X.B., Liu Y.Q., Lai X.N. et al. (1990). The changes in tissue repiratory enzyme activities following gunshot wounds and their significance in determining the area of damaged tissue. *J. Trauma (China)*, **6**, (suppl.), 132–4.

Hagelin K.W. (1989). Optical Properties of Viable and Devitalized Skeletal Muscle Tissue. Doctorial thesis, University of Göteborg, Sweden.

Haljamäe H., Almskog B., Jennische E. et al. (1979). Cellular transmembrane potential registrations for continuous mapping of the areas of cellular injury caused by high velocity missiles. *Acta Chir. Scand. Suppl.*, **489**, 165–72.

Harger J.H., Huelke D.F. (1970). Femoral fractures produced by projectiles – the effect of mass and diameter on target damage. *J. Biomechan.*, **3**, 487–93.

Harvey E.N., Korr I.M., Oster G. et al. (1947). Secondary damage in wounding due to pressure changes accompanying the passage of high velocity missiles. *Surgery*, **21**, 218–39.

Harvey E.N., McMillen J.H., Butler E.G. et al. (1962). Mechanism of wounding. In *Wound Ballistics* (Coates J.B., ed.). Washington, D.C: US Army Surgeon General, pp. 143–235.

Heaton L.D., Hughes C.W., Rosegay H. et al. (1966). Military surgical practices of the United States in Vietnam. *Curr. Probl. Surg.*,

Huelke D.F., Darling J.H. (1964). Bone fractures produced by bullets. *J. Forensic. Sci*, **9**, 461–9.

Huelke D.F., Harger J.H., Buege L.J. et al. (1968). An experimental study in bio-ballistics: femoral fractures produced by projectiles. *J. Biomechan*, **1**, 97–105.

Janzon B. (1983). *High Energy Missile Trauma. A Study of the Mechanisms of Wounding of Muscle Tissue*. Gothenburg, published by author (Engwalls Väg 10, S-147 63.

Janzon B., Seeman T. (1985). Muscle devitalization in high-energy missile wounds, and its dependence on energy transfer. *J. Trauma*, **25**, 138–44.

Janzon B., Schantz B., Seeman T. (1988). Scale effects in ballistic wounding. *J. Trauma*, **28**, (suppl.), S29–32.

Kokinakis W., Neades D., Piddington M. et al. (1979). A gelatin methodology for estimating vulnerability of personnel to military rifle systems. *Acta Chir. Scand. Suppl.*, **489**, 35–56.

Lei P., Zhu C., Zhang G.J. et al. (1990). An experimental study of craniocerebral injury caused by 7.62 mm bullets in dogs, comparison with the characteristics of penetrating craniocerebral, tangential brain and skull injuries. *J. Trauma (China)*, **6**, suppl., 187–91.

Lewis D.H. (1990). The effect of missile wounding on the regulation of the microcirculation in skeletal muscle. *J. Trauma (China)*, **6**, suppl., 25–31.

Liu Y., Cheng X., Li S. et al. (1988). Wounding effects of small fragments of different shapes at different velocities on soft tissues of dogs. *J. Trauma*, **28**, (1 suppl.), S95–8.

Liu G.J., Wang Z.G., Zhu P.F. et al. (1990a). Observations on the inner surface of the wound track inflicted by high-velocity bullets: a scanning electron microscopic study. *J. Trauma (China)*, **6**, suppl., 140–3.

Liu Y.Q., Chen Y., Chen L. et al. (1990b). Mechanism, explorations and characteristics of the remote effects of projectiles. *J. Trauma (China)*, **6**(2), suppl., 16–20.

Loh Y, Lee J.S. (1990). Study of pig femoral fractures in vitro induced by missiles. *J Trauma (China)*, **6**, 2, Supplement, pp. 79–81, May 1990.

Ma Y.Y. (1990). Pressure effects of gunshot wounds in the spinal canal. *J. Trauma (China)*, **6**, suppl., 21–4.

Ma Y., Feng T., Fu R., Li M. (1988). An analysis of the wounding factors of four different shapes of fragments. *J. Trauma*, **28**, (1 suppl.), S230–5.

Owen-Smith M. (1981). *High Velocity Missile Wounds*. London: Arnold.

Peters C.E. (1990a). A mathematical model of wound ballistics. *J. Trauma (China)*, **6**, (suppl.), 303–18.

Peters C.E. (1990b). Common misconceptions about the physical mechanisms in wound ballistics. *J. Trauma (China)*, **6**, (suppl.), 319–26.

Ragsdale R.D., Josselson A. (1988). Experimental gunshot fractures. *J. Trauma*, **28** (1 suppl.), S109–15.

Rich N.M. (1978). Military surgery: 'Bullets and blood vessels'. *Surg. Clin. North Am.*, **58**, 995–1003.

Rich N.M., Manion W.C., Hughes C.W. (1969). Surgical and pathological evaluation of vascular injury in Vietnam. *J. Trauma*, **9**, 279–91.

Röckert H., Berlin R., Dahlgren B. et al. (1979). Cell damage at different distances from wound channels caused by spherical missiles with high impact velocity. *Acta Chir. Scand. Suppl.*, **489**, 151–8.

Rybeck B. (1974). Missile wounding and hemodynamic effects of energy absorption. *Acta Chir. Scand. Suppl.*, 450.

Sun D.R., Wang C.R., Hua J. et al. (1990). Investigation of indirect fracture of long bones using strain gauges. *J. Trauma (China)*, **6**, (suppl.), 335, 336.

Suneson A. (1989). Distant Pressure Wave Effects on Nervous Tissues by High-energy Missile Impact. Doctorial thesis, University of Göteborg, Sweden.

Tikka S.A. (1989). Missile Injury. Observations on the Mechanism of Trauma and Revision Surgery of Soft Tissue Gunshot Wounds. Doctorial thesis, University of Helsinki, Annales Medicinae Militaris Fenniae, LXIV, 3a.

Wang D.W., Liu X.T., Wang C.R. et al. (1990a). The effect of injury to organs adjacent to the wound channel in 44 swine shot with steel balls and 22 wounded soldiers. *J. Trauma (China)*, **6**, (suppl.), 101–4.

Wang Z.G., Feng J.X., Liu Y.Q. (1982). Pathomorphological observations of gunshot wounds. *Acta Chir. Scand. Suppl.*, **508**, 185–95.

Wang Z.G., Tang C.G., Chen X.Y. et al. (1988). Early pathomorphological characteristics of the wound track caused by fragments. *J. Trauma*, **28**, (suppl.), S89–94.

Watkins F.P., Pearce B.P., Stainer M.C. (1988). Physical effects of the penetration of head simulants by steel spheres. *J. Trauma*, **28**, (suppl.), S40–53.

Whelan T.J. Jr, Burkhalter W.E., Gomez A. (1968). Management of war wounds. *Adv. Surg.*, **3**, 227.

Zhang D.C., Qian C.W., Liu Y.G. et al. (1988). Morphopathologic observations on high-velocity steel bullet wounds at various intervals after wounding. *J. Trauma*, **28**, (suppl.), S89–94.

FURTHER READING

Committee on Trauma of the American College of Surgeons (1988). *Advanced Trauma Life Support Program*. Chicago: American College of Surgeons Publication.

Cooper G.J., Ryan J.M. (1990). The interaction of penetrating missiles with tissues – some common misapprehensions, and the implications for wound management. *Br. J. Surg.*, **77**, 905–9.

Eiseman B., Swan K. (1988). Military strategy in trauma. In *Trauma* (Mattox et al., eds). Connecticut: Appleton and Lange, pp. 781–8.

Fackler M.L. (1988). Wound ballistics: a review of common misconceptions. *JAMA*, **259**, 2730–6.

Fackler M.L., Surinchak J.S., Malinowski J.A., Bowen R.E. (1984). Bullet Fragmentation: A Major Cause of Tissue Disruption. *J Trauma*, **24**, 35–9.

Fackler M.L., Breteau J.P.L., Courbill L.J. et al. (1988). *Open Wound Drainage Versus Wound Excision on the Modern Battlefield*. Letterman Army Institute of Research: Report 256.

Friedrich P.l. (1898). *Antiseptic Treatment of Fresh Wounds. Report on animal experiments carried out to establish the incubation period of infective agents in fresh wounds*. Leipzig: Leipzig University Press (translated from German).

Heggers J.P., Robson M.C., Doral E.T. (1969). Quantitative assessment of bacterial contamination of open wounds by a slide technique. *Trans. R. Soc. Med.*, **63**, 532–4.

Lindsey D. (1980). The idolatry of velocity, or lies, damn lies, and ballistics. *J. Trauma*, **20**, 1068–9.

Odling-Smee G.W. (1970). Ibo civilian casualties in the Nigerian Civil War. *Br. Med. J.*, **1**, 592–6.

Ogilvie H. (1956). Lessons of the war that are already being forgotten. *Guy's Hosp. Gaz.*, October, 401–5.

Robens W., Küsswetter K. (1982). Fractures typical to human bone by assault missile trauma. *Act Chir. Scand.*, Suppl. 508, 223–7.

Ryan J.M. (1990). An Enquiry into the Nature of Infection in Fragment Wounds – With particular reference to the role of contamination. Thesis for Master of Surgery, University College Dublin.

Ryan J.M., Cooper G.J., Maynard R.L. (1988). Wound ballistics: contemporary and future research. *J.R. Army Med. Corps*, **134**, 119–25.

Ryan J.M., Cooper G.C., Milner S., Haywood I.R. (1991). Field surgery on the modern battlefield – strategy and wound management. *Ann. R. Coll. Surg. Eng.*, **73**.

5. Penetrating Head Injury

R. L. Maynard, I. V. Allen and J. B. Hull

INTRODUCTION

Penetrating head injury is an impact on the head in which the dura is breached, allowing communication between the cranial contents and the exterior (Crockard, 1982). This definition includes injuries where a missile perforates the head or lodges in the cranial cavity. It also includes tangential impacts leading to fracture of the skull and laceration of the dura by bone fragments.

Compared with the extensive studies undertaken on the pathogenesis of closed or blunt head injury (see Chapter 9), the biophysical principles of penetrating head injury have not been extensively studied. In 1973, Clemedson observed that:

> No systematic, qualitative or quantitative studies of cranial injuries caused by high velocity ammunition have yet been published, even though military interest has mainly involved this type of ammunition.... (Clemedson et al., 1973)

The reasons for the limited interest in the problem include the lack of a suitable animal model and a feeling of pessimism regarding the likely outcome of penetrating injuries to the brain, particularly from high-velocity rifle bullets. Until recently, the incidence of penetrating head injury in civilian practice was low by comparison with closed injury. Less emphasis has therefore been placed on penetrating injury.

In war, the majority of penetrating head injuries are caused by antipersonnel fragments, and not by bullets. In the Korean War, Meirowski (1965) reported 879 cases of penetrating head injuries, of which 46.5% were due to fragments and 30% to bullets. In the Second World War the ratio was 4:1 in favour of fragments (Small and Turner, 1947).

Developments in the design of military helmets have significantly reduced the incidence of penetrating fragment wounds but protection of the head against high-velocity rifle bullets is not possible with present lightweight materials.

In parallel to the high incidence of penetrating head injuries in war, such injuries are now seen very frequently in civilian practice in many parts of the world. For example, in Harris County, Texas, craniocerebral gunshot wounds were responsible for 16% of deaths from 'external causes' in the early 1980s. Half of the deaths were suicides and the remainder assaults (Kaufman et al., 1986).

The expanding civilian experience of gunshot wounds has led to a greater interest in management, including rapid evacuation. The appreciation of the need for early intensive care, including airway control and ventilation, has improved survival. In Northern Ireland, 80% of the casualties during the early 1970s, arrived at hospital within 60 minutes of wounding, many having received effective resuscitation in the ambulance (Byrnes et al., 1974). An interval of less than an hour between wounding and admission had been previously achieved in the USA (Jett et al., 1972); recent figures from Phoenix (USA) showed that in a recent analysis of 100 consecutive craniocerebral gunshot wounds, there was a mean interval of 23 minutes between wounding and admission to hospital (Grahm et al., 1990).

Despite more rapid transport of casualties to hospital and an improved understanding of optimal management, the prognosis for these patients remains poor. In the cases from Northern Ireland and Phoenix, 56% and 59% respectively died. The poor outlook for severe penetrating head injuries is underscored by the view that the likely mortality for a patient with a penetrating head injury and a score on the Glasgow Coma Scale of less than 5 is 100% (Hubschmann et al., 1979). Surgical intervention is probably not warranted in patients with a post-resuscitation score on the Glasgow Coma Scale of less than 5 and without evidence on computerized tomography (CT) scan of an intracranial haematoma (Grahm et al., 1990).

INTERACTION OF PROJECTILES WITH THE HEAD

In the following account, only the effects of missiles impacting upon the cranium will be considered. Maxillofacial injury, ophthalmic injury or extracranial soft tissue injury will not be discussed. The consequences of injury to soft tissues including major arteries and the cranial nerves, both inside and outside the skull, will also not be considered.

Missiles impact the skull in three ways: a tangential strike without penetration but with injury to soft tissues and occasionally fracture of the skull; penetration and lodgement sometimes with a complex track caused by rebound from the inner table of the skull; perforation of the skull.

The mechanical interaction of missiles with the head will be considered in terms of the covering of the skull, the cranium and the brain.

The covering of the skull

The scalp comprises five layers: skin, subcutaneous fatty tissue, the epicranial muscle (comprising the occipitofrontalis and the temporoparietalis and its aponeurosis), loose subepicranial connective tissue and the pericranium. The penetration mechanics of

TABLE 5.1
PENETRATION OF SKIN BY PROJECTILES. (MODIFIED FROM DI MAIO, 1981)

Reference	Tissue	Missile	Missile diameter (mm)	Missile weight (g)	Velocity (m/s)	E/a (m-kg/cm²)	J/cm²*	Comments
Journee, 1907	Skin and muscle	Lead ball	11.25	8.5	60	1.56	15.3	Superficial skin damage
					70	2.13	20.9	Perforated skin penetrated into muscle
Grundfest et al., 1945	Skin	Steel sphere	3.17	0.13	51.8	0.23†	2.26	Velocities obtained by extrapolation of data
			6.35	NS‡	38.1	–	–	
		Lead ball	4.37	NS‡	82.9	–	–	'Cut' in skin surface
Sperraza and Kokinakis, 1968	Skin	Steel sphere	6 §	1	60	0.6	6.3	Half the missiles striking at these velocities perforated the skin
				2	52	–		
				3	40	–		
Mattoo et al., 1974	Skin and muscle	Lead ball	8.5	4.5	61.6	1.53	15.0	Abraded the skin
					71.3	2.06	20.30	Perforated skin penetrating into muscle

* This column has been derived from Di Maio's column headed E/a (m-kg/cm²) using the conversion factor
  1 kg(F)·m = 9.8 Joules.
† This figure calculated from data in original article.
‡ Not stated in original article.
§ Calculated from missile weight and density of steel.

the individual layers are not known. The muscle is thin and it is unlikely that it contributes significantly to the resistance offered by the scalp to penetration.

Studies of the capacity of skin to resist penetration by projectiles have been conducted (Journee, 1907; Grundfest et al., 1945; Sperrazza and Kokinakis, 1968; Mattoo et al., 1974). The subject was reviewed by Di Maio, in 1981 and Table 5.1, modified from this contribution, summarizes the results.

The velocity at which a projectile has a 50% probability of penetration of skin (V_{50}) can be related to the ratio of the presented area of the projectile and its mass (Sperrazza and Kokinakis, 1968). The relationship for the penetration of isolated skin and combat clothing is shown in Figure 5.1.

Subcutaneous tissue and muscle offer very much less resistance to penetration than does skin, and this can be assumed to apply to the scalp.

The contribution made by the skin to mitigating skull fracture was stressed by Tedeschi (1977), who pointed out that without the scalp the skull could be fractured by as little as 40 psi (280 kPa), whereas the intact head could withstand 425–900 psi (2.9–6.2 MPa).

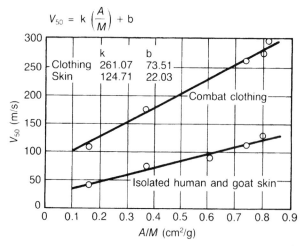

Figure 5.1 Ballistic limit (V_{50} – velocity predicted to result in a 50% probability of penetration) versus fragment area/mass for combat clothing and isolated human and goat skin. A = cross-sectional area of missile (cm²); M = mass of missile (g); k, b = constants. (Reproduced from Sperrazza and Kokinakis, 1968.)

The skull

In his classic work on head injuries, Rowbotham (1945) began his account of the mechanical properties of the skull by referring to the observation of Von Bruns in 1854, that if the skull was a uniform elastic sphere, the lines of fracture resulting from

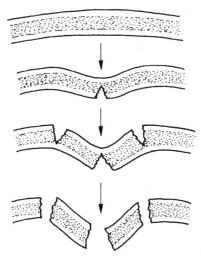

Figure 5.2 The sequence of events in fracture by local deformity. (Reproduced from Rowbotham, 1945.)

the application of force could be calculated mathematically.

However the skull is irregular in terms of curvature and thickness and, although ideas derived from a study of oversimplified models of skull biomechanics are useful in considering probable effects of various impacts, the precise effects of specific impacts arc impossible to prcdict for both penetrating and blunt injury.

The vault of the skull is composed of two layers of compact bone, the inner and outer tables, linked by a layer of cancellous bone, the diploe. The radius of curvature of the inner table is less than that of the outer. The inner table is more brittle than the outer. Impacts upon the outer table transmit force and a stress cone through the two tables. Fracture of the inner table may occur despite the outer table being undamaged. The probable explanation is that bone is stronger in compression than tension and when the outer table is compressed by an impact the inner table is under tensile forces and could break (Rowbotham, 1945). This phenomenon, and the effects of the application of greater force over a small area, are illustrated in Figure 5.2. This feature had also been discussed by Treves in 1883 with reference to the effects of a sabre cut. The greater damage to the inner table produced at the impact site is mirrored by a greater degree of injury to the outer table at an exit site if the projectile retains sufficient energy to leave the skull.

The thickness of the skull is not uniform. It is thin at the centre of the squamous temporal bone and thick at the occipital protuberances. Racial differences in skull thickness have also been described, with Negroid skulls tending to be thicker than Caucasian. Rowbotham reported the observation allegedly made by Herodotus that Egyptian skulls were thick and tough whereas Persian skulls were thin and brittle.

Detailed study of the thickness of the regions of the skull has led to the concept of a number of thickenings or buttresses linked by strengthened arches. Between these strong areas, panels of thinner bone are found. Six regions where the skull is strengthened and from which arches run upwards to the apex of the vault becoming thinner have been described (Le Count and Apfelbach, 1920), and are illustrated in Figure 5.3.

1. In front from the root of the nose and glabella.
2. One behind including the inion and the external and internal crests of the occipital bone.
3. On each side from the external angular process of the frontal bone projecting obliquely back to the sphenoid in the base of the skull.
4. One on each side formed by the petrous temporal bones and continuing externally as the mastoid process.

Rowbotham added arches at the supraorbital ridges, the temporal crests and the curved lines (superior nuchal lines) of the occiput.

Fractures which occur in the vault of the skull tend to run 'up into the vault and down into the bones of the base of the cranium between the arches' (Le Count and Apfelbach, 1920). Fractures which run through the posterior and middle cranial fossae are probably deflected towards the apex or basc of the petrous, depending on their angle of approach to this thickened region, and Le Count and Apfelbach pointed out that the application of force sufficient to fracture the middle part of the petrous temporal bone is likely to be fatal.

Though essentially strong, the base of the skull is weakened by foramina – the hypoglossal foramina in the posterior cerebral fossa, the foramina of the greater wing of the sphenoid and the foramen lacerum may be involved in fractures. Figure 5.4 shows fracture lines running towards the hypophyseal fossa.

The impact of penetrating projectiles of high momentum upon the skull leads to the high acceleration of the head. In addition to the penetrating wound, injury to the brain from acceleration may also occur. This phenomenon is often overlooked in analyses of the pathogenesis of penetrating head injury. A tangential impact upon the vault of the skull will impart rotatory momentum to the head. However, bullets and fragments are generally of low mass and high velocity. Their kinetic energy may be high, but the momentum of such projectiles is low and they would not be expected to produce high acceleration of the skull as a whole, though damage to the brain produced by the transfer of energy occurring during penetration may be great. The importance of rotary acceleration of the head during blunt impacts as an important mechanism of injury was established during the Second World War (Holbourn, 1945) and has since been extensively studied (Gennarelli *et al.*, 1971, 1979; Hume

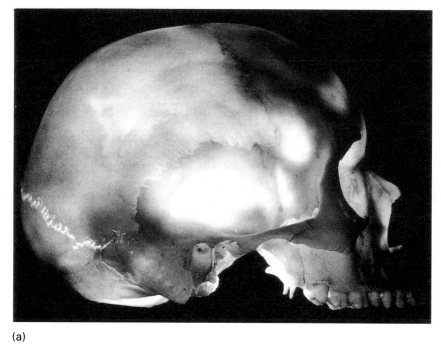

(a)

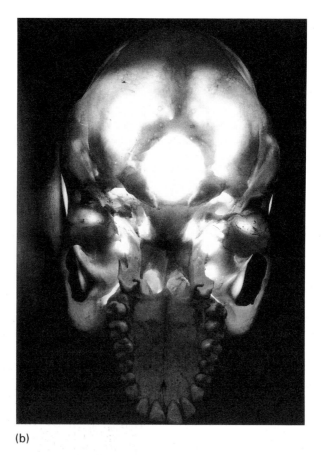

(b)

Figure 5.3 (a), (b) The weak panels and strong buttresses of the vault and base.

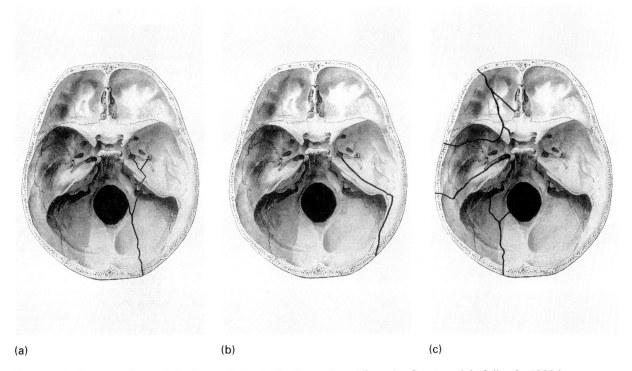

(a)   (b)   (c)

Figure 5.4 Fracture lines of the base of the skull. (Reproduced from Le Court and Apfelbach, 1920.)

Adams *et al.*, 1981). Non-penetrating impact to the head is described in Chapter 9.

Penetration of the skull by projectiles may leave fractures that indicate the angle of impact. Bevelling of the edges of the entrance wound on the outer surface of the skull and of the edges of the exit wound on the inner surface of the skull has been described. The production of elliptical entrance wounds with asymmetrical bevelling has also been reported (Knight, 1977). There is variation in the effect of a projectile according to the density of the bone struck. In a case recorded by Knight, a high-available-energy bullet that struck in line with the external auditory meatus decelerated rapidly in the petrous temporal bone, transferred high energy and caused complete destruction of the head.

INTERACTION OF PROJECTILES WITH THE BRAIN

The extent of temporary cavitation around the track of a projectile through soft tissue is largely dependent upon the amount of energy transferred from the projectile to the tissue (see Chapter 4). Many handgun bullets and most fragments with low available energy produce injury largely confined to the track of the projectile. In brain injuries, this type of wound is exemplified by an airgun pellet which, having penetrated a child's skull, retained sufficient velocity to traverse the brain but not to leave the cranium (Figure 5.5).

High-velocity rifle bullets have high available kinetic energy. As they decelerate in tissue, the energy transfer to the skull and brain is substantial. Deceleration is principally dependent upon the presented area of the projectile (for non-fragmenting projectiles) and a bullet with very low yaw will not decelerate as quickly as a large antipersonnel fragment. With most wound tracks traversing the brain, bullets will increase their yaw and the change in presented area will increase the rate of energy

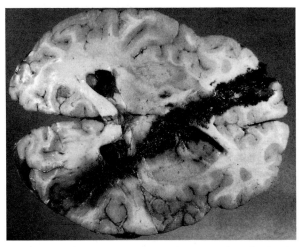

Figure 5.5 A low-energy-transfer wound to the brain of a child. A 0.177-in. airgun slug can just be seen in the occipital cortex. (Reproduced from Knight, 1977.)

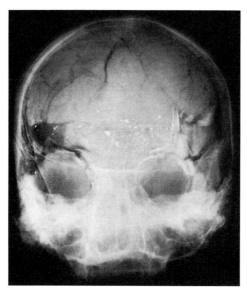

Figure 5.6 Gelatin-filled human skull showing damage produced by impact of a 7.62-mm high-available-energy rifle bullet. The projectile has fragmented.

transfer. Bullets with high initial yaw resulting from impact upon materials such as a helmet, will decelerate more rapidly in the initial part of the track and transfer a greater proportion of their energy in the early stages of penetration.

Fragmentation of a bullet or the deformation of its nose or base as it passes through tissue, also leads to a very high energy transfer.

As a projectile decelerates in the brain and gives up energy, tissue is displaced outwards forming a temporary cavity. Details are discussed in Chapter 4, but the special characteristics of the skull–brain system require further consideration here. The brain is rather like water and can be considered incompressible (Holbourn, 1945), though some compressibility had previously been suggested on the assumption that escape of fluids from the brain would occur (Flexner *et al.*, 1932). However, in most injuries this does not happen, particularly in rapid pressure changes produced by the expansion of a temporary cavity.

Expansion of the temporary cavity leads to the development of very high pressures within the skull and outward fracture of the cranium. The extensive fracturing produced by the formation of a large temporary cavity in a gelatin-filled skull simulant is shown in Figure 5.6. The rapid pressure rise within a skull by the passage of a projectile and the formation of the temporary cavity is shown in Figure 5.7. The initial fast-rising pressure peak is probably a stress wave generated within the skull by the passage of the projectile; the second peak results from the production of a temporary cavity.

Complex patterns of pressure changes have also been revealed by the use of human skulls filled with 20% gelatin and covered with two layers of chamois leather soaked in gelatin (Watkins *et al.*, 1988). Pressure transducers were mounted inside the skull via the foramen magnum and a series of studies undertaken with different projectiles. The

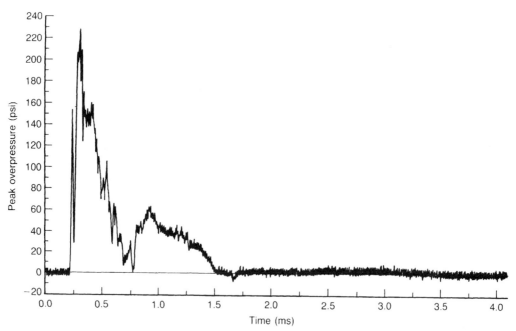

Figure 5.7 Pressure–time curve recorded within the skull of a baboon during impact of a 4.8-mm steel sphere. 1 psi = 6.89 kPa.

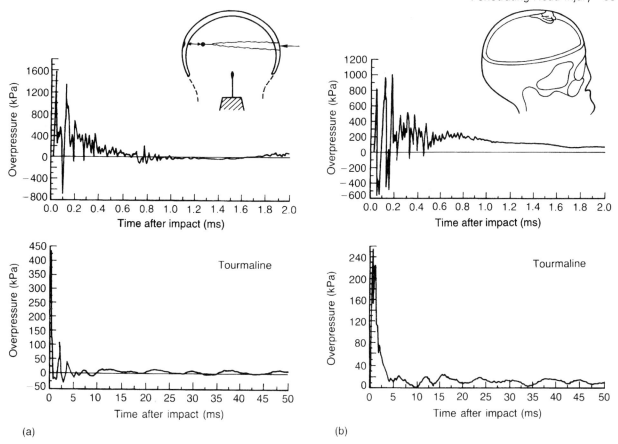

Figure 5.8   Pressure–time curves recorded within a gelatin-filled human skull following penetration by a 6-mm steel sphere at an impact velocity of 450 m/s (a) and a tangential impact at 838 m/s (b).

pressure traces from two experiments are shown in Figure 5.8.

The relative contributions to brain injury of the direct stress wave and the temporary cavitation produced by the passage of a projectile through the brain are poorly understood. The high peak pressures are often quoted as capable of causing damage, though there is little direct evidence to support this. In addition to the pressure pulses generated in the brain, cavitation may produce marked and rapid differential movement of its different parts. The edges of the lesser wings of sphenoid, the crista galli, the clinoid processes, the edges of the foramen magnum, the falx cerebri and the tentorium cerebellae are all likely to damage brain which impacts against them (Tedeschi, 1977). Whether this plays a part in brain injury produced as a result of penetrating head injury is not clear. Some changes may be the consequence of an increase in intracranial pressure after injury because of bleeding and herniation of the uncus and tips of the temporal poles at the tentorium, together with downward displacement of the brain stem against the edges of the foramen magnum.

PATHOLOGY OF PENETRATING HEAD INJURY

Despite the fact that penetrating head injury is common in war, there are few detailed studies of the pathology of this injury. In the First World War, only the gross brain change in fatalities were described in detail (Cushing, 1918). Subsequent to the Second World War, the macroscopic findings were extended but histological details were lacking (Freytag, 1963) until a series of experiments were undertaken in which anaesthetized dogs were injured by military rifle bullets (Clemedson *et al.*, 1973). Brain fixation was undertaken by vascular perfusion but the histological examination reported was incomplete (Allen *et al.*, 1982). The incorrect assumption that the pathological effects of penetrating head injury were likely to be similar to the those seen in non-penetrating head injury seems to have retarded work in this area.

A series of studies on anaesthetized monkeys began in the late 1970s, and a number of observations of light and electron microscopic changes were made (Allen *et al.*, 1982, 1983a, b, 1985). The experiments were based on transfrontal injury with or without a preliminary burr hole to avoid the

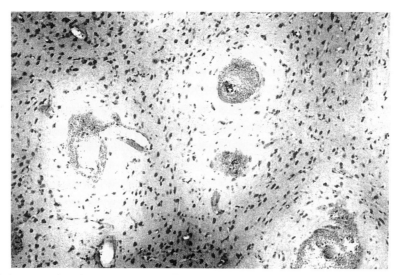

Figure 5.9 Area of decreased staining intensity. H&E, × 45. (Reproduced from Allen *et al.*, 1982.)

complicating effects of bone fragments. Two standard spherical steel projectiles were used: a 3.22-mm with a nominal impact velocity of 1000 m/s (Rhesus monkeys) and a 4.8-mm with an impact velocity between 181 and 364 m/s (Baboons).

Extensive tissue destruction and haemorrhage were found along the track of the projectile. There was extensive subarachnoid haemorrhage and bleeding into the lateral ventricles. In those animals in which the sphere had penetrated bone, fragments were found along the wound track.

With light microscopy, lesions could be categorized into those anatomically in continuity with the missile track and more disseminated ones outside the missile path. A zone of pallor and oedema was often noted adjacent to the wound, and blood vessels in this area were disrupted. Three types of disseminated lesion were consistently observed:

1. Ring haemorrhages occurring adjacent to the missile track but also frequently seen at a distance from the primary wound. They were particularly prominent in the hypothalamus, mid brain, pons and cerebellum.
2. Areas of decreased staining density, often associated with perivascular ring haemorrhages but also observed in areas without haemorrhage. Within these areas nuclear density was reduced, suggesting inter- or intracellular oedema (Figure 5.9).
3. Areas of increased staining density in association with areas of haemorrhage.

The classic changes seen in non-penetrating head injury, such as destruction of neurones and diffuse axonal injury with microglial reaction, were not found. This may be due to the short survival time (for the Rhesus monkey group a maximum of 169 minutes). The widespread ring haemorrhages are a less prominent feature of closed head injury, though they had previously been described in penetrating injuries in man (Freytag, 1963). It has been suggested that the respiratory failure sometimes seen in penetrating injury which has not obviously involved the brain stem may be related to these widely disseminated lesions.

The unexpected finding seen on electron microscopy was the presence of swelling of the astrocyte foot processes (Figure 5.10). This was widespread and, though there was some suggestion that it was associated with the pale areas described at light microscopy, this was not conclusive. In some areas, rupture of swollen foot processes was observed. The cause of this lesion is obscure. Similar changes have been described in spinal cord injury (Griffiths *et al.*, 1978), in cerebral ischaemia (Jenkins *et al.*, 1979) and in response to lateral head acceleration (Maxwell *et al.*, 1988). Such lesions have not been previously described in either experimental work

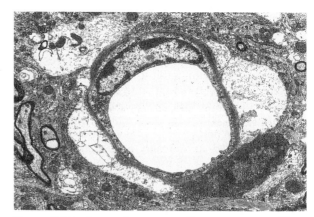

Figure 5.10 Area of astrocyte foot process swelling. Electron micrograph: × 6545. (Reproduced from Allen *et al.*, 1982.)

or in patients with penetrating injury. The swelling may reflect damage to the blood–brain barrier produced either as a direct effect of tissue distortion, local ischaemia or the release of chemical mediators. A similar response follows increased levels of potassium and adenosine (Bourke *et al.*, 1981) and is of particular interest in that the adenosine-induced change could be inhibited by a non-diuretic acylaryloxyacid derivative. The implications for the management of physiological disturbance following penetrating head injury could be considerable.

PHYSIOLOGICAL DISTURBANCES FOLLOWING PENETRATING HEAD INJURY

Disturbances of the cardiorespiratory systems are common. The exact mechanisms are obscure and few studies in experimental animals have been reported. Respiratory failure following experimental head injury is common (Gerber and Moody, 1972; Crockard *et al.*, 1977; Brown *et al.*, 1979). Cardiovascular disturbances occur within seconds of injury: bradycardia, conduction abnormalities and ST segment depression. A linear relationship between depression of cardiac output 30 minutes after injury and the impact energy of the projectile was demonstrated, though at 1 hour postinjury the correlation was less evident (Maynard *et al.*, 1983, unpublished observations). Prediction of survival has been quantified by means of a multiple regression analysis of 10 physiological variables (Crockard *et al.*, 1977). Of those studied, cerebral blood flow and mean arterial blood pressure at 30 minutes postinjury proved the most useful for the prediction of a survival period. In penetrating head injuries, the normal autoregulation of cerebral blood flow is lost and blood flow becomes dependent upon cardiac output and systemic blood pressure.

Further investigations of the mechanisms underlying the cardiovascular changes has shown that pretreatment of animals with atropine prevents postinjury bradycardia but not the fall in cardiac output, though the ganglionic blocker hexamethonium seemed to prevent both effects (Levett *et al.*, 1980a, b). These findings have given rise to speculation regarding malfunction of the hypothalamus even when the wound track does not obviously involve this part of the brain. There is also evidence that hypothalamic lesions can occur in cases of transfrontal head injury.

REFERENCES

Allen I.V., Scott R., Tanner J.A. (1982). Experimental high-velocity missile head injury. *Injury*, **14**, 183–93.

Allen I.V., Kirk J., Maynard R.L. et al. (1983a). Experimental penetrating head injury: some aspects of light microscopical and ultrastructural abnormalities. *Acta Neurochir. Suppl. (Wien)*, **32**, 99–104.

Allen I.V., Kirk J., Maynard R.L. et al. (1983b). An ultrastructural study of experimental high velocity penetrating head injury. *Acta Neuropathol. (Berl.)*, **59**, 277–82.

Allen I.V., Crockard A., Maynard R.L., Cooper G.J. (1985). In *Trauma of the Central Nervous System* (Dacey R.G. Jr, ed.), New York: Raven Press.

Bourke R.S., Waldman J.B., Kimelberg H.K. et al. (1981). Adenosine-stimulated astroglial swelling in rat cerebral cortex *in vivo* with total inhibition by a non-diuretic acylaryloxyacid derivative. *J. Neurosurg.*, **55**, 364–70.

Brown F.D., Johns L.M., Jafar J.J., Crockard H.A. (1979). Detailed monitoring of the effects of manitol following experimental head injury. *J. Neurosurg.*, **50**, 423–32.

Byrnes D.P., Crockard H.A., Gordon D.S., Gleadhill C.A. (1974). Penetrating craniocerebral missile injuries in the civil disturbances in Northern Ireland. *Br. J. Surg.*, **61**, 169–76.

Clemedson C.J., Falconer B., Frankenberg L. et al. (1973). Head injuries caused by small calibre, high velocity bullets. An experimental study. *Z. Rechtsmed.*, **73**, 103–14.

Crockard H.A. (1974). Bullet injuries of the brain. *Ann. R. Coll. Surg. Engl.*, **55**, 111–23.

Crockard H.A. (1982). Early management of head injuries. *Br. J. Hosp. Med.*, **29**, 635–8, 641–4.

Crockard H.A., Brown F.D., Calica A.B. et al. (1977). Physiological consequences of experimental cerebral missile injury and the use of data analysis to predict survival. *J. Neurosurg.*, **46**, 784–94.

Cushing H. (1918). A study of a series of wounds involving the brain and its enveloping structures. *Br. J. Surg.*, **5**, 558–684.

Di Maio V.J.M. (1981). Penetration and perforation of skin by bullets and missiles: a review of the literature. *Am. J. Forensic Med. Pathol.*, **2**, 107–10.

Flexner L.B., Clark J.H., Weed L.H. (1932). The elasticity of the dural sac and its contents. *Am. J. Physiol.*, **101**, 292–303.

Freytag E. (1963). Autopsy findings in head injuries from firearms. *Arch. Pathol.*, **76**, 215–25.

Gennarelli T.A., Ommaya A.K., Thibault L.E. (1971). Comparison of linear and rotational acceleration in experimental cerebral concussion. In *Proceedings of the 15th Stapp Car Crash Conference*. New York: Society of Automotive Engineers, pp. 797–803.

Gennarelli T.A., Abel J., Hume Adams J., Graham D.I. (1979). Differential tolerance of frontal and temporal lobes to contusion induced by angular acceleration. In *Proceedings of the 23rd Stapp Car Crash Conference*. New York: Society of Automotive Engineers, pp. 797–803.

Gennarelli T.A., Hume Adams J., Graham D.I. (1981). Acceleration induced head injury in the monkey. I. The model, its mechanical and physiological correlates. *Acta Neuropathol. Suppl. (Berl.)*, **7**, 23–5.

Gerber A.M., Moody R.A. (1972). Craniocerebral missile injury in the monkey: an experimental physiological model. *J. Neurosurg.*, **36**, 43–9.

Grahm T.W., Williams F.C., Harrington T., Spetzler R.F. (1990). Civilian gunshot wounds to the head: a prospective study. *Neurosurgery*, **27**, 696–700.

Griffiths I.R., McCulloch M., Crawford R.A. (1978). Ultrastructural appearances of the spinal cord microvasculature between 12 hours and 4 days after impact injury. *Acta Neuropathol. (Berl.)*, **43**, 205–11.

Grundfest H., Korr I.M., McMilen J.H., Butler E.G. (1945). *Ballistics of the Penetration of Human Skin by Small Spheres*. Committee on Medical Research of the Office of Scientific Research and Development, Minor Casualties Report No. 11.

Hammon W. (1971). Analysis of 2187 consecutive penetrating wounds of the brain from Vietnam. *J. Neurosurg.*, **34**, 127–31.

Holbourn A.H.S (1945). The mechanics of brain injuries. *Br. Med. Bull.*, **3**, 147–9.

Hubschmann O., Shapiro K., Baden M., Shulman K. (1979). Craniocerebral gunshot injuries in civilian practice: prognostic criteria and surgical management experience with 82 cases. *J. Trauma*, **19**, 6–12.

Hume Adams J., Graham D.I., Gennarelli T.A. (1981). Acceleration induced head injury in the monkey. II. Neuropathology. *Acta Neuropathol. Suppl. (Berl.)*, **7**, 26–8.

Jenkins L.W., Povlishock J.T., Becker D.P. et al. (1979). Complete cerebral ischaemia: an ultrastructural study. *Acta Neuropathol. (Berl.)*, **48**, 113–25.

Jett H.H., Van Hoy J.M., Hamit H.F. (1972). Clinical and socioeconomic aspects of 254 admissions for stab and gunshot wounds. *J. Trauma*, **12**, 577–80.

Journee C. (1907). Rapport entre force vive des balles et la gravite Blessures qu'elles peuvent Causer. *Rev. Artillerie*, **70**, 81–120.

Kaufman H.H., Makela M.E., Lee K.F. et al. (1986). Gunshot wounds to the head: a perspective. *Neurosurgery*, **18**, 689–95.

Knight B. (1977). Firearm injuries. In *Forensic Medicine*. (Tedeschi C.G., Eckert W.G., Tedeschi L.G., eds). Philadelphia: W.B. Saunders Company, pp. 510–26.

Le Count E.R., Apfelbach C.W. (1920). Pathological anatomy of traumatic fractures of cranial bones and concomitant brain injuries. *JAMA*, **74**, 501–11.

Levett J.M., Johns L.M., Replogle R.L., Mullan S. (1980a). Cardiovascular effects of experimental cerebral missile injury in primates. *Surg. Neurol.*, **13**, 59–64.

Lewelt W., Jenkins L.W., Miller J.D. (1980b). Autoregulation of cerebral blood flow after experimental fluid percussion injury of the brain. *J. Neurosurg.*, **53**, 500–11.

Mattoo B.N., Wani A.K., Asgekar M.D. (1974). Casualty criteria for wounds from firearms with special reference to shot penetration. II. *J. Forensic Sci.*, **19**, 585–9.

Maxwell W.L., Irvine A., Adams J. et al. (1988). Response of cerebral microvasculature to brain injury. *J. Pathol.*, **155**, 327–35.

Meirowski A.M. (1965). Penetrating wounds of the brain. In *Neurological Surgery of Trauma* (Meirowski A.M., ed.). Washington DC: US Government Printing Office, pp. 103–30.

Rowbotham G.F. (1945). *Acute Injuries of the Head*. Edinburgh: E & S Livingstone Ltd.

Small J.M., Turner E.A. (1947). Surgical experiences of 1200 cases of penetrating brain wounds in battle, NW Europe 1944–1945. *Br. J. Surg.* (War Surg. suppl. 1), 62–74.

Sperrazza J., Kokinakis W. (1968). Ballistic limits of tissue and clothing. *Ann. N.Y. Acad. Sci.*, **152**, 163–7.

Tedeschi C. (1977). The wound: assessment by organ systems, I. The head and spine. In *Forensic Medicine* (Tedeschi C.G., Eckert W.G., Tedeschi L.G., eds). Philadelphia: W.B. Saunders Company, pp. 29–75.

Treves F. (1883). *Surgical Applied Anatomy*. London: Cassell.

Von Bruns P. (1854). *Die Chirurgischen Krankheiten und Verletzungen des Gehirns und seiner Umhullungen. Handbuch der praktischen Chirurgie fur Arzte und Wundarzte*. Tubingen.

Watkins F.P., Pearce B.P., Stainer M.C. (1988). Physical effects of the penetration of head simulants by steel spheres. *J. Trauma*, **28**, (suppl.), S40–54.

6. Penetrating Injury of Bones

M. Mars and R. F. Spencer

Penetrating injuries of bone are increasing in frequency and severity as the availability and sophistication of both firearms and ammunition increases. In less 'advanced' societies, penetrating bone injuries are still inflicted with axes, knives and spears.

Bone injury can only occur after a missile has passed through skin and soft tissue. The overall effect of the injury and its outcome are influenced by both soft tissue and bone damage. The response of bone to trauma may be divided into two categories: those occurring immediately and resulting from the forces applied, and the subsequent inflammatory and reparative events which ultimately lead to union. An understanding of the former requires a knowledge of the basic structure of bone, its biomechanical properties and the forces producing the injury, while the latter involves the pathophysiological events which follow. These will be reviewed.

BONE STRUCTURE

Bone consists of an outer shell of compact cortical bone of variable thickness. Within this shell are varying amounts of spongy cancellous bone forming a network of trabeculae, which follow the lines of stress and tension within the bone. In long bones, the widened metaphyseal ends are filled with cancellous bone which disperses the forces generated around joints.

The basic building block of compact bone is the osteon or haversian system. This consists of a central canal, 3–9 mm long, containing blood vessels. The walls of the canal are lined with osteogenic cells and around the canal are a series of thin concentrically arranged lamellae. Canaliculi pass radially from the central canal to lacunae containing osteocytes. The lacunae within an osteon are connected by a further network of canaliculi. These interconnecting canaliculi are filled with protoplasmic extensions of osteocytes forming a functional cellular syncytium within the matrix of bone. The canaliculi are the path by which nutrients from the central vessel reach the osteocyte. The osteons are usually orientated with their long axis roughly parallel to the long axis of the bone. Between the haversian systems are irregularly arranged layers of interstitial lamellae.

The internal and outer surfaces of compact bone are composed of lamellae circumferentially ori- entated to the long axis of the bone. The inner endosteal surface is lined with osteogenic cells. A periosteum of dense fibrous and elastic tissue surrounds the compact bone. It is divided into an outer fibrous layer and an inner more vascular cambium layer consisting of loosely arranged osteogenic cells.

Penetrating the inner and outer circumferential lamellae are Volkmann's canals carrying nutrient arteries feeding the haversian systems. These canals traverse the cortex forming connecting channels linking periosteal, haversian and medullary blood vessels.

Bone matrix and cells

Bone matrix consists of collagen and ground substance, in which are embedded crystals of hydroxyapatite. Type 1 collagen constitutes about 90% of the dry weight of demineralized bone. It is synthesized on the ribosomes of osteoblasts and is structurally and genetically different to the collagen found in hyaline cartilage and skin. Ground substance is a complex viscous interfibrillar cement in which collagen is embedded. It is produced by osteoblasts and consists of covalently bonded protein-polysaccharides known as proteoglycans.

Osteoblasts produce bone matrix and are present at sites of ossification. They are found in the inner cambium layer of the periosteum, lining the endosteum, and may arise from blood vessel walls and the reticulum of bone marrow. When bone is being formed, they come to lie adjacent to the layer of unmineralized osteoid bone. Both the nucleus and cytoplasm have high concentrations of alkaline phosphatase. This may have a role in calcification.

Osteocytes lie buried in lacunae in the matrix of bone and are derived from the osteoblasts which laid down the surrounding bone matrix. They are considered to have a function in calcium homeostasis and may play a part in osteolysis.

Osteoclasts are multinucleate giant cells usually found lying in depressions on the surface of bone – Howship's lacunae. They contain acid phosphatase and have a well-developed Golgi apparatus. The region of plasma membrane adjacent to bone has many folds and has been termed a brush border. Bone resorption occurs at this brush border, by mechanisms that have not been fully elucidated. They are important in the normal process of bone remodelling and resorption of necrotic bone following fracture.

Blood supply

Bone necrosis occurs in all fractures and early reconstitution of the blood supply to the injured area facilitates healing. The blood supply of mature long bone is derived from three sources: (i) the

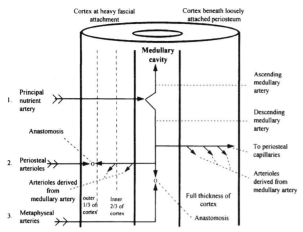

Figure 6.1 The arterial blood supply to mature long bone.

metaphyseal vessels; (ii) the nutrient artery and its branches and (iii) periosteal vessels (Figure 6.1).

The metaphyseal vessels arise from the rich arterial anastomoses around joints. Many vessels penetrate the thin cortical bone forming an extensive anastomotic network within the trabeculae of the cancellous bone of the metaphyseal region. At the junction of the metaphysis and the diaphysis, the metaphyseal arteries converge and anastomose with the medullary arteries.

The medullary arteries are branches of the nutrient artery of the bone, which traverses the cortex and divides into ascending and descending branches. The medullary arteries supply the endosteal surface and its branches ramify through cortical bone in Volkmann's canals, supplying vessels to the central canals of the haversian systems. The extent of this collateralization is such that no osteocyte in its lacuna is more than a few millimetres from a capillary.

Periosteal vessels are considered to be of two types: a capillary network in the periosteum and larger periosteal vessels which enter at the insertions of intermuscular septae to bone, for example the linea aspera in the femur. These larger vessels send branches into the cortex. It was generally held that medullary vessels supply the inner two-thirds of the cortex and periosteal vessels the outer third. In microangiographic studies of untraumatized canine long bones, Rhinelander (1968) demonstrated that periosteal vessels are only involved with cortical blood supply in regions immediately adjacent to their entry point at the insertion of muscular septae. Medullary artery derived vessels supply the full thickness of the cortex in most of the bone.

Arterial pressure is higher in medullary vessels than in periosteal vessels and blood flow is centrifugal (Brookes *et al.*, 1961). It has been suggested that under certain pathological conditions, flow reversal may occur (Brookes, 1971).

A fourth blood supply arises during fracture healing. New vessels derived from surrounding soft tissue supply the periosteal callus and detached bone fragments. These vessels penetrate the callus and may extend into the cortex.

Venous drainage of cortical bone is also considered to be centrifugal and the periosteal capillary network has been described as venous (Brookes, 1971). There is, however, evidence from *in vivo* studies in a rabbit model of centripetal flow from some haversian systems back into sinusoids within the medulla (Branemark, 1961).

Venous drainage of the metaphyseal region can be via metaphyseal veins passing through the cortex with metaphyseal arteries or via medullary veins draining into the veins accompanying the nutrient artery and the emissary veins. However, Hungerford could not demonstrate venous drainage into the diaphyseal region when contrast medium was injected into the metaphysis during venography (Hungerford, 1980).

BIOMECHANICS

The response of bone to applied force is dependent on extrinsic and intrinsic factors. Extrinsic factors are the magnitude and direction of the applied force and the duration of its application. Intrinsic factors are the capacity of bone to absorb energy and its modulus of elasticity.

The following terms are those most commonly used in relation to the biomechanics of bone. *Load* is the force applied to a body. *Stress* is the term applied to a force acting within a solid object when a load is applied to the object. The effects of the force are confined to the interior of the object and no visible deformity is present. *Strain* refers to any deformation which may occur following the application of a load. A stress threatening to crush the structure is *compression*. Conversely, a stress threatening to pull it apart is *tension*. A *shear force* results from an external load or *shear stress* producing an angular deformity. This occurs across a solid structure. These stresses may result in local deformations of the bone.

Figure 6.2 shows a standard stress–strain curve of a bone loaded in tension. The straight line portion is known as the *elastic region* and the curved portion the *plastic region*. The point where the graph becomes curved is known as the *yield point*. The stress required to reach the yield point is the *elastic limit*, beyond which permanent deformation occurs. The slope of the straight part of the graph and the elastic region is referred to as the *modulus of elasticity* or 'Young's modulus'. When loads are removed in the elastic region the structure returns to the original shape. This is not so of the plastic region, where permanent deformation occurs. The modulus of elasticity is also sometimes referred to as the *stiffness*. Strength is the maximum stress at the point of

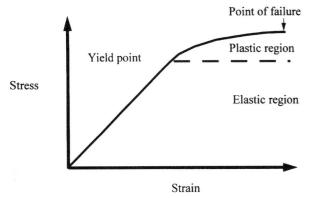

Figure 6.2 Standard stress–strain curve of a bone loaded in tension.

failure. In tensile loading this is known as the *ultimate tensile strength*. The strain at the point of failure is the *ductility* and represents the extent of permanent deformity. The area under the curve is the *strain energy* and represents the energy absorbed by bone under loading. The total strain energy stored at the point of failure is the *toughness* of the material.

Some materials display no intervening plastic region between the yield point and ultimate strength, and these are referred to as *brittle*. The mechanical properties of bone are also influenced by different rates of loading. This property is referred to as *viscoelasticity*. Bone also displays *anisotropy*. This term refers to the variable biomechanical properties of bone dependent on the direction of loading. This may take place in tension, compression and shear. Bone behaves differently in different sections, due to variations in architecture, and also with different loads. The result is, for example, that plastic deformation of cortical bone is diminished with transverse loading but such bone is strong in compression, less so in tension. Trabecular bone also demonstrates anisotropy, depending on the alignment of trabeculae (Einhom, 1988).

Fractures

From a biomechanical viewpoint, bone usually breaks in tension or shear, and occasionally in compression. This certainly applies insofar as cortical bone is concerned. Bone is neither very plastic nor very brittle, possessing the properties of a fibrous composite (Currey, 1984). Collagen contributes to the tensile strength of bone, and the ground matrix and hydroxyapatite impart strength against compressive forces. Cracks are propagated from one weak area to the next in a stepwise fashion. In this respect, the haversian systems and nutrient vessels represent points of failure. The propagation of these cracks under tension provides the characteristic fracture patterns. Because the spreading damage occurs at the sites of vascular supply, a

theoretical price is paid in terms of healing potential. Compression forces may also initiate fractures but they do so more rarely than tension forces. Under such circumstances the propagation of shear forces leads to eventual buckling and disintegration. Compression forces have a far greater predilection for vascular channels than do tension forces.

Penetrating injury

The severity of penetrating bone injury is dependent on the extent of associated soft tissue injury and the nature of the fracture produced. These in turn relate to the kinetic energy of the missile, the rate at which the kinetic energy is transferred to bone and soft tissue and the size of the contact area between the missile and the body. The kinetic energy of an object is expressed as $KE = mv^2/2$, where m is the mass of the object and v its velocity.

In most societies gunshot injuries are the commonest cause of penetrating bone injury. The missile is not however always a bullet. In less developed countries incised injuries produced by assault with machettes, bushknives or axes predominate. Industrial accidents with rivet guns, staple guns, bandsaws and fan blades have been reported. The patient too can become the projectile and impale himself.

Gunshot injury

With the kinetic energy of a bullet related to the square of its velocity, the bullet's speed is an important variable in its potential to cause damage. Distinction is made between high-and low-velocity injuries, as this influences the degree of both bone and soft tissue damage and their subsequent management. High velocity is arbitrarily defined as a bullet with a muzzle velocity greater than 2000 ft/s (600 m/s). The importance of velocity has been overemphasized and management options should not be dictated by muzzle velocity alone as the severity of the injury is not solely dependent on bullet velocity. The shape and construction of the bullet, its orientation and flight characteristics during passage through tissue and the ease with which it deforms or fragments in tissue all influence the extent of bone and soft tissue damage (Fackler, 1988) (see also Chapter 4).

Bullets damage tissue by direct and indirect mechanisms. They crush tissue with which they make direct contact, leaving a path or permanent cavity in the tissue. The amount of direct trauma can be increased by the degree of yaw or 'tumbling' of the bullet that occurs in the tissue. A bullet travelling with its longitudinal axis parallel to its line of flight will cause about one-third as much direct trauma as a bullet which has tumbled or yawed 90 degrees. Soft-nose and hollow-point bullets are designed to deform and flatten on impact. This increases their diameter between two and five times, thereby enlarging the volume of tissue injured. Bullets which fragment on impact or within soft tissue also increase the volume of tissue damaged (Hollerman *et al.*, 1990).

Military bullets usually have an outer metal jacket to prevent fragmentation and deformation. Hunting bullets are however designed to deform and fragment. This increases the tissue damage, raising the chances of a kill and lessening the likelihood of a wounded animal escaping to suffer. This should be borne in mind when managing injuries caused by civilian rifles (Fackler *et al.*, 1984; Hollerman *et al.*, 1990).

Indirect injury is caused by temporary cavitation. Temporary cavitation occurs after the bullet has passed through the tissue and the extent of the cavitation is related to the kinetic energy of the bullet, the degree of yaw and the rate at which the energy is transferred. Cavitation is increased by yaw and is maximal in the regions in which the long axis of the bullet was at 90 degrees to its flight path.

What is the effect of cavitation on bone? Bone is denser than muscle with a specific gravity of 1.11. The critical velocity for bone to fracture is approximately 200 ft/s (60 m/s) (Amato *et al.*, 1989). High-velocity injury to bone may be due to direct hit or occur indirectly when the force of the pressure wave causing temporary cavitation fractures the bone.

The effects of a direct hit by a high-velocity bullet on bone have been filmed by Amato *et al.* (1989). The model consisted of a femur embedded in gelatin with a specific gravity similar to muscle. The bullet passes through the bone forming the initial permanent cavitation. The size of this hole is similar to the diameter of the bullet. Rapid transfer of kinetic energy occurs. Within 10 μs of the bullet exiting the bone this transferred energy causes maximal temporary cavitation of the bone. The bone 'explodes', with fragmentation occurring over several centimetres. Soft tissue recoil returns the fragments to the vicinity of their original position. Secondary and subsequent oscillations of the temporary cavity appear to then drive the bone fragments forward, after the bullet. These bone fragments become secondary missiles which cause further soft tissue and neurovascular damage.

The effect of temporary cavitation on the severity of the bone injury is the result of both soft tissue and bone cavitation. Soft tissue may be stripped from periosteum, removing an important source of blood supply during fracture repair, and the medullary blood supply is disrupted with some of the fragments rendered avascular. Moreover, fragments may be lost from the wound. Soft tissue injury, avascular bone and bone deficit impair the healing process.

The efficiency of low-velocity hand guns in producing fractures is related to the thickness of soft tissue the bullet must penetrate to reach the bone, and the resultant velocity at impact with bone.

Bullets may deflect off bone causing splintering, they may flatten and fragment on impact with bone, or they may pass through bone with minimal comminution. Certain larger hand guns loaded with deforming ammunition can cause bone fragmentation and significant soft tissue damage (Figures 6.3–6.6).

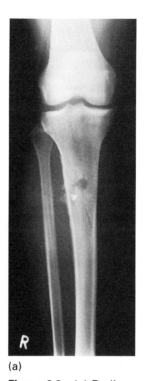 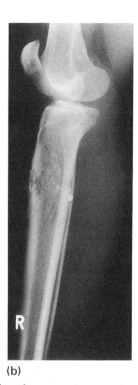

(a) (b)

Figure 6.3 (a) Radiograph showing an antero posterior view of the tibia and fibula with a cavity produced by a bullet tracking through the proximal third of the tibia. (b) Lateral view of bullet track through the tibia.

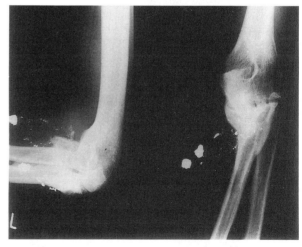

Figure 6.4 Radiograph showing lateral and antero posterior views of the left elbow. The olecranon is fractured and the radial head dislocated. Bullet fragments and debris are seen at, and tracking away from, the fracture site.

Shotgun wounds are low-velocity injuries in which the pellets of low mass rapidly dissipate their kinetic energy in the soft tissue. Close-range shotgun injuries are however different. The pellets and wadding used to propel them form a shot cloud which can act as if it is a large bullet. The shot cloud may pass through bone with little temporary cavitation, but still leave a large defect. Wadding provokes a marked inflammatory response in soft tissue, and may become embedded in soft tissue or bone.

Incised injuries

Knife, axe and spear injuries are low-velocity injuries in which soft tissue damage usually exceeds that of bone. The bone injury may involve only one surface of bone, a slice fracture, or may extend through both cortices as a hairline crack fracture or a transverse fracture (Figures 6.7–6.10).

EFFECT OF ASSOCIATED SOFT TISSUE INJURY

Soft tissue trauma influences the prognosis of these injuries. Open fractures have been classified by Gustilo into three groups based on the mechanism of injury, the extent of soft tissue damage, the configuration of the fracture and the amount of contamination (Gustilo and Anderson, 1976; Gustilo *et al.*, 1990). A Type I open fracture has a skin wound of less than 1 cm. It is usually a clean wound

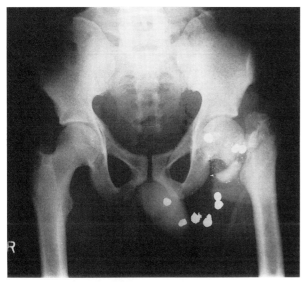

Figure 6.5 Radiograph of the pelvis with fractures of the head and neck of the left femur caused by large shotgun pellets.

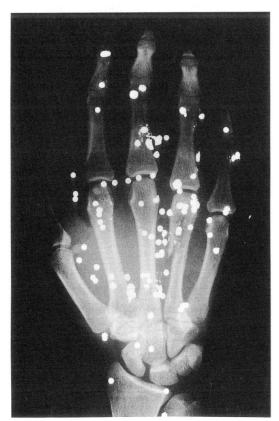

Figure 6.6 Radiograph of the hand showing a 'cloud' of small shotgun pellets and a fracture of the shaft of the fourth metacarpal.

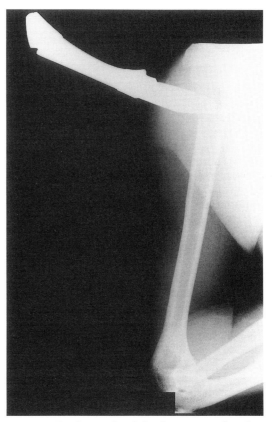

Figure 6.7 Radiograph of the humerus, showing an embedded knife.

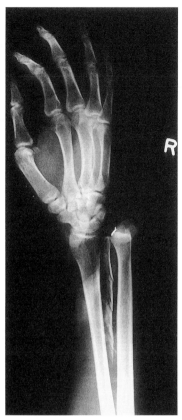

Figure 6.8 Radiograph of the wrist and forearm showing a slice fracture of the radius along the radial metaphysis with splaying of the radius and ulna caused by assault with a sugarcane cutter's knife.

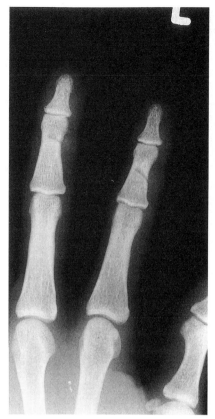

Figure 6.9 Radiograph of the index and middle fingers of the left hand, showing an incised injury through one cortex of the middle phalanges, caused by the blunt side of a butcher's bandsaw.

caused by a spike of bone penetrating the skin. Type II open fractures have skin wounds larger than 1 cm, with a slight or moderate crushing injury, moderate comminution of the fracture and moderate contamination. Type III injuries are characterized by extensive soft tissue injury and severe comminution. They are further subdivided into three subgroups. Type IIIa fractures have adequate soft tissue cover of the fractured bone. Type IIIb fractures have massive contamination, extensive soft tissue damage with loss of soft tissue or periosteal stripping requiring tissue flaps to gain soft tissue cover of the bone. Type IIIc injuries are any open fractures with an associated vascular injury.

The classification correlates the extent of the soft tissue injury with subsequent infection. The infection rate for Type I fractures is 2–7%, Type II 7%, Type IIIa 7%, Type IIIb 10–50% and Type IIIc 25–50%. The overall non-union rate for all Type III fractures is 20–30% and the amputation rate associated with Type IIIc fractures ranges from 25 to 90%.

Using this classification, low-velocity injuries are usually Type I or Type 11 fractures (Woloszyn *et al.*, 1988). Incised wounds are low velocity but, because of the larger wound and greater contamination, are usually Type II injuries. High-velocity injuries are by definition Type III wounds and most fall into the Type IIIa subcategory, with concomitant vascular trauma converting any fracture to Type IIIc.

The foundation of management of these injuries is to optimize the healing milieu by:

1. Reducing the chances of infection by early initiation of appropriate antibiotic therapy (Thoresby and Darlow, 1967; Patzakis *et al.*, 1974), antitetanus prophylaxis and immediate debridement of the wound with copious irrigation, followed by second-look debridement of Type III fractures after 24–72 hours.
2. Fracture stabilization.
3. Wound grafting.
4. Early bone grafting.
5. Prompt revascularization of arterial injuries.

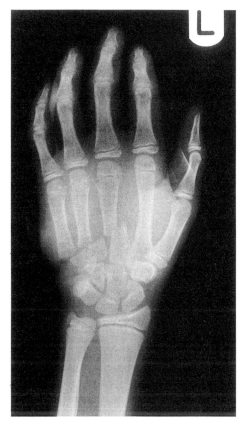

Figure 6.10 Radiograph of the left hand showing transection of the third, fourth and fifth metacarpals and associated soft tissue trauma, following assault with a sugarcane cutter's knife.

FRACTURE HEALING

Healing of bone occurs by a process of *regeneration*, the cells involved being capable of proliferation. The process should therefore not be confused with that of *repair*, which occurs in such structures as the spinal cord and is characterized by fibrous tissue formation.

The majority of fractures heal by secondary repair. Following a fracture in a hollow long bone, bleeding occurs into the periosteal area and between the bone ends. A haematoma is formed within the tissues, producing a collar around the bone at the site of fracture. If the fracture is displaced or if there has been extensive soft tissue damage, bleeding extends into soft tissue planes and a litre of blood may be extravasated in fractures of the femur. This fibrin clot has been considered as a scaffold for fibrocellular invasion and repair. Sevitt questioned this: fibrovascular invasion of the clot is not a prominent histological feature (Sevitt, 1981).

Necrosis of the cortex and marrow at the site of the fracture is a consistent feature, as the medullary blood vessels and haversian blood supply are disrupted. The extent of cortical necrosis ranges from a few millimetres in undisplaced fractures to several centimetres in displaced fractures with periosteal stripping.

An aseptic inflammatory phase then commences and lasts several days. It is characterized by local hyperaemia with the formation of a protein-rich exudate and the arrival and proliferation of inflammatory cells. As this is usually an aseptic response, polymorphs are not abundant. Multinucleate giant cells are found in disrupted areas, as are mast cells and other mononuclear cells. The first evidence of increased cell division is detectable about 8 hours after the injury and is initially extensive. The repair process begins away from the necrotic tissue and involves ingrowth and proliferation of osteogenic granulation tissue consisting of new blood vessels, osteogenic and connective tissue cells. It becomes more localized to the region of the fracture 2–3 days after injury, and by this stage the proliferating cells are those of osteogenic capacity, arising from the periosteum and medullary cavity.

Periosteal callus is derived from osteogenic cells in the inner cambium layer. The osteogenic granulation tissue advances towards the fracture gap and forms an external bridge across the fracture site. The bases of the bridge are initially trabecular bone with the advancing granulation tissue laying down cartilage and fibrous tissue. This subsequently undergoes endochondral ossification. The blood supply of the external callus is derived from new vessels from the surrounding soft tissue. The callus gap under the arch is filled with clot and debris. Histiocytes and fibroblasts invade this area and the tissue laid down may be fibrous, cartilagenous or osseous. Cartilage production in the periosteal callus is increased by fracture instability and ischaemia. The maturing external callus becomes a network of cancellous bone which is progressively remodelled into compact bone.

Between the bone ends the medullary callus forms. Medullary callus begins with a foundation of reticulin and collagen fibres laid down in viable bone marrow. Osteogenic granulation tissue then advances towards the fracture gap. The new vessels finally cross the gap and medullary circulation is re-established. Behind the advancing granulation tissue, osteogenesis occurs. Medullary callus may initially plug the medulla but is gradually resorbed and replaced by haemopoetic fatty tissue.

The first radiologically visible healing tissue is the primary callus, which advances on both sides of the fracture to produce the external bridging callus around the fracture gap.

Architectural remodelling continues and final return to previous strength is referred to as *consolidation* and may take 6 months or more.

Primary bone healing

Modern internal fixation techniques occasionally achieve a situation where absolute immobility is obtained at the fracture site. A good example of this is plating of forearm bones. When slight compression is applied to the fracture ends, the circumstances for healing between cortices, otherwise known as primary bone healing, are created.

In this situation, and provided the gap remains small, healing occurs in the same fashion as normal bone turnover, culminating in realignment of haversian systems. Although apparently ideal in some respects, this microscopic process takes a long time to achieve. During this period, bone is liable to refracture and the strength of the fixation device is all important for stability.

Cellular contact theory

External callus orientates itself towards the opposite fragment and does not proliferate indifferently. The controls imposed on the process may be many but the cellular contact effect observed by Charnley and based on the work of Ham (1930) has considerable appeal, and is doubtless of significance at a local level (Charnley, 1961).

Following observations of the healing of fractures and the fate of bone stumps and amputees, it was suggested that the proximity of other bone cells acts as both an initial stimulant and later as a limiting influence. Callus first grows towards the opposite side of a fracture gap and then ceases production on making contact with its partner growing the opposite way. Following amputation this process is not initiated, no callus forms and the area becomes biologically inactive, despite the presence of all or many of the necessary ingredients for reparative osteogenesis.

Cancellous bone healing

Much of the work on fracture healing has concentrated on cortical bone, with the result that little is understood to date about the processes involved in healing cancellous bone. Despite this, it has been widely suggested that cancellous bone does not heal by external callus production. There is evidence that this is not entirely true. Recent work by Finnigan and Uhthoff has identified several types of cancellous bone healing, based on the vascularity of the fragments and the rigidity of immobilization (Finnigan and Uthoff, 1987). Fronts of ossification become visible both histologically and radiologically between fractured bone ends which ultimately become united. In some cases the fracture line remains visible for some time, and is ultimately replaced by endochondral ossification. When movement between the bone surfaces is present, external callus formation is indeed observed, although this is generally much less exuberant than around cortical bone. This may be due to the fact that the periosteum in the metaphyseal area is very much thinner than along the diaphysis.

In general, the front of ossification between fractured cancellous bone surfaces leads to union more rapidly than the combined efforts of external and medullary callus in the diaphysis. However, under conditions of gross mobility, non-union may occur.

Factors affecting fracture healing

Movement and micromovement

It has been seen that a certain amount of movement at the fracture site encourages the production of external bridging callus. When this is abolished, as in primary bone healing, union takes longer to achieve. When gross movement occurs, non-union may result. Consequently, surgeons have frequently sought to encourage what is commonly termed micromovement at the fracture site. This consists of shifts between the fractured bone ends which are not gross in nature but are sufficient to stimulate osteogenesis. The precise reasons for this are unclear, but there is increasing evidence that a number of locally active substances, such as prostaglandin E_2 and growth factor beta, may be activated under conditions of strain. Therefore, when osteoblastic columns and sheets are produced and subjected to strain, the local production of these substances further enhances the reparative process.

The extreme example of this is possibly the so-called 'secondary injury phenomenon'. Chapman and others have described a prostaglandin-dependent effect which may occur 2 weeks after initial injury, and which results in exuberant callus formation (Chapman, 1987). This was first observed by Smith, who performed delayed internal fixation of a number of different types of diaphyseal fracture, and noted a considerable amount of callus when surgical intervention took place at this stage (Smith, 1964).

In many instances modern fixation devices seek to produce a certain amount of movement at the fracture site. Although interlocked nailing of the femoral shaft is said to splint the fracture site rigidly, this is not invariably so, and a great degree of movement both in a rotatory and mediolateral plane takes place. Similarly, external fixation devices applied to the tibia are deliberately designed to allow a certain amount of movement at the fracture site. Alterations in pin arrangements and diameter can be planned in order to maximize this effect.

Local and systemic mediators

A great deal of attention has been focused in recent years on possible local and systemic mediators of bone healing. Although initial interest centred on possible systemic effects, little evidence has emerged to support the existence of any centrally released endocrine or para-endocrine substance which actually mediates fracture healing.

In a variety of endocrine disturbances, fractures heal remarkably normally and, even in growth hormone-deficient states, there is a satisfactory response.

As in other tissues, excess circulating corticosteroids delay healing, as does a deficiency of vitamin C. Vitamin A in excessive doses predisposes to fracture by weakening the bony structure. Vitamin D is important in calcium absorption and osteoclastic activity. Recent evidence has shown high circulating levels of vitamin K follow multiple fractures, but the precise significance of this is unknown (Bitensky *et al.*, 1988).

There has been some speculation regarding the possible importance of endocrine substances following neural injury, a situation in which it is stated that fractures may heal faster with more callus production. Recent evidence suggests the presence of a circulating somatomedin-related substance (Bidner *et al.*, 1990). However, there is no evidence that such compounds are produced centrally. In fact, they are much more likely to be produced locally, since the overwhelming weight of evidence indicates that it is the local effects of neural injury which stimulate osteogenesis (Spencer, 1989).

Far more important than systemically released substances appear to be the locally released polypeptides and other compounds which arise from the fracture gap. Bone marrow itself is known to be highly osteoinductive, and the work of Urist and colleagues over the years has identified a low-molecular-weight polypeptide (bone morphogenetic protein) which will induce bone formation in soft tissues (Urist *et al.*, 1982). In addition, prostaglandin E_2 and growth factor beta are both osteoinductive and have been found in the region of healing fractures. Further substances, such as interleukins, cytokines and interferon, have all been shown to have some mediating effect in local bone production (Canbrella *et al.*, 1991). The observations of Currey indicate a locally mediated feedback mechanism which is neurally regulated and controls the formation, healing and remodelling of every bone on a predetermined scale (Currey, 1984). It seems quite possible that the response to injury is mediated through this local feedback mechanism.

Soft tissue trauma

The influence of soft tissue trauma on the outcome of compound fractures has been previously outlined. It is thought that soft tissue damage retards healing because of the extent of local vascular injury. Soft tissue stripping may reduce the soft tissue blood supply to the periosteal callus and may injure the nutrient vessels. Dispersion of the fracture haematoma and mesenchymal cells in damaged tissue planes occurs and this has been suggested as a possible mechanism for the delay in healing.

Bone loss

Bone loss predisposes to fibrous union. As new bone is produced at a rate of 5 mm per year, bony union may be prolonged or impossible if the gap exceeds 1 cm (Sevitt, 1981).

REFERENCES

Amato J.J., Syracuse D., Seaver P.R., Rich N. (1989). Bone as a secondary missile: an experimental study in the fragmenting of bone by high velocity missiles. *J. Trauma*, **29**, 609–12.

Bidner S.M., Rubins I.M., Desjardins J.V., Zukor D.J., Goltzman D. (1990). Evidence of a humoral mechanism for enhanced osteogenesis after head injury. *J. Bone Joint Surg.*, **72A**, 1144–9.

Bitensky L., Hart J.P., Catterall A. et al. (1988). Circulating vitamin K levels in patients with fractures. *J. Bone Joint Surg.*, **70B**, 663–4.

Branemark P.I. (1961) Experimental investigation of microcirculation in bone marrow. *Angiology*, **12**, 293–306.

Brookes M. (1971). *The Blood Supply of Bone*. London: Butterworths.

Brookes M., Elkin A.S., Harrison R.G., Heald C.B. (1961). A new concept of capillary circulation in bone cortex. *Lancet*, **i**, 1078–81.

Canbrella M., McCarthy T.C., Canalis E. (1991). Current concepts review: transforming growth factor-beta and remodelling of bone. *J. Bone Joint Surg.*, **73A**, 1418–28.

Chapman M.W. (1987). Prostaglandins and the secondary injury phenomenon. In *Fracture Healing* (Lane J.M., ed.) pp. 87–96. New York: Churchill Livingstone.

Charnley J. (1961). *The Closed Treatment of Common Fractures*, 3rd edn. Edinburgh: Livingstone.

Currey J. (1984). *The Functional Adaptations of Bones*. Princeton, NJ: Princeton University Press.

Einhom T.A. (1988). Biomechanical properties of bone. Triangle : 2. *New Frontiers Bone Res.*, **27**, (1/2), 27–36.

Fackler M.L. (1988). Wound ballistics. A review of common misconceptions. *JAMA*, **259**, 2730–6.

Fackler M.L., Surinchak J.S., Malinowski J.A., Bowen R.E. (1984). Bullet fragmentation: a major cause of tissue disruption. *J. Trauma*, **24**, 35–9.

Finengan M.A., Uthoff H.K. (1987). Healing of trabecular bone. In *Fracture Healing* (Lane J.M., ed.) pp. 33–8. New York: Churchill Livingstone.

Gustilo R.B., Anderson J.T. (1976). Prevention of infection in the treatment of one thousand and twenty-five open fractures of long bones. *J. Bone Joint Surg.*, **58A**, 453–8.

Gustilo R.B., Merkow R.L., Templeman D. (1990). The management of open fractures. *J. Bone Joint Surg.*, **72A**, 299–304.

Ham A.W. (1930). An histological study of the early phases of bone repair. *J. Bone Joint Surg.*, **12**, 827.

Hollerman J.J., Fackler M.L., Coldwell D.M., Ben-Menachem Y. (1990). Gunshot wounds: bullets, ballistics, and mechanisms of injury. *Am. J. Radiol.*, **155**, 685–90.

Hungerford D.S. (1980). Bone marrow pressure and intramedullary venography. In *Scientific Foundations of Orthopaedics and Traumatology* (Owen R., Goodfellow J., Bullough P. eds) pp. 357–61. London: Heinemann.

Patzakis M.J., Harvey J.P., Ivler D. (1974). The role of

antibiotics in the management of open fractures. *J. Bone Joint Surg.*, **56A**, 532.

Rhinelander F.W. (1968). Circulation in bone. In *The Biochemistry and Physiology of Bone*, 2nd edn (Bourne, G.H. ed.) pp. 2–76. London: Academic.

Sevitt S. (1981). *Bone Repair and Fracture Healing in Man*. Edinburgh: Churchill Livingstone.

Smith J.E.M. (1964). The results of early and delayed internal fixation of fractures of the shaft of the femur. *J. Bone Joint Surg.*, **46**, 28–31.

Spencer R.F. (1989). The Effect of Head Injury on Fracture Healing – Clinical and Experimental Studies. Doctor of Medicine Thesis, University of Edinburgh.

Thoresby F.P., Darlow H.M. (1967). The mechanism of primary infection of bullet wounds. *Br. J. Surg.*, **54**, 359–63.

Urist M.R., Lietze A., Mizutana H. et al. (1982). A bovine low molecular weight bone morphogenic (BMP) fraction. *Clin. Orthop. Rel. Res.*, **162**, 219–32.

Woloszyn J.T., Uitvlugt G.M., Castle M.E. (1988). Management of civilian gunshot fractures of the extremities. *Clin. Orthop. Rel. Res.*, **226**, 247–51.

7. Penetrating Injury of Blood Vessels

J. V. Robbs

Injury to the major blood vessels may result in dramatic pathophysiological changes which mandate early diagnosis and correction if life or limb is to be salvaged. It is essential that a practising surgeon have an understanding of the pathology and the pathophysiological changes consequent on the injuries in order to treat them adequately and rationally.

ARTERIAL INJURY

Mechanisms of injury

Mechanisms of injury are summarized in Table 7.1. Stab wounds, whether caused by a knife or other sharpened implement, will cause damage confined to the track of the implement. It should, however, be remembered that the mobility of various fascial planes in relation to the posture of the victim at the time of the stabbing may make probing of the skin wound an unreliable pointer to the depth or direction that the implement had taken through the tissues. This type of wound will usually result in a simple laceration or perforation of the blood vessel. Missile wounds, in contrast, not only disrupt the tissue but the kinetic energy inherent in a fast-moving missile is dissipated in the surrounding tissues. The resultant tissue destruction is proportional to the amount of energy transmitted to the tissues by the missile – a matter discussed in detail on page 38. In summary, small increases in velocity create a great increase in energy dissipation. Tissue damage is found along the local track of the missile. Other associated effects are hydraulic shock waves set up in the surrounding fluid-containing tissues and a temporary cavitation

TABLE 7.1

MECHANISMS OF VASCULAR INJURY

Stab
Missile
   Low velocity
   High velocity (>600 m/s)
Blast
   Shotgun
   Bomb
Blunt
   Direct
   Indirect
Iatrogenic

effect due to the energy transfer from the missile. Finally, damage may be compounded by secondary missiles from fragmentation of bone or the missile itself. A small-calibre hand gun, such as a 0.32 or up to 0.38, may result in little more tissue damage than its track through the soft tissue. Once a muzzle velocity of 600 m/s or more is reached, the effects caused by remote shock waves and the cavitation effect become increasingly severe. The possibility of delayed thrombosis in the vessel due to intimal damage then arises. Extensive tissue necrosis and the drawing into the cavity of contaminating foreign material further compound the issue (Levien, 1989).

Open blast injuries such as those caused by close-range shotgun discharge, are characterized by extensive destruction of tissue which contains a large number of foreign bodies, particularly if the smaller calibre birdshot (about 2 mm) has been used. In addition, clothing and even cartridge wadding may be found. An additional and frequent finding is that there are multiple sites of perforation within a segment of blood vessel. Embolization of the small missiles distal to the site of perforation is also occasionally seen. Bomb blasts result in extensive local tissue trauma but the situation is compounded by the fact that many of the fragments are jagged, high-velocity missiles. The injuries are then complex.

Blunt trauma may be direct or focal. An example of this would be a kick impinging the popliteal artery against the bone. Indirect injury results from shearing and distraction forces. A typical example is the injury to an artery adjacent to a joint which dislocates, such as the knee or the elbow or in association with long bone fractures. It should, however, be borne in mind that an added dimension to arterial injuries associated with fractures is the lacerating effect of bony fragments. Specific consideration must be given to partial or complete vascular disruption following shearing forces associated with rapid deceleration. This applies particularly to the aorta but may also be found in the vascular pedicles of solid organs, in particular the renal arteries. The usual circumstances in which this situation obtains is in automobile collisions or aviation accidents, where the shear is in an anteroposterior direction. Vertical deceleration may result from falls from a height. With regard to the aorta, anteroposterior deceleration usually results in damage to the aortic isthmus just distal to the origin of the left subclavian artery. Vertical deceleration causes disruption just above the aortic valve. The classic reason for rupture at these sites is the difference in rate of deceleration of the mobile descending thoracic aorta and heart and the relatively fixed arch of the aorta. The junction of the two areas at the aortic isthmus where the ligamentum arteriosum is attached and the area just above the aortic valve is thus subjected to shear strain. This is the most frequent finding. Another possible explanation for tears close to the aortic valve is the sudden ejection of the contents of the heart by the compression force (Carmack *et al.*, 1959; Spencer *et al.*, 1961).

In our own practice, traction injury to the left subclavian artery is being seen with increasing frequency as a consequence of motor vehicle accidents (Costa and Robbs, 1988). In most cases passenger-restraining devices could be regarded as the likely cause. In each instance, a shoulder-harness seat belt with a lap strap (three-point fixation) had been used. The usual finding was that the diagonal component (shoulder strap) had been loose fitting, allowing considerable play between the chest wall and the belt. This had been a consequence of either faulty adjustment of the older (non-inertia reel) belts which require manual tightening or the individual had taken up the slack on the inertia reel by means of a peg or clip to relieve pressure across the shoulder. Probably at the moment of impact the forward acceleration of the torso pivoting on the lap strap component is suddenly arrested by the strap across the shoulder girdle which allows the torso to continue its anterior movement with the shoulder as a fixed point. The resultant distraction and shearing forces result in disruption of the neurovascular bundle and bony structures around the shoulder girdle. This experience is in contrast to previous reports which have highlighted skeletal complications of the use of motor vehicle passenger restraining devices; few reports of vascular injuries have appeared (Williams and Kirkpatrick, 1971; Woelfel *et al.*, 1984).

Iatrogenic injury warrants independent consideration and the most frequently encountered is that caused by catheterization of an artery whether during diagnostic procedures, for example cardiac catheterization, or for the purpose of monitoring using arterial pressure lines. The injury is always structural and related to local trauma; the development of an ischaemic limb following arterial catheterization, for whatever reason, is *never* due to spasm on its own. Over-distention of the vessel by balloon embolectomy catheter causing vessel rupture is invariably a result of using fluid to distend the balloon, which creates a hydraulic system which is capable of generating high pressures. It is preferable to inflate the balloon with air to avoid this complication (Hirschberg *et al.*, 1988). An additional important cause of iatrogenic injury is the inadvertent intra-arterial injection of noxious substances. Important agents are those which are lipid soluble and become fixed in the walls of small vessels, thus causing local endothelial damage with superimposed thrombosis. Examples are diazepam and thiopentone (Schulenberg *et al.*, 1985).

Pathology

Perforation or transection of an artery by penetrating trauma may cause a variety of pathological situations. Partial or complete severance of an artery may result in ongoing free haemorrhage. If the bleeding is contained by the surrounding tissues, a false aneurysm (pulsating haematoma) is formed (Figure 7.1(a)). In the majority of cases this situation is associated with a partial transection or lateral perforation in the vessel wall. Often total

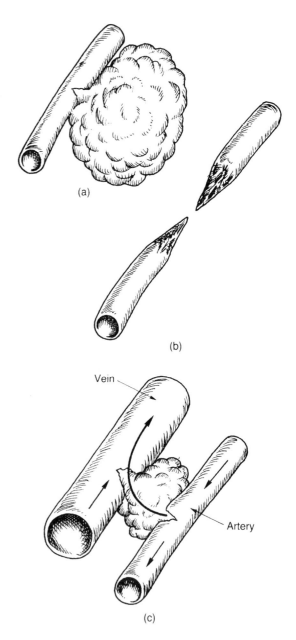

Figure 7.1 (a) Partial laceration of artery with false aneurysm formation. (b) Total disruption with thrombosis. (c) Partial laceration of artery and vein with formation of arteriovenous fistula.

interruption of the vessel results in spasm of the ends with superimposed thrombosis. This may result in initial brisk haemorrhage which subsequently stops (Figure 7.1(b)). An important consideration is that the clots may subsequently lyse due to endogenous fibrinolytic processes or, more likely low-grade infection, resulting in haemorrhage. If this occurs within 24 hours it is usually a result simply of spasm passing off and the thrombus being dislodged or lysed. Low-grade infection, on the other hand, results in delayed or secondary haemorrhage between 5 and 10 days later. Simultaneous perforation of an adjacent artery and vein results in the formation of an acute arteriovenous fistula (Figure 7.1(c)) with or without a false aneurysm.

The intima is the least elastic component of the arterial wall when compared to the media and adventitia. Therefore if distraction or shearing forces occur the intima is the most vulnerable to disruption, with the result that the vessel tears from inside out (Figure 7.2(a)). The range of injury therefore varies from isolated intimal disruption leaving an intact media and adventitia to total disruption of all layers of the vessel wall. Partial disruption exposes an area of denuded media

which is thrombogenic, resulting in platelet adhesion with initiation of thrombosis which may then result in partial or more frequently complete occlusion of the artery at this level. In addition, a distally based intimal flap may develop which further compounds the issue by partially occluding the lumen or even acting as the entry point of a dissection. It is, however, more likely that the major component of traumatic thrombosis in the smaller vessels is the denuded media rather than dissection. In a larger vessel such as the aorta, circumferential intimal destruction with some media and adventitia remaining intact may result, with the passage of time, in the development of an aneurysm (Figure 7.2(b)). In the presence of total disruption the consequences already outlined may occur.

An extremely important consideration with regard to intimal disruption with secondary thrombosis is the shock wave associated with high-velocity missile trauma, which may cause intimal disruption due to distortion caused by pressure waves without any obvious macroscopic injury to the vessel. It is also extremely important to realize that, particularly in the presence of distraction-type forces, a small intimal tear may only become manifest as a thrombosis several hours after the initial injury (Robbs and Baker, 1984).

Iatrogenic catheter trauma may result in all the consequences of penetrating injury that have just been described. In addition, retrograde passage of the catheter may cause dissection between layers of the arterial wall with the formation of an intimal flap which acts in turn as a nidus for thrombus formation (Figure 7.3). This is particularly likely to

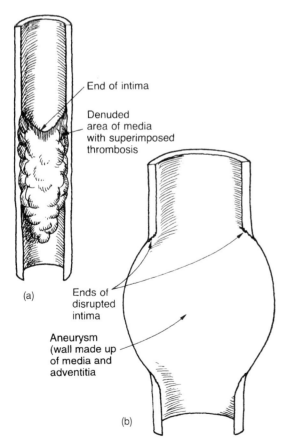

Figure 7.2 (a) Intimal disruption with superimposed thrombosis. (b) Intimal disruption with the formation of true aneurysm.

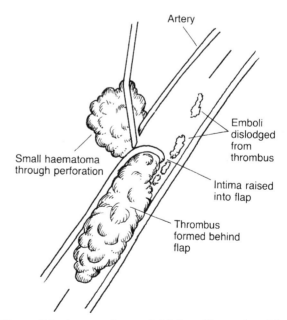

Figure 7.3 Iatrogenic arterial injury illustrating false aneurysm formation, intimal flap with supraimposed thrombosis and distal embolization.

occur in the upper limb vessels such as the brachial and radial, which are frequently used for pressure monitoring and less frequently for diagnostic catheterization. Atheroscelerotic vessels are far more vulnerable to this type of injury and plaque may be dislodged or elevated resulting in thrombosis or distal embolization. Post-catheterization thrombosis is often mis-diagnosed as 'spasm' or 'embolism' and treatment frequently is either expectant or by simple passage of a balloon embolectomy catheter. The latter can either aggravate the clinical situation or result in temporary improvement only. Correct management requires a full understanding of the underlying pathology with appropriate local surgical correction (Mills and Robbs, 1991).

Spasm

Spasm in an artery complicates any trauma to the vessel whether penetrating or blunt, and occurs at the site of the injury. In the arterial tree distal to the injured area, unopposed action of the normal sympathetic vasomotor tone results in vasoconstriction as this is no longer countered by intraluminal pressure. Spasm *per se* acting in isolation will very rarely, if ever, result in peripheral ischaemic manifestations, and as the cause of an absent pulse is a retrospective diagnosis made at operation or on good quality angiography. It must, however, be noted that in children, in view of the small calibre of their arteries, spasm will frequently result in a peripheral pulse being inpalpable, but here again the principle applies that spasm will never cause manifest ischaemia in an extremity (Mills and Robbs, 1991).

Pathophysiology

Laceration or complete transection of the artery may result in massive exanguinating haemorrhage. This may occur freely through the entry or exit wounds or into one or other body cavity such as the pleura or peritoneum. The consequences of this are obviously the effects of hypovolaemia, which in turn depends upon the rate and quantity of blood loss. This is dealt with in some detail in other sections of this book (see Chapter 40). If the haemorrhage is contained by surrounding tissues, a false aneurysm or pulsating haematoma forms. Frequently, however, as has been mentioned, significant haemorrhage is not a consequence of complete transection because the ends of the vessel develop spasm with thrombosis. In these circumstances delayed haemorrhage may occur due to lysis of the clot. As described earlier, this may either be a consequence of low-grade sepsis or due to spontaneous lysis of the thrombus. The latter usually occurs within a 24-hour period once spasm has passed off. Haemorrhage due to low-grade infection (secondary haemorrhage) is usually delayed by a period of 5–7 days or more.

The effects of false aneurysm are those of compression. Particularly vulnerable in this regard are nerves, and we have seen compressive neuropraxias involving the brachial plexus as well as the sacral plexus. The prognosis for these compression injuries is variable but, in our experience, if brachial plexus compression occurs at root level resulting in paralysis of the intrinsic muscles of the hand, there is little chance of recovery. This applies particularly when there is overt infection. This serves to emphasize the importance of early diagnosis and treatment of penetrating vascular injury (Robbs and Naidoo, 1984).

Arteriovenous fistula

A particular and not uncommon result of penetrating injury is the formation of an arteriovenous shunt between closely adjacent vessels. The hemodynamic effects are directly proportional to the extent of the communication and it follows that the more proximal the fistula is sited in relation to the heart and the greater its size, the more significant its effects will be. The immediate effect is to reduce the peripheral resistance as the arterial tree distal to the communication is short circuited. This results in a fall in diastolic blood pressure thus increasing pulse pressure and pulse rate and there is a marked increase in cardiac output due to the increased venous return (Sako and Varco, 1970). The blood volume also increases for reasons which are not understood but are probably related to hormonal changes (Warren *et al.*, 1951). The net effect of this hyperdynamic state may be cardiac decompensation with dilatation of the ventricles and congestive heart failure, though this usually takes some time to develop.

However, in our experience in young patients even with longstanding fistulas of many years duration this is an uncommon complication unless there is an underlying cardiomyopathy. A further complication is subacute bacterial endarteritis and it is an important late complication of large untreated fistulas (Hook *et al.*, 1957). Damaged endothelium is rendered susceptible to infection when bacteraemia occurs. Possibly the high-velocity jet of blood flowing through the fistula and impinging on the endothelium may be responsible for the endothelial injury. Another possibility is that the rapid flow from a high- to low-pressure area may cause subendothelial ischaemia by a Venturi effect. These changes are reversible with closure of the fistula (Weinstein, 1980).

At a local level there is dilatation of the artery leading to the fistula and in the vein that drains it. These vessels eventually undergo degenerative and permanent aneurysmal changes. An extensive collateral network also develops. In the tissues distal to the shunt there is a marked increase in venous pressure, which in the extremities will produce a picture of venous insufficiency with oedema and dilatation and hypertrophy of superficial veins. In the lower extremity, superficial varicosities may develop together with typical venous ulceration. The arterial tree distal to the fistula becomes deprived of blood and peripheral ischaemia may occur accompanied by muscle wasting and other trophic changes (Sako and Varco, 1970). Most post-traumatic arteriovenous fistulas are diagnosed and treated shortly after injury and the typical changes described apply only to longstanding fistulation. In the acute injury, the only obvious manifest sign is likely to be the classical machinery murmur. It must be emphasized, however, that unless this is specifically sought at the time of presentation the diagnosis may be missed as haemorrhage is frequently not a major feature as the artery 'bleeds into the vein'.

Aortic tears and other shearing injuries

The aortic tear associated with a deceleration injury is transverse and, as described earlier, may extend through the intima and media with preservation of the adventitia, or it may extend through all layers. This results in either free rupture or false aneurysm formation. Dissection between the layers of the aortic wall rarely occurs and is usually associated with some underlying disease process such as cystic mucoid degeneration. If immediate death does not occur from haemorrhage, secondary fatal haemorrhage may occur within 4 weeks of injury. Beyond that time haemorrhage rarely occurs and the aneurysm may remain stable for many years, although progressive late enlargement and rupture have been described (Warren *et al.*, 1951).

Typical shearing trauma resulting from blunt injury results in disruption of the intima with superimposed thrombosis, and the mechanisms of this have already been described. Once the thrombotic process has been initiated and total occlusion of the vessel occurs at that site, proximal and distal propagation of clot takes place within the stagnant intraluminal column of blood until a point of entry of collateral flow is reached (Figure 7.4). In the arterial tree distal to the site of obstruction, the reduction in the intraluminal pressure results in an initial clampdown of muscular arteries and arterioles due to unopposed resting sympathetic tone. This further reduces distal flow because of an increase in peripheral resistance and thus sets up a vicious cycle. The distal tissues are rendered ischaemic, which results in a combination of anaerobic metabolism with failure of the sodium–potassium pump at cell membrane level. There is an accumulation of lactic acid, potassium and various intracellular enzymes such as CPK, LDH and SGOT. These are powerful vasodilators and result in local vasodilatation with consequent reduction in the peripheral resistance.

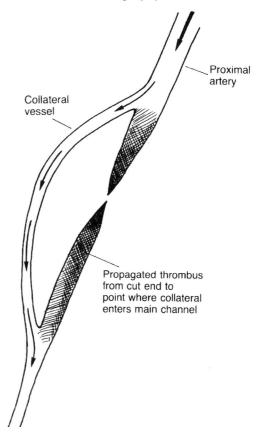

Figure 7.4 Consequences of arterial disruption with propagation of thrombus proximally and distally to the sites of collateral flow. Note: distal vessel collapse.

There is an increasing appreciation of the damage caused by free radicals generated during the reperfusion of ischaemic tissue, whether by collaterals or otherwise. Free radicals are created by the process of gaining or losing an electron and once this occurs the compound becomes unstable and highly reactive as an oxidizing or reducing agent (McCord, 1985; Clark, 1986). The pathways are summarized in Figure 7.5. To acquire an extra electron and regain stability the free radical pulls

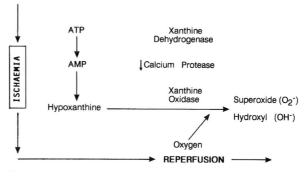

Figure 7.5 Free radical production.

an electron from adjacent molecules. These radicals thus have the ability to participate in chain reactions and create general molecular chaos with loss of function. Oxygen is particularly susceptible to free radical conversion and gaining one electron converts it to superoxide, the second to hydrogen peroxide, the third forms an hydroxyl group and the fourth forms water. Superoxide and hydroxyl are powerful oxidizing agents and are responsible for perpetuation of cellular damage. It would appear that the process is initiated when the decreasing blood flow to tissue is sufficient to limit oxygen availability for the production of ATP – the major energy source for cellular metabolism. Depletion of ATP results in elevated levels of AMP, which is catabolized to hypoxanthine which accumulates in the tissue. While this ATP depletion is occurring the cell is unable to maintain normal ion gradients across membranes and calcium accumulates in the cell cytoplasm and activates a protease which in turn activates xanthine dehydrogenase to xanthine oxidase. When oxygen is reintroduced into the system by reperfusion, the xanthine oxidase mediates the production of free oxygen radicals which then potentiate tissue damage. Naturally occurring defences against the activity of the free oxygen radicals are certain enzymes such as superoxide dismutase, catylase and glutathione peroxidase. Other scavengers of free radicals are iron-binding proteins, vitamin E, beta carotene and ascorbic acid. Mannitol has also been shown to have some free radical scavenging properties. Experimentally allopurinol, which is a xanthine oxidase inhibitor, has been shown to modify the rate at which oxygen free radicals are produced. The susceptibility of various tissue to ischaemia seems to be proportional to the rate at which the inactive xanthine dehydrogenase is activated prior to reperfusion.

Factors influencing limb survival (Figure 7.6)

The time scale for the progression of an ischaemic process to an irreversible state is dependent on three major factors:

1. The development of collaterals.
2. The ability of the circulating blood to deliver oxygen to the tissues.
3. The metabolic demands of the ischaemic tissue.

Collaterals depend upon the rate at which occlusion occurs and the extent of occlusion, that is, the degree to which thrombus propagates. The more rapid this process the less time there is for collaterals to develop. Cardiac output is an extremely important factor, as is the patency of the inflow vessels, the outflow vessels and the collaterals themselves. The cardiac output in turn depends on myocardial contractility and the circu-

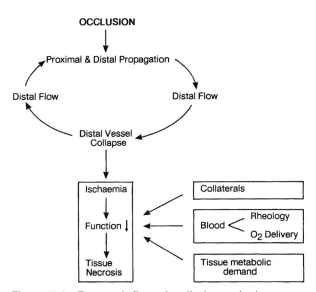

Figure 7.6 Factors influencing limb survival.

lating blood volume. Hypovolaemic shock can very severely aggravate the local situation. Oxygen delivery to the tissues depends on haemoglobin concentration and the flow characteristics of blood. Anaemia, for example, results in diminished oxygen transport and delivery. From the point of view of rheology the most important factor is viscosity. A marked increase in viscosity results from polycythaemia from whatever cause and a diminishing plasma volume resulting from, for example, extra cellular fluid volume deficiency. The metabolic rate of tissues, and hence their demand for oxygen and nutrients, varies from tissue to tissue, with nerve tissue having the highest demand and skin the lowest. These metabolic demands may be increased by the stress of exercise and decreased by cooling or rest. The vulnerability of different tissues within a limb to ischaemia varies. If a situation of total ischaemia to an extremity is created by, for example, applying a pneumatic tourniquet at very high pressures, peripheral nerves are most vulnerable and cease to function within 10–15 minutes. Muscles will become irreversibly damaged within 3–4 hours, and the least vulnerable is the skin and appendages which show irreversible changes only after about 12 hours. In humans it is not known at what stage the totally ischaemic peripheral nerve becomes irreversibly damaged, as all these statements are based on clinical observation. It is thus clear that limb survival following trauma that renders the limb acutely ischaemic depends upon a large number of interacting factors. No absolute time interval can be given within which revascularization should not be attempted. Each individual case must be carefully assessed on its merits whatever the duration of the acute ischaemia.

Clinical considerations

It is outwith the scope of this account to discuss in detail the clinical presentation, but the cornerstone of diagnosis is clinical awareness. The possibility of vascular injury must be considered in every patient with penetrating injury. It is also essential to consider the possibility of an arterial injury in any long bone fracture and in particular dislocations around the elbow and knee. Careful history must be taken to establish whether significant haemorrhage occurred at the time of injury. For reasons which have already been outlined, probing the wound has little value but the site of injury must be carefully assessed for signs of a pulsating haematoma. The area of the wound must be auscultated, because the only sign of an arteriovenous fistula may be a machinery murmur. The peripheral pulse must be carefully assessed and if there is any pulse differential on comparison with the other limb the possibility of arterial injury must be considered. It must be emphasized, however, that the presence of a pulse does not exclude a partial transection of the vessel. Unexplained hypovolaemia or a low haemoglobin level in a patient presenting some time after injury may all point towards significant blood loss. Local clinical signs of ischaemia must also be assessed, these include pallor or cyanosis, marked reduction in temperature, hypoaesthesia and diminution in voluntary movement. Signs suggestive of grave ischaemia are total anaesthesia, paralysis and increase in tissue turgor, particularly within the extensor compartment which is the most vulnerable muscle compartment in the leg. Signs suggestive of irreversible ischaemia are fixed skin staining or total muscle rigidity in all compartments (Robbs and Baker, 1979; Meek and Robbs, 1984).

The definitive diagnosis of vascular injury is made by good quality angiography. The presence of a Doppler signal does not exclude vascular injury and this investigation can only serve to confirm the physical findings.

Once the decision has been made to restore arterial continuity this can be done by lateral suture, patch angioplasty, end to end anastomosis or replacement of an autogenous interposition graft.

Compartment syndrome

Compartment syndrome is a condition in which fluid accumulation causes a high pressure within a closed fascial space, such as a muscle compartment, reducing capillary blood perfusion below a level necessary for tissue viability. In the context of trauma, raised intercompartmental pressure may occur in the presence of gross associated soft tissue trauma with haemorrhage into the compartment, prolonged ischaemia resulting in intracellular

oedema and revascularization oedema when blood flow is restored to a critically ischaemic muscle (Matsen et al., 1977, 1980; Mubarek and Hargens, 1983). The condition is also a feature of prolonged crushing, such as in the collapse of buildings. In the situation of arterial occlusion with some collateral circulation, there is a positive hydrostatic pressure within the capillary bed but insufficient circulation to relieve tissue anoxia. This leads to transcapillary leakage into the interstitial tissues as cell membrane function is arrested, with oedema and increasing intracompartmental pressure.

Restoration of arterial flow to a critically ischaemic limb may also precipitate this situation. In these circumstances the vessels are maximally dilated and the sudden increase of perfusion pressure into an excessively permeable capillary bed and the compartment pressure rises rapidly (revascularization syndrome).

The build-up of pressure within the muscle compartment is not easily dissipated because of the inelastic nature of the fascia investing muscle. The local ischaemia produced must be relieved by decompressing the muscle compartment in order to prevent muscle and nerve necrosis. Decompressive fasciotomy allows the muscles to expand out of their tight fascial enclosure. The four muscle compartments of the leg, and the two compartments of the forearm, are involved most frequently. If pressure remains sufficiently high for a significant period of time, normal function of the muscles and nerves is jeopardized and myoneural necrosis eventually results. Volkmann's contracture follows: permanent loss of function with fibrosis and fibrous contraction of the necrotic muscle bellies.

The diagnosis is suggested when a palpable increase in tissue turgor is felt, particularly in the extensor compartment of the leg when compared with the opposite normal side. Sensory nerve fibres are more sensitive to hypoxia than muscle and paraesthesia and pain develop early in the course of the condition. Motor fibres are more resistant and paralysis of muscles is a later phenomenon (Whitesides et al., 1975). However, loss of sensation and absent pulses can be complications of nerve or vascular injury and as such are non-specific. The definitive diagnosis can be made by measurement of the intracompartmental pressure. A variety of wicks and catheters have been described in order to make these measurements. The normal intramuscular pressure ranges from 0 to 8 mmHg. Decompressive fasciotomy should be considered for pressures greater than 30 mmHg if there is clinical suspicion of a compartment syndrome in the traumatized limb (Whitesides et al., 1975; Mubarek et al., 1978).

Operative decompression must include all fascial compartments. In the lower limb this includes the extensor peroneal flexor and deep flexor compartments. It is also preferable to perform open fasciotomy and not to rely on subcutaneous decompression via small incisions.

Late revascularization (Robbs and Baker, 1979)

During the period of ischaemia, when there is minimal collateralization a combination of anaerobic metabolism, failure of the sodium potassium pump at cell membrane level and muscle necrosis, the venous effluent from an ischaemic limb contains a high level of lactate and an increased P_{CO_2} resulting in a fall in pH. Potassium levels are also high, as well as various intracellular enzymes such as CPK, LDH and SGOT. Myoglobin is also released from necrotic muscle cells following reperfusion of an ischaemic limb. This bolus of 'metabolic debris' enters the systemic circulation and the patient may develop acidosis, hyperkalaemia and myoglobinuria. Myoglobin crystals precipitate out in the renal tubules, particularly in an acid urine and at low tubular flow rates, causing blockage which may result in oliguria and lead to renal failure. This is the syndrome known as the myonephropathic metabolic syndrome or crush syndrome (see also p. 285). The effects of myoglobulinuria are compounded by episodes of hypotension consequent on hypovolaemia which may have already caused some damage to the renal tubules. Profound hypotension may also occur, due to a combination of diminution in cardiac contractility and peripheral vasodilatation resulting from the acidosis, hyperkalaemia and the release of other vasoactive substances. Within the limb itself endothelial damage results in severe interstitial oedema, the extent of which depends upon the degree and duration of the ischaemia. As already described, oedema within the muscle compartments may result in compartment syndrome.

Prevention of these profound effects involves gradual and intermittent release of the occluding clamps at the time of reperfusion. It is also important to ensure that the patient is normovolaemic as measured by the central venous pressure and to induce an osmotic diuresis to facilitate flushing away of the myoglobin crystals, increase the flow rate in the tubules and dilute the urine in the distal nephron. This is best effected by the use of mannitol administered to the normovolaemic patient prior to initial release of the clamps. The recommended dosage is 10 mg per kg body weight. It is also advisable to administer bicarbonate in order to render the patient alkalotic. In this type of situation it is also advisable to routinely perform fasciotomy in the affected limb. During the postoperative period, until such time as myoglobinuria has resolved, a urine output of 200 ml/h should be maintained by crystalloid infusion. In our clinical experience if this regimen is adhered to, the myonephropathic syndrome does not occur even though myoglobulinuria is a frequent finding (Baxter, 1966; Rowland and Penn, 1972).

VENOUS INJURIES

The venous system is injured by exactly the same mechanisms described under mechanisms of arterial injury. Although obviously venous injuries may occur in isolation, they are frequently associated with arterial damage. The major problem presented by injuries to the venous system is that reconstruction does not yield results equivalent to arterial repair, particularly when the injuries are complex with loss of vessel wall. This applies whether autogenous or prosthetic material is used for replacement. The reasons for this are that the vessels are delicate and thin walled, which makes repair technically difficult. In addition, the flow rates through the vessel are much slower and the pressures much lower. Therefore any narrowing or lack of congruity of the intimal surface creates an ideal nidus for thrombus formation.

The initiation of thrombosis in this way eventually results in cessation of flow in the vessel with proximal and distal propagation of the thrombus to the point of collateral flow – a similar occurrence as in the arterial system. The sequelae with regard to the extremity or tissue drained by the particular venous system then depend upon the degree of obstruction and the efficacy of collateralization. In general, there is initial venous hypertension with tissue oedema. Should efficient collaterals develop this resolves, though long-term dysfunction may result. In certain circumstances thrombus propagation may occur into the small venous radicles, and in this way totally occlude all venous outflow. The resultant rising interstitial tissue pressure will eventually cause cessation of arterial inflow and tissue necrosis. Obviously in the longer term specific manifestations will differ, depending on what region is involved. Should the thrombus dislodge, particularly if the great veins are involved, this may be carried to the right side of the heart and thence into the pulmonary vasculature (pulmonary embolism).

Air embolism is a well-described complication of venous injury particularly when the great veins of the neck and mediastinum are breached (Schaff and Brawley, 1977; Robbs and Reddy, 1987). This may also occur with vena caval injury when the peritoneal cavity is opened (Kudok and Bongard, 1984; Robbs and Costa, 1984). A significant quantity of air may lead to the formation of an 'air lock' within the ventricle with resultant ineffective cardiac function. Multiple emboli into the cerebral circulation may result in transient or permanent neurological deficit. Of particular importance is the presence of multiple air emboli into the coronary vessels. There is an increasing awareness of this phenomenon, which is associated with concomitant penetrating lung injury and, in particular, tension pneumothorax, and in patients with these combinations of injuries on positive pressure ventilation. Special autopsy techniques are required to conclusively demonstrate this phenomenon and it may well be a cause of many unexplained cardiogenic deaths in polytrauma patients in the intensive care unit (King et al., 1984).

Meticulous technique is required if venous reconstruction is to be successful and there is little debate that this should be performed when a simple laceration is found. In the presence of complex injuries when an interposition graft is required, attempts to increase flow through the graft by creating arteriovenous fistulase have met with mixed success. The major consideration in these circumstances is whether the patient would not benefit more by simple ligation of the particular vessel rather than submitting them to lengthy fruitless attempts which may further aggravate a deteriorating clinical situation. Most is known about obstruction of large veins in the neck and mediastinum and an outcome of phlebographic studies that have been made of the collateralization that develops in patients with superior mediastinal fibrosis (Barrett, 1958). It has been shown that when a single brachiocephalic vein is obstructed, a ready collateral pathway to the superior vena cava develops through the anterior jugular system and the anterior communicating veins in the neck. With obstruction of the superior vena cava cephalad to the azygos vein the main alternative pathways are the superior intercostal veins which carry blood to the azygos and semi-azygos systems and on to the heart. The superficial veins on the chest wall do not dilate or become prominent, indicating that these collaterals are adequate in such circumstances. When the azygos vein becomes involved the superficial veins on the chest wall dilate and, together with the azygos system, drain into the inferior vena cava. Possibly the internal and external vertebral plexus play a major part in the development of collaterals. These collateral pathways are made possible largely because of the absence of valves in the great veins of the neck and mediastinum. Ligation of one or both internal jugular veins is well tolerated. Collateral flow occurs through the visceral plexuses, vertebral plexuses and the superior intercostal veins (Robbs and Reddy, 1987).

Ligation of the inferior vena cava caudal to the renal veins is surprisingly well tolerated and may have minimal sequelae. The major collaterals are the gonadal veins and the lumbars. Cephalad to the renal veins, inferior vena caval interruption may result in gross sequelae, ascites and gross lower extremity oedema. Similarly, the renal veins may be ligated with no adverse effects on the kidney provided that the suprarenal and gonadal venous collaterals are preserved (Conti, 1982). With regard to the visceral vessels, portal venous ligation has been well tolerated, as has the ligation of the superior mesenteric vein (Mattox et al., 1975). It should, however, be emphasized that whenever feasible repair should be carried out. With regard to the lower limbs there have been mixed reports in relation to interruption of the major venous trunks (Rich et al., 1970, 1977a, b). It would appear that if the profunda collateral remains intact the sequelae are minimal following ligation, although the principle applies that reconstruction should be attempted if possible (Mullins et al., 1980). In the upper limb venous injuries assume a far less important role from the point of view of long-term morbidity. It would appear that these veins may be ligated with impunity. In our own experience, the only problems with limb oedema which has resolved within a matter of days have followed ligation of the distal subclavian and proximal axillary vein cephalad to the profunda brachiae (Robbs and Reddy, 1984). In essence, the management of venous injuries has not been as comprehensively studied as that of arterial trauma, and the sequelae present less threat to life or limb; however, the principle remains that continuity should be restored whenever possible by simple suture or reanastomosis.

REFERENCES

Barrett N.R. (1958). Idiopathic mediastinal fibrosis. *Br. J. Surg.*, **46**, 207–18.

Baxter C.R. (1966). Acute renal insufficiency complicating traumatic surgery. In *Care of the Trauma Patient* 2nd edn (Shires, G.T. ed.). New York: McGraw Hill, pp. 508–20.

Cammack K., Rapport R.L., Paul R.J. et al. (1959). Deceleration injuries of the throracic aorta. *Arch. Surg.*, **79**, 90–4.

Clark I.A. (1986). Tissue damage caused by free oxygen radicals. *Pathology*, **18**, 181–6.

Conti S. (1982). Abdominal venous trauma in abdominal trauma. In *Trauma Management*, vol. 1 (Blaisdell L.L., Trunkey D., eds). New York: Thieme-Stratton, pp. 364–71.

Costa M., Robbs J.V. (1988). Non-penetrating subclavian artery trauma. *J. Vasc. Surg.*, **8**, 71–5.

Hirschberg A., Thomson S.R., Robbs J.V. (1988). Vascular complications of diagnostic angiography via limb arteries. *J.R. Coll. Surg. Edinb.*, 1988; 33: 196–8.

Hook E.W., Wainer H.S., McGee T.J. et al. (1957). Acquired arterio-venous fistula with bacterial endarteritis and endocarditis. *JAMA*, **164**, 1450–5.

King M.W., Aitchison J.M., Nel J.P. (1984). Fatal air embolism following penetrating lung trauma – an autopsy study. *J. Trauma*, **24**, 2–4.

Kudok K.A., Bongard F. (1984). Determinants of survival after vena-caval injury. *Arch. Surg.*, **119**, 1009–15.

Levien L.J. (1989). Ballistics of bullet injury in operative Athedic surgery. In *Rob & Smith's Operative Surgery Part 1 – Trauma Surgery* 4th edn. (Champion H.R., Robbs J.V., Trunkey D.D., eds). London: Butterworths, pp. 106–10.

Matsen III F.A., Mayo K.A., Krugmire R.B. et al. (1977). A model compartment syndrome in man with particular reference to the quantification of nerve function. *J. Bone Joint. Surg.*, **59A**, 648–53.

Matsen III F.A., Winquist R.A., Krugmire R.B. (1980). Diagnosis and management of compartmental syndromes. *J. Bone Joint Surg.*, **62A**, 286–91.

Mattox K., Espada R., Beall A.C. (1975). Traumatic injury to the portal vein. *Ann. Surg.*, **18**, 519–24.

McCord J.M. (1985). Oxygen derived free radicals in post-ischaemic tissue injury. *New Engl. J. Med.*, **312**, 159–63.

Meek A.C., Robbs J.V. (1984). Vascular injury with associated bone and joint trauma. *Br. J. Surg.*, **71**, 341–44.

Mills R.P., Robbs J.V. (1991). Paediatric arterial injury – management options at the time of injury. *J.R. Coll. Surg. Edinb.*, **36**, 13–17.

Mubarak S.J., Hargens A.R. (1983). Acute compartment syndromes. *Surg. Clin. N. Am.*, **3**, 539–64.

Mubarak S.J., Owen C.A., Hargens A.R. et al. (1978). Acute compartment syndromes: diagnosis and treatment with the aid of the Wick catheter. *J. Bone Joint Surg.*, **60A**, 1091.

Mullins R.J., Lucas C.E., Ledgerwood A.M. (1980). The natural history following venous ligation for civilian injuries. *J. Trauma*, **20**, 737–41.

Rich N.M., Hughes C.W., Bough J.H. (1970). Management of venous injuries. *Ann. Surg.*, **171**, 724–9.

Rich N.M., Collins G.J., Anderson C.A., McDonald P.T. (1977a). Autogenous venous interposition grafts in repair of major venous injuries. *J. Trauma*, **17**, 512–20.

Rich N.M., Collins G.J., Anderson C.A. et al. (1977b). Venous trauma: successful venous reconstruction remains an interesting challenge. *Ann. Am. J. Surg.*, **134**, 226–9.

Robbs J.V., Baker L.W. (1979). Late revascularization following acute arterial occlusion. *Br. J. Surg.*, **6**, 129–31.

Robbs J.V., Baker L.W. (1984). Cardiovascular trauma. *Curr. Prob. Surg.*, **21**, 32–4.

Robbs J.V., Costa M. (1984). Injuries to the great veins of the abdomen. *S. Afr. J. Surg.*, **22**, 223–8.

Robbs J.V., Naidoo K.S. (1984). Nerve compression injuries dues to traumatic false aneurysm. *Ann. Surg.*, **200**, 80–2.

Robbs J.V., Reddy E. (1987). Management options for penetrating injuries to the great vein of the neck and superior mediastinum. *Surg. Gynec of Obstet*, **165**, 323–6.

Rowland L.P., Penn A. (1972). Myoglobinuria. *Med. Clin. N. Am.*, **56**, 1233–56.

Sako Y., Varco R.L. (1970). Arterio-venous fistula – results of management of congenital and acquired forms, blood flow observations on proximal arterial degeneration. *Surgery*, **67**, 40–7.

Schaff H.V., Brawley R.K. (1977). Operative management of penetrating vascular injuries of the thoracic outlet. *Surgery*, **82**, 182–91.

Schulenburg C.E., Robbs J.V., Rubin J. (1985). Intra-arterial diazepam – a report of 2 cases. *S. Afr. Med. J.*, **68**, 891–3.

Spencer F.C., Guerin P.F., Blake H.A. (1961). A report of fifteen patients with traumatic rupture of the thoracic aorta. *J. Thorac. Cardiovasc. Surg.*, **41**, 1–7.

Warren J.V., Elkin D.C., Nickerson J.L. (1951). The blood volume in patients with arteriovenous fistulas. *J. Clin. Invest*, **30**, 220–5.

Weinstein L. (1980). Pathogenesis of infective endorcarditis. In *Heart disease – A Text Book of Cardiovascular Medicine* (Braunutilde, ed.) Philadelphia: WB, Sanders, pp. 1181–90.

Whitesides T.E., Haney T.C., Marimoto K. et al. (1975). Tissue pressure measurements as a determinant for the need of fasciotomy. *Clin. Orthop. Res.*, **113**, 43–6.

Williams J.S., Kirkpatrick J.R. (1971). The nature of seat belt injuries. *J. Trauma*, **11**, 207–18.

Woelfel G.F., Moore E.E., Goghill T.H. et al. (1984). Severe thoracic and abdominal injuries associated with lap-harness seat belts. *J. Trauma*, **24**, 166–8.

8. Protection Against Penetrating Injury

T. A. Abbott and
R. G. Shephard

INTRODUCTION

The use of protective garments to prevent both blunt and penetrating injury certainly goes back to prehistoric times and, although the popular conception of armour or body armour is of a medieval suit made up of steel plates or chain-mail, the reality encompasses a much wider range of materials and forms. In the earliest times, natural materials such as textiles, leather and wood were used to prevent sharp-edged weapons or missiles from penetrating the body and to spread the impact load and cushion its effect. It should be noted that all these natural materials are fibrous in character and that such materials, particularly strong ones such as silk, have been appreciated throughout history as having special protective properties. Indeed today, with the introduction of synthetic fibres of very high specific strength, fibrous materials represent a major part of the protective materials field.

The advent of metallurgy, first bronze and later iron and steel, enhanced not only the capabilities of weapons but also those of armours. Indeed, metallic armours were often necessary to counter the sharp edges of metallic weapons. However, until recent times when mass production became available, metal working was a very specialized art, its products represented a very high financial investment and were available only to the few. For this reason the use of natural fibrous materials continued in parallel with the use of metallic ones.

Another misconception is that the use of firearms immediately made steel armours obsolescent. This is not the case, as medieval armours were used for protection against the firearms of the day and indeed were proof-tested against them. However, it is certainly true that advances in firearms technology during the eighteenth and nineteenth centuries, together with the need for greater mobility of armies, meant that personnel armour technology could no longer keep pace with the requirements of protection and light weight with the material available at the time and such armour therefore fell largely into disuse.

The renaissance in work on personnel armour arose from the trend in the First World War towards more static warfare and the great advances that had been made in materials technology – particularly that of steel. The first modern steel helmets were developed in 1915, and with the rapidly accelerating advances in materials technology the science of protection against penetrating injury has gradually caught up with weapons technology to a point where effective protection can be given in many circumstances and where body armour and helmets are an accepted part of military and police equipment. The use of such equipment has led to a significant decrease in numbers of casualties. The range of materials used today includes not only metallic alloys but also, increasingly, polymeric materials in sheet or fibrous form and even brittle ceramics.

The problems of providing personal protection against bullets or fragments are those of removing substantial amounts of energy from high-velocity projectiles within a very short distance and doing this with the very low weights of material that can be carried by an individual. Removing energy within the short distance of separation of the armour from the body plus the degree of deformation that the body will tolerate without injury, means that the armour must exert very large forces on the projectile and must therefore be made of high-strength materials. In addition, the projectile energy will usually be concentrated over a very small cross-sectional area, and it is necessary to increase this, so that the energy is dissipated in a larger volume of material. Such an approach will also make the impact more tolerable. Finally, the material used must not hinder the wearer's movements unduly or lead to excessive physiological stress. The latter restriction means that flexible materials must be used where possible, areas of rigid plates limited and some means of ventilation provided. In practice, the weight per unit area (areal density) of a body armour covering the entire torso cannot exceed $5–10 \, kg/m^2$, while the maximum areal density of a rigid breast- or backplate can range up to $35 \, kg/m^2$ depending on the area covered. The shell of a helmet stands off some way from the head to accommodate transient deformation on impact and allow for the skull's lack of tolerance to it. The effect of areal density on helmet weight, on stability and the perceived effect on the head is therefore disproportionate and helmet shells rarely exceed $10 \, kg/m^2$. The need for flexibility and the relative tolerance to injury of the limbs means that arm or leg armour is rarely used, except in special cases of extreme threat such as the disposal of explosive ordnance (usually bombs).

The principles underlying the design of body armour are discussed below. Because the approach adopted depends so much upon the challenge which is to be countered, a short account of various projectiles (ballistic threats) is also provided.

BALLISTIC THREATS

Apart from those due to hand-wielded weapons such as knives and bayonets, which represent a relatively small percentage of injuries (though of

83

increasing prominence in civil life) the vast majority of penetrating injuries sustained in wartime or during police operations are caused by bullets fired from small-arms weapons or by fragments from shells, grenades and mortar bombs. These missiles can be broadly divided into three categories, fragments, high-velocity bullets and low-velocity bullets but, more recently, a subcategory known as flechettes has appeared and injury is also possible from the blast effects of fragmenting weapons (see p. 247).

Fragments

Fragmentation weapons are devices packed with high explosive contained in a relatively thin cast iron or steel case. Their detonation breaks the case into very large numbers of small fragments travelling at high velocities in all directions. A typical grenade might produce 1000 fragments, while the number would be nearer 10 000 for a shell. The initial velocities of these fragments range from 1000 to 2000 m/s. The initial velocity of a fragment depends on the particular point on the case from which it originated, and in projectiles, which are travelling at substantial velocities when they detonate, this terminal velocity is added vectorially to that of the fragment to form a forward-thrown spray enhanced by hundreds of metres per second.

The numbers and sizes of fragments will vary widely from a few of many grams weight to very large numbers which are little more than fine metallic dust. This is particularly true of cast-iron-cased weapons. However, there are so few large fragments produced that they stand very little chance of hitting a human target on the battlefield. Fragmentation weapons are thus 'area weapons' depending for their effects on the random chance of hitting a target; when they do they may deliver far more energy than is required to produce incapacitation. Fine metallic dust is rapidly slowed up by air resistance and is unlikely to produce significant injury even if it does reach a target. For this reason, modern weapons are designed to control the size of the fragments and yield fragments of sufficient size to retain the capacity to injure and of sufficient numbers to ensure a high probability of an impact. The optimum fragment size selected appears to be approximately 0.1 g in mass.

Many naturally fragmenting rather than specially designed munitions still exist, but recent introductions are usually of the controlled fragmentation type. In either case, fragments are generally of approximately equal length and breadth and even when they do have a significant long axis, or are plate-like, their stable position in flight is with their maximum area presented to the direction of motion. After initial tumbling, therefore, these fragments are neither aerodynamically designed to retain their velocity nor particularly good penetrators when they meet a target. Most fragments, therefore, lose velocity quite rapidly as they travel away from the point of detonation and, while individuals near to that point may encounter many high-velocity fragments, the larger numbers in the weapon's potential area of effect will in general risk impact from only a few fragments with a velocity of a few hundreds of metres per second. This is borne out by the fact that casualties struck by fragments have only one or two wounds and, while these may be still severely incapacitating and potentially lethal, they are of such a size and velocity that they can be stopped by modern lightweight armour.

Typical examples of fragments are shown in Figure 8.1, together with values for mass, velocity, energy and momentum per unit cross-sectional area. The latter is a better guide to armour-penetrating capability, representing as it does impulse (force × time), than is energy per unit area, which places too great an emphasis upon velocity as compared with mass. Fragments are invariably made from ferrous metals, which is important to those who design armour because such materials have a hardness of the order of 600 HV (HV = 'Vickers Hardness', a scale of hardness used by metallurgists) if steel or 400 HV if iron. This is of little importance with soft armours which cause virtually no fragment deformation but can affect the performance of hard armours. The ferrous composition of fragments also means that material density is close to 7.9 g/cm^3.

	Fragments	HIGH-VELOCITY BULLETS	LOW-VELOCITY BULLETS
1 cm [	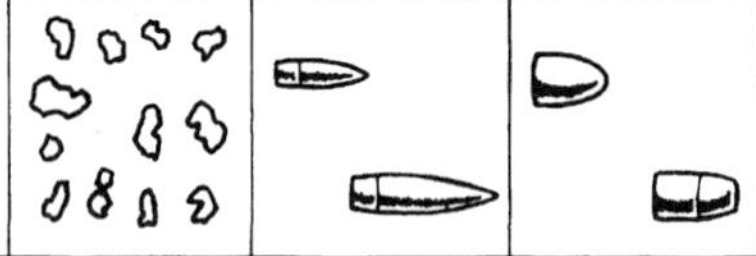		
CALIBRE (mm)	1–10	5.56, 7.62	9, 0.38 in.
MASS (g)	0.1–1.0	3.5, 9.3	7.4, 10.2
VELOCITY (m/s)	1000	970, 820	390, 350
ENERGY (J)	5.0–500	1660, 3140	570, 640
MOMENTUM/AREA (kg m/s/mm^2)	0.02–0.04	0.14, 0.17	0.05, 0.05

Figure 8.1 Examples and typical parameters of ballistic threats.

Flechettes

The ballistic shortcomings of fragments described above have led to the production of weapons which contain large numbers of small preformed steel darts or flechettes. These weigh a few grams at most, have a length of 1–2 cm, a cross-section of a few square millimetres, a point at one end and three or four small fins at the other. Thousands may be ejected from a weapon on its detonation. Though their initial velocity may be no more than a few hundred metres per second, once they are stabilized by their fins, flechettes undoubtedly lose less velocity due to air drag than do fragments. They are also more difficult to stop, particularly with soft textile armours, in that their long thin shafts can separate the yarns of the weave. The low terminal velocity of flechettes may mean their wounding power is reduced. For the design of armour, flechettes are a potentially difficult threat to counter but they are currently not in common use.

Low-velocity bullets

Bullets fired from hand and submachine guns are usually categorized as low velocity. At the lower end of the range such as 0.22-in. or 0.38-in. calibres, they may be entirely made of a lead alloy. However, lead alone will not withstand higher accelerations in the gun barrel and on impact tends to flatten and have little penetration, so that higher-powered guns invariably use lead alloy bullets jacketed or half jacketed (round the base) with a thin coating of a copper alloy. Low-velocity bullets usually have relatively low length to diameter ratios, rounded or even flat noses and are stabilized in flight by spin imparted to them in the rifled barrel. They are relatively massive, weighing up to 10 g, and rely on this rather than velocity for their range and penetration capabilities. The velocity at which they leave the muzzle depends on the length of the barrel, and thus the velocity of a given round will be higher if fired from a submachine rather than a hand gun. The short length of hand-gun barrels and the relatively low muzzle velocity imparted means that these weapons are relatively inaccurate and ranges of engagement rarely exceed 30 m. They are, therefore, used much more in police work than in warfare and the number of low-velocity wounds on the battlefield is fairly small.

Figure 8.1 lists the characteristics of a number of low-velocity bullets and demonstrates that while they are much more massive than fragments, their penetrating power, as measured by momentum per unit cross-sectional area, is very similar. They therefore represent a similar challenge to the skill of the designer of body armour, though the much greater energy they deliver may cause other problems.

Two new classes of low-velocity bullet are worthy of mention:

1. KTW rounds have a low friction polyfluoro-ethylene (PTFE) coating and also usually non-deformable brass cores, both features designed to increase penetration. Some similar rounds have hard noses of steel or more rigid jackets.
2. 'Tres haute vitesse' (THV) bullets, as their name implies, are specially designed to achieve higher velocities for a given cartridge or barrel length.

High-velocity bullets

A much more common weapon on the battlefield, carried by every soldier, is the high-velocity rifle. It is designed for accuracy at ranges up to 500 m or more, though most engagements are closer to 100 m. The greater range is achieved by higher muzzle velocities (800–1000 m/s) and relatively long bullets with ogival noses and boat-tailed rear ends which reduce aerodynamic drag (see Chapter 2). The normal construction is again a lead alloy core with a metal jacket, but energies are much higher than for fragments or low-velocity bullets and, in particular, the penetrating power, as measured by the momentum per unit cross-sectional area, is three to four times greater (Figure 8.1). The high-velocity bullet is, therefore, more able to pierce armour and can be even more effective if special armour piercing bullets are used. These have tough, hardened steel cores specifically designed to survive impact with and penetrate steel armours but, although there are methods of combating them, they are not usually used specifically against personnel. However, there is a tendency to manufacture even the soft bullet with a mild steel insert in the core, which decreases deformation and enhances armour penetration. Despite the fact that hard armour is necessary to stop high-velocity bullets, the modern trend (for logistic and other reasons) towards the lighter high-velocity bullets weighing about 3.5 g has eased the problem. Light bullets of a high velocity are easier to stop than heavy ones.

Blast

Injury and protection from blast are dealt with in another part of this book (see Chapter 21). This threat is mentioned here only because it is an ancillary effect in fragmentation weapons because of their explosive fillings. However, blast is a very much shorter range effect than fragmentation and any individual near enough to such a weapon to suffer blast injury is very much more at risk from multiple, high-velocity fragment injury.

Ballistic limit velocity measurement

In order to assess the performance of armours it is necessary to measure the velocity at which they are able to stop specified projectiles. However, reference to Figure 8.2 shows that for a given projectile and armour there is no single velocity below which there is no penetration and above which every projectile penetrates. Rather, there is a sigmoid penetration probability curve rising gradually from zero to unity as velocity increases. With fragment-protective armours, it is usual to estimate the velocity at which the probability of penetration is 50% – V_{50} ballistic limit velocity (V_{50}). This can be done by firing a large number of rounds at the armour, over a range of velocities, and plotting the complete penetration probability curve. However, such a procedure would require hundreds of rounds to be fired and is both expensive and time consuming. It can be shown that a good estimate of the V_{50} is obtained by firing a relatively small number of rounds at velocities close to estimated V_{50}, raising the velocity after a partial penetration and lowering it after a complete one. A complete penetration is deemed to have occurred when any particle penetrates a thin 'witness' sheet placed a certain distance behind the armour: this criterion equates to the so-called 'protection' ballistic limit. If the three lowest velocities with and the three highest without penetration are averaged, this provides a good estimate of V_{50} given that all six velocities are within a bracket of $40\,\text{m/s}$. This has become the standard method of measuring V_{50} and is relevant to fragment protection where protection can never be guaranteed but is a matter of increasing its probability.

With bullets, however, the wearer would like to know that the armour worn *will* stop a given bullet at a given velocity. This can be achieved by firing a series of bullets at a fixed velocity until the desired degree of confidence of non-penetration is reached. More information is gleaned, however, if ballistic limit velocity (V_{o}) is measured. To do this using the penetration probability curve with any degree of confidence, would require the firing of even more rounds than for the determination of V_{50} but we can achieve a useful result by using the equation:

$$V_{R} = A(V_{I}^{2} - V_{o}^{2})^{1/2}$$

In this equation, V_{I} is the initial velocity of the bullet before impacting the armour, V_{R} is its residual velocity or that of its debris after penetrating the armour (measured if necessary with a ballistic pendulum), A is a constant for the particular armour and bullet and V_{o} is the ballistic limit velocity. By firing bullets at the armour in a range of velocities above the ballistic limit and fitting the results to this equation, a reasonable estimate of V_{o} may be obtained with a relatively small number of shots.

Incidence of threats

Because the number of casualties produced during warfare is so much more than that produced during police or even antiterrorist activity, the major threat addressed by designers of body armour is that posed on the battlefield. The relative importance of different weapons as causes of injury may be determined by consulting casualty statistics from various wars (Beebe and de Bakey, 1952; Coates and Bayer, 1962; Kovaric et al., 1969). They show that the percentages vary markedly from one theatre to another and depend upon the types of warfare, terrain and the combatants. It is clear, however, that in nearly all wars, fragments account for the majority of battlefield casualties.

The percentage of wounds caused by fragments can vary from 60 to 90% (Figure 8.3). High-velocity bullets account for the next largest number but

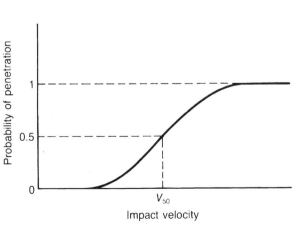

Figure 8.2 Penetration probability–velocity curve.

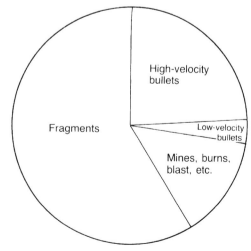

Figure 8.3 Sources of casualties in recent wars.

rarely exceed 25% of the total, and low-velocity bullets are a relatively minor cause. The remaining miscellaneous category in Figure 8.3 covers mines, burns and blast injury and, because of differences in reporting, may actually contain a proportion of fragment injuries from mines. The clear conclusion is that protection against fragments is likely to contribute most, followed by protection against high-velocity bullets.

PROTECTION AGAINST FRAGMENTING WEAPONS

Materials

The choice of materials used for personal protection down the centuries has been dominated by weight and the difficulty and encumberance caused. Consequently, most modern effort has been directed at finding materials or other means of offering the maximum protection at a minimum weight. An excellent summary of materials is given by Laible and Barron (1980). In recent years, attempts to completely protect the whole of the body from fragments have given way to selective protection of areas which, if injured, could be life threatening, at the expense of leaving the extremities exposed. As already mentioned, only in very special circumstances – bomb disposal and mine clearance – have the limbs been protected with a consequent penalty of threefold increase in weight.

In the early twentieth century most military armours, helmets or breastplates were commonly made of metal, often a steel such as a 'Hadfield' containing approximately 12% of manganese. It was not until the Second World War that substantial improvements began in protective levels of lower-weight armours. Initially, some of the aluminium alloys offered slight weight advantages over steel; later more expensive titanium-based alloys became available, but cost precluded their extensive use. Then new polymer-based synthetic materials, glass-reinforced plastics, proved very effective in anti-fragmentation armours and as a flexible armour, nylon 66 in textile form offered substantial weight savings over metals. One major factor which has undoubtedly enhanced the ballistic resistance of these polymeric materials, particularly those in fibrous form, is the specific strength which is markedly greater than that of even the toughest steels. There is one area where metallic armours are still of some importance in personal protection, namely in defeating very sharp or narrow projectiles such as flechettes, by the use of thin sheet metals, particularly titanium.

Testing

Over the last 30 years a great deal of work, much of it empirical, has been carried out on a very wide range of lightweight materials. The usual test method employed has been to determine the V_{50} of

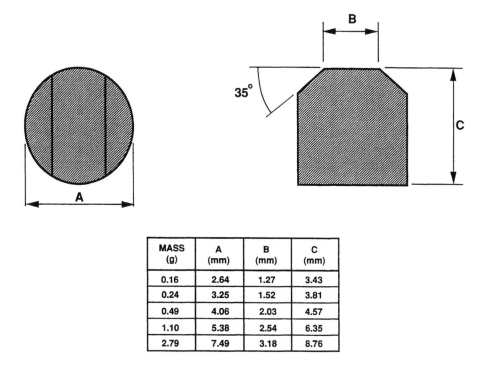

MASS (g)	A (mm)	B (mm)	C (mm)
0.16	2.64	1.27	3.43
0.24	3.25	1.52	3.81
0.49	4.06	2.03	4.57
1.10	5.38	2.54	6.35
2.79	7.49	3.18	8.76

MATERIAL: High carbon bright steel Rockwell C30

Figure 8.4 Fragment simulating projectile (chisel-nosed cylinder).

each candidate material at a variety of areal densities (weight/unit area). For the majority of work, a 1.1-g (17-grain) fragment simulator representative of the average size of actual fragments has been used. The shapes of the simulated fragments have included spheres, cubes and cylinders, but the shape currently accepted in most countries is the chisel-nosed (35 degree angle) cylindrical fragment (Figure 8.4). These are usually fired from a rifled barrel using, in the UK, a high-density polyethylene sabot which is discarded in flight. In the USA the rear of the simulated fragment has a small skirt, or obturator ring, to ensure a close fit within the barrel. Either compressed gas (usually helium) or a solid propellant can be used to vary velocity. Careful comparisons between these two types of simulators have shown that there is very little difference between the V_{50} values determined for most commonly used materials. However for a number of reasons, the test is subject to variability and results should be carefully assessed, bearing in mind all relevant details of sample preparation and test procedure.

In spite of possible uncontrolled factors, practical testing of material with fragment simulators is reasonably accurate and the results reproducible. Research into other simulators continues (e.g. Prosser, 1988).

Fibres

As has been mentioned, one of the earliest naturally occurring materials to be used for fragment protection was silk and in the early part of the twentieth century it was surprisingly effective. It was not until the Second World War that new high-tenacity synthetic fibres, particularly the polyamides, began to be used for vests to protect against fragments. These materials, particularly nylon 66, were carefully evaluated and employed as multiple layers of closely woven textile during the Korean and Vietnam conflicts. There was clear evidence that they markedly reduced both the number of casualties and deaths. Other than the physical tensile strength of nylon 66, there was no obvious reason why these materials were particularly good at resisting penetration. However by studies of energy absorption it rapidly became obvious that the specific strength of a yarn (tensile strength/density) was a very important factor but also that the yarn modulus (stiffness) was critical, although its effect was difficult to quantify. It was believed that a high modulus would ensure that the energy of the impact was rapidly dissipated as a longitudinal shock wave, some of which would be transferred to other yarns by frictional contact, along with some back reflections (Figure 8.5). This was undoubtedly true but the behaviour of carbon fibre, which became available at about this time, showed that a material of very high modulus was not necessarily good for

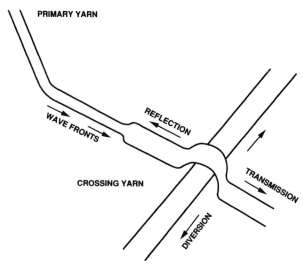

Figure 8.5 The effect of a crossing yarn on wave propagation.

ballistic resistance because such fibres had a poor shear strength at high rates of strain. More recent work by Prosser (1988) suggests that it is the force needed to shear the yarns which absorbs the majority of the energy.

The introduction of PRD 49 (now Kevlar 49) by the Du Pont Company in the early 1970s, with a tensile strength nearly three times that of nylon, provided a significant advance in lightweight protective materials. The basic strength of these aromatic polyamides (commonly known as 'aramids' and including Twaron (AKZO) and Technora (Teijin)) lay in their highly orientated structure which is the consequence of the process whereby they are spun from a liquid crystalline solution. In recent years modified and improved yarns with even higher tenacities and moduli have been produced, but the effects of these on ballistic properties have been marginal and microscopic studies of their structure suggest that they are now at the limit of their orientation and performance.

Polyethylene fibres with very high molecular weight and carefully controlled orientation of the fibres with a high degree of crystallinity and a minimum number of defects were introduced in the early 1980s and also have high tenacities and moduli.

Application to lightweight armour has been limited, but in some areas of protection they may prove superior to the aromatic polyamides though they have disadvantages.

Textiles

Much work has been devoted to evaluate different weaves, knits, sewing and spot bonding of multiple layers of these specialist yarns. A plain woven structure usually gives the best ballistic performance.

Ballistic performance of multiple layers against fragments does not appear to be improved by sewing or spot bonding the layers together, by the use of special high-tenacity threads or by pleating. Surface contamination of the textile by spinning oils, sizes or lubricants has an adverse effect.

Non-woven materials based on the same high-performance fibres are made by a variety of processes, many of which involve adhesive or surface 'melding' techniques to keep the structures coherent. Although these processes are cheaper than weaving, they produce materials with inferior ballistic resistance. There is, however, one important exception – needle-punched felt produced from nylon or polypropylene. These are particularly efficient at low areal densities, less than $4.0 \, kg/m^2$, but suffer from being thick and bulky. Both nylon and aramid-based felts have been evaluated, and although prototype vests which incorporate felt backed with woven textile were found to be ballistically effective and light weight, they were considered too bulky and stiff for military use. Interfibre friction may be important but the large deformation cone produced as the fragment is retarded can itself be hazardous if the armour is worn close to the body.

Textile treatments

Many manufacturers of soft armour employ textiles which have been treated to produce a water-repellent finish. Water greatly reduces ballistic protection offered by textile armours – a 30% loss in V_{50} is not unusual. The precise mechanism and cause of this degradation has not been clearly established but it is thought to be due to a lubricating action both between the fragment and the textile and between the yarns. Most water-repellent agents are either waxes or fluoropolymers, and it is essential that application is minimal, otherwise they may act as lubricants. Normally the water repellents only reduce ballistic performance slightly, though some have claimed that they actually enhance resistance. The efficacy of the repellent is a matter of considerable variation depending on the textile being treated, the agent being used, the amount added and the nature and length of exposure to water. Exposure by total immersion for brief periods (15–30 minutes) has little effect on the better agents but long periods (24 hours) can severely degrade performance although this recovers when the armour has dried. In military armours in use in the UK, it has been the practice to ensure the ballistic performance is unimpaired by water by encapsulating the whole of the textile in a sealed waterproof envelope of reinforced plasticized PVC or polyurethane which is sealed around the textile filler during manufacture and inserted into a removable textile cover which can be cleaned. Most other military and commercial armours rely solely on water-repellent treatment. The two main problems with an impermeable envelope are the added weight and the difficulty of adapting the filler to its cover, as obviously the envelope must not be sewn through or punctured in any way.

Many other textile structures have been considered, in particular combinations or hybrids, in order to enhance performance or to reduce weight and costs. It appears that some of these structures have advantages but their selection is largely a matter of empirical experiment. During the last quarter century attempts have been made to establish a theory of energy absorption by such fibres, yarns, textiles and multilayer structures at high rates of strain. Better understanding would make it much easier to design the ideal structure with a capacity for optimum energy absorption over very brief time intervals. A full understanding has been slow to appear. Many models and theories have been put forward and substantiated for particular cases, but there have always been anomalies and exceptions which do not fit with theory. Part of the difficulty lies in the anisotropic behaviour of different fibres and the structures into which they may be converted. The importance of friction in absorbing energy is difficult to establish and treatment of aramid though not polyethylene yarns to decrease their surface friction has made little difference to ballistic performance. It has been claimed that only textiles with high melting points are ballistically satisfactory, presumably because of their decreased tendency to melt when impacted. High-speed video-thermography during ballistic impact (Shenton and Bashford, 1989) indicates that temperatures seldom rise by more than 45°C, but that material in a considerable area around the impact point does increase in temperature, but by only a few degrees.

Films

The other class of flexible materials evaluated for use in ballistic protection is that of thin films. These materials, highly orientated in one direction only and laid with alternate orientation of each layer, have been effective in stopping fragments at similar areal densities to the textiles already described. These materials are difficult to produce, shape and mould into personal armour.

Composite materials

The other very important class of lightweight materials extensively used for fragmentation protection is that of the composites which give essentially rigid armours of particular value for helmets. It should be pointed out that virtually all military helmets offer very little protection against bullets and are essentially designed to protect only against fragments. However it is a strange anomaly that for many years the quality assurance test for UK steel combat helmets was carried out using 0.303 rifle bullets – admittedly downloaded to simulate a very long range!

The earliest of these composites to be used for personal armour was glass-reinforced plastic (GRP). Glass fibres alone, however, gave poor textile-based armour, but, when bonded with resin (usually unsaturated polyester resin) can form useful and fairly cheap protection against fragments. Performance is markedly improved if the glass fibre is woven rather than a random mat. The standard 'E' glass was mostly used for armours, but an improvement in performance can be achieved by using the more recently available 'S'.

'E' glass is the common form of glass fibre available in the UK. 'S' glass is said to be superior as a component of the body armour because of its different tensile properties. The precise differences in properties have not been disclosed. However most of the recent work on composite materials has concentrated on the use of high-tenacity nylon- or aramid-based textiles. Many resin systems have been tried but the dominant one, which gives excellent adhesion to nylon, is the phenolic/polyvinyl butyral (50/50) system using a maximum resin content of 20% of the total weight. As with textile armours, a great deal of experimental work has been done to optimize these composites and again many theories have been put forward, with limited success, to predict their ballistic performance. The presence of the resin does not enhance the textile performance in any way but merely provides a rigid structure. The use of polymeric plasticizer enhances the ballistic performance by increasing the resilience of the composites on impact. Other resin systems, such as epoxy resin with chlorinated rubber plasticizers, perform equally well but are usually more expensive.

The strength of the bond required between the textile and the resin has been the subject of considerable investigation. It is often claimed that the energy absorption of a composite during impact is enhanced if the composite delaminates extensively and many attempts to surface-treat textiles to achieve this have been made. However such treatments can make the composite weak so that it fails in normal use or during routine handling – a compromise is required to achieve adequate general performance while sufficiently enhancing ballistic properties. For helmets the textile/resin bond strength is only just adequate in the usual aramid composites, while that in the nylon composites is excellent. Ultra-high-molecular-weight polyethylene textiles in composites are presently under intensive investigation because they might offer a substantial saving in weight for rigid armours or, alternatively, enhancement of ballistic protection.

As with textile materials, there are considerable possibilities of mixing, blending or hybridizing different fibres into a composite structure. By such a means it would be possible to combine the excellent bonding properties of nylon with the ballistic resistance of an aramid to give a structure which is extremely tough yet gives good protection

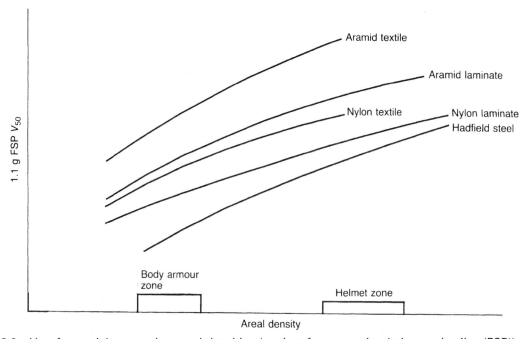

Figure 8.6 V_{50} of materials at varying areal densities (against fragment simulating projectiles (FSP)).

from fragments. However, in the final analysis, composite materials are less efficient than textiles in fragment-protective armours (Figure 8.6). Attempts to make composite materials from needle-punched felts have met with limited success and it still appears that moderately long continuous filament textiles are the basis for the best composites.

Ceramics

Although ceramic materials are excellent at stopping high-velocity bullets, they are seldom used in fragmentation protective armour. In the future they may have some applications against high-velocity or large fragments. Ceramics tend to be considerably heavier than other materials, partly because they require a composite backing. They are also rigid and uncomfortable.

Transparent materials

Transparent personal armours for fragment protection are very important in protection of the eyes and face. They are commonly employed in glasses, goggles and visors usually worn attached to, or in conjunction with, a helmet. Until 30 years ago they were usually made from cellulose acetate or polymethyl methacrylate, which although moderately hard and very clear, cannot be considered ideal because it suffers from brittle failure when impacted. Cellulose acetate can be plasticized to varying degrees to reduce its brittleness but then becomes too flexible. However, polycarbonates have greatly improved protection. The materials are ductile even when struck at high velocities. They appear to fail by displacing a discrete plug of

materials, a mechanism similar to that of metals, and do not produce secondary fragments. Even at moderately low temperatures (−20°C), at which most plastics behave in a brittle manner, polycarbonate behaves in a ductile way. The fragment-stopping efficiency of polycarbonate, however, does not compare very favourably with that of opaque materials such as textiles or composites, and in order to offer a similar level of protection to that given by these materials a much higher areal density is required.

Figure 8.7 gives some comparisons of the ballistic properties of transparent materials. It is clear that all transparent visors offer a much lower level of protection to the face than that available for other areas, unless the visors are much thicker than opaque armours. This thickness would render the visors excessively heavy and out of balance with the rest of the system. The only practical solutions are to find better materials than polycarbonates, or to restrict the area of vision provided by the visor.

Polycarbonate does suffer from two further major defects: it is comparatively soft and easily scratched and is very prone to attack by agents applied to its surface, particularly if these contain organic solvent. Coatings can be applied to make it scratch resistant but in many cases this makes it more brittle, especially at low temperatures. Similarly solvents, or adhesives which contain them, produce microcrazing of the polycarbonate which leads to brittle failure on impact.

Many attempts have been made to find an alternative but success has been limited. However, there are now coating materials available which give a marked increase in the scratch hardness of the surface without any appreciable effect on

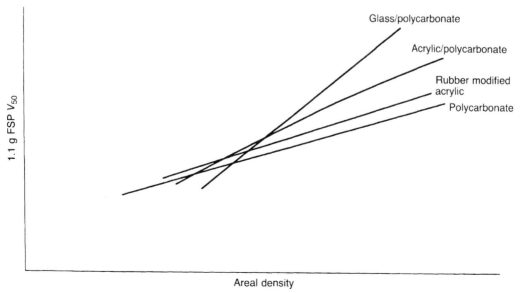

Figure 8.7 V_{50} of some transparent materials at varying areal densities (against fragment simulating projectiles (FSP)).

brittleness. Alternative approaches to the use of a polycarbonate have been to add various rubbery polymers to the more brittle polymers such as polymethyl methacrylate and polyvinyl chloride, but these efforts produce their own problems.

Glass itself is a good agent for stopping fragments but obviously suffers very badly from brittleness necessitating a spall (fragment release from the inner aspect of the material) protective backing. However, when combined with polycarbonate, with the right adhesive, excellent armours can be produced for protection against higher-velocity fragments. The density of glass means that a rather thin layer is needed and the inherent fragility is a severe disadvantage for military use. Using borosilicate as opposed to soda glass, with a polyurethane adhesive and a polycarbonate backing, a good eye protector or visor can be produced but if curvature, especially double curvature, is required production costs rise.

It seems likely that some of the newer 'engineering' polymers which are now being produced could offer improvements over polycarbonate in the near future. There are undoubtedly many applications within industry, especially in aerospace, for this class of materials.

CONCLUSION

Some of the lightweight materials now being used in fragment-protective armours have been discussed. They have been selected largely for their ability to stop fragments. In many cases there are other factors, such as bulk, thickness or deformation, which make them rather less satisfactory. The textile-based structures deform to a large degree on impact with large fragments, although it is not generally considered that this is likely to cause blunt injury. The head is, of course, at particular risk if the helmet permits considerable deformation and this is one reason for having a minimum clearance of some 18 mm between the shell of the helmet and the head.

Most of the materials used for fragmentation protection have been assessed for toxicity if they are carried into a wound, as has their aggravating effects from melting or burning. Fortunately in most instances the thickness of materials in personal armour means that burning takes place slowly and thermal insulation is good. However some doubt has been expressed about the use of polyethylene-based armours which melt and burn at modest temperatures, whereas the aramid fibres are inherently flame retardant and present little hazard.

PROTECTION AGAINST LOW-VELOCITY BULLETS

As defined, low-velocity bullets have maximum velocities in the range of 500–600 m/s with the lower-powered weapons giving only 200 m/s. Mass varies between 2 and 15 g and one of the most useful indices for comparison is the muzzle energy per cross-sectional area of the bullet. Table 8.1 lists a variety of types of bullet commonly encountered but is not comprehensive. The most common low-velocity round in military use is probably the 9-mm fired by many machine-guns and pistols. In the USA the different types of bullet are placed in four main categories by the National Institute of Justice (NIJ) depending on their relative penetrating energy. More recently the Personal Protection Armour Authority (PPAA) has proposed a slightly

TABLE 8.1

THE PROPERTIES OF TYPICAL LOW-VELOCITY BULLETS. (ACTUAL VELOCITIES AND ENERGIES WILL VARY WITH THE PROPELLANT USED AND THE BARREL LENGTH.)

Bullet	Mass of Bullet (g)	Muzzle		Muzzle energy per cross-sectional area (J/mm^2)
		Velocity (m/s)	Energy (J)	
0.30	7.1	610	1321	29.0
0.44	15.6	448	1565	15.9
9 mm Norma	11.8	362	773	12.2
0.357	10.2	390	776	12.0
9 mm 2Z	7.5	395	580	9.1
9 mm Parabellum	8.0	380	578	9.1
0.22 High velocity	2.6	400	208	8.5
0.45 ACP	14.5	280	568	5.5
0.22 Service	2.6	317	131	5.3
0.38 Norma special	10.2	265	358	4.9
0.38 2Z	11.5	204	239	3.3
0.22 Short	1.84	266	63	2.6

different method of categorizations. However, the objective in both classifications is to proffer advice on different types of armour which are able to give protection. In the UK these categories have not been recognized and each manufacturer declares the protective capabilities against each type of bullet.

Essentially the types of material used for protection against a low-velocity bullet are similar to those used for protection against fragments. While in the past metallic and other rigid materials have been used, textiles have now established themselves as the preferred materials. Their great advantage, in addition to low weight, is the fact that they are similar to normal clothing, can conform reasonably comfortably to a wide variety of body shapes and can be easily handled and manufactured by conventional textile techniques. Having said this, it must be recognized that the very high strength yarns and textiles used do need careful handling to minimize damage during manufacture.

The methods used for testing of armours against fire from small arms are different from those employed for fragmentation. Although the V_{50} technique described above can be used, it is not particularly convenient or very meaningful. Usually the capacity of the armour to stop a given bullet at muzzle velocity is determined. Consequently most tests are carried out at a range of some 3 m – the normal distance between the muzzle and target which permits the use of a timing system. The NIJ standards which are used by many test authorities and the German DIN standards, usually specify that three rounds shall be fired spaced at least 5 cm apart and all these should be stopped by the armour. These standards are used in the UK, but for research more stringent procedures are adopted.

Textiles

Empiricial assessment of small-arms rounds on lightweight armour has been the basis of protection. A full understanding of the mechanisms of protection by both textile and composite has not been achieved and only a partial interpretation of the mechanism, on a non-quantitative basis, is possible. Again the tensile strength and modulus of the yarns used are two of the critical parameters but shear strength is probably less important. Examination of textile armours and of the lead bullets used to test them shows that comparatively few yarns are sheared and the pattern of the textile weave is clearly impressed onto the lead which itself is grossly deformed. The toughness of the textile causes the bullet to flatten so that its presented area makes it easier to arrest. This is true to a lesser extent for a cased bullet, dependent on the thickness and shape of the jacket. There are, however, a number of factors which can enhance the level of ballistic protection offered by textile armour against

low-velocity bullets which are different from the same effects against fragments. One is to keep the multiple plies of the textile in close contact by stitching or quilting.

Spot bonding of the layers with small amounts of adhesive has a very similar effect.

To date all materials tested with fragment simulators or bullets have always, as expected, shown the poorest ballistic performance when struck orthogonally by the test missile. Recently some have claimed that with some low-velocity bullets striking aramid textiles this is not necessarily so – at certain oblique angles there is a greater chance of penetration. This unexpected finding is believed to apply only to certain open structures when the layers are not held close together during test and can deform.

Blunt trauma

One of the major differences between small-arms bullets and fragment simulators is the greater energy of the former which can result in a considerable risk of blunt trauma. Blunt injury over some of the vital organs, especially the heart, can be serious. There are two main solutions which are used by most manufacturers: either the back layers of the armour are made more rigid to spread the load or the armour is held away from the body by a spacer. Typical materials used to increase the stiffness are thin membranes of polycarbonate or resin applied to the inward layers. A wide variety of materials, such as foam and feathers, have been used and are usually described by the manufacturers as 'trauma packs'. These are not in common military use as they greatly increase bulk, and rigid layers negate some of the merit of textile-based protection and greatly reduce comfort. Consequently, it is usual in these circumstances to incorporate more layers of the ballistic protective material which acts as its own trauma pack and at the same time enhances performance, admittedly at some slight increase in cost.

Composites

The use of composites to resist penetration by low-velocity bullets is largely restricted to those missiles of low energy and by the use of heavier composites. Consequently, as with fragment protection, the efficiency of composites is limited; helmets which are truly bullet protective tend to be heavy. However, for rounds with moderate energy such as the 9-mm 2z (the standard 9-mm round used by UK armed forces) aramid composites can be used with areal densities between 6 and 8 kg/m^2. The higher-energy rounds, such as the 0.44-in. magnum, require a much greater areal density to defeat them, whereas low-energy rounds, such as the 0.22-in. or 0.38-in., can be

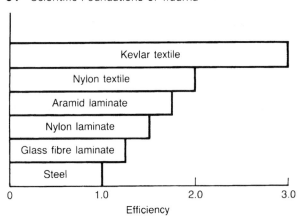

Figure 8.8 The relative efficiency (by weight) of materials protecting against 9-mm rounds.

stopped with ease by nylon composites. Figure 8.8 shows the relative efficiency of some composites and textile materials against 9-mm rounds compared with steel at identical weights. Compared with steel the aramid- and nylon-based composites are respectively about 1.8 and 1.5 times more effective. The indentation, however, in a helmet shell made of these materials can be quite deep and a stand-off of at least 25 mm from the head is essential to avoid damage to the skull even though penetration does not occur. Recently it has been claimed that woven polyethylene laminates and uniaxial polyethylene laminates are effective in resisting bullet penetration but this awaits confirmation in the military field. The major problem with polyethylene, as has been recounted in protection from fragments, is its poor adhesion which can in a helmet shell permit severe deformation or delamination. Enhancement of bonding methods may overcome this problem. It is unusual to employ composite plates for armours against low-velocity bullets because textiles are so much more efficient. However plates are sometimes used in combination with textiles to offer protection against multiple threats. Similarly the use of ceramic-faced armours is unnecessary if only low-velocity threats are likely but they are employed where there is also a possibility of high-velocity impact.

Transparent materials

As in fragment protection, transparent materials are not as efficient as opaque materials against low-velocity rounds. Consequently visors or goggles which are truly bullet protective are heavy and are difficult to support even when attached to a helmet. Most of the materials used are based on polycarbonate, often in combination with glass or acrylic sheet – similar to systems used for transparent security-glazing. If a wide field of view is needed such eye protectors are not suitable for continuous wear.

Conclusions

In conclusion it is obvious that the low-velocity rounds differ greatly in their ability to penetrate lightweight armour materials. Below an energy of 5 J/mm^2 the rounds are fairly easy to stop, between 5 and 10 J/mm^2 they can be stopped with moderate ease, but above this figure blunt injuries are a threat even though the round is arrested.

PROTECTION AGAINST HIGH-VELOCITY BULLETS

Because high-velocity bullets bring much greater energy and momentum to bear per unit area of the armour than do fragments and low-velocity bullets, much heavier armours are required for their arrest. In general, high-velocity-bullet protective armours have areal densities in the range 20–80 kg/m^2 but only the lower end of this is practicable for use in body armour.

Metals

The mechanism by which high-velocity bullets usually penetrate homogeneous sheets of metals used in body armour is described as plugging, which involves the punching out of a cylindrical plug of material of the same diameter as the impacting projectile from the armour (Figure 8.9). It is characteristic of flat-nosed projectiles where the loading on the metal plate leads to very high shear stresses below the periphery of the projectile. However, the pointed noses of high-velocity bullets

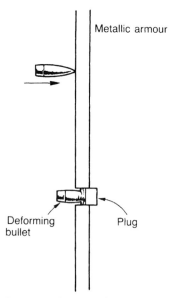

Figure 8.9 Plugging failure of armour.

flatten rapidly on impact with a rigid armour sheet and then present a flat nose leading to the same form of failure. Plugging occurs because it is the minimum energy form of failure in plates of this thickness, energy being absorbed by shear over a very small cylindrical surface measuring only a few square millimetres around the periphery of the plug. The well localized energy absorption can lead to very high local temperatures which soften the metal by phase transformation or even possibly melting, so that less resistance is offered and further deformation can occur. In steels, deformation often takes the form of adiabatic shear banding, the bands appearing as microscopic white zones.

Plugging is, therefore, a very inefficient means of absorbing projectile energy. Bullets which impact a metal plate very close to the ballistic limit velocity may also cause plastic deformation in the form of 'dishing' over a rather larger area and consequential greater energy absorption. However, at a few tens of metres per second above that limit velocity plugging only occurs. The net result is that metals are not very efficient protective armours and, furthermore, when penetrated they do not remove much energy from the bullet.

Constraints on weight mean that metals used in body armours tend to be only a few millimetres in thickness and thus only the very highest specific strength materials are likely to be of any use. In practice this limits the field to steels and aluminium or titanium alloys, and the penetration mechanism described above further limits the scope for the application of the various strength levels available in many of the latter. Although aluminium alloys have been used extensively in light vehicle armour where they have the added advantage of providing structural stiffness, they have no such advantage for personnel. Titanium alloys also show little performance advantage and are, in addition, very expensive so the use of metals in bullet-protective personnel armour has mostly been confined to high-strength, high-hardness steels.

Even high-manganese Hadfield's steel, much used in fragment protective armours and helmets, offers little advantage against bullets, and the best results have been obtained with medium carbon, silicon-containing, martensitic steels such as AISI 4340, Compass B or EN 40C. If these steels are given a range of quenching and tempering treatment, a definite increase in ballistic limit velocity with increasing hardness is seen up to about 650 HV. However, above this level the steel plates become too brittle and begin to shatter on impact.

This behaviour has led to the investigation of materials known as dual hardness steels which have a high-hardness steel front plate firmly bonded to a softer but less brittle backing plate. The concept is that the front plate destroys the projectile and prevents penetration while the backing holds the relatively brittle front plate together. The bond

between the two plates is of great importance: a poor bond invariably leads to poor ballistic performance.

Dual hardness steels may, in some circumstances, have a small advantage over monolithic ones but the difference in performance is small.

The dual hardness concept has also been extended to other means of hardening the front surface of the steel armour including laser glazing and the deposition of weld metal coatings containing a variety of high-hardness metal carbides. None of these techniques has led to any significant performance advantage, and no metallic armour yet devised will effectively stop high-velocity bullets at an areal density below $40 \, \text{kg/m}^2$ which is above the useful limit for personnel armour plates. There is, therefore, little use for metallic materials in modern bullet-protective body armours.

Textiles

While, as we have seen, textiles have an almost complete monopoly for lightweight protection against fragments, they have a basic defect against high-velocity bullets. This arises from the fact that they are made up from discrete fibres or yarns which are pushed to one side by a pointed projectile; high-velocity bullets are thus able to find an easy route through a textile. Another factor that may possibly be relevant is that textile fibres always have a critical transverse impact velocity above which they shear through without transverse wave propagation or energy absorption. High-velocity bullets almost always impact above this critical velocity and, unlike fragments, will not lose velocity rapidly in the armour. Textiles are not, therefore, good at stopping high-velocity bullets and, in adequate areal densities, are far too bulky to be worn as a garment. Such materials have however found some application in the protection of equipment from impacts by high-velocity small-arms bullets. The use of textiles, particularly woven aramids, behind hard-plate armours to catch the debris of bullets broken up by the plates is accepted practice, and they are very effective in this role, being used behind ceramic plates in body armour and steel in some helicopters.

Laminates

In contrast to the situation with textiles, textile laminates have played a significant part in lightweight protection against high-velocity bullets both in their own right and as backings for ceramic armours. The invention during the Second World War of a woven glass-reinforced plastic laminate armour called Doron was largely in response to a bullet threat, albeit a rather lower velocity one, and glass and aramid fibre laminates continue to show some promise in this role: at least equivalent to that of the best steels.

The mechanisms involved are similar to those in fragment-protective laminate armours: delamination and the conventional textile absorption of energy by transmission of longitudinal and transverse waves along the yarns and from yarn to yarn. While the bonding resin prevents sideways slipping of the yarns and easy penetration of the pointed projectile, the delamination, particularly towards the back face of the armour, is almost certainly effective in releasing the yarns for more effective energy absorption rather than in absorbing energy itself. In the thicker laminates used against bullets there is greater resistance to bending, penetration may commence on the front face by plugging before transitioning to a textile failure mode and there is a marked increase in the area of delamination from the front to the back of the laminate, probably reflecting more efficient energy absorption in the later layers.

Laminate armours are outstripped in performance by ceramic armours and, where weight is at a premium, they are encountered usually as the backing component of these.

Ceramic armours

Although largely developed in the 1960s during the Vietnam War, the concept of ceramic armour is not entirely new. Ceramics have been used as armour by primitive peoples in the past, the hard coating of steels has a long history and the glass-faced, Doron-backed armour already referred to was developed during the Second World War.

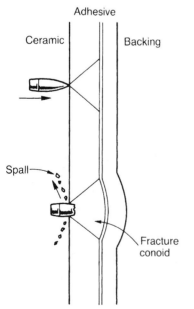

Figure 8.10 Principle of operation of ceramic armour.

A ceramic armour (Figure 8.10) consists of a monolithic front face of a low density but hard and brittle ceramic, adhesively bonded to an energy-absorbing backing of metal or composite. When a bullet or other projectile impacts the ceramic front face (Frechette and Cline, 1970), a fracture conoid is broken out of the ceramic. The armour backing supports this conoid and holds it in place while the bullet is comminuted by the hard ceramic. At the same time the load in the backing is spread over the base area of the conoid which is much wider than the calibre of the bullet. Thus a much greater volume of backing material is available for energy absorption. Finally, when the bullet debris has worked its way through the ceramic, it is caught by the backing material acting as armour in its own right.

The best ceramic materials have high hardness, in order to comminute the bullet material effectively, and low density in order to maximize the thickness of the ceramic layer at a given areal density. The ceramics used must be brittle because the formation of a fracture conoid is an essential part of the protective mechanism and ductile materials, such as metals and fibre-reinforced plastics, do not fail in this way. The cone crack is actually an adjunct of typical hertzian cracking and there are in fact a series of concentric cones rather than a single one. The cone that actually bears the load depends on geometry more than material properties, and the cone angles in different materials vary very little. For this reason the base area of the conoid and amount of backing material taking part in energy absorption are directly proportional to the thickness of the ceramic, and low-density materials such as boron carbide and glasses with densities below 2.5 g/cm^3 therefore have a significant advantage. High hardness is achieved mainly in covalently bonded ceramics such as boron and silicon carbides but other materials such as alumina also have strong bonding and high hardness leading to high shock-wave velocity in them. Indeed, it has been suggested that armour performance is correlated with this velocity, which is a function of the elastic modulus and density of the material, though no comprehensive theory has developed out of this hypothesis. What is true is that the best ceramics can deal almost as easily with armour-piercing bullets with hardened steel cores as they can with ball rounds. They do this partly by fragmenting the bullet via a reflected shock wave, which travels through the bullet core and breaks off its back end. With soft-cored ball rounds even relatively soft glassy materials can comminute the lead or mild steel which is converted into a fine powder.

The final failure of the ceramic cone arises from an axial crack which grows from the back face of the ceramic towards the apex. The back face is in tension and the ceramic fails in bending mode. The stiffer the backing material, the more support it will give to the ceramic and the longer this bending failure can be delayed. While the ceramic conoid remains intact it continues to comminute the bullet, and computer modelling has shown that a few microseconds delay in failure will significantly enhance the ballistic limit velocity. Stiff backings are, therefore, a great advantage and indicate the use of high-modulus fibre-reinforced materials such as aramid laminates.

The other two functions of the backing, those of deforming to absorb energy over the conoid base area and catching the bullet and ceramic debris, are however best achieved by more flexible materials. Again, textile laminates though perhaps not those best suited for the support function, can fill this role. A compromise needs to be struck and it has been shown in practice that, at a given weight, either an aluminium backing with better stiffness or a glass-reinforced plastic backing with better energy absorption can give the same performance. Aramid laminates actually perform better than either of these, though the degree of stiffness is open to debate, and there are ceramic armours with almost pure aramid textile backings which perform quite well.

The degree of bonding between ceramic and backing can also be quite significant. It is not essential to have any bond at all at this interface, providing that both faces are accurately machined to match. However this does not happen in practice and a filler medium is essential to transfer the stress across the gaps caused by irregularities. Voids at the interface reveal themselves in reduced performance when an impact occurs over them and for practical purposes, to overcome rough handling and to give multiple impact performance, the bond is usually made with a tough, flexible resin such as a polysulphide or silicone.

A common criticism of ceramic armours concerns their failure to withstand multiple impacts. The area of the base of the first fracture conoid may be that of a circle of diameter 10 cm and a second impact within or overlapping this area will certainly not be met with the original level of armour performance. For this reason some ceramic armours are built up from small ceramic tiles, the argument being that an impact in one tile will leave adjacent ones unaffected and improve the multi-hit capability. However this view is not necessarily valid, because an impact near the edge of a tile will not allow the whole of the fracture cone to develop and will therefore reduce performance. Also poor multi-hit capability is as much to do with delamination of the backing as fracture of the ceramic and the former will usually be much more extensive than the latter. In practice, a well-constructed ceramic armour with a monolithic ceramic face, a tough interface bond and a flexible resin such as a thermoplastic in the backing can give quite good multi-hit performance against shots as little as

7.5 cm apart. Also, while multi-hit capability may be important in vehicles and helicopters, the individual soldier when hit by a bullet on an armour plate usually moves sufficiently quickly to avoid a closely spaced second hit.

The final component of a ceramic armour is a single layer of glass fibre, aramid or nylon textile, bonded to the front face of the ceramic and known as a spall shield. When struck by a projectile, a bare ceramic face emits a shower of high-velocity debris and this has been known to cause injury, particularly to the eye, in the wearer or others in the vicinity. The adhesion of a spall shield to the ceramic dramatically reduces this and also helps in keeping the armour in one piece after an impact. On the debit side, there are some reports that spall shields reduce the performance of the armour but this effect, if it exists, is a relatively minor one.

Ceramic armours at areal densities of $20-35$ kg/m^2 are effective in stopping high-velocity bullets and outperform all other armour types by a substantial margin (Figure 8.11). The most expensive varieties with boron carbide facings and aramid laminate backings have been used by helicopter pilots and can provide coverage of most of the thorax at tolerable weights. Less costly

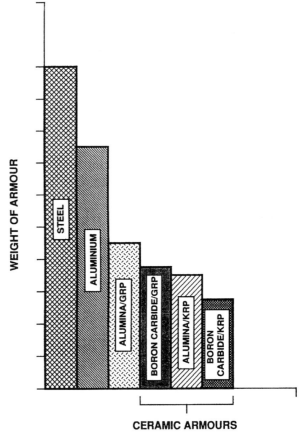

Figure 8.11 Comparative weights of high-velocity bullet protective armours.

versions which substitute alumina for the boron carbide, but with the disadvantage of higher ceramic density (3.8 g/cm^3), can be used to cover more limited areas.

Transparencies

The scope for protecting against high-velocity bullets with transparent materials is very limited. Laminates of polycarbonate have been used in bullet-proof glazing, as have laminated glass constructions, but the weights of such materials necessary to stop a high-velocity bullet are far in excess of the weight that can be carried on the head to give any but the most limited field of vision. The most efficient practical transparent armour is borosilicate glass bonded to a polycarbonate backing with a suitable transparent polymeric interlayer, and this is outperformed only by the exceedingly expensive, single crystal sapphire on a polycarbonate backing developed during the Vietnam War for helicopter transparencies. Neither of these armours performs as well as opaque ceramic and neither is really viable for facial protection of an individual. This is, therefore, an area of protection where no satisfactory solution is yet available.

Blunt trauma protection

The amount of energy imparted by a high-velocity bullet is substantially greater than that available from a low-velocity bullet or fragment. It may be, therefore, that even though the bullet is stopped by an armour, the transient deformation might cause damage. The problem is likely to be alleviated by the fact that all useful armours against high-velocity bullets are rigid plates; the greater the rigidity the less the problem. Any residual effect can be dealt with by the use of suitable cushioning or rigid sheet, load-spreading materials, as with low-velocity protective armours. Rigid sheets, although effective, further reduce the flexibility of the garment behind the armour plate and it is probably better either to add additional layers to the ceramic armour backing or to the body armour in which the plate is worn. These will not only reduce the transient deformation effects but also increase the ballistic protection limit.

HUMAN FACTORS

Many problems arise when protective materials which offer good resistance to fragmentation weapons and small arms are converted into military hardware such as body armour and helmets. Even after a great deal of effort to produce ergonomic designs, the items invariably cause problems of comfort and compatibility. The final design is always a compromise between the protective level sought and the requirements of the user to carry out all duties, many under extremely arduous conditions.

The first and major constraint is always that of weight, although bulk is also important. The second is provided by the contours of the human body and particularly by the large surface area of the extremities. Complete coverage of the legs, feet, arms and hands requires an area nearly twice that of the torso alone. The third, which can have a gross effect on comfort, is the comparative rigidity of many of the protective materials. To a certain extent this is related to their weight and bulk.

In general, in order to produce items which offer protection despite these constraints, the following criteria are commonly accepted in the design of military equipment:

1. Fragmentation protection is easier to achieve than rifle bullet protection at tolerable weight and comfort.
2. Fragmentation armours are usually made to protect only the critical organs of the thorax and upper abdomen, extending from the waist to the neck, with a helmet covering the upper and rear parts of the head.
3. The protection of the remainder of the head and face are largely dependent on compatibility with other items of military equipment such as respirators, hoods, eye protectors, hearing protectors, communications headsets and weapon sights. No doubt many of these latter items will gradually be either miniaturized or integrated into a full head protection system.

Bullet-protective armours are an even greater problem as the ceramic plates now commonly used to stop high-velocity rounds are considerably heavier than fragmentation armours and, because of their rigidity, much more uncomfortable. No satisfactory bullet-protective helmet has yet been devised, as the weight of the ceramic needed is still a factor of three greater than can be tolerated on the head for continuous wear. Many rigid plates for protecting the various organs of the body have been devised but even the smallest ones, designed to protect just the heart and associated vessels, weigh about a kilogram. Even when these plates are curved, to approximate to bodily contours, they cause considerable discomfort. Larger plates to protect the liver, spleen and lungs can weigh up to 3 kg, which tends to be excessive for continuous wear.

However, despite weight and discomfort, both fragment- and bullet-protective armours are worn for many hours at a time. Depending on climatic conditions and what is to be done, they greatly impair efficiency and can easily lead to problems of heat stress which are further severely aggravated when other equipment such as respirators or suits to protect against chemical weapons are also worn. The matter is made worse by the inherent impermeability of armour systems which do not readily allow perspiration to evaporate. Some military experts would claim that there are many circumstances when the use of armour is counterproductive, maximum mobility being essential. One difficulty lies in the marked difference between training exercises, when performance is monitored but no real risk exists, and in real battle, when the risks are all too evident.

In the long term, unless armour systems can be made substantially lighter and less rigid, it will be essential to produce integrated protective 'ensembles' which control body temperature and local humidity as well as offering protection against all the expected military threats.

CASUALTY REDUCTION ANALYSIS

Assessment of the expected reduction in casualties as a consequence of wearing low-velocity bullet-protective body armour is not, in principle, difficult. Particularly in a police scenario, all that is necessary is an analysis of previous shooting incidents according to the weapon used and the part of the body hit and comparison of this with parts of the body covered by the proposed armour and the ability of the armour to protect against the various weapons. Naturally, this procedure is dependent on data being available, and there may be further complications such as assailants who recognize the presence of body armour firing at different parts of the body, however, the basic analytical problem is fairly simple.

This is not the case with fragment-protective armours worn by soldiers in combat. Then the size and velocity of the fragments encountered will vary widely and the armour can not be expected to protect against every fragment. In addition, a soldier protected from one or more fragments may be wounded or killed by other fragments hitting unprotected areas. One way to overcome this difficulty is to carry out a casualty reduction analysis using a computer model of the actual situation on a battlefield. In the past, analyses have been carried out using practical trials with a fragmentation weapon detonated in the middle of an arena on which body armours are arrayed on dummies. The difficulties are that the terminal velocity of a shell is almost impossible to simulate, dummies may shield one another, no information on the degree of wounding can be collected and the procedure is extremely expensive.

The equivalent computer simulation starts with the fragmentation weapon being considered and deals individually with each of its zones, usually annular regions about the main weapon axis, within which the distribution of fragment sizes and initial velocity has been predetermined. With a grenade, a random orientation and static detonation at ground level might be considered, whereas with a shell a typical burst height, terminal velocity and angle of descent would be simulated. Each of the sizes, velocities and numbers of fragments are considered independently and followed on their way to potential targets on the ground over the whole area of effect of the weapon. The slowing down of each class of fragments from air drag is calculated, as is the shielding of the potential targets by the terrain. Undulations in the ground can shield the lower part of the body from a ground burst and this effect is greater as range increases, on rougher terrain and when targets are squatting, in the prone position or in trenches rather than standing. The effect will be less for air burst weapons. The part of the body hit by each fragment class is determined and, if armour is present, the residual velocity after penetration is determined. The residual velocity and fragment mass are then used in an experimentally determined formula to assess the degree of wounding in that part of the body and, in the case of multiple wounds, these degrees of wounding combined to give an overall assessment of the degree of injury or incapacitation. The total number of casualties over the whole of the weapon's area of effect are then summed, assuming a uniform distribution of troops or possibly some other distribution which peaks at the point of aim.

Clearly there are many uncertainties in this procedure, including the actual weapon used, the position, orientation and velocity at time of burst, the accuracy of air drag formulae and of weapons data, the type of terrain and distribution, the orientations of the body and the precision of data on armour and of formulae for assessing the degree of wounding. The analysis can never be an accurate predictor of the number of casualties in a given scenario. What it can do, however, is to compare what is likely to happen if armour is worn with what will happen if it is not. It can also give some idea of the relative efficacy of helmets and body armour and of the relative performance of different armours using different materials or different areas of coverage at a given weight.

Typical results obtained suggest that while helmets are very important for reducing fatalities, body armour is much more effective at reducing overall casualties. Also that the wearing of both helmet and body armour can substantially reduce the number of casualties sustained in combat even with relatively light weights.

A rather different analysis can be carried out for high-velocity bullets. It will be remembered that these are in the form of relatively heavy, rigid plates which can never cover the whole of the body. It is therefore necessary to assess their optimum size, shape and position to give maximum protection, which can again be done by computer modelling by building up geometrical simulations of the human body and its vital organs. Various sizes and shapes of armour plate are overlayed and statistical analysis carried out of possible shot lines through the body to see whether the plates will give protection.

Overall, mathematical analysis and particularly computer analysis is playing an increasing part in the development of personal protection against ballistic threats. The methods used are still capable of considerable refinement but even in their present state can give very useful information to the developer of body armour.

REFERENCES

Beebe G.W., de Bakey M.E. (1952). *Battle Casualties – Incidence, Mortality and Logistic Considerations*. Chas C Thomas.

Coates J.B., Beyer J.C., eds (1962). *Wound Ballistics*. Washington, DC: Office of the Surgeon General, Department of the Army.

Frechette V.D., Cline C.F. (1970). Fractography of ballistically tested ceramics. *Bull. Am. Ceramic Soc.*, **49**, 994–7.

Kovaric J.J., Aaby G., Hamit H.F., Hardaway R.M. (1969). Vietnam casualty statistics. *Arch. Surg.*, **98**, 150–2.

Laible R.C., Barron F. (1980). *Ballistic Materials and Penetration Mechanics*. Amsterdam: Elsevier Scientific.

Prosser R.A. (1988). Penetration of nylon ballistic panels by fragment simulating projectiles. *Textile Res. J.*, **58**, 161–5.

Shenton S.P., Bashford D.P. (1989). *The Assessment of Frictional Effects in Lightweight Textile Armours using Thermal Imaging*. Fulmer Research Ltd (MOD Contract 3L 31b/3151).

9. Non-penetrating Injuries of the Head

R. Bullock and D. I. Graham

INTRODUCTION

Brain damage after head injury constitutes a major health problem throughout the world. In the UK with a population of about 55 million, it has been estimated that some 1500 patients per 100 000 population per year report to accident and emergency departments because of head injury, of whom between 200 and 300 are admitted to hospital. There are about nine deaths per 100 000 population per year – 1% of all deaths. Head injury is now the most important cause of death and severe disability in children and adults under 45. Recent estimates from the USA have put the annual cost of head injury and the consequent loss of earning capacity at \$35 billion. Some 25% of deaths from trauma and almost 50% of those caused by road traffic accidents are the outcome of head injury. The accumulating population of disabled survivors after head injury is so large now that one family in 300 has a member with such a disability.

Multicentre outcome studies have shown that about 35% of severely head-injured patients will die and between 1 and 5% will remain vegetative. Between 5 and 18% are left severely disabled 6 months after their injury. Among both the severely and more mildly disabled survivors of severe head injury, long-term psychological disorders, such as impairment of memory and intellect, personality disintegration and learning disorders are very frequent, so that premorbid levels of employment and social function are seldom achieved. Given this high prevalence, it is not surprising that the economic and social consequences of head injury have stimulated much research in many countries into its incidence and causes, the nature of the injury sustained and how the morbidity and mortality may be prevented by improved methods of clinical management and of accident prevention.

Descriptive human neuropathological studies, and dynamic pathophysiology studies in a variety of animal models, have now given a clear understanding of the mechanisms of immediate 'primary' damage and the consecutive forms of secondary, delayed damage, which are responsible for death in up to 40% of those who die under medical care. This group is a particular focus of interest for therapy because secondary damage may be preventable (Jones *et al.*, 1994).

Dynamic pathophysiology studies have also led to advances in head-injury prevention, via legislation (e.g. seat belts, helmets) and the design of vehicles. However, our understanding of the mechanisms which allow recovery and regeneration within the injured nervous system are still very poor, despite extensive current research.

The purpose of this chapter is to review the mechanisms of brain damage due to head injury and to relate them to the aims of current and future forms of therapy and research.

Dr Murray Goldstein, head of the National Institute for Neurological Disorders and Stroke, of the National Institute of Health, has recently described head injury as 'the silent epidemic' which has killed more young people in the USA than all the wars in that country's history. He has declared head injury to be the highest priority for future research in the field of neurological disorders, in the hope that brain damage may eventually become both more easily preventable and treatable.

Mechanisms of brain damage

The forces acting on the brain during head injury produce complex movements and deformation. When the freely mobile head is struck by a blunt object, an *acceleration* injury occurs. If the moving head suddenly strikes a blunt object a *deceleration* injury occurs. Sharply focused blows, in contrast, usually produce open brain injuries as a result of penetrating wounds of the skull, especially in the frontobasal region. Various analytical and physical models have made major contributions to the understanding of the mechanisms involved in head injury and have been extensively reviewed (Thibault and Gennarelli, 1985).

Anatomical factors

The human brain weighs about 1.2 kg, and is poorly supported by the falx and·tentorium within the skull. Its soft consistency and absence of intrinsic fibrous supporting structures make it especially vulnerable to shearing forces. The brain is restrained only by the cranial nerves and brain stem at the base, and by the parasagittal bridging veins along the interhemispheric convexity. It 'floats' within the cerebrospinal fluid (CSF) and is thus free to move within its large cranium in relative contrast to the brain of lower mammals. Cerebral atrophy develops at the rate of about 2–3% of brain mass per decade after the age of 40 years, and further increases the mobility of the brain within the skull.

It has been known for many decades that concussion can be reproduced in the laboratory by delivering controlled blows to the freely movable head by a pendulum (*acceleration concussion*), but that this is much more difficult if the head is fixed (*compression concussion*). Following a blow to the head, there may be either *linear* (translational) or *angular* (rotational) movement of the skull. If the blow is directed eccentrically, the result is a combined translational and rotational acceleration type of injury (the classical 'uppercut' in boxing). Pure translational acceleration creates intracranial pressure gradients, while pure rotational acceleration produces rotation of the skull relative to the brain and is particularly likely to tear parasagittal bridging veins.

There are two main hypotheses that have been advanced to account for brain damage incurred at the moment of injury – the *skull distortion/head rotation* hypothesis and the *head translation/cavitation* hypothesis. Holbourn (1945) explained *coup* lesions (contusions that occur directly below the site of injury) and *contrecoup* lesions (contusions located on the side of the brain diametrically opposite the point of injury) on physical principles elaborated by experiments on gelatin models. He postulated that brain damage was due to *rotational acceleration forces*. The main requisite for contrecoup damage was rotational movement of the head in the coronal, sagittal or horizontal plane, or a combination of these, the movement being translated to the brain which collides with its dural compartment, the surfaces of which may be rough, especially in the orbital and temporal areas. At these sites *shear strains* develop to cause *contusion* of the brain and tearing of blood vessels.

This theory was supported by direct observations of brain movement in monkeys fitted with transparent lucite calvaria. It was found that when the head was free to move, blows to the head caused swirling rotational movements of the brain within the cranium. Brain damage may also occur as a result of cavitation (bubble formation) because of short duration reductions in intracranial pressure.

Recent work has shown that skull distortion and rotation of the head are more important in the production of coup and contrecoup injuries than either rotation alone or translation/cavitation. Concussion is produced much more readily by angular acceleration than by translation or acceleration. Even though various experimental models have provided a substantial body of knowledge about the immediate physiology of cerebral concussion, many of the animals in these experiments were either only briefly unconscious or died rapidly; the very common clinical condition of prolonged post-traumatic unconsciousness (caused by diffuse injury) was notably absent. In the last few years attempts have been made to mechanically reproduce the prolonged coma seen in patients after head injury in the absence of intracranial haematomas. These non-human primate experiments used the Penn I (Adams *et al.*, 1982) and Penn II (Gennarelli and Thibault, 1982) devices, which are based on inertial, that is *non-impact*, controlled angular acceleration of the head through 60 degrees

in the sagittal/lateral plane. Initial work showed that at low and moderate acceleration levels, cerebral concussion with and without contusions in the frontal and temporal lobes was readily produced, but at high acceleration, the animals died rapidly from massive subdural haematomas. It is now possible to reproduce experimentally almost all of the types of brain damage which occur in man as the result of a non-missile head injury (Gennarelli, 1994).

There are remarkably close similarities in the principal neuropathological findings in patients who die as a result of a blunt head injury and in non-human primates subjected to angular acceleration as described above. These studies have shown that all the principal neuropathological features of head injury can be induced by the two phenomena – *contact* and *acceleration*. Features due to contact result from an object striking the head, and produce local effects such as scalp laceration, skull fracture, extradural haematoma, and some types of cerebral contusion and intracerebral haemorrhage. Acceleration, in contrast, results in movement of the brain which leads to intracranial and intracerebral pressure gradients as well as shear, tensile and compressive strains. Such inertial mechanisms are responsible for the two most important types of damage encountered in man – *acute subdural haematoma* resulting from tearing of subdural bridging veins and *diffuse damage to axons*.

An understanding of these dynamic pathophysiological events has led to major improvements in the design of motor vehicle interiors, seat belts, crash helmets and aerospace equipment such as aircraft ejection seats.

CLASSIFICATION OF BLUNT HEAD INJURY

Many approaches to the classification of brain damage due to head injury have been proposed. The distinction between *primary* and *secondary* damage has been emphasized in an attempt to provide clinicopathological correlation and to exploit options for therapy. This approach helps to identify potentially preventable secondary effects in patients who either 'talk and die' or 'talk and deteriorate' – the clearest hallmarks of delayed damage (Reilly *et al.*, 1975; Jennett and Carlin, 1978). This also emphasizes that an apparently trivial head injury may set in motion a cascade of events leading to death or severe persistent disability. Primary damage, occurring at the moment of injury, usually takes the form of cortical surface contusions, haematomas and lacerations, diffuse axonal injury and damage to cranial nerves. Secondary damage is usually produced by complicating processes that are *initiated* at the moment of injury but do not present clinically for a period of time after the injury. The major causes are intracranial haemorrhage, brain swelling, ischaemic

TABLE 9.1

<small>DATA FROM A CONSECUTIVE SERIES OF 635 FATAL NON-MISSILE HEAD INJURIES OVER A 15-YEAR PERIOD (1968–82) ON WHOM POST-MORTEM EXAMINATIONS WERE UNDERTAKEN IN THE INSTITUTE OF NEUROLOGICAL SCIENCES, GLASGOW. FOR DEFINITION OF TYPES OF DAMAGE, SEE TEXT</small>

Sex:

497 males		(78%)
138 females		(22%)

Type of injury:

Road traffic accident	335	(53%)
Falls	222	(35%)
Assaults	31	(5%)
Other	47	(7%)

Incidence of:

Fracture of the skull		75%	
Surface contusions*		94%	(mild in 6%, moderate in 78%, severe in 10%)
Gliding contusions		31%	
Intracranial haematoma[†]		60%	
Extradural	10%		
Subdural	18%		
Intracerebral	16%		
'Burst lobe'	23%		
Diffuse axonal injury[‡]		29%	
Brain stem damage secondary to a raised intracranial pressure		53%	
Hypoxic brain damage[§]		55%	
Brain swelling		53%	(34% unilateral, 17% bilateral)
Intracranial infection		4%	

Note: Some of the figures are approximate, since full histological studies were undertaken on only 434 of the 635 cases.
* Measured quantitatively using the contusion index technique (see Adams *et al.*, 1985).
† Some patients had more than one haematoma.
‡ 122 cases (see Adams *et al.*, 1989).
§ Cases with hypoxic damage in arterial boundary zones, and of diffuse type.

brain damage, infection and raised intracranial pressure. Both primary and secondary factors coexist in most patients with severe injury, and Table 9.1 and Figure 9.1 show the incidence and overlap of the causes of damage found in a series of 635 head-injury patients in Glasgow who died and underwent detailed neuropathological evaluation (Adams and Graham, 1988; Adams, 1990).

Computerized tomography (CT) has played a very important role in the diagnostic evaluation of head-injured patients and magnetic resonance imaging (MRI) has provided important information for the diagnosis and classification of traumatic shearing lesions during life (Jenkins *et al.*, 1986; Gentry *et al.*, 1988). It is however important to realize that neither hypoxic damage nor diffuse axonal injury can be diagnosed with certainty in life, nor by macroscopic examination of the brain,

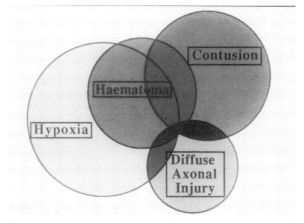

Figure 9.1 Venn diagram to show the mechanisms of brain damage in patients who die after severe head injury, and the extent to which they overlap.

which may appear entirely normal; detailed histological study is always necessary. Diagnosis in life thus rests upon deductions based on the history, clinical features and imaging.

Primary damage: contact phenomena

The principal lesions are scalp lacerations, skull fracture and surface contusions (Adams, 1990).

Scalp lacerations

These are of medicolegal importance, as an indicator of the site of injury. They are important sources of blood loss, particularly in children and, if there is an associated fracture of the skull, they may be potential routes for intracranial infection.

Skull fractures

In general, the more severe the injury the greater the likelihood of skull fracture. The frequency of fracture therefore varies according to the head-injury population that is studied. A frequency of 3% has been reported among accident/emergency attenders, rising to 65% of patients admitted to a neurosurgical unit and to 80% in fatal cases (Jennett and Teasdale, 1981). The vault is involved three times more often than the base but there may be fractures in both sites. Skull fracture is however by no means an invariable finding in fatal head injury. Post-mortem experiments have shown that the skull may deform inwards for up to several centimetres at the moment of impact, before springing back to its normal position, with or without fracturing (Ford and McLaurin, 1963; Bullock and Teasdale, 1990a,b). Considerable underlying damage may thus be incurred, the most obvious example being the development of an extradural haematoma (see below). The importance of a skull fracture cannot be overemphasized because patients with a fracture have a high incidence of intracranial haematoma (about 1 in 10). With radiological evidence of skull fracture, *and* any impairment of consciousness, some 1 in 4 of patients in an accident and emergency department or primary surgical ward will be shown to have an intracranial haematoma; without fracture and with normal consciousness the risk is 1 in 6000 (Mendelow *et al.*, 1983). The presence of a skull fracture is thus an important factor in triage of those patients who remain conscious after their injury; all such patients should undergo a CT scan and should be treated with prophylactic antibiotics (Servadei *et al.*, 1988; Bullock and Teasdale, 1990a).

In about 10% of patients the fracture of the vault is *depressed* and is classified as *compound* if there is an associated laceration of the skull and *penetrating* if there is also a tear of the dura. Both are very important as potential sources for intracranial infection. Depressed fracture is also associated with an increased incidence of post-traumatic epilepsy

(Jennett, 1974). Intracranial infection may be a complication of fractures of the base of the skull, because the fracture line passes through the air sinuses or the middle ear; hence the clinical importance of CSF rhinorrhoea, otorrhoea and of intracranial aerocele. Basal fractures complicate about 17% of severe head injuries and they are frequently associated with cranial nerve damage, producing anosmia (9%), unilateral blindness, deafness, diplopia and swallowing or speech disorder.

In very severe head injuries there may be a *hinge* fracture that extends across the base of the skull, usually in the region of the posterior part of the pituitary fossa and the adjacent flat parts of the temporal bones. If a patient falls on the occiput there may be an associated *contrecoup* fracture of the roof of the orbits and ethmoid plates.

CSF leak into the middle ear usually closes spontaneously (Jennett and Teasdale, 1981; Cooper, 1987). Other leaks that persist beyond 7–14 days should be managed by surgical repair.

Surface cerebral contusions and lacerations

The pia-arachnoid is intact over contusions but torn in cortical lacerations. Both have long been considered an indication of the severity of injury. Nevertheless, patients with diffuse axonal injury may die from their head injury, yet display only minimal or even no surface contusions.

Surface contusions are most severe at the crests of gyri but may also extend through the cortex into the subcortical white matter. Initially, they are haemorrhagic and swollen, consisting of punctate haemorrhages or streaks of haemorrhage at right angles to the cortical surface (Figure 9.2(a)). If the patient survives they are converted in the long term into shrunken brown scars at the crest of the gyri with loss of cortical substance (Figure 9.2(b)). With the exception of early infancy where contusions appear as tears in the subcortical white matter and in the inner layers of the cortex, particularly in the frontal and temporal lobe, contusions present similar features in all age groups.

Surface contusions have a very characteristic distribution affecting particularly the frontal poles, the orbital surfaces of the frontal lobes, the temporal poles, the lateral and inferior surfaces of the temporal lobes and the cortex above and below the Sylvian fissures. Contusions of the parietal and occipital lobes and of the cerebellum are uncommon unless they are directly related to a fracture of the skull. Because the damage is focal, patients with quite severe contusions may make a smooth and uneventful recovery provided there are no other types of brain damage or complications of the original injury. However, contusions may be responsible for widespread focal cerebral atrophy; when they affect the orbital frontal and temporal regions, they are frequently the cause of the memory loss and personality disintegration which

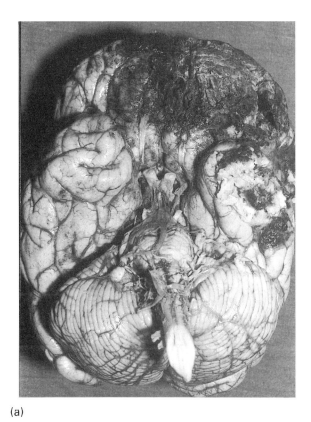

(a)

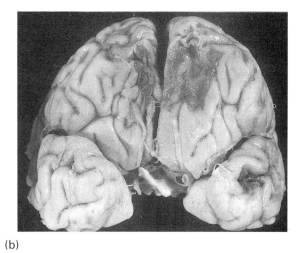

(b)

Figure 9.2 Cerebral contusions. (a) Massive frontal and left temporal contusions are seen in the formalin-fixed brain of a patient who died 3 days after injury. (See Graham, 1990.) (b) Shrunken atrophic cortex on the orbital surface of the frontal lobes and tip of the left temporal lobe due to healed contusions – from a patient who made an apparently complete recovery from a head injury sustained many years previously. (See Graham, 1990.)

are common neuropsychological sequelae of head injury. Healed contusions have been found incidentally in some 2.5% of autopsies in a general hospital (Figure 9.2(b)).

Different categories of surface contusions may give clues to the dynamic mechanisms of injury. They are common beneath the site of a fracture and are most severe when a blow is delivered to the stationary head. Their size depends on the area of contact between the striking object and the skull. By contrast, contrecoup contusions are due to sudden deceleration of the moving head, and the classical example is a fall on the occiput which results in severe contusions to the frontal and temporal poles. Coup and contrecoup contusions must be differentiated from *gliding* ones which are focal shear-induced haemorrhages in the cortex and subjacent white matter, occurring at the superior crests of the cerebral hemispheres. They are a common finding in cases of diffuse axonal injury (see below).

Cerebral contusions may be quantified by the *contusion index* which takes into account the depth and extent of contusions in various parts of the brain (Adams *et al.*, 1985). The use of this index has established that contusions are significantly more severe when a skull fracture is present and are significantly less severe in patients who die with diffuse axonal injury. Contusions are also more severe in patients who do not experience a lucid interval during life than in those who do.

Pathogenesis Surface contusions and lacerations are due mainly to contact between the surface of the brain and the rough and irregular bony surfaces of the base of the skull as a result of sudden deceleration of the skull in which the brain has been rotating.

Histologically, cerebral contusions are characterized by three features:

1. Streaky haemorrhages which are usually peri-vascular and which may be as small as a few hundred red cells or several centimetres in extent. Obvious tears in vessels and thrombi are both surprisingly infrequent. Red blood cells have been shown to pass through the apparently intact walls of small capillaries, after contusions in humans.
2. Swelling and vacuolation of the neuropil – this is chiefly due to gross swelling of astrocytes especially perivascular astrocytic foot processes. This may progress to cause compression of the lumens of capillaries and small arterioles (Figure 9.3). This process causes pallor of staining of the cortex and is cytotoxic oedema.
3. Vacuolation, and later pyknosis, shrinkage and death of neurones.

Astrocytic swelling and neuronal pyknosis extend many millimetres beyond the margins of the haemorrhagic focus. Shear stress with deformation of neuronal and glial membranes, may cause loss of

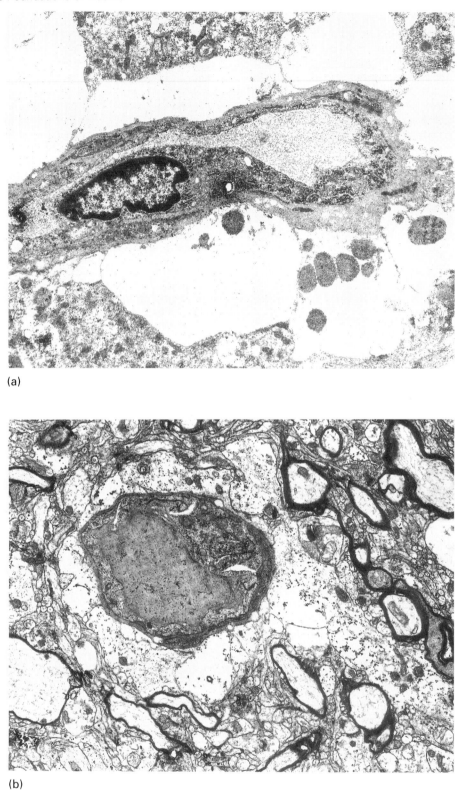

(a)

(b)

Figure 9.3 Transmission electron micrographs after human cerebral contusion. (a) Thin section through a cortical capillary to show flattening of the vessel lumen and massive swelling of the perivascular astrocytic foot processes (a); the lumen is narrowed so that passage of red cells would be impossible. Magnification × 10 500. (b) A cortical capillary, day 5 after injury – note that the perivascular astrocytic swelling is less marked. The tight junctions between the endothelial cells, however, remain intact. Magnification × 8200.

ionic homeostasis, with efflux of K$^+$ and entry of Na$^+$ into neurones. Harmful neuromodulators and transmitters, such as excitatory amino acids, free radicals, polyamines and free Ca^{2+}, may be released, to exacerbate damage in adjacent neurones.

Mapping studies of blood flow and blood–brain barrier with single photon emission computed tomography (SPECT) have also shown in every case studied that zones of profoundly reduced cerebral blood flow are present around focal contusions. In about a third of cases, a halo of blood–brain barrier breakdown develops in the 2–5 days after injury, and in such instances represents a potential mechanism for delayed vasogenic cerebral oedema and swelling of the contused brain which will cause secondary elevation in intracranial pressure (ICP) and brain shift (Figure 9.4) (Bullock and Teasdale, 1990a). Delayed swelling is an important complication which may cause death 3–10 days after injury even in those with focal contusions at presentation, who may have been fully lucid. Features on CT scan, such as effacement of basal cisterns (an indicator of brain swelling), midline shift and prominent mass effect and oedema, then become an indication for such contusions to be prophylactically resected, or managed by intracranial pressure monitoring, even in those who are conscious (Galbraith and Teasdale, 1981; Bullock and Teasdale, 1990a).

In the future, therapy with drugs which may limit secondary neuronal necrosis by blocking the effects of excitatory amino acids, cytokines or free radical species may limit brain damage due to contusion. Agents which stabilize the blood–brain barrier may be beneficial by preventing delayed swelling. Unfortunately, several trials with corticosteroids, even in very high doses have failed to show clinical benefit.

Primary damage: acceleration/deceleration phenomena

Principal consequences are diffuse axonal injury and diffuse vascular injury.

Diffuse axonal injury

Immediate prolonged unconsciousness unaccompanied by an intracranial mass lesion occurs in almost 50% of patients with severe head injury and is the chief clinical indicator of diffuse axonal injury. It is the major neuropathological finding in about 35% of all deaths. Diffuse axonal injury was first described by Strich (1956) in a series of patients with post-traumatic dementia as 'diffuse degeneration of white matter'. This type of brain damage is now widely recognized and has been referred to by a variety of names and more recently as 'diffuse axonal injury – DAI' (Adams, 1990). The degeneration of white matter was attributed by Strich to shearing injury affecting nerve fibres at the time of the original injury. The concept that DAI is indeed a form of primary brain damage has, however, not remained unchallenged. Thus, some have suggested that this form of damage to white matter is due to hypoxia, oedema or is secondary to damage to the brain stem resulting from an intracranial expanding lesion. Diffuse axonal injury identified by silver impregnation was present in varying degrees of severity in about 30% of the cases in the Glasgow Database (Adams *et al.*, 1989). By immunohistochemistry using an antibody to the precursor protein of amyloid (Blumbergs *et al.*, 1994) DAI can be identified in about 90% of fatal cases of head injury (Gentleman *et al.*, 1995).

Anatomical and histological findings To make a diagnosis of DAI post mortem, the brain must be properly fixed. In severe cases, two of the three distinctive features may be identified macroscop-

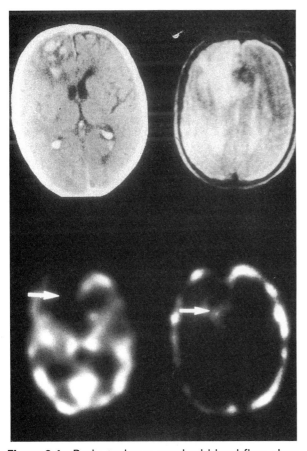

Figure 9.4 Brain oedema, cerebral blood flow changes and blood–brain barrier changes 10 days after focal left frontal contusion. Top left – CT scan. Top right – T$_2$-weighted MRI scan; note the extensive oedema in relation to the contusion. Bottom left – ^{99}Tc^m-labelled HMPAO blood flow map; note the zone of profoundly reduced blood flow (arrowed). Bottom right – ^{99}Tc^m-labelled pertechnetate SPECT map to show blood–brain barrier changed; note the barrier breakdown in relation to the contusion (arrowed).

ically. In milder cases, the diagnosis of DAI may only be possible if appropriate histological studies are undertaken. In severe DAI the three most distinctive features are: a focal lesion in the corpus callosum which usually extends over several centimetres; lies to one side of the midline; often involves the interventricular septum; and is associated with intraventricular haemorrhage (Figure 9.5); small focal lesions in the dorsolateral quadrant of the rostral brain stem adjacent to the superior cerebellar peduncles: and microscopic evidence of widespread damage to axons. The appearances of the individual lesions depend on the length of survival after injury: in a patient surviving for only a few days, the lesions in the corpus callosum and brain stem are usually haemorrhagic.

The histological features of the axonal injury also depend upon the length of survival. If a few days, there are numerous axonal bulbs (reactive axonal swellings) seen in haematoxylin and eosin sections as eosinophilic swellings on nerve fibres in silver-stained preparations and as argyrophilic swellings (Figure 9.6(a). These axonal bulbs are widely distributed, although neither uniformly nor symmetrically. For example, they are particularly common in the parasagittal white matter, in the corpus callosum (both adjacent to and remote from the focal lesions noted above), in the internal capsule, in deep grey matter and in various tracts in the brain stem including the medial lemnisci, the medial longitudinal bundles, the central tegmental tracts and the corticospinal tracts. In addition to typical axonal swellings, coarse varicosities in axons may also occur. If the patient survives weeks, multiple clusters of microglia are seen throughout the white matter of the brain (Figure 9.6(b)); in addition there are enlarged astrocytes and lipid-filled macrophages. Survival for 2–3 months is associated with the detection of myelin breakdown products by the Marchi technique in the white matter of the cerebral hemispheres, cerebellum, ascending and descending fibre tracts of the brain stem and in the descending tracts of the spinal column (Figure 9.6(c)).

In those who survive months or years, external abnormality may be minimal and may be limited to small healed surface contusions, and ventricular enlargement because of reduction in the bulk of white matter (Figure 9.7). Indeed, naked-eye abnormalities may be difficult to identify, so that a pathologist, unaware of the syndrome, may find it hard to reconcile the apparently normal appearances of the brain with the persistent post-traumatic vegetative state of the patient.

Clinical features There are few specific clinical, radiological or biochemical features of DAI which make it easy to establish the diagnosis during life and the clinical and radiological picture in an individual patient is usually the result of a number of coexisting pathological processes. Patients with 'pure' DAI form a distinct group characterized clinically by a high incidence of injury due to road traffic accidents and infrequent lucid intervals. They have a lower incidence of fracture of the skull, cerebral contusions, intracranial haematomas; when compared to patients without this type of brain damage high intracranial pressure is infrequent. Gliding contusions are frequent, as are haematomas in the deep grey matter (basal ganglia

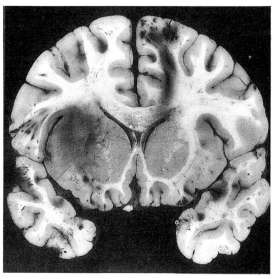

(a)

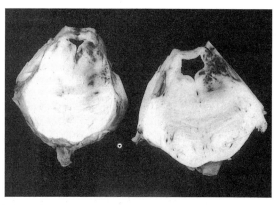

(b)

Figure 9.5 Diffuse axonal injury. (a) Section through the formalin-fixed brain of a patient who died 32 hours after injury. Note the 'gliding contusion' at the apex of the parasagittal cortex. There is also a lesion of the corpus callosum and petechial haemorrhage, and a deep basal ganglia haematoma is apparent on the contralateral side. (See Graham, 1990.) (b) Sections through the brain stem of a patient who survived 6 days after a head injury. There is a haemorrhagic lesion in the dorsolateral quadrant of the rostral pons. (See Graham, 1990.)

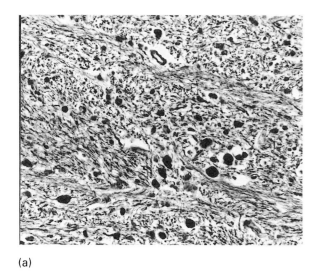

(a)

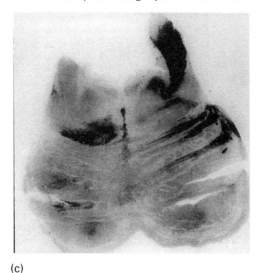

(c)

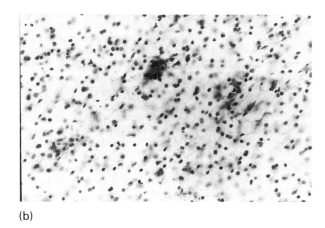

(b)

Figure 9.6 Histological features of diffuse axonal injury. (a) Many black, oval or circular axonal swellings (axonal bulbs) can be seen in the brain stem of a patient who survived 5 days after a head injury. Palmgren × 190. (See Graham, 1990.) (b) 'Microglial stars' forming within the white matter tracts 6 weeks after severe head injury. Cresyl Violet × 76. (See Graham, 1990.) (c) Section through the midpons in a patient who died 7 months after severe diffuse axonal injury. Degeneration (seen as black staining) can be seen in the superior cerebellar peduncle, medial lemniscus and corticospinal tracts. Marchi × 2.5. (See Graham, 1990.)

haematomas) of the cerebral hemispheres and the hippocampus. Typical DAI has also been described in a small number of patients who have fallen from a height (Adams, 1990) or have been assaulted (Graham *et al.*, 1992). Occasional patients demonstrate the classical macroscopic features of DAI on CT scan or MR imaging; in such instances the prognosis is uniformly poor (Figure 9.8) (Jenkins *et al.*, 1986).

DAI may be one of the most important factors which determines outcome after head injury and, in particular, it may be the cause of delayed recovery of intellectual function after minor head injury (Blumbergs *et al.*, 1994). It is of interest that microglial stars have been identified in the white matter of patients after even minor head injury, when weeks later death has occurred because of an unrelated cause. It therefore seems likely that the incidence of DAI – particularly the milder grades – is much higher than published figures suggest.

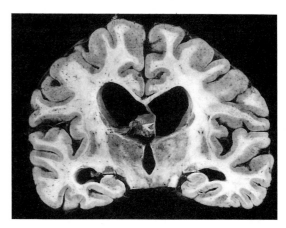

Figure 9.7 Diffuse axonal injury and persistent vegetative state. Coronal section through the brain of a patient who died 21 months after a severe head injury. There is marked enlargement of the ventricular system. (See Graham, 1990.)

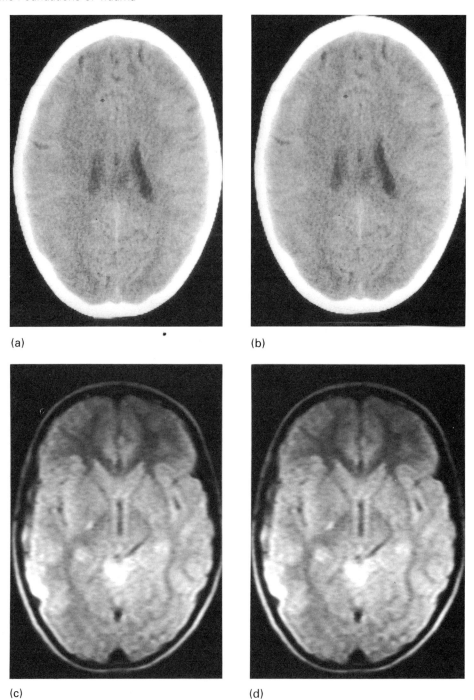

(a)

(b)

(c)

(d)

Figure 9.8 The appearances of diffuse axonal injury on MRI and CT scanning. (a), (b) Magnetic resonance image ((a), left; (b), right) – T$_2$-weighted scan to show the dorsolateral quadrant brain stem lesion, corpus callosum haematoma and deep white matter shearing injury. (c), (d) CT scan cuts ((c), left; (d), right) to show diffuse axonal injury.

Pathogenesis New insights into the pathogenic mechanisms by which mechanical shear stress cause damage to axons and dendrites has recently been provided by studies in a number of animal models. These concepts have been reinforced by observations in man. There is now support for the hypothesis that both functional and anatomical interruption of axons (*axotomy*) may not occur instantaneously at the moment of injury: axotomy may require up to 24 hours to be complete and there is now some early evidence from experimental studies that this process may be influenced by pharmacological manipulations (Povlishock and Jenkins, 1995).

Classic neurohistological techniques have long established that reactive axonal swellings (axonal bulbs) require 18–24 hours of survival to appear in the human brain, although such patients will usually manifest ongoing or transient loss of consciousness which implies functional interruption of axonal function. Evidence in support of delayed or secondary axotomy has been obtained from post-mortem studies. For example, in a recently documented series of patients with DAI found at post-mortem one-third were able to speak after injury prior to death (Blumbergs et al., 1989). Within the Glasgow head injury database, 17 patients of the 122 with histological evidence of DAI also demonstrated a lucid interval by being able to speak after injury.

DAI, with a pattern remarkably similar to that seen in humans, has been achieved in non-human primates using the PENN II acceleration device. Good correlation was found between the duration of the acceleration impulse and the severity of the DAI. High-energy acceleration with longer impulse times tended to cause the most severe DAI, particularly when a lateral rotational component was used rather than purely sagittal acceleration. More sudden brief deceleration forces were associated with tearing of the parasagittal bridging veins and formation of acute subdural haematoma, especially when the head was rotated obliquely. Although the PENN model studies have unequivocally demonstrated that DAI is the result of shear forces applied to the brain, the biomechanical complexity of the model and the severity of the injuries sustained has limited its usefulness for studying the metabolic and biochemical correlates.

A fluid percussion injury model has been devised to transmit shear forces to the brain while the cranium is kept stationary. A brief impact of measured duration and energy may be transmitted to the brain of an anaesthetized animal by hydraulically coupling a fluid-filled cylinder and piston system to the closed skull. The model has been modified and refined to eliminate focal contusion at the site of impact. It has been used for both cats and rats and produces unconsciousness of variable duration, depending upon the magnitude of injury. Histological studies have demonstrated axonal bulbs and microglial stars within the deep white matter, particularly the brain stem near the ponto-mesencephalic junction. Although such models lack the ability to faithfully reproduce the primate patterns of injury as seen in the PENN II device, they have been important in improving our understanding of the mechanism of post-traumatic brain damage (Povlishock, 1992; Marmarou et al., 1994).

Erb and Povlishock (1988) have performed carefully time-sequenced electron-microscopical studies in cats and non-human primates after fluid percussion injury. These have shown that the first abnormality to develop within a few minutes of injury is swelling within the laminae of the myelin sheath at the node of Ranvier, maximal near points of angulation in the course of an axon. Membrane-bound blebs of extruded axoplasm occur within which there is an accumulation of axoplasmic organelles and cytoskeletal components at the site of swelling. In some axons these changes progress and anterograde axonal transport ceases. The axoplasm is then gradually 'pinched off' so that the reactive axonal swelling begins to form proximal to the site of the abnormality and axoplasm distally shrinks and becomes metabolically inactive. By 18–24 hours, a fully developed axonal bulb forms proximal to the discontinuity which then becomes complete. Distal degeneration of the axon then develops, followed weeks or months later by Wallerian degeneration of the axon and neurone as a whole.

Biochemical studies have been performed by Faden et al. (1989) and Katayama et al. (1990) using the microdialysis technique to continuously monitor fluxes in ions and neurotransmitters within the extracellular space immediately after fluid percussion injury. Their studies in anaesthetized rats have shown that deformation of neural tissue by a shear stress results in the immediate massive efflux of K^+ into the extracellular space, together with concomitant release of excitatory amino acids, particularly glutamate. In the rat fluid percussion model, the ion flux persists for only about 5–10 minutes, and K^+ efflux may be substantially reduced by tetrodotoxin – an agent which selectively blocks ion flux through voltage gated channels.

It is likely that deformation of axonal or dendritic membranes in response to a shear stress results in instant depolarization and massive ion flux, which is followed by localized peri-axonal swelling and cessation of axonal function. Excitatory amino acids may open agonist-operated ion channels to exacerbate this process and allow calcium entry into the axoplasm which could initiate damage to intra-axonal organelles and disaggregation of the microtubular system.

The behavioural correlates of fluid percussion injury have been studied in rats by using different types of maze to test memory and beam walking and rotating rod tasks so as to test motor control. A close correlation was shown between the magnitude of injury and duration of memory defects and motor disturbance (Lyeth et al., 1992). These authors have also investigated the effect of pretreatment with muscarinic cholinergic antagonists (scopolomine) and potent glutamate antagonists (MK-801 and CGS 19755) and demonstrated that they are able to ameliorate the effects of fluid percussion injury. These observations suggest that ion flux (particularly calcium) in response to excitatory neurotransmitter release may constitute the major *functional* substrate for shear injury to the nervous system and, moreover, that ion flux of this type is a major factor in determining the transient functional neurological disturbances which are so apparent in human shear injury (Bullock and Fujisawa, 1992).

Primary damage to the brain stem

Although cases with primary focal damage to the midbrain and the pontomedullary junction have been reported (Adams, 1990), we still maintain the view that primary damage to the brain stem does not occur in isolation but rather is part of the clinicopathological entity of diffuse axonal injury. This view is supported by the studies carried out in non-human primates subjected to the Penn I and Penn II devices. The lower brain stem may, however, be focally injured in traumatic hyperextension of the head or fracture-dislocations of the atlanto-occipital joint, or in complex basal skull fractures. Most patients who sustain sufficiently severe head injuries to damage the brain stem do not survive long enough to reach hospital care.

Diffuse shear injury to the cerebral vasculature

Multiple petechial haemorrhages have been referred to as 'diffuse vascular injury'. Such lesions are seen particularly in patients dying within hours or even minutes of injury. They are particularly prominent in the rostral brain stem, especially in the floor of the aqueduct under the rostral part of the fourth ventricle, but they may also occur throughout the brain. In rapidly fatal injuries haemorrhages into the rostral brain stem are usually more numerous and severe than in the medulla, but there have been many examples

where these petechial lesions are limited to the rostral brain stem, the lower stem being normal. Although the pathogenesis of this type of brain damage remains to be established, it does seem possible that acceleration/deceleration impulses can selectively damage blood vessels in the brain. Certainly this type of brain damage is virtually restricted to road traffic accidents.

Diffuse vasomotor paralysis and brain swelling

In addition to causing frank petechial haemorrhage, shear forces appear to cause transient loss of vasomotor control of the cerebral vasculature. In normal physiological circumstances, cerebral vasomotor control is a highly complex process, occurring in pial regulatory arterioles, such that cerebral blood flow is kept constant over the 'autoregulatory range' of mean systemic blood pressure 40–150 mmHg (Figure 9.9). This is mediated predominantly by peptidergic adventitial neural networks with their cell bodies in the brain stem and trigeminal ganglia.

After severe diffuse shear injury, this vasomotor control may be lost, or deranged, so that the brain loses the ability to control its own blood flow in response to changes in systemic blood pressure, $PaCo_2$ and PaO_2 (Lewelt et al., 1982; and see Figure 9.9). This has three major consequences:

1. A mild or moderate fall in systemic blood pressure (eg. to 50–60 mmHg mean), which would normally be compensated for by autoregulation, may severely jeopardize cerebral blood flow, especially in the presence of raised intracranial pressure (ICP), and a secondary ischaemic injury may be induced (see below).

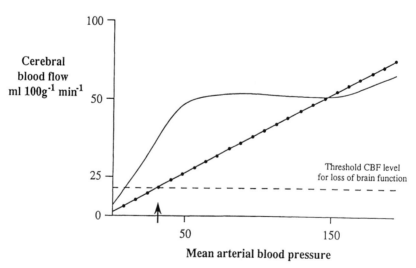

Figure 9.9 The normal cerebral autoregulation curve (solid line) and changes which occur after head injury (dotted line). Note that in the conscious, healthy individual a mean arterial blood pressure of 50–60 mmHg will produce only minimal change in cerebral blood flow (CBF), but in the unconscious head-injured patient the same mean arterial blood pressure may be associated with profoundly reduced cerebral blood flow – sufficient to impair neurological function, or structure.

2. An uncontrolled surge in systemic blood pressure, such as that which always occurs after the moment of injury, or that which may occur in response to pain, vomiting or the Cushing's reflex (see below), may damage the unresponsive vascular bed, to cause massive vasodilatation and consequent brain swelling, or frank petechial haemorrhage, which increases brain bulk (Langfitt *et al.*, 1964).

3. Sudden changes in physiological parameters, such as $PaCo_2$, PaO_2 (as caused by respiratory obstruction) and ICP (e.g. upon removal of a haematoma) may induce massive, uncontrolled vasomotor changes, which may manifest as acute brain swelling, with transtentorial herniation – discussed below (Miller *et al.*, 1978).

Enhanced vulnerability to ischaemic brain damage after axonal shear injury

In a recent series of experiments with the rat fluid percussion injury model, Jenkins *et al.* (1989) have demonstrated that a mild shear injury, insufficient on its own to cause either axonal bulbs or neuronal damage, was able to cause extensive hippocampal neuronal necrosis when an equally mild ischaemic injury (6 minutes of hypotension and carotid occlusion) was added, either 1 or 24 hours later. This enhanced ischaemic vulnerability was abolished by pretreatment with a cholinergic (scopolamine) or glutamatergic (phencyclidene) antagonist, which suggests that the process is receptor mediated.

The clinical implications of these effects on both the cerebral circulation and the neurones themselves are considerable; the injured brain is highly vulnerable to even mild and transient secondary ischaemic injury and rapid changes in blood pressure, PaO_2 and $PaCo_2$ (Miller *et al.*, 1978; Manon *et al.*, 1992; Jones *et al.*, 1994).

Injury to large cerebral vessels

The cavernous part of the carotid artery may be damaged, resulting in a *carotico-cavernous fistula*. Injury to the dura may lead to thrombosis of meningeal arteries and veins and *venous infarction*, and in rare instances *traumatic intracranial aneurysms* or a *dural arteriovenous fistula* may develop. Massive subarachnoid haemorrhage due to traumatic rupture of a vertebral artery may rarely occur, from shearing forces (Adams, 1990). A bruise or laceration below and behind one ear is usual in these cases and most of the victims die very soon after injury.

Damage to cranial nerves

In particular, the olfactory, optic and acoustic nerves may suffer contusion directly or may be torn at the time of injury.

Other types of injury

The *hypothalamus* and *pituitary gland* may also be damaged. There is no doubt that the pituitary stalk can occasionally be torn at the time of head injury and massive infarction of the anterior lobe of the pituitary gland inevitably results. However, most of the damage sustained by the hypothalamus and pituitary stalk is probably secondary to raised ICP and shift and distortion of the brain. Clinically, diabetes insipidus develops rapidly in such cases and may be difficult to control.

Secondary damage

The most important categories are ischaemia, haematomas, brain swelling and infection.

Mechanisms of secondary damage: physiological considerations The adult brain is especially vulnerable to secondary ischaemic damage because of particular physiological, biochemical and anatomical characteristics. There is now evidence that many of the processes concerned with maintenance of energy homeostasis are massively disturbed after severe head injury. The adult brain is totally dependent upon continuous oxygen delivery to maintain its aerobic metabolism. In normal circumstances the brain is predominantly dependent upon aerobic glucose breakdown, although anaerobic glycolysis can occur for brief periods and results in the accumulation of large quantities of lactate and hydrogen ions. Neuronal energy metabolism is directed towards maintenance of the resting membrane potential, ionic homeostasis, and neurotransmitter production and delivery. When oxygen delivery or substrate supply are interrupted for more than a few seconds, the resting membrane potential cannot be maintained and impulse conduction and neurotransmitter function cease. Consciousness is rapidly lost if oxygen and substrate delivery ceases to the whole brain.

Because of the importance of oxygen and substrate delivery to neurones for the brain and therefore the organism as a whole, blood flow to grey matter is the highest for any organ in the body and is precisely regulated to match metabolic demand, which is in turn determined by levels of cerebral function. About 60–70% of cerebral capillaries are perfused during normal mammalian function but this may increase in response to demand; for example, during an epileptic seizure or, to a lesser extent, during a repetitive motor task or abstract mental function. Both the intrinsic peptidergic cerebral vasoregulatory system and 'myogenic', vascular smooth muscle responses to metabolic mediators, such as carbon dioxide and hydrogen ion concentration and the level of adenosine diphosphate (ADP) are important in maintaining this close coupling between flow and metabolism. The responses are lost following diffuse shearing head injury and also after many severe cerebral insults, such as subarachnoid haemorrhage, status epilepticus and global ischaemic cerebral events.

The cerebral cortex requires a continuous perfusion of about 80 ml/100 g/min, in contrast to white matter which requires about 25 ml/100 g/min in the awake human. When cortical cerebral blood flow falls to levels around 20 ml/100 g/min energy metabolism rapidly falls, membrane potential is lost and neurotransmitter function ceases. A further fall to levels below about 18 ml/100 g/min results in a failure of ionic homeostasis and a massive efflux of K^+ and influx of Na^+ into neurones takes place. Extracellular K^+ is buffered by uptake into astrocytes which then swell to produce cytotoxic oedema which may be seen ultrastructurally within minutes after a severe ischaemic event. If blood flow falls to levels around 14–15 ml/100 g/min, intracellular organelles sustain permanent damage (see below) and permanent structural damage with cellular necrosis (pyknosis on light microscopy) will then be seen. The duration of an ischaemic event is also crucial in determining outcome (Figure 9.10). A hierarchy of sensitivity to ischaemia exists within various brain regions – the hippocampus, cerebral cortex, cerebellum and basal ganglia being the most vulnerable; within these regions certain cell types, for example the pyramidal cells of CA1 of the hippocampus, are particularly at risk (Ng *et al.*, 1989).

Several mechanisms may operate after head injury to jeopardize substrate and oxygen delivery to the brain (Marion *et al.*, 1992):

1. Systemic hypotension may reduce CBF below the autoregulatory range.
2. Normal autoregulatory processes may be abolished.

3. Unconsciousness may cause failure to maintain the airway. Aspiration pneumonia, pneumothorax and pulmonary contusion are fairly frequent consequences of severe injury, particularly motor vehicle accidents. All may produce hypoxaemia, sometimes in addition to hypotension.
4. Because the brain is within the closed skull, an expanding intracranial mass (usually in excess of 40 ml) may cause intracranial pressure to approach mean arterial pressure. A cerebral perfusion pressure of 40 mmHg is necessary to maintain adequate CBF when autoregulation is normal; but when autoregulation is impaired, CBF may be reduced even when cerebral perfusion pressure is around 50–60 mmHg (Langfitt *et al.*, 1964; and see below).

Ischaemic damage

This is a most important mechanism of brain damage after severe head injury. In the Glasgow database for the period 1968–72, ischaemic damage was found in 92% of 151 patients who died after head injury (Table 9.2). It was assessed as severe in 27%, moderately severe in 43% and mild in 30%. The highest incidence was in the hippocampus (80%) and the basal ganglia (79%); it was less frequent in the cerebral cortex (46%) and in the cerebellum (44%) (Graham *et al.*, 1978).

Damage in the cerebral cortex took several forms. In the commonest type it was centred on the boundary zones between the distributions of the major cerebral arterial territories, particularly between those of the anterior and middle cerebral arteries. In the majority it was bilateral. This 'watershed' or boundary zone pattern is thought to be largely attributable to a failure of cerebral perfusion. The second most common pattern was diffuse damage in the cortex of both cerebral hemispheres. In the third, it was centred on the territory supplied by the anterior and/or middle cerebral arteries.

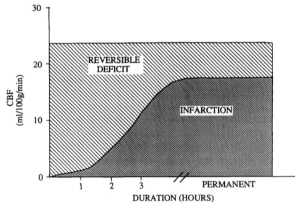

Figure 9.10 The relationship between duration of ischaemia, level of cerebral blood flow (CBF) and cerebral infarction. The data was obtained from healthy, young primates with middle cerebral artery occlusion under anaesthesia. This curve is shifted to the 'left' in humans after head injury where autoregulation is lost and shear damage to membranes may predispose tissues to infarction. (Data redrawn after Jones *et al.*, 1981.)

TABLE 9.2

ISCHAEMIC BRAIN DAMAGE AFTER FATAL HEAD INJURY, OVER TWO TIME PERIODS. (MODIFIED FROM GRAHAM *ET AL.*, 1989A.)

	1968–72	1981–2
Overall incidence	92%	88%
Incidence of haematoma	21%	46%
Incidence of ischaemic damage in the hippocampus	86%	84%
High ICP present during life	26%	49%
Patterns in cortex		
Focal	32%	59%
Boundary zone	8%	8%
Diffuse	9%	24%

The knowledge that much of this ischaemic brain damage could be attributed to a critical reduction in regional cerebral blood flow has led to increased recognition and treatment of hypoxia and hypotension at the scene of the accident, during interhospital transfer and in critical care units. It has given further emphasis to the need for speed in the detection and relief of cerebral compression due to traumatic intracranial haematoma (Bullock and Teasdale, 1990a,b).

As an audit for the effectiveness of such changes in management, a further detailed analysis of a second consecutive series of 112 fatal head injuries in the 2-year period 1981–2 was undertaken. Ischaemic damage was found in the brains of 88%. There was no statistical difference in the proportion of cases with severe or moderately severe ischaemic damage in the two groups, thus emphasizing that ischaemic brain damage is still very frequent and further efforts are required. The available evidence suggests that this type of brain damage occurs soon after injury, and it remains an important cause of mortality and morbidity (Graham *et al.*, 1989a). Indeed, ischaemic brain damage was, after diffuse axonal injury the second most common finding in patients who remain severely disabled or vegetative.

Clinicopathological correlates of ischaemic brain damage

Ischaemic damage is correlated with the following major clinical factors:

1. A known episode of hypoxia (a systolic arterial pressure known to have been less than 80 mmHg for at least 15 minutes or a PaO_2 less than 6.5 kPa (50 mmHg) at some time after the injury).
2. A sustained increase in ICP (> 30 mmHg).

In some instances, the cause of damage can be suspected from the pattern and distribution of the lesions, especially in the cerebral cortex. For example, in over half of the patients in Glasgow where there was diffuse ischaemic damage there had been either an episode of cardiac arrest or status epilepticus. The majority of ischaemic lesions in the cerebral cortex or elsewhere were focal, suggesting that the ischaemic damage was due to a critical reduction in *regional* cerebral blood flow. Cerebral perfusion may be altered not only by systemic hypotension and local factors such as vasospasm, contusions and haematomas, but also by an increase in intracranial pressure. The contribution of relatively small variations in systemic arterial pressure in such circumstances of high ICP and marginal cerebral perfusion pressure may be crucial.

Using established histological criteria (Adams, 1990) ICP at some time during life was assessed as having been high in 125 (83%) of the original series of 151 head-injury deaths and in 97 (87%) of the subsequent series of 112 cases. Evidence of increased ICP is therefore very common in fatalities. However, extensive ischaemic damage can also occur in the absence of high ICP, especially when secondary to status epilepticus or cardiorespiratory arrest. This may reflect activation of excitatory neuronal systems which project into the hippocampus and may contribute to the high frequency of ischaemic damage found in the hippocampus in fatal human head injury.

The frequency and distribution of damage in the hippocampus were studied in a consecutive series of 112 fatal human non-missile head injuries; damage to the hippocampus was noted in 94 (84%) and the lesions always involved the CA1 subfield and were bilateral in 70 (Kotapka *et al.*, 1992). Traditionally, such damage has been considered to be secondary to decreased cerebral perfusion pressure and/or raised ICP; however, hippocampal damage has also been noted in fatal human head injury *without* evidence of a high ICP. This pattern is very similar to that observed in experimental head injury in non-human primates in which the monitoring procedures established with considerable likelihood that the damage was not related to high ICP, hypotension, hypoxia or a significant reduction in cerebral perfusion pressure. Therefore hippocampal damage, which appears on histological examination to be 'ischaemic' in nature, may occur *without* a prior hypoxic/ischaemic episode. Several authors have recently proposed that the mechanism which accounts for the selective vulnerability of the hippocampus in traumatic brain injury involves pathological neuronal activation via excitatory amino acid neurotransmitters, such as glutamate. The increases in glutamate concentration in the extracellular fluid of the hippocampus following fluid percussion brain injury in the rat (Faden *et al.*, 1989) and after subdural haematoma accord with this view. Treatment of rats prior to fluid percussion injury with glutamate receptor antagonists attenuated the hippocampal damage produced in this model, and the same was true of subdural haematoma in the rat (Chen *et al.*, 1991, and see below).

Intracranial haematoma

Intracranial haematoma is a common complication of head injury. Haematomas were present in 55% of the cases in the Glasgow Neuropathology Database, although almost all had been surgically evacuated before death. It is the most common cause of clinical deterioration and death in patients with a lucid interval after injury. Even an apparently trivial head injury can be transformed into a threat to life by the development of an intracranial haematoma. In several series of patients in whom death after head injury might have been prevented by more effective management, almost two-thirds were found to have an intracranial haematoma (Bullock and Teasdale, 1990a).

Neuroradiological investigations have shown that intracranial haematomas are often present long before they produce clinical deterioration. Although some undoubtedly enlarge, the main effects are delayed. The reasons for this are not fully understood. Associated swelling of the brain, and shifts and herniation are probably largely responsible.

Following trauma there may be bleeding into the extradural, subdural or subarachnoid space; into the brain parenchyma; or into the ventricles. Some degree of subarachnoid haemorrhage invariably occurs as a result of surface cerebral contusions and, if the amount is large, it may be a causative factor for vasospasm which is seen in about a third of patients, if a carotid angiogram is done after severe injury. If recovery is slower than expected or if there is late clinical deterioration, hydrocephalus may have developed following a subarachnoid haemorrhage. Intraventricular haemorrhage commonly occurs in patients with diffuse axonal injury (see above) but it is extradural, subdural and intracerebral haematomas that are by far the most important causes of intracranial mass lesions.

Extradural haematoma

Extradural haematoma complicates about 5–15% of fatal head injuries and was recorded in 8% of patients in the Glasgow Database. An overlying fracture of the skull was present in 90% of adult patients (Table 9.3; Marshall et al., 1991; Bullock and Teasdale, 1990a).

Pathogenesis Extradural haematoma is a 'fracture haematoma', which forms because of bleeding from the vascular supply to the dura, and which accumulates in the space created when the dura is stripped from the inner surface of the skull as a consequence of impact deformation. It has shown that the skull deforms inward on impact and springs back to its normal positions thus, separating from the dura. Extradural clots are commonest in young adults, in whom the dura is easily stripped from the calvaria, and rarer in children and the elderly, in whom the dura is densely adherent to the bone. It most commonly develops in relation to a bleed from a meningeal artery – usually the middle meningeal. As the haematoma develops, arterial bleeding may gradually strip off

TABLE 9.3
INCIDENCE AND TYPE OF ACUTE INTRACRANIAL HAEMATOMA AFTER HEAD INJURY.

Author	Population studied	n	Overall haematoma incidence (%)	Type of haematoma (%)				
				Extradural only	Extra and intradural	Subdural only	Subdural and intracerebral	Intracerebral only
Strang et al. (1978)	Emergency room attenders (Scotland)	3568	0.2					
Miller and Jones (1985)	Admission to a neurosurgical unit providing primary care (Edinburgh, UK)	1919	4	22%		34%	44%	
Brocklehurst et al. (1987)	Admission to a neurosurgical unit providing primary care (Hull, UK)	4011	2	29%		53%		18%
Teasdale et al. (1982)	Transfers to Neurosurgery (Glasgow, UK)	Pre CT 223 Post CT 492	34 26	27%	8%	25%	26%	13%
Stone et al. (1983)	Patients in neurosurgical centre (Chicago, USA)	486		8%	5%	70%		17%
Turazzi et al. (1987)	Patients in coma in neurosurgical centre (Italy)	Pre CT 1000 Post CT 385	35 33	25%		41%	34%	
Marshall et al. TCDB (1991)	Patients in four neurosurgical centres (USA)	746	40	12%		60%		28% (including contusions)

more dura mater from the skull and the space occupied by the clot increases (Ford and McLaurin, 1963). A large ovoid mass progressively distorts the adjacent brain. In those who have experienced a lucid interval, there is frequently little evidence of other types of brain damage (Figure 9.11(a)). If, however, the patient has been in coma from the time of the original injury, other types of brain damage are likely to be present.

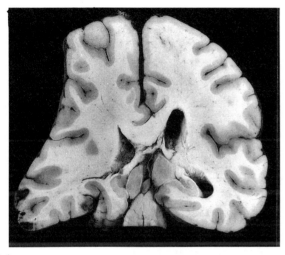

(a)

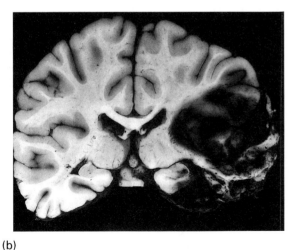

(b)

Figure 9.11 Extradural and intradural haematoma. (a) Section through the formalin-fixed brain of a patient who died with an extradural haematoma *in situ*. Coronal slice of fixed brain showing distortion by the extradural haematoma (left), a shift of the midline structures, asymmetry of the lateral ventricles, a supracallosal hernia and a tentorial hernia. There is a contusion at the crest of the left inferior temporal gyrus. (See Graham, 1990.) (b) 'Burst lobe'. The haematoma in the right temporal lobe was in continuity with an acute subdural haematoma. (See Graham, 1990.)

Extradural haematomas occur most commonly under the thin bone of the squamous part of the temporal bone, but in some 20–30% the haematoma is elsewhere, such as the frontal and parietal regions or within the posterior fossa, and in some of these sites bleeding is from venous sinuses. Occasionally extradural haematomas are multiple.

Extradural haematomas may coexist with intradural ones: between in 5 and 11% of patients in various series (Table 9.3).

It is unusual for an extradural haematoma, on its own, to cause a deterioration in conscious level or focal neurological signs when its volume is less than 40 ml. Small extradurals organize, liquefy, and usually resorb and disappear by 6 weeks after injury. Occasionally, they may calcify (Bullock and Teasdale, 1990a).

Clinical features There is considerable variation in the pattern of presentation, as is the case for intracranial haematomas in general. There seems to be little relationship between the site, size and nature of an intracranial haematoma, and neurological function. Despite extensive study the effect of a haematoma upon brain function remains relatively poorly understood. Larger haematomas, and those in the temporal fossa, tend to cause more fulminant signs; rapidly deteriorating conscious level, contralateral hemiparesis and ipsilateral dilatation of the pupil being the classic features. At the opposite end of the spectrum, several series of chronic extradurals, and extradural haematomas which were sufficiently asymptomatic not to require surgery, have now been reported.

The variable clinical features, and the dire consequences of failure to diagnose an extradural haematoma – the most eminently treatable clinical entity in head injury – means that management of head-injured patients must be by strictly applied algorithms or protocols, to ensure that all those at risk of a haematoma undergo a CT scan as early as possible after injury (see below).

Subdural haematoma
Subdural haematomas which are sufficiently large to act as significant intracranial expanding lesions, complicate between 26 and 63% of severe head injuries (Table 9.3). Most occur together with a 'burst lobe' (Figure 9.11(b)) but 'pure' subdural haematomas were found in 13% of the patients in the Glasgow Database. In that the blood spreads freely throughout the subdural space they may develop very rapidly. The haematoma tends to cover the entire hemisphere, so that the volume of a subdural haematoma is usually greater than that of an extradural one. Thin bilateral acute subdural haematomas are common in acutely fatal injuries. The mortality and morbidity are far greater in patients with subdural haematoma than in those with an extradural haematoma because of asso-

ciated focal and diffuse shear-induced brain damage. Only about 30–40% of patients who have a subdural evacuated make a good recovery, while 70–80% do so after an extradural has been removed (Jennett and Teasdale, 1981; Cooper, 1987; Tyson, 1987).

Clinical studies have shown that, in 72% of patients with an acute subdural haematoma, the injury is produced by a fall or an assault, whereas only 24% result from a road traffic accident. This is in marked contrast to patients without mass lesions who are in coma for more than 24 hours; 89% are from road traffic accidents and only 10% from falls and assaults (Gennarelli and Thibault, 1982). The reason for this pattern of aetiology is apparent from studies in animal models (see below).

Pathogenesis Acute subdural haematomas are caused by rupture of the bridging veins, or by a small tear in a cortical artery. When caused by the former mechanism, there may be very little evidence of other brain damage. This is the pattern most often seen in boxers. The latter may be an isolated event, often seen in elderly patients and occurring in response to a relatively minor head injury. Tearing of vascular adhesions between the cortical artery and the dura have been demonstrated. When acute subdural haematoma is associated with massive contusions, usually of the temporal or frontal poles, the pial surface becomes pulped and lacerated and small arteries may tear causing bleeding both into the contused brain and subdural space. The term 'burst lobe' is then used. In the Glasgow Database a burst lobe was found in 26% of patients who died after head injury.

Studies with the Penn I and Penn II models of head injury have shown that the subdural bridging veins are sensitive to the rate at which they are deformed by acceleration/deceleration (i.e. they are strain-rate sensitive). A rapidly applied, low-energy deceleration force caused large acute subdural haematomas, which were rapidly fatal as a result of brain swelling. With the Penn II device where the duration of acceleration impulse is longer, and the energy greater, the bridging veins did not rupture but prolonged coma and DAI were produced. This explains the frequency of acute subdural haematoma in patients who fall, in whom the period of deceleration is shorter than in patients who are involved in road traffic accidents.

A number of aspects of the pathophysiology of acute subdural haematomas remain poorly understood. For example, it is difficult to understand how bleeding from a low-pressure venous source can continue until the brain is compressed, and midline shift is produced.

Swelling of the hemisphere under an acute subdural haematoma is a frequent CT finding even when the haematoma is thin. Such swelling often persists after the haematoma is evacuated so that

ICP remains high postoperatively. It may develop peroperatively over a few minutes, once the haematoma has been removed and perfusion has been restored (Figure 9.12). This swelling is probably due to dilatation of a vascular bed with severely deranged autoregulation. It may be one of the most difficult complications for the neurosurgeon to manage (Bullock and Teasdale, 1990a).

Neuropathological studies have shown that ischaemic brain damage is present in about two-thirds of the hemispheres where an overlying acute subdural haematoma had been present, which suggests that the presence of the blood may

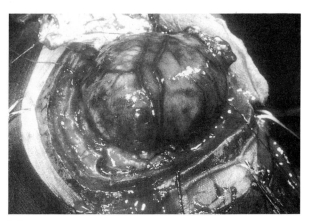

(a)

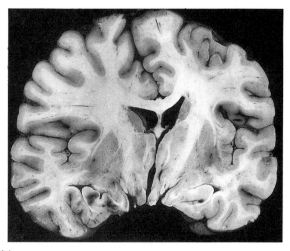

(b)

Figure 9.12 Acute hemispheric swelling. (a) Massive intraoperative swelling of the left cerebral hemisphere after removal of an acute subdural haematoma. Note the discoloration of the cortex due to petechial haemorrhage. (b) Coronal section at the level of the foramen of Munro. There is diffuse swelling of the left hemisphere, i.e. on the same side from which an acute subdural haematoma had been evacuated. (See Graham, 1990.)

be locally harmful. There are similar findings in studies with a rat model of acute subdural haematoma. In this, a severe reduction in local cerebral blood flow developed within the cortex under the haematoma, together with a massive increase in glucose metabolism, seen in the 'peri-ischaemic' cortex, and the hippocampus (Miller *et al.*, 1990). This increase in metabolism was associated with a sevenfold increase in extracellular glutamate, suggesting that an 'excitotoxic' process may be implicated in the brain damage which is so frequent in patients who develop an acute subdural haematoma (Chen *et al.*, 1991). We have recently mapped cerebral blood flow distribution in patients with acute subdural haematomas *in situ* and shown marked reductions in flow in the hemisphere under the clot which support the experimental findings.

Clinical features As for extradural haematoma, the clinical features are extremely variable. Between 60 and 70% of patients who demonstrate an acute subdural clot on CT scanning will have a skull fracture, and from 55–70% will have been lucid at some time, emphasizing the importance of *secondary* (and thus avoidable) brain damage in the 60% of patients who fail to make a good recovery after removal of the clot.

Many authors have proposed classifications for acute subdural haematoma, depending on the time which has elapsed between injury and diagnosis, and upon the appearances at surgery. However, with increasing use of CT scanning early after injury, such approaches have become less relevant. An acute clotted subdural haematoma has high CT density compared to brain for about 7–10 days, after which liquefication progressively occurs, with a change to isodensity and later hypodensity. Isodense and hypodense collections are now generally termed chronic subdurals – more usually haematomas (black, tarry liquid; 'old engine oil'), but sometimes hygromas (clear yellow, proteinaceous fluid).

The relationship between acute and chronic subdural haematomas remains poorly understood. Many patients with small, asymptomatic acute subdural haematomas unassociated with mass effect on CT, have now been followed by serial CT scanning and, in most of these, the haematoma disappears within 2–3 weeks. Recent clinical studies have shown that this almost always occurs when the haematoma is less than 10 mm thick, while larger subdurals tend to become chronic requiring burr hole drainage of a liquefied and enlarging chronic haematoma (Matthew *et al.*, 1995).

During the process of resorption, acute inflammatory changes are seen on the dural and pial surfaces adjacent to the clot and neutrophil and fibroblast activity together with neovascularization are very prominent. At this stage, blood–brain barrier mapping studies have shown a 'band' of barrier breakdown on both the pial and dural surfaces.

Clinical features: chronic subdural haematoma and hygroma These lesions may cause a wide range of neurological manifestations, ranging from headache, vomiting and papilloedema, to hemiparesis, transient ischaemic attacks, progressive dementia, akinetic mutism, meningism and behaviour disturbances (Cooper, 1987). Despite increasingly early diagnosis by CT, they are still found unexpectedly at post-mortem. Although management by burr hole drainage and copious washing of the subdural space is effective in the majority, recurrences develop in at least a third of patients, and may occasionally necessitate craniotomy (Tyson *et al.*, 1980).

Chronic subdural haematoma These may present weeks or months after a head injury that may have seemed at the time to have been trivial. In 50% of cases, there is no history of injury at all. The haematoma becomes encapsulated in a vascular membrane and slowly increases in size, possibly as a result of repeated small haemorrhages into it until it becomes large enough to produce symptoms attributable to distortion of the brain and raised ICP. Chronic subdural haematoma is particularly common in older age groups in whom there is already some cerebral atrophy, in infants with non-accidental injury and those with shunts *in situ* for hydrocephalus. As the haematoma expands slowly the period of spatial compensation may be so long that there may be considerable distortion of the brain before there is any significant rise in ICP. Death is usually due to herniation secondary to the increased ICP in untreated cases. Recent studies using radiolabelled red cells have shown chronic subdural haematomas to be dynamic lesions with a turnover of 10% of their volume per day (Ito *et al.*, 1976). Two major factors appear to be responsible for the ongoing haemorrhage: production of fibrin degradation products in the fluid and friable new vessel formation in the capsule, with a widely patent blood–brain barrier, which may allow passage of red cells in and out of the haematoma (Bullock and Teasdale, 1990a).

Subdural haematoma of infancy A haematoma may develop after a traumatic delivery or a fall. It is also the most common type of intracranial injury found in infants subjected to non-accidental injury, particularly the 'shaking injury' (Leestma, 1988); other evidence of injury should be sought and it is advisable to undertake a skeletal survey. The haematoma may contain clotted blood but often it is chronic and consists of encapsulated xanthochromic fluid – a subdural hygroma.

Intracerebral haematoma

These were found in some 15% of patients in the Glasgow Database. They may be single or multiple and occur principally in the subfrontal and temporal regions or less commonly in the cerebellum (Figure 9.13).

It may be difficult to clearly differentiate a post-traumatic intracerebral haematoma from a 'burst lobe', or severe focal contusion. In Glasgow the term 'haematoma' is applied to a CT lesion which is chiefly of high density (clotted blood) while a lesion of predominantly low density, or patchy, mixed density, is termed a contusion, or 'burst lobe'. At post-mortem, the distinction may be much clearer. In general, the pathophysiological consequences of both intracerebral haematoma and contusions are similar and many simply classify haematomas as

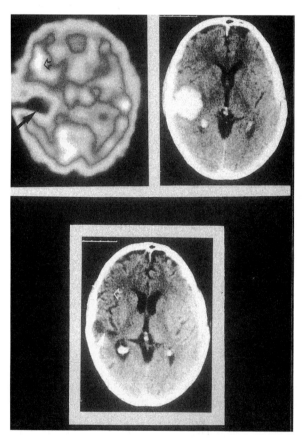

Figure 9.13 Post-traumatic intracerebral haematoma. Top right – CT scan demonstrating a right temporoparietal intracerebral haematoma. Top left – ^{99}Tc^m-labelled HMPAO cerebral blood flow mapping study demonstrating a profound flow defect extending around the intracerebral haematoma (solid arrow). There is also a zone of increased cerebral blood flow in the parietal cortex adjacent to the haematoma – focal hyperaemia (open arrow). Bottom – CT scan made 3 months after haematoma evacuation. Note the small tissue defect at the site of the haematoma (solid arrow), and preservation of tissue at the site of pre-existing hyperaemia (open arrow).

extradural and intradural, the latter being five times more frequent than the former.

Studies in animal models have shown that expansion of an intracerebral haematoma continues until a pressure gradient of about 40 mmHg develops between the haematoma core and surrounding brain, to limit further expansion (Langfitt, 1968). This in turn induces an ischaemic zone surrounding the lesion, in which cytotoxic oedema is very prominent, and probably worsens over the first few days. A delayed, vasogenic oedema component has been shown to develop in two-thirds of a group of 22 patients with contusions and haematomas, maximal between the fifth and tenth day after injury (Bullock and Teasdale, 1990a). This accords with animal studies, and may explain the delayed deterioration which is seen in some patients, a week or more after a focal brain injury.

Delayed haematomas have been reported to occur in between 1.5 and 7% of patients with a severe head injury. A delayed traumatic intracerebral haematoma is now usually defined as a lesion of increased attenuation on CT scanning, developing in a part of the brain or intracranial cavity which the admission CT scan had suggested was initially normal or near-normal.

As a result of CT scanning there is an increasing awareness of relatively small haematomas in the basal ganglia of patients who have otherwise sustained severe diffuse brain injury (Adams, 1990). These lesions occurred in 3% of a series of severely injured patients undergoing CT scanning. Patients with such haematomas have a reduced incidence of a lucid interval and an increased incidence of gliding contusions and diffuse axonal injury. Post-traumatic basal ganglia haematomas on CT scan are thus an indicator of severe diffuse brain damage and carry a poor prognosis. The pathogenesis and prognosis for post-traumatic intraventricular haemorrhage is similar.

If a solitary haematoma is found in the brain of a patient who has suffered a head injury, the possibility that it was due to hypertension or a ruptured intracranial aneurysm must be considered, the latter having precipitated the injury. Interpretation of the findings at post-mortem can be difficult. If the haemorrhage is in the subfrontal or temporal regions, it is more likely that the intracranial haematoma is traumatic than spontaneous.

Brain swelling

After removal of an intradural lesion, raised ICP is present in 60% of patients (Becker *et al.*, 1977). In one series, ICP rose uncontrollably to cause death in a third of patients. Such high ICP is usually the result of brain swelling: this remains one of the most lethal, yet poorly understood complications of severe brain injury. In 85% of cases of severe swelling, it follows evacuation of acute subdural haematoma (Lobato *et al.*, 1988).

The causes of brain swelling are not clear. In general, it may be due either to an increase in the cerebral blood volume (*congestive brain swelling*) or to an increase in the brain water content (*cerebral oedema*). Three main types of brain swelling are encountered in patients who have sustained a head injury: focal swelling adjacent to contusions; diffuse swelling of one cerebral hemisphere; and diffuse swelling of both cerebral hemispheres.

Swelling adjacent to contusions This is common and is due to physical disruption of tissue, frank haemorrhage, early massive cytotoxic oedema and later vasogenic oedema, the outcome of damage to the blood–brain barrier. Swelling of such focal lesions may cause progressive shifts of the lobes or midline of the brain. It is usually maximal several days after injury, when the vasogenic component of the oedema is prominent and it spreads rapidly into adjacent white matter.

Hemispheric swelling This is most often seen in association with ipsilateral acute subdural haematoma as discussed above.

The experimental studies of Langfitt have shown that this form of swelling is due to engorgement of a non-reactive vascular bed secondary to cerebral ischaemia, produced by high ICP (Langfitt *et al.*, 1965). The extent to which ischaemia contributes to this vasomotor paralysis remains uncertain. The rapidity of onset of such swelling after a subdural haematoma suggests that the swelling is due in the first instance to vasodilatation with or without significant pre-existing ischaemia. The development of vasogenic oedema from subsequent breakdown of the blood–brain barrier may occur much later. However, neither barrier breakdown nor 'oedema' as seen by MRI imaging has yet been established in this condition.

Diffuse brain swelling This occurs mainly in children and adolescents (Graham *et al.*, 1989b). At post-mortem the brain is uniformly swollen and the ventricles are small and symmetrical. In some cases the swelling may be associated with widespread ischaemic brain damage or be secondary to post-traumatic status epilepticus or cardiorespiratory arrest.

The cause is also not clear. Loss of vasomotor tone and consequent vasodilatation with increased cerebral blood volume probably contribute to the swelling (Bruce *et al.*, 1981). After diffuse head injury widespread cerebral oedema has not been demonstrated on magnetic resonance imaging or by direct measurements of brain water content. Reduced intracranial compliance due to failure of CSF absorption mechanisms has also been proposed (Marmarou *et al.*, 1987). Possibly astrocyte swelling, caused by uptake of extracellular K^+, and neuronal swelling, from Na^+ entry, may contribute.

Whatever the mechanism, its rapidity of onset, variable clinical pattern and association with prior ischaemic events make brain swelling a major focus for future clinical study.

Infection

Meningitis complicates 5–9% of severe non-missile head injuries. Microorganisms (usually paranasal pneumococci or cutaneous staphylococci) enter the cranium through an open fracture of the skull or through a fracture of the base of the skull, bringing the subarachnoid space into continuity with major air sinuses. The latter is often associated with CSF rhinorrhoea or otorrhoea or an aerocele. If there is a small defect in the dura at the base of the skull meningitis may be delayed for many months or even years; a small traumatic fistula may also be a cause of recurrent episodes of meningitis (Jennett and Teasdale, 1981).

Occasionally, an intracerebral abscess or subdural empyema forms following a compound depressed fracture.

Brain damage secondary to high intracranial pressure

Using the structural criterion of pressure necrosis in one or both para-hippocampal gyri (which allows the pathologist to state with some certainty whether ICP has been high during life), it was found that ICP had been high at some time during life in 324 of the 434 cases (75%) of the series of fatal head injuries in Glasgow (Graham *et al.*, 1978). The importance of intracranial haematoma in these fatal head injuries is reflected in the fact that a large proportion of such patients die due to distortion and herniation of the brain and secondary haemorrhage into the brain stem. Post-traumatic brain swelling and widespread ischaemic damage with consequent swelling may also initiate herniation.

In a unilateral supratentorial mass lesion of whatever nature (haematoma, swelling, abscess), one cerebral hemisphere enlarges or is compressed. The sulci are narrowed and the gyri flattened. The ipsilateral ventricle and the third ventricle are compressed and there is displacement of structures across the midline. A *supracallosal* hernia develops when the ipsilateral cingulate gyrus becomes displaced beneath the falx (Figure 9.14). A *tentorial* hernia develops when the medial part of the ipsilateral temporal lobe becomes displaced through the tentorial incisura. This is of great clinical significance as the hernia not only displaces but also compresses the midbrain. The ipsilateral third nerve becomes stretched and distorted, producing the characteristic dilatation of the pupil (Figure 9.15). When the condition is advanced, the hypothalamic structures are displaced backwards and downwards and come to lie below the level of

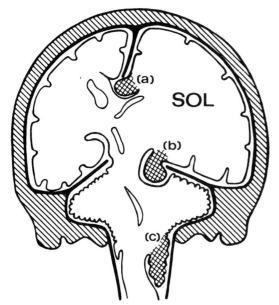

Figure 9.14 Raised intracranial pressure. Diagramatic representation of distortion and herniation of the brain caused by a space-occupying lesion (SOL) in one cerebral hemisphere. There is displacement of the midline structures and ventricles, and supracallosal (a), tentorial (b) and tonsillar (c) herniae have developed. (See Graham, 1990.)

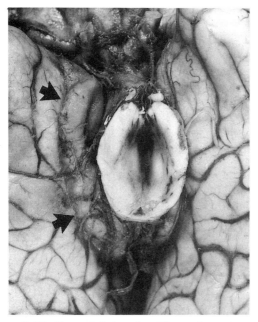

Figure 9.15 Tentorial hernia. There is a tentorial hernia almost the full length of the parahippocampal gyrus (black arrows). There is also angulation of the occulator nerves, extensive secondary haemorrhage in the midline of the upper brain stem and haemorrhagic necrosis in the contralateral cerebral peduncle (white arrow). (See Graham, 1990.)

the tentorial opening. Eventually, the supratentorial expanding mass exerts sufficient pressure on the brain stem to produce ischaemia and initiate the Cushing's response – bradycardia, an increase in pulse pressure and mean arterial pressure, and changes in respiration. Eventually, terminal haemorrhage and infarction in the central portion of the midbrain and upper pons are produced. As a result of brain distortion and internal herniation, the circulation through the pericallosal, anterior choroidal and posterior cerebral arteries may become severely impaired with widespread infarction in the structures they supply (see above).

A *tonsillar* hernia occurs when the cerebellar tonsils are displaced through the foramen magnum. This may also take place with a supratentorial mass lesion. When the herniation is consequent upon a large or diffuse supratentorial mass lesion, there is often a combination of tentorial and tonsillar herniation.

If the ICP remains high after a craniotomy, then an external *hernia* may develop through the defect in the skull. This may simply amount to protrusion of small pieces of brain through burr holes but, if an external decompression has been undertaken, or the bone flap has not been replaced, a large part of the cerebral hemisphere may herniate through the defect. Such herniated tissue may undergo infarction as a result of compression of cortical arteries and veins against the edges of the defect, so the prognosis is usually worse in patients in whom the bone flap has been left out after a craniotomy for a traumatic mass lesion.

Mass lesions in the posterior fossa rapidly produce obstruction to the flow of CSF which in turn leads to dilatation of the ventricular system and a rapid increase in ICP. *Tonsillar* herniation is inevitably more severe than with supratentorial masses and the low medulla becomes compressed against the anterior margin of the foramen magnum. Occasionally the posterior inferior cerebellar arteries may be compressed to such an extent that infarction occurs in the cerebellar hemisphere. The cerebellum may also very rarely be displaced upwards through the tentorial opening by a posterior fossa mass to produce a *reversed tentorial* hernia.

Most patients who manifest established brain stem changes from transtentorial herniation die. In a series of 36 persistently vegetative patients who survived for more than 4 weeks and were subject to a comprehensive neuropathological analysis, there was not one case in whom the clinical state could be attributed solely to this form of secondary damage to the brain stem. The two common causes were DAI and diffuse ischaemic damage (McLellan *et al.*, 1986).

Pathogenesis In a recent review of the underlying pathophysiology of raised intracranial pressure, Miller and Adams (1992) emphasized the impor-

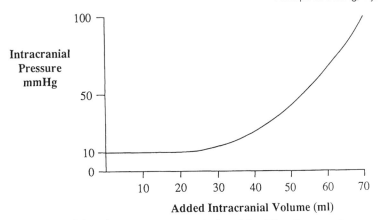

Figure 9.16 Theoretical intracranial volume pressure relationship. The time scale may be from minutes to months, but once compensating mechanisms have been exhausted (after a volume of about 40 ml), a small increase in volume will produce a large increase in pressure. When intracranial pressure is above 50 mmHg for a prolonged period, the likelihood of reduced cerebral perfusion and ischaemic brain damage becomes very high. (See Graham, 1990.)

tance of the *rate of development* of an intracranial expanding lesion and the concept of the pressure–volume curve, first introduced by Langfitt. As an intracranial mass lesion develops within the rigid confines of the adult skull, a compensatory reduction in other intracranial contents can, for a time, prevent any increase in ICP. This is brought about by a reduction in the volume of intracranial CSF by shifts of CSF into the distensile spinal theca. Later, a reduction in intracranial blood volume may occur and, in certain circumstances, some reduction in the volume of brain tissue, achieved by reducing the volume of extracellular fluid. Once this compensatory capacity has become exhausted, ICP must rise, slowly at first but then rapidly to levels approaching that of the systemic arterial pressure. This is clearly shown by the pressure–volume curve (Figure 9.16). In general, the more slowly a focal lesion expands, the more likely it is to produce distortion of the brain without an early increased ICP. In elderly patients where there is some cerebral atrophy and increased volume of CSF, a slowly expanding lesion such as a chronic subdural haematoma may attain a considerable size before leading to a significant increase in the intracranial pressure. If by contrast the focal lesion is expanding rapidly, death occurs quickly as a result of a high ICP before much distortion and herniation of the brain has taken place.

HEAD INJURY PATHOPHYSIOLOGY: IMPLICATIONS FOR MANAGEMENT

The first part of this chapter reviewed the advances in pathophysiology which have led to a clearer understanding of the mechanisms which damage the human brain during and after head injury. Over the last 20 years in the light of these findings, the management of head-injured patients has evolved

considerably. Technological advances in brain imaging (CT scanning) and neurological intensive care have also been important influences on management.

There is as yet no form of drug therapy which is effective in limiting brain damage after human head injury, although many agents have been tried both empirically and in structured clinical trials. An important advance in management over the past few years has been the recognition that some forms of therapy may be harmful – corticosteroids and barbiturates are examples.

Improvements in head-injury management have clearly led to improvements in outcome. Data from Glasgow in the 'pre-CT scan era' (1973–9) indicates that patients who were persistently in coma 6 hours or more after severe head injury had an incidence of death or persistent vegetative state of 43% (Jennett and Teasdale, 1981). A recent North American study (The Traumatic Coma Data Bank Study) collected outcome data from 1984 to 1987. Four centres with a special interest in head injury pooled data from 746 severely head-injured patients. For this group, the overall mortality rate was 36%. Severely-injured patients, however, only comprise 5% or so of the total of head-injured patients who present to an accident and emergency department.

The most significant improvements in head-injury outcome over the last decade have come from changes in management of the less severely injured. Evidence for this was seen in a study of 8000 head injuries managed in 41 different hospitals in the USA (Klauber *et al.*, 1989). Seventy per cent of these were classified as 'mild and moderate' injuries with an expected mortality rate of 10% or less. The 41 hospitals, all with similar levels of technology and types of treatment, managing this large sample were stratified on the basis of the mortality achieved in relation to that expected. The best hospitals reported a mortality nine times lower than expected and the worst hospitals reported mortality rates eight times higher. This enormous difference in outcome was attributed largely to the speed with which the diagnosis was made and to variations in management policy. In the same study, the difference in outcome for patients with *severe* head injury was only 1.2-fold between the best and the worst hospitals.

The enormous variation in injury severity creates a major problem in management. In Britain about 10% of the patients who present to an accident and emergency department will have sustained a head injury – about 5000 patients per year for a district general hospital serving a population of 250 000. However, only about 1% of this group of patients will need to be transferred to a specialist neurosurgical unit (Bullock and Teasdale, 1990b). The spectrum of head injury thus extends from those who have sustained a mild episode of transient unconsciousness ('concussion') to those who remain deeply unconscious with evidence of severe brain damage. Management algorithms must take account of the fact that even those with mild injuries may occasionally rapidly deteriorate because of an intracranial haematoma.

Aims of management

Because the management of head injury is multi-disciplinary, and involves personnel across a spectrum from police, ambulancemen and paramedics, to accident and emergency personnel, general surgeons, trauma surgeons, intensivists and neurosurgeons, the aims of management need to be general. These can be briefly summarized as follows:

1. To prevent ongoing hypoxic/ischaemic damage after head injury by rapid resuscitation and optimizing brain perfusion and oxygenation as soon as possible.
2. To identify patients at risk for the development of an intracranial haematoma and to diagnose this by CT scan as quickly as possible *before* secondary brain damage takes place.
3. To operate as speedily as possible after injury upon those patients with significant intracranial haematomas. Ideally this should be *prophylactic* before deterioration has taken place. The decision to operate may in some cases be difficult: ICP monitoring may be useful to identify those who need an operation.
4. To provide optimal conditions for recovery from brain damage in those patients who have continued disturbance of consciousness. This will usually be by neurological intensive care.

The emphasis on head-injury management has shifted away from 'observation of patients until they deteriorate then referral to the neurosurgeon'. It is now possible to identify those patients who are at risk of brain damage and intracranial haematoma and to *prophylactically* screen them for an intracranial haematoma using CT scanning. This change has come about because of several factors. CT scanners are now much more widely available in district and community hospitals. The cost of a CT scan is now less than the cost of a 24-hour hospital stay. The risk factors for an intracranial haematoma are now well established so that it is possible to predict, with acceptable accuracy, those patients who will require a CT scan.

Neurological observation in a district hospital is a relatively poor technique for detection of an intracranial haematoma because the 'pick-up' rate for intracranial haematomas in conscious patients who are neurologically normal without a skull fracture is low, so that the levels of vigilance by the observers are often poor.

With carefully applied guidelines, it should be possible to reduce dramatically the numbers of patients kept in hospital for neurological observation and to increase the numbers who are observed at home by a responsible adult, such as a family member (Mendelow *et al.*, 1983).

REFERENCES

Adams J.H. (1990). Brain damage in fatal non-missile head injury in man. In *Handbook of Clinical Neurology.* Vol. 13 (57). *Head Injury* (Braakmann R., ed.). Amsterdam: Elsevier Science, pp. 43–63.

Adams J.H., Doyle D., Graham D.I. et al. (1985). The confusion index: a reappraisal in man and experimental non-missile head injury. *Neuropathol Appl Neurobiol*, **11**, 299–308.

Adams J.H., Doyle D., Ford I. et al. (1989). Diffuse axonal injury in head injury: Definition, diagnosis and grading. *Histopathology.* **15**, 49–59.

Adams J.H., Graham D.I. (1988). *An Introduction to Neuropathology.* Edinburgh: Churchill Livingstone, p. 119.

Adams J.H., Graham D.I., Gennarelli T.A. (1982). Neuropathology of acceleration-induced head injury in the sub-human primate. In *Head Injury: Basic and Clinical Aspects* (Grossmann R.G., Gildenberg P.L., eds). New York: Raven, pp. 141–50.

Becker D.P., Miller J.D., Ward J.D. et al. (1977). The outcome from severe head injury with early diagnosis and intensive management. *J. Neurosurg.*, **47**, 491–502.

Blumbergs P.C., Jones N.R., North J.B. (1989). Diffuse axonal injury in head trauma. *J. Neurol Neurosurg Psychiat.*, **52**, 838–41.

Blumbergs PC, Scott G., Manavis J. et al. (1994). Staining of amyloid precursor protein to study axonal damage in mild head injury. *Lancet*, **344**, 1055–6.

Brocklehurst G., Gooding M., James G. (1987). Comprehensive care of patients with head injuries. *Br Med J.* **294**, 345–7.

Bruce D.A., Alavi A., Bilaniuk L. et al. (1981). Diffuse cerebral swelling following head injuries in children: the syndrome of malignant brain edema? *J. Neurosurg.*,

54, 170–8.

Bullock R., Fujisawa J. (1992). The role of glutamate antagonists for the treatment of CNS injury. In Proceedings of Ninth Annual Meeting, Neurotrauma Society. New Orleans, USA. *J. Neurotrauma*, **9** (suppl. 2), S443–62.

Bullock R., Teasdale G.M. (1990a). Surgical management of traumatic intracranial haematomas. In *Handbook of Clinical Neurology*. Vol. 13 (57). *Head Injury* (Braakmann R., eds). Amsterdam: Elsevier Science.

Bullock R., Teasdale G.M. (1990b). ABC of major trauma – head injury. I and II. *Br. Med. J.*, **300**, 1515–18, 1576–9.

Chen M-H., Bullock R., Graham D.I. et al. (1991). Ischaemic neuronal damage after acute subdural haematoma in the rat: effects of pretreatment with a glutamate antagonist. *J. Neurosurg.*, **74**, 944–50.

Cooper P.R. (1987). *Head Injury*. Baltimore: Williams and Wilkins.

Erb D.E., Povlishock J.T. (1988). Axonal damage in severe traumatic brain injury: an experimental study in the cat. *Acta Neuropathol.*, 347–58.

Faden A.I., Demediuk P., Hunter S.S., Vink R. (1989). The role of excitatory amino acids and NMDA receptors in traumatic brain injury. *Science*, **244**, 798–800.

Ford L.E., McLaurin R.L. (1963). Mechanisms of extra-dural haematomas. *J. Neurosurg.*, **20**, 760–9.

Galbraith S., Teasdale G.M. (1981). Predicting the need for operation in a patient with an occult traumatic intracranial haematoma. *J. Neurosurg.*, **55**, 75–81.

Gennarelli T.A., Thibault L.E. (1982). Biomechanics of acute subdural haematoma. *J. Trauma*, **22**, 680–6.

Gennarelli T.A. (1994). Animate models of human head injury. *J. Neurotrauma*, **11**, 357–68.

Gentleman S.M., Roberts G.W., Gennarelli T.A. et al. (1995). Axonal injury: a universal consequence of fatal closed head injury? *Acta Neuropathol*, **83**, 537–43.

Gentry L.R., Godersky J.C., Thomson B. (1988). MR imaging of head trauma: review of the distribution and radiopathologic features of traumatic lesions. *Am. J. Neuroradiol.*, **9**, 101–10.

Graham D.I., Adam J.H. and Doyle D. (1978). Ischaemic brain damage in fatal non-missile head injuries. *J. Neurol. Sci.*, **39**, 213–34.

Graham D.I., Ford I., Adams J.H. et al. (1989a). Ischaemic brain damage is still common in fatal non-missile head injury. *J. Neurol. Neurosurg. Psychiat.*, **52**, 346–50.

Graham D.I., Ford I., Adams J.H. et al. (1989b). Fatal head injury in children. *J. Clin. Pathol.*, **42**, 18–22.

Graham D.I., in *Trauma in Systemic Pathology*. Third edn, Vol. 4. *Nervous System, Muscle and Eyes* (Weller R. ed.). Edinburgh: Churchill Livingstone, pp. 125–50.

Graham D.I., Clark J.C., Adams J.H. et al. (1992). Diffuse axonal injury caused by assault. *J Clin. Pathol.*, **45**, 840–1.

Holbourn A.H.S. (1945). The mechanics of brain injuries. *Br. Med. Bull.*, **3**, 147–9.

Ito H., Yamamoto S., Komai T. et al. (1976). Role of local hyperfibrinolysis in the etiology of chronic subdural hematoma. *J Neurosurg.*, **45**, 26–31.

Jenkins A., Teasdale G., Hadley M.D.M. et al. (1986). Brain lesions detected by magnetic resonance imaging in mild and severe head injury. *Lancet*, **ii**, 445–6.

Jenkins L.W., Moszynski K., Lyeth B.G. et al. (1989). Increased vulnerability of the mildly traumatised rat brain to cerebral ischaemia: the use of controlled secondary ischaemia as a research tool to identify common or different mechanisms contributing to mechanical ischaemic brain injury. *Brain Res.*, **477**, 211–24.

Jennett B. (1974). Early traumatic epilepsy: incidence and significance after non-missile injuries. *Arch. Neurol.*, **30**, 394–8.

Jennett B., Carlin J. (1978). Preventable mortality and morbidity after head injury. *Injury*, **10**, 31–9.

Jennett B., Teasdale G. (1981). *Management of Head Injury*. Philadelphia, PA: FA Davis.

Jones T.J., Morawetz R.B., Crowell R.M. et al. (1981). Thresholds of focal cerebral ischaemia in awake monkeys. *J. Neurosurg.*, **54**, 773–82.

Jones P.A., Andrews P.J.D., Midgeley et al. (1994). Measuring the burden of secondary insults in head-injured patients during intensive care. *J. Neurosurg. Anaesthesiol.*, **6**, 6–14.

Katayama Y., Becker D.P., Tamura T., Hovda D.A. (1990). Massive increases in extracellular potassium and the indiscriminate release of glutamate following concussive brain injury. *J. Neurosurg.*, **73**, 889–900.

Klauber M.R., Marshall L.F., Luerssen T.G. et al. (1989). Determinants of head injury mortality: importance of the low risk patients. *Neurosurgery*, **24**, 31–6.

Kotapka M.J., Graham D.I., Adams J.H., Gennarelli T.A. (1992). Hippocampal pathology in fatal non-missile human head injury. *Acta. Neuropathol.*, **83**, 530–4.

Langfitt T.W. (1968). Increased intracranial pressure. *Clin. Neurosurg.* **16**, 436–71.

Langfitt T.W., Weinstein J.D. and Kassel N.M. (1964). Transmission of increased intracranial pressure, part 2, within the supratentorial space. *J. Neurosurg.*, **21**, 998–1005.

Langfitt T.W., Weinstein J.D. and Kassell N.F. (1965). Cerebral vasomotor paralysis is produced by intracranial hypertension. *Neurology*, **15**, 641–62.

Leestma J.E. (1988). *Forensic Neuropathology*. New York: Raven Press.

Lewelt W., Jenkins L.W., Miller J.D. (1982). Effect of experimental fluid percussion injury to the brain on cerebrovascular reactivity to hypoxia and to hypocapnia. *J. Neurosurg.*, **56**, 332–7.

Lobato R.D., Sarabia R., Cordobes F. et al. (1988). Post traumatic cerebral hemispheric swelling. Analysis of 55 cases studied with computed tomography. *J. Neurosurg.*, **68**, 417–23.

Lyeth B.E., Ray M., Hamm R. et al. (1992). Post injury scopolamine administration in experimental traumatic brain injury. *Brain Res*, **569**, 281–6.

Marion D.W., Darby J., Yonas H. (1992). Acute regional cerebral blood flow changes caused by severe head injuries. *J. Neurosurg.*, **74**, 407–14.

Marmarou A., Masset A.L., Ward J.D. et al. (1987). Contribution of CSF and vascular factors to elevation of ICP in severely head injured patients. *J. Neurosurg.*, **66**, 883–90.

Marmarou A., Foda M.A.A.-E., van den Brink W. et al. (1994). A new model of diffuse brain injury in rats. *J. Neurosurg.*, **80**, 291–300.

Marshall L. F., Kauber M. R. et al. (Traumatic Coma Data Bank Study Group) (1991). Outcome after severe head injury. *J. Neurosurg.*, **75**, (suppl.) 528–36.

Marshall L.F., Marshall S.B., Klauber M., Clark M., Eisenberg H., Jane J.A., Luerssen T., Marmarou A., Foulkes M.A. (1991). A new classification of head injury based on computerised tomography. *J. Neurosurg.*, **75**, 514–20.

Mathew P., Oluoch-Olunya D.L., Condon B.R., Bullock R. (1995). Acute sub-dural haematoma in the conscious patient: outcome with initial non-operative management. *Acta Neurochir. (Wein)*, **121**, 100–8.

McLellan D.R., Adams H.J., Graham D.I., Kerr A.E. and Teasdale G.F.M. (1986). The structural basis of the vegetative state and prolonged coma after non-missile head injury. In *La Coma Traumatique*. (Cohabon F. and Massarot M. eds). Padua: Liviana Editrice, pp. 165–85.

Mendelow A.D., Teasdale G.M., Jennett B. et al. (1983). Risks of intracranial haematoma in head injured adults. *Br. Med. J.*, **287**, 1173–6.

Miller J.D., Jones P.R. (1985). The work of a regional head injury service. *Lancet*, **i**, 1141–4.

Miller J.D., Bullock R., Graham D.I. et al. (1990). Ischemic brain damage in a model of acute subdural hematoma. *Neurosurgery*, **27**, 433–9.

Miller J.D. and Adams J.H. (1992). The pathophysiology of raised intracranial pressure. In: *Greenfield's Neuropathology*. 5th edn (Adams J.H. and Douchen L.W., eds) London: Edward Arnold, pp. 69–105.

Miller J.D., Sweet R.C., Narayan R., Becker D.P. (1978). Early insults to the injured brain. *JAMA*, **240**, 439–42.

Ng, H.K., Graham D.I., Adams J.H. et al. (1989). Changes in the hippocampus and the cerebellum resulting from hypoxic insults: frequency and distribution. *Acta Neuropathol.*, **78**, 438–43.

Povlishock J.T. (1992). Traumatically induced axonal injury: pathogenesis and pathobiological implications. *Brain Pathol.* **2**, 1–12.

Povlishock J.T., Jenkins L.W. (1995). Are the pathobiological changes evoked by traumatic brain injury immediate and irreversible? *Brain Pathol.*, **5**, 415–26.

Reilly P.L., Adams J.H., Graham D.I., Jennett B. (1975). Patients with head injury who talk and die. *Lancet*, **ii**, 375–7.

Servadei F., Ciucci G., Morichetti A. et al. (1988). Skull fracture and factors of increased risk in minor head injuries: indications for broader use of cerebral computed tomography. *Surg. Neurol.*, **30**, 364–9.

Stone J.L., Rifai M.H.S., Sugar O. et al. (1983). Subdural hematomas. 1. Acute subdural hematoma: progress in definition, clinical pathology and therapy. *Surg Neurol.*, **19**, 216–31.

Strang L., MacMillan R. and Jennett B. (1978). Head injuries in accident and emergency departments in Scottish hospitals injury. *Injury*, **10**, 154–9.

Strich S.J. (1956). Diffuse degeneration of the cerebral white matter in severe dementia following head injury. *J. Neurol. Neurosurg. Psychiatr.*, **19**, 163–85.

Teasdale G.M., Galbraith S., Murray L. et al. (1982). Management of traumatic intracranial haematoma. *Br Med J.* **285**, 1695–7.

Thibault L.E., Gennarelli T.A. (1985). *Biomechanics and Craniocerebral Trauma. Central Nervous System Trauma. Status Report*. pp. 379–90.

Turazzi S., Bricolo A., Pastut M.L. et al. (1987). Changes produced by CT scanning in the outlook of severe head injury. *Acta Neurochir. (Wien)*, **85**, 87–95.

Tyson G., Strachan W.E., Newman P. et al. (1980). The role of craniectomy in the treatment of chronic subdural hematomas. *J Neurosurg.*, **52**, 776–81.

Tyson G.W. (1987). *Head Injury Management for Providers of Emergency Care*. Baltimore, MA: Williams and Wilkins.

10. Non-penetrating Injury of the Thorax
A. A. Vlessis and
D. D. Trunkey

INTRODUCTION

Blunt injuries to the upper torso or thorax are a major cause of overall mortality and morbidity following injury. According to Besson and Saegesser (1983), there are 12 thoracic injuries per one million population per day, of which four require hospitalization, with one severe case every other day. Many investigators have shown that 50% of fatal accidents are associated with chest trauma and in half of these the chest injury is the primary cause of death. In 25% of the deaths where thoracic injury contributes to the primary cause of mortality (usually brain injury), the pathophysiology is either hypovolaemia from associated chest injuries, hypoxia, aspiration or other injuries impairing oxygen transport.

This chapter emphasizes the following concepts to explain the mortality and morbidity of thoracic trauma and shock. These include:

1. Injuries to the chest wall and thoracic viscera can directly impair oxygen transport mechanisms.
2. Hypoxia and hypovolaemia as a consequence of thoracic injuries may cause secondary injury to patients with brain injury or may directly cause cerebral oedema.
3. Conversely, shock and/or brain injury can secondarily aggravate thoracic injuries and hypoxaemia by disrupting normal ventilatory patterns or by causing loss of protective airway reflexes and subsequent aspiration.
4. The lung is also a target organ for secondary injury following shock and remote tissue injury. Microemboli formed in the peripheral microcirculation can lead to ventilation-perfusion mismatch and right heart failure.
5. Tissue injury and shock can activate the inflammatory cascade which may contribute to pulmonary injury.

These concepts are explored in the first part of this chapter; the pathophysiology and management of specific thoracic injuries is then discussed.

OVERVIEW OF PATHOPHYSIOLOGY

Death following blunt thoracic impacts is often secondary to some impairment in oxygen delivery and/or transport, usually hypovolaemic shock. Unfortunately, the human organism is somewhat limited in its compensatory reactions to shock associated with serious blunt chest trauma. These can be broadly categorized into three groups: blood-flow redistribution, oxygen transport components and plasma refill.

Redistribution of blood flow is achieved by arterial vasoconstriction and venoconstriction, as well as increased adrenergic discharge. Blood-flow redistribution manifests as the classic clinical signs of shock. Factors determining oxygen transport capacity are pulmonary gas exchange, cardiac output, haemoglobin concentration and oxygen-haemoglobin affinity. Following traumatic shock, some of these oxygen transport components are intrinsically exhausted but lend themselves to clinical augmentation. The final compensatory mechanism is plasma refill which is initiated by the reduction in hydrostatic pressure in the capillary bed and hormonal action on the kidney and splanchnic bed. The therapeutic goal of the clinician is to augment or supplement these compensatory mechanisms whenever possible during acute resuscitation.

Failure to restore homeostasis during the compensation phase results in cell distress and decompensation. With the aid of the clinician, the patient will either reach the recovery phase or continue to decompensate, culminating in death. Discussed below are the three phases of hypovolaemic shock as they relate to blunt thoracic trauma: compensation, cell distress and decompensation, and recovery phases.

Compensation phase

Hypovolaemia results in an immediate redistribution of blood flow. The response is mediated by neuronal (sympathetic division of the autonomic nervous system) and endocrine (epinephrine and norepinephrine from the adrenal medulla) components (Chien, 1967; Vatner, 1974). Sympathetic fibres converge on arterioles, precapillary sphincters and venules of the non-coronary and non-cerebral circulation. Their synaptic discharge elevates peripheral vascular resistance and blood pressure, allowing perfusion of the myocardium and brain at the expense of the skin, skeletal muscle and, as shock progresses, the viscera. Sympathetic fibres also innervate the adrenal medulla and their stimulation causes large quantities of epinephrine and norepinephrine to be released into the circulation. The alpha adrenergic action of these contributes to the peripheral arterial vasospasm and resultant increase in vascular resistance and blood pressure. Neuronal- and endocrine-induced venoconstriction increases cardiac preload by contracting the intravascular space and expediting return of blood to the heart. The net effect of the sympathetic response is a reduction in functional intravascular space and redistribution of systemic blood flow from the periphery to the heart and brain.

The clinical manifestations of hypovolaemic shock are a direct reflection of blood-flow redistribution. The skin and extremities become cool and pale. Peripheral pulses are thready or absent and oliguria is evident. Electrocardiographic evidence of myocardial ischaemia may become evident as ST segment elevation or depression on the rhythm monitor. As shock progresses and cerebral perfusion pressure drops, decreased mentation or coma may intervene. It is important to recognize that alcohol intoxication can mask these clinical signs of hypovolaemia by inducing a generalized vasodilatation which can nullify the effects of the adrenergic system (Malpas *et al.*, 1990). Hypotension then ensues at an earlier stage.

The compensatory changes in the oxygen-transport components are graded according to the degree of tissue hypoxia. Responses are effected through increased pulmonary gas exchange as well as alterations in blood flow and oxygen-haemoglobin affinity. Physiological hypoxia is detected as a decrease in oxygen tension within the carotid and aortic bodies located in the bifurcations of both common carotid arteries and along the aortic arch (Guz, 1975). Afferent signals from carotid and aortic body chemoreceptors pass to the medulla through the glossopharyngeal and vagal nerves to the central respiratory centre, resulting in tachypnoea. Likewise, acidosis which often accompanies hypovolaemic shock can stimulate the central respiratory centre. Tachypnoea increases pulmonary alveolar oxygen tension and reduces carbon dioxide tension, thereby facilitating more complete saturation of available haemoglobin while simultaneously accelerating carbon dioxide disposal. Tachypnoea is one of the easiest ways of increasing oxygen flow to body tissues as well as counteracting systemic acidosis. However, injury to the upper torso, particularly the chest wall, may impair the respiratory response to hypoxia and acidosis. It can also be appreciated that the surgeon who wishes to take advantage of tachypnoea during resuscitation may do so by increasing the inspired oxygen concentration either by nasal prongs or bag-mask.

The next compensatory mechanism, cardiac output, can be augmented by two mechanisms. First, adrenergic discharge from the adrenal medulla stimulates beta receptors on the myocardium which increases the rate and force of contraction. Secondly, parasympathetic activity mediated via vagal pathways to the sinoatrial and atrioventricular nodes is reduced, further increasing heart rate. The overall result is an increase in heart rate, stroke volume and hence cardiac output.

In hypovolaemia, however, volume loss may limit stroke volume so that the product of stroke volume and heart rate fail to increase cardiac output. In fact, most studies of pure hypovolaemic shock demonstrate that cardiac output falls from the inception of the shock (Guyton and Crowell, 1961). Therefore, the cardiac response to blood volume reduction dampens, but does not completely reverse, the effects of hypovolaemia on blood flow. This is especially evident in the elderly patient who lacks the cardiac reserve necessary to increase blood flow after volume loss (Schlag *et al.*, 1988).

Finally, changes in haemoglobin concentration and oxygen-haemoglobin affinity can have profound effects on oxygen transport to the body tissues. Haemorrhage results in the loss of red blood cell mass as well as plasma volume. Initially, haemoglobin concentration does not change appreciably. However, volume resuscitation and plasma refill proceed, haemodilution ensues. Tissue oxygen delivery – the product of blood flow and oxygen content – is influenced, in that at a given oxygen tension, blood oxygen content is almost directly proportional to haemoglobin concentration. Oxygen-haemoglobin affinity also affects oxygen delivery to tissues. Elevated hydrogen ion and carbon dioxide concentrations in hypoxic or ischaemic tissues facilitate release of oxygen from haemoglobin by decreasing its affinity for oxygen (Kilmartin and Rossi-Bernardi, 1973). As red blood cells pass through the pulmonary capillary, carbon dioxide is lost and blood pH rises, haemoglobin affinity for oxygen increases and oxygen binding to haemoglobin is encouraged. If hypoxic conditions persist for several hours, red blood cell 2, 3-diphosphoglycerate levels increase (Keitt *et al.*, 1974). This also decreases oxygen-haemoglobin affinity and promotes oxygen release in systemic tissues. Unfortunately, the continued presence of excess 2, 3-diphosphoglycerate also hinders oxygen-haemoglobin association in the lungs. Therefore, the benefits of elevated 2, 3-diphosphoglycerate after prolonged hypoxia are questionable.

Plasma refill following mild to moderate haemorrhage in man has been extensively studied by Moore *et al.* (1965). Blood-volume restoration occurs by both haemodynamic and endocrine mechanisms (Skillman *et al.*, 1967a, b). As already mentioned, haemorrhage initiates constriction of arterioles and precapillary sphincters. Pressure in the postcapillary venule declines despite venoconstriction. Because osmotic pressure remains the same, fluid moves intravascularly from the interstitial space. During the first 2 hours, plasma refill occurs rapidly (at rates up to 90–170 ml/hour) and then tapers off gradually until blood volume is restored to normal. Total circulating protein mass increases with contributions from all molecular sizes, including most globulins; albumin plays a major role, contributing up to four grams an hour initially. The source of albumin is predominantly extravascular but anabolism and decreased catabolism also contribute.

The endocrine influence on blood-volume restoration is substantial (Lefer, 1982). Renin activity increases in response to decreased renal arterial pressure and/or perfusion. Renin forms angiotension I from angiotensinogen. Angiotensin-converting enzymes cleave this decapeptide to the more active octapeptide, angiotensin II. Angiotensin II is a strong cardiac inotrope and a potent vasoconstrictive substance, even in the coronary vasculature. Vasopressin, or antidiuretic hormone, is released from the hypothalamus and functions to increase free water resorption from the renal collecting tubules. Its vasoconstrictive properties on the splanchnic circulation also aid extravascular plasma recruitment from the viscera. Cortisol increases extracellular osmolality which may shift intracellular fluid into the interstitium (Pirkle and Gann, 1976). As interstitial pressure increases, interstitial protein and fluid movement into the vascular space accelerates via the lymphatics.

In mild to moderate haemorrhage (10–20% of blood volume), these mechanisms can maintain cardiac output and blood pressure at acceptable levels and restore blood volume to normal within 36 hours. More extensive haemorrhage necessitates therapeutic intervention to avoid cellular distress and further decompensation.

Cell distress and decompensation phase

The human organism has an intrinsic ability to compensate for haemorrhage. When the severity of the shock insult exceeds these intrinsic compensatory capabilities, cell distress and decompensation ensue.

During severe or prolonged shock, substrate delivery and waste product removal from systemic tissues is insufficient to maintain cell viability. Oxygen drives aerobic metabolism by supporting oxidative phosphorylation of cellular adenine nucleotides (ATP). As oxygen becomes limited, the combustion of reduced carbon fuels slows. Some usable cellular energy can be captured via anaerobic pathways which primarily utilize glucose and contribute to the systemic metabolic acidosis associated with shock. Cellular ATP levels drop, limiting the activity of membrane-bound, ATP-driven ion pumps. Plasma membrane potential declines as ions continue to passively diffuse down transmembrane electrical and concentration gradients. The net result is a loss of intracellular potassium and an accumulation of intracellular sodium, calcium and water (Trunkey et al., 1976; Hansen, 1985). At this point, cell functions have ceased and impending cell demise is irreversible. Organ failure becomes clinically apparent as individual cells within underperfused tissues expire.

Recovery phase

Blood-volume restoration with normalization of haemodynamic parameters is essential to survival and eventual recovery from the injury. The recovery phase, however, can contribute to the overall pathophysiology depending on the degree of shock and tissue injury. Fluid resuscitation during the compensation phase will reverse the autonomic and hormonal effects on the microcirculation rescuing ischaemic cells in the peripheral and splanchnic circulations. With the emergence of trauma centres and the rapid, effective techniques of resuscitation, it has become clear that the resuscitation itself can induce additional host injury which occurs as a result of the reperfusion of ischaemic tissues as well as pulmonary microcirculatory damage induced by remote injuries. These two phenomenon, termed reperfusion injury and shock lung, will be discussed briefly below.

Reperfusion injury

Reperfusion injury is an additional tissue injury produced during the reperfusion of a previously ischaemic tissue which exceeds the injury induced by the period of ischaemia alone (McCord, 1985) and has been described in most tissues, including bowel, kidney, liver, heart and brain.

It is largely attributable to the formation, after the reintroduction of oxygen, of so-called *reactive oxygen species* such as hydrogen peroxide and superoxide (O_3) because of the presence of high levels of xanthine oxidase in ischaemic cells. If the normal cellular capacity to detoxify the reactive molecules is inadequate, hydroxyl radicals form and alter membrane fluidity and transmembrane flux (Bruch and Thayer, 1983).

Other sources of reactive oxygen during reperfusion include accelerated eicosanoid metabolism (Van Blisen et al., 1989) and autoxidation of semiquinone (Demopoulos et al., 1982).

Polymorphonuclear leucocytes also contribute to reperfusion injury *in vivo* (McCord, 1987) by adhering to the damaged endothelium of ischaemic tissues (Mullane et al., 1984). Chemotactic factors, including a superoxide-dependent factor, released during reperfusion, promote leucocyte infiltration into the tissues (Petrone et al., 1980).

Shock lung

The shock lung syndrome was first described by Brewer et al. (1946) after their experience with Second World War casualties. They noted an increase in lung water content following severe trauma to the chest or to other remote areas of the body. The injury was often associated with shock and occurred without myocardial failure. Patients experienced progressive hypoxia culminating in respiratory failure and death.

The initial defect in shock lung syndrome appears to be injury to the endothelium of the pulmonary capillary, with increase in permeability and non-cardiac pulmonary oedema. Although the cause remains unknown, two cytokines, interleukin-1 (IL-1) and tumour necrosis factor (TNFα), are likely mediators. They both directly increase pulmonary endothelial permeability *in vivo* (Goldblum *et al.*, 1988; Horvath *et al.*, 1988) as well as in isolated pulmonary artery endothelial monolayers (Hennig *et al.*, 1987; Goldblum *et al.*, 1989). The TNFα-induced increase in endothelial permeability may be mediated by arachidonic acid metabolites in that cyclo-oxygenase and lipoxygenase inhibition can block the effect *in vitro* (Clark *et al.*, 1988). Besides acting separately to induce pulmonary endothelial damage, simultaneous administration of IL-1 and TNFα synergistically induce pulmonary injury in rabbits (Okusawa *et al.*, 1988).

IL-1 and TNFα also lead to endothelial injury indirectly by facilitating interactions between the endothelium and granulocytes. Both substances induce cell-surface expression of endothelium-leucocyte adhesion molecules (Pohlman *et al.*, 1986; Broudy *et al.*, 1987) and TNFα that of adhesion molecules (CDw18) which promote recognition of endothelial surfaces (Gamble *et al.*, 1985; Berger *et al.*, 1988). In this manner, granulocytes become adherent to the pulmonary vascular endothelium and, once stimulated, release toxic substances which damage the endothelial barrier and result in pulmonary oedema. Evidence in support of this mechanism comes from a study of haemorrhagic shock in rabbits in which neutrophil adherence to endothelium was blocked with a monoclonal antibody to adhesion molecule CDw18; survival was enhanced to 100% from 29% by pretreatment with the anti-CDw18 antibody (Vedder *et al.*, 1988).

Microembolism following remote musculoskeletal injury also contributes to pulmonary dysfunction after trauma (Saldeen, 1976; Jansson *et al.*, 1985). Platelet and fibrin aggregates released from the peripheral circulation during resuscitation become lodged in the pulmonary vasculature. Release of tissue thromboplastin into the venous circulation from sites of remote injury can also activate the extrinsic coagulation pathway and cause pulmonary microthrombi (Jansson *et al.*, 1988). Vasoactive and immunoreactive substances are liberated from the embolic aggregates and the adjacent endothelium to cause pulmonary vasoconstriction as well as leucocyte chemoattraction, adherence and infiltration. The microemboli and resultant pulmonary vascular response can elicit a significant right to left shunt (Figures 10.1–10.3) which compounds the diffusion-related hypoxia induced by the concomitant pulmonary endothelial leak and further impairs oxygen delivery to the peripheral tissues. If the embolic shower is extensive, pulmonary hypertension may develop

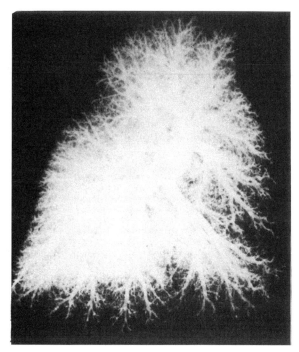

Figure 10.1 Pulmonary artery casting from normal human cadaver. (Reproduced with permission from Marcel Dekker, Inc, New York, 1985.)

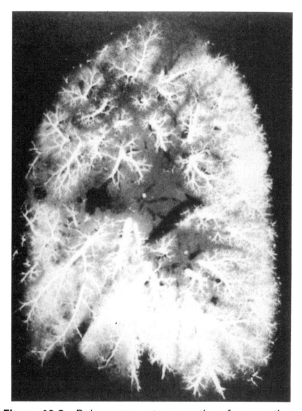

Figure 10.2 Pulmonary artery casting from patient with ARDS secondary to blunt trauma. (Reproduced with permission from Marcel Dekker, Inc, New York, 1985.)

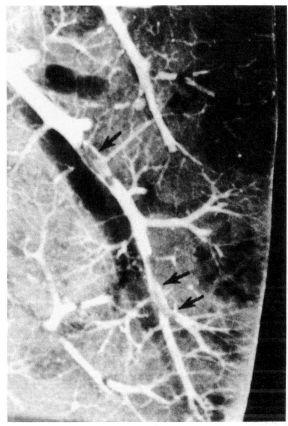

Figure 10.3 Close-up of pulmonary artery casting from patient with ARDS showing macro-filling defects in pulmonary circulation and 'pruning' of vascular tree. (Reproduced with permission from Marcel Dekker, Inc, New York, 1985.)

TABLE 10.1
DISTRIBUTION OF INJURIES FOLLOWING MOTOR VEHICLE ACCIDENTS. (FROM BESSAN AND SAEGESSER, 1983).

Encephalon	43%
Chest	12%
Abdomen, pelvis	9%
Upper extremities	13%
Lower extremities	23%

CHEST WALL INJURIES

Physical forces

Blunt injury to the thorax can be caused by a number of physical forces, the most common of which follow automobile accidents. There are at least five different types of collisions that are encountered: frontal, lateral, rear, rotational and rollover. Table 10.1 presents the most common sites of injury for motor vehicle accidents. Ejection, steering assembly impact, windshield impact, instrument panel impact and rear collision account for the majority of injuries.

Compressive crush injury of the chest wall can be devastating, and in one recent study crush injury caused flail chest or multiple rib fractures in 59% of the patients with significant chest injury and an additional 12% had fractured the sternum. Shock was present in 40% of the cases and nearly 10 units of blood were required in each case (Besson and Saegesser, 1983).

Studies using human cadavers to evaluate chest wall trauma have been carried out (Patrick *et al.*, 1967). The cadavers were subjected to deceleration impacts on a 6-in. (152-mm) pad on the anterior chest surface. At a sled velocity of 16.8 mph (7.5 m/s), four rib fractures were caused at impact. At 18.5 mph (8.3 m/s) chest deflection was increased, resulting in extensive fractures. Other studies have confirmed these findings and have shown that the older the patient the more extensive the damage to the chest wall. Newman and Jones (1984) studied impact, restraint use, and severity of injury after frontal, side and rollover impact. Unrestrained drivers had an incidence of four or more rib fractures of 47.4, 59 and 75% respectively for the three types of impact. The comparative figures for restrained drivers were 8.7, 77.7 and 50%. There was a corresponding high association of intrathoracic injuries. Not surprisingly, the same study showed a very close relationship between chest injuries (Abbreviated Injury Scale >2) sustained in frontal impacts and the speed of the automobile. In restrained occupants, rib fractures and sternal fractures were not seen until the car was travelling faster than 15 mph (6.7 m/s), whereas rib fractures were common in unrestrained occupants when the speed of

followed by right ventricular failure. As the right ventricle dilates, the interventricular septum deviates to the left and hinders left ventricular filling and thus reduces stroke volume (Qvist *et al.*, 1988). At this point, the decreased arterial oxygen content and impaired cardiac output are often irreversible and the patient succumbs to cardiopulmonary failure.

Finally, hypovolaemic shock severe enough to depress cerebral oxygenation can impair central epiglottic reflexes, making the patient susceptible to aspiration and chemical injury to the lungs.

In summary, blunt chest trauma, or remote musculoskeletal trauma, can lead to cardiopulmonary dysfunction secondary to cytokine-mediated endothelial injury, microembolism syndrome and/or aspiration pneumonitis. The clinician must be conscious of these potential secondary injuries provoked by the resuscitation which may require additional intensive care management subsequently.

the automobile was <10 mph (4.5 m/s). Significant rib fractures did not occur in the restrained persons until speeds of around 30 mph (13.5 m/s). In contrast, multiple rib fractures and significant intrathoracic injuries were quite common in unrestrained persons at speeds of 10–20 mph. In this series there was only one death in restrained occupants, whereas seven deaths occurred in unrestrained occupants. Most of the deaths were secondary to associated lung contusions or rupture of the aorta or heart. These data are consistent with other investigative work (Paris *et al.*, 1975; Hobbs, 1981; Huelke, 1982). Thus, injury to the chest wall as a consequence of blunt trauma is directly related to type of impact, speed of impact, age of the patient, and whether or not the occupant is restrained. The incidence of injuries to specific thoracic structures in automobile accidents is shown in Table 10.2.

TABLE 10.2
INCIDENCE OF CHEST INJURIES FOLLOWING BLUNT TRAUMA

	Kemmerer et al. (1961) (%)	Besson and Saegesser (1983) (%)
Rib fractures	39	47
Haemothorax	28	24
Lung laceration	10	21
Ruptured great vessel	10	4
Lung contusion	6	12
Lacerated diaphragm	5	7
Myocardial injury	6	7
Sternal fractures	5	22 *
Lacerated trachea	1	5

* Steering wheel injuries.

As a contrast to compressive forces, shear forces can be associated with motor vehicle accidents and may produce degloving types of injuries on the chest wall, which most often occur when the patient is run over by a large vehicle or one with lugs on the wheels. As the vehicle passes over the body, the skin and subcutaneous tissues are pushed ahead, tearing the nutrient blood vessels which emerge from muscle; subsequent extensive soft tissue loss is common. Associated fractures of the ribs may become open to create further problems.

There are other types of trauma that can cause chest wall injury, including sport injuries, assaults and falls from modest heights. Blast injury is a special type of force that may cause compressive type of injury or result in the generation of stress waves within the chest, but is most often associated with underlying visceral damage; rib fractures are uncommon.

A special type of injury is impalement, usually caused by a blunt object which may create a very large hole in the chest wall with surrounding soft tissue and bony injury. By definition there is an open pneumothorax and the injury has the features of both blunt and penetrating trauma.

Pathophysiology

Fractures to the clavicle, sternum and scapula
Fractures to the clavicle are very common and rarely cause major pathophysiological changes. Although painful, they usually do not embarrass ventilation and only rarely are associated with major vessel lacerations.

Fractures to the sternum (Figure 10.4) are being reported with increasing frequency and constitute 5–10% of all thoracic injuries. Part of this increased incidence may be due to better recognition of the close association with injury from the steering column. Isolated sternal fractures are uncommon and do not usually cause major problems, except pain. Sternal fractures are rare, usually associated with other significant chest wall damage including flail chest. The most common associated internal injury is myocardial contusion, which can lead to very significant arrhythmias and haemodynamic instability (discussed below).

The scapula is not commonly fractured in that it is covered by a relatively thick coat of muscle. The presence of a fracture implies the application of a large amount of kinetic energy to that portion of the body and should make the clinician suspicious of significant associated injuries. Fractures which involve the glenoid fossa and acromion, however, may give rise to considerable orthopaedic problems.

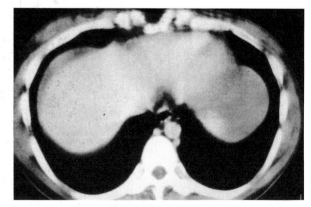

Figure 10.4 CT scan of a patient who sustained a steering wheel crush injury to the chest following a head-on motor vehicle accident. Note the complex sternal fracture. This patient also suffered a myocardial contusion.

Injuries to the ribs, including flail chest

There is a high correlation between impact velocity and severity of injury to the chest wall (Huelke, 1982; Besson and Saegesser, 1983). There appears to be a linear relationship between ribs fractured and the pathophysiological consequences. Other factors include age, location of the rib fractures, the presence of a flail segment and associated injuries.

The one thing in common with almost all injuries involving the bony thorax is pain. Pain can lead to decreased ventilation, decreased vital capacity, inability to clear secretions and retention of carbon dioxide. As more ribs are fractured, there is a progression of pathophysiological findings, including ventilation-perfusion abnormalities, increase of respiratory work, hypoxaemia and a decrease in the functional residual capacity. All of these become especially common when multiple rib fractures result in a flail chest. If the flail segment is large enough, it may move inward during inspiration, so comprising ventilation, causing shift of the mediastinum toward the contralateral side and a concominant obstruction to venous return to the heart. Negative intrathoracic pressure is reduced, contributing to decreased ventilation.

Several articles have pointed out the significance of associated injuries (Craven *et al.*, 1979; Besson and Saegesser, 1983; Landercasper *et al.*, 1984). Some investigators feel that it is the associated injury which is the primary disorder of flail chest (Table 10.3). Clearly, they do contribute, but our opinion is that they are not necessarily primary. The most common associated injury is pulmonary

contusion, which is accompanied by ventilation perfusion abnormalities; however, this may be less than previously appreciated (Craven *et al.*, 1979). There is an associated atelectasis and shunting of blood in the larger contusions of either the chest wall or the lung. Compliance decreases and airway resistance rises, and there is an associated decline in pulmonary diffusion and increase in respiratory work that is additive to that contributed by the chest wall damage.

Ultimately, the combination of pain, the decrease in ventilation, and the sequelae of the associated injuries lead to retention of carbon dioxide, hypoxaemia, and respiratory insufficiency. Although isolated rib fractures in the young, healthy patient may be of little consequence, isolated rib fractures in the elderly or those with pre-existing pulmonary disease can lead to fatality through the mechanisms that have been described.

Diagnosis

The diagnosis and management of injury to the chest follows standard lines for the evaluation and treatment of serious injury. History is of prime importance, especially that obtained from those involved at the scene such as paramedics, who can give valuable information on mechanisms of injury and the need, for example, to extract the victim from behind a steering wheel. Clinical features of ventilatory insufficiency are sought and supplemented by routine blood-gas analysis. Associated injuries are evaluated and lower rib fractures should call attention to the possibility of abdominal injury.

Concurrent haemodynamic instability and/or unconsciousness is optimally managed by immediate intubation and ventilation. Pain is relieved as soon as diagnosis is complete and by methods in which the team is experienced, though epidural anaesthesia is currently preferred (Wisner, 1990; Mackersie *et al.*, 1991). Operative treatment of chest wall instability is not often needed.

Treatment of ventilatory insufficiency

Ventilatory insufficiency can be categorized as minor, moderate or severe. Most importantly from a treatment standpoint, treatment can be divided into ventilatory and non-ventilatory support. The indications for ventilatory management are shown in Table 10.4. If at all possible, it is best to avoid ventilatory therapy, since chronic intubation and the use of ventilators sets the stage for major complications, primarily pulmonary sepsis. If the patient meets the criteria outlined in Table 10.4, however, there is often no other recourse. Aggressive conservative management may prevent the patient with moderate ventilatory insufficiency from falling into the severe category. Treatment includes adequate pain relief, nasotracheal suction,

TABLE 10.3

INJURIES ASSOCIATED WITH MULTIPLE RIB FRACTURES (n = 542) AS REPORTED BY BESSON AND SAEGESSER (1983)

	Incidence %	Mortality %
Intrathoracic		
Pulmonary injury	33	35
Left haemothorax	32	37
Right haemothorax	24	39
Left pneumothorax	23	27
Right pneumothorax	16	27
Diaphragmatic injury	10	34
Cardiac contusion	8	58
Tracheobronchial injury	3	36
Aortic injury	2	71
Intra-abdominal		
Kidney	23	21
Liver	18	53
Spleen	15	44
Hollow viscus	4	47
Pancreas	3	33
Mesentery	3	70
Adrenal gland	3	70

Clinical signs of progressive fatigue or deterioration

- Respiratory rate > 35/min or < 8/min
- Pao_2 < 60 mmHg at Fio_2 > 0.5
- $Paco_2$ < 55 mmHg at Fio_2 > 0.5
- Pao_2/Fio_2 ratio < 200
- Vital capacity < 15 ml/kg
- Forced expiratory volume in 1 second (FEV_1) < 10 ml/kg
- Inspiratory force > −25 cmH$_2$O
- Alveolar – arterial oxygen gradient > 450 with F_iO_2 of 1.0
- Shunt fraction (Q_s/Q_t > 0.2)
- Dead space tidal volume ratio (V_a/V_t) > 0.6

Additional indications for mechanical ventilation:

- Clinical evidence of severe shock
- Associated severe head injury with lack of airway control or need to hyperventilate
- Severe associated injury requiring surgery
- Airway obstruction
- Significant pre-existing chronic pulmonary disease

incentive respirometers, chest physiotherapy and supplemental oxygen to maintain the arterial oxygen tension above 60 mmHg (Table 10.4).

There are some controversial adjunctive measures advised in treating ventilatory insufficiency, such as restriction of intravenous fluids, steroids, diuretics and salt-poor albumin (Trinkle *et al.*, 1975). It is not necessary to use any of these. The resuscitation of the trauma patient should be based on maintaining flow to the critical organs, and this is best determined by keeping atrial filling pressures as near normal as possible, maintaining adequate urinary output (>0.5 ml/kg/hr) and reversing the clinical signs of shock. Keeping the patient 'dry' will not selectively reduce oedema in the chest wall nor in parenchymal lung injuries. The efficacy of diuretics in treating chest wall injuries and underlying pulmonary contusions is unproven. It is unrealistic to think that contusions of the chest wall or the lung can be selectively 'dehydrated'. The administration of salt-poor albumin is equally controversial, and in one randomized study (Lucas *et al.*, 1980) was shown to adversely affect mortality and morbidity.

TRACHEOBRONCHIAL INJURY

Physical forces

Tracheobronchial injuries constitute less than 1% of all major thoracic injuries. They are most often seen after high-speed motor vehicle accidents or falls from significant heights. Occasionally they follow crush injuries to the chest but this is most often associated with traumatic asphyxia although injury to the tracheobronchial tree is possible, particularly lacerations to the trachealis muscle.

The forces involved are typically deceleration injuries causing shear to one or the other main stem bronchus. Eighty-five per cent of lacerations are within 2 cm of the carina. If the injury involves the distal trachea, there is typically a linear laceration of the trachealis muscle which implies increased pressure such as that that might come from a closed glottic injury and compressive forces to the thorax. Injuries involving the main stem bronchus are usually circumferential and complete.

Pathophysiology

The most immediate effect of a tracheobronchial injury is the release of air into potential spaces. If the air dissects into the pleural cavity, this may lead to immediate pneumothorax and not infrequently to a tension pneumothorax. Depending on its size a pneumothorax can cause immediate hypoxia and respiratory embarrassment. A tension pneumothorax is usually associated with complete collapse of one lung with increased intrapleural pressure and shift of the mediastinum towards the opposite hemithorax. The latter causes further ventilatory embarrassment because of contralateral lung compression and obstruction of venous return, either from kinking of the great veins or increased intrapleural pressure.

Air may also dissect into the mediastinum and be at sufficient pressure to obstruct the venous return. Rarely air can also dissect into the pericardial sac where it may contribute to pericardial tamponade and obstruction of venous return. The authors have seen at least one instance where air dissected into the subcutaneous tissue and was of sufficient magnitude to cause a decrease in chest wall compliance.

As soon as the pleural cavity has been decompressed with tube thoracostomy the most common pathophysiological effect is 'wasted' ventilation. This is associated with constant bubbling from the underwater seal and can make positive-pressure ventilation extremely difficult.

Diagnosis

Disruption of the tracheobronchial tree is suggested by significant haemoptysis, airway obstruction, progressive mediastinal air, subcutaneous emphysema, tension pneumothorax and persistent air leak after placement of a chest tube. Chest roentgenograms typically show mediastinal air, subcutaneous air and obvious pneumothorax (Figure 10.5). Bronchoscopy is essentially mandatory in all cases of suspected tracheobronchial injury, not only to

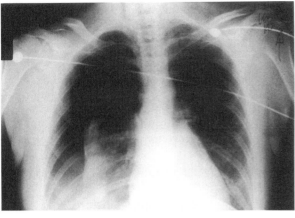

(a)

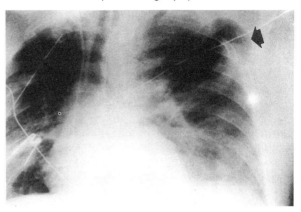

Figure 10.6 Lung herniation (arrow) through a traumatic chest wall defect.

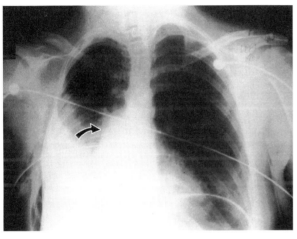

(b)

Figure 10.5 Bronchial disruption. Initial chest roentgenogram (a) showing large right pneumothorax. After chest tube placement (b) the right lung remained collapsed (arrow).

confirm the diagnosis, but also to direct the surgeon to the proper haemithorax. Since the injuries are typically near the carina, air may dissect into the opposite pleural cavity confusing the surgeon.

LUNG INJURY

Physical forces

The most common cause of lung injury is a motor vehicle accident. Frontal crashes can produce lung injury by direct impact with the steering column, dashboard or other hard surfaces. Lateral crashes or 'T bone' injuries are commonly associated with lung injury secondary to intrusion into the vehicle by the other vehicle and direct compressive forces on the lateral bony thorax (Figure 10.6). Rotational and rollover accidents can result in lung injury by shear forces. Injury can also occur as a sequelae of

crush, either by direct compressive forces or shear. Falls may cause lung lacerations as a consequence of direct forces when the victim lands, or from shear- or deceleration-type forces. Injuries resulting from assaults are usually direct compressive forces transmitted through the chest wall.

Traumatic asphyxia is a particular type of direct compression to the chest and is usually associated with a closed glottis or high pressures suddenly transmitted to the tracheobronchial tree. This compressive force is sufficient to cause a sudden rise in the pressure in all the great veins in the upper half of the body with a similar high pressure in the capillaries of the head and neck and associated rupture and extravasation of blood into the tissue. The pressure may also be transmitted into the alveoli resulting in pneumatocele and extravasation of blood.

The final physical force that may injure the lung is blast. Although blast injury can also cause thermal burns and injury by penetration due to secondary missiles, the primary effect is due to the blast wave propagating through the body as a stress wave. The stress wave loses energy (and thus produces injury) at air–tissue interfaces (see p. 216).

Pathophysiology

Injury to the lung may result in: parenchymal laceration, systemic air embolism, contusion, haematoma and pneumatocele. The most common features shared by all these injuries are haemothorax and pneumothorax. Haemothorax can be caused by injuries to the chest wall with laceration of the parietal pleura or injuries to the lung parenchyma or vessels with a tear of the visceral pleura. Haemothorax can also occur as a consequence of mediastinal visceral injury which breaches the parietal pleura lining the mediastinum. Because of the relatively low intra-alveolar and tracheobronchial pressures, significant bleeding can occur into the pleural space as the lung collapses.

Pneumothorax most commonly occurs after disruption of the visceral pleura with communication to the alveolar sacs or bronchi. Air escapes from the tracheobronchial tree and cannot return, usually as a consequence of a tissue flap valve created by the injured pulmonary parenchyma or pleura. Pneumothorax can also occur as a result of direct injury to the trachea and/or main stem bronchi with dissection into the mediastinum and penetration into the pleural cavity. Occasionally, pneumothorax can develop as a result of chest wall defects where the tissue serves as a flap valve for air.

Lung lacerations are more common than appreciated 20 years ago. CT examination now shows that these occur in approximately one-third of significant thoracic injuries where there is visible contusion on plain chest X-rays. The cause is typically from direct compression of ribs onto the parenchyma causing shear injury, or by direct penetration of the rib that has been fractured.

Systemic air embolism is the consequence of a bronchopulmonary vein fistula and occurs in approximately 4% of all major thoracic injuries (Yee *et al.*, 1983). Two-thirds of cases are from penetrating trauma and a third from blunt trauma. When systemic air embolism occurs from blunt trauma it is usually due to a laceration of the lung from a fractured rib or from pneumatocele formation within the pulmonary parenchyma. With spontaneous ventilation the pressure differential is typically from the pulmonary vein to the bronchus which may result in haemoptysis. Once positive-pressure ventilation has been started or the patient grunts or performs a Valsalva manoeuvre as a result of resuscitation, the pressure differential is from the bronchus into the pulmonary vein thus causing air to flood the systemic circulation.

Pulmonary contusions with extravasation to the interstitium and alveolar sacs are the most common injury to the lung following blunt trauma. Contusions can also occur around lacerations from any cause or as a consequence of blast injury. Pneumatoceles are the outcome of internal lacerations of the pulmonary parenchyma either from shear injury or violent explosive increases in tracheobronchial airway pressures, which result in disruption of alveolar septa and coalescence of injured alveoli (Figure 10.7). A pulmonary haematoma results from the same forces that cause a pneumatocele but, instead of filling with air, the space fills with blood.

Diagnosis

Clinical signs permit diagnosis of massive haemothorax and tension pneumothorax. Small amounts of blood (less than 250–300 ml) and air may not be seen on X-ray but can be detected on CT, which is also the best way of identifying lung laceration especially at the periphery of the lung where there may also be a pneumatocele. A laceration involving the visceral pleura gives rise to a continuous air leak.

Systemic air embolism requires a strong index of suspicion in any major chest injury. Neurological features without the presence of head injury imply the condition unless proven otherwise. Air in the retinal vessels, sudden cardiac collapse after intubation and positive-pressure ventilation (probably the result of air in the coronary arteries), froth on arterial puncture and the characteristic sound from a Doppler probe over a peripheral artery are all diagnostic. At emergency thoracotomy for cardiac arrest air may be seen in the coronary arteries.

About a third of pulmonary contusions are not diagnosed on an initial chest X-ray but become visible at 18–24 hours as fluid accumulates after

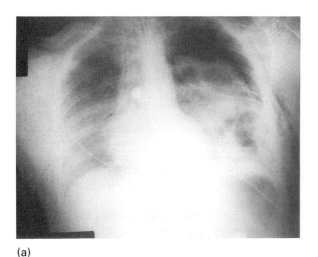

(a)

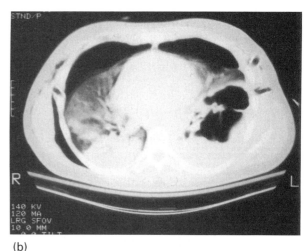

(b)

Figure 10.7 Large left pneumocoele and bilateral pneumothoraces demonstrated on chest roentgenogram (a) and computed tomography (b).

initial resuscitation. CT is more sensitive and permits classification into three grades – mild, moderate and severe.

Management

Tube thoracotomy is the routine treatment for collections of blood and air, though in a tension pneumothorax it may be preceded by needle puncture in the second intercostal space. Careful attention to detail is required to avoid persistent blood and fibrin in the pleural space which as they organize form a constricting layer which must later be removed by decortication. Bleeding from a lung laceration can be tamponaded by re-expansion of the lung in 85% of cases but in the remainder thoracotomy and direct suture is required. Persistent bleeding is more often from intercostal or internal mammary vessels and requires thoracotomy.

Systemic air embolism is managed by thoracotomy and clamping of the hilum of the damaged lung to stop the continued passage of air into the blood vessels. Physical removal of air from the heart and pharmacological removal from the systemic circulation by tracheobronchial administration of adrenalin are followed by repair of the lung injury.

The recent more common demonstration of pulmonary contusions by CT has led to controversy over their management. Most do not require specific treatment but the 10% classified as severe are often associated with a significant flail component in the chest wall and carry a mortality of 40% (Clark *et al.*, 1988). Rarely in such patients whose respiratory function deteriorates it may be appropriate to resect the damaged lobe to reduce right to left shunt and improve oxgenation. In moderate or minor contusions the authors find no evidence that adjunctive measures such as restricted hydration or steroids are of value. Routine chemoprophylaxis has been suggested as valuable (Grover *et al.*, 1977; Locurto *et al.*, 1986) but a randomized trial failed to confirm their efficacy (LeBanc and Tucker, 1985).

Pneumatoceles are treated non-operatively unless infection and abscess supervene. Truamatic asphyxia and blast injuries are managed on conventional lines and for the degree of respiratory impairment and injury with which they present.

CARDIAC INJURY

Physical forces

Cardiac injury is the cause of death in up to 70% of motor vehicle accident fatalities (Sigler, 1945; Parmley *et al.*, 1958). Injuries sustained reflect the forces incurred upon impact (Nirgiotis *et al.*, 1990; Fulda *et al.*, 1991). Heart compression between the sternum and vertebral column can lacerate or rupture the myocardium. Rapid compression during late diastole may rupture chordae, papillary muscles and valve leaflets. Impalement by fractured ribs or sternal fragments may also accompany compressive injury. Direct precordial impacts can induce myocardial contusion, coronary artery laceration and/or coronary thrombosis. Acute compression of the abdomen and lower extremities can raise intrathoracic venous pressures to the point of right atrial or ventricular rupture. An understanding of the physiology associated with each of these injuries helps to guide the clinician to proper diagnosis and therapy.

Pathophysiology

The presentation of cardiac tamponade depends on the underlying cause. When it is secondary to myocardial rupture or coronary artery laceration, it occurs abruptly. Slow extravasation of blood from a minor laceration or contusion may lead to tamponade over hours or days and can often be confused with pulmonary embolism because external compression of the right atrium by pericardial blood prevents diastolic filling of the right atrium and ventricle, central venous pressures rise, cardiac output falls and clinical features of shock become evident. Blood within the pericardium which does not cause these haemodynamic effects can still lead to sterile pericarditis and its long-term sequelae.

Cardiac contusion is a spectrum of injury ranging from localized ecchymosis to frank infarction. Animal studies demonstrate poor contractility in the area of contusion which may require 2–5 weeks to resolve (Sabbah *et al.*, 1989). The localized impairment of function diminishes overall cardiac performance. Depending on cardiac reserve, contusion may precipitate circulatory collapse, which is particularly common in the elderly patient with a limited cardiac reserve and heightened haemodynamic demands because of other injuries. Contusion and subsequent oedema impair blood flow locally leading to ischaemia and possibly infarction. Ectopic electrical activity originating in the injured and ischaemic myocardium predisposes to arrhythmias (Snow *et al.*, 1982). Conduction abnormalities, including bundle branch block, may also occur in 6–20% of patients (Snow *et al.*, 1982); (Fabian *et al.*, 1988).

Persistent murmur or development of congestive failure after blunt trauma may signify valvular or interventricular septal rupture. The aortic valve, particularly the non-coronary cusp, is most susceptible followed by the mitral valve (Liedtke and Demuth, 1973). The classic clinical signs of valvular insufficiency lead the clinician to the diagnosis.

Diagnosis

Shock disproportionate to blood loss should make the clinician suspicious of cardiac laceration or rupture with tamponade. Beck's triad – paradoxical pulse, decreased heart tones and neck vein distension – is a common clinical occurrence, but cannot be completely relied upon. The presence of a pericardial rub, valvular insufficiency murmur or chest wall contusion are also suspicious physical findings.

Cardiospecific enzymes are often elevated. Serum creatinine phosphokinase measured in isolation is insensitive for diagnosis (Keller and Shatney, 1988) but its elevation is strongly correlated with the development of cardiac complications (Healy *et al.*, 1990). A globular appearance of the cardiac shadow on chest X-ray is present in tamponade. Electrocardiography may demonstrate a local area of ischaemia/infarction but ECG abnormalities may also be the consequence of anaemia or electrolyte imbalance.

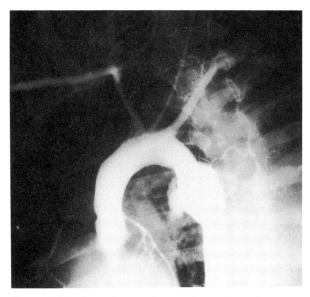

Figure 10.8 Contained descending thoracic aorta transection at the level of the ligamentum arteriosus.

Management

The management approach to cardiac injuries is dictated by the urgency of the situation. Myocardial rupture is the most acute lesion. The overwhelming majority of these patients die at the scene (Parmley *et al.*, 1958). The patient who has obtainable vital signs in the field, but arrives at the emergency room without vital signs, has a poor prognosis. In one study only 2% of these patients benefited from emergency room thoracotomy (Esposito *et al.*, 1991). The patient with rupture who arrives in the emergency room with vital signs and presents in tamponade has an excellent prognosis if the diagnosis is quickly recognized.

Valvular disruption can have an acute presentation and requires immediate therapy. Mitral valve rupture may precipitate acute congestive failure. Aortic leaflet, chordae and papillary ruptures are much less acute. The only physical sign may be persistent murmur.

Management of cardiac contusion remains a subject of controversy, but is directed at the haemodynamic problems caused by myocardial insufficiency. Recovery from significant contusion may require several weeks. Late complications include aneurysm formation, endomyocardial thrombosis with distal emboli and myocardial rupture.

INJURY OF THE AORTA AND GREAT VESSELS

Physical forces

The most common site of vascular injury following blunt chest trauma is the descending aorta at the level of the ligamentum arteriosum (Figure 10.8). During rapid horizontal deceleration, the momentum of the mobile heart carries it in an anterior direction away from the fixed thoracic aorta posteriorly. The descending aorta then tears at its ligamentous attachment to the left pulmonary artery. Vertical deceleration secondary to falls induces acute lengthening of the proximal subclavian and innominate artery as the heart and arch move inferiorly. This is the second most common thoracic great vessel injury. Deceleration forces less commonly lead to injury of the aortic root and ascending aortic. Acute hyperextension of the neck with rotation of the head can avulse the great vessels to the head as they branch off the aorta. Direct compressive forces to the anterior chest wall may shear off the innominate or left common carotid arteries as they are pushed passed the vertebral column (Figure 10.9).

Pathophysiology

Haemorrhage associated with aortic rupture is usually fatal. Only 10–20% survive long enough to reach the emergency room because the disruption of intima and media is contained by the adventitia. Forty per cent of those have a major haemorrhage within 24 hours and an additional 30% within the next several days (Parmley *et al.*, 1958). The remaining 30% develop false aneurysms and are at risk for late rupture. Rapid fluid resuscitation with restoration of blood pressure may precipitate haemorrhage and death and if a lesion has been diagnosed, it is important to avoid hypertension, especially during induction of anaesthesia. Eventual disruption is accompanied by massive haemothorax or retropleural haematoma. Haemothorax is

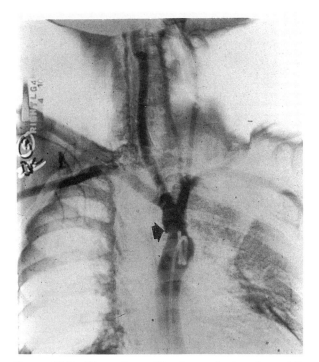

Figure 10.9 Disruption of the innominate artery at its takeoff from the aorta as demonstrated by digital subtraction angiography. Repair was done with a bypass graft from the ascending aorta to the distal innominate artery.

rare in innominate and subclavian disruption; apical or retropleural haematomas, however, are common. Symptoms secondary to an expanding haematoma such as hoarseness, superior vena cava syndrome and stridor may develop. Vascular occlusion will cause features distal to the injury such as anuria, stroke, paraplegia or upper extremity ischaemia.

Diagnosis

The mechanism of injury coupled with the physical examination should alert the clinician to the possibility of great vessel disruption. Table 10.5 summarizes warning signs of great vessel injury. A large collective review demonstrated that 93% of patients with great vessel injury had an abnormal mediastinum on initial chest X-ray (Woodring, 1990). In the remaining 7% the history and physical examination as well as serial chest X-rays may direct the clinician to obtain an aortogram which is the current gold standard for diagnosis. In addition, it is indispensable in planning the surgical approach. A small percentage of normal patients will have a ductus diverticulum which must not be confused with a contained rupture. Computed tomography has little or no role in evaluation of thoracic great vessel after blunt trauma (McLean *et al.*, 1991).

TABLE 10.5

WARNING SIGNS OF AORTA AND GREAT VESSEL INJURY

History	Physical examination
Ejection from vehicle	Significant chest wall contusion
High-speed deceleration	Fracture of ribs, clavicle, sternum or scapula with or without impalement by bony fragments
Paraplegia with or without bony spine deformity	Base of neck haematoma
Co-occupant killed in accident	Superior vena cava syndrome
Fall from significant height	Pulse disparity between extremities
	Posterior murmur
	Tamponade
	Tracheal deviation
	Anuria

Management

Although conservative medical management of thoracic aortic disruption has been reported (Wigle and Moran, 1991), most trauma surgeons advocate immediate repair. This stems from the fact that a significant percentage of patients will experience an exsanguinating haemorrhage or dissection in the immediate postinjury period (Parmley *et al.*, 1958).

If patients have significant associated injuries which preclude repair, a period of conservative management aimed at rigid blood pressure control is an acceptable mode of treatment.

Surgical repair of innominate and proximal subclavian disruptions should be preceded by bronchoscopy and oesophagonscopy to rule out associated airway and oesophageal injury.

Disruptions of the aortic root and ascending aorta require cardiopulmonary bypass.

DIAPHRAGM

Physical forces

Invariably the force that causes rupture of the diaphragm is direct compressive, either by direct action on the bony thoracic cage or by increasing intra-abdominal pressure to the extent that it causes a 'blow-out' of the diaphragm. Lateral impacts in car accidents create a particular high risk in that they cause compression of the thorax towards the vertebral body which then tends to stretch and tear the diaphragm.

Pathophysiology

It must be emphasized that if enough kinetic energy has been applied to the torso so as to rupture the diaphragm, there are often significant associated injuries as well. Small ruptures may not cause immediate difficulty with ventilation but do create a problem in diagnosis and prevention of late sequelae such as incarceration or strangulation of abdominal viscera. If the injury is a moderate or severe rupture, there can be associated ventilatory insufficiency and hypoxaemia. Part of this insufficiency is the consequence of ineffective bellows action of the bony thorax, particularly if the left hemidiaphragm has been ruptured. In many instances rupture of the right hemidiaphragm will not be noticed because the liver serves as an immediate 'patch' to the diaphragmatic hole. If the liver has been injured, bleeding may occur into the right hemithorax. If the hole is large enough for abdominal viscera to enter the pleural cavity, there may be considerable immediate ventilatory embarrassment. In some instances there may be shift of the mediastinum with resultant venous obstructive symptoms and hypoxaemia. If there has been hollow viscus injury within the abdominal cavity, contamination of the pleural cavity is inevitable.

Diagnosis

The diagnosis of diaphragmatic injuries is problematical (Figure 10.10). It has been the authors' experience that approximately one-third of plain X-rays fail to show significant disorder that would lead to the diagnosis. In contrast, Besson and Popovici (1991) state that 90% of plain chest X-rays are abnormal but this statement is qualified in that their series was of diaphragmatic hernia. Adjunctive studies such as barium enema (gastrografin), CT scan, diagnostic peritoneal lavage also have a high false-negative rate (Brown and Richardson, 1985; Harms *et al.*, 1987). Laparoscopy has been used successfully in diagnosing rupture of the diaphragm but does run the risk of causing tension pneumothorax when air is insufflated into the peritoneal cavity. Conversely, thorascopy appears to have a high rate of positive diagnosis with minimal complications (Jackson *et al.*, 1975; Jones *et al.*, 1981).

Management

Surgical repair is always indicated. Lacerations tend to be radial and lend themselves to primary suture. Those caused by avulsion of the diaphragm from the rib cage are also repaired by suture. The authors have not found it necessary to use synthetic prosthesis to repair large defects because the diaphragm tends to be redundant and apposition of tears is usually relatively easy.

OESOPHAGEAL INJURIES

Physical forces

Rupture of the oesophagus due to blunt impact is a rare injury because of the protected nature of the oesophagus. The cervical oesophagus is relatively

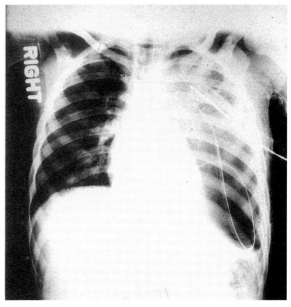

(a)

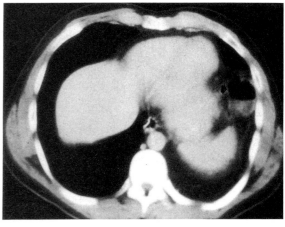

(b)

Figure 10.10 Traumatic diaphragmatic hernias demonstrated by chest X-ray and computed tomography. In (a), note the presence of the nasogastric tube above the inferiorly displaced left hemidiaphragm. A hollow fluid-filled viscus is clearly seen above the left hemidiaphragm in (b).

short and can rarely be injured by direct forces (top of the steering wheel or clothes line injury) which push it directly against the vertebral body. Such a force would invariably also be associated with either carotid artery injury or spinal cord transection. The thoracic oesophagus lies along the anterior part of the vertebral bodies or to the left side as it descends into the chest and is again protected from significant blunt forces. An area where the oesophagus is vulnerable is at the thoracic inlet (Figure 10.11). We have seen one case where the

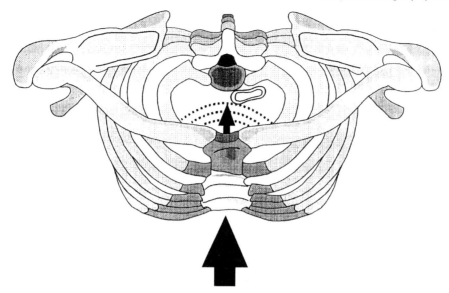

Figure 10.11   Direct compressive force at the manubrium against the vertebral column can lacerate the oesophagus. Other structures in the thoracic outlet are also vulnerable to injury.

manubrium was pushed directly back against the vertebral body causing a 7 cm longitudinal rent in the oesophagus with subsequent mediastinitis. Case reports also exist documenting intra-abdominal pressure increases as a cause of oesophageal rupture which is not dissimilar from postemetic rupture.

Diagnosis

Conscious patients who present with cervical oesophageal injuries will invariably have pain on swallowing and cervical subcutaneous emphysema. Those with injury to the thoracic oesophagus may have immediate acute chest pain, vomiting, rapid respirations and subcutaneous emphysema. If the laceration is small, clinical and physical findings may be late and primarily related to mediastinitis.

Plain films of the chest often reveal mediastinal emphysema, subcutaneous emphysema, haemopneumothorax and later evidence of air-fluid levels within the mediastinum or microbubbles associated with infection. Contrast studies will show leak of contrast usually within the mediastinum or into the deep cervical fascia. Oesophagoscopy is not usually necessary.

Management

Surgical exploration and repair is the treatment of choice for cervical oesophageal rupture.

Injuries to the thoracic oesophagus are usually not appreciated until later in the patient's course when complications develop – mediastinitis or increasing mediastinal or subcutaneous emphy-

sema. If the diagnosis is made within 6 hours of injury, primary repair is done. Between 6 and 12 hours the surgeon will have to use judgement as to whether or not there is established mediastinitis or infection of the oesophageal wounds. After 12 hours the authors prefer some type of drainage procedure and consideration for oesophageal exclusion.

REFERENCES

Berger M., Wetzler E.M., Wallis R.S. (1988). Tumor necrosis factor is the major monocyte product that increases complement receptor expression on mature human neutrophils. *Blood*, **71**, 151–8.

Besson A., Popovici Z. (1991). Diaphragmatic injury in thoracic surgery. In *Surgical management of chest injuries*, Vol 7, (Webb W., Besson A., eds). St Louis: Mosby Year Book, 1991.

Besson A., Saegesser F. (1983). *Color Atlas of Chest Trauma and Associated Injuries*. New Jersey: Med Economic Book.

Brewer L.S., Samson P.C., Burbank B. et al. (1946). The wet lung in war casualties. *Ann. Surg.*, **123**, 343.

Broudy V.C., Harlan J.M., Adamson J.W. (1987). Disparate effects of tumor necrosis factor-α/cachectin and tumor necrosis factor-β/lymphotoxin on hematopoietic growth factor production and neutrophil adhesion molecule expression by cultured human endothelial cells. *J.Immunol.*, **138**, 4298–302.

Brown G.L., Richardson J.D. (1985). Traumatic diaphragmatic hernia: a continuing challenge. *Ann. Thoracic Surg.*, **39**, 170–5.

Bruch R.C., Thayer W.S. (1983). Differential effect of lipid peroxidation on membrane fluidity as determined by electron spin resonance probes. *Biochim. Biophys. Acta*, **733**, 216–22.

Chien S. (1967). Role of the sympathetic nervous system in hemorrhage. *Physiol. Rev.*, **47**, 214.

Clark G.C., Schecter W.P., Trunkey D.D. (1988). Variables affecting outcome in blunt chest trauma: flail chest versus pulmonary contusion. *J. Trauma*, **28**, 298–303.

Clark M.A., Chen M-J., Crooke S.T., Bomalaski J.S. (1988). Tumor necrosis factor (cachectin) induces phospholipase A_2 activity and synthesis of phospholipase A_2-activating protein in endothelial cells. *Biochem. J*, **250**, 125–32.

Craven K.D., Oppenheimer L., Wood L.D.H. (1979). Effects of contusion and flail chest on pulmonary perfusion and oxygen exchange. *J. Applied Physiol.*, **47**, 729–33.

Demopoulos H.B., Flamm E., Seligman M., Pietronigro D.D. (1982). Oxygen-free radicals in central nervous system ischemia and trauma. In *Pathology of Oxygen* (Autor A.P., ed.). New York: Academic Press, pp. 127–55.

Esposito T.J., Jurkovich G.J., Rice C.L., et al. (1991). Reappraisal of emergency room thoracotomy in a changing environment. *J. Trauma*, **31**, 881–6.

Fabian T.C., Mangiante E.C., Patterson C.R. et al. (1988). Myocardial contusion in blunt trauma: clinical characteristics, means of diagnosis and implications for patient management. *J. Trauma*, **28**, 50–7.

Fulda G., Brathwaite G.E.M., Rodriguez A. et al. (1991). Blunt traumatic rupture of the heart and pericardium: a ten year experience (1979–1989). *J.Trauma*, **31**, 167–73.

Gamble J.R., Harlan J.M., Klebanoff S.J., Vadas M.A. (1985). Stimulation of the adherence of neutrophils to umbilical vein endothelium by human recombinant tumor necrosis factor. *Proc. Natl. Acad. Sci. USA*, **82**, 8667–1.

Goldblum S.E., Yoneda K., Cohen D.A., McClain C.J. (1988). Provocation of pulmonary vascular endothelial injury in rabbits by human recombinant interleukin-1β. *Infect. Immun.*, **56**, 2255–63.

Goldblum S.E., Henning B., Jay M. et al. (1989). Tumor necrosis factor α-induced pulmonary vascular endothelial injury. *Infect. Immunol.*, **57**, 1218–26.

Guyton A.C., Crowell J.W. (1961). Dynamics of the heart in shock. *Fed. Proc.*, **20**, 51.

Guz A. (1975). Regulation of respiration in man. *Ann. Rev. Physiol.*, **37**, 303.

Hansen A.J. (1985). Effect of anoxia on ion distribution in the brain. *Physiol Rev*, **65**, 101–48.

Harms B., Helgerson R., Starling J. (1987). Diaphragmatic injuries following blunt trauma. *Am. J. Surg.*, **53**, 325–30.

Healy M.A., Brown R., Fleizer D. (1990). Blunt cardiac injury: is diagnosis necessary? *J. Trauma*, **30**, 137–46.

Hennig B., Goldblum S.E., McClain C.J. (1987). Interleukin-1 (IL-1) and tumor necrosis factor/cachectin (TNF) increase endothelial permeability in vitro. *J. Leukoc. Biol.*, **42**, 551–2.

Hobbs C.A. (1981). Car occupant injury patterns and mechanisms. *Supplementary Report* 648, Crowthorne: Transport and Research Laboratory.

Horvath C.J., Ferro T.J., Jesmok G., Malik A.B. (1988). Recombinant tumor necrosis factor increases pulmonary vascular permeability independent of neutrophils. *Proc. Natl. Acad. Sci. USA*, **85**, 9219–23.

Huelke D.F. (1982). Steering assembly performance and driver injury severity in frontal crashes. SAE 820474. In *Proceedings of the International Congress and Exposition*, Detroit, pp. 1–30.

Jackson A.M., Ferreira A.A. (1975). Thoroscopy as an aid to the diagnosis of diaphragmatic injury and penetrating wounds to the left lower chest: a preliminary report. *Injury*, **7**, 213.

Jansson I., Loven L., Rammer L., Lennquist S. (1985). Pulmonary trapping of platelets and fibrin after musculoskeletal trauma: an experimental model. *J. Trauma*, **25**, 288–98.

Jansson I.G., Hetland O., Rammer L.M. et al. (1988). Effects of phospholipase C, a tissue thromboplastin inhibitor, on pulmonary microembolism after missile injury of the limb. *J. Trauma*, **28**, (suppl. 1), S5222–5.

Jones J.W., Kitahama A., Webb W.R. et al. (1981). Emergency thoroscopy: a logical approach to chest trauma management. *J. Trauma*, **21**, 280–4.

Keitt A.S., Hinkes C., Block A.J. (1974). Comparison of factors regulating red cell 2, 3 diphosphoglycerate in acute and chronic hypoxia. *J. Lab. Clin. Med.*, **84**, 275–80.

Keller K.D., Shatney C.H. (1988). Creatine phosphokinase-MB assays in patients with suspected myocardial contusion: diagnostic test or test of diagnosis? *J. Trauma*, **28**, 58–63.

Kemmer W.T., Eckert W.G., Gathright J.B. et al. (1961). Patterns of thoracic injuries in fatal traffic accidents. *J. Trauma*, **1**, 595.

Kilmartin J.V., Rossi-Bernardi L. (1973). Interaction of hemoglobin with hydrogen ions, carbon dioxide and organic phosphates. *Physiol. Rev.*, **53**, 836.

Landercasper J., Cogbill T.H., Lindes-Smith L.A. (1984). Long term disability after flail chest injury. *J. Trauma*, **24**, 410–15.

LeBanc K.A., Tucker W.Y. (1985). Prophylactic antibiotics in closed tube thoracostomy. *Surg. Gynecd. Obstet.*, **160**, 259–64.

Lefer A.M. (1982). Vascular mediators in ischemia and shock. In *Pathophysiology of Shock, Anoxia and Ischemia* (Couley R.A., Trump B.E., eds). Baltimore: Williams & Wilkins, pp. 165–81.

Liedtke A.J., DeMuth W.E. (1973). Non-penetrating cardiac injuries: collective review. *Am. Heart J.*, **86**, 687–97.

LoCurto J.L., Tischler C.D., Swan K.G. et al. (1986). Tube thoracostomy in trauma – antibiotics are not. *J. Trauma*, **26**, 1067–72.

Lucas C.E., Ledgerwood A.M., Higgins R.F., Weeber D.W. (1980). Impaired pulmonary function after albumin resuscitation from shock. *J. Trauma*, **20**, 446–51.

Mackersie R.C., Karagianes T.G., Hoyt D.B., Davis J.W. (1991). Prospective evaluation of epidural and intravenous administration of fentanyl for pain control and restoration of ventilatory function following multiple rib fractures. *J. Trauma*, **31**, 443–51.

Malpas S.C., Robinson B.J., Maling J.B. (1990). Mechanism of ethanol-induced vasodilation. *J. Appl. Physiol.*, **68**, 731–4.

McCord J.M. (1985). Oxygen derived free radicals in post ischemic tissue injury. *N. Engl. J. Med.*, **312**, 159–63.

McCord J.M. (1987). Oxygen-derived radicals: a link between reperfusion injury and inflammation. *Fed. Proc.*, **46**, 2402–6.

McLean T.R., Olinger G.N., Thorsen M.K. (1991) Computed tomography in the evaluation of the aorta in patients sustaining blunt chest trauma. *J. Trauma*, **31**, 254–6.

Moore F.D. (1965). The effects of hemorrhage on body composition. *N. Engl. J. Med.*, **273**, 567–77.

Mullane K.M., Read N., Salmon J.A., Moncada S. (1984). Role of leukocytes in acute myocardial infarction in anesthetized dogs. *J. Pharmacol. Exp. Ther*, **228**, 510–22.

Newman R.J., Jones I.S. (1984). A prospective study of 413 consecutive car occupants with chest injury. *J. Trauma*, **24**, 129–34.

Nigriotis J.G., Colon R., Sweeney M.S. (1990). Blunt trauma to the heart: the pathophysiology of injury. *J. Emerg. Med*, **8**, 617–23.

Okusawa S., Gelfand J.A., Ikejima T. et al. (1988). Interleukin-1 induces a shock-like state in rabbits. Synergism with tumor necrosis factor and the effect of cyclooxygenase inhibition. *J. Clin. Invest.*, **81**, 1162–72.

Paris F., Tarazona V., Blasco E. et al (1975). Surgical stabilization of traumatic flail chest. *Thorax*, **30**, 521–6.

Parmley L.F., Manion W.C., Mattingly T.W. (1958). Non-penetrating rupture of the heart. *Circulation*, **18**, 371–96.

Patrick L.M., Mertz H.J. Jr, Croelle C.K. (1967). Cadaver, knee, chest, and head impact wounds. In *Proceedings of the 11th Stapp Car Crash Conference*. New York: Society of Automotive Engineers.

Pirkle J.C., Gann D.S. (1976). Restitution of blood volume after hemorrhage: role of adrenal cortex. *Am. J. Physiol.*, **230**, 1683–7.

Petrone W.F., English D.K., Wong K., McCord J.M. (1980). Free radicals and inflammation: superoxide-dependent activation of a neutrophil chemotactic factor in plasma. *Proc. Natl. Acad. Sci. USA*, **77**, 1159–63.

Pohlman T.H., Stanness K.A., Beatly P.G. et al. (1986). An endothelial cell surface factor(s) induced *in vitro* by lipopolysaccharide, interleukin-1 and tumor necrosis factor-increases neutrophil adherence by a CDw 18-dependent mechanism. *J. Immunol.*, **136**, 4548–53.

Qvist J., Mygind T., Crottogini A. et al. (1988). Cardiovascular adjustments to pulmonary vascular injury in dogs. *Anesthesiology*, **68**, 341–9.

Sabbah H.N., Moyhi J., Hawkins E.T. (1989). Longitudinal evaluation of left ventricular performance in dogs following nonpenetrating cardiac trauma. *J. Trauma*, **29**, 175–9.

Saldeen T. (1976). The microembolism syndrome. *Microvasc. Res.*, **2**, 227–59.

Schlag G., Krosl P., Redl H. (1988). Cardiopulmonary response of the elderly to traumatic and septic shock. In *Perspectives in Shock Research*, Vol. II (Passmore J.C., ed.) Inc., New York: Alan R. Liss, pp. 233–42.

Sigler L.H. (1945). Traumatic injury of the heart – incidence of its occurrence in forty-two cases of severe bodily injury. *Am. Heart J.*, **30**, 459–78.

Skillman J.J., Awwad H.K., Moore F.D. (1967a). Plasma protein kinetics of the early transcapillary refill after hemorrhage in man. *Surg. Gynecol. Obstet.*, **125**, 983–96.

Skillman J.J., Lauler D.P., Hickler R.B. et al. (1967b). Hemorrhage in normal man: effect of renin, cortisol, aldosterone and urine composition. *Ann. Surg.*, **166**, 865–85.

Snow N., Richardson J.D., Flint L.M. (1982). Myocardial contusion: implications for patients with multiple traumatic injuries. *Surgery*, **92**, 744–50.

Trinkle J.K., Richardson D.J., Franz J.L. et al. (1975). Management of flail chest without mechanical ventilation. *Ann. Thorac. Surg.*, **19**, 355–61.

Trunkey D., Holcroft J., Carpenter M.A. (1976). Calcium flux during hemorrhagic shock in baboons. *J. Trauma*, **26**, 633–8.

Van Blisen M., Engels W., Vander Vusse G.J., Reneman R.S. (1989). Significance of myocardial eicosanoid production. *Mol. Cell Biochem.*, **88**, 113–21.

Vatner S.F. (1974). Effects of hemorrhage on blood flow distribution in dogs and primates. *J. Clin. Invest.*, **54**, 225.

Vedder N.B., Winn R.K., Rice C.L. et al. (1988). A monoclonal antibody to leukocyte adherence-promoting glycoprotein, CD18, reduces organ injury end improves survival from hemorrhagic shock in rabbits. *J. Clin. Invest.*, **81**, 939–44.

Wigle R.L., Moran J.M. (1991). Spontaneous healing of traumatic aortic tear: case report. *J. Trauma*, **31**, 280–3.

Wisner D.H. (1990). A stepwise logistic regression analysis of factors affecting morbidity and mortality after thoracic trauma: effect of epidural analgesia. *J. Trauma*, **30**, 799–805.

Woodring J.H. (1990). The normal mediastinum in blunt traumatic rupture of the thoracic aorta and brachiocephalic arteries. *J. Emerg. Med.*, **8**, 467–76.

Yee E.S., Verrier E.D., Thomas A.N. (1983). Management of air embolism in blunt and penetrating thoracic trauma. *J. Thorac Cardiovasc. Surg.*, **85**, 661–7.

11. Non-penetrating Injury of the Abdomen

A.K.C. Li and
S. Paterson-Brown

INTRODUCTION

Blunt abdominal trauma (BAT) is a common problem for the emergency surgeon. However, as a result of concomitant injuries, which are often multiple, the overall picture can be complex and confused with other injuries disguising the underlying abdominal problem. Associated injuries are also major factors in mortality and morbidity (Cox, 1984). Death which is the direct consequence of BAT is either from exsanguination or subsequent sepsis and multiorgan failure. Because of these two major events, delay in diagnosis and treatment remains the most important contributing factor. Early resuscitation followed by precise diagnosis of the injury or injuries is the key to a successful outcome. However, a correct decision at exploration of the abdomen about the choice of treatment – resection, repair, bypass or drainage – may make the ultimate difference between survival and death or between a speedy or a prolonged and complicated recovery. For this, a detailed understanding of the mechanism, distribution, natural history and pathology of injuries which can be sustained in BAT is of assistance in the improvement in outcome in a number of ways:

1. In deciding whether surgery should be undertaken.
2. The appropriateness of a procedure, given the overall condition of the patient and the presence of other injuries.
3. The likelihood of post-traumatic complications, their recognition and correct management.

AETIOLOGY

It is now well recognized that road traffic accidents (RTA) are the most common cause of BAT although personal confrontations, industrial and animal accidents and sporting injuries are other causes. In some reported series, RTAs account for up to 90% of BAT (Cox, 1984) and this figure has risen steadily over the past 40 years in direct relationship with the increase in traffic on ever more congested roads. Modern warfare produces few cases of BAT, and those which do occur tend to be from vehicle accidents of one form or another. Large studies of trauma in North America have demonstrated that 13% of trauma admissions require surgery for BAT

(Cox, 1984) and figures from Britain suggest that 2–3% of all RTA victims sustain abdominal injuries (Department of Transport, 1986).

The introduction of compulsory wearing of seat belts has had a major effect in reducing the incidence of severe injuries from head-on collisions in RTAs, although restraints appear to provide little or no protection from lateral impacts (Newman, 1986). The same may be true of the air bag but information is so far lacking. However, seat belts do appear to have altered the incidence of abdominal injuries and some studies have actually shown an increase in injuries to the small bowel and mesentery (Appleby and Nagy, 1989; and see also below).

DISTRIBUTION OF INJURIES

Although insignificant injury to the small bowel and mesentery seem to be the most common injury from BAT found at laparotomy, the spleen is the most common organ damaged (42%) followed by the liver (36%) and the bowel and mesentery (17%) (Cox, 1984). Injuries to other structures are less common, though distension of the stomach and urinary bladder make their rupture more likely. Retroperitoneal structures are better protected and are therefore less susceptible to blunt injury unless this is severe, although there is some experimental data which suggests that the kidney is particularly at risk from lateral impacts. Diagnosis in blunt injury to retroperitoneal structures may often be delayed.

MECHANISM OF INJURY

Experimental studies in the early part of this century, initially using cadavers and later anaesthetized animals, combined with clinical observation and knowledge of the type of injury, have helped to demonstrate the mechanisms which underlie damage following blunt impact to the abdomen. It is now accepted that there are four main mechanisms: crushing; shearing; bursting; and penetration from bony spicules.

Crushing

The abdomen may be crushed on an anteroposterior or lateral axis and those underlying organs that cannot be easily displaced mainly because of their peritoneal attachments – such as the liver, spleen and retroperitoneal structures are more likely to be injured. In RTAs the steering wheel is a leading source of injury and experimental studies have demonstrated that its stiffness is an important determinant of the severity of the injury sustained (Lau et al., 1987). The duodenum and pancreas may be particularly vulnerable in central anteroposterior crush such as by a heavy impact with a boot or club which drives the abdominal wall inwards and may drive the structures against the lumbar spine (see below). Although small bowel is highly mobile except at its proximal and distal ends, it may still suffer crushing injury to its wall or mesentery, particularly if it is brought in direct or indirect contact with bone. Penetrating injuries to the liver, spleen, bladder and rectum may follow crushing injuries to the overlying ribs and pelvis when bony spicules penetrate their substance.

Crushing impacts produce a wide spectrum of injuries in both solid and hollow organs which can include rupture, haematoma within the wall or retroperitoneal space, and the creation of areas of devitalized tissue which are the result of either direct contusion or associated vascular disruption. Some of these are considered in more detail below (see pp. 146–8) for individual organs.

Shearing

This form of injury is produced either by sudden deceleration force or one applied across the points of attachment of an organ. Intra-abdominal structures can be subjected to shearing when this is applied between their fixed and mobile points, and a rent or tear can result. When solid organs such as the liver or spleen continue to move – usually in a forward direction – shearing may cause tears at the hilum or other points of vascular attachment such as that of the hepatic veins, with consequential haemorrhage. Tears in the small bowel at or near the duodenojejunal flexure or the ileocaecal region can also be attributed to shearing forces, as are those colonic injuries which are found in the sigmoid and transverse areas at or adjacent to their junction with the more rigid ascending, descending and rectal parts. Shearing during rapid deceleration can also explain the increase in incidence of small and large bowel injuries from RTAs after the introduction of seat belts (Appleby and Nagy, 1989).

Rents to the mesentery or even detachment of it from the bowel are also the outcome of shear and lead to both haemorrhage and devitalization. Blood loss may be considerable if the superior mesenteric vein or other large tributaries of the valveless portal venous system are involved (Donahue and Strauch, 1988). Acute dissection of the aorta in association with the use of seat belts is similarly thought to be related to shearing forces (Dajee *et al.*, 1979).

Deformation of the external abdominal wall, such as occurs with disruption of the pelvic girdle or lower thoracic rib cage, results in deformation shear to attached structures. Tears in the bladder may be the outcome of such a shearing element and the male urethra is also susceptible to this force where it traverses the perineal membrane, as are the venous and arterial plexuses in the same region. A similar mechanism associated with lower thoracic compression may also contribute to diaphragmatic rupture (Johnson, 1988).

Bursting

A bursting injury follows a sudden rise in intra-luminal pressure, possibly related to some form of functional and temporary closed loop; as for example, closure of the oesophago-gastric and pyloric sphincters. Although bursting injuries are the direct consequence of an external crushing force, the nature of the injury is different from that of a direct compressive effect. First, they may occur at some distance from the site of compression; for example, when rupture of intestinal contents takes place in an external hernia after blunt trauma to the abdominal wall. A similar mechanism also produces the 'blow-out' injuries of hollow viscera such as the small bowel, colon, urinary bladder, stomach and gall bladder, especially if they are distended. The mechanisms underlying diaphragmatic rupture which are predominantly a paroxysmal rise in intra-abdominal pressure are considered on page 139.

ASSOCIATED INJURIES

Blunt trauma does not have respect for precise anatomical boundaries and thoracoabdominal trauma may produce injuries both above and below the diaphragm. In one study, 35 of 70 patients with liver injuries required entry into the thoracic cavity (Grasberger *et al.*, 1985). The same is true in the lower abdomen where injuries to the pelvic ring are often associated with visceral damage, such as rupture of the bladder. Extensive pelvic fracture may lead to considerable blood loss which of itself, and associated with lower abdominal signs, can mimic intra-abdominal visceral injury.

Visible associated injury to the abdominal wall – such as abrasions and bruises – is highly characteristic of violent deceleration in patients wearing seat belts and provides a clinical clue to the likelihood of BAT. Furthermore, in rapid deceleration such as occurs in head-on collisions, continued forward movement of the upper torso accompanied by flexion may cause either a characteristic crush fracture of a vertebral body or a distraction injury of the lumbar spine – Chance fracture-dislocation (Gumley *et al.*, 1982) which is highly characteristic. In one series there was a 19% incidence of lumbar spine injury in patients who required laparotomy for BAT after motor car accidents, with an increased risk in those wearing lap as distinct from three-point anchorages (Appleby and Nagy, 1989).

In liver injury, as in many other intra-abdominal injuries, the chief determinant of survival other than the extent of tissue damage is the simultaneous occurrence of other injuries (Pretre *et al.*, 1988), particularly head injury (Davis *et al.*, 1976).

Injury to individual structures and organs

Diaphragm
See page 139.

Solid structures
The most important of these are the liver, spleen and pancreas.

The first two share some common features in that closed injuries are characterized by capsular laceration, intraparenchymal haematoma or both. In the presence of laceration, there is a varying amount of free bleeding into the peritoneal cavity depending on the severity of the underlying injury. A haematoma with an intact capsule may (more commonly in the spleen than the liver) expand eventually, leading to capsular rupture – the so-called delayed presentation which occurs in a small number of patients estimated at approximately 1.5% (Dang et al., 1990). There is considerable evidence from scanning studies of the resolution of small haematomas in both organs with minor features of blood loss and the absence or non-progression of local signs (Delius et al., 1989). The widespread use of ultrasonography and CT scanning in the diagnosis of BAT may uncover such lesions but should not necessarily result in active treatment.

Spleen
In addition to the general features described, there are some particular matters which are worthy of note. The severity of the injury varies widely from a small capsular tear, through severe laceration which may divide the organ down to its hilum into two or more fragments, to complete avulsion from the vascular pedicle (Buckman et al., 1989). A careful appraisal of the extent of splenic injury by either scanning or laparotomy is helpful in deciding the tactics of treatment – whether it is possible or not to preserve the spleen. There is also ample clinical experience which suggests that a diseased spleen is more susceptible to violence (Pearce et al., 1988), though it is possible (if unlikely) that a diseased organ can also undergo 'spontaneous' rupture. Infectious mononucleosis, malaria and other disorders that cause changes in splenic size and texture have all been reported to be associated with an increased risk of rupture.

A further interesting though not very well documented late outcome of splenic rupture is intraperitoneal 'splenosis' in which there is seeding of cells throughout the peritoneal cavity. This occurrence has been used as the justification of deliberate splenic autotransplantation after injury, in the hope that some aspects of function of the organ will be preserved (see below).

Maintenance of splenic function is of special importance in childhood where there is a well-recognized occurrence of serious postsplenectomy infection principally with encapsulated gram-positive organisms, such as *streptococcus pneumoniae* and meningococci. The exact mechanism is not well understood but there are a number of theories which are considered in a recent review (Shaw and Print, 1989). Evidence for an increased risk of infection in adults is also present, though the occurrence is much less. The possibility of post-splenectomy infection has prompted attempts to preserve a damaged spleen, either by adopting a non-operative approach which is now commonly used in children, by repair (often with the supplementary use of absorbable meshes (Lange et al., 1988)) or by autotransplantation. Splenorrhaphy is a safe procedure and provided it is technically feasible appears to have less complications than either splenectomy or non-operative management (Rappaport et al., 1990). However, there is no objective evidence to support the use of auto-transplantation (Shaw and Print, 1989).

Both the liver and spleen are essential components of the reticuloendothelial system (RES). In an experimental model splenectomy has been shown to reduce both the clearance of gram-negative bacteria from the blood and the ability to survive a severe septic challenge (Cheslyn-Curtis et al., 1988). Experimental partial hepatectomy has a similar effect, with the extent of the reduction in RES function being proportional to the amount of liver removed (Vo and Chi, 1988).

Though in the past the rise in platelet count after splenectomy has been regarded as benign, there is some evidence that there is an increased risk of subsequent thromboembolic episodes (Pimpl et al., 1989).

Liver
As with the spleen, the degree of damage varies from small capsular lacerations, to large contusions and avulsion of great veins. Possibly as a consequence of deceleration of lateral movement of the trunk with continued rotation of the liver, the most severe injury in terms of outcome is avulsion of hepatic venous channels that enter the vena cava including either of the main veins (Beal, 1990). Though such injury may be immediately fatal it is sometimes tamponaded by abdominal pressure or by the use of antishock G-suits (Aberg et al., 1986), and severe blood loss occurs only when the abdomen is opened. Preoperative recognition of the presence of this type of injury may allow pre-emptive cross clamping of the aorta before the abdomen is opened (Feliciano et al., 1986). In laceration-contusion of the parenchyma tearing of large veins is also the major cause of bleeding and often poses significant problems for arrest. Damage to bile ducts is relatively uncommon but crush injury may be the cause of bile duct transection. In this injury, an impact coming from the front compresses the upper abdomen and forces the liver in a cranial direction, thus stretching the structures

in the portal triad and tearing the duct in the free edge of the lesser omentum just above its fixed part within the pancreas (Rydell, 1990).

Within the liver substance a haematoma may, after a delay of some days, rupture into the biliary tree and cause haemobilia usually accompanied by episodes of obstructive jaundice from clot in the common duct. With non-operative management of a liver contusion this complication should be carefully borne in mind; its occurrence is initially best managed by arteriography and embolization but open procedures may be required.

Pancreas

Closed pancreatic injuries are relatively uncommon. Minor haematomas are probably often subclinical. The characteristic major injury is transection of the gland and duct just to the left of the midline, which is thought to be the outcome of anteroposterior force driving the gland against the left side of the vertebral bodies. Leakage of pancreatic secretion from the severed duct causes a picture which resembles acute pancreatitis but, unlike this condition, surgical management is nearly always necessary to arrest progression. Occasionally a duct transection leads not to spreading retroperitoneal inflammation but to a collection of pancreatic secretion – one form of 'pseudocyst'. In such a patient presentation may be delayed and take the form of a slowly expanding mass in the abdomen. Stricture of the duct may also be a late sequel of injury and presents with recurrent attacks of acute pancreatitis, as chronic pancreatitis or pancreatic abscess (Carr et al., 1989).

Hollow viscera

Stomach Closed injury is relatively rare, perhaps because the organ is partially protected by its relatively thick wall. Bursting of the oesophago-gastric junction has been described in compression injuries and may also take place down the line of the lesser curvature. A special form of iatrogenic injury takes place when an endotracheal tube is accidentally inserted into the oesphagus and used for 'positive-pressure ventilation'.

Duodenum Closed rupture of the duodenum is relatively common and, as previously mentioned, may be associated with delayed diagnosis. As with transection of the pancreas it has been postulated that the duodenum is driven against the lumbar spine, and to a certain extent this is confirmed by the site which is usually posterior in the second part. Blood loss into the retroperitoneum is not often severe but intestinal content causes a spreading retroperitoneal cellulitis with systemic disturbance and the onset of ileus. Late intervention to close the tear is often difficult and the mortality remains at around 10%. Duodenal injury may be combined with damage to the head and uncinate

process of the pancreas, and such injuries are difficult to treat and may require complex surgical manoeuvres (Mansour et al., 1989).

Small bowel Mention has already been made of the tendency for the small bowel to rupture either in the proximal jejunum or distal ileum where the segment is less mobile than elsewhere. The distal ileum is also the most susceptible to traction injury of the mesentery. If a mesenteric arcade is torn then progressive ischaemia with rupture is inevitable. However, it is usual for the lesion to call attention to itself because of bleeding before gangrene develops. Very occasionally the process is sufficiently slow for the damaged gut to become wrapped in omentum, and in such circumstances it may be weeks or months before the patient presents with features of small bowel obstruction.

Contusions of the bowel may progress to delayed perforation though recent experimental studies suggest that those contusions whose size is less than the circumference of the bowel wall have a very low incidence of delayed perforation and should usually be left alone (Paterson-Brown et al., 1990). A similar rule of thumb applies to mesenteric injury, which must be greater than twice the circumference of the bowel before ischaemic complications develop.

Large bowel The greater part of the large bowel is surprisingly rarely damaged by BAT but the caecum is the most susceptible to rupture, presumably because of its frequent gaseous distension. Injuries may take the form of lacerations or contusions.

Retroperitoneal haematoma

These are sometimes classified as *central* or *peripheral*. The presence of the former, particularly if it is expanding, often implies some damage to the great vessels such as may occur in acute flexion and their identification should lead to further studies in an attempt to identify the cause and to decide whether there is progressive bleeding. The latter are either the consequence of diffuse injury or of fracture of the pelvis, with blood tracking upwards through the retroperitoneal space.

One of the interesting and confusing features of all retroperitoneal effusions, including that of blood, is their tendency to cause intestinal ileus. Diagnostic confusion may result. It is thought that the cause may lie in stimulation of the sympathetic-parasympathetic imbalance with dominant activity of the sympathetic component, which is known experimentally to cause a picture of intestinal atony (Neely and Catchpole, 1967).

Urological injury

Kidney Compression from a blow in the flank or from anteriorly may drive the kidney against the twelfth rib. Severe force from behind may damage the pedicle. Such kidney injury is not uncommon in violent contact sports such as rugby football. As with the spleen and liver, the damage varies. There may be only a slight capsular tear with minor bleeding. Either the cortex or the medulla may sustain an isolated injury. In the former, a perinephric haematoma forms; in the latter, there is bleeding into the renal pelvis with haematuria. More severe injuries are extensions and combinations of these with leakage of urine into the perinephric space. Finally the kidney may be sheared off its pedicle, either in part or totally – usually known as a critical injury and encountered in less than 2% of all kidney injuries. Leakage of urine is rarely of importance except as an indication of the severity of injury because, apart from rare circumstances, the urine is sterile.

Injury to an abnormal kidney (usually cyst or hydronephrosis) is well recognized and has a particular importance in that the contralateral organ may share the disease process.

Bladder Rupture is either *intra-* or *extraperitoneal*. The former is relatively rare and is said to be usually encountered in those who have a distended bladder and are subject to a blow on the lower abdomen – a combination of circumstances likely to take place in a drunken brawl. The bladder is usually split on its upper or posterior surface. Extraperitoneal rupture is nearly always the outcome of a fractured pelvis with severe disruption of the pelvic ring. The mechanisms are two: most commonly tearing at the bladder–urethral junction as the pubic bones are moved away from the anterior aspect; less frequently puncture by a spicule of bone at the same site. The effects are usually dominated by the pelvic fracture, and it is only as urinary extravasation into the extraperitoneal plane takes place that the injury is detected unless a high index of suspicion is maintained.

Extraperitoneal rupture merges into injury of the prostatic urethra in which the bladder and prostate are torn away from and often lacerated by a severe pelvic disruption. There may be severe bleeding from a concomitant tear of the blood vessels passing through the pelvic diaphragm. The clinical features are the same but the specialized urological management is different.

Obstetric injury

The uterus – normally well protected by the bony walls of the pelvis – becomes at risk of injury during pregnancy as it rises above the pelvic brim and becomes distended. Outcome for the mother is related to blood loss from a laceration of the uterine wall or from placental abruption. For the fetus it is influenced by both the injuries sustained by the mother and any additional direct injury (Drost *et al.*, 1990). In a series of 315 pregnant women who suffered a traumatic incident, 25 (8%) were suffi-

ciently injured to require hospital admission irrespective of the pregnancy. There was only one maternal death, four pregnancies were lost and one neonate died as a result of direct injury.

CLINICAL SCIENTIFIC BASIS OF MANAGEMENT

The principles of management are the same for BAT as for any other injury – adequate initial resuscitation with attention to the supply of oxygen via an adequate airway and volume replacement, precise diagnosis and definitive surgery to correct intra-abdominal abnormalities.

An element of logic can be applied to the diagnostic process by a careful consideration of the mechanism of injury and its likely consequences in terms of internal damage. This may be supplemented by external signs of injury, for example, the appearances of seat-belt signs on the abdominal wall.

In recent years a considerable effort has been made to supplement clinical diagnosis by the use of a number of techniques, most of which have been subjected to moderately rigorous evaluation. These are considered briefly below:

Peritoneal lavage

Detection of abnormalities such as blood or intestinal content by instilling and withdrawing a measured quantity of saline is the definitive non-operative test for BAT. With standard criteria (Table 11.1) a positive result is associated with the presence of intra-abdominal injury in 95% of patients and conversely less than 5% of patients with a negative lavage have internal damage (Velanovich, 1990). The main problem is that its sensitivity in detection of injury is such that exploration may be undertaken for intra-abdominal injuries that prove trivial or the blood found may be the consequence of contiguous injury – such as a retroperitoneal haematoma or a pelvic fracture. Where possible further studies such as CT or ultrasonographic scanning should be used.

Conventional radiology

Though an upright chest X-ray can detect free air under the diaphragm and may draw attention to features of thoracoabdominal trauma, it is often difficult to obtain in the critically ill patient. Similarly, though abdominal X-rays are sometimes valuable and detect subtle signs of BAT, they lack sensitivity. Contrast studies of the upper gastrointestinal and renal tracts are indicated in specific circumstances, as occasionally is arteriography, but they are not of general value as screening procedures.

TABLE 11.1
EVALUATION OF PERITONEAL LAVAGE EFFLUENT

I. Positive Criteria	
(a) Macroscopic Evaluation	— Frank blood on initial opening
	— Bile or intestinal contents in effluent
	— Unable to read newspaper print through the *tubing* of the effluent bag
	— Lavage fluid in chest-drain or urinary catheter
(b) Microscopic criteria	— RBC concentration >100 000/m^3
	— WBC concentration >500/mm^3
	— Amylase concentration >200 units/100mm^3
	— Positive gram stain for bacteria
II. Equivocal Results	— RBC concentration 50–100 000/mm^3
	— WBC concentration 100–500/mm^3
	— Amylase concentration 75–200 units/100mm^3
III. Negative Criteria	— RBC concentration <50 000/mm^3
	— WBC concentration <100/mm^3
	— Amylase concentration <75/100mm^3

Key: RBC = Red blood cell
WBC = White blood cell

Ultrasonography

The increasing experience of high-resolution scanning over the last few years has made this a very useful investigation. The presence of free intra-peritoneal blood or other fluid can be detected with a high degree of accuracy, as can damage to the liver and spleen (Jones *et al.*, 1983). In particular, when a CT scanner is not available the use of ultrasonography is valuable in the follow-up of lesions that are managed non-operatively.

CT scanning

There is little doubt that the introduction and widespread availability of CT scanning has had a major impact on the management of BAT. Its role in immediate assessment is now established (Sorkey *et al.*, 1989). However injuries – especially those of the gastrointestinal tract – may still go undetected and this can be hazardous when there is a lesion of a solid organ which is suitable for non-operative treatment. The demonstration that gastrointestinal disruption is more commonly associated with hepatic and splenic injury in adults (26%) than in children (7%) suggests that, particularly in the former, CT should be combined with peritoneal lavage when the former detects a solid organ injury. CT is also extremely helpful in retroperitoneal injuries and, as with ultrasonography, in continued assessment of injuries treated non-operatively.

Blood tests

For obvious reasons these are not that applicable in differential diagnosis in BAT. Serial observations in specific circumstances may be useful in evaluation.

Laparoscopy

Although, as already mentioned, the sensitivity of peritoneal lavage is high, its specificity and ability to detect gastrointestinal injuries that mandate surgery is low. In an effort to reduce the unnecessary laparotomy rate after peritoneal lavage, mini-laparoscopy under local anaesthesia has been used (Sherwood *et al.*, 1980). Preliminary reports suggest that specificity is increased without affecting sensitivity (Cuschieri *et al.*, 1988).

REFERENCES

Aberg, T., Steen S., Othman K. et al. (1986). The effect of pneumatic antishock garments in the treatment of lethal combined hepatic and caval injuries in rats. *J. Trauma*, **26**, 727–32.

Appleby J.P., Nagy A.G. (1989). Abdominal injuries associated with the use of seatbelts. *Am. J. Surg.*, **157**, 457–8.

Beal S. (1990). Fatal hepatic haemorrhage: an unresolved problem in the management of complex liver injuries. *J. Trauma*, **30**, 163–9.

Buckman, R.F., Dunham C.M., Kerr T.M., Militello P.R. (1989). Hypotension and bleeding with various anatomic patterns of blunt splenic injury in adults. *Surg. Gynecol. Obstet.*, **169**, 206–12.

Carr N.D., Cairns S.J., Lees W.R., Russell R.C.G. (1989). Late complications of pancreatic trauma. *Br. J. Surg.*, **76**, 1244–6.

Cheslyn-Curtis S., Aldridge, M.C., Biglin, J.E.J. et al. (1988). Effect of splenectomy on gram-negative bacterial clearance in the presence and absence of sepsis. *Br. J. Surg.*, **75**, 177–80.

Cox E.F. (1984). Blunt abdominal trauma. *Ann. Surg.*, **199**, 467–74.

Cuschieri A., Hennessy, T.P.J., Stephens R., Berci, G. (1988). Diagnosis of significant abdominal trauma after road traffic accidents: preliminary results of a multi-centre trial comparing minilaparoscopy with peritoneal lavage. *Ann. RCS Engl.,* **70**, 153–5.

Dajee H., Richardson, I.W., Iype M.O. (1979). Seat belt aorta: acute dissection and thrombosis of the abdominal aorta. *Surgery,* **85**, 263–7.

Dang C., Schlater T., Bui H., Oshita T. (1990). Delayed rupture of the spleen. *Ann. Emerg. Med.,* **19**, 399–403.

Davis J.J., Cohn I., Nance F.C. (1976). Diagnosis and management of blunt abdominal trauma. *Ann. Surg.,* **183**, 672–7.

Delius R.E., Frankel W., Coran A.G. (1989). A comparison between operative and nonoperative management of blunt injuries to the liver and spleen in adult and pediatric patients. *Surgery,* **106**, 788–93.

Department of Transport (1986). *Road Accidents Great Britain. The casualty report.* London: HMSO.

Donahue T.K., Strauch G.Q. (1988). Ligation as definitive management of injury to the superior mesenteric vein. *J. Trauma,* **28**, 541–3.

Drost T.F., Rosemurgy A.S., Sherman H.F. et al. (1990). Major trauma in pregnant women: maternal/fetal outcome. *J. Trauma,* **30**, 574–8.

Feliciano D.V., Mattox K.L., Burch J.M. et al. (1986). Packing for control of hepatic haemorrhage. *J. Trauma,* **26**, 738–43.

Grasberger R.C., Scott C.M., McCormick J.R. et al. (1985). Pericardial complications in hepatic trauma. *J. Trauma,* **25**, 322–5.

Gumley G., Taylor T.K.F., Ryan M.D. et al. (1982). Distraction fractures of the lumbar spine. *J. Bone Joint Surg.,* **64B**, 520–5.

Johnson C.D. (1988). Blunt injuries of the diaphragm. *Br. J. Surg,* **75**, 226–30.

Jones T.K., Walsh J.W., Maull K.I. (1983). Diagnostic imaging in blunt trauma of the abdomen. *Surg Gynecol. Obstet.,* **157**, 389–98.

Lange D.A., Zaret P., Merlotti G.J. et al. (1988). The use of absorbable mesh in splenic trauma. *J. Trauma,* **28**, 269–73.

Lau I.V., Horsch J.D., Viano D.C., Andrzejak D.V (1987). Biomechanics of liver injury by steering wheel loading. *J. Trauma,* **27**, 225–35.

Mansour M.A., Moore J.B., Moore E.E., Moore F.A. (1989). Conservative management of combined pancreatoduodenal injuries. *Am. J. Surg.,* **158**, 531–5.

Neely J., Catchpole B.N. (1967). An analysis of the autonomic control of gastrointestinal motility in the cat. *Gut,* **8**, 230–41.

Newman R.J. (1986). A prospective evaluation of the protective effect of car seat belts. *J. Trauma,* **26**, 561–4.

Paterson-Brown S., Francis N., Whawell S. et al. (1990). Prediction of the delayed complications of intestinal and mesenteric injuries following experimental blunt abdominal trauma. *Br. J. Surg.,* **77**, 648–51.

Pearce W.H., Moore E.E., Moore F.A. (1988). Injury to the spleen. In *Trauma* (Mattox K.L., Moore E.E., Feliciano D.V., eds.) California: Appleton and Lange, pp. 443–57.

Pimpl W., Dapunt O., Kaindl H., Thalhamer J. (1989). Incidence of septic and thrombolic-related deaths after splenectomy in adults. *Br. J. Surg.,* **76**, 517–21.

Pretre R., Mentha G., Huber O. et al. (1988). Hepatic trauma: risk factors influencing outcome. *Br. J. Surg.,* **75**, 520–4.

Rappaport W., McIntyre K.E., Carmona R. (1990). The management of splenic trauma in the adult patient with blunt multiple injuries. *Surg. Gynecol. Obstet.,* **170**, 204–8.

Rydell W.B. (1970). Complete transection of the common bile duct due to blunt abdominal trauma. *Arch. Surg.,* **100**, 724–8.

Shaw J.H.F., Print C.G. (1989). Postsplenectomy sepsis. *Br. J. Surg.,* **76**, 1074–81.

Sherwood R., Berci G., Austin E., Morgenstern L. (1980). Minilaparoscopy for blunt abdominal trauma. *Arch. Surg.,* **115**, 672–3.

Sorkey A.J., Farnell M.B., Williams H.J. et al. (1989). The complementary roles of diagnostic peritoneal lavage and computed tomography in the evaluation of blunt abdominal trauma. *Surgery,* **106**, 794–801.

Velanovich V. (1990). Bayesian analysis of the reliability of peritoneal lavage. *Surg. Gynecol. Obstet.,* **170**, 7–11.

Vo N.M., Chi D.S. (1988). Effect of hepatectomy on the reticulo-endothelial system of septic rats. *J. Trauma,* **28**, 852–4.

12. Epidemiology of Road Traffic Accidents

M. Waters and D. W. Yates

INTRODUCTION

An accident is defined as a completely unforeseen event occurring by chance, but the study of road traffic accidents over many years has shown that most are avoidable. Only a very small minority of accidents are truly the outcome of chance. Epidemiological principles, used to study a disease in a community at a particular time, can be employed to investigate the true incidence of accidents, predisposing factors and the nature and severity of injuries sustained. Audit of the effectiveness of preventative measures can also be undertaken.

Epidemiology can be used to pursue primary road accident prevention such as the identification of problems which could be addressed by changing behaviour by education, by law enforcement and by road engineering. Human error has been assessed as a prime factor in 70% of accidents, and a highly significant contributory factor in 95% (Department of Transport, 1987).

Human error can never be eliminated but its consequences can be minimized by making vehicles intrinsically safer. Biomechanics provides a scientific basis for such improvements, which may lead to a reduction in the severity of injuries sustained as a result of a given impact – the secondary approach to road accident prevention.

Road traffic accidents can result in untimely death, disfigurement and permanent disability, and the costs may be devastating to family life, in that accident rates in most countries are highest in men in the second and third decades of life. The impact on health-care resources is also immense. Particularly high accident rates occur in countries where walking and cycling are the main modes of transport. Paradoxically these countries usually have less money to spend on health care (Table 12.1).

There has been a steady decline in road-user deaths and injuries in the UK since around 1960 (Table 12.2). The number of licensed two-wheeled motor vehicles (TWMV) has fallen by more than one-third over the last 9 years, as have the deaths of their users. In contrast, despite the continuing rise in the numbers of other licensed motor vehicles (by approximately 30% over the same period of time), the number of other road-user deaths has fallen. The UK has the lowest rate of road fatalities currently in the European community but has a disappointingly high pedestrian fatality rate, particularly between the ages of 5 and 14. In 1990, this was 32% of all road traffic accident fatalities, twice that found in the Netherlands, Norway, Luxemburg and Sweden (Parliamentary Advisory Committee for Transport and Safety (PACTS), 1990; Ackroyd, 1990).

This chapter begins by highlighting some of the difficulties inherent in the collation of data on road accidents and goes on to describe the legislative approach to reducing road trauma-related morbidity and mortality, using the UK as the main example.

DATA COLLECTION

Accurate data collection is essential for assessment of the size of the problems relating to road traffic accidents and for monitoring the effects of changes in behaviour and the environment, brought about by education or legislation. Definitions which are

TABLE 12.1

INTERNATIONAL COMPARISON OF DEATH FROM MOTOR VEHICLE ACCIDENTS AT DIFFERENT AGES (1985). (DERIVED FROM ICD E CODES 810–819, 9TH REVISION AND HUTCHINSON, 1987)

		Age (yr)			
	Total	0–14	15–24	25–64	65+
Australia	2933	248	1033	1260	392
Austria	1518	79	523	606	310
Federal Republic of Germany	7978	437	2682	3221	1638
Hong Kong	291	24	47	125	95
Japan	12 456	724	3142	5660	2923
Kuwait	464	108	61	268	17
Portugal	2597	206	592	1310	489
Thailand	4315	456	1210	2347	238

TABLE 12.2

RELATIONSHIPS BETWEEN THE NUMBER OF LICENSED MOTOR VEHICLES AND TRAFFIC FATALITIES UK: 1930–94. (DERIVED FROM ROAD ACCIDENTS GREAT BRITAIN, 1994)

	TWMV		All Other Vehicles	
	Licences held × 10³	Fatalities	Licences held × 10³	Fatalities
1930	712	1832	1588	5473
1940	278	1270	2022	7339
1950	729	1129	3671	3883
1960	1796	1743	7604	5227
1970	1048	761	13 952	6378
1980	1372	1163	17 828	4842
1990	833	659	23 867	4558
1994	630	444	24 570	3206

TWMV = two-wheeled motor vehicles.

internationally recognized and understood must be used. Sources of bias should be identified where possible.

Definitions

Three categories of severity of injury are used by the police in the UK. These are 'fatal', 'serious' and 'slight'.

A fatal accident is one in which at least one person is killed and death occurs at the time of the accident or during a variable period afterwards. The UK and the USA both use the World Health Organization (WHO) recommendation of 30 days for this time. However, in Japan death must have occurred within 24 hours of the accident. In Canada, death occurring within 12 months is recorded as a road accident fatality. Thus interpreting fatal accident statistics depends on the country of origin.

A serious injury in the UK is anything which necessitates the patient being detained in hospital. Thus a patient with a minor head injury who requires overnight observation is put in the same category as a patient with multiple injuries who needs surgery and intensive care and who later dies more than 30 days from the time of the accident.

A slight injury is one which does not require inpatient hospital treatment, for example, abrasions and minor sprains, but can also include complex and disabling knee injuries which are initially treated on an outpatient basis. This severity classification is subject to the vagaries of hospital admission policies.

In the USA, most of the police forces use a classification known as the K,A,B,C,O code recommended by the National Safety Council:

K = Death occurring up to 30 days after injury.
A = Incapacitating injury, i.e. one that prevents the individual from normally continuing the activities that he or she was capable of before the accident.
B = Non-incapacitating injury (evident). Any injury which is not severe enough to be incapacitating but which is evident at the scene to any observer, for example, bumps, bruises and minor lacerations.
C = Possible injury. Including a momentary loss of consciousness and non-evident but possible injuries, i.e. complaints of pain, nausea and limping.
O = No indication of personal injury, a 'damage-only' accident.

This system allows considerable difference in interpretation, in the same way as the British system. Some countries use the length of hospitalization to differentiate serious, minor or non-incapacitating injuries. Hong Kong uses admission for as little as 12 hours and Japan uses admission for 30 days to describe a serious injury. France, Belgium and West Germany use 6 days (Hutchinson, 1987). Serious injury, as defined by the police forces of many countries, encompasses a group of patients who after *medical* assessment, would be regarded as having relatively minor injuries. For detailed analysis and research purposes, the exact definitions of severity must be known for each country studied. Ideally, there should be a medical assessment of severity of injury, using ICD codes (currently ninth revision) or the Injury Severity Score (ISS). The latter is derived from the Abbreviated Injury Scale (AIS) manual, which was developed by the Association for the Advancement of Automotive Medicine.

The Occupant Injury Classification (OIC) is a system used by the United States National Accident Sampling System (NASS) and uses the AIS to code severity. The New York State Injury Coding Scheme (NYSICS) is a more detailed system based on the location and type of the physical complaints and the victim's physical or emotional state, which is used by the police and has been shown to be more effective than the KABCO scale.

SOURCES OF INFORMATION

The police

In most countries the police accident reports provide the basis of accident data collection. Standardized coded forms which are designed to allow computerization of the collective data for rapid analysis have been developed and validated. Because the individual states of the USA and Australia are responsible for traffic safety, their respective forms vary in some of the details. However, there is enough common information to make the fatal accident reporting system in the United States (FARS) and the Australasian fatal accident reporting form (NAASRA) fairly comprehensive. The Stats 19 form has been used by the Department of Transport in Great Britain since 1978. It was last revised in February 1991.

All these forms record: accurate location of the accident; details of persons involved and their injuries; vehicle movements and damage sustained; and, where possible, estimates of crash speed. Details of road conditions in terms of class of the road, the type of junction (if any) involved, and both weather and lighting conditions are also required. The American National Highway Traffic Safety Administration (NHTSA) samples data from 60 sites nationwide and reviews crashes reported by the police. In 1988, it introduced the General Estimates System (GES) to examine a sample of crashes in more detail on an annual basis.

There are problems associated with police data:

1. Information is collected by police officers, who are not road engineers and cannot make

informed comments on crash speed, vehicle movements and damage sustained in relation to vehicle design. Report forms can include diagrams to represent sequential vehicle movement. It is difficult to assign computer codes to a sequence of vehicle movements, especially when more than one vehicle has been involved in an accident.

2. Witnesses and victims of accidents may well be heavily biased against providing accurate information to the police.
3. There is known to be marked under-reporting of low-velocity accidents which result only in damage to vehicles or very minor injuries that usually involve pedestrians or cyclists (GES, 1990; Road Accidents Great Britain, 1990).
4. It may not always be possible to complete the form; for example, in 'hit and run' accidents. If the deformation of a vehicle is severe, it may not be possible to determine the seating position of the occupants or whether seat belts were worn. If a report originates at the scene, it can be very difficult to ascertain whether drugs or alcohol contributed to the accident.
5. The more complex the design of the report form, the greater the temptation not to record information at the scene and to rely upon memory.
6. Location of accidents can be difficult to document accurately, especially in urban areas undergoing rapid development. Map revision seldom keeps pace with new building programmes.
7. The General Estimate System is helpful in demonstrating trends but year-to-year variations could also be due to differences in the sample used.

Several studies have been undertaken comparing police data with that of a research team, notably in Southern Australia and Indiana in the USA (Howard et al., 1979; Daltrey, 1983; Shinar et al., 1983). Errors of omission and commission have been consistently demonstrated, not only with respect to vehicle make, pre-existing defects and damage sustained, but also relating to the road and conditions prevailing at the time of the accident. One of the recommendations which arose from these studies is that there should be a regular audit of information given on police accident report forms.

Other sources of accident data

Hospital records
Hospital records are subject to confidentiality laws, so access is often either limited or time consuming to obtain. Emergency department records could be a useful source of information about 'slight' accidents which may not have been reported to the police. A study in Birmingham (Bull and Roberts, 1973) showed that the police were aware of all the fatalities during the study period but that only 71% of road traffic accidents known to the hospital were also known to the police. The remaining incidents had involved a single vehicle, pedal cyclists or pedestrians. Accidents not resulting in obvious injury will be even less likely to be reported and more difficult to trace. All apparently trivial incidents are worthy of study because they form part of a wider spectrum and because severity of injury can be influenced by many factors which merit individual attention.

The Association of British Insurers conducted a 'snapshot' study of all claims reported on one day in 1989 (Broughton, 1990). By comparing claim forms with Stats 19 data, it appeared that 12.5% of accident claims would have been reported by police as injury accidents but only 7.5% of accident claims mentioned injury. Injury to pedestrians and pedal cyclists were least well reported.

Some of these problems could be overcome if police and hospital data were matched. In Scotland, accident data has, since 1981, been collected through the Scottish Hospital Inpatient Study (SHIPS), and matched with Stats 19 data at the Transport and Road Research Laboratory (TRRL). The National Accident Sampling System (NASS), under the auspices of the NHTSA, is an equivalent system in the USA. It does not provide and trace data for all accidents, although these initiatives do provide same useful information.

A further issue is the quality of medical care – efficient and prompt hospital treatment has been shown to influence outcome, especially for the severely injured. Fatality statistics may therefore reflect the varying quality of resuscitation. This is particularly important when comparison is to be made between centres and over time.

Coroners records and death certificates
Clearly these are only useful for fatalities but in some countries they are the major source of information. *Transport Statistics Great Britain* is an annual publication that uses this type of information, together with vehicle registration data.

Insurance claims
It might be expected that insurance companies would receive claims for single vehicle and low-velocity accidents which have not caused injury and which have not been reported to the police. In contrast to police data, the vehicle details provided by the claimant should be reasonably accurate. Insurance claims have been studied and compared with police statistics. At the time of the study, any crash should have been reported to the police. However where there had not been any injury, only 25% of accidents were known to them and, even where there had been an injury, only 65% of accidents were known (Searles, 1980).

Thus insurance companies could provide data complementary to but not as comprehensive as official statistics. In the USA, the Highway Loss Data Institute (HLDI) gathers and publishes road accident statistics based on insurance claims. The Motor Accidents Board in Victoria, Australia, is an equivalent body that also publishes annually (Trinea *et al.*, 1988).

Vehicle licensing centres

In the UK the Driver and Vehicle Licensing Centre (DVLC) keeps a record of all driving convictions, including those associated with alcohol, together with a vast amount of data on motor vehicles, all of which is available through the Home Office (Jones, 1989a).

Traffic census

These are useful for calculating traffic flow, although in the UK only major roads are studied – a restriction which fails to recognize that most pedestrian and pedal cyclist injuries in children under 10 years of age occur on quiet, unassessed, residential roads.

In conclusion, road accident statistics can best be collated by collaboration and cooperation between official sources and between organizations in the public and private sectors. Where information is duplicated, it can be compared for accuracy but the real value of different bodies which facilitate information flow is that each has a different interest which, when integrated, helps to create an overall picture.

ADDRESSING BEHAVIOURAL AND ENVIRONMENTAL PROBLEMS FOR THE ROAD USER

Introduction

Data collected are analysed annually in order to identify particular areas of need and difficulty. A road traffic accident can be considered to be the result of interaction between human behaviour and the environment. Causation may be addressed by attempting to change inconsistent human behaviour, or by changing the environment. Although education increases knowledge, it does not necessarily directly change behaviour. Legislation may be necessary. The following section will consider how these interrelated issues have been addressed.

Education

A vital ingredient to improved road safety is appropriately targeted, attractively and persuasively packaged public-information campaigns, which should be tightly controlled and audited. Vague exhortations about good behaviour are ineffective and even counterproductive.

Driving instruction

It takes time to acquire the skills required to drive a car and misplaced confidence may be present at all ages but especially in the young. Instructors in the UK are not rigorously assessed and it is not compulsory to receive pretest tuition from an 'approved' instructor. Additionally, there are no facilities for the identification of special problems and subsequent special training.

With a wide spectrum of driving abilities and no national guidelines for instruction, it is inappropriate to have a test which merely passes or fails. Instruction should have a standard content which could be modified to aid individuals with learning difficulties. The use of road simulator techniques has been proposed but the equipment is very expensive.

In 1991 the Parliamentary Advisory Committee for Transport and Safety (PACTS) recommended changes in driving instruction as an outcome of research at the Transport and Road Research Laboratory (TRRL). The results of a special driving test taken 2 years after the standard driving test were examined. Less than 50% passed, most failing on faults such as driving too quickly for the road conditions, approaching junctions too fast and not anticipating the action of other drivers. These are all problems which are prominent in accident causation and are not addressed by current driving instruction. The feasibility of introducing a probationary period after passing the standard road test, during which there is restriction on the speed at which the driver may travel, has been investigated in New Zealand and Australia. Video instruction techniques have been introduced into general training and, in New Zealand, an early evaluation of the scheme suggests that it has been successful in reducing the accident rate (Gloag, 1991).

Motor cyclists

This group of road users has, over the last few years, been declining in numbers in many countries. Driving instruction is now based on preparation for a two-part test – technical skills and road sense. In the UK, 15 year olds are now restricted to riding motorcycles of less than 50 cc capacity. Some lives have been saved by improvements in both vehicle and motorbike design: for example, front and side underrun guards on lorries; and anti-lock braking and leg guards on motorcycles. The areas of the body still most frequently seriously injured are the head, cervical spine and legs. Despite increased public awareness about the risks of head injury, it took legislation in the UK and the USA to enforce the wearing of standardized helmets and to increase the previously low compliance rate.

Pedal cyclists

Training in the UK has been available for many years through the Royal Society for the Prevention of Accidents (RoSPA) National Cycle Proficiency Scheme and their recent initiative 'Cycleway'. These courses are targeted at 9–10 year olds and are promoted in conjunction with local education authorities. Evidence from 1970 onwards suggests that children experience lasting benefit from cycling training and tuition in road skills (Risk *et al.*, 1976). Appropriate education packages should also be targeted at parents. The use of safety helmets and high visibility clothing at all times of the day has been shown to be effective. Parents must be convinced of the importance of these measures, whether their child is playing or cycling to school. Some schools, in conjunction with local road safety departments, are encouraging the sale of reduced-price helmets but it will take more governmental and parental support to ensure that helmets are routinely used. Extrapolation of American data suggests that, if helmets were always worn, there would be a 75% reduction in head injuries to children in the UK (Pless, 1991).

Pedestrians

Children usually receive tuition at primary school about crossing the road safely. Teaching is given by police or road safety officers and takes the form of single talks, rather than a structured training programme. However, young children are limited in their ability to recognize danger and an evaluation of the effectiveness of this type of tuition in Scandinavia and the Netherlands showed that it is ineffective under the age of 8. Although young children can be taught to look in both directions at the edge of the road, they are not capable of effectively processing the information acquired, and translating it into safe actions (Aviary and Aviary, 1982). Educational television is widely accepted by children. This has been used successfully in the UK's 'Mind How you Go' since 1982 and 'Play it Safe' in 1992.

Traffic clubs have been extensively developed in some countries, for example, Sweden and the Netherlands, and with some benefit. The UK Tufty Clubs aimed at 2–5 year olds have been popular for some years. In Greater London, a scheme aimed at older children, called the 'Streetwise Kids Scheme', is being evaluated. It is hoped that this will develop into a National Traffic Club.

The relationship of alcohol to accidents

The relationship of alcohol to performance was reported in the classical case-controlled Grand Rapid Study (Borkenstein *et al.*, 1964). Further analysis of the original data (Allsop, 1966) demonstrated that the risk of accident rose with the blood alcohol concentration (BAC) for every age group and especially for women and infrequent drinkers. There was a high incidence of single vehicle accidents amongst drinking drivers.

For any given BAC, different individuals will experience different degrees of effect. The rate at which alcohol is consumed and absorbed affects the speed of onset and duration of any adverse effects. Most people consistently exhibit a change in behaviour at 50 mg/100 ml BAC.

Vision is affected by low concentrations of alcohol. There is difficulty in focusing and following moving objects, difficulty in recovering from the glare of headlights and impaired discrimination between light and sounds of varying intensities. For driving on the left-hand side of the road, studies with a simulator have demonstrated a decrease in steering accuracy with a tendency to overcorrect on left-hand bends. There is an increased tolerance of bends to the right as the main driving line shifts towards the crown of the road (Drew *et al.*, 1958). These effects lead to decreased ability to 'interpret the road' rather than to impaired motor ability. The driver who drinks is less likely to comply with standard safety protocols, such as the use of seat belts and to conforming to the highway code, possibly due to a reduced perception of risk. This renders the drinking driver more likely to cause, or to be involved in a crash (Mayhew *et al.*, 1987).

It has been claimed that alcohol would be protective in the event of an accident because the victim is more relaxed on impact and thus would suffer less severe injuries. However, a study of 1 million motor vehicle accidents and the relationship between the risk of death or serious injury and alcohol demonstrated the converse; after allowing for the use of seat belts, impact speed, vehicle weight and driver's age, the conclusion was that the risk of death or serious injury increased for the drinking driver and vehicle occupant compared to the non-drinker (Waller *et al.*, 1986).

The size of the problem

Drinking and driving remains a serious problem. In the UK in 1988, 840 deaths (1 in 6) and 5650 serious injuries (1 in 11) were associated with the use of alcohol. This figure has been adjusted to account for deaths which occurred after the 30-day limit and for those who do not have their blood alcohol measured on arrival at hospital because they are so seriously injured that resuscitation is the main priority. The blood alcohol concentration is calculated for all patients who are killed outright.

The figures in Table 12.3 show that the proportion of fatalities with BACs of greater than 80 mg/100 ml fell from 30.7% in 1982–85 to 20% in 1988 though in the latter period considerably more than half those killed had a level in excess of 150 mg/100 ml. Nevertheless, since 1982 there has been a significant downward trend in fatalities associated with the BAC higher than the legal limit in the UK both for car drivers and TWMV riders. The majority of such fatalities occur between the hours of 10 p.m. and 4 a.m. (Table 12.4). Most fatalities occur at weekends.

TABLE 12.3

RELATIONSHIP BETWEEN DRIVER FATALITIES AND BLOOD
ALCOHOL CONCENTRATION (BAC). (DERIVED FROM BRITISH
MEDICAL ASSOCIATION, 1988)

%Driver fatalities	BAC (mg/100ml)						
	0–9	10–50	51–80	81–100	101–150	151–200	>200
1982–5	60.1	6.5	2.8	2.3	8.8	8.3	11.3
1988	69.9	8.1	2.0	2.0	4.0	6.0	8

TABLE 12.4

RELATIONSHIPS BETWEEN DEATH ASSOCIATED WITH BAC
>80 MG/100 ML BLOOD AND TIME OF DAY FOR DIFFERENT
CATEGORIES OF ROAD USER IN THE UK, 1993. (DERIVED FROM
ROAD ACCIDENTS GREAT BRITAIN, 1994)

Category of road user	% Fatalities with illegal BAC	
	10 p.m. to 3.59 a.m.	4 a.m. to 9.59 p.m.
Motorcycle riders	59	6
Other vehicle drivers	49	11
Passengers	42	10
Pedestrians	74	17
Cyclists	—	4

n = 1724.

Table 12.5 also highlights the vulnerability of pedestrians and cyclists late at night. Alcohol-related accidents are particularly a problem of young people, not just in the UK (Jones, 1989a) but also in the USA and Ireland (Hutchinson, 1987). In some industrialized countries, the life expectancy of 15–24 year olds is now less than it was 20 years ago because of motor vehicle accidents associated with the use of alcohol (Havard, 1988).

It has been postulated that drinking and driving is just part of risk-taking behaviour patterns in a subset of young people who engage in many forms of high-risk activity associated with adolescent lifestyle (Jessor, 1987). The further suggestion is that young people may have a special sensitivity to and less experience of alcohol which may be linked with a greater willingness to accept risk (Mayhew, 1987). The conclusion is that the young should be the subject of further detailed psychosocial research, so that countermeasures could be appropriately targeted to behaviour as a whole, rather than just problems with alcohol.

Legal limits and enforcement measures
The United Kingdom Road Safety Act of 1967 established a blood alcohol concentration (BAC) of 80 mg per 100 ml as the legal limit, a level chosen

following a European Conference of Ministers of Transport and which was subsequently adopted by Austria, Belgium, Denmark, Luxemburg, Switzerland, Spain and West Germany. The Nordic Countries and some Australian States had already accepted 50 mg/100 ml blood, while Eastern European countries and Turkey set the limit at nil. Some American states chose the far higher level of 150 mg/100 ml blood but the American Medical Association has recently recommended that it should be reduced to 50 mg/100 ml (Gloag, 1987). Blood tests have largely replaced urine testing, which is less accurate in reflecting the total body load of alcohol.

In 1983, testing for the concentration of alcohol in the breath was introduced in the UK, a level of 35 mg/100 ml corresponding to a BAC of 80 mg/100 ml. In order to be an effective deterrent, blood and breath alcohol limits must be adequately enforced. The 1981 Transport Act allowed the police to test 'at their discretion' persons of whom they had reasonable suspicion might have committed or were likely to commit a traffic offence while under the influence of alcohol. The Act did not specifically permit random breath testing. It did however stimulate debate about the benefit which might accrue from the imposition of random testing under legislation.

During the last 15 years, high-profile random breath testing checkpoints have been introduced in Australia, New Zealand, Finland and some American states. In New South Wales, such measures have been associated with a fall of 37% in the numbers of drivers killed with an illegal alcohol level and constituted a saving of at least 177 million Australian dollars over 3 years, which more than offset the initial costs to the state of 8 million dollars on police equipment, manpower and advertising. Public acceptance showed an increase from 42% before random testing, to 91% two years later, which presumably reflects a recognition of the effectiveness of increased enforcement in turn resulting in increased deterrence and saving of life. The chances of being stopped and tested in New South Wales were once per driver per year, compared in Britain to once for every 100 drivers per year (Gloag, 1986). Recent opinion polls in Britain (by the National Opinion Poll and the Consumers Association) have suggested that attitudes are changing as each showed that more than 70% of the population surveyed were in favour of random testing. This was also strongly supported by PACTS, in combination with a plea for reduction of the legal BAC to 50 mg/100 ml, and a further reduction to 20 mg/100 ml in due course (Parliamentary Advisory Committee for Transport and Safety, 1990).

In 1974 the Blennerhasset Committee made a number of recommendations, especially with respect to alcohol, which were included in the 1981

Transport Act. An important new concept was that of the 'high-risk offender', defined as a person having two convictions for drink-driving within 10 years, with a BAC of more than 200 mg/100 ml on one occasion, or one such offence combined with a refusal to give a specimen on another occasion. It was hoped that deterrence would be effected by instant disqualification for 3 years, following which the high-risk offender was obliged to undergo full medical examination by a practitioner appointed by the Minister for Transport. This was aimed at making recidivists seek help and thus preventing danger to the public. The outcome has not yet been fully evaluated because relatively few offenders have achieved reinstatement of their driving licence since the scheme began in 1983 (British Medical Association, 1988).

The use of legislation to change the environment

Education increases knowledge but does not always lead to a change in behaviour. Legislation has proved particularly effective in enforcing a change in behaviour on the issues of seat belts and motor cycle helmets. Their use is thought to be chiefly responsible for the substantial reductions in death and serious injury rates which must be weighed against 'the loss of personal freedom of choice'.

Major milestones in legislation affecting road safety are listed in Table 12.5. Most entries refer to the UK but significant developments in other countries are also presented.

INJURY REDUCTION THROUGH IMPROVED DESIGN

It is worth summarizing some basic principles of safe car design before reviewing developments in seat-belt legislation.

1. There should be a reinforced safety-cage construction around the passenger area to withstand the effects of rollover.
2. The front of the car should be designed to absorb a frontal collision force – the so-called 'crumple zone'.
3. There should be a survival space between the front seats and the dashboard, the size of which is calculated from knowledge of the biomechanics of impact – the 'ride-down area'.

Better steering wheel design, padded dashboards, elimination of sharp edges and laminated windscreens have all made the car interior a safer place. However these are of very limited value without the use of seat belts, because the unbelted occupant is projected against the interior wall of the passenger compartment, negating the effect of the deceleration of the occupant cage produced by the

crumple zone and the protective effect of the ride-down area. Additionally, the risk of ejection from a vehicle is high where belts are not used.

Whilst improvements in the interior design of vehicles are very successful in reducing severity of injury, bioengineering research has also to address the safety aspects of external car design. More than half the deaths associated with cars are the result of being struck by the exterior of a vehicle. Clearly the speed of impact is very relevant but significant improvements can be made, for example the abolition of sharp edges on car bumpers and wings and anti-underrun bars along the sides and rear of lorries.

Seat belts for front seat vehicle occupants

Seat-belt wearing was first suggested by C.L. Straith in the USA as long ago as the 1930s. The three-point safety belt was developed in Sweden and became a standard fitting to Volvo cars from 1959 onwards but it was 1975 before Sweden made seat-belt use by drivers and front seat passengers compulsory. Before the introduction of the law, the voluntary user rate was 51%; after introduction it became 93%. There was a 51% reduction in serious and fatal injuries, and this was more marked for front-seat passengers than for drivers (Nordin, 1985). Although there was an increase in minor chest injuries (AIS 1–2) of 8%, there was a decrease in more serious injuries (AIS 3–6) of 54%. Similarly, there was an increase in mild head injuries (AIS 1–2) of 43% and a reduction in more serious injuries (AIS 3–6) of 64%.

The UK was one of the last countries with high motor vehicle usage, to introduce seat-belt legislation. When the Transport Act of 1981 became effective in early 1983, the rate of seat-belt wearing jumped from 30% to more than 92% in October 1984. It was concluded that between 200 and 440 lives were saved and 7000 serious injuries were prevented each year (Gloag, 1987). The Department of Health commissioned a study to assess the medical effects of seat-belt legislation in the UK which revealed a dramatic change in the numbers, severity and spectrum of injuries (Rutherford et al., 1985). Eye injuries and facial lacerations had been reduced dramatically. There was a decline in serious head injury for belted front-seat passengers, but not for drivers. This was attributed to the fact that inertia seat belts facilitate contact between the head and the steering wheel at certain speeds. There were fewer deaths from serious lung, heart and aortic injuries, but among survivors, there was a 100% increase in fractures of the sternum. There had been fewer fatal liver, spleen and renal injuries but an increase in bowel perforations which are usually attributed to incorrect seat-belt usage resulting in 'submarining' below the lap section of the belt on impact. Survivors less frequently sus-

TABLE 12.5
MAJOR MILESTONES IN PROGRESS AND LEGISLATION RELATING TO ROAD SAFETY (UK UNLESS SPECIFIED)

Date	Legislation	Chief features	Organizations established	Other events
1903–4	Motor Car Act	Driving licences. Braking requirements		
1930	Road Traffic Act	Facilitation of conviction for being under the influence of alcohol		
1931				Highway Code
1950s			Traffic Accident Prevention HQ (Japan)	Encouragement of road research by Department of Science and Industry
				Three-point seat belt developed (Sweden).
1960	Compulsory use of helmets for motorcyclists (Victoria, Australia)		Australian Road Research Board set up	Learner motorcyclists restricted to machines of less than 250 cc
1962	Road Traffic Act	Possible conviction if inability to drive under influence of alcohol proven. Use of alcohol levels as evidence		
1964–5			TRRL and National Highway Bureau (USA) established	Trial motorway speed limit of 70 mph. 'Don't Drink and Drive' publicity campaign
1967	Road Safety Act	Blood/breath alcohol limits. Mandatory road-testing on suspicion. Seat-belt fittings on new cars. Permanent 70 mph limits on some roads		
1968–9	Working hours for drivers limited Compulsory seat-belt wearing (Queensland, Australia)			Pelican crossings introduced. Update on Highway Code State of emergency declared in Japan by National Police Agency
1970	Heavy Goods Vehicle driving tests and instructor registration		Parliamentary Advisory Council for Transport and Safety Federal Office of Road Safety (Australia)	
	Fundamental Law on Traffic Safety (Japan)		Central Council on Traffic Safety and Head Office for Traffic Policy (Japan)	
1971			National Road and Traffic Institute (Sweden) reorganized and expanded	Green Cross Code for Children
1972	Road Traffic Act	Sixteen year olds limited to 'mopeds' (less than 50 cc). Better definition of 'reasonable cause' to take blood alcohol sample. Magistrates allowed to report drug or alcohol dependence	Traffic Safety Research Division added to Federal Highway Research Institute (Federal Republic of Germany)	
1973	Compulsory Safety helmets for motorcyclists		National Road Safety and Standards Authority (Australia)	Blennerhasset Committee to investigate cause of static casualty figures
1975	Compulsory wearing of front seat belts (Sweden)			
1976	Random breath-testing (Victoria, Australia)			

Date	Legislation	Chief features	Organizations established	Other events
1977	State legislation for child safety seats (USA)			
1978	High-intensity rear fog lights compulsory			Highway Code updated
1981	Transport Act (see 1983)			WHO International Conference on RTAs in developing countries
1982	Two part motorcycle test	Machine handling off road first; road awareness skills second. Time limit of 2 years for provisional licence for machines greater than 50 cc		
1983	Transport Act 1981 becomes effective	Compulsory use of front seat belts. Children confined to back seats unless restrained in front. Breath tests accepted as evidence. Concept of 'high risk offender'		
1984	Standards for instructor tests and registration increased			Pedal cycles must meet British Safety Standards
	Zero blood alcohol levels for drivers with a provisional licence (Australia)			
	Universal safety laws for child back-seat passengers (USA)			
1985				Traffic cones and other warning devices for broken-down vehicles
1986	Dim–dip headlights for all new vehicles			
1987	Fitted rear seat belts on new cars			Highway Code update. New 'Don't Drink and Drive' campaign. Target for accident casualties set for AD 2000 (UK 33% reduction; WHO 25% in Europe)
1988	Extended opening hours for drink licensed premises			'Don't Drink and Drive' Campaign again
1989	Compulsory wearing of seat belts by children			Further publicity campaigns
1990	Helmets for cyclists compulsory (Victoria, Australia)			Policy document from Departments of Transport and Education on 'Children and Roads: a safer way'
	Safety audit for development of new road schemes			
1991	Compulsory use of rear seat belts			Consultative document from Department of Health includes accident prevention as target area

TABLE 12.6

COMPARISON OF THE EFFECT OF SEAT-BELT USAGE ON SEVERITY OF INJURY ON FRONT-SEAT PASSENGERS IN GREAT BRITAIN, FINLAND AND OHIO. (DERIVED FROM ROAD ACCIDENTS GREAT BRITAIN 1985, RTAS 1984 HELSINKI, CENTRAL STATISTIC OFFICE OF FINLAND AND 1984 OHIO TRAFFIC ACCIDENT FACTS, COLOMBUS, OHIO DEPARTMENT OF ROAD SAFETY)

	Great Britain 1985		Finland 1984		Ohio, USA 1984	
	No belt	Belt	No belt	Belt	No belt	Belt
Fatal	7	1	9	4	0.2	0.05
Serious	30	17	91	96	24	19
Slight	63	82			76	81
No. in group	3002	104 718	587	2566	433 538	108 031

tained long bone fractures but their distribution was similar to those who were unbelted.

A substantial increase in the incidence of cervical and lumbar sprains was found and it was recognized that the onset of symptoms could be delayed by 1–2 days. The injuries usually resulted from rapid deceleration or low-speed frontal or rear impacts, resulting in hyperflexion followed by hyperextension of the cervical spine. The use of head restraints was proposed to prevent the hyperextension component of the injury. There has been debate as to their effectiveness because it is now thought that hyperflexion is the principle cause of injury. The number of patients with cervical fractures had been reduced but those with thoracic and lumbar fractures remained the same. In terms of the need to admit to hospital and subsequent length of stay, front-seat passengers enjoyed a shorter stay and fewer admissions twice as often as drivers (Table 12.6).

Similar patterns of injury have been shown by other workers (Tolonan et al., 1986; Otremski et al., 1990). The risk of whiplash or more serious cervical spine injury increased in the front-seat passenger position and increased with age greater than 60 years (although for women this increase starts earlier, in the fifth decade). The risk of potentially fatal head, cervical spine or intrathoracic injury increases with speed, especially over 80 km per hour (50 mph) because of impacts of exceptional severity (Arajavi and Santaverta, 1989).

Australia introduced a series of compulsory front-seat-belt laws from 1969. In the USA, New York State became the first to do likewise in 1984. The pre-law user rate was 16% and by 1985 it had levelled out to about 57%. Although enforcement and compliance have proved more difficult than in the UK, within the first 6 months, there was an 18% reduction in occupant fatalities. If the user rate could be increased further, the cost-benefit in terms of lives and money saved would be appreciable (Petrucelli, 1985).

Rear seat belts

The danger for both child and adult rear-seat passengers was highlighted as long ago as 1975 (Christian, 1975). Just before the moment of impact, the victim moves forwards into the back of the front seat at the speed of the car injuring the head and the face. At impact, the body is thrown forwards into the front passenger area with further injury to the head and fractures of the limbs. There is a risk of ejection, which increases significantly if the car overturns. In Christian's series of 185 patients, 81% were injured at speeds of 64 km per hour (40 mph) or less. Fourteen per cent were seriously injured, 36% moderately and 50% sustained injuries which, although minor, warranted immediate hospital attention. In a follow-up study (Christian and Bullimore, 1989) there was a marked reduction in severity of injury among restrained subjects despite the low numbers of the study. All deaths occurred in the unrestrained group (see Table 12.7).

In 1988 there were nearly 25 000 unrestrained rear-seat casualties in the UK, 4000 of whom were killed or seriously injured. It was estimated that

TABLE 12.7

REDUCTION IN ISS FOR UNRESTRAINED AND RESTRAINED REAR-SEAT PASSENGERS. (DERIVED FROM CHRISTIAN AND BULLIMORE, 1989).

ISS score range	Unrestrained	Restrained
0	5	5
1–3	230	23
4–7	116	2
8–11	29	0
12–15	15	0
16	1	0
Total	396	30

70% of rear-seat and 6% of front-seat fatalities could have been prevented by use of rear seat belts (Parliamentary Advisory Committee for Transport and Safety, 1990). However the user rate in October 1989 in the over-14 age group was only 11%, the lowest rates being in rear-seat passengers of old cars which did not have rear seat belts fitted as standard. In the 0–13-year age group, the rate was 70% in 1989 irrespective of the age of the car (Broughton, 1989). This wide difference reflected the change in the law in September 1989, which required children up to 14 years of age to use rear-seat restraints where these were fitted. The Parliamentary Advisory Committee for Transport and Safety (1990) estimated that 50% of licensed vehicles were by then fitted with rear-seat restraints. The compulsory use of rear seat belts for all adults and children was eventually introduced in 1991. It is too early for official statistics to demonstrate the anticipated benefit.

It is expected that the compliance rate amongst adults for rear seat belts will increase with the passage of time as the number of cars which have not had them fitted during manufacture falls. There have been extensive publicity campaigns on television and by posters in public places advising of the dangers to children of travelling unrestrained. In addition, encouragement has been provided by loan schemes which offer types of car restraint appropriate for the age of the child, at a reasonable cost. This work was largely pioneered by the Child Accident Prevention Trust (CAPT). In Australia, New Zealand and the USA, general practitioners, paediatricians and nurses have encouraged the use of car restraints for children; child seat loan schemes are run by hospitals and child health clinics as well as by parent groups and other interested bodies (Gloag, 1987).

Priority in the USA has been given to children's safety before that of the driver and front-seat passenger. Between 1977 and 1984, all 50 states had enacted child passenger safety laws requiring children under the age of 10 to use a seat belt in the rear of a car. Just as in the UK, passengers on school buses do not have to comply (Petrucelli, 1985).

Risk compensation hypothesis

The argument that seat-belt use constituted a severe loss of personal freedom was mitigated by the sound evidence of benefits obtained. A subtle 'risk compensation hypothesis' has now been proposed which suggests that the gain from improvement in road safety will be offset or lost by a compensatory increase in driver's risk-taking behaviour. For example, provision of better braking systems can lead to later braking or better street lighting which may encourage faster night driving in towns. Such trends, it is argued, might result in increased injuries to other road users, such as pedestrians

(Gloag, 1987). Indeed, examination of the numbers of fatally and seriously injured pedestrians and pedal cyclists in 1983–4 did show an increase following the introduction of the seat-belt law but traffic had increased by 7% compared to 1981–2, and over the same period of time 'BMX' bicycles had rapidly gained in popularity. This resulted in increased exposure of under 15 year olds to 'stunt riding' and therefore risk-taking behaviour. McKay (1985) concluded that there was no evidence to support the validity of the risk compensation hypothesis when applied to the seat-belt law.

THE VULNERABLE ROAD USER

Pedestrians and pedal cyclists are most at risk of injury. Amongst these, children and the elderly are particularly vulnerable. In many developing countries, pedestrians, pedal cyclists, van and bus occupants are injured far more frequently than are car occupants, which is partly a reflection of the number of motorized vehicles in use in relation to the population at risk. It is instructive to break down overall casualty rates into age-group rates. It should be noted that changes in the numbers within sections of the population may, over a period of time skew age-related casualty rates. In the USA the population-based traffic accident death rate decreased from 21.3 per 100 000 population in 1975 to 19.1 in 1984 but 10% of this reduction was the result of natural ageing.

In the UK the total amount of motorized traffic has doubled since 1970 but the number of pedestrians killed has fallen by 42%. Between the years 1988 and 1989, pedal-cyclist deaths increased by 30% though the total numbers of casualties rose by only 10%. In 1990, the numbers of fatally, seriously and slightly injured had all fallen by approximately 10%. Pedal-cycle traffic in Britain makes up less than 1% of all traffic, and assessments of yearly changes are subject to wide sampling errors. In the Netherlands, there is a much higher use of pedal cycles and that country has the highest cycle fatality rate in Europe for both children over 6 years and adults. Table 12.8 gives an international comparison of current pedestrian death rates and it can be seen that the young and the very old are the most vulnerable. This clear demarcation suggests an urgent need for investigation into the place, time and nature of such accidents.

The Green Cross Code was introduced to the UK in 1971, to improve children's behaviour at pedestrian crossings, but 78% of pedestrian accidents in 1989 occurred more than 50 m from such a crossing. In the 0–4-year age group, an accident is most likely to occur near to the home, an observation also reported from Norway and Japan (Hutchinson, 1987; Jones, 1989c). As a child grows up, most accidents occur on the way to school. The number of pedal-cyclist accidents similarly rises with age,

TABLE 12.8

INTERNATIONAL COMPARISON OF PEDESTRIAN AND PEDAL CYCLISTS' DEATH RATES. (DERIVED FROM ROAD ACCIDENTS GREAT BRITAIN, 1990)

	Pedestrians (1989)		Pedal cyclists (1986–8 average)	
	Death rate per 100 000 population	Peak incidences (yr)	Death rate per 100 000 population	Peak incidences (yr)
UK	3.1	5–14, > 70	0.5	10–14
Netherlands	1.3		2.0	10–14
Sweden	1.8		0.8	10–14
USA	2.6		0.4	10–14

peaking in the senior school age group and reflecting the child's increased freedom to ride unsupervised on busy roads. Many of the more minor cycling accidents involve stunt riding and play on quiet roads. The TRRL has studied the numbers of cycling accidents in hospital records and concluded that only 68% of cycling accidents are reported to the police. Thus accidents which involve play, though potentially serious, often go unnoticed by collectors of statistics (Taylor, 1989) (Table 12.9).

The peak times for both pedestrian and cycling accidents are between 8–9 a.m. and 3–6 p.m. on weekdays, with a small peak for adults between midnight and 2 a.m. At weekends, the last peak is much higher and the incidence of accidents for all ages is spread out over daylight hours more evenly between 10 a.m. and 8 p.m. Ninety-five per cent of

TABLE 12.9

CHARACTERISTICS OF PEDAL CYCLE CASUALTIES IN THE UK: 1989. (DERIVED FROM ROAD ACCIDENTS GREAT BRITAIN, 1994)

	Casualties	
	% Children (0–15 yr)*	% Adults (> 15 yr)[†]
Accident on road (speed Limit > 40 mph)[a]	9	12
Casualties on built-up roads[a] (speed Limit < 40 mph)	91	88
Casualties in daylight[b]	88	78
Casualties at a junction[b]	69	75

* n = 5445.
† n = 20 279.
[a] = 1994 data
[b] = 1989 data

cycling accidents which involve children under 10 years old and 75% of those in adults occur during daylight hours. There are also seasonal variations. Pedestrian accidents are commonest between October and December – an indication of poor lighting, poor visibility and adverse road conditions. Cycling accidents are most common in better weather between May and August which includes the school summer holidays. There is a marked preponderance of male to female casualties, especially in younger age groups. A boy cyclist has a six times greater risk of being involved in an accident than does a girl. The TRRL has studied this and concluded that more boys have bikes and play out on the street than do girls. They also undertake risky behaviour in both cycling and crossing the road more often than do girls of an equivalent age. Night accidents and those on roads with a speed limit greater than 64 km per hour (40 mph) tend to be associated with more severe injuries. Seventy-two per cent of cycling accidents involving a car occur as the cyclist is travelling straight ahead. This suggests that motorists fail to notice pedal cyclists or misjudge their speed as they drive across or into their path. Eleven per cent of accidents in 1989 involved the cyclist's failure to negotiate a right-hand turn.

Studies of children's accidents have resulted in the development of schemes which involve traffic calming, such as the redirection of the main traffic flow around residential areas which are then subjected to speed restrictions – 32 km per hour (20 mph) in the Netherlands, Japan and Sweden. Entry and exit to these areas has been made more difficult to ensure that most of the traffic does not pass through them inadvertently. The Netherlands and Japan have both substantially reduced their child casualty rates by the provision of protected areas for pedestrians. Japan has 9000 residential and 28 000 school zones and special play areas of the type already described. The Netherlands has 3000 'Woonerven' or residential yards. Ninety per cent of new residential areas are designed on the same principle (Plowman and Hillman, 1984).

Great Britain has been slow to benefit from this Scandinavian experience. Early results from limited and experimental schemes in Britain do show promising results in reducing the numbers of both pedestrian and cycling accidents. The Parliamentary Advisory Committee for Transport and Safety (1990) and the Child Accident Prevention Trust (1991) have both given strong support to such schemes.

Another safety measure currently being introduced is the cyclist's safety helmet which offers a large amount of protection and should result in a significant reduction in morbidity in that head injury is the cause of death or serious disability in 70% of accidents. Initially attempts to introduce these in Australia encountered a significantly surprising amount of opposition. Fortunately this has mostly been overcome and, in Victoria at least, most children wear safety helmets.

FIRES IN CARS

The Transport and Road Research Laboratory in the UK is currently investigating claims from the British Fire Brigade that an increasing number of crashes involve fire. There are also an increasing number of fires which develop spontaneously both while the car is stationary and being driven. A surprising 10–12% of fire deaths each year in the UK are caused by fires in cars but about half of these are instigated by a crash (World in Action, 1991). Many of the substances used in car upholstery would be illegal in the home because of a high degree of flammability and consequent production of toxic smoke. A suggestion has been made that every car should carry a fire extinguisher. However, death is often due to people being trapped within their vehicle, who may not be able to get to and use the fire extinguisher. This is an issue which should be investigated urgently.

CONCLUSION

The epidemiology of road traffic accidents uses statistics to define the causes of death and injury. Improvements can be achieved by changes in legislation, by well-organized enforcement of the law, by education of appropriately targeted groups of the public and by better road engineering and car design. Although the numbers of deaths and serious injuries have declined steadily over the last decade there is still a vast amount of work to be done to ensure that this downward trend both continues and accelerates.

More international cooperation is needed, matched by realistic funding, for collection of comparable data, perhaps with the United Nations and World Health Organization taking the initiative. Much more research should be done on setting up and evaluating educational programmes for each category of road user. Vehicles can be made safer still for both the occupants, pedestrians and pedal cyclists. Poor road surfaces and accident black spot areas should be identified and improvements coordinated by local road traffic safety officers. Realistic goals should be set with target dates for achievement both nationally and globally. This may be expensive, but the long-term benefits in terms of lives saved and the reduction in health-care bills and rebuilding costs will be far greater still.

REFERENCES

Ackroyd, R. (1990). *General review of road traffic accidents in 1990. Road Accidents Great Britain. The Casualty Report.* London: HMSO.

Allsop R. (1966). *Alcohol and Road Accidents: a discussion of the Grand Rapid Study: RRL6.* Crowthorne: Transport and Road Research Laboratory.

Arajavi E., Santaverta S. (1989). Chest injuries sustained in severe traffic accidents by seat belt wearers. *J. Trauma,* **29,** 37–41.

Aviary J.G., Aviary P.J. (1982). Scandinavian and Dutch lessons in childhood road traffic accident prevention. *Br. Med. J.,* **285,** 621–6.

Borkenstein R., Crowther R., Schumate R. et al. (1964). *The Role of the Drinking Driver in Traffic Accidents.* Department of Police Administration, Indiana University.

British Medical Association, Board of Science and Education (1988). *Report: The Drinking Driver.* London: BMA.

Broughton J. (1989). *Seat Belt Use by Car Occupants. Road Accidents of Great Britain.* London: HMSO.

Broughton J. (1990). The ABI *'Snapshot' of motor insurance claims, Road Accidents Great Britain.* London: HMSO.

Bull J., Roberts B. (1973). Road accident statistics; a comparison of police and hospital information. *Accid. Analysis Prevent,* **5,** 45–53.

Child Safety Review (1991). Child Accident Prevention Trust (1991). London. Fact sheet.

Christian M. (1975). Non-fatal injuries sustained by back seat passengers. *Br. Med. J.,* **1,** 320–2.

Christian M., Bullimore D. (1989). Reduction in accidents, injury and severity in rear seat passengers using restraints. *Injury,* **20,** 262–4.

Daltrey R. (1983). *Accident Data: The Report Form. Traffic Engineering Evaluation* (Anreassend D., Gipps P., eds). Caulfield, Australia: Monash University.

Department of Transport (1987). *Road Safety. The Next Steps.* London: Department of Transport and Road Safety.

Department of Transport (1989). *Road Accidents Great Britain, The Casualty Report.* London: HMSO.

Drew G. C., Colquhoun, W. P., Long, H.A. et al. (1958). The effect of small doses of alcohol on a skill resembling driving. *Br. Med. J.,* **2,** 993–9.

Gloag D. (1987). *Colloquium on Strategies for Accident Prevention: A Review of the Present Position.* Medical Commission on Accident Prevention, The Royal College of Surgeons of England, London.

Gloag D. (1991). Road hazards and safer driving. *Br. Med. J.,* **303,** 1090.

Havard J. (1988). Drunken driving among the young. *Br. Med. J.,* **293,** 774.

Howard B., Young M., Ellis J. (1979). *Appraisal of the Existing Traffic Accident Data Collection and Recording System – South Australia.* Report No: CR6. Office of Road Safety, Commonwealth Department of Transport.

Hutchinson T.P. (1987). *Road Accident Statistics.* Rumsby Scientific Publishing, Adelaide.

Jessor R. (1987). *Risky Driving and Adolescence Problem Behaviour, Theoretical and Empirical Linkage.* International Congress and Symposium Series 116, London: Royal Society of Medicine, pp. 97–110.

Jones D. (1989a). *Drinking and Driving in Great Britain. Road Accidents Great Britain.* London: HMSO.

Jones D. (1989b). *The New Child Seat Belt Legislation. Road Accidents Great Britain.* London: HMSO.

Jones D. (1989c). *Child Casualties in Road Accidents. Road Accidents of Great Britain.* London: HMSO.

Mayhew D., Beirness D., Donelson A., Simpson H. (1987). *Why are Young Drivers at Greater Risk of Collision?* International Congress and Symposium Series, 116. London: Royal Society of Medicine, pp. 97–110.

McKay M. (1985). Seat belts and risk compensation. *Br. Med. J.*, **291**, 757–8.

Mondon J.M. (1966). *An Experiment in Enforcing the 30mph Speed Limit*. RRL report no. 24. Harmondsworth: Road Research Laboratory.

Nordin H. (1986). *The Seat Belt Wearing Law in Sweden and its Effect on Occupant Injuries in Volvo Cars*. Volvo Car Corporation, Götenborg, Sweden.

Otremski I., Wilde B., Marsh J., et al. (1990). Fracture of the sternum in motor vehicle accidents and its association with medio-sternal injury. *Injury*, **21**, 81–3.

Parliamentary Advisory Committee for Transport and Safety (PACTS) (1990). Parliamentary Briefing Report, November, St Thomas' Hospital, London.

Petrucelli E. (1985). The medical effects of seat belt legislation in the United Kingdom: one Viewpoint from the USA. *Arch Emerg. Med.*, **2**, 234–6.

Pless I.B. (1991). Accident prevention. *Br. Med. J.*, **303**, 462–4.

Plowden, H. (1984). *Danger on the Road: the needless scourge*. London: Policy Studies Institute.

Risk A., Raymond S., Preston B., (1976). Child cyclists accidents and cycling proficiency training. *Accid. Analysis Prevent.*, **12**, 31–40.

Road Accidents Great Britain. *The Casualty Report* (1990). London: HMSO.

Road Accidents Great Britain. *The Casualty Report* (1994) London: HMSO.

Rutherford W., Greenfield T., Hayes H., Nelson J. (1985). *The Medical Effects of Seat Belt Legislation in the United Kingdom*. DHSS Research Report no. 13. London: HMSO.

Searles B. (1980). Unreported traffic crashes in Sydney. In *Proceedings of 10th Conference of Australian Road Research Board*, Part 4, pp. 62–74.

Shinar D., Treat J., McDonald S. (1983). The validity of police reported accident data. *Accid. Analysis Prevent.*, **15**, 175–91.

Taylor S. (1989). *Road Accidents Great Britain: pedal cyclists casualties*. London: HMSO.

Tolonan S.L., Santavirta S., Kiviloto O., Linqvist C. (1986). Fatal cervical spine injuries in road traffic accidents. *Injury*, **17**, 154–8.

Trinea G.W., Johnston I.R., Campbell B.J. et al. (1988). *Reducing traffic injury – a global challenge*. Royal Australasian College of Surgeons.

Waller P., Stuart R., Hansen A. et al (1986). The potentiating effects of alcohol on driver injury. *JAMA*, **256**, 1461–6.

World in Action (1991). *Chariots of Fire*. Granada Television, April.

13. Road Traffic Accidents: Injury Criteria

D. C. Viano

The design of occupant protection systems requires understanding of both the mechanisms of injury and human impact tolerance. Injury mechanisms are the physical processes that result in tissue damage or functional impairment, while human impact tolerance refers to the extreme loads that the human system can withstand with little or no injury. This field of research is injury biomechanics and focuses on non-penetrating injuries that can occur in restrained and unrestrained occupants of motor vehicles involved in crashes, during sport or military conflict, and in other activities (Viano, 1988; Viano et al., 1989). With sufficient information about injury mechanisms and tolerance, engineers can develop systems that maximize human protection. This is achieved through the development of realistic anthropomorphic test devices (dummies) and criteria to evaluate their engineering measurements, which in turn are used to assess the effectiveness of protective systems in the development stage, as well as in actual impacts.

TRAUMA MECHANISMS

Impact between the human body and an external object can cause compression, stretching, and other deformation of tissues beyond their recoverable limits. In some cases, there may be no apparent gross physical damage but functional changes may occur none the less.

Two basic mechanisms are associated with blunt, non-penetrating impact injuries: localized deformation of tissues and acceleration in the direction of loading. In the automotive environment, the primary collision between the vehicle and whatever it may strike is followed by an impact between the occupant and the inside of the vehicle. This local loading of a part of the body against the instrument panel or even a seat belt is often referred to as the 'second collision'. There is also, however, a 'third collision' between soft tissue and skeletal structures that takes place inside the body as it is being retarded by the vehicle interior or restraint system. The contribution of these types of impacts to the injury process differs depending on the body region, degree of restraint and the severity of impact. The basic function of protection systems is to reduce the severity of impacts and their injury potential.

Impact of the face can directly cause laceration from both blunt and sharp surfaces and severe blows can result in skull fracture. At the same time, however, the impacted head experiences abrupt deceleration during which the rigid skull may slow down faster than soft brain tissue. This results in relative motion between the brain and skull. With a sufficiently severe impact, these processes result in vascular and neural damage arising from compression, stretching and shearing of tissues. The greatest concern in closed head injury is impact acceleration. In the abdominal region, injuries from blunt impact may result from either direct deformation of soft tissues or the relative motion of internal organs to their points of fixation. Major laceration of the liver at the vascular junction is evidence of the latter mechanism. Injuries from local deformation are more common, however, and can occur before significant whole-body deceleration (Lau et al., 1987).

The primary mechanism of thoracic injury in vehicle occupants is direct compression of the rib cage in combination with deformation and stretching of internal organs and vessels during impact (Kroell et al., 1973). When chest compression exceeds the tolerance of the rib cage, ribs fracture and internal organs and vessels can be injured. In some impacts, however, internal injury can occur without skeletal damage – this principally occurs in high-velocity loadings such as exposure to blast. When the organs or vessels are loaded slowly, the input energy is absorbed gradually through deformation. By contrast, when loaded rapidly, the viscous tissues cannot deform rapidly enough. Instead they develop high internal pressures and undergo deformation that can cause damage before the ribs have deflected to any degree. The ability of an organ or other system to absorb such energy rapidly without failure under compression is called its 'viscous tolerance'. Internal organs and vessels can also be torn from their points of attachment during thoracic acceleration and an associated rapid motion of the undamaged rib cage but this is rare.

For non-penetrating impacts to a specified body region, the primary factors that determine the type and severity of injury are the contact area over which the impact energy is spread and the speed of the impacting object. In the motor vehicle accidents, effective restraint systems not only spread the impact energy over the strongest body structures but markedly reduce the contact velocity between the body and the interior surfaces. To assist in the design of such systems, efforts have been made to quantify levels of injury and to establish numerical relationships between injury severity, and measurable engineering parameters such as force, acceleration or deformation. These relationships are known as injury criteria.

ACCELERATION TOLERANCE CRITERION

Rocket sled experiments demonstrated the effectiveness of belt-restraint systems in achieving high tolerance to long-duration, whole-body acceleration and thus improved the protection of military personnel exposed to rapid but sustained deceleration (Stapp, 1970). Whole-body tolerance to deceleration increased as the duration of the exposure decreased (Figure 13.1), linking information generated in regimens differing by orders of magnitude in duration of deceleration. This tolerance curve was based, however, on peak sled accelerations and total time duration rather than an average of peak accelerations measured on the test subjects themselves. Even with this limitation, the data did provide useful early guidelines limiting acceleration to 60 g for the development of crash-restraint systems for both military and civilian personnel.

The basis for the whole-body acceleration tolerance is Newton's second law: that the acceleration (a) of a rigid mass is in proportion to the force on the mass (m), or $F = ma$. (Although the human body is not a rigid mass, a well-distributed restraint system such as the harness used in the rocket sled test makes the thorax at least respond as though it was fairly rigid.) Thus, the greater acceleration, the greater the force on the body and the greater the risk of injury. Ability to withstand higher accelerations of shorter duration implies that tolerance relates to the transfer of momentum because an equivalent change in velocity (v) can be achieved by increasing the acceleration and decreasing its duration (t) or vice versa because $v = at$. The implication for occupant protection systems is that the risk of injury can be decreased for a particular impact if the crash deceleration can be extended over a longer period of time. This can be achieved by increasing the body's stopping distance through the use of crushable structures, safety belts and airbags.

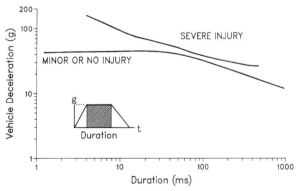

Figure 13.1 Whole-body human tolerance to vehicle deceleration based on impact duration. (Reproduced from Viano, 1988, with permission.)

FORCE TOLERANCE CRITERION

In the early 1960s motor-vehicle safety engineers were seeking information on the tolerance of the thorax to force. This information was needed for the development of the energy-absorbing steering system, which included a device that limited the force that could be applied to it before the structure would deform and absorb energy as it compressed.

Available human tolerance data did not provide information on the appropriate yield force, so sled tests were conducted with embalmed cadavers to simulate the response of an unrestrained occupant interacting with load-measuring surfaces (Patrick *et al.*, 1965). Head, chest and knee contacts against padded load-cells provided the first information on human tolerance to impact force. The resulting data on force tolerance of the rib cage provided the necessary information to design the energy-absorbing element in the steering column on a biomechanical basis.

Subsequent experiments with a prototype energy-absorbing steering system confirmed that a 3.3 kN (740 lb) maximum force on the sternum from the wheel hub and an 8.0 kN (1800 lb) maximum distributed load on the shoulders and chest resulted in steering column compression with only minor risk of rib fracture to the cadavers (Gadd and Patrick, 1968). These load levels were thus considered conservative thresholds of injury in situations with well-centred impacts.

COMPRESSION TOLERANCE CRITERION

In the course of the cadaver experiments, it was observed that the concept of whole-body deceleration and force did not adequately describe the tolerance of the chest to blunt impact nor the risk of internal organ injury. This is because force acting on a deformable human body generates two simultaneous responses: compression of the thoracic structure and acceleration of its masses. The neglected mechanism of injury was compression of the chest which caused the sternum and ribs to bend and possibly fracture when their bending tolerance was exceeded. Force is therefore not a sufficient indicator of injury risk by impact because it cannot discriminate between the two potential responses. In addition, the acceleration mechanism is less relevant to thoracic injury than is compression.

This fact was confirmed in a series of thoracic impacts where maximum acceleration of the thoracic spine was found to be a poor indicator of injury potential. Chest compression, in terms of maximum percentage change in thoracic anteroposterior depth, was a better predictor of injury (Kroell, 1976). Tests with human volunteers showed that chest compression up to 20% during moderately long-duration loading produced no detectable injury and was fully reversible. Impact tests with human cadavers at levels of compression greater than 20% showed that, as the compression increased, so did the risk of rib fractures. At 40% compression, multiple skeletal injuries occurred, to produce flail chest. As the protective capability of the rib cage was destroyed, direct loading of vital organs produced injury to the heart, lungs and great vessels.

VISCOUS TOLERANCE CRITERION

Research on the mechanisms of soft tissue injury has made it increasingly evident that the body cannot be considered a rigid structure, and thus an injury criterion based on whole-body acceleration is not an appropriate predictor of injury risk. The body is deformable. At low-impact speeds ($< 5\,\mathrm{m/s}$ or 11 mph), rib-cage tolerance and risk of crush injury can be evaluated using a compression criterion. This is particularly applicable to belt-restrained occupants in frontal crashes, in which the relative velocity between the occupant and a reasonably snug restraint system is small, and therefore the rate of chest compression is also small. However, for high thoracic compression rates ($> 5\,\mathrm{m/s}$), which are typically experienced by unrestrained occupants or those in side impacts, the maximum compression criterion does not adequately address the viscous properties of the chest and thus risks of soft tissue injury. For these impacts, both the percentage compression and the velocity of deformation are important parameters relating to injury.

Insight into the mechanism of soft tissue injury in high-speed impact can be obtained from research on abdominal injury using a velocity range of $5\text{--}20\,\mathrm{m/s}$ (11–45 mph) (Lau and Viano, 1981a). These speeds are typical of body impacts in high-speed automotive, military and sports injury environments. The liver was the target organ, and the test was set up to attain a maximum 16% abdominal compression, well within the range of tolerable compression for a human volunteer in low-speed (0.4 m/s or 0.9 mph) loading. Using a varying rate of abdominal compression, the experiments verified an increasing severity of liver injury as the velocity of abdominal compression increased. Thus rate of compression is an important factor in soft tissue injury. Subsequent blunt thoracic impact experiments on other organ systems substantiated the interrelationship between magnitude and velocity of chest compression (Jonsson *et al.*, 1979; Lau and Viano, 1981b). These two factors were found critical to the severity of both skeletal and internal thoracic injury, including the likelihood of ventricular arrhythmia and fibrillation (Lau *et al.*, 1981; Stein *et al.*, 1982).

The previous observations led to the concept of a viscous tolerance criterion, which addressed the combined influence of compression percentage and velocity of tissue deformation on soft tissue injury (Viano and Lau, 1983). The relationship between deformation velocity (V) and compression (C), defined as $VC = [V(t) \times C(t)]$, is the viscous response and is a measure of the energy dissipated by rate-dependent or viscous elements in the thorax. Tests were conducted with velocities of compression in the range of $5\text{--}22\,\mathrm{m/s}$ (11–49 mph) and maximum thoracic compression of 4–55%. Using a threshold of critical injury, the experiments confirmed a velocity and compression sensitivity in tolerance to chest impact.

Further analysis of biomechanical data showed that the maximum of the time varying product of V and C was the best predictor of injury (Lau and Viano, 1986; Viano and Lau, 1988). This product ($VC_{\max}$) is the maximum viscous response, and a tolerance of $VC_{\max} = 1.0\,\mathrm{m/s}$ is now widely used in safety testing. The combined criteria indicate that although the chest can withstand 35% compression for slow rates of deformation to avoid crushing injury, the tolerable compression decreases significantly to 10% at a deformation velocity of $10\,\mathrm{m/s}$ to assure $VC_{\max} = 10\,\mathrm{m/s}\,(0.10) = 1.0\,\mathrm{m/s}$ (Figure 13.2).

In more recent experiments on upper-abdominal injury from steering wheel contact, the maximum viscous response proved the best predictor of liver injury severity as well as time of injury occurrence (Lau *et al.*, 1987). It also described more clearly the important biomechanical responses of the abdomen during steering wheel contact and airbag interactions. These studies showed that liver injury by steering wheel contact occurred at the same time as the peak abdominal viscous response, which was

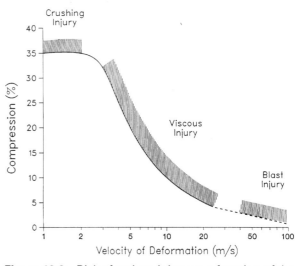

Figure 13.2 Risk of serious injury as a function of the maximum compression and velocity of deformation based on a crushing or viscous mechanism of injury. (Redrawn from Viano *et al.*, 1988, with permission.)

before maximum compression of the abdomen or maximum acceleration of the spine.

INJURY ASSESSMENT

Injury-assessment procedures have been refined as the scientific basis for safety engineering has evolved. Fundamental to the accurate assessment of injury risk is a requirement that the test device or mathematical model has biofidelity. Given the geometric and inertial similarity of dummies to people, the device must also deform under impact force in a human-like manner and experience joint articulations under forces and moments that are realistic. Several test devices or dummies are available which have biofidelity in various body regions.

The Hybrid III dummy is the state-of-art frontal-impact dummy developed primarily for automotive injury assessment with the capability of simulating the human response to impact loading (Foster *et al.*, 1977). More recently, Harry G. Armstrong (Aerospace Medical Research Laboratory) has developed ADAM, the Advanced Dynamic Anthropomorphic Manikin (Rasmussen and Kaleps, 1989) which simulates responses of the spine and extremities to the forces of ejection and wind blast. There is also BioSID, a side-impact test device, with flexible ribs to assess injury risks in the chest and abdomen during impact. All of these dummies have an array of transducers which measure key impact responses (Table 13.1). These include deflection and acceleration measurements as well as the forces, moments and deformation across joints.

Procedures are well established to handle the instrumentation, including signal conditioning, fil-tering, analogue to digital sampling requirements, and on-board and off-board data acquisition. Much of the capabilities of dummies are duplicated in mathematical simulations which include whole-body models using body segments with inter-connecting joints for two-dimensional and three-dimensional response assessment. There are also specific body region models, such as spinal and brain response simulations. The dynamic response of body regions as measured in dummies or mathematical simulations can be used to interpret the potential for injury by comparison of responses to injury probability functions or against a set of tolerance levels. These approaches provide the opportunity to interpret injury risks for particular blunt impact or acceleration exposures.

RISK ASSESSMENT

A scientific basis for safety engineering includes determination of injury risk by a probability distribution function, the assessment over a range of exposure severities, and interpretation of the relative performance of safety systems against those in use. The background for these procedures has been described by Horsch (1987) as approaches to increase the safety of systems that interface with occupants who show a distribution of tolerance to impact acceleration and who are exposed to a potential range of loading severities.

The key to an accurate interpretation is understanding that situations which have very low risk of injury but happen very frequently, may result in as much injury as severe exposures that are infrequent. Thus, balancing the safety design over the actual distribution in impact severities that result in field injury provides the basis for optimizing safety designs.

An example of current risk assessment capabilities in the automotive industry is shown in Figure 13.3 where the safety of a base-line steering system is compared to a self-aligning steering wheel (Horsch *et al.*, 1985). With impact loading of the chest and abdomen in a frontal crash, the modified steering wheel produces lower viscous responses over the entire range of impact exposures in which drivers experience injury. The safety analysis converts the viscous response from the Hybrid III dummy to probabilities of injury using a Logist function, which is a sigmoidal representation of the probability of injury as a function of the viscous response.

An injury probability function has three distinct regions. For very low levels, there is a very low, essentially zero, probability of injury. Similarly, for very high values, the probability of injury is essentially 100%. Between these two regions is a transition zone in which the probability of injury is proportional to a change in the biomechanical response. This type of sigmoidal function is typical

TABLE 13.1
MECHANISM OF BLUNT IMPACT AND ACCELERATION INJURY.
(REPRODUCED FROM VIANO, 1991, WITH PERMISSION)

Body region	Injury biomechanics
Head	Force on skull. Viscous mechanism, compression of brain
Face	Force
Neck/spine	Flexion moments. Extension forces. Shear forces
Chest	Viscous mechanism. Compression. Spinal acceleration
Abdomen	Viscous mechanism. Compression
Extremities/ Joints	Flexion moments Extension/shear force. Rotation
Soft tissue	Viscous mechanism. Compression
Long bones	Force/moments

Effectiveness of Self-Aligning Wheel

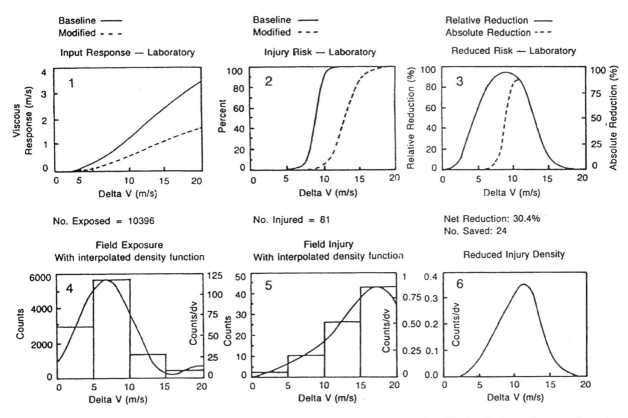

Figure 13.3 Risk assessment using a computer program providing a scientific basis for safety engineering analysis: (1) viscous response for crash speeds (Delta V) up to 20 m/s with the baseline and modified steering system design; (2) conversion of viscous response to injury risk using an established injury risk function; (3) calculation of the relative and absolute reduction in the injury risk with the modified design; (4) field exposure data on the distribution of frontal crashes; (5) field injury data for drivers with critical chest injury; (6) distribution of drivers saved from injury with the modified design. This example gives a projected 30.4% reduction in injury with the modified design. (Reproduced from Viano, 1991, with permission.)

of human tolerance which involves a distribution of biological responses dependent on the strength of the human frame.

Since injury risks are related to the severity of the impact for the baseline and modified steering system, a risk reduction can be determined with the new design. The laboratory tests with the systems can be related to field exposures, and the reduction in risk with the modified design can be interpreted as a potential reduction in field injuries. The new design reduces field injury according to the reduced risk and results in a distribution of occupants who are protected by the modified design. In this situation, the greatest protection occurs at approximately 12 m/s exposure. The benefit of the new system would be 30.4% in real-world crashes. The keys to this type of risk assessment are the interpretation of laboratory tests using an injury probability function, analysis of the safety system over the range of expected exposures and inter-

pretation of benefits based on current field injury experiences.

Further research is needed to develop and refine injury probability functions for specific body regions and injury types. However, Table 13.2 provides statistical parameters and thresholds for serious-critical injury based on a 25% probability of occurrence (Viano, 1991). The risk functions were computed using Logist, which relates the probability of injury to the magnitude of a biomechanical parameter.

A major goal of biomechanics research is to quantify the response and tolerance of humans during impact in order to develop an understanding of how the body can best be protected using established principles of load distribution and energy absorption (Viano, 1988; Viano *et al.*, 1989; Cooper *et al.*, 1991; Viano, 1991). This information is transferred to the laboratory, where simulations of crashes and humans in the form of

TABLE 13.2

AVAILABLE STATISTICAL PARAMETERS AND THRESHOLDS FOR SERIOUS-CRITICAL INJURY BASED ON A 25% PROBABILITY OF OCCURRENCE ($ED_{25\%}$). THE RISK FUNCTIONS RELATE THE PROBABILITY OF INJURY OCCURRENCE $P(x)$ TO THE PROBABILITY OF MAGNITUDE OF THE BIOMEDICAL PARAMETER, x, BASED ON A STATISTICAL FIT TO $P(x) = [1 + \exp(\alpha - \beta x)]^{-1}$. GOODNESS OF FIT IS QUANTIFIED BY CHI-SQUARED (χ^2), P-VALUE (p) AND CORRELATION COEFFICIENT (R). (REPRODUCED FROM VIANO, 1991, WITH PERMISSION)

Body region	$ED_{25\%}$	α	β	χ^2	p	R
Frontal impact						
Head (skull fracture)						
HIC	560	2.048	0.0017	12.7	0.000	0.38
A	160 g	2.859	0.0112	6.0	0.015	0.23
Chest (AIS 4+)						
VC	1.0 m/s	11.42	10.56	25.6	0.000	0.68
C	34%	10.49	0.277	15.9	0.000	0.52
Femur (fracture)						
F	6.0 kN	7.590	0.0011	4.9	0.028	0.39
Lateral Impact						
Chest (AIS 4+)						
VC	1.5 m/s	10.02	6.08	13.7	0.000	0.77
C	38%	31.22	0.79	13.5	0.000	0.76
Abdomen (AIS 4+)						
VC	2.0 m/s	8.64	3.81	6.1	0.013	0.60
C	47%	16.29	0.35	4.6	0.032	0.48
Pelvis (pubic ramus fracture)						
C	27%	84.02	3.07	11.5	0.001	0.91

anthropomorphic test devices and mathematical models are used to develop, assess and refine countermeasures that reduce the risk of impact injury.

REFERENCES

Cooper G.J., Townend P.J., Cater S.R., Pearce, B.P. (1991). The role of stress waves in thoracic visceral injury from blast loading: modification of stress transmission by foams and high density materials. *J. Biomech.*, **24**, 273–85.

Foster J.K., Kortge J.O., Wolanin M.J. (1977). Hybrid III – A biomechanically-based crash test dummy. In *Proceedings of the 21st Stapp Car Crash Conference*. SAE Technical Paper no. 770938. Warrendale, PA: Society of Automotive Engineers, pp. 973–1014.

Gadd C.W., Patrick L.M. (1968). Systems versus Laboratory Impact Tests for Estimating Injury Hazard. Society of Automotive Engineers Paper no. 680053, Warrendale, PA; January.

Horsch J.D. (1987). Evaluation of occupant protection from responses measured in laboratory tests. In *Restraint Technologies: Front Seat Occupant Protection (SP-690)*. SAE Technical Paper no. 870222. Warrendale, PA: Society of Automotive Engineers, pp. 13–32.

Horsch J.D., Lau I.V., Andrzejak D.V., Viano D.C. (1985). Mechanism of abdominal injury by steering wheel loading. In *Proceedings of the 29th Stapp Car Crash Conference*. SAE Technical Paper no. 851724. Warrendale, PA: Society of Automotive Engineers, pp. 69–78.

Jonsson A., Clemendson C.J., Sundquist A.B., Arvebo E. (1979). Dynamic factors influencing the production of lung injury in rabbits subjected to blunt chest wall impact. *Aviat. Space Environ. Med.*, **50**, 325–37.

Kroell C.K. (1976) Thoracic response to blunt frontal loading. In *The Human Thorax-Anatomy, Injury and Biomechanics*. SAE Publication P-67. Warrendale, PA: Society of Automotive Engineers, pp. 49–78.

Kroell C.K., Gadd C.W., Schneider D.C. (1973). Biomechanics in crash injury research. In *19th International ISA Aerospace Instrumentation Symposium*. Las Vegas May.

Lau I.V., Viano D.C. (1981a). Influence of impact velocity on the severity of non-penetrating hepatic injury. *J. Trauma*, **21**, 115–23.

Lau I.V., Viano D.C. (1981b). Influence of impact velocity and chest compression on experimental pulmonary injury severity in an animal model. *J. Trauma*, **21**, 1022–8.

Lau I.V., Viano D.C. (1986). The viscous criterion – bases and applications of an injury severity index for soft tissues. In *Proceedings of the 30th Stapp Car Crash Conference*. SAE Technical Paper no. 861882. Warrendale, PA: Society of Automotive Engineers, pp. 123–42.

Lau I.V., Viano D.C., Doty D.B. (1981). Experimental cardiac trauma-ballistics of a captive bolt pistol. *J. Trauma*, **21**, 39–41.

Lau I.V., Horsch J.D., Viano D.C., Andrzejak D.V. (1987). Biomechanics of liver injury by steering wheel loading. *J. Trauma*, **27**, 225–35.

Patrick L.M., Kroell C.K., Mertz H.J. (1965). Forces on the

human body in simulated crashes. In *Proceedings of the Ninth Stapp Car Crash Conference*, Society of Automotive Engineers, Warrendale, PA; October, pp. 237–64.

Rasmussen R.R., Kaleps I. (1989). The USAF Advanced Dynamic Anthropomorphic Manikin – ADAM. In *Proceedings of the AGARD Conference – Implications of Advanced Technologies for Air and Spacecraft Escape*. France: Advisory Group for Aerospace Research and Development, pp. 9.1–9.7.

Stapp J.P. (1970). Voluntary human tolerance levels. In *Impact Injury and Crash Protection* (Gurdjian E.S., Lange W.A., Patrick L.M., Thomas L.M., eds). Springfield, IL: Thomas, pp. 308–49.

Stein, P.D., Sabbah H.N., Viano D.C., Vostal J.J. (1982). Responses of the heart to nonpenetrating cardiac trauma. *J. Trauma*, **22**, 34–73.

Viano D.C. (1988): Causes and control of automotive trauma. *Bull. N. Y. Acad. Med.*, **64**, 376–421.

Viano D.C. (1991). Live fire testing: assessing blunt impact and acceleration injury vulnerabilities. *Milit. Med.*, **156**, 589–95.

Viano D.C., Lau I.V. (1983). Role of impact velocity and chest compression in thoracic injury. *Aviat. Space Environ. Med.*, **54**, 16–21.

Viano D.C., Lau I.V. (1988). A viscous tolerance criterion for soft tissue injury assessment. *J. Biomech.*, **21**, 387–99.

Viano D.C., King. A.I., Melvin J.W., Weber K. (1989) Injury biomechanics research: an essential element in the prevention of trauma. *J. Biomech.*, **22**, 403–17.

14. Aviation: Injuries and Protection

D. J. Anton

This chapter deals with the type and the bio-mechanical principles of injury arising from inertial and impact loads in fixed and rotary wing (helicopter) aircraft. It also discusses standards for injury protection. Specific injury modes in military aircraft associated with airborne escape and head-mounted equipment are also addressed.

HISTORY

The first documented powered aviation accident was in 1908 when Lt Thomas Selfridge of the US Army Evaluation Board was killed whilst flying with Orville Wright in a 'Wright Flyer'. Selfridge died of skull fractures and his autopsy was the first recorded incident in aviation pathology. Little appears to have been learnt from Selfridge's accident and a high toll in death and injury continued to be exacted in the early years of aviation. The concept of personal protection was almost completely ignored in the quest for improved aircraft control and structural reliability. The emerging requirement to restrain the pilot to the airframe arose more from examples of unrestrained individuals fouling controls or falling from the aircraft during flight manoeuvres, than from considerations of preventing impact injury.

The importance of adequate restraint was, in part, overlooked because of the lack of crashworthiness in early types of aircraft. Wooden-frame structures frequently broke on impact impaling the occupant. The problem was compounded in 'pushers' where the occupant was at risk of being crushed by the engine at the rear if he was restrained.

The First World War did little to advance impact protection. Parachutes were developed to save airmen's lives from crashes although few aircrew carried them routinely. Restraint systems were adopted but with the principal objective of securing the pilot against flight loads which were particularly important in the absence of lateral control trim. Some studies were, however, directed towards crash injury protection; Chandler (1990) refers to observations made in 1919 that, in one aircraft type, cutting 20.3 cm (8 in.) away from the cowl to allow clearance for the pilot's head, practically eliminated head injuries. The same report also referred to the use of a simple shock absorber between the aircraft and the restraint system: 'this decidedly reduced the number and extent of injuries to the upper abdomen and ribs'. Chandler also refers to the following rules made in 1918 under the heading 'General Rules and Regulations Governing Flying on Individual Fields'. These state that:

1. All machines must be equipped with safety belts for pilot and passenger.
2. Always use safety belts. In case of accident, do not release the belt until after the accident. It will probably save injury, especially if the machine turns over.

Little real progress was made until the Second World War, which brought fresh problems because of the advent of metal monocoque airframes and aeroengines of greater power. These advances substantially increased the speed of aircraft and pilots could no longer abandon a stricken aircraft manually because of the increase in aerodynamic load and the risk of striking the fin of the airplane. Although a patent for an aircraft escape system had been filed in the USA in the 1920s, it was research in Germany and Sweden that led to the first practical ejection seats. Whilst working at Ernst Heinkel AG between 1939 and 1945, Arno Goetz (1954) was closely involved in ejection-seat development and conducted what were probably the first modern biomechanical studies on the strength of the human body. He made the important observation that 'an acceleration can be of any magnitude from the point of view of skeletal strength if its duration is correspondingly brief'.

In North America De Haven, who had been seriously injured in an aircraft crash in the First World War, reported the results of the first systematic analysis of injuries in aircraft accidents (De Haven, 1945). He concluded that:

1. In accidents where the cabin structure was distorted but remained substantially intact, the majority of serious and fatal injuries were caused by cabin installations.
2. Crash force, sufficient to cause partial collapse of the cabin structure, was often survived without serious injury.
3. The head was the first and often the only vital part of the body exposed to injury.
4. Causes of head injury were heavy instruments, solid instrument panels, seat backs and unsafe design of control wheels.
5. The probability of severe injuries of the head, extremities and chest was increased by failure of safety-belt assemblies or anchorages.
6. Failure of the 454-kg (1000-lb) (breaking strain) safety belt occurred in 94 cases among 260 survivors of these crashes. Only seven survivors showed evidence of injury to the abdominal viscera; two of these were classified as serious.
7. The tolerance of crash forces by the human body had been grossly underestimated.

8. If spin-stall dangers were lessened and safer cabin installations used, fatal or many serious injuries should be rare in the types of aircraft studied, except in extreme accidents.

De Haven's study was a forerunner of the systematic, combined engineering and medical/pathological scrutiny that now characterizes accident investigation in many countries. Other accident studies were conducted, and Stapp and others explored the field of human tolerance to short-duration accelerations. Eiband (1959) summarized the literature on human tolerance to impact. He indicated that adequate torso and extremity restraint was the principle variable in establishing tolerance limits. Survival of impact forces increased with wider distribution of force to the entire skeleton for all impacts from all directions.

The general principles for improving impact survivability may be summarized thus:

1. A protective shell, free of intrusion, must be maintained around the periphery of the flail envelope of the occupants.
2. The seat and its attachments should be as strong as the airframe to which they are attached.
3. The occupant should be restrained in the seat in such a way as to minimize flail.
4. Aircraft structures should be designed to crush and yield in such a way as to limit the load applied to the occupant.

In 1967 the first issue of the *Crash Survival Design Guide* was produced. It was an organized compendium of the research conducted on both human tolerance to impact and crashworthiness. The 1971 revision was the basis of the United States Army's first standard for aircraft crashworthiness. The 'Design Guide', whilst enunciating principles applicable to all aircraft, was specifically concerned with rotary wing and light fixed wing aircraft (defined by a mission gross weight of 5675 kg (12 500 lb) or less).

PROTECTION IN COMMERCIAL AIRCRAFT

Fixed wing aircraft

Civil transport aircraft rarely crash, although when they do large numbers of people may be killed or injured. From 1955 onwards, a number of studies were conducted on the crash environment of these aircraft, culminating in 1984 in the Federal Aviation Administration (FAA) Controlled Impact Demonstration Crash Test of a Boeing 720 Aircraft. This test, though not an unqualified success, confirmed the results of previous investigation that in survivable accidents, the aircraft structure remains substantially intact and provides a volume within which the occupants can remain intact throughout the impact sequence. It

was also found that seat detachment was usually related to cabin-floor displacement and excessive lateral inertial loads.

The orientation of passenger seats has been a matter of discussion, occasionally vigorous. Eiband (1959) suggested that a rearward-facing passenger seat would offer the best protection in an impact but he cautioned that such a seat should include a lap and chest strap, a winged back with full head rest, load-bearing arm rests with recessed hand holds and provision to prevent arm and leg flail. For forward-facing seats he recommended full body restraint and full-height seat back with integral head support.

The theoretical performance of forward- and rearward-facing seats in transport aircraft was analysed by Pinkel (1959). He assumed that passenger restraint forces were applied through the seat-back attachment points on the forward-facing seats, and for rearward-facing seats through the seat back, at a point twice the distance of the seat-belt attachments to the floor. Using these assumptions he calculated that rearward-facing seats would have half of the design strength of forward-facing seats, if the increase in weight due to the need for a stronger seat back was ignored. Although he recognized the lack of actual crash data for reaching a firm decision on seat orientation, he discussed the relative merits of forward- and rearward-facing seats in the following terms:

> In crashes involving fire or ditching, it is important that the passengers survive the actual crash with only minor injuries, so that they can evacuate the aeroplane. Rearward-facing seats should provide better protection from injury, and appear to have an advantage under these conditions.

> In crashes which do not involve fire or ditching, rapid and unassisted evacuation of the airplane is not so critical, and a higher level of injury might be acceptable. The forward-facing seat should have greater strength than a rear-facing seat of equivalent weight, and thus restrain the passenger in more severe crashes. Since a passenger who is held in place by his seat generally fares better than one who breaks free, a forward-facing seat appears to have an advantage under these conditions.

Mason (1962) reviewed practical experience with rearward-facing seats. He quotes one series of investigations in which 18.9% of forward-facing passengers died compared with 5.3% of rearward-facing occupants. In another study, 11.1% of passengers in forward-facing seats were killed and 84.4% uninjured. The comparable figures for rearward-facing seats were 1.0% killed and 98.3% uninjured.

Notwithstanding the obvious biomechanical advantages of a rearward-facing seat, the overwhelming number of passengers in commercial aircraft travel facing forwards, restrained only by a lap belt. There are several reasons for this:

1. On a material-for-material basis, Pinkel's (1959) work indicated that rearward-facing seats are heavier than forward-facing ones if the same impact performance is required. Increased floor strength, and hence mass, is also required if the increased loads on impact with rearward-facing seats are to be transmitted into the structure, without failure. The cost implications of mass increase were addressed by the FAA, which calculated that each 0.454-kg (1-lb) weight increase in an aircraft can cause 56.78 litres (15 US gallons) of additional fuel burn per annum.

2. There is a considerable reluctance by airlines to fit rearward-facing seats. It is claimed that passengers do not like them, which has been borne out by apparent passenger preference for forward-facing seats in those aircraft where both seat types are fitted. Regrettably, many rearward-facing seats have not been correctly designed and are uncomfortable. Experience in those aircraft fitted only with correctly designed rearward-facing seats shows that passengers are frequently not aware of seat orientation.

3. There is evidence to suggest that passengers in rearward-facing seats are at risk from being struck in the face by objects falling from overhead bins during impacts. The risk of head and facial injury is considered to be less when seats face forward.

In 1983 the FAA reviewed crash injury protection in survivable US Civil Air Transport Accidents between 1970 and 1978. The purpose of the report was to:

1. Compile a database on passenger seat and restraint system performance in survivable accidents.

2. Determine if a correlation existed between occupant, seat and restraint system performance, airframe and floor deformation, and passenger injuries and fatalities.

The review indicated that:

although injuries and fatalities seem to be decreasing in the more recent survivable crashes, seat performance continues to be a factor in these crashes. Failures ranging from seat pan collapse to complete break-away of the seat assembly from the floor are reported. Floor or cabin deformation is frequently a cause of seat failure. Flailing injuries, due to either bending over the restraint system or secondary impact with the aircraft interior, appear to be common.

The study listed 327 fatalities and 294 serious injuries to passengers involved in accidents with US carriers where seats could have been a contributing factor, and indicated four areas that had to be addressed to improve protection:

1. The survivable crash environment required definition so that crash loads and displacements could be established.

2. An understanding of structural component and whole aircraft response to the crash environment is required.

3. Validated analytical modelling and test engineering methods require development.

4. Human factors and injury mechanisms for occupants of transport aircraft require definition.

As a result of the study, the FAA announced its intention to introduce new seat and restraint standards for new type certificate passenger aircraft. The new and old requirements are compared in Table 14.1. A safety factor of 1.33 is also applied to the shown loads. Seat manufacturers are allowed to demonstrate compliance with the load and safety factors by static testing. The standards also apply to the supporting structure of each item of mass that could injure an occupant if it came loose in a minor crash landing.

Additionally, two dynamic tests were defined, using instrumented 50-percentile 49 CFR Part 572 anthropomorphic test dummies to simulate seat occupants. Test 1 approximates to a near vertical impact, with some forward speed, applying a minimum of 14 G deceleration from a minimum velocity of 10.67 m/s, canted aft 30 degrees from the vertical axis of the seat. Test 2 approximates a horizontal impact with some yaw, applying a minimum 16 G deceleration from a minimum of 13.41 m/s, the seat yawed 10 degrees from the direction of deceleration. To simulate the effects of cabin-floor deformation, the parallel floor rails or fittings in test 2 are misaligned by at least 10 degrees in pitch, and 10 degrees in roll before the dynamic test. The tests require that the seat remains attached, although it may yield to a limited extent. The tests also include a requirement limiting the pelvic load to 6.672 kN (1500 lbf), head deceleration to a HIC ≤ 1000

TABLE 14.1
FAA SUSTAINABLE STATIC LOAD FACTORS OF SEATS AND
SAFETY BELTS ASSUMING A MINIMUM SEAT OCCUPANT WEIGHT
OF 77.2 KG (170 LB)

	Pre-1988	*Post-1988*
Forwards	$-9.0\ G_x$	$-9.0\ G_x$
Rearwards	–	$+1.5\ G_x$
Sidewards	$+/-1.5\ G_y$	$+/-3.0\ G_y$ airframe, $4.0\ G_y$ seats/attachments
Downwards	$+4.5\ G_z$	$+6.0\ G_z$
Upwards	$-2.0\ G_z$	$-3.0\ G_z$

(Head Injury Criterion) and axial femoral load to 10.008 kN (2250 lb).

Of these two tests, Test 2 is considered the more stringent. The peak deceleration (16 G) and the velocity change (13.41 m/s) were chosen as the result of a study of crash dynamics and the levels were also considered to be compatible with existing floor strengths in the current fleet of transport aircraft. Subsequent to the promulgation of these rules, the FAA issued a Notice of Proposed Rule Making (NPRM) to cover the installation of the upgraded seats in new aircraft of current type and within the existing fleet; all transport category aircraft would be required to have seats installed, meeting the new criteria, by June 1995.

The first transport aircraft accident involving seats tested, but not certificated, to the new standards occurred in January 1989 when a Boeing 737–400 crashed on the M1 motorway in England. A combined medical and engineering, structural crashworthiness and survivability study was undertaken. The aircraft suffered two major structural failures on impact, one slightly forward of the wing leading edge and one aft of the trailing edge. It did not catch fire. The failures left the structure in three principal sections. The forward section sustained considerable crushing in the lower flight deck area and the belly skin disintegrated along the length of the passenger cabin. The floor of this part of the passenger cabin was entirely disrupted with separation of the seats from their attachments. The centre section was intact, although all of the overhead lockers and cabin furnishings failed on impact. Fourteen of the triple passenger seats remained attached to the floor in this area. The tail section separated from the main fuselage and came to rest partially inverted over the rear of the centre section. Seven passenger seat triples remained attached to the floor in this region.

The fact that the centre section is a particularly rigid structure and that nearly all the seats were retained in this area, meant that the occupants were all subjected to a broadly similar impact pulse. Considerable effort was therefore made to model the impact conditions and relate those conditions to passenger injuries.

The impact pulse was defined using the computer program KRASH which solves the coupled Euler equations of motion for 'n' interconnected lumped masses. Each mass has a maximum of six degrees of freedom defined by inertial coordinates and eulerian angles. The concentrated masses interact through interconnecting beams which are appropriately attached and have specifiable stiffnesses. The modelling indicated that the best fit conditions for the acceleration environment of the centre section of the aircraft were a peak longitudinal deceleration of -26.1 G_x superimposed upon a -17.8 G_x plateau which represented the plastic deformation pulse transmitted to the seats. The

pulse shape indicated that the initial impulse in the major impact was primarily longitudinal, followed by a $+23$ G_z vertical pulse, when the engine nacelles and fuselage centre section struck the ground.

One hundred and twenty-six passengers and crew were on board. The types of injuries seen were typical of such accidents, although the fitment of tougher seats almost certainly saved lives at the price of a greater number of more serious injuries. Thirty-nine passengers died at the scene of the accident and eight more in hospital at times up to 22 days later. Seventy-nine survived. Injuries were classified and coded using the Injury Severity Score (ISS). The worst occurred in the regions of greatest structural damage – where the seat attachments failed.

It was known that some, but not all, of the passengers adopted a brace position before the aircraft hit the ground. Subsequent analysis of the head injuries showed that there was a statistically significant relationship between failure to adopt a brace position and suffering an episode of impairment of consciousness. It also appeared probable that the injuries sustained to the back of the head were related to the failure of the overhead bins, or to the liberation of bin contents. No causal relationship was, however, demonstrated. Facial injury was caused by striking the back of the seat in front, the face then following a trajectory down the back of the seat until coming to rest when the subject's torso was arrested on the knees.

Significant injuries were caused to the upper limbs and shoulders during the impact and were the result of a variety of mechanisms. Some passengers attempted to shield or protect those next to them by placing an arm around them which caused dislocation of the shoulder. Others braced themselves by putting their arms out in front with the same result. There was evidence to suggest that some forearm fractures were due to head impact when the arms were held up in protection. Other major injuries were caused to the pelvis and lower limbs. Only 18 surviving passengers and six fatalities did not have injury in this area. There was an excess of femoral fracture in the centre seat of the triples. The front-seat spar in this seat type and position is supported on either side by the legs and consequently cannot deform under load. The observation of an excess of femoral fractures in this position suggests that femoral bending, rather than femoral axial loading, might have been the fracture mechanism. This hypothesis has been tested in a series of computer reconstructions.

Simulation of the response of the occupants to the impact was carried out using the program MADYMO. Using a 50-percentile Hybrid III dummy dataset and the results of the KRASH simulation, femoral axial and bending loads were calculated for both the upright and the braced occupant. This showed that axial loads of 3.4 kN and bending loads of 1.3

kN were induced in the femurs of simulated upright occupants, and axial and bending loads of 2.3 kN and 2.7 kN respectively in the femurs of simulated braced occupants. The greater bending loads in the braced occupant resulted from the effects of the shift of body mass. These findings are of considerable interest and, if confirmed, have regulatory importance as the current FAA requirements deal only with femoral axial loads as a limiting factor in the acceptability of seats when dynamically tested.

The detailed biomechanics of the mechanisms for pelvic, lower leg, ankle and foot fracture when an aircraft impacts have still to be investigated. Leg flail on impact may be responsible for some tibial fractures and for hyperextension injuries to the knee. All of the injuries detailed above were found in occupants restrained by a lap belt in a forward-facing seat. Most of the injuries would have been prevented (subject to the seats staying attached to the floor and the overhead bins and their contents staying attached to the roof) if the occupants had been fully restrained with a shoulder harness or if the seats had been facing backwards.

Considerable scope exists for injury research in passenger aircraft. Studies in the automotive environment have some application but the addition of a significant G_z acceleration component to the impact pulse which is absent from car crashes considerably changes injury mechanisms. This is particularly true in helicopters.

Helicopters

Although the same principles of impact protection apply, substantial differences exist between fixed wing and rotary wing aircraft impact. Helicopters (rotorcraft) fly much more slowly than fixed wing aircraft and generally have very substantial vertical velocity change components on impact. They also have a higher accident rate than fixed wing aeroplanes. The figures are difficult to compare because of the differences in operating methods. The United Kingdom Civil Aviation Authority has quoted figures of approximately 0.7 reportable accidents per 100 000 revenue hours for all passenger operations by UK operators of fixed wing aircraft over 2300 kg for the decade 1980–89. UK helicopter operators averaged 2.6 reportable accidents per 100 000 hours flown for the same period. In contrast, the FAA has quoted accident rates for transport rotorcraft (those over 2724 kg (6000 lb) gross weight) of eight accidents per 100 000 flight hours and 14.3 accidents per 100 000 flight hours for normal category rotorcraft. Because of the higher seating capacity, transport helicopters are said to have a higher relative risk of serious injury than normal category rotorcraft despite the lower accident rate.

The risk of serious injury is enhanced by the lower standards for seat strength that have been applied in the past to helicopters. Current requirements for existing rotorcraft specify that the seats should resist combinations of inertial forces up to a maximum of 6 G using components relative to the rotorcraft of:

Forwards $-4\,G_x$
Rearwards $+3\,G_x$
Downwards $+6\,G_z$
Upwards $-3\,G_z$
Sidewards $+/- 0{-}3\,G_y$

These load factors are applicable to the weight of the seat and a 76-kg (170-lb) occupant. The strength requirements are factored by 1.33 and also apply to the harness and its local attachments.

For transport rotorcraft in particular, these strength requirements are low and may not exploit the available strength of the airframe. In consequence, accidents are encountered where the airframe may stay substantially structurally intact yet the seats fail. When this happens passengers may sustain gross injuries as a consequence of secondary collisions.

During the 1980s the FAA and the helicopter industry cooperated in studies to improve the crashworthiness of civil helicopters. This work was based on that conducted by the US Army and codified in the US Army Aircraft Crash Survival Design Guide. As a result of this work the FAA issued an NPRM recommending:

1. A shoulder harness for each occupant.
2. An increase in the static load factors.
3. The definition of two dynamic tests.

The increase in the static load factors was substantial:

Upwards $-4.0\,G_z$
Forwards $-16\,G_x$
Sidewards $+/- 8\,G_y$
Downwards $+20\,G_z$ (after any stroking of the attenuation system)

The dynamic tests were defined using similar instrumented anthropomorphic test dummies to those required for use in fixed wing aircraft.

Test 1 approximates a near-vertical impact, with some forward speed, applying a minimum of 30 G deceleration from a minimum velocity of 9.14 m/s (30 feet per second (fps)), canted aft 30 degree from the vertical axis of the seat.

This test reflects the considerable vertical velocity component present in many helicopter accidents. In the same series of accidents studied, the US Army Aircraft *Crash Survival Design Guide* gives the median of the distribution of the survivable vertical velocity change as being 7.3 m/s (24 fps). Ninety-five per cent of accidents were stated to incur vertical velocity changes of less than 12.8 m/s (42 fps). These two values are the equivalent of a body in free fall from 2.72 m and 8.4 m (8ft. 11in. and 27ft. 5in.) respectively.

Test 2 approximates a horizontal impact with some yaw, applying a minimum of 18.4 G deceleration from a minimum of 12.8 m/s (42 fps), with the seat yawed 10 degree from the direction of travel.

The *Crash Survival Design Guide* gives figures for survivable longitudinal velocity changes of a median of approximately 8.5 m/s (28 fps), with 95% of accidents incurring a velocity change of less than 15.2 m/s (50 fps).

It can be appreciated that the significant vertical velocity changes impose accelerations that require attenuation before transmission to an occupant. In most modern helicopters this is provided by a combination of planned deformation and energy absorption in the fuselage as well as energy attenuation, usually by the seat stroking, in the seat itself. Adequate coupling of the occupant to his seat is essential if flailing is not to negate the effects of the attenuation, and for this reason a shoulder harness must be fitted.

The recommendations detailed above were subsequently embodied as final rules for both normal and transport category rotorcraft but applying only to new type certificate aircraft and not to existing types or their derivatives. Subsequent to the new rules the FAA issued a further NPRM requiring the installation of shoulder harnesses in all newly manufactured rotorcraft even if they have a Type Certificate which precedes December 1989.

ESCAPE FROM MILITARY AIRCRAFT

The speed and altitude at which combat aircraft fly dictate the use of airborne escape systems. The majority of such systems are of the so-called 'open' variety where the crew member is propelled clear of the aircraft by a gun or rocket, or a combination of both. Such escape systems, though life-saving, pose a number of specific injury hazards.

Ejection gun acceleration

Thoracolumbar spinal injury

Vertebral compression fracture on ejection was initially observed on the first seats designed and produced in Germany. Early prototype versions produced peak accelerations of 12 g and rates of rise of acceleration of 1100 gs. Other workers suggested that tolerance to short-duration accelerations was most dependent upon the rate of rise of acceleration (jolt) and it was thought that when the onset was too rapid, reflex contraction of the spinal extensors could not occur with sufficient rapidity and spinal wedge fractures resulted.

It was not until after the war that much work was directed towards defining the physiological limits of jolt and peak acceleration. Different propulsive charges and types of ejection gun to produce accelerations that were subjectively tolerable to human volunteers were investigated. The importance of rigid coupling between the body and the ejection seat was recognized and further work led to the development of an electronic analogue for assessing the variables involved in seat ejection. The outcome of this effort was the setting of limiting values of peak acceleration and jolt to 25 g and 250 gs, these values applying solely to accelerations in the vertical plane. These were not 'no injury' levels but rather represented values at which complicated or unstable vertebral fractures are rare.

Ejection seats manufactured by the Martin Baker Aircraft Company began to be installed in Royal Air Force (RAF) and Royal Navy (RN) combat aircraft from the late 1940s onwards, but it was not until the late 1950s that sufficient experience in their use, in the UK, had accrued to permit a clear-cut analysis of injury. An analysis of RAF and RN experience between 1949 and 1960 showed that there was an increase in vertebral fracture rates from 10 to 35% with the change to the 80 fps telescopic ejection gun from the earlier guns with velocities of 53–60 fps. This increase in gun velocity was the result of improving the safe escape envelope of the ejection seat. Differences also emerged in the spinal injury rates for RAF and RN ejections, that for the RN being lower. No clear explanation was forthcoming for this difference, although it was suggested that closer attention to the adjustment of the restraint harness, which is imperative for catapult launch and deck landing, may have lead to improved spinal alignment at the time of ejection. Other workers have also emphasized the importance of adequate harness restraint to ensure optimal spinal and pelvic alignment with the thrust axis of the ejection seat, and the avoidance of static loading of the spine by an incorrectly designed and adjusted shoulder harness. The faceblind handle which is pulled down to initiate the ejection sequence also improved spinal alignment by preventing forward flexion of the head and reducing the load carried by the lower thoracic vertebrae.

During the 1960s considerable technical development of the ejection seat took place, driven by the dual requirement to automate the ejection sequence and further to enlarge the safe escape envelope. Development in the latter area led to the introduction of the rocket-assisted ejection seat which permitted the derating of the ejection gun from 80 to 64 fps. The effect of the rocket was to augment the ejection-seat thrust, the ignition of the rocket being timed to coincide with the full extension of the ejection gun. Careful attention to the thrust characteristics and ignition of the rocket not only resulted in considerable improvement in the seat escape envelope but also in the shape of the force/

time profile of the early part of the ejection sequence.

While these changes were being made it was recognized that, although the use of the faceblind handle improved spinal alignment, initiation by this method was neither as reliable nor as quick as initiating by a seat-pan handle. This was of significance in that aircraft were operating at a lower altitude and ejections were therefore taking place closer to the ground offering less time to prepare for escape. To avoid time being wasted in deciding which handle to use, RAF teaching changed in the early 1970s to emphasize the use of the seat-pan handle as the primary method. Use of the faceblind handle was relegated to well-foreseen medium-level ejection. As a consequence, new ejection seats in the RAF inventory (Martin Baker Mk 9 seats onwards) incorporated only a seat-pan handle, although no retrospective modifications were carried out.

In an attempt to remedy the deleterious effects of seat-pan handle initiation on spinal loading and alignment, powered shoulder retraction was incorporated on some types of rocket ejection seat. It has been reported that this resulted in a significant decrease in the incidence of vertebral fractures on US Navy F4 ejections.

Further attempts were made to produce a mathematical model from ejection-seat test data which would allow predictions to be made of vertebral fracture rates. The advantages of such an approach are that it provides, in theory at least, a method for judging the acceptability of the accelerations on an escape system, without having to wait for injury data to accrue. Proposals for such a model were first put forward by staff at the Aerospace Medical Research Laboratory in 1967, but it was not until 1973 that agreement was reached by the five nations of the Air Standardisation Co-ordinating Committee on the adoption of the model known as the Dynamic Response Index (DRI).

The single axis DRI can be determined as a function of the $+G_z$ acceleration time history of the first part of the operation of the escape system. It is said to be representative of the maximum dynamic compression of the lower thoracic and lumbar vertebral column and provides a means of estimating the probability of spinal injury for those who are at risk. It does not attempt, however, to predict the precise location or severity of the injury. In physical terms, the DRI is calculated by describing the human body in terms of an analogous lumped-parameter mechanical model. The DRI has been validated against United States Air Force operational experience of ejection, and since 1978 has been calculated for RAF escape systems.

Subsequent work by Brinkley (1985) on the DRI has expanded its use to assessing the effect of accelerations perpendicular to the chest and parallel to the shoulders. Similar assumptions are made

about the body response in the x and y axes as in the +z axis, although different natural frequency and damping ratios are used for each. Work has not yet been undertaken to compare the three axis DRI predictions with data on RAF spinal injury.

The RAF experience showed that spinal injury was common on ejection. For later types of seat it is generally not well predicted by the use of the DRI. Table 14.2 shows the observed and DRI-predicted

TABLE 14.2

OBSERVED AND DRI-PREDICTED SPINAL FRACTURE RATE FOR MARTIN BAKER EJECTOR SEATS USED IN 223 EJECTIONS IN THE RAF BETWEEN 1968 AND 1984

Ejection seat type	DRI predicted	Observed rate
Mk 2	80–100%	69%
Mk 3	80–100%	65%
Mk 4	40%	39%
Mk 5	NR	67%*
Mk 6	4%	65%
Mk 7	4%	50%
Mk 9	4%	29%

NR = Not recorded.
* n = 6 ejections only.

TABLE 14.3

DISTRIBUTION OF SPINAL FRACTURES FOR EJECTIONS PRESENTED IN TABLE 14.2

Vertebral level	Ejection seat type			
	2/3	4/5	6/7	9
D1	0	0	0	0
D2	0	0	0	0
D3	1	0	0	0
D4	2	1	0	1
D5	1	3	0	1
D6	2	1	1	3
D7	7	3	2	0
D8	6	1	3	3
D9	7	3	3	1
D10	5	7	0	0
D11	9	8	7	1
D12	19	12	9	4
L1	10	7	8	4
L2	4	2	1	2
L3	0	1	1	0
L4	0	1	1	0
L5	0	0	0	0
Sacral	0	0	2	0
Not recorded	0	1	1	1
Total	73	51	39	21

Note: Numbers beneath ejection seat types denote total numbers of fractures for that vertebral level. Because, frequently, more than one vertebra was involved, the sum of the fractures is greater than the sum of the injuries.

TABLE 14.4

EFFECTS OF HARNESS TYPE ON INCIDENCE OF INJURIES WITH POOLED MKS 6–9 MARTIN BAKER EJECTION SEATS

	Injured	*Not injured*	*Total*
Harness			
Torso harness	23	40	63
Simplified combined harness	14	13	27
Total	37	53	90

spinal fracture rate for Martin Baker Marks 2–9 ejection seats used in 223 'within envelope' RAF ejections between 1968 and 1984. The majority of the injuries were anterior wedge compression fractures, with the preponderance occurring at the thoracolumbar hinge (D11-L1). Table 14.3 shows the distribution of fractures along the vertebral column for the same series of ejections. Not all the spinal fractures may be attributable to the effects of ejection gun acceleration. Table 14.4 examines the effect of a change in harness on the Martin Baker Marks 6, 7 and 9 ejection seats. For convenience the data for the three seats have been pooled.

The difference in injury rates between the two types of harness fails to achieve statistical significance because of the relatively few ejections with the simplified combined harness (SCH). Figure 14.1(a) and (b) show the difference in $-G_x$ impact restraint afforded by the two types. It can be seen that the simplified combined harness does not give as good restraint as the torso harness and the trend indicated in Table 14.4 accords with expectation.

Cervical spinal injury
Cervical spinal fracture occurring as a result of ejection-gun acceleration is almost unknown. In an analysis of 237 'within envelope' UK MOD peace-time ejections between 1968 and 1981, the Advisory Group for Aerospace Research and Development (AGARD) Aerospace Medical Panel Working Group 11 (WG11) (1984) reported two minor fractures, one an anterior wedge of C5 and the other a minor flake detachment from the upper anterior surface of C5. These injuries may not, however, have occurred as a result of ejection-gun acceleration.

The same source reported German Air Force (GAF) experience, and details one fatal case that was attributed to forces in the early part of the escape sequence. An ejection took place from an aircraft that was inverted after uncontrolled oscillations. The pilot died of an extensive circular fracture at the skull base and rupture of the atlanto-occipital ligament. The skull fracture resulted in extensive trauma to the mid brain, hind brain and cerebellum. The fracture mechanism was distraction due to forward flexion. Forensic evidence indicated that this occurred in the first 0.6 seconds of the ejection sequence.

Soft tissue cervical spinal injury is more common, occurring in approximately 30% of cases. As with many other ejection injuries it is difficult to be certain whether the injury arises as a result of initial or later accelerations in the escape sequence.

Femoral fracture
Rarely, mid-shaft femoral bending fracture is seen as a complication of the initial gun acceleration. Brinkley (1991, personal communication) stated that USAF experience with the F105 aircraft indicated that if the feet were withdrawn from the rudder pedals before ejection there was a serious risk of fracture. Subsequent parachute landing carries a risk of exacerbating the fracture and cases have been reported of aircrew dying from loss of blood before rescue. The risk of fracture is increased in individuals with large buttock/knee dimensions and also where overall stature gives a sitting

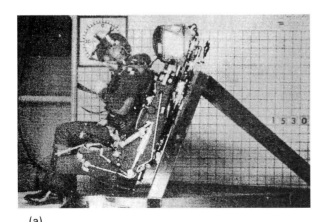

(a)

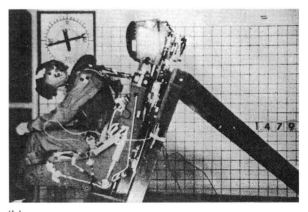

(b)

Figure 14.1   (a) Impact restraint afforded by Torso harness. (b) Simplified combined harness.

position where part of the upper leg is no longer supported by the top of the personal survival pack (PSP) even when the feet are on the rudder pedals. Current RAF practice is to reject individuals who have 50-mm clearance between the underside of the thigh and a point 50 mm rearwards from the top of the front horn of the PSP. Recent work at the RAF Institute of Aviation Medicine, using a 50-percentile Hybrid III anthropomorphic dummy equipped with 6 degree of freedom femoral load cells, has indicated that the dummy femur is subjected to bending strains on ejection that are approximately 75% of the quoted bending strain to failure of the isolated femur of a young adult. The 50-percentile Hybrid III dummy has a buttock knee dimension that equates to the 30-percentile RAF aircrew; actual femoral bending loads on ejection may therefore be higher in the majority of military aircrew.

Clearing the ejection path

Through-canopy ejection

In reviewing Martin Baker experience, the statement was made that: 'The use of correctly matched canopy penetrators, a powerful catapult (ejection gun), secure harness, stable low resonance sitting platform, adequate seat to canopy clearance and cast acrylic (canopies) up to 9 mm thick will enable safe, injury free ejections to be made through the canopy. This is confirmed by a wealth of test data and some 1000 emergency through canopy ejections made without significant canopy penetration related injury' (Miller, 1982). Miller concluded that, with the above design considerations, direct canopy penetration has proved to be a most satisfactory method of crew escape.

Through-canopy ejection has been used extensively, as Miller indicates, as the system is both cheap and incurs the minimum time delay in getting aircrew out of the aircraft. Historically, through-canopy ejection has been said to be associated with an increased incidence of vertebral compression fracture because the ejection seat slows momentarily as it passes through the canopy, thus allowing the occupant to start to separate from the seat. Having penetrated the canopy the seat accelerates and catches up with the man, who in turn has started to slow as he passes through the canopy. The net effect is to impart an additional rapid-onset acceleration to the occupant, so increasing the probability of a spinal compression fracture.

A further disadvantage is apparent in the front seat of tandem aircraft. To enable the rear pilot to have an adequate forward view the front pilot is generally positioned lower down and further away from the canopy, which itself curves downwards fairly steeply. When a front-seat ejection is initiated, the ejection seat has further to travel before hitting the canopy; the pilot's head has more time to nod forward and therefore hits the canopy in a forward flexed position. In one ejection from the front seat of a T2 Harrier, the pilot sustained unstable cervical spinal fractures of C4, 5 and 6 that required fusion. Similar problems have been encountered in the front seat of other tandem aircraft, a finding at variance with Miller's observations.

Impairment of consciousness

Consciousness may be impaired. Recent RAF experience provides examples. One pilot, ejecting through the canopy of the front seat of a tandem aircraft, suffered a chin/sternum injury and was unconscious for 10 minutes. Another ejecting from the same type over water, failed to complete any of his postejection drills and drowned; at autopsy there was evidence of a chin/sternum contact. Because of these instances, and concern over possible increase in the incidence of spinal injury, through-canopy ejection was abandoned in the RAF. Miniature detonating cord systems have been fitted to canopies to ensure their complete disruption.

AGARD WG 11 (1984), assessing the incidence of impairment of consciousness on UK MOD ejections, found that six survivors from 237 'within envelope' ejectees (2.5%) were assessed as having suffered a head injury, as judged by post-traumatic amnesia lasting from 1 minute to 4 hours. Eight fatalities were also noted in this series, one of which showed unequivocal and three circumstantial evidence of impairment of consciousness, to give an overall incidence estimate of 4.2%. Ejection forces (a loose term embracing ejection-seat instability, drogue and parachute forces, and including both direct and inertial trauma) were deemed to be responsible for half of the fatalities related to impairment of consciousness and a third of the injuries in the survived group.

Windblast

Entry into the airstream exposes aircrew to aerodynamic forces usually referred to as windblast. The forces are proportional to the air density and the square of the aircraft velocity, and at high speed are severe and produce characteristic injury patterns. Entry into the airstream causes the ejected man and seat to decelerate as a function of drag and mass. Drag in turn is a function of dynamic pressure, the drag coefficients and the frontal area.

Unrestrained limbs and head will decelerate more rapidly than the trunk/ejection seat complex, since they have a greater ratio of surface area to mass. Ring et al. (1975) reviewing USAF noncombat ejection experience state that flail starts to become a significant problem above 300 knots (kt), with leg flail predominating at the lower speeds. At around 600 kt at sea level the probability of some form of flail injury occurring reaches 100%. Combat experience has shown that ejection speeds are higher than in peacetime and that flail injury is a significant cause of major aircrew injury and loss under wartime conditions.

The RAF requires the fitment of leg restraints on all its ejection seats and has fitted arm restraints to the escape system in the Tornado aircraft. It is much more difficult to engineer a satisfactory restraint for the arm than the leg. A study of the incidence of arm injury on Tornado ejections demonstrated three injury mechanisms:

1. Clavicular fractures, thought to be due to an interaction with the CO_2 canister in the lifepreserver.
2. Soft tissue injuries – mild to moderate bruising, with or without elbow effusion, after apparently normal arm restraint line retraction.
3. Severe bruising, upper limb fracture and shoulder dislocation.

Matching the Tornado ejections against other fast jet ejections for speed and height showed no significant difference in the incidence of injury, which suggests that the Tornado arm restraint system was not functioning correctly.

At very high ejection speeds (circa 550 kt+ at sea level) head flail becomes a significant problem, either because it is driven back into the headbox of the ejection seat, or because of the development of excessive lifting forces with consequent neck distraction injury.

Interactions between the head and the headbox of the ejection seat first became of serious concern in the RAF during the high-speed ejection testing of the Martin Baker Mk 10A ejection seat used in the Tornado aircraft. Analysis of the high-speed cine film from a 628-kt test ejection showed that, during the initial rise of the seat, the inertial reaction to the +Gz acceleration forced the dummy's head forward onto its chest. As the head and the top of the seat emerged into the air flow, the head was driven forcibly back into the front of the headbox. Substantial damage was caused to the helmet. Calculations, based on the aerodynamic loading, indicated a maximum impact velocity between head and headbox of 13.6 m/s. Assuming a slightly lower impact velocity of 12 m/s and a 6.8-kg combined head/helmet mass, gave an energy of impact of approximately 460 J rather more than twice the 200 J design criterion then laid down in British Standard 2495:1960. As a consequence of this incident the ejection-seat headbox of the Mk 10A seat was modified to improve its ability to attenuate impact. Following modification, the headbox/helmet successfully attenuated impact energies up to 570 J without exceeding either 20 kN transmitted force, or a peak acceleration of 310 G. Regrettably, the principle of specifying headbox attenuation was not carried over to other ejection seats, and operational experience began to accrue indicating that

helmet/headbox impacts, however occasioned, were a cause of impairment of consciousness on escape.

A review of aircrew helmet performance on ejection from RAF fast jets showed that 17 out of 200 aircrew who ejected successfully suffered helmet impacts. Sixteen of these helmets were available for inspection, and the cause of the impact damage was attributed to the ejection seat (usually headbox) in seven.

Ejection-seat instability

It has been known for some time that unless ejection seats are stabilized they have a tendency to pitch, roll, and/or yaw, during rocket burn shortly after initial entry into the airstream. As a result of this instability, subsequent drogue and parachute deployment vectors can be markedly 'off axis', giving rise, on occasion, to unacceptably high forces on the seat occupant.

Two fatal ejections with evidence of lateral parachute extraction caused by seat instability triggered an investigation into the stability of the particular type of ejection seat concerned. Initial information from the films of trials indicated that yaw rates in excess of 2000 degrees/s could occur early in the ejection sequence. These data had been obtained by a simple single axis analysis of progressive frames of 35-mm film and were in excess of any that had been measured using angular rate gyros on other, similar ejection seats. Since angular rate gyro data were not available for this particular mark of seat, a mathematical solution was developed. This, in conjunction with an ejection-seat model and a computer program for the derived instantaneous angular positions of the ejection seat, as seen in progressive film frames, gave results that compared reasonably well with rate gyro data obtained from other ejection-seat tests. Reprocessing of the original seat qualification data using the new method revealed peak yaw rates occurring during rocket burn, of between 950 and 1000 degrees/s. These values were consistently obtained across the speed range from 340 to 600 kt. It should be noted that although these yaw rates were high, they had historically been deemed acceptable.

The significance of such yaw rates lies in the indication of the degree of ejection-seat instability, occurring early in the ejection sequence, with consequential effects on subsequent drogue and parachute deployment vectors, particularly at low altitude.

Ejection-seat stabilization and parachute deployment

During the ejection sequence the seat is, generally, first stabilized by a 'drogue' parachute before deployment of the main parachute. Significant forces may be encountered in these phases of the ejection.

Drogue deployment

Loads occur during drogue deployment at so-called 'drogue snatch' and at drogue inflation. Drogue snatch occurs at line stretch and is caused by the mass of the drogue system being suddenly accelerated to the velocity of the seat. On many ejection seats, this is characterized by a sharp peak and a short-duration acceleration. A typical example is seen in Figure 14.2. The snatch load is the first triangular spike of 1362 kgf (3000 lbf) with a 30 millisecond time base. Figure 14.3 is an analysis of data from a number of ejection seat test shots at low altitude and shows that the acceleration vector with respect to the seat can act in almost any direction.

Drogue opening

Drogue snatch is followed by drogue opening, and considerable loads can be encountered. Figure 14.4 is an acceleration trace from a test ejection of a new type of parachute headbox – a 45 Gy peak can be seen on an approximately triangular pulse of 140 milliseconds duration. Also shown is a significant difference between the magnitude of the y axis (L/R) accelerations for the head and torso. Lack of fidelity in the response of the dummy neck makes the evaluation of such data problematical but head and neck accelerations of this magnitude are highly undesirable and exceed the requirements of the ASCC standard. Such accelerations at drogue opening are not unusually high however, when compared with other seat test data. Modern escape systems produce more consistent application of such loads because of earlier and more reliable deployment of the drogue.

Parachute opening forces

The parachute snatch force is produced at line stretch as the mass of the parachute is accelerated to the velocity of the seat occupant. The orientation of the force vector to the crewman is dependent upon how long the ejection seat has had to align under the drogue and is thus most random for ejections

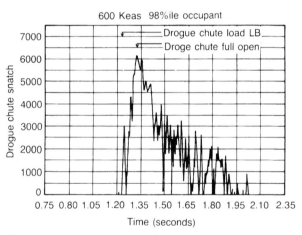

Figure 14.2 Drogue chute load.

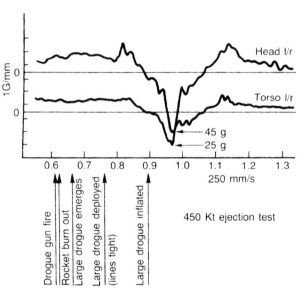

Figure 14.4 Acceleration trace from a 450 kt test ejection of a new type of parachute headbox.

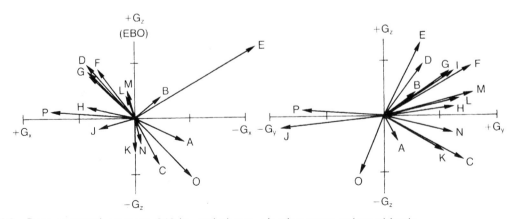

Figure 14.3 Drogue snatch vectors, 240 kt, and above, ejection tests at low altitude.

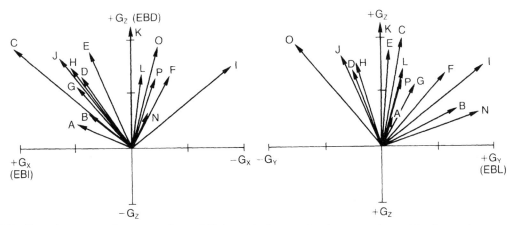

Figure 14.5 Parachute snatch vectors from 240 kt and above, ejection tests low-altitude mode.

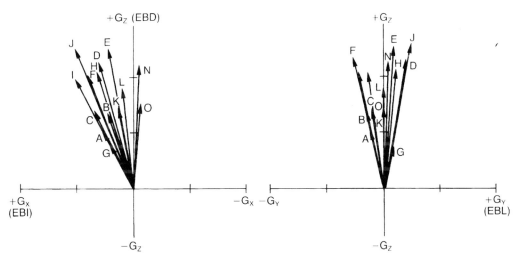

Figure 14.6 Parachute opening vectors from 240 kt and above, ejection tests low-altitude mode.

occurring at low altitude (below barostat height), or below the switchover point for the barometrically controlled G stop (Figures 14.5, 14.6). Where the scissor shackle release time is barometrically extended on high-altitude ejections, seat alignment has time to occur and the deployment vectors are therefore much closer to the ideal, and snatch and opening loads are reduced.

Helmet–parachute riser interactions
Placing the parachute in the headbox of the ejection seat has a number of important benefits. It also has one significant drawback in that, for parachute deployments in vectors forward and/or to the side of the seat occupant, the parachute risers have to sweep around the helmet as the parachute risers go 'lines tight'. One RAF fatal accident has occurred where there was some evidence to indicate that the helmet came into contact with the parachute risers with sufficient force to leave marks on both the helmet and the visor assembly. The individual

concerned died of a subarachnoid haemorrhage but without evidence of any focal injury. Subsequent laboratory experiments, conducted at forces well below those encountered on escape, demonstrated the capacity for the parachute risers deployed in the forward hemisphere of the seat to interact with protrusions on the helmet. This qualitative experiment showed not only the importance of helmets having smooth external profiles, but also the need to ensure that ejections are as stable as possible, so that acceptable parachute deployment vectors can be achieved.

Parachute landing
Spinal injury may be attributable to the effects of a parachute landing and some have suggested that up to 30–40% of total injury is attributable to this phase of the ejection sequence (Shannon, 1970). A review of RAF experience failed to show a statistically significant difference between the spinal injury rates over land compared with those over

water, suggesting that spinal injury occurred predominantly as a result of ejection-gun acceleration (Anton, 1986). This finding is supported by the incidence of spinal fracture of only 0.5 per 10 000 jumps in French military parachutists (Leger and Delahaye, 1982).

Other injuries, such as sprains of the knee and sprains and fractures of the ankle, are associated with parachute landing. Late ejection frequently also means that aircrew have insufficient time to lower their personal survival pack (PSP). Recent RAF experience suggests that this is associated with fractures of the tibia and fibula when the lower leg is bent under the PSP on landing.

Neck injury in high-performance aircraft

Neck injury of all types is a hazard of flight in fast jet and other aircraft. The risk arises from a variety of causes. The accelerations that are produced in air combat flight may mean that the helmeted head which weighed 6 kg in the 1-G environment, increases to up to 60 kg during combat manoeuvring and substantially more on ejection or during a crash. Developments in the mounting of equipment on helmets have meant that the overall mass has increased yet further. To compound the problem, some of the mass additions are substantial and eccentrically mounted. The neck is therefore exposed to considerable additional loads which may exceed its structural strength.

The 1984 Report of AGARD Working Group 11 concluded that: 'there was little reliable evidence to suggest that head and neck injury was a significant problem on "within envelope" ejections on modern ejection seats'. As a consequence, however, of the background work to the WG 11 report, instances were discovered of cervical fracture occurring in flight which usually involved a member of crew who was unaware of injury during application of high manoeuvring loads as part of air combat, or to avoid birds or terrain. These observations were made in a number of NATO Air Forces, which suggests that the problem is more common than had previously been realized.

With the deployment of aircraft capable of sustained high-G, complaints about acutely stiff and painful necks became more common. Anxiety was expressed by clinicians involved with the treatment of aircrew that repetitive vertebral trauma might lead to an increased incidence of cervical spondylosis, and that this in turn might lead to the affected crew being withdrawn prematurely from fast jet flying.

Soft tissue neck injury arising in-flight

Some information is available on the incidence of soft tissue neck injury in aircrew. Aghina (1985) has reported that F16 pilots had eight times more neck symptoms than F104 pilots, and that during an observation period of 6 months, 67% of the F16 pilots had experienced neck symptoms. In that these reports relate to a group flying with relatively lightweight helmets, it is clear that increasing helmet mass was likely to increase both the intensity and frequency of neck symptoms. The problem of neck injury in the F16 aircraft may be exacerbated by the pilot's sitting position which, because of the reclination of the ejection seat, requires a compensatory flexion of the cervical spine.

A study of 437 pilots flying three types of aircraft showed that increased aircraft performance was associated with increased neck injury prevalence, and that increased age was associated with increased prevalence of major neck injury (Vanderbeek, 1988).

Soft tissue injury to the neck occurring as a result of high-G flying may be an important cause of loss of aircrew effort applied to the flying task. Knudson *et al.* (1988) surveyed high +Gz induced neck pain and injury in aviators from the United States Navy Pacific Light Attack Wing. They found that 74% of F/A18 aviators surveyed, reported neck pain with high +G_z. Out of 37 pilots reporting neck injury, 11 required removal from flight status for, on average, 3 days. The inability to function effectively during high G flight, and the impact of lost pilot days, highlighted the need for further studies into the prevalence of, and solutions for, +G_z induced neck injury.

Schall (1989) reported on a series of F15 and F16 aircrew, two of whom sustained a herniated nucleus pulposus at the C5/6 level, and one of whom sustained a similar injury at C6/7. A further patient sustained an interspinous ligament injury between C6/7. Three of the four patients were flying a defensive basic fighter manoeuvre at the time of onset of their symptoms. A common feature was either having the head moved from the centreline at the time of the manoeuvre or being caught unawares by the other pilot manoeuvring.

Some authors recommend that aircrew should conduct neck strengthening exercises as a routine, and also engage in neck 'warm-up' exercises immediately before high-G flying. This advice has apparently been adopted in some air forces, although data validating the usefulness of neck-strengthening and neck 'warm-up' techniques are lacking.

Neck fracture occurring during flight

This subject is of considerable interest in that the fractures that have been reported have occurred at very much lower acceleration levels than are conventionally assumed necessary to provoke injury.

Two reliably documented instances have occurred in the RAF. In the first, a student flying a Hawk jet was looking down and to his left at his hand-held map when the aircraft encountered a downdraft. At this moment the instructor called for the student to execute a snatch pull, which was achieved, but he was unable to maintain his head in an erect position, and sustained compression fractures of C5 and 6 and bruising to the left of the midline of his upper thorax where his chin contacted his chest. There was a neurological injury attributable to either injury of the brachial plexus or nerve root. In the second, a student suffered an undisplaced crack fracture of the pedicle of C6 as a result of an undocumented flight manoeuvre. Schall also reported three fractures of the cervical spinal (Schall, 1989). Two were compression fractures (one C7 and one C5) occurring during basic fighter manoeuvring; the third was fracture of the spinous process of C7 which occurred when an F16 instructor was caught unawares by the student's manoeuvre.

The Royal Norwegian Air Force has reported a cervical fracture in a pilot sustained during air combat manoeuvring. A flight surgeon flying in the back seat of a F16B in a mixed exercise which included an interception, handed over control of the aircraft to the pilot in the front seat. He then relaxed in his seat and turned his head maximally over his left shoulder to look for the opponent; as he did this the pilot in the front seat abruptly instituted an 8G climbing turn. The flight surgeon was caught completely unawares, momentarily losing consciousness. His next recollection was being jacknifed in the cockpit under sustained high G. The flight was continued but in the ensuing hours after landing, nausea and neck pain developed. Equivocal radiographic evidence of a C6 compression fracture was obtained, together with evidence of C5/6 ligamentous injury – widening of the disc space and minor posterior slippage of C6 on C5.

It is surprising that, if injuries such as this can occur as a result of in-flight loads, they do not occur more commonly as a result of emergency escape. The peak G and the onset rate for the instances described do not significantly exceed 8G, or an onset rate of 6–10 Gs, values that are well below those associated with use of the escape system, although the durations are far greater.

Schmorl and Junghanns (1971) considered the question of lumbar vertebral fracture following minor trauma. He noted that, at times, quite minor trauma may cause collapse of a healthy vertebra. Uncoordinated contraction of various groups of back muscles with resulting paradoxic fixation and rotation of the spine appears to be the mechanism responsible. Given this underlying mechanism, the neck injuries may be caused by a combination of acute loading under high G, and reflex muscle contraction, coupled with an off-axis position of the neck. Schmorl also noted that pain, and other neurological symptoms, appeared some time after the injury, perhaps because of the detachment of an impacted fragment or the gradual development of a haematoma.

Chronic injury

The relationship between trauma and what has been termed spondylosis deformans (osteophytosis) has also been described (Schmorl and Junghaans, 1971). In summary, there does appear to be a relationship between either single or repeated injury and the development of chronic change in the lumbar spine of both animals and man, but it is not clear to what extent the findings can be applied to the neck.

Degenerative changes of the intervertebral discs of the cervical spine are common after the age of 40 and affect 70% of patients over 70, so at the moment it is impossible to answer the question whether cervical spondylosis is caused or exacerbated by exposure to manoeuvring loads of high-performance aircraft. However, in a review of 31 pilots and 15 age-and sex-matched controls for evidence of osteophytic spurring, disk space narrowing and changes in neck range of motion, significant differences in the incidence of osteophytic spurring at C5 and C6 were found between the pilots and the control group and similar trends were apparent for disc space narrowing (Gillen and Raymond, 1989).

If it can be demonstrated that flying high-performance aircraft produces an increased incidence of radiologically diagnosed cervical spondylosis, the question of the clinical significance of the finding still has to be addressed. X-ray changes frequently occur without clinical symptoms and, except in the case of large posterior osteophytes which could theoretically fracture under load and compromise the integrity of the spinal cord, the X-ray findings should not of themselves be a reason for rejection of crew from high-performance aircraft flying.

The evidence suggests that the incidence of radiologically diagnosed cervical spondylosis (spondylosis deformans) is higher in RAF pilots than in the civil population (MacKenzie Crooks, 1970). This author also observed that the incidence of radiological changes of cervical spondylosis (70%) was much higher in aircrew who had ejected, than in a reported series in civilians and in a control series of pilots who had not ejected. This finding of an increased incidence of change in the group who had ejected suggests that trauma to the cervical spine on ejection can result in long-term sequelae.

Prediction of neck tolerance to injury

It is clearly important to be able to predict neck tolerance to injury, although there are considerable practical difficulties in doing this. Tolerance criteria for neck injury are not well established – a situation which contrasts with head injury. There are four reasons for this state of affairs (Goldsmith and Ommaya, 1984):

1. There are fewer investigations of neck injury, because the cervical region is less frequently injured than the head.
2. Neck injuries do not exhibit a well-defined spectrum of injuries as is seen in head injury; neck injuries are either minor or catastrophic.
3. Neck response is crucially dependent upon the orientation of the head and neck and also upon the direction of load.
4. No effective scaling relationship from animal data has been developed for the neck.

It should also be noted that data available from analysis of automobile accidents indicates that catastrophic neck injury rarely occurs in the absence of head injury, which suggests that it is the added loading of the neck by the torso which is crucial, rather than the simple response of the neck to inertial loading by the head.

Volunteer and cadaver experiments have yielded some information on the tolerance of the neck to injury. There is a large database on the response of the human neck, to predominantly $-G_x$ impacts, within the range of accelerations that are tolerable to volunteers. Unfortunately, extrapolation of these data to higher levels of acceleration is limited by the non-linear response of the neck and the difficulty in predicting its position at the start of the impact. Mertz and Patrick (1971) undertook a series of experiments in which human volunteers were subjected to static and dynamic environments which produced non-injurious neck responses for neck extension and flexion; cadavers were then used to extend the data into the injury region. Analysis of the data from both sources indicated that the magnitude of the moment about the occipital condyles was the critical injury variable for both extension and flexion.

Some work has been undertaken to assess the safety aspects of the addition of helmets and other masses to the head. Muzzy et al. (1986) describe a series of $-G_x$ acceleration exposure experiments using United States Navy volunteers, in which the dynamic response of the head was measured as a function of mass distribution variations. The kinematic response was measured for each subject: without addition of mass; with a helmet and weight carrying frame; and with a helmet with weights positioned on the frame mid-sagitally. There was approximately a 30% addition to the head mass with these weights. Computer modelling of the head-neck response was used to predict the severity of exposure with the addition of mass. The results are said to have validated the models used for predicting mass effects and showed that

maximum angular travel was the first safety variable to approach the established threshold of limits.

An important finding of the investigation was the fact that because of variability of response between subjects, it was not possible to define discrete figures for safety. The authors suggest that a series of safety parameters have to be adhered to, as some of their subjects reached angular displacement and torque limits whereas others did not.

Computer modelling

Because of the limitations of volunteer experiments, increasing attention has been directed towards the use of computer models such as the head-spine model used at the United States Air Force Armstrong Aerospace Medical Research Laboratory (USAF AAMRL). The version currently in use represents the neck by two parallel three-dimensional beam elements: one has non-linear viscoelastic axial load deformation characteristics which represents the cervical spine; the other non-linear bending behaviour and is used to account for the stiffening effects of the soft tissues of the neck.

Validation of the head-spine model has been undertaken using both data from spinal injuries from operational duties and the comparison of information from model prediction experiment. Much of this validation has, however, been centred around the response of the thoracolumbar spine, which is constrained anatomically to a much more limited range of motion than is the neck.

A different approach to modelling the behaviour of the cervical spine has been adopted by Snijders and Roosch (1990). In an attempt to analyse the load on neck structures which arises from exposure to high-G manoeuvring flight, a biomechanical model was developed that permits the calculation of forces in a number of neck muscles and in the joints of the cervical spine. This has been applied to the calculation of loads to the cervical spine in air-combat manoeuvring F16 aircraft and has yielded useful insights into the stresses of the neck.

Mechanical dummies

An alternative to modelling is to use dummies well instrumented for effects on the neck. One such example is the Hybrid III anthropomorphic dummy fitted with transducers in the upper and lower neck. These transducers measure forces along the three orthogonal axes and the moments about these axes, and enable forces to be measured under a variety of impact conditions and with a variety of head-mounted equipment. There are difficulties in the interpretation of such data because of the limited biofidelity of the Hybrid III neck.

Seemann *et al.* (1986) compared the standard Hybrid III neck response with that of human volunteers to $-15\,G_x$ impacts, and also to impacts with vector components $+_y$, $+_z$, and $-_{x'}$, $+_{y'}$, using the database of the United States Navy Biodynamics Laboratory. They concluded that the Hybrid III neck was much too stiff to respond in a human-like manner to $-_x$ and $+_{z'}$, but had a remarkable and unexpected similarity to human neck motion for $+_y$ and $-_{x'}$, $+_y$ impacts. Modifications to the linkage between the Hybrid III head and neck were mathematically modelled. This indicated that a physical relocation of the neck/torso joint would result in much improved dummy $-G_x$ neck response.

Before that, the same group had compared human versus manikin head and neck response to $+G_z$ acceleration, by exposure of subjects to peak accelerations ranging from 3 G to 12 G at onset rates from 100 to 1200 Gs. The human head response appeared to be very sensitive to initial orientation and position. Two types of response were observed in man: one was primarily flexion of the head and neck; in the other the head exhibited significant extension followed by flexion. The dummy head response was only in flexion. It was concluded that further work was required to analyse the effect of the initial position on head-neck response.

Considerable work remains to be done to understand neck response to acceleration and to predict neck tolerance to injurious forces. The requirement for, and the application of, this knowledge is not confined to the aviation world. The apparent rise in soft tissue neck injuries in car accidents following the introduction of shoulder restraint provides but one example of this.

Copyright (c) Controller HMSO London 1992.

REFERENCES

AGARD WG 11 Report of the Working Group on The Clinical and Biomedical (1984). *Evaluation of Trauma and Fatalities Associated with Aircrew Ejection and Crash*. AGARD Advisory Report No. 194. Paris: AGARD.

Aghina, J.C.F.M., reported in van Dalen A., van den Biggelaar H.H.M. (1985). Systematic radiographic examination of the spine for selection of F16 pilots: a preliminary report. In *Medical Selection and Physiological Training of Future Fighter Aircrew*. AGARD Conference Proceedings No. 396. Paris: AGARD pp. 41-1, 41-4.

Aircraft Crash Survival Design Guide (1980). USARTL-TR-79-22 US Army AVRADCOM. Virginia: Fort Eustis.

Anton D.J. (1986). *The Incidence of Spinal Fracture on Royal Air Force Ejections 1968-1984*. Aircrew Equipment Group Report No. 529. *Royal Air Force Institute of Aviation Medicine*.

Brinkley J.W. (1985). Acceleration exposure limits for escape system advanced development. *J. SAFE Assoc.*, **15**, (2), 10-16.

Chandler R.F. (1990). *Occupant Crash Protection in Military Air Transport*. AGARDograph No. 306. Paris: AGARD.

De Haven H. (1945). '*Relationship of Injuries to Structure in Survivable Aircraft Accidents*', Report No. 440. Washington, DC: National Research Council.

Eiband A.M. (1959). Human Tolerance to Rapidly Applied Accelerations: A Summary of the Literature, NASA, Memo 5-19-59E. Cleveland, Ohio: NASA, Lewis Research Centre, June.

FAA Report DOT/FAA/CT-82-118 (1983). *Crash Injury Protection in Survivable Air Transport Accidents – US Civil Aircraft Experience from 1970-1978*, March.

Gillen M.H., Raymond D. (1990). Progressive cervical osteoarthrosis in high performance aircraft pilots. In *AGARD Conference Proceedings No. 471*. Paris: AGARD.

Goetz A. (1954). 'Limits and Special Problems in the use of Ejector Seats' D. Ing Dissertation, University of Rostock.

Goldsmith W., Ommaya A.K. (1984). Head and neck injury criteria and tolerance levels. In *The Biomechanics of Impact Trauma* (Aldman B., Shapon A., eds). Amsterdam: Elsevier Science.

Knudson R., McMillan D., Doucette D., Seidel M. (1988). A comparative study of G-induced neck injury in pilots of the F/A-18, A-7, and A-4. *Aviat. Space Environ. Med.*, **59**, (8), 758-60.

Leger A., Delahaye R.P. (1982). Parachuting. In *Physiopathology and Pathology of Spinal Injuries in Aerospace Medicine*. AGARDograph No. 250 (Eng.). Paris: AGARD.

MacKenzie Crooks L. (1970). Long term effects of ejecting from aircraft. *Aerospace Med.* July. **41**., 803-4.

Mason J.K. (1962). *Aviation Accident Pathology*. London: Butterworths.

Mertz H.J., Patrick L.M. (1971). Strength and response of the human neck. *SAE Trans.* **80**, Technical Paper 710855.

Miller B.A. (1982). *Unassisted Through Canopy Ejection Experience*. Higher Denham, Middlesex: Martin Baker Aircraft Company.

Muzzy W.H., Bittner A.C., Willems C. (1986). Safety evaluation of helmet and other Mass to the head. In *Thirtieth Annual Workshop of Human Factors Society*, Dayton, OH, 3 October.

Pinkel I.I. (1959). *A proposed Criterion for the Selection of Forward and Rearward Facing Seats*. Paper Number 59-AV-28. New York: The American Society of Mechanical Engineers, January.

Report on the Accident to Boeing 727-400, G-OBME near Kegworth, Leicestershire on 8 January 1989 (1989). Department of Transport Aircraft Accident Report 4/90. London: HMSO.

Ring W.S., Brinkley J.W., Noyes F.R. (1975). USAF Noncombat ejection experience 1968-1973, distribution, significance and mechanism of flail injury. Biodynamic Response to Windblast. In *AGARD Conference Proceedings*, No. 170. Paris: AGARD.

Schall D.G. (1989). Non ejection cervical spine injuries due to +Gz in high performance aircraft due to +Gz. *Aviat. Space Environ. Med.*, **60**, (5), 445-56.

Schmorl G., Junghanns H. (1971). *The Human Spine in Health and Disease*, 2nd edn. (trans. Besemann E.F.). New York: Grune & Stratton.

Seemann M.S., Muzzy W.H., Lustick L.S. (1986). Comparison of human and hybrid III head and neck dynamic response. In *Proceedings of Thirtieth Stapp Car Crash Conference*, San Diego, CA. SAE Publication, P189. 22–27 October.

Shannon R.H. (1970). Analysis of injuries incurred during emergency ejection. Extraction combat and non-combat. *Aerospace Med.*, **41**, 799–803.

Snijders C.J., Roosch E.R. (1990). Analysis of the biomechanic and ergonomic aspects of the cervical spine under load. In *AGARD Conference Proceedings* No. 471. Paris: AGARD.

Vanderbeek R.D. (1988). Period prevalence of acute neck injury in US Air Force pilots exposed to high G forces. *Aviat. Space Environ. Med.*, **59**, No(12).

SECTION 3
BLAST OVERPRESSURE INJURY

15. Physics of Detonations and Blast-waves

M. J. Iremonger

NOTATION

b	Coefficient in Friedlander equation
C_D	Drag coefficient
c_E	Sound speed in shocked explosive
c_o	Ambient speed of sound in air
D	Detonation wave velocity
E	Shock-wave energy density
γ	Heat capacity ratio
I^+	Specific positive-phase impulse
I^-	Specific negative-phase impulse
P_E	Detonation pressure
P_d	Peak dynamic pressure
P_m	Peak overpressure for shock-wave in water
$P_m(t)$	Overpressure in water as a function of time
P_o	Ambient atmospheric pressure
P_r	Reflected peak static overpressure
P_s	Peak static overpressure
$P_s(t)$	Static overpressure as a function of time
R	Range from centre of explosion
ρ	Air density behind shock front
ρ_E	Density of compressed explosion products
ρ_o	Ambient air density ahead of blast-wave
t	Time
t_a	Time of arrival of air blast-wave
t^+	Positive-phase duration
t^-	Negative-phase duration
T_o	Ambient air temperature
T_s	Air temperature immediately behind shock front
θ	Time decay constant for shock-wave in water
u	Particle velocity (wind speed) of air
u_E	Particle velocity of gaseous explosion products
V	Shock front velocity of blast-wave in air
V_r	Shock front velocity of reflected blast-wave
W	Weight (energy) of explosion
Z	Scaled distance

INTRODUCTION

Explosions

Detonations and blast-waves are associated with explosions. In essence, an explosion is a process involving a rapid release of energy. High-pressure shock-waves are generated which propagate into and through the surrounding medium.

Explosions may arise naturally, for example from lightning or volcanoes or be artificial – accidental or intentional. Examples of accidental events include the failure of pressurized gas containers, and explosions in dust or vapour clouds. Explosions may be physical, chemical or nuclear in origin. The latter two categories provide the most common examples of intentional explosions, namely high explosives and nuclear weapons.

Explosives

The energy of explosives is liberated by either burning or detonation and most release energy by either process.

Burning or deflagration produces a 'low' explosive. Examples include gunpowder and modern propellants. The explosive reaction occurs at the surface as material is heated above its decomposition temperature: heat and gas are released as the surface recedes. The reaction propagates at a velocity less than the speed of sound in the explosive material.

Detonating or 'high' explosives such as trinitrotoluene (TNT) are activated either by burning or by mechanical forces which initiate a shock (detonation) wave. This wave, with high temperature and pressure gradients at the shock front, causes chemical reactions to propagate supersonically through the explosive.

If an explosive is in contact with a solid material an intense shattering effect, proportional to the detonation pressure, occurs, known as *brisance*. In contact with air, the violent expansion of the gaseous products of a chemical or nuclear explosion produces a shock-wave (*blast-wave*) in the surrounding air. The peak pressure and velocity of the blast-wave decays as it propagates but its effects can be felt at considerable distances. Detonation of an explosive in water produces both a shock-wave and an underwater bubble, the latter being caused by the expanding gaseous products of the explosion.

DETONATION OF HIGH EXPLOSIVES

Initiation

For reasons of both safety and reliability, it is usual for an explosive device to contain both a primary charge (the initiator) and a secondary (main) charge. Safety is achieved because it is possible to break the chain between the main charge which is insensitive to detonation, and the initiator. The system is reliable because the primary charge is sensitive, that is, it is easy to detonate. A booster charge may be used between the initiator and the main charge to make an explosive 'train' with increased safety and reliability.

As the temperature of an explosive is raised, it decomposes. The decomposition rate increases rapidly as the ignition point of the explosive is reached. Most common explosives ignite at temperatures between 150 and 350°C. If the heat liberated by decomposition is not dissipated by conduction or radiation, the charge can decompose spontaneously. Confinement leads to higher pressures that may greatly increase the rate of burning. Detonation is achieved if the flame front accelerates to sonic velocity and a shock-wave is formed.

Whereas the primary charge is usually initiated by burning to detonation, the main or receptor charge is most commonly set in train by the shock-wave generated in the primary or donor charge, which is transmitted across the boundary between the two. The main charge is compressed and heated, thereby liberating chemical energy and accelerating the wave. Energy continues to be released and the wave accelerates until it reaches the velocity of sound in the compressed explosive. Detonation of the main charge is then achieved. If the shock-wave from the donor is too weak, the wave decelerates and decays in the receptor leaving the bulk of it chemically unchanged.

Propagation

Once formed, the detonation wave front propagates into the explosive that has yet to react. The increases in temperature and pressure behind the shock front promote an explosive chemical reaction, the energy of which maintains the propagation of the shock. A full analysis of this detonation process is complex. Equations can be established from a consideration of the conservation of mass, momentum and energy and the equations of state of the explosive medium. A one-dimensional theory by Chapman (1899) and Jouguet (1905) is often quoted. This assumes a steady plane wave in a non-viscous medium. Baker et al. (1983), Johansson and Persson (1970), Taylor (1952) and other authors of accounts of detonation theory give details of these theories.

Conservation of momentum across the shock front relates the pressure change to the density of the explosive ρ_E, the detonation wave velocity D and the particle velocity of the gaseous products u_E. This pressure change approximates to the detonation pressure p_E. Thus

$$p_E = \rho_E D u_E \qquad (3.1)$$

As u_E is proportional to D and, for a given explosive, D, rises with increasing density, it follows that both the detonation pressure and its rate of propagation are very dependent on the initial density of the explosive. This in turn is affected by the method of consolidation used in its manufacture (e.g. casting or sintering) as well as by the intrinsic density of the material. The velocity of detonation D is also modified by the degree of confinement and, if not confined, the initial detonation cannot be maintained in a small-diameter charge because of lateral dissipation. For detonation of the explosive device, it is necessary for the initiating charge to transmit an adequate shock-wave to the main charge. It is possible for a nitroglycerine-based explosive to achieve a detonation velocity as low as 2000 m/s instead of more than 6000 m/s if too weak a detonator is used.

The Chapman–Jouguet analysis contains the following relationship between detonation wave velocity D, particle velocity of the gaseous products

TABLE 15.1
COMPARATIVE DATA FOR SOME HIGH EXPLOSIVES

Explosive	Density (kg/m³)	Mass specific energy (kJ/kg)	TNT equivalent	Detonation velocity (m/s)	Detonation pressure (N/m²)
C-4 (91% RDX, 9% plasticizer)	1580	4870	1.08	–	–
Comp B (60% RDX, 40% TNT)	1690	5190	1.15	7990	29.5
HMX	1900	5680	1.26	9110	38.7
Nitroglycerin	1590	6700	1.48	–	–
PETN	1770	5800	1.28	8260	34.0
Pentolite 50/50 (50% PETN, 50% TNT)	1660	5110	1.13	7470	28.0
RDX	1650	5360	1.19	8700	28.0
Tetryl	1730	4520	1.00	7850	26.0
Torpex (40% RDX, 40% TNT, 18% A1)	1760	7540	1.67	–	–
TNT	1600	4520	1.00	6730	21.0

u_E and the speed of sound in the shocked material c_E.

$$D = u_E + c_E \qquad (3.2)$$

where c_E is about a third higher than the speed of sound of the uncompressed explosive. For TNT, c_E is approximately $5400\,m/s$ and u_E is about $1500\,m/s$. This gives a detonation velocity of $6900\,m/s$. Typical figures for a range of high explosives are given in Table 15.1.

Explosive effectiveness

The effectiveness of an explosive depends on both the amount of energy available within the explosive and the rate of its release. Various parameters are used as a measure of effectiveness.

Much of the energy stored in an explosive is released as heat. When measured under adiabatic conditions, the constant volume *heat of explosion* is a measure of the work capacity of the explosive. *Explosive power* is defined as the product of the heat of explosion and the volume of gas generated per unit mass of explosive. For primary explosives such as lead azide, a high *detonation pressure*, which is a measure of the initiating ability of an explosive, is more important than explosive power. Detonation pressure is also the main factor in determining brisance.

In air, the expansion of the gaseous products of an explosion generate the blast-wave in the surrounding air. In determining blast over pressures, detonation pressure and velocity are unimportant compared to the explosive power. The most common means, however, of comparing the blast effects of different explosives (see 'Scaling' below) is to relate them to an equivalent weight of TNT. The equivalence is based on relative heats of explosion in the form of *mass specific energy* measured in kJ/g or kJ/kg. Table 15.1 gives typical values for a range of explosives.

The explosion process is described in detail by Bailey and Murray (1989).

BLAST-WAVES IN AIR

Formation

The violent expansion of gases in a chemical explosion with the associated detonation shock front, pushes back the surrounding air. A pressure pulse is formed. Because air is compressible the temperature increases and the propagation speed increases. In consequence the initial pressure pulse rises more steeply and a supersonic shock front is formed. Figure 15.1 shows a simple example of this steepening process. The pressure in the surrounding air increases from ambient to a peak almost instantaneously as the shock front passes. The term *overpressure* is used to describe the rise in pressure above ambient. This steep-fronted pressure pulse – the blast-wave – develops a similar shape whatever is the configuration of the initial pressure pulse and is produced by physical, chemical and nuclear explosions. At a sufficient distance from the centre of the explosion the magnitude of the blast-wave depends only on the energy released.

Blast-waves in free air

As the blast-wave propagates away from the centre of the explosion (Figure 15.2) its energy is spread through an increasing volume and the magnitude of the peak overpressure is rapidly attenuated. For a spherical explosive the shock front in free air lies on a spherical surface. Near to the source the peak overpressure decreases with the cube of the distance from the centre of the explosion. At greater distances it attenuates more slowly and far from the centre, the shock front becomes nearly planar and the peak pressure reduces almost linearly with range. The shock front velocity also declines until at very low overpressures it is moving at the speed of sound. Behind the shock front the pressure decays rapidly for high peak overpressures, more slowly for lower values. Inertial effects cause overexpansion and a consequent rarefaction with pressures below that of the atmosphere (*underpressure*). The

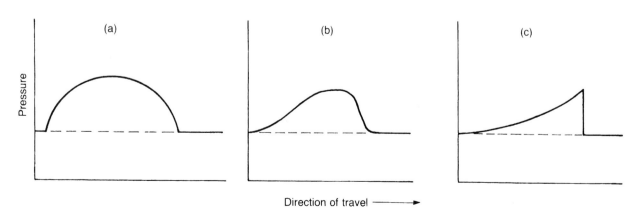

Figure 15.1 Steepening of pressure pulse to form a shock-wave. Illustrative pressure vs. distance relationships at successive times (a), (b) and (c).

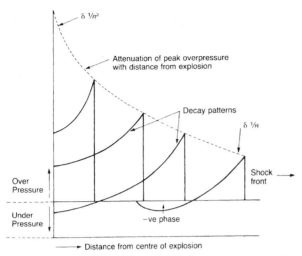

Figure 15.2 Blast-wave profiles at increasing distances from centre of explosion showing attenuation with range.

cycle of compression and rarefaction is repeated with decreasing amplitudes but the oscillations are quickly damped in air and only a single cycle is usually considered.

In addition to causing the pressure changes described above, passage of the shock front also sets the air in motion. This causes a blast wind and its associated *dynamic pressure*. The maximum wind velocity is at the shock front blowing away from the explosion source and during the underpressure phase a reverse wind blows back toward the source.

Blast-wave parameters

It is useful to consider the passage of the blast-wave through a particular position in space at some distance from the explosion centre. A typical curve showing the variation in pressure with time is in

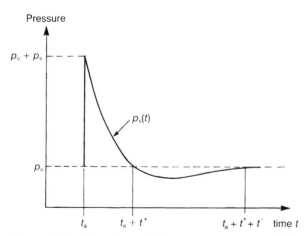

Figure 15.3 Variation of blast-wave pressure with time at a fixed location.

Figure 15.3 which indicates some of the parameters which characterize the blast-wave.

The shock front reaches the position at a *time of arrival* t_a before which pressure is at the ambient atmospheric value p_o. At time t_a the pressure rises almost instantaneously to a peak value $p_o + p_s$, where p_s is called the *peak static overpressure* or *peak overpressure*. The pressure immediately falls from its peak value and decays as a function of time, $p_s(t)$, to p_o. This region of the blast-wave in which the pressures are above the ambient values is the *positive phase*. Its duration, the *positive phase duration* t^+, is an important parameter of the blast-wave because it governs the area of the positive-phase time-history – the *positive-phase impulse*. Structural damage and injuries to personnel can often be related to the impulse magnitude. The duration of the positive phase increases with the energy yield and the distance from the explosion. Measured as an impulse per unit area, the *specific positive-phase impulse* I^+, is:

$$I^+ = \int_{t_a}^{t_a+t^+} P_s(t)\mathrm{d}t \qquad (3.3)$$

Similar parameters are associated with the negative phase which follows the positive one. Here, pressures are below ambient with the primary parameters being *negative-phase duration* t^- and *specific negative-phase impulse* I^-, where:

$$I^- = \int_{t_a+t^+}^{t_a+t^++t^-} P_s(t)\mathrm{d}t \qquad (3.4)$$

Similar parameters are associated with the dynamic pressure p_d. Its positive-phase duration is longer than that for the static overpressure because the motion of the air behind the shock front keeps the wind blowing in the same direction after the overpressure decays to zero and becomes negative. The dynamic pressure is related to air density ρ and the air particle velocity (wind speed) u by the expression

$$P_d = \frac{1}{2}\rho u^2 \qquad (3.5)$$

which represents the kinetic energy per unit volume of air immediately behind the shock front.

Mathematical relationships

Consider a spherically symmetrical explosion in a still homogeneous atmosphere producing an instantaneous pressure rise at the shock front. The mathematical analysis of such an ideal blast-wave is extremely complex. Non-ideal waves, with, for example, significant pressure rise-times or variations caused by ground effects, are not amenable to analysis. The Rankine–Hugoniot equations for the shock front of an ideal blast-wave provide some useful relations which agree well with experimental observations. These equations are based on a consideration of the conservation of mass, momentum and energy at the shock front.

The shock front velocity V can be expressed as:

$$V = c_o \left(1 + \frac{\gamma + 1}{2\gamma} \cdot \frac{p_s}{p_o}\right)^{1/2} \qquad (3.6)$$

where c_o is the ambient speed of sound ahead of the blast-wave, p_s is the peak static overpressure, p_o is the ambient pressure ahead of the blast-wave and γ is the ratio of the constant pressure and constant volume heat capacities (specific heats) of the medium. With γ taken as its usual value for air of 1.4, the shock front velocity becomes:

$$V = c_o \left(\frac{7p_o + 6p_s}{7p_o}\right)^{1/2} \qquad (3.7)$$

The density of the air behind the shock front ρ is related to the air density ahead of the shock front ρ_o by

$$\rho = \rho_o \left(\frac{2\gamma p_o + (\gamma + 1)p_s}{\gamma P_o + (\gamma - 1)p_s}\right) \qquad (3.8)$$

hence, with $\gamma = 1.4$ for air

$$\rho = \rho_o \left(\frac{7p_o + 6p_s}{7p_o + p_s}\right) \qquad (3.9)$$

The peak wind (particle) velocity behind the shock front is given by

$$u = \frac{c_o p_s}{\gamma p_o} \left(1 + \frac{\gamma + 1}{2\gamma} \cdot \frac{p_s}{p_o}\right)^{-1/2} \qquad (3.10)$$

With $\gamma = 1.4$ for air, this becomes

$$u = \frac{5p_s}{7p_o} \cdot \frac{c_o}{(1 + 6p_s/7p_o)^{1/2}} \qquad (3.11)$$

The dynamic pressure p_d is defined in terms of u by Equation (3.5). By substituting the Rankine–Hugoniot equations for ρ and u given above, a relationship can be found between the peak dynamic pressure in air, the peak static overpressure and the ambient pressure. Thus:

$$p_d = \frac{5p_s^2}{2(7p_o + p_s)} \qquad (3.12)$$

Taking p_o as 101 kPa or kNm^{-2} (14.7 psi), the normal ambient pressure at sea level, dynamic pressure can be calculated for a range of peak static overpressures:

p_s kPa	(psi)	p_d kPa	(psi)
50	(7.3)	8.3	(1.2)
100	(14.6)	31	(4.5)
150	(21.8)	66	(9.5)
200	(29.1)	110	(16.0)
250	(36.4)	163	(23.8)
300	(43.7)	223	(32.5)
350	(50.9)	290	(42.2)

Behind the shock front, the static and dynamic pressures decay with time. Various models for the pressure-time histories have been proposed. Only the positive phase is usually considered. The simplest model of a blast-wave profile assumes a linear decay with time (Figure 15.4). With the appropriate initial peak pressure and a 'positive-phase duration' modified to give the correct impulse for the real waveform (i.e. the same area under the pressure–time curve), such an approximation is often used for designing structures to resist blast. More complex models based on an exponential decay with typically three or four parameters allow a number of the blast-wave characteristics to be matched. The modified Friedlander equation, for example, allows the matching of any three of the following four characteristics: peak overpressure, positive-phase duration,

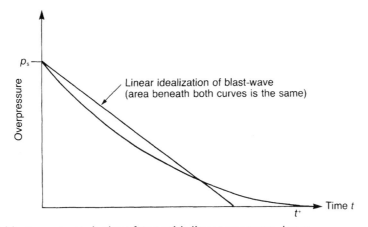

Figure 15.4 Idealized blast-wave: equivalent form with linear pressure decay.

specific impulse and the initial decay rate of the blast-wave. It predicts static pressures as:

$$p_s(t) = p_s(1 - t/t^+)e^{-bt/t^+} \qquad (3.13)$$

where t is time measured from the time of arrival t_a to the end of the positive phase at time $t_a + t^+$ and $p_s(t)$ is the static overpressure at time t. The coefficient b increases with p_s, the peak overpressure. It equals 1 for overpressures less than 70 kPa (10 psi).

The reader is referred to the works of Baker (1973) and Kinney and Graham (1985) for a fuller treatment of the mathematical analysis of blast-waves. Brode (1955) gave the first full solution to the equations representing an ideal blast-wave.

Reflections

It is assumed above that the blast-wave propagates through free air without obstruction; in reality, reflection of blast-waves from surfaces occur. An explosion may detonate on the ground with immediate reflection or a large above-ground explosion may have effects at ranges where ground-reflected waves merge with the incident waves. It should also be borne in mind that the main interest in blast-waves is their interaction with a structure or person – the target of an intentional explosion.

Normal reflection

The simplest case is the normal reflection of a plane blast-wave from a plane rigid surface. This case of normal or 'side-on' reflection in which the angle of incidence is zero is illustrated in Figure 15.5. The incident wave is shown just before its impact with the wall. Its shock front (parameters: overpressure p, density ρ, temperature T and particle velocity u with a subscript s) is moving into a medium at ambient conditions (subscript o), which is still. The particles are stopped at the surface and a new or reflected wave is generated which propagates back through the medium. Reflection increases the pressure, density and temperature above their incident values because the reflected wave (subscript r) is

moving into a medium which is not at ambient conditions. The shock-front velocity changes from V for the incident wave to V_r for the reflected wave.

For normal incidence the reflected peak overpressure p_r is given by

$$p_T = 2p_s + (\gamma + 1)p_d \qquad (3.14)$$

Substituting for p_d from Equation 3.12 with $\gamma = 1.4$ for air gives

$$p_r = 2p_s \cdot \frac{7p_o + 4p_s}{7p_o + p_s} \qquad (3.15)$$

Note that for very weak shocks, where $p_s << p_o$, p_r approaches $2p_s$. For strong shocks, in which $p_s >> p_o$, p_r approaches $8p_s$, a theoretical upper limit for air. In practice, however, air does not act as ideal gas under strong shock conditions and reflection coefficients (the ratio p_r/p_s) of more than 20 can occur.

The reflected overpressure gives the instantaneous loading on any object side-on to the path of the blast-wave.

Regular oblique reflection

The reflected overpressure is also enhanced when the blast-wave meets a surface at an angle. Unlike sound-waves, the angle of reflection does not equal the angle of incidence (Figure 15.6). Up to angles of incidence of about 39 degrees for air the angle of reflection is smaller than the angle of incidence. The reflected overpressures are similar to the values generated by normal reflection, with some reduction in reflection coefficients with angle for strong shocks. There is a critical angle of incidence above which regular reflection cannot occur. For strong shocks in air this angle is between 39 and 40 degrees. Higher critical angles are possible for weak shocks. Kinney and Graham (1985) give a more detailed account of this subject.

In this region of regular oblique reflection, the conditions at the reflecting surface itself change directly from ambient to reflected. However an object away from the surface, which is initially at

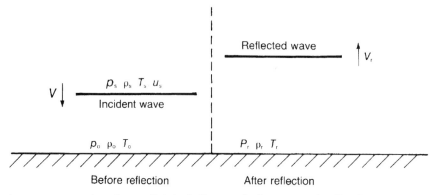

Figure 15.5 Blast-wave parameters immediately before and after normal reflection.

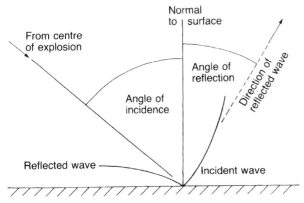

Figure 15.6 Oblique reflection terminology.

15.7). The triple point (which is in reality a circular line) follows a concave path of increasing height.

The Mach Stem region is of particular importance for nuclear and fuel-air explosives when detonated at optimum height above the ground, in order to maximize the destructive area of the explosive. Since the Mach Stem is nearly vertical, the blast overpressures and winds act horizontally with magnitudes greater than the radiating incident waves.

Surface bursts

When detonated against a surface such as the ground there is an immediate reflection. For a perfect reflector, the blast parameters correspond to those from a free-air spherical burst of twice the source energy. In practice some energy is absorbed in producing a crater and ground-shock. This reduces the resulting enhancement coefficient to about 1.8.

Surface bursts produce horizontal blast forces at ground level, as in the Mach Stem region discussed above.

Internal (confined) explosions

When an explosion is detonated within a confined space such as a building there are multiple reflections from the walls and enhanced pressures result. Similar internal reflections occur when the blast-wave from an external explosion enters a room through vents such as doors or windows. The magnitudes of the reflected pressures are highly dependent on position in relation to the walls, corners and vents.

For an internal explosion, the short-duration shock oscillations dissipate to leave an overpressure created by the heated gas in the structure. The

ambient pressure, is subject to successive loading from first the incident wave and then the reflected wave.

Mach reflection

Regular reflection does not occur for angles of incidence above the critical value mentioned above. Instead, for strong shocks, the incident and reflected waves coalesce to form a third shock-wave – the Mach Stem. The geometry and terminology of Mach reflection is shown in Figure 15.7.

The reflected wave travels through air which has been heated and compressed by the passage of the incident wave. As a result, it moves faster than the incident wave and, beyond the region of regular oblique reflection, catches the incident wave to form the Mach Stem. As the range increases, the reflected and incident waves merge at increasing heights. The junction of the incident, reflected and Mach Stem waves is called the 'triple point' (Figure

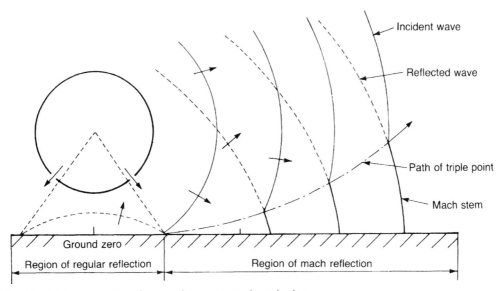

Figure 15.7 Mach Stem creation for an above-ground explosion.

decay of this gas-pressure phase depends on the openings in the structure. It is usually assumed to be quasi-static in relation to its loading on the structure. Internal explosions in vented buildings cause outside air blast of diminished magnitudes compared to free air blast. The quantification of these effects is discussed by Baker *et al.* (1983).

Scaling

The scaling of blast-wave parameters is based on principles of geometric similarity. The 'cube root' scaling law formulated by Hopkinson (1915) states that the magnitudes of distance and time are scaled in proportion to the relative dimensions of explosive charges detonated in the same atmosphere. The relative volumes of two spheres are proportional to the cubes of their diameters. For free air detonations, the weight (yield or energy) of a homogeneous explosive is proportional to its volume. It follows, therefore, that scaled distances and times are proportional to the cube root of the explosive weight.

It is useful to introduce the notion of a scaled distance Z, where:

$$Z = \frac{R}{W^{1/3}} \qquad (3.16)$$

with R representing the distance from the centre of the explosion and W the energy of the explosive. This 'energy' usually represents the weight of a standard explosive such as TNT. By expressing the yield of an explosive in terms of an equivalent weight of TNT (Table 15.1), it is possible to obtain blast-wave parameters for a range of explosives from a single graph (see Baker *et al.*, 1983). Almost 100% of the energy liberated in a chemical explosion is converted into blast energy. Note, however, that only 50% of the energy of a nuclear explosion is released into the blast-wave and the remainder as thermal and nuclear radiation. This must be taken into account when scaling from a chemical to nuclear explosions or vice versa. The report by Kingery and Bulmash (1984) is an authoritative source of airblast data.

At the same scaled distance each explosion produces identical static and dynamic peak pressures and shock-wave velocities. The time of arrival, positive and negative phase durations and specific impulses are all scaled in proportion to the cube root of the explosive weight.

The cube root 'law' implies that there is a single curve of peak pressure versus scaled distance for explosions of varying magnitude. Figure 15.8 shows that this is not exactly true. Cube root scaling does, however, give reasonable correlation with a wide range of experimental data and is used almost universally.

Other scaling laws are discussed by Baker (1973).

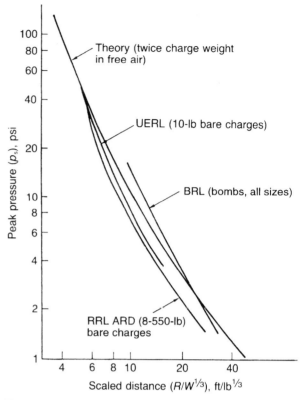

Figure 15.8 Pressure vs. distance curves for ground burst of bare charges. (Reproduced from Kennedy, 1946.)

Blast loading

The interaction of a blast-wave and an object in its path is complex. The loading across the surface of the object will vary unless the shape of the shock front matches that of the surface. This is unlikely unless both can be considered to be plane – a reasonable assumption for the shock front at some distance from the explosion and in the Mach Stem region.

Consider the interaction of a plane shock front with, for the sake of simplicity, a solid box-shaped object (Figure 15.9). At time t_1 the object is at ambient pressure and is unloaded. At time t_2 the

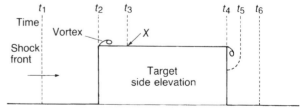

Figure 15.9 Interaction of blast-wave with a solid box-shaped object.

shock front of the blast-wave encounters the front face of the object and is reflected from it. The face is subjected to a lateral load from both the reflected static overpressure p_r and the drag pressure. Drag pressure equals $C_D p_d$ where p_d is the dynamic pressure and C_D is a drag coefficient. C_D is about 2 for an unstreamlined object such as a wide box. As the blast-wave front traverses the object (time t_3), the static overpressure exerts a force on the sides of the box. That on the front face lessens as the blast-wave decays. When the shock front reaches the rear of the box at time t_4, it diffracts around the edges and travels down the back surface (time t_5). By t_6 the shock front has fully passed and continuity is restored – the object is completely affected by the static overpressure. There is an overall crushing pressure on the object but the overpressure decays rapidly with time. The net sideways force on the box (acting towards the right in Figure 15.9) reduces to near zero as it is encompassed by the blast-wave. The dynamic pressure, however, continues to exert a net sideways force to the right for the full extent of the positive-phase duration as the wind gives a negative suction force on the rear face of the box. For nuclear explosions, which have long positive-phase durations measured in tenths of seconds or greater, the dynamic pressure loading far exceeds the static overpressure loading for small targets such as personnel and vehicles. For conventional explosions the 'drag' loading caused by the dynamic pressures is generally less than the 'diffraction' loading caused by the static overpressures. The quantification of blast loading is considered in detail by Glasstone and Dolan (1977) and Baker *et al.* (1983).

The response of an object to blast loading depends upon the relation between the loading time and the natural period of vibration of the object. If the loading time is relatively short, it is reasonable to treat the loading as impulsive. The positive-phase impulse is the important loading variable. If the loading time is long compared to its natural period, the object is subject to quasi-static loading and peak overpressure is important. Analysis techniques for these limiting cases are described by Baker *et al.* (1983). The treatment is significantly more complicated for intermediate loading times and for problems which cannot be idealized as systems with a single degree of freedom. Numerical analysis techniques are then required.

Blast loading causes an overall structural response as described above. A blast-wave can also be directly transmitted through a surface into a material as a stress-wave. The proportions of the loading that are transmitted and reflected depend on the density and the speed of sound in the two media.

Blast loading and the consequent response of structures to such loading are described in detail by Smith and Hetherington (1994).

UNDERWATER EXPLOSIONS

An explosive detonated under water produces a shock-wave which is not fundamentally different from the blast-wave in air. The gaseous products of the explosion form a bubble, the subsequent expansion and contraction of which produces additional and longer-term pressure fluctuations in the water. Cole (1965) and Kaye (1983) consider these phenomena in depth.

Primary shock-wave

The detonation wave in a high explosive charge is directly transmitted to the surrounding water. The acoustic impedance of water, the product of its density and sound velocity, is less than half that of the detonation products. In water, therefore, the initial velocity and pressure of the shock-wave are significantly less than the corresponding values for the detonation products. Thus a detonation velocity of about 7500 m/s is transmitted into the water at an initial velocity of some 5000 m/s which decreases rapidly to the speed of sound in water – about 1500 m/s. The shock loses energy as it propagates away from the explosion and the peak shock pressures reduce, though at a lesser rate than in air. Durations are, however, shorter than in air so that impulse values are not excessive compared to the same charge weight detonated in air. Cube root scaling can be used in a similar way to that for air blast.

A typical overpressure–time plot is shown in Figure 15.10. The initial overpressure decay is exponential and it is usually assumed to be of the form

$$p_m(t) = p_m e^{-t/\theta} \qquad (3.17)$$

where p_m is the peak overpressure, and θ is a time decay constant which equals the time taken for the pressure to decay to the value p_m/e. Both time t and θ are measured from the time of arrival of the shock-wave. After this the pressure falls more slowly than the exponential decay. The area under the overpressure–time curve gives positive specific impulse. Integration is normally taken to a time 5θ.

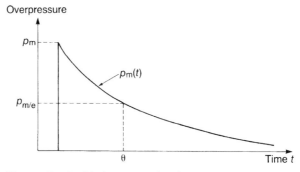

Figure 15.10 Underwater shock-wave parameters.

A shock-wave energy density E can be defined. Its basic form is:

$$E = \int_0^t p_m^2(t)dt \qquad (3.18)$$

where time t is measured from the time of arrival of the shock-wave.

When the shock-wave strikes a solid object which has a higher acoustic impedance than that of water, the wave reflection is similar to that for air blast. The compressive pressure is reflected. However, if the shock-wave reaches the surface of the water it reflects from the air, which has a lower acoustic impedance than that of water. The compressive pressure then reflects as a rarefaction or tensile pressure wave. Below the surface the reflected shock-wave interacts with the initial shock-wave to cause a pressure drop, possibly to values below ambient hydrostatic water pressure.

Bubble effects

The hot gases from a spherical charge detonated under water create a spherical gas bubble which expands rapidly. The inertia of the surrounding water allows it to expand beyond the point of pressure equilibrium and its internal pressure falls significantly below ambient hydrostatic pressure. Motion is then reversed and the bubble contracts. When it reaches its minimum size the gas pressure will have increased significantly and, as it starts to expand again, an acoustic pulse is transmitted to the water. More than ten such oscillations may occur. The pulses, which are transmitted to the water at points of maximum re-compression, progressively weaken because of energy losses and only the first few are significant. The bubble rises in the water during each period of contraction though its depth remains constant during the expansion phases. Compared with the shock-wave, the bubble pulses produce low pressures of long duration.

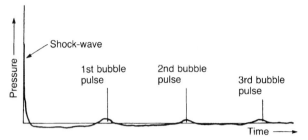

Figure 15.11 Pressure profiles of underwater primary shock-wave and bubble pulses.

Figure 15.11 indicates the relative magnitudes and time-scales of the shock-wave and bubble pulses. Table 15.2 gives data measured at 60 ft from a 300-lb TNT charge detonated in 100 ft of water. The 'Direct' bubble pulse refers to the first oscillation. The 'Composite' bubble pulse is the combined effect of the first and all subsequent bubble oscillations. The impulse and energy values for the shock-wave were obtained by integration to 2 ms after the shock front and, for the bubble pulses, by integration over times of pressure in excess of hydrostatic. Note that the bubble pulses produce significant impulses and energy densities because of their long duration.

REFERENCES

Bailey A., Murray S.G. (1989). *Explosives, Propellants and Pyrotechnics*. London: Brassey's (UK).

Baker W.E. (1973). *Explosions in Air*. Austin, TX: University of Texas Press.

Baker W.E., Cox P.A., Westine P.S. et al. (1983). *Explosion Hazards and Evaluation*. Amsterdam: Elsevier Science.

Brode H.L. (1955). Numerical solutions of spherical blast waves. *J. Appl. Phys.*, **26**, 766–75.

Chapman D.L. (1899). On the rate of explosion in gases. London, Dublin and Edinburgh. *Philosophical Magaine*, **213**, series 5 (47), 90.

TABLE 15.2

SHOCK-WAVE AND BUBBLE-PULSE PARAMETERS FROM AN UNDERWATER EXPLOSION. (REPRODUCED FROM COLE, 1965.)

	Depth (ft)	Peak pressure (lb/in^2)	Positive impulse (lb-s/in^2)	Energy density (in-lb/in^2)
Shock-wave	40	1770	1.15	170
	Bottom	1940	1.41	250
Direct bubble pulse	20	428	1.1	47
	26	71	0.84	5.9
	45	56	1.5	9.5
	65	84	4.0	18
	96	81	1.2	11
Composite bubble pulse	20	555	2.9	130
	26	106	2.1	16
	45	79	2.6	19
	65	93	3.4	28
	96	68	1.2	7

Cole R.H. (1965). *Underwater Explosions*. New York: Dover Publications.

Glasstone S., Dolan P.J. (1977). *The Effects of Nuclear Weapons*, 3rd edn. US Departments of Defense and Energy.

Hopkinson B. (1915). British Ordnance Board Minutes 13565.

Johansson C.H., Persson P.A. (1970). *Detonics of High Explosives*. London: Academic Press.

Jouguet E. (1905). Sur la propagation des reactives chimiques dans la gaze. *Journal of Pure and Applied Mathematics*, **70**, Series 6(1), 347.

Kaye S.M. (1983). Underwater explosions. In *Encylopaedia of Explosives and Related Items* PATR Vol. 10. Dover, NJ: US Army R & D Command, Large Calibre Weapons Laboratory.

Kennedy W.D. (1946). Explosions and explosives in air. In *Effects of Impact and Explosion*, Vol. 1. Summary Technical Report of Division 2. Washington, DC: NDRC, chap. 2.

Kingery C.N., Bulmash G. (1984). *Airblast Parameters for TNT Spherical Air Burst and Hemispherical Surface Burst*. Technical Report ARBRL-TR-02555. Maryland: US Army Armament Research and Development Center, Ballistic Research Laboratory.

Kinney G.F., Graham K.J. (1985). *Explosive Shocks in Air*, 2nd edn. Berlin: Springer-Verlag.

Smith P.D., Hetherington J.G. (1994). *Blast and Ballistic Loading of Structures*. Oxford: Butterworth-Heinemann.

Taylor J. (1952). *Detonation in Condensed Explosives*. Oxford: Clarendon Press.

16. Blast Biology

J. T. Yelverton

INTRODUCTION

A basic understanding of the mechanics, pathogenesis and treatment of blast injury developed during and just after the Second World War (Zuckerman, 1940; Cameron *et al.*, 1943; Goligher *et al.*, 1943; Williams, 1943; Wakely, 1945; Corey, 1946; Clemedson, 1948; Benzinger, 1950; Desaga, 1950; Rossle, 1950; Schardin, 1950). Continued research over the past 40 years has added to the understanding of the effects of free-field blast-waves (Clemedson, 1956; White and Richmond, 1960; Von Gierke, 1964; Richmond *et al.*, 1968; Jonsson, 1979) and to the evidence that gas-containing organs are more vulnerable to direct blast than are solid ones (Kolder and Stockinger 1957; Chiffelle, 1966; Clifford *et al.*, 1984; Moe *et al.*, 1987). This has led to the development of damage risk criteria for primary blast injury in man (Bowen *et al.*, 1968; Richmond *et al.*, 1986). These criteria define the tolerance of the lung alone.

Damage to the lung by a blast-wave can lead to upper airway obstruction from haemorrhage, changes in blood-gas parameters due to increased venous/arterial shunting, and pulmonary hypertension with possible congestive heart failure. At higher overpressures, the formation of alveolar-venous fistulae in the lung parenchyma permits air to enter the circulation and can result in early death from coronary and cerebral air embolism. Contusions and/or ruptures of the lining of the gastrointestinal tract are also frequently described following blast exposure. However, the onset of effects from these lesions may be delayed. Additional criteria have been established relating the severity of eardrum rupture to blast overpressure and duration (Richmond *et al.*, 1989), which may be useful in establishing combat casualty criteria in the future.

Recent studies have shown that damage to the upper respiratory tract can be important as an indication of the presence of other non-auditory blast injuries (Dancer *et al.*, 1981; Yelverton *et al.*, 1983; Dodd *et al.* 1990). It was observed that demonstrable haemorrhagic changes tend to occur in the upper respiratory tract, either before or concurrent with injuries to the gastrointestinal tract and/or the lungs.

This chapter will outline the human tolerance to classical free-field blast-waves (Friedlander waves), and how these criteria may be applied to the complex waves arising from explosions within confined spaces or close to multiple reflecting surfaces.

PHYSICAL CHARACTERISTICS OF BLAST-WAVES

A brief discussion of some of the basic physical characteristics of both free-field and complex blast-waves is essential to the understanding of the bioeffects of the various waveforms.

Free-field waves The classical free-field blast-wave occurs in an open environment. As Figure 16.1 demonstrates, it is characterized by a simple nearly instantaneous rise in pressure to a peak value, followed by an exponential decay to a subatmospheric value before a return to ambient pressure.

Complex waves Complex waves are frequently described as a series of non-uniform shocks separated by varying time intervals. They are produced in many ways, some of which are described in the following text.

Interaction with obstacles

A classical blast-wave can interact with an obstacle in the open to produce a complex wave (Figure 16.2) (Vassout *et al.*, 1978). The wave here strikes the leading edge of a semicylindrical shield, creating a reflection that diffracts around the shield producing vortices along the edges at the top and sides of the shield. This causes a temporary sharp drop in pressure and an increase in its duration. During this time the wave is re-formed to reach a more or less steady-state value – the stagnation pressure which is the algebraic sum of the incident overpressure and the drag (dynamic) pressure. In this case the dynamic pressure has a negative value because air flow causes a reduction in loading at the top and sides of the shield (Glasstone, 1957).

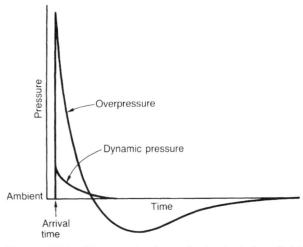

Figure 16.1 Characterization of classical free-field blast-wave with associated dynamic pressure component. (From Glasstone, 1957.)

200

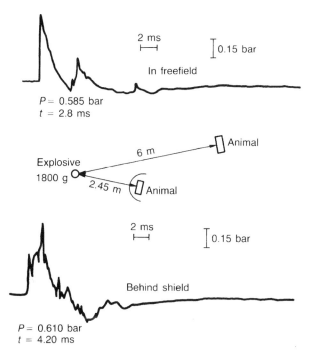

Figure 16.2 A classical blast-wave recorded in the free-field compared to one of equivalent peak overpressure recorded behind a shield (1 bar = 100 kPa). (Reproduced from Vassout *et al.*, 1978.)

Entry into enclosures

A complex wave can also form when a classical wave enters a structure, compartment or enclosure through an opening. The features are to a large extent dependent on the ratio of the volume of the structure to the area of the way of entry (White *et al.*, 1957; Richmond *et al.*, 1959; Richmond and Kilgore, 1970), as well as to the geometry of the enclosure and its material composition (Clemedson and Jonsson, 1976a,b). Structures with large volume-to-area (V/A) ratios have waveforms with low-amplitude incident and reflected shock fronts in the early part of the wave – called the diffraction phase. The latter is followed by a slow-rising fill phase peaking at a pressure well below that of the outside incident wave (Richmond, 1971; Richmond and Kilgore, 1972). During the fill phase, the static pressure converts to a high-velocity flow through the entryway with dynamic pressures that are greater than that in the incident blast-wave (Richmond *et al.*, 1980). The pressure-time records illustrated in Figure 16.3 are examples of complex waves resulting from the entry of a 40-psi (276-kPa) incident wave into an underground shelter with two compartments of identical dimensions but with V/A ratios of 66 and 175 units respectively (Richmond *et al.*, 1959).

As the V/A ratio decreases, the intensity of the incident and reflected shocks increase, the fill phase peak pressure can approach half that of the outside wave, and the time to peak becomes shorter. The

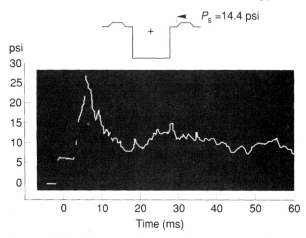

Figure 16.3 Pressure–time patterns recorded inside open underground personnel shelters during Operation Plumbbob. T is gauge location. Number 1 is the incident wave. (Adapted from Richmond and Kilgore, 1972.)

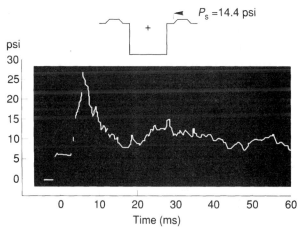

Figure 16.4 Pressure–time patterns recorded in a rectangular two-man foxhole, one-seventh scale model, in a shocktube. + = gauge location. (Reproduced from Richmond, 1971.)

waveform illustrated in Figure 16.4 is that of a 14.4-psi (99-kPa) incident wave entering a two-man rectangular foxhole (Richmond, 1971).

Firing from an enclosure

Complex waves can result from the firing of large-calibre weapons or the launching of rockets from enclosures. The blast-wave from a Carl-Gustaf recoilless weapon fired from a $4.2 \times 5.5 \times 2.5\,m$ enclosure (Figure 16.5) is an example. It consists of a reverberant pressure-field of more than 300 ms duration with a low-amplitude incident wave, a small negative phase and no quasi-static pressure component (Clemedson and Jonsson, 1976a,b). The frequency and amplitude of the pressure oscilla-

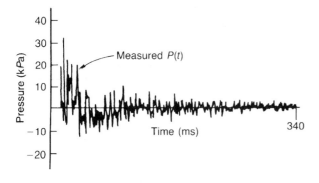

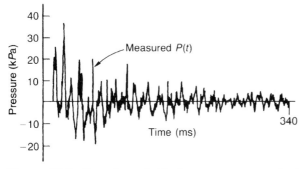

Figure 16.5 Reverberant blast-waves measured at two different locations in a 4.2 × 5.5 × 2.5 m enclosure which were generated by firing a recoilless rifle in the enclosure. (Reproduced from Clemedson and Jonsson, 1976a,b.)

tions following the incident wave vary with the location of the recording apparatus within the enclosure (Figure 16.5).

Explosions in an enclosure

Complex waves are also produced by the penetration of armoured vehicles by high-explosive anti-tank rounds or by the detonation of a high-explosive charge in an enclosed space (Sewell *et al.*, 1972; Blacksten and Schecter, 1979; Richmond *et al.*, 1985). The pressure-time profile of an explosion in an enclosed space has an initial blast phase followed by a hydrostatic pressure rise sustained for a short period followed by a prolonged decay phase (Sewell *et al.*, 1972). The hydrostatic phase is also termed the 'quasi-static pressure'.

The initial blast phase consists of the incident shock followed by reflections from the walls of the enclosure. Since scaling laws still apply, a detonation occurring in the centre of a confined space results in an incident wave that is the same as if the event had occurred in the open air (Sewell *et al.*, 1972). The effective yield could be a factor of two, four or eight times higher if the explosion occurred respectively against a wall, at the junction of two walls or in a corner. For a given charge weight, incident pressure levels within the compartment would be multiplied by a factor of $2^{1/3}$, $4^{1/3}$ or $8^{1/3}$

if the charge was detonated at one of these three locations (Taylor, 1968; Cooper, 1989). Depending upon the location in the room, some of the reflections could interact to produce a pressure about five times that of the incident wave (Blacksten and Schecter, 1979).

The reflections from the walls superimpose on the hydrostatic pressure rise which starts at the end of the incident wave. The pressure rise is a product of the energy released and additional gases generated during the explosion. Rise time depends on the type of explosive, the amount of oxygen available, ambient pressure, temperature, ignition conditions, degree of turbulence in the flame front and the volume of the structure. Peak value of the hydrostatic pressure is mainly a consequence of the maximum temperature reached by the gases in the confining volume (Sewell *et al.*, 1972).

The equation

$$P = 2410 \, (W/V)^{0.72}$$

where P = mean pressure (psi), W = explosive weight (lb) and V = volume of enclosure (ft^3), which was derived to calculate the average blast load on enclosure walls (Weibull, 1968), has also been used (rather contentiously) to estimate the residual overpressure. This assumes that the term 'residual' refers to the peak quasi-static pressure (Blacksten and Schecter, 1979).

At the end of the hydrostatic pressure rise there is a short period of sustained pressure followed by a decay phase. The sustained period is the outcome of, on the one hand, the cooling effect of heat transfer to the walls of the enclosure and, on the other hand, the energy released during recombination of the constituents of the combustion flame

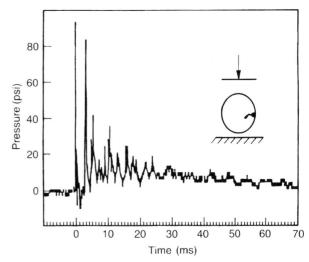

Figure 16.6 Pressure–time pattern recorded by the side-on gauge in an instrumentation cylinder against a wall and at 3 ft (0.9 m) from a 1-lb (0.45-kg) C-4 charge detonation in the centre of a 10 × 10 × 8 ft (3.0 × 3.0 × 2.4 m) enclosure.

front into stable molecules. The decay phase begins as a result of continued heat transfer to the surrounding walls and mass discharge of pressurized gases if vents are present. Ambient downstream pressure (usually atmospheric) and vent geometry have little or no influence on venting rate but the total available vent area is of significance. Though the rate of cooling and mass discharge are slow enough not to have an effect on the initial blast phase or the hydrostatic pressure rise and only a

moderate effect upon the sustained pressure phase, they appreciably affect phase of decay (Sewell *et al.*, 1972). Peak hydrostatic pressure is nearly always reached, even when containing walls ultimately fail because structural inertia is high compared to the time-course of explosion events (Blacksten and Schecter, 1979).

The pressure–time history from the explosion of a small high-explosive charge in an enclosure is shown in Figure 16.6. The recording was made in a

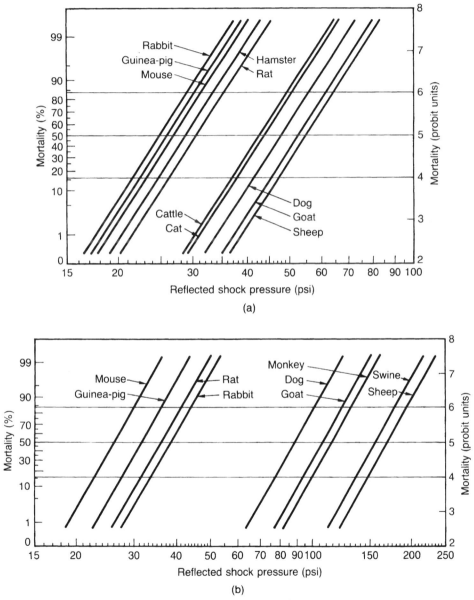

(a)

(b)

Figure 16.7   (a) Mortality curves for animals exposed to 'long-duration' reflected pressures while mounted side-on against the endplate of a shock tube. Probit regression equation: $y = a + b \log x$, where y is the percentage of mortality in probit units, a and b the intercept and slope constants, and x the pressure. All measurements were made at ambient pressure of 12 psi. (Reproduced from Richmond *et al.*, 1968.) (b) Mortality curves for animals exposed to 'short-duration' reflected pressures from high-explosive charges detonated overhead while mounted prone on a concrete pad. Probit regression equation: $y = a + b \log x$, where y is the percentage mortality in probit units, and b the intercept and slope constants, and x the pressure. All measurements were made at ambient pressure of 12 psi. (Reproduced from Richmond *et al.*, 1968.)

vented $10 \times 8 \times 8$-ft underground bunker using an instrumentation cylinder located 3 ft from a 1-1b C-4 explosive.

BIOLOGICAL EFFECTS

Damage risk criteria for primary blast effects from free-field waves were established in 1968 (Bowen *et al.*, 1968). Attempts to use the same criteria for a complex wave environment are complicated by the variability of the dynamic components of the waves. The tolerance of mammals to classical and complex blast-waves is discussed below.

Free-field blast-waves

Mammalian mortality studies have demonstrated that tolerance to classical free-field blast-waves is dependent upon the animal species, the peak overpressure and positive-phase duration of the blast-wave (Damon *et al.*, 1966a and b; Bowen *et al.*, 1968; Richmond *et al.*, 1968). Mortality curves for animals exposed on reflecting surfaces are shown in Figure 16.7. Probit analysis (Finney, 1964) of the mortality illustrates three important points: first, for a given species and classification of wave duration, there is a linear relationship between the probit of mortality and the logarithm of reflected overpressure; second, all the probit lines have a common slope, which suggests a common mechanism of lethality; and, third, the data tend to separate into 'small' and 'large' mammal groups. The probit transformation used in these and the forthcoming analyses is simply the addition of five to the normal distribution of the deviate to eliminate negative values; thus, a probit value of 5 is equal to 50% mortality.

By combining scaling laws derived from dimensional analysis with additional probit analyses of the mortality data used to derive Figure 16.7, the blast loading to a mammal can be used to calculate the equivalent overpressure, P^* (psi), that would be expected to produce the same mortality in a 70-kg mammal exposed to a long-duration blast-wave (i.e. square wave) at sea level:

$$P^* = P/(1 + 6.76T^{-1.064})$$

where $P = P_r(14.7/P_0)$ and $T = t^+(70/m)^{1/3}(P_0/14.7)^{1/2}$. P_r(psi) is the experimental peak reflected pressure and P_0(psi) is the ambient pressure.

The duration, T, is derived from the experimental duration, t^+, and m (kg) is the body mass.

Using the equivalent overpressures, both individual and parallel probit analyses were carried out for all the species listed in Figure 16.7 except that the guinea-pig was excluded from the parallel analyses. Figure 16.8 is an illustration of the mortality data for sheep treated in this manner.

The equivalent square wave pressures resulting in 50% mortality (P_{sw} values) for the various species

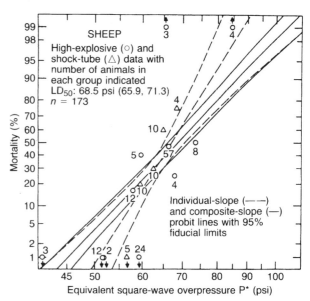

Figure 16.8 Results of the parallel-probit analysis for the sheep in terms of equivalent square-wave overpressure, defined by $P^* = P/(1 + 6.76T^{1.064})$. Results of an individual analysis for sheep are shown for comparison. (Reproduced from Bowen *et al.*, 1968.)

can be considered as indices of blast tolerance which are independent of body mass (Bowen *et al.*, 1968). The P_{sw} values for the eight 'large' animal species ranged from 50.0 (345 kPa) to 71.9 psi (496 kPa), with a geometric mean of 61.4 psi (423 kPa), and those for the five 'small' animal species ranged from 30.8 (212 kPa) to 36.9 psi (254 kPa) with a geometric mean of 33.1 psi (228 kPa) (Figure 16.9). The large/small separation is supported by the fact that the ratio of lung volume to body mass is distinctly different in large and small animals. Data on lung volume and density, as well as tolerance to whole-body impact, clearly suggest that man belongs to the 'large' animal group (White *et al.*, 1971). Assuming this to be the case, the tolerance for man was arbitrarily taken to be the geometric mean of this group ($P_{sw} = 61.5$ psi (424 kPa)).

Figure 16.9 contains five survival curves giving peak reflected overpressure vs positive overpressure duration, scaled to an ambient pressure of 14.7 psi (101 kPa) and a 70-kg mammal with a P_{sw} of 61.5 psi (424 kPa), and are therefore assumed to apply to man at sea level. The curves derived from the equation:

$$P = 61.5 (1 + 6.76T^{-1.064}) e^{0.1788(5-z)}$$

where z is the survival in probit units.

The equivalent overpressure was made applicable to various levels of lethality by the transformation:

$$P^* = P_{sw} e^{c(y-5)}$$

where y is the mortality in probit units and c is the reciprocal of the probit slope (which is 0.1788 in this

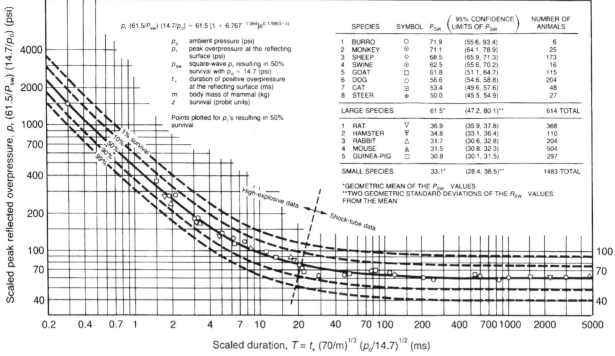

$$p_r (61.5/P_{sw}) (14.7/p_o) = 61.5 [1 + 6.76T^{-1.064}]e^{0.1788(5-z)}$$

p_o	ambient pressure (psi)
p_r	peak overpressure at the reflecting surface (psi)
P_{sw}	square-wave p_r resulting in 50% survival with $p_o = 14.7$ (psi)
t_+	duration of positive overpressure at the reflecting surface (ms)
m	body mass of mammal (kg)
z	survival (probit units)

Points plotted for p_r's resulting in 50% survival

SPECIES	SYMBOL	P_{sw}	95% CONFIDENCE LIMITS OF P_{sw}	NUMBER OF ANIMALS
1 BURRO	○	71.9	(55.6, 93.4)	6
2 MONKEY	⊙	71.1	(64.1, 78.9)	25
3 SHEEP	◇	68.5	(65.9, 71.3)	173
4 SWINE	⊕	62.5	(55.6, 70.2)	16
5 GOAT	□	61.8	(51.1, 64.7)	115
6 DOG	○	56.6	(54.6, 58.8)	204
7 CAT	⊡	53.4	(49.6, 57.6)	48
8 STEER	⊛	50.0	(45.5, 54.9)	27
LARGE SPECIES		61.5*	(47.2, 80.1)**	614 TOTAL
1 RAT	▽	36.9	(35.9, 37.8)	368
2 HAMSTER	▼	34.8	(33.1, 36.4)	110
3 RABBIT	△	31.7	(30.6, 32.8)	204
4 MOUSE	▲	31.5	(30.8, 32.3)	504
5 GUINEA-PIG	□	30.8	(30.1, 31.5)	297
SMALL SPECIES		33.1*	(28.4, 38.5)**	1483 TOTAL

*GEOMETRIC MEAN OF THE P_{sw} VALUES
**TWO GEOMETRIC STANDARD DEVIATIONS OF THE P_{sw} VALUES FROM THE MEAN

Figure 16.9 Survival curves (24-hour) applicable to sharp-rising blast-waves, derived from the analysis of data for 12 mammalian species (excluding guinea-pig). (Reproduced from Bowen *et al.*, 1968.)

case). Since the curves are presented in terms of survival, the term $e^{c(y-5)}$ becomes $e^{c(5-Z)}$ where Z is the survival probit. The overpressure scaling factor, $61.5/P_{sw}$, seen in the figure accounts for differences in species tolerance. This technique allows all points to be compared to the 50% survival curve derived from man (Bowen *et al.*, 1968).

The damage–risk curves for humans (illustrated in Figures 16.10–16.12) were derived directly from this set of curves. In all cases, it can be seen that the longer the duration the lower the pressure required to produce injury. From about 50 ms, the probability of survival from blast lung injury is independent of overpressure duration.

As seen in the figures, the peak pressure necessary for the production of lung injury depends on the orientation of the individual with respect to the blast. Subjects in a prone position, with the long axis of the body parallel to the blast wind, are more resistant to lung injury than those that are standing or prone broadside with the long axis of the body perpendicular to the blast wind. If the long axis of the body is perpendicular to the shock front, the incident pressure is the blast load, but if the axis is parallel to the oncoming wave, the load is the stagnation pressure (i.e. incident plus the dynamic pressure). Individuals near a reflecting surface that is parallel to the shock front are the most vulnerable if the positive-phase duration of the wave is

spatially longer than the width of the body (Bowen *et al.*, 1968). In this case, the incident wave produces, upon striking the reflecting surface, a reflected wave with a peak overpressure which is more than twice the original value (Glasstone, 1957).

Studies using guinea-pigs exposed to long-duration waves generated by shock tubes have demonstrated that, as long as the thorax was near a reflecting surface, the LD_{50} pressure did not vary with change in orientation of the animal (Clare *et al.*, 1962). However, if the positive-phase duration is spatially shorter than body width, the decay rate of the blast-wave is such that the most severe loading occurs on the side of the body closer to the oncoming wave. The impulse of the shock front at the leading edge of the body and not the reflected pressure, becomes the effective dose (Bowen *et al.*, 1968).

Complex waves

The response of animals and man to complex blast-waves is more difficult to predict. Subjects may be more or less tolerant to complex waveforms than to free-field waves. The rate of rise, the number and intensity, and the frequency of oscillation of the pressure pulses are among the additional features that are important in determining biological tolerance to complex waves.

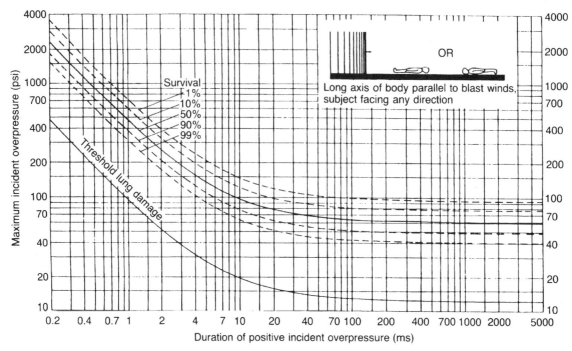

Figure 16.10 Survival curves predicted for a 70-kg man applicable to free-stream situation where the long axis of the body is parallel to the blast winds. (Reproduced from Bowen *et al.*, 1968.)

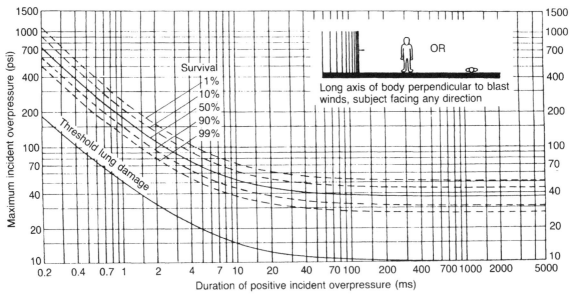

Figure 16.11 Survival curves predicted for a 70-kg man applicable to a free-stream situation where the long axis of the body is perpendicular to the blast winds. (Reproduced from Bowen *et al.*, 1968.)

Wave interaction with obstacles

An incident which occurred during the Second World War has been reported by Desaga (1950). Thirteen men occupying an anti-aircraft gun emplacement were exposed to the detonation of a 2000-1b high-explosive bomb which contained a 550-kg (1210-1b) explosive charge. The bomb exploded 9.2 m from the 4 × 6 m emplacement which was open at the top and surrounded by a 1.6-m high rampart with a single entryway. The location of eight of the men during the blast exposure was known and is shown in Figure 16.13. Subjects 7 and 8 were killed and Subjects 3, 4, 5 and 6 suffered

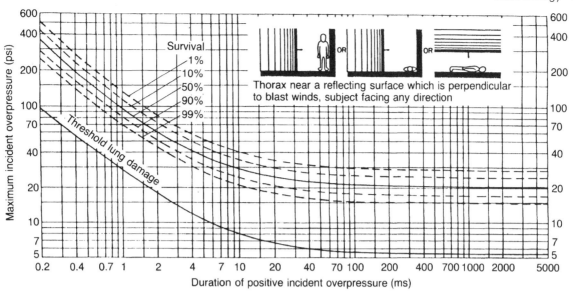

Figure 16.12 Survival curves predicted for a 70-kg man applicable to blast situations where the thorax is near a surface against which a blast-wave reflects at normal incidence. (Reproduced from Bowen *et al.*, 1968.)

moderate or extensive trauma. Subjects 1 and 2 sustained only slight injuries. The two men who were fatally injured were crouched against a wall in the corner farthest from the blast and both died 45 minutes after exposure. Bloody froth at the mouth, marked lung haemorrhage, and bilateral eardrum ruptures were marked at post-mortem. The reflected overpressure was estimated to be 235 psi (1620 kPa). Two of the men, 3 and 4, who sustained extensive lung injuries and bilateral eardrum ruptures were standing on the gun platform. Their upper bodies were above the level of the rampart and for them an incident pressure load of 81 psi

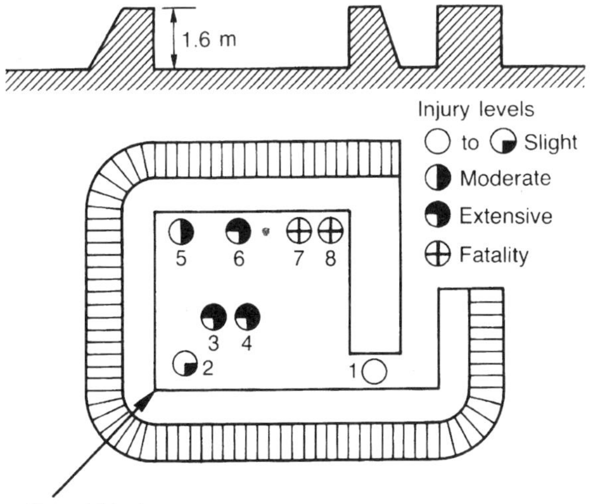

(558 kPa) was estimated in that they were fully exposed to the blast. Subjects 5 and 6 were partially sheltered by the ramparts. Subject 5 had moderate lung injury but not eardrum ruptures; however, Subject 6 had extensive lung haemorrhage and rupture of one eardrum. The two who had slight injuries and no eardrum ruptures were near the upstream wall and were probably in a relatively low pressure region created by the vortex that was formed as the blast-wave swept over the rampart. This example serves to emphasize the difficulties in predicting biological effect in even simple geometric shapes.

In an experimental study, rats were subjected to the blast from a 1.8-kg high-explosive explosion. They were exposed free-field and behind a semi-cylindrical shield, of the kind shown in Figure 16.2 (Vassout *et al.*, 1978). Animals were divided into two groups, orientated either end-on or side-on to the shock front. Exposure distances were adjusted so that the mean values of the peak overpressures in the free-field and behind the shield were virtually the same (about 8.5 psi (59 kPa)). The positive-phase durations were 2.8 and 4.2 milliseconds, respectively. Comparison of the amplitude spectra indicated a higher energy level between 40 and 125 Hz for the pressure–time profile recorded behind the shield and a yet higher level from 250 to 1000 Hz for the profile recorded in the free-field. There was a 60% incidence of lung injuries in the rats exposed either side-on or end-on to the shock front in the free-field. The lack of any orientation effects is probably due to the fact that, at these low overpressures, the dynamic pressure, calculated to be 1.6 psi (11 kPa), does not add significantly to the side-on blast load. In contrast, for rats that were

Figure 16.13 Anti-aircraft gun emplacement and distribution of the crew when exposed to the blast from a 2000-lb bomb. (Reproduced from Desaga, 1950.)

exposed in the free-field to 58 psi (400 kPa) during the same experiment, the calculated dynamic pressure was 52 psi (358 kPa). One hundred per cent of the side-on and only 20% of the end-on animals were killed by the blast. For animals that were behind the shield, only 50% of the side-on while over 80% of the end-on rats sustained lung injuries compared to the free-field rats exposed to the same peak overpressure. A possible explanation for the lessening of the side-on effects behind the shield is that the thoraces of the side-on subjects were in the low-pressure region of the vortex created as the shock-wave passed over and around the shield. The increase in effects in the end-on animals behind the shield is that they were exposed to both the direct and indirect waves of the 4.2 ms duration complex wave created by the interaction of the free-field wave with the shield.

Wave entry into enclosures

During above-ground nuclear weapons tests, several species of animals were exposed to the complex waves formed in the fast and slow fill underground shelters illustrated in Figure 16.3 (White *et al.*, 1957; Richmond *et al.*, 1959). Except for eardrum rupture, there was no direct relationship between primary blast injuries and the pressure–time patterns recorded in the shelters. For these long duration waves, the incidence of eardrum rupture was simply related to maximum overpressure without regard to the waveform (Zalewski, 1906; White *et al.*, 1957; Richmond *et al.*, 1959; Richmond and White, 1962). The P_{50} (pressure required for 50% incidence of eardrum rupture) pressures for dogs, rabbits and guinea-pigs were estimated to be 28, 15 and 8 psi (193, 103 and 55 kPa), respectively. These values compare favourably to the respective P_{50} pressure of 29.8, 9.3 and 7.4 psi (205, 64 and 51 kPa) recently reported for complex waves (Richmond *et al.*, 1989). The incident and reflected pressure spikes associated with the diffraction phase were either not large enough individually or the time intervals between shocks were long enough, so the rates of pressure rise in the gas-containing organs were too slow to produce significant levels of nonauditory injuries (Richmond and White, 1962).

Dogs were also exposed to smooth-rising overpressure levels ranging from 4.2 to 113 psi (29 to 779 kPa) with four different rise-times of 14 to 15, 30 to 34, 80 to 94 and 238 to 403 ms (Figure 16.14). Eardrum rupture was seen at levels as low as 9.4 psi (65 kPa) but lung haemorrhage was not evident until 106 psi (731 kPa) (Richmond and Kilgore, 1972). This is quite remarkable when one considers that, in dogs, the threshold for lung haemorrhage is 9 psi (62 kPa) and the LD_{50} is 46 psi (317 kPa) for exposure to a square wave at an ambient atmospheric pressure of 12 psi (83 kPa) (Bowen *et al.*, 1968).

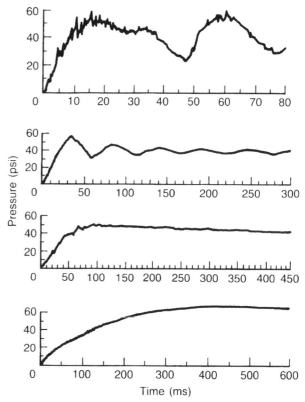

Figure 16.14 Pressure–time patterns generated in a shocktube to evaluate the influence of the rate of rise to peak pressure on the response of dogs to blast. (Reproduced from Richmond and Kilgore, 1972.)

The high-velocity flow through the entryway of the fast-fill chamber posed the most significant hazard to the test subjects. On two separate field studies, dogs that were placed near the entryway of the fast-fill chamber were either killed or sustained serious injuries from violent displacement and subsequent impact with the rear wall of the chamber. Blast jetting through open hatches and firing ports, and not the complex wave formed thereafter, is also the major direct airblast hazard to personnel inside an armoured vehicle. Studies with sheep indicated that slight crushing type injuries began at jet flow stagnation pressure levels above 10.3 psi (71 kPa) and that severe injuries would be predicted at stagnation pressure levels over 20.6 psi (142 kPa). These criteria were limited to jetting through either circular openings of 15–48 cm in diameter or equivalent-area rectangular openings having length/width ratios of 1.0–2.5 (Richmond *et al.*, 1980).

In structures with small V/A ratios, such as foxholes, the direct overpressure effects of the diffraction phase predominate because of the multiplication of the incident shock front reflecting from the walls and floor of the foxhole. There is little or no fill-phase associated with these relatively open structures. The magnitude of the reflected shocks, which represent the peak overpressure, can be more than twice the pressure in the incident wave. The results of laboratory studies with rats in one-seventh scale model foxholes and on field tests with sheep in full-scale two-man rectangular foxholes demonstrated that response tended to vary with the time interval between incident and reflected shock for a given incident overpressure (Richmond, 1961; Richmond and Fletcher, 1970; Richmond *et al.*, 1971). These findings related quite well to the results from experiments in which the pressure loading was done in a step-wise fashion by exposing subjects to shocks at various distances from the endplate of a shock tube (Froboese and Wunsche, 1959; Richmond, 1971). As the distance from the endplate and correspondingly the time between the incident and reflected shocks increased, the lethal peak reflected overpressure rose to about 1.8 times that for classical free-field blast-wave. The critical time delay for increased tolerance varied with species size. It is approximately 0.13 ms for rats and 1 ms for sheep.

The protective effects of 'long-duration' pressure loading was also demonstrated by pressurizing animals to increasingly higher ambient pressure levels before exposure to blast (Damon *et al.*, 1966). Resistance to blast injury increased with the ambient pressure.

Firing from an enclosure

The results of a study conducted in 1976 suggested there was a significant risk of non-auditory injury associated with firing large calibre weapons from within enclosures (Clemedson and Jonsson, 1976a,b). Rabbits were exposed from one to three times to reverberant pressure waves at various locations inside a nearly closed room. The approximately 500-ms duration waves were generated by firing the Carl-Gustaf recoilless gun (Clemedson and Jonsson, 1976a,b). The interval between shots for the animals that were repeatedly exposed was 1 minute. Nearly 35% sustained moderate to severe injuries from peak overpressures that never exceeded 5.8 psi (40 kPa). This pressure level is about one-fifth that required to produce the same level of injury in rabbits exposed to free-field blast-waves (Richmond *et al.*, 1966). Frequency analysis of the waveforms at the various locations suggests that the more severely injured animals were exposed to waveforms with the strongest pressure components in the 150–500 Hz range, which matches the natural frequency of the rabbit thoracicoabdominal complex (Clemedson and Pettersson, 1956; Clemedson and Jonsson, 1964; von Gierke, 1964). The authors suggest that the first 50 ms of exposure to such a waveform would be enough to excite resonance and thereby enhance injury (Clemedson and Jonsson, 1976a).

In experiments investigating tolerance to dual blast loadings at the author's laboratory, sheep were exposed to blasts from two 8-lb charges. The intervals between blasts were varied from 0 to 14 ms in 2-ms increments. Lung haemorrhage did not change significantly as a function of the time between blasts. Results from another series of tests suggested that lung haemorrhage might be more severe when the interval between blasts was 9.6 ms and less severe when it was 3.7 ms.

Explosions in an enclosure

Direct blast effects produced by shaped charge warheads and by detonating bare explosive charges inside enclosures have been the subject of recent investigations by the author of this chapter. The LAW, DRAGON and TOW warheads have been fired through various thicknesses of armour into enclosures, and 0.125-, 0.25-, 0.50-, 1.0- and 3.0-lb charges have been detonated in the centres of four different enclosure volumes of 194, 200, 300, and 640 ft^3 each. Injuries sustained by sheep placed at various locations in these volumes were evaluated in terms of existing damage risk criteria (Bowen *et al.*, 1968; Richmond *et al.*, 1986) and enclosure volume. Attempts were made to correlate the injuries produced with the mean overpressure predicted for a given charge weight and chamber volume (Weibull, 1968), the 'effective peak' overpressure obtained by curve smoothing of the complex wave, or the summated impulse of the first few milliseconds of the waveform. The results of these various methods were plotted against the damage risk criteria iso-damage curves. Even though no definitive conclusions could be drawn, the data obtained suggest that:

1. Of the damage correlates examined, the effective peak overpressure appears to be most effective in relating injury levels to the iso-damage curves.
2. The frequency content of a complex blast-wave is important in determining the extent of injury because animals at different ranges from a detonation in a given enclosure tend to sustain equivalent damage.
3. For a given charge weight detonated in the centre of an enclosure, the response of a subject near a wall varies with the volume of the enclosure.
4. Subjects in corners sustained more severe injuries than subjects along a wall at the same distance.

Theoretical aspects

The response of a mammal to classical blast-waves is dependent upon the overpressure impulse and/or direct transmission of the shock into the body, given that the wave duration is short compared to the natural period of the subject. The compressive effects of overpressure become important if the wave duration is long compared to the natural period (Schardin, 1950). Reported critical natural resonant frequencies for man are between 40 and 60 Hz (von Gierke, 1964, 1968). The gross response of the thoracoabdominal system can be characterized as an implosion process during which the chest wall is accelerated inward during the initial blast loading of the subject (Clemedson and Jonsson, 1964; Bowen *et al.*, 1965, 1966; White and Richmond, 1960). Intrapulmonary pressure will increase, and this dissipates the momentum gained by the acceleration of the chest wall. The maximum pressure in the lungs can reach values several times higher than the loading pressure because of lung inertial effects (Figure 16.15) (Clemedson and Jonsson, 1976b).

With short-duration waves, the chest wall undergoes severe acceleration but travels only a short distance before the impulse load is relieved. With long-duration waves, the maximum intrathoracic pressure (ITP) is reached while the load is still being applied. It then tends to oscillate about the mean value of the loading pressure. In this case, the maximum pressure of the wave engulfing the animal and the damping rate of the thoracic system determine the amplitude of the ITP (Schardin, 1950).

The dynamic reactions of the thoracoabdominal system can be described by mathematical models. Model studies have been conducted with various species of mammals by assigning values to mass density, bulk modulus and shear modulus con-

stants for different tissues and organs. These studies have shown that increases in the mass or area of the thorax increase the injury response to blast loading from long-duration waves. Increases in lung volume or tissue resistance decrease the injury; the effective area of the airways or the stiffness of the rib cage have little effect on blast response, and it has also established that the abdomen exerts little if any influence on intrathoracic response, because the motion of the abdomen is much slower than that of the chest wall during blast loading (Holladay and Bowen, 1963; Bowen *et al.*, 1965, 1966; Fletcher, 1970; Stuhmiller, 1988). The resonant frequency of the abdomen is only about 1/20 of that of the chest (von Gierke, 1964, 1968).

The air in the lungs acts as a nonlinear spring. For long-duration waves, the intensity of the blast load affects the response time or time-to-peak internal pressure (T_p). The larger the blast load the shorter the response time and the higher the peak intrapulmonary pressure and injury potential.

The T_p is related to the mass of the animal and can be expressed as $T_p = 0.6 \, m^{1/3} \, (12/P_0)^{1/2}$, where m is the mass in kilograms and the term $(12/P_0)^{1/2}$ corrects for the local ambient pressure. With classical pressure waves, it has been demonstrated empirically in several species of animals that the partial impulse (I_p) in the portion of the incident wave occurring before the time, T_p, can be correlated with injury production (Bowen *et al.*, 1968).

Lung injury resulting from exposure to rapidly decaying short-duration waves with spatial lengths less than a body width is frequently localized on the side facing the oncoming wave. This effect is probably related in part to the low speed of sound through lung tissue. Reported speed of sound measurements for inflated rabbit and calf lungs range from 10 to 30 m/s (Clemedson and Jonsson, 1962), while a value of 30 m/sec has been predicted for sheep lungs (Stuhmiller, 1988). Some recent work supports the idea that most of the lung injury produced from short-duration blast loading is from direct transmission of stress waves into the lung while direct compression and/or shear contributes little to the mechanism of injury production (Cooper *et al.*, 1989; Bell *et al.*, 1990).

The dynamic pressure variations which occur in the lungs during exposure to complex blast-waves probably differ sufficiently from those described for classical waves that the criteria that have been established for estimating man's tolerance to air blast could be adjusted downward. The results from one study suggest that a reduction in tolerance levels of up to 25% would be reasonable (Clemedson and Jonsson, 1976a). Attempts have been made to develop an analytical method to relate the response of a thorax loaded by a complex blast-wave to that obtained from exposure to a classical blast-wave (Josephson and Tomlinson,

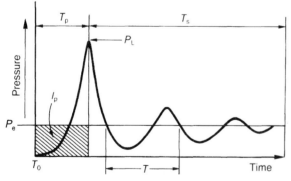

P_e = effective pressure against the chest from time T_0
T_p = time to first peak pressure P_L in the lung
I_p = partial impulse transferred to the chest for the time T_p
P_L = maximum pressure in the lung during the entire process
T = period of oscillation
T_s = time from the first peak pressure until the pressure waves cease

Figure 16.15 Intrathoracic pressure–time pattern resulting from exposure to a short-duration classical wave. (Reproduced from Clemedson and Jonsson, 1976b.)

1988; Axelsson and Richmond, 1989), using either a one-lung or two-lung model previously developed for evaluating the response to classical waveforms (Holladay and Bowen, 1963; Bowen et al., 1965, 1966; Fletcher, 1970). Intrathoracic pressure and the effect of the frequency content of the complex wave on internal pressure as well as chest wall velocity and acceleration, were evaluated as indicators of injury. Both studies concluded that the models could be used to correlate the injury potential of complex blast-waves with the injury potential for classical waves, and that the frequency content of a complex wave is extremely important in determining the risk of injury.

More recent studies indicate that there is a good correlation between injury and calculated chest wall velocities, using a single degree of freedom mathematical model, for sheep exposed to complex blast-waves (Axelsson and Yelverton, 1966; Yelverton, Johnson, Axelsson, 1996). A good correlation was also demonstrated between these findings and the previously established injury prediction curve (Bowen et al., 1968).

REFERENCES

Axelsson H., Richmond D.R. (1989). The Non-auditory Effects of Complex Blast Waves on Personnel Inside an APC Attacked by Shaped Charge Warheads. FOA Report, C 20773–2.3 Sweden: National Defence Research Establishment.

Axelsson H., Yelverton J.T. (1996). Chest Wall Velocity as a Predictor of Nonauditory Blast Injury in a Complex wave Environment. *The Journal of Trauma: Injury, Infection, and Critical Care,* **40**, (35), 51–7.

Bell S.J., Iremonger M.J., Smith P.D. (1990). A Shock tube simulation of personnel blast protection. In *Proceedings of the Eleventh International Symposium on Military Applications of Blast Simulations (MABS 11). Albuquerque, NM, 10–15 September,* pp. 713–22.

Benzinger T. (1950). Physiological effects of blast in air and water. In *German Aviation Medicine, World War II,* vol. 2. Washington, DC: US Government Printing Office, pp. 1225–59.

Blacksten H.R., Schecter G. (1979). *Wall Breaching Devices/ Concepts Technologies,* KFR254–79, US. Naval Surface Weapons Center, Contract No. N60921–79-C-A118. Submitted by Ketron Inc., Arlington, VA, December.

Bowen, I.G., Holladay, A., Fletcher E.R., Richmond, D.R., White C.S. (1965). *A fluid-Mechanical Model of the Thoraco-Abdominal System with Applications to Blast Biology.* Technical Progress Report, DASA-1675. Washington, DC: Defense Atomic Support Agency, Department of Defense, June.

Bowen I.G., Fletcher E.R., Richmond D.R. et al. (1966). *Biophysical Mechanisms and Scaling Procedures Applicable in Assessing Responses of the Thorax Energized by Air-Blast Overpressures or by Nonpenetrating Missiles.* Technical Progress Report, DASA-1857. Washington, DC: Defense Atomic Support Agency, Department of Defense, November. (Also in *Ann. N.Y. Acad. Sci. 152* (Art. 1): 122–46, 1968.)

Bowen I.G., Fletcher E.R., Richmond D.R. (1968). *Estimate of Man's Tolerance to the Direct Effects of Blast.* Technical Progress Report No. DASA–2113. Washington, DC: Defense Atomic Support Agency, Department of Defense.

Cameron G.R., Short R.H.D., Wakely C.P.G. (1943). Pathological changes produced in animals by depth charges. *Br. J. Surg.,* **30**, (117–20), 49–64.

Cameron G.R., Short R.H.D., Wakely C.P.G. (1944). Abdominal injuries due to under water explosion. *Br. J. Surg.,* **31**, (121–4), 51–66.

Chiffelle T.L. (1966) *Pathology of Direct Air Blast Injury,* Technical Report No. DASA-1778. Washington, DC: Defense Atomic Support Agency, Department of Defense, April.

Clare V.R., Richmond D.R., Goldizen V.C., Fischer C.G., Pratt D.E., Gaylord C.S., White G.S. et al. (1962). *The Effects of Shock Tube Generated, Step-Rising Overpressures on Guinea Pigs Located in Shallow Chambers Oriented Side-On and End-On to the incident Shock.* Technical Progress Report No. DASA-1312. Washington, DC: Department of Defense, Defense Atomic Support Agency.

Clemedson C-J. (1948). On Undervattensdetonations-Skador. *Sartryck ur Tidskrift I Militar Halsovard, Arg.,* **73**.

Clemedson C-J. (1956). Blast injury. *Physiol. Rev.,* **36** 336–54.

Clemedson C-J., Jonsson A. (1962) Distribution of extra- and intrathoracic pressure variations in rabbits exposed to air shock waves. *Acta Physiol. Scand.,* **54**, 18–29.

Clemedson C-J., Jonsson A. (1964). Dynamic response of chest wall and lung injuries in rabbits exposed to air shock waves of short duration. *Acta Physiol. Scand.,* **62**, (suppl. 233).

Clemedson, C-J., Jonsson A. (1976a). Effects of the frequency content in complex shock waves on lung injuries in rabbits. *Aviat. Space Environ. Med.,* **47**, 1143–52.

Clemedson, C-J., Jonsson A. (1976b). Determination of serious health risks to personnel as a result of the firing of recoilless weapons in a confined space. *Forsvarets Forskningsanstalt,* FOA Report Stockholm, Sweden, 141 pp.

Clemedson C-J., Pettersson H. (1956). Propagation of a high-explosive air shock wave through different parts of an animal body. *Am. J. Physiol.,* **184**, 119–26.

Clifford C.B., Jaegar J.J., Moe J.B. et al. (1984). Gastrointestinal lesions in lambs due to multiple low-level blast overpressure exposure. *Milit. Med.,* **149**, 491–5.

Cooper G.J., Pearce B.P., Cater S.R., Kenword C.E. et al. (1989). Augmentation by foam materials of lung injury produced by blast waves – the role of stress waves in thoracic visceral injury at high rates of energy transfer. In *Proceedings of the International Research Council of the Biokinetics of Impacts (IRCOBI), Stockholm, Sweden,* 13–15 September.

Cooper P. (1989). Effects of surfaces adjacent to explosions. Presented at *First EG&G International Blast Biology Meeting,* Boston, Mass., 15–16 June.

Corey E.L. (1946). Medical aspects of blast. *US Naval Med. Bull.,* **46**, 623–52.

Damon E.G., Gaylord C.S., Hicks W. et al. (1966a). *The Effects of Ambient Pressure on Tolerance of Mammals to Air Blast.* Technical Progress Report No. DASA-1852. Washington, DC: Department of Defense, Defense Atomic Support Agency.

Damon E.G., Gaylord C.S., Yelverton J.T. et al. (1966b). *The Tolerance of Cattle to 'Long'-Duration Reflected Pressures in a Shock Tube*, Technical Progress Reports No. 1855. Washington, DC: Department of Defense, Defense Atomic Support Agency.

Dancer A., Parmentier G., Vassout P. (1981). *Etude des Effets D'une Onde de Choc Forte Sur le Porc, Influence du Nombre D'Expositions*; Rapport S-R 904/81. Saint-Louis, France: Franco-German Institut.

Desaga H. (1950). Blast injuries. In *German Aviation Medicine, World War II*, vol. 2. Washington, DC: US Government Printing Office, pp. 1274–93.

Dodd K.T., Yelverton J.T., Richmond D.R. et al. (1990). The non-auditory injury threshold for repeated intense freefield noise. *J. Occup. Med.*, **32**, 260–6.

Finney D.J. (1964). *Probit Analysis. A Statistical Treatment of the Sigmoid Response Curve*. Cambridge: Cambridge University Press.

Fletcher E.R. (1970). A model to simulate thoracic response to air blast and to impact. In *Symposium on Biodynamic Models and Their Applications*, Report No. AMRL-TR-71–29. Ohio Aerospace Medical Research Laboratory, Aerospace Medical Division, Air Force Systems Command, Wright-Patterson Air Force Base, pp. 27–70.

Froboese M., Wunsche O. (1959). *Todlichkeitsgrenzen fur Albinoratten bei Luftstossbelastung in Abhangigkeit von der Strossrichtung und Druckverlaufsform*, Rapport Bericht, Band I: Text 2/59. St. Louis, France: French-German Research Institute.

Glasstone S. (1957). *The Effects of Nuclear Weapons*. Prepared by the Department of Defense. Washington, DC: United States Atomic Energy Commission, US Government Printing Office, 730 pp.

Goligher J.C., King D.P., Simmons H.T. (1943). Injuries produced by blast in water. *Lancet*, 119–23. **ii**.

Holladay A.E., Bowen I.G. (1963). A mathematical model of the lung for studies of mechanical stress. In *Proceedings of the San Diego Symposium for Biomedical Engineering*, pp. 39–50.

Jonsson A. (1979). *Experimental Investigations on the Mechanisms of Lung Injury in Blast and Impact Exposure*, Linkoping University Medical Dissertation No. 80. Stockholm: Department of Surgery, Linkoping University and National Defence Research Institute.

Josephson, L.H., Tomlinson P. (1988). Predicted thoraco-abdominal response to complex blast wave. *J. Trauma*, **28**, (Suppl. 1), S116–24.

Kolder H.J., Stockinger L. (1957). Feinstrukturelle Veranderungen in der Lunge nach Explosiver Dekompression and Kompression. *Arch. Exp. Pathal. Pharmakol.*, **32**, 23–33.

Moe B., Clifford C.B., Sharpnack D.D. (1987). Effects of blast waves on nonauditory epithelial tissues. In *Basic and Applied Aspects of Noise-Induced Hearing Loss* (Salvi R.J. eds). New York: Plenum Press, 73–85.

Richmond, D.R. (1961). *Notes of the Canadian Biomedical Experiments Carried Out in Conjunction with the 100-Ton Explosion at Suffield Experimental Station Near Ralston, Alberta, Canada*, Technical Progress Report No. DASA-1261. Washington, DC: Department of Defense, Defense Nuclear Agency.

Richmond D.R. (1971). Blast protection afforded by foxholes and bunkers. In *Probleme Des Baulichen Schutzes Kolloquiem beim Schutzkommission beim Bundesministerium des Innern, in Weil/Rhein*, June, pp. 9–36.

Richmond D.R., Fletcher E.R. (1970). The effects of air blast on sheep in two-man foxholes – Project LN401. In *Operation Prairie Flat Symposium Report*, Vol. 1 – Part II, 420–441 DASA–2377–1 (DASIAC SR-92). Santa Barbara, CA: DASA Information and Analysis Center, January.

Richmond D.R., White C.S. (1962). A tentative Estimation of man's tolerance to overpressures from air blast. In *Proceedings of the Symposium on Effectiveness Analysis Techniques for Non-Nuclear Warheads Against Surface Targets, October 30–31, 1962*, Vol. 1: L-L-34. Dahlgren, VA: US Naval Weapons Laboratory. (Also in Technical Report No. DASA-1335. Washington, DC: Department of Defense, Defense Atomic Support Agency.)

Richmond D.R., Kilgore D.E. (1970). Blast effects inside structures. In *Proceedings of the Second Conference on Military Applications of Blast Simulators, November 2–5, 1970*, Dahlgren, VA. pp. 781–804. (Also in Technical Report No. DNA-2775P. Washington, DC: Department of Defense, Defense Nuclear Agency. 1972.)

Richmond D.R., Taborelli R.U., Bowen I.G., Chiffelle T.L., Hirsch F.G., Longwell B.B., Riley J.G., White C.S. et al. (1959). *Blast Biology – A Study of the Primary and Tertiary Effects of Blast in Open Underground Protective Shelters*, USAEC Civil Effects Test Group Report, WT-1467. Washington, DC: Office of Technical Services, Department of Commerce, 30 June.

Richmond D.R., Damon E.G., Bowen, I.G. et al. (1966). *Air-Blast Studies with Eight Species of Mammals*, Technical Progress Report No. DASA-1854. Washington, DC: Department of Defense, Defense Atomic Support Agency.

Richmond D.R., Damon E.G., Fletcher E.R., Bowen I.G., White C.S. et al. (1968). The relationship between selected blast wave parameters and the response of mammals exposed to air blast. *Ann. N.Y. Acad. Sci.*, **152**, 103–21. Also Technical Progress Report DASA 1860. Washington DC: Department of Defense, Defense Nuclear Agency.

Richmond, D.R., Fletcher E.R., Jones R.K. (1971). *The Effects of Airblast on Sheep in Two-Man Foxholes*, Technical Progress Report No. DASA-2711. Washington. DC: Department of Defense, Defense Nuclear Agency.

Richmond, D.R., Fletcher E.R., Saunders K. et al. (1980). *Injuries Produced by the Propagation of Airblast Waves Through Orifices*, Topical Report No. DNA-5618T. Washington, DC: Defense Nuclear Agency, March.

Richmond, D.R., Yelverton J.T., Fletcher E.R., Phillips Y.Y. et al. (1985). Biologic response to complex blast waves. In *Proceedings of the Ninth International Symposium Military Applications of Blast Simulations (MABS 9), Oxford, England*, Paper No VII. 7. PP. VII. 7.1 to VII. 7.20. Foulness, Southend-on-Sea, Essex: Atomic Weapons Establishment, September.

Richmond D.R., Yelverton J.T., Fletcher E.R. (1989). New airblast criteria for man. Presented at the *Twenty-Second DoD Explosives Safety Seminar, Anaheim, CA, 26–28 August 1986*.

Richmond, D.R., Yelverton J.T., Fletcher E.R. et al. (1989). Physical correlates of eardrum rupture. *Ann. Otol., Rhinol. Laryngol.*, **98** (No. 5, Part 2, S140), 35–41.

Rossle R. (1950). Pathology of blast injuries. In *German Aviation Medicine, World War II*, Vol. 2. Washington, DC: US Government Printing Office, pp. 1260–73.

Schardin, H. (1950). The physical principles of the effects

of a detonation. In *German Aviation Medicine, World War II*, Vol. 2. Washington, DC: US Government Printing Office, pp. 1207–24.

Sewell G.S., Kinney G.F., Sinclair J.E. (1972). Internal Explosions in vented and unvented chambers. In *Minutes Fourteenth Annual Explosives Safety Seminar, Marriott Hotel, New Orleans*, Vol. 1. Washington, DC: Department of Defense Explosives Safety Board, pp. 87–98.

Stuhmiller J.H., Chuong C.J., Phillips Y.Y., Dodd K.T. (1988). Computer modeling of thoracic response to blast. *J. Trauma*, **28** (Suppl. 1). S132–9.

Taylor W.J. (1968). Blast behavior in confined regions. *Ann. N.Y. Acad. Sci.*, **152**, (Art. 1), 339–56.

Vassout P., Parmentier G., Dancer A. (1978). *Influence due Nombre D'Expositions a unde de Choc Forte sur les Lesions Pulmonaires et les Taux de Mortalite Chex le Rat*, Saint-Louis, France: Rapport Bericht Institute Franco-Allemand de Recerches de Saint Louis.

Von Gierke H.E. (1964). Biodynamic response of the human body. *Appl. Mech. Rev.*, **17**, 951–8.

Von Gierke, H.E. (1968). Response of the body to mechanical forces and overview. *Ann. N.Y. Acad. Sci.*, **152** (Art. 1) 172–86.

Wakely C.P.G. (1945). Effect of underwater explosions on the human body. *Lancet*, **i**, 715–18.

Weibull H.R.W. (1968). Pressures recorded in partially closed chambers at explosion of TNT charges. *Ann. N.Y. Acad. Sci.*, **152** (Art. 1) 357–61.

White C.S., Richmond D.R. (1960). Blast biology. In *Clinical Cardiopulmonary Physiology* (Gordon B.L., Kory R.C., eds). New York: Grune and Stratton, pp. 974–92.

White C.S., Chiffelle T.L., Richmond O.R., Lockyear W.H., Bowen I.G., Goldizen V.C., Meredith H.W. et al. (1957). *Biological Effects of Pressure Phenomena Occurring Inside Protective Shelters Following Nuclear Detonation*, USAEC Civil Effects Test Group Report, WT-1179, Office of Technical Services. Washington, DC: Department of Commerce, October.

White C.S., Jones R.F., Damon E.G. et al. (1971). *The Biodynamics of Air Blast*, Technical Progress Report, DNA 2738T. Washington, DC: Defense Nuclear Agency, July.

Williams E.R.P. (1943). Blast effects in warfare. *Br. J. Surg.*, **30**, (117–120), 38–49.

Yelverton J.T., Richmond D.R., Fletcher E.R.et al. (1983). Bioeffects of simulated muzzle blasts. In *Proceedings MABS-8, Eighth International Symposium on Military Application of Blast Simulation, Spiez, Switzerland*, pp. VI. 6–6 VI. 6–25, 20–24 June.

Yelverton J.T., Johnson O.L., Axelsson H. (1996). Review of Nonauditory Effects of Blast overpressure. In *Scientific Basis of Noise-Induced Hearing Loss*, Chapter 36, pp. 447–61. (Axelsson A., Borchgrevink H.M., Hamernik R.P., Hellström P.A., Henderson O., Salvi R.J., eds) New York: Thieme Medical Publishers, Inc.

Zalewski T. (1906). Experimentelle Untersuchungen uber die Resistenzfahigkeit des Trommelfells. *Z. Ohrenheilkd.*, **52**, 109–28.

Zuckerman S. (1940). Experimental study of blast injuries to the lungs. ii, *Lancet*, 219–35.

17. Blast Injury of the Lung

R. L. Maynard, D. L. Coppel and K. G. Lowry

INTRODUCTION

In a detailed survey of early work on the effects of blast-waves on the lungs, Clemedson (1949) cites a report of Jars in 1768 that suggested that the death of a miner in an explosion was caused by 'la grande et prompte dilatation d'air'.

The specific pulmonary effects of blast were first noted in the late nineteenth century. Experimental work on the effects of blast was undertaken by Hooker (1924) in an attempt to clarify the syndrome of 'shell shock' reported extensively during the First World War. Confusion had arisen during this war regarding the physical and psychological effects of shelling and exposure to blast, and this had caused a variety of similar terms to be invented (Clemedson, 1949). The confusion has persisted.

Shell shock, shock lung and blast lung are commonly used terms but they describe very different clinical entities. Blast lung (Williams, 1942), blast chest (Thomas, 1941) and pulmonary concussion (Osborn, 1941) are synonymous. It should be noted that although the blast-wave produced by explosions plays a key part in producing the primary injury, the term 'shock lung' conventionally relates to the effects of hypovolaemic and other types of shock, for example septic shock, upon the lung. It is synonymous with post-traumatic pulmonary insufficiency (PTPI) and the adult respiratory distress syndrome (ARDS) (Moore *et al.* 1969; Blaisdell and Lewis, 1979). The injuries in the lung exposed to blast closely resemble those seen in pulmonary contusion and the term 'blast contusion', indicating both the pathological mechanism and the consequences, might be adopted as more helpful than some of those listed above.

In terms of the distribution of lesions, blast-induced lung injury differs from contusions induced by blunt impacts upon the chest, but in terms of pathophysiological changes the two types of injury are similar.

Patients suffering from blast lung and those suffering from impact-induced pulmonary contusions are often found to have sustained other serious injuries. The pulmonary injuries, combined with the effects of the intravenous administration of fluids and the reduced capacity of the damaged lung to resist bacterial invasion, may lead to deterioration in lung function and a clinical picture which is indistinguishable from ARDS. This deteriorating state is due only in part to the primary blast-induced damage to the lung.

In addition to the effects of explosions upon the lung, several authors have examined the changes in respiratory function which commonly follow such injuries and have attributed these to the consequences of blast upon the central nervous system. Neurogenic pulmonary oedema has been described and suggested to be related to a change in the functioning of the autonomic nervous system (Cassen and Kistler, 1954).

Changes in the functioning of the respiratory and cardiovascular systems after exposure to blast have been attributed by some to the effects of air emboli (Clemedson and Hultman, 1954).

BLAST LUNG

Blast lung is a term used to describe the direct damage to the lung produced by the interaction with the body of the blast-wave generated by an explosion. The blast-wave comprises the shock front, and the dynamic overpressures (blast wind) resulting from motion of the air and combustion products. Injuries produced by the latter and those produced by the casualty being thrown by the blast wind against a hard surface are not included in this classification, though they may have pulmonary consequences. Blast lung is produced principally by the interaction of the shock-wave with the thorax.

It is accepted that the damage may increase in severity in the period immediately following the initial exposure. The pulmonary effects of distant lesions which produce, for example, fat emboli or lead to septicaemia are excluded by this term. Also excluded are the effects on the damaged lung of the inappropriate administration of intravenous fluids.

This limited definition allows a more precise and consistent description of changes, particularly pathophysiological ones. Considerable difficulties are experienced in distinguishing between the direct effects of the blast or shock-wave and the crush or displacement injury arising from the effects of the blast wind. In some of the early experimental work on blast this distinction was not recognized and all effects were ascribed to the 'blast'. The distinction will be reviewed later.

The first detailed experimental investigation of the effects of blast upon the body was undertaken by Hooker (1924). Since his work, comparatively few groups have examined the effects of blast in detail.

The major historical landmarks of experimental investigations of the effects of blast-waves upon the body are given below:

1. Work done during the Second World War in the UK on the pathology and pathophysiology of

blast injury (Zuckerman, 1940, 1941; Krohn *et al.*, 1942) identified the critical importance of lung damage as a cause of death in blast injuries. At the same time, important contributions were made by Wilson and Tunbridge (1943), Tunbridge and Wilson (1943) and by Hadfield (1941).

2. German investigation during the Second World War (Benzinger, 1950; Rossle, 1950).

3. Swedish studies after the Second World War in the 1940s and 1950s (Clemedson, 1949; Clemedson and Hultman, 1954; Clemedson, 1956). Clemedson's reviews of 1949 and 1956 should be consulted for further guidance to the literature.

4. Wide-ranging investigations at the Lovelace Foundation for Medical Education and Research, Albuquerque during the 1950s, 1960s and 1970s. A large series of reports dealing with many aspects of blast injury were produced, culminating in prediction of human susceptibility to blast lung expressed in terms of peak overpressure and overpressure duration (see Chapter 16). Two papers relating particularly to lung injury are important sources of information (Chiffelle, 1966; Richmond and White, 1966).

5. Underwater blast research at the Admiralty Marine Technology Establishment (AMTE) during and after the Second World War. The work was reported in a long series of official reports, concluding in an invaluable compilation and bibliography (Bebb *et al.*, 1981).

This list of research efforts is not exhaustive but the references provided will allow interested readers to follow the major advances and disagreements in the area. More modern research is addressed by other chapters in this volume.

Despite the considerable amount of work done on the pathological effects of blast upon the lung, the mechanism by which blast-waves of different duration interact with the thorax and lung to produce pulmonary damage is not fully defined. Chapters 16 and 19–21 discuss this further.

Action of blast-waves upon the lung

During the First World War, it was known that explosions could rupture the eardrum and throw casualties violently to the ground, but the mechanism by which blast could interact with internal organs was not understood. Reports of casualties succumbing to the effects of explosions during the Spanish Civil War had placed great emphasis on the observation that death could occur without leaving external signs of injury (Haldane, 1938). In these reports, the distance at which blast alone could kill was probably exaggerated.

In 1940 Zuckerman listed three possible mechanisms to explain the production of lesions in the lung:

1. A lowering of the intra-alveolar pressure as a result of the subatmospheric component of a blast-wave which follows the initial overpressure. The reduction in pressure could act via the airways and produce sudden expansion and rupture of the capillaries of the alveolar walls (Logan, 1939).

2. Distension of the lungs by air being forced down the airways by the fast rise in overpressure produced by the blast (J. Barcroft, 1941, unpublished work).

3. Direct impact of the blast-wave upon the chest wall leading to a sudden compression of the chest and contusion of the lung. This was the view advanced by Hooker (1924), who suggested that the air might not be expelled from the lung during the rapid thoracic compression.

Zuckerman (1940) discredited the concepts of overexpansion (1) and movement of air down the trachea (2). In a series of studies using rabbits, he demonstrated that protection of the animal's chest with a steel cylinder, whilst leaving the head exposed and the airway open, prevented the lung being damaged by blast of an intensity which, in unprotected animals, produced severe damage and death. He also pointed out that whether the glottis was open or closed could have made little difference to the outcome, as the duration of ambient pressure elevation was so short that no mass movement of air via the trachea would occur.

However, some support for the theory that subatmospheric pressure effects were important has been provided by other experiments on mice which showed that rapid decompression could produce lung damage (Latner, 1942; Topliff, 1976). It was further suggested from these studies that the uniform expansion of the lungs produced by the subatmospheric pressure phase of a blast-wave could explain the rather uniform distribution of haemorrhage sometimes seen in blast lung (see below). However, the Lovelace Foundation showed that lesions may be produced by long-duration, slowly declining, overpressures within shock tubes that do not have a subatmospheric phase. Latner's original suggestion that the subatmospheric phase could increase the severity of the damage produced by the positive wave has not been disproven but the extent of the contribution to lung injury made by the subatmospheric pressure wave is not considered to be significant.

Two of the observations made by Zuckerman supported the theory that lung damage was produced by the direct impact of the blast-wave upon the body – blast contusions were often largely confined to the lung facing the blast, and 'rib markings' were frequently present on the injured lung.

Zuckerman exposed animals to blast produced by the detonation of balloons filled with hydrogen and oxygen. The records of blast overpressure resembled those obtained close to explosions of high explosive, though the rise time of the shock-wave was longer in the balloon studies. When animals were placed very close to the explosion, lung lesions were severe and tended to be most marked on the side facing the blast. At greater distances, lesions were less severe but were more evenly distributed throughout both lungs. It was concluded that the predominantly unilateral lesions provided further evidence to suggest that damage could not be dependent upon the sudden inflow of air via the trachea – if this had occurred, the lesions would be bilateral. It was also observed that the mainly unilateral lesions could be reduced by protecting the side of the animal facing the explosion with a suitable layer of sponge rubber. In contrast, recent work by Jonsson (1979) and Cooper et al. (1991) has shown that various foamed materials placed upon the chest wall can make lesions produced by exposure to blast more severe (see Chapter 21).

Zuckerman's observations supported the theory that impact of the blast upon the body was responsible for the lung damage, but failed to explain why bilateral lesions were produced when the animals were placed at greater distance from the explosion.

In the studies described above, the presence of 'rib markings' on the pleural surfaces of the lungs was noted. These lesions were interpreted as further evidence of the impact of blast upon the chest wall. The supposition was that the ribs had been driven forcibly inwards and had damaged the lung.

Rib markings have been described by many other workers, including Chiffelle (1966) who reported that they could be found on the surfaces of both lungs and also on those parts of the lung in contact with other comparatively hard structures such as the vertebral column and the heart. It is particularly interesting to note that in Chiffelle's illustration of rib markings they are most marked on the posterior surface of the less damaged of the two lungs. It has been clearly demonstrated that the so-called rib markings were more closely related to the intercostal spaces than the ribs (Greaves et al., 1943; Clemedson, 1949; Bebb et al., 1981). Clemedson injected Indian ink into the superficial parts of the lung via the intercostal spaces and found that the ink clearly marked the lines of haemorrhage on the surfaces of the lungs. Wright showed that if small segments of rib were resected, bridges of haemorrhage linked the linear ones in the intercostal spaces (quoted by Bebb et al., 1981).

In Clemedson's studies, the linear haemorrhages were most commonly seen on the surface of the lung most distant from the explosion. He argued that a compression wave passing through the body would attain a greater velocity through bone (rib) than through the soft tissues of the intercostal space and that the difference in velocity would account for the damage to the lung adjacent to the intercostal space.

Bebb concluded that the true rib markings described by Zuckerman were produced as a result of the impact of the blast wind upon the chest and were therefore understandably more marked on the side facing the explosion. In a later publication, Zuckerman reported that 'in lesser degrees of injury the lines of haemorrhage followed the lines of the spaces between the ribs' (Zuckerman, 1952). In this account the transmission of energy through the body was referred to: 'and in the boundary zones between tissues and air, and thus between media of acoustically different properties, the tissues are torn'.

Local forces in the lung

The discussion so far has outlined the interaction of blast with the thoracic cavity. At the level of the lung parenchyma there are three favoured hypotheses for the damage to lung tissue:

1. Damage to epithelial surfaces within the lungs as a result of a stress wave passing through the parenchyma and encountering interfaces of different density. The phenomena of 'spalling' or 'scabbing' may occur.
2. The transmission of pressure pulses and subsequent flow of blood from the great vessels of the abdomen to the pulmonary vessels leading to rupture of pulmonary capillaries. This theory was developed by The Lovelace Foundation workers and has been outlined by Chiffelle (1966).
3. Compression and subsequent violent re-expansion of small air spaces in the lung as a result of the passage of the shock-wave.

Mechanism (1) is founded on the principle that when a stress wave encounters an interface between media of differing acoustic impedance (the product of density and the speed of sound in the material), some of the energy of the wave is reflected from the surface and a proportion is coupled through the surface into the second medium. The distribution between reflected and coupled stress depends on the relative acoustic impedances of the materials. When a stress wave passes from a dense to a less dense medium the incident stress wave is reflected as a tensile wave. Tensile forces at the interface could damage the epithelium. As a shock-wave passes through the lung it encounters a series of tissue/air and air/tissue interfaces, and on each occasion when the wave leaves tissue and enters air these tensile forces may occur. The forces produced will be dependent upon the magnitude of the stress wave. To what extent these forces at tissue/air interfaces explain the damage produced in the lung by blast-waves is unknown; recent work discussed by Cooper (outlined in Chapter 21) has suggested that the *rate* of rise of the stress wave is a major determinant of the forces across the interface, and thus the severity of haemorrhagic contamination.

The theory (2) above (Richmond and White, 1966) rested upon an analysis of the behaviour of a model of the thorax and abdomen when exposed to shock-waves of differing characteristics. In the model, the thorax contained both a gas phase (air spaces in the lung) and a liquid phase (blood in the pulmonary vascular system). The gas phase was connected to the exterior by the trachea. The liquid phase was connected to the abdomen which contained *only* a liquid phase.

The effects of impact of a range of different pressure waveforms upon the model were considered: the external pressure, the pressure in the gas phase and the pressure in the liquid phase being modelled.

With impact by a short-duration blast with an effectively instantaneous rise in pressure, the following consequences were predicted (Figure 17.1):

1. Deformation of the walls of the thorax.
2. A pressure pulse transmitted to the abdominal liquid phase would be transmitted to the thoracic liquid phase before the pressure had risen in the thoracic gas phase.
3. Significant gas flow down the trachea would not occur.

As a result of (2), a marked though transient pressure differential would be established across the pulmonary blood vessels, leading to their distension and rupture. The predicted pressure changes with respect to time are shown in Figure 17.1. Note that in this model, bulk flow of liquid from abdomen to thorax is not predicted, though with slower rising pressure pulses this could occur and exacerbate the damage in the pulmonary circulation.

This theory has been challenged (Bebb *et al.*, 1981). If injury were dependent upon the delay between the arrival of the shock-wave via the air route across the lung and the liquid route via the abdomen, then animals subjected to underwater

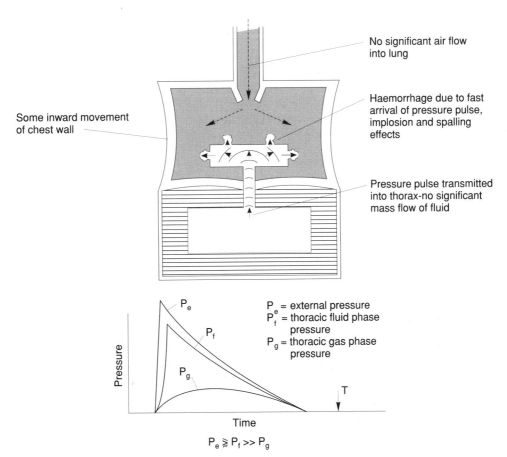

Some inward movement of chest wall

No significant air flow into lung

Haemorrhage due to fast arrival of pressure pulse, implosion and spalling effects

Pressure pulse transmitted into thorax-no significant mass flow of fluid

P_e = external pressure
P_f = thoracic fluid phase pressure
P_g = thoracic gas phase pressure

$P_e \gtrsim P_f \gg P_g$

Figure 17.1 Response of the torso to fast-rising blast overpressure. P_g = pressure in gas phase of lung; P_f = thoracic fluid pressure; P_e = external pressure. (Reproduced from Richmond and White, 1966.)

explosion and immersed completely in water should sustain less, rather than more, damage than animals immersed only to the diaphragm. Rawlins argued that:

> For since the shock wave must impinge simultaneously on the abdomen and thorax of an immersed animal, the lag time of the shock wave traversing the gaseous phase of the chest and tending to counteract the shock wave travelling in the liquid phase from the fluid compartment of the abdomen, must at least be shorter than the lag time of the airborne shock wave, if any, impinging upon the thorax of an animal immersed only to its diaphragm.

Experiments had shown that animals were invariably more severely injured when totally immersed than when immersed only to the diaphragm, and that therefore the theory was not supported.

The last hypothesis listed above, (3) suggested that implosion of alveolar spaces could play a role in the way in which shock-waves produce lung injury. It is known that when a stress wave passes through a liquid containing small gas bubbles, they are compressed. A very marked rise in the pressure and temperature in the bubble occurs and there is a subsequent forcible re-expansion. It is tempting to propose that similar phenomena occur in alveoli but the significance of this in blast-induced lung injury is unknown.

PATHOLOGICAL FEATURES OF BLAST LUNG

Accounts can be found in a wide range of papers and reports (Hooker, 1924; Falla, 1940; Zuckerman, 1940, 1941; Hadfield, 1941; Williams, 1942; Greaves et al., 1943; Wilson and Tunbridge, 1943; Savage, 1945; Clemedson, 1949; Benzinger, 1950; Rossle, 1950; Chiffelle, 1966; Coppel, 1976; Marshall, 1977; Bebb et al., 1981; Cooper et al., 1983). This list is not exhaustive and many authors who have reported single cases or series of cases of blast injury have included details of the pathological changes found at post-mortem examination.

In general terms a consistent pattern of injuries has been described, though in detail different authors have stressed different findings.

Upper respiratory tract: nasal cavity, paranasal sinuses and larynx

Comparatively little attention has been paid to this area. Zuckerman (1940) reported finding blood-stained fluid or froth in the nose, mouth and upper respiratory passages of animals exposed to blast. Close examination of the mucous membrane of the upper respiratory tract was not reported either by Zuckerman (1940, 1941) or by Tunbridge and Wilson (1943); it is therefore not possible to judge how much of the fluid had been generated by local damage. Chiffelle (1966) reported damage to the upper respiratory tract; his comments are reproduced below:

> The mucosal lining of the trachea, larynx and nasopharynx may have patchy areas of ecchymosis which, in the case of the trachea, often show a transverse linear configuration corresponding to the underlying cartilaginous rings or plates. Some focal loss of epithelial lining may be found in microscopic sections of the haemorrhagic areas, not unlike that found in the bronchi. Haemorrhage into the paranasal sinuses is another frequent finding, and splotchy areas of haemorrhage are found in the mucous lining of the nasal passages and of the turbinate bones.

Ecchymoses of the laryngeal mucous membrane have been reported by Buffe et al. (1987), who argued that the acceleration of the cartilaginous structures and their subsequent impact upon soft parts of the larynx and trachea might explain the findings.

Lungs

Macroscopic findings (Figure 17.2)
Before considering the lungs in detail, a brief description of changes produced in the chest wall and visible at post-mortem examination is warranted.

Most workers have ignored the chest wall in considering the effects of blast-waves. Chiffelle, for example, makes no mention of damage to the chest wall (Chiffelle, 1966). O'Reilly (see Zuckerman, 1941) reported a case in which extensive bruising was found in the inner surface of the chest wall and in the intercostal spaces. Zuckerman, commenting on this, observed that similar haemorrhages were sometimes seen in animals, following the course of the intercostal nerves and being continuous with the haemorrhages around the spinal roots.

Rib fractures are not common. If very severe blast loads occur, fractures in the posterior angle may be

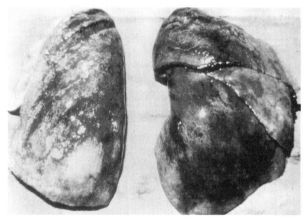

Figure 17.2 Post-mortem appearance of the lungs of a patient following a bomb explosion.

evident though blast loads of the required severity usually produce lung injury incompatible with life.

Examination of blast-damaged lungs shows areas of macroscopic haemorrhage. These may range from slight spotting of the pleural surface to confluent haemorrhages involving whole lobes or even lungs. The distribution of haemorrhage has been commented upon by many workers and a variety of deductions drawn on the likely mechanisms of injury. Zuckerman (1940, 1941) reported that very slightly damaged lesions were found just beneath the pleura. A careful post-mortem study of 30 victims reported an even distribution of small haemorrhages throughout the lungs (Savage, 1945).

Falla (1940) also drew attention to the even distribution of haemorrhages:

> The cut surfaces of the lungs were most striking, since innumerable bright red points of haemorrhage were to be seen wherever a cut was made in either lung. The condition was unlike any I have met, and may perhaps best be described as a miliary condition of unmistakable fresh haemorrhages.

Zuckerman examined histological sections from Falla's case and confirmed the latter's observations and commented that, at a microscopic level, the changes did not correspond to those seen in severe damage in experimental animals (see below).

Chiffelle (1966) reported that lesions were more marked in areas where the lung abutted upon hard structures and where pinching of the lung or stress concentration might be expected; for example, at the costo-phrenic angles. The anterior borders of the lower lobes and the azygous lobe in experimental animals were common sites of haemorrhage. Recent work by Cooper *et al.* (1991) has suggested that stress concentration of waves coupled into the thorax produces greater haemorrhagic contamination adjacent to reflecting surfaces such as the mediastinum, than in peripheral parenchyma close to the body wall (Figure 17.3) (Cooper and Taylor, 1989). Tearing of the pleura has been recorded with the formation of superficial bullae. Pneumothoraces and haemopneumothoraces have also been reported (Chiffelle, 1966).

The weight of the damaged lung is increased due both to haemorrhage and to the oedema. The increase is frequently used experimentally to grade the severity of lung injury.

Microscopic changes (Figure 17.4)
Zuckerman (1940, 1941) described areas of lung in which the alveoli and small airways were filled with blood. Disruption of the alveolar walls was often seen with bleeding from torn capillaries. In more severely damaged areas, disruption of the

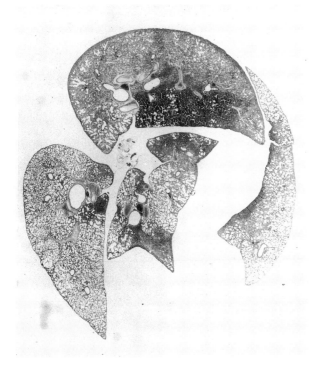

Figure 17.3 Transverse section of lung from rat exposed to blast overpressure. The blast-wave approached the lung from the top of the picture. Contusions are most severe in the lung lobe abutting the mediastinum *in vivo*.

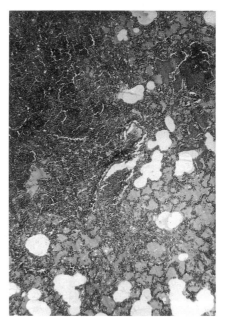

Figure 17.4 Primary blast lung. This is the periphery of an area of confluent haemorrhage. Intra-alveolar haemorrhage, blood in bronchioles, oedema and dilated alveolar ducts are evident.

normal lung architecture was observed and filling of the larger airways with blood noted. There was no mention of capillary congestion.

Hadfield (1941) drew attention to the capillary congestion which had been observed in sections of blast-damaged human lung and speculated on the source of the blood seen in the alveolar spaces. Diapedesis was suggested. Hadfield commented: 'We find it difficult to believe, having in mind the histological picture of these lungs, that the capillary rupture does account for all the capillary bleeding', and later: 'It seems to us that the major clinical manifestations are more probably due to capillary dilatation of the lung than to actual bleeding into the lung, which may be a consequence of capillary dilatation.' Congestion was also noted by Savage (1945).

Zuckerman examined histological sections from Falla's case and commented:

> Microscopically the lesions do not correspond to the severer cases seen in the experimental material . . . The lungs show signs of old bronchitis and pleural thickening; the acute changes are a fairly generalised arteriolar dilatation, and intense capillary dilatation, with exudation of fluid into many alveoli.

Widespread capillary dilatation was also reported by Wilson and Tunbridge (1943). The cause of the capillary dilatation remains unknown.

Several other histological features of blast damage of the lungs of experimental animals have been recorded (Chiffelle, 1966). A 'wide separation' of alveolar tissue from more rigid structures such as bronchovascular bundles has been described and attributed to the application of shearing forces between structures of different densities. The suggestion that the spaces could arise as a result of a sudden and violent distension of the larger pulmonary vessels was also made but seems less plausible. In experimental pulmonary contusions, one of the present authors (R.L.M.) has observed that bleeding into alveoli is often more marked in the alveoli which border secondary lobules and abut upon interlobular septae. Bleeding into perivascular and peribronchial connective tissue spaces gives rise to ring haemorrhages and can track for considerable distances along these connective tissue channels. This is also a common finding in pulmonary contusions. Dilatation of lymphatic vessels by fluid and blood has also been seen in peribronchovascular connective tissue spaces.

Damage to the bronchial wall can follow blast injury (Cameron et al., 1943; Cohen and Biskind, 1946; Rossle, 1950). Flattening, fraying and stripping of the normal ciliated epithelium have been reported, as has the loss of cilia. At more severe levels of injury considerable intramural bleeding may occur and damage to the tunica muscularis and the cartilaginous plates (tunica conjunctivo-cartilaginea) have been reported.

Air emboli may have an important role in the causation of early death in blast injury. In severe lung damage, fistulas may be seen between air spaces and thin-walled pulmonary veins.

Ultrastructural changes

There is only one reported ultrastructural study (Brown et al., 1993). Anaesthetized rats lying in the left lateral position were subjected to a blast-wave directed normally to the surface of the right chest wall. Lungs of surviving animals were examined at 30 minutes and at 24 hours postinjury. At 30 minutes, damage was limited to the right lung which showed extensive haemorrhage. The left lung was normal to macroscopic examination and showed only some congestion and minor haemorrhage on light microscopy.

On electron microscopy, an increase in endothelial and epithelial pinocytosis was noted. This change is not uncommon in the early stages of lung injury produced by a variety of insults. It may be that it reflects increased fluid transport, the hypothesis being that an initial increase in permeability and subsequent increased leakage of fluid is compensated by increased pinocytosis. An increase in the frequency of blebbing of the epithelial cell membrane and ballooning of the endothelial cell membrane was also noted (Figure 17.5). These changes may indicate intracellular oedema and a local change in membrane permeability. Such changes are infrequently seen in lungs from controls. The mechanisms underlying these changes are not understood. Cellular organelles showed no signs of damage in the blast-exposed animals or in the controls (Figure 17.6).

It would be interesting to know the effect of shock-waves upon intercellular junctions in the lung. In areas of marked damage, cells were widely

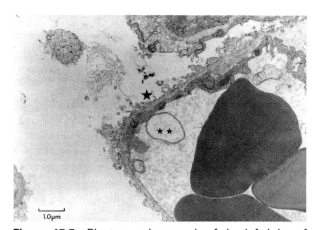

Figure 17.5 Electron micrograph of the left lobe of rat lung. The animal was killed 24 hours after blast injury to the right lateral thorax showing an area of Type I epithelial cell necrosis(*) and endothelial cell 'Ballooning'(**). (× 14 175.)

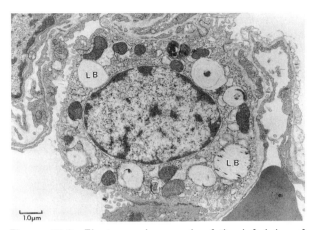

Figure 17.6 Electron micrograph of the left lobe of rat lung. Animal killed 24 hours after blast injury to the right lateral thorax showing loss of lamellated body structure from a Type II pneumocyte. LB = Lamellated body. ($\times$ 11 900.)

separated but it was not possible to differentiate between 'general damage' to the tissue and specific damage to intercellular junctions.

At 24 hours postinjury, bruising was macroscopically visible on the left lung. The ultrastructural changes recorded above were more marked at 24 hours than they had been at 30 minutes postinjury.

It was suggested by the authors that the initial blast-induced damage was more widespread than generally appreciated and that might account for the apparently progressive changes.

PATHOPHYSIOLOGICAL EFFECTS OF BLAST INJURY OF THE LUNG

To understand the associated changes in lung-function, blast lung may be thought of as a diffuse pulmonary contusion. Extensive studies have been undertaken on the effects of pulmonary contusion but very few on the effects of blast lung. Blockage of airways with blood while blood flow to damaged parts of the lung continues creates a shunt, with blood of low partial pressure of oxygen entering the pulmonary veins. Later as blood flow to the damaged areas decreases, the shunt fraction also declines. In the miliary haemorrhage described above, the capacity of the lung to divert blood flow away from damaged areas may be markedly reduced and improvement in arterial oxygenation consequently slow.

There have been two principal studies of the pathophysiological effects of blast: indirect studies designed to identify reflex changes dependent upon lung damage (Krohn *et al.*, 1942) and studies of lung function in blast-injured dogs and sheep (Damon *et al.*, 1971).

The indirect studies were mainly on rabbits, with a few experiments on cats and monkeys. Only the data on the respiratory system will be considered here. Records of diaphragmatic electromyograms and afferent activity in the vagus nerves were recorded using implanted silver electrodes. In rabbits exposed to a pressure close to that known to kill 50% of animals, a period of apnoea lasting from 5 to 20 seconds was observed to follow the explosion and was followed by slow deep breathing which gradually accelerated until it reached some 10 times the normal rate after about 30 minutes. The rate returned to return to normal over a period of several hours.

Bilateral section of the vagus nerves prevented the acceleration of respiration. It was felt that blast-induced damage stimulated receptors in the lung and that this accounted for the changes in respiratory rate. Receptors sensitive to irritants in the airways and juxta-pulmonary-capillary (J receptors) might certainly be expected to be stimulated by blood leaking into the airways and into the interstitial spaces of the interalveolar septae.

The work of Damon *et al.* (1971) involved the exposure of extensively instrumented animals to blast-waves. The unique nature of these difficult experiments makes them of great interest. The following physiological variables were determined: venous-arterial shunt ($\dot{Q}s/\dot{Q}$); alveolar–arterial oxygen gradient (A–a O_2); arterial–alveolar CO_2 gradient (a–A CO_2), alveolar dead space ventilation, arterial oxygen tension (Pa_{O_2}), and arterial carbon dioxide tension (Pa_{CO_2}).

Animals, each acting as its own control, were exposed to long-duration blast-waves designed to simulate the effects of nuclear weapons. At these long durations, lung injury is effectively duration independent. It was noted that post-exposure there was a marked increase in the venous–arterial

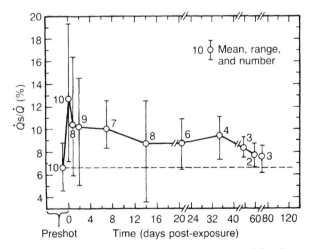

Figure 17.7 Percentage pulmonary shunt ($[\dot{Q}s/\dot{Q}] \times 100$) after blast injury in sheep. (From Damon *et al.*, 1970.)

shunt, rising to 0.3 in those animals exposed to an overpressure of 40 psi (276 kPa).

In further studies changes in the shunt fraction were followed over periods of up to 120 days postinjury (Damon *et al.*, 1970). The pattern of recovery measured by the decrease in the shunt fraction is shown in Figure 17.7. Initially recovery on day 1 was rapid but reduced in rate thereafter. It was suggested that the former might be dependent on diversion of blood away from areas of injury and the latter upon repair of damaged tissue.

HEALING PATTERN OF BLAST CONTUSIONS

Experimental studies of the pattern of healing of the blast-damaged lung are few. Chiffelle (1966) reported that pulmonary haemorrhages 'melt away' rapidly – over a period of 3–4 weeks. Rapid clearance of blood from the lungs has also been observed in a study in which pigs were killed at intervals up to 3 weeks after a blunt impact injury to the lower lobe of the right lung (Maynard *et al.*, 1984). By 72 hours postinjury, the centres of secondary lobules were macroscopically cleared of blood though the periphery of lobules was still heavily laden.

Chiffelle (1966) reported that emphysematous changes and fine scarring remained after the blood had cleared from the lungs and that these features were unchanged at 2 months postinjury. Severely damaged areas of lung are heavily infiltrated by fibrous tissue and abnormal air spaces lined by a low cuboidal epithelium (Figure 17.8) (Maynard *et al.*, 1984). The effect of fibrosis on lung function in the long term has not been studied in blast-injured casualties.

There is a wide variation in the extent of bleeding found in the lungs of patients dying as a result of blast injury and some authors have discussed the importance of pneumonia in the apparent progression of lesions (Hadfield, 1941; Osborn, 1941; Zuckerman, 1941). In clinical practice the degree of progression can be markedly influenced by concomitant therapy, particularly the injudicious use of crystalloid infusions. The additional development of infection, fat embolism syndrome, oxygen toxicity and left ventricular failure can cause a potentially curable phase to become irreversible.

DIAGNOSIS OF BLAST INJURY OF THE LUNG

Blast injury must always be considered in patients who have been in close proximity to an explosion. Signs and symptoms are usually obvious from the outset but may be delayed. It is this delay that makes it so important to observe and monitor patients at risk for at least 48 hours. Respiratory symptoms of late onset may be due to secondary complications which compromise pre-existing but unrecognized primary blast lung injury. It is these secondary effects in some patients that very often make the diagnosis confusing.

The severity of the blast effects are related to the size of the explosive device involved and the patient's position and proximity to the explosion. It has been frequently noted that explosions in a confined space are much more likely to result in multiple injuries and death than those in the open.

Penetrating wounds, traumatic amputations of limbs and extensive soft tissue injuries are not uncommon and necessitate urgent resuscitation and treatment. They take precedence over the diagnosis of blast lung which, although rare (2% of all patients admitted to hospital following bomb explosion), must not however be neglected. The

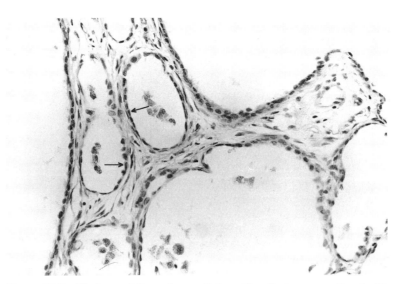

Figure 17.8 Pig lung at 3 weeks postinjury. Small air spaces lined with cuboidal epithelium (arrows) are seen surrounded by fibrosis.

clinical pattern is inconsistent and patients with severe injuries do not always develop blast lung whilst others with minor injuries may.

The presenting symptoms of blast lung are dyspnoea, a dry cough which may develop into frothy sputum and haemoptysis, chest pain or retrosternal discomfort. The patient is often restless and confused. On examination there may be cyanosis and tachypnoea. Auscultation of the lungs reveals diminished air entry in both lungs, coarse crepitations and marked bronchoconstriction with inspiratory and expiratory wheeze. The chest X-ray shows diffuse lung infiltrates and pulmonary oedema. This is usually bilateral but may be unilateral, depending on the patient's posture at the time of the blast. Pneumothoraces, haemothoraces and pneumomediastinum occur frequently and are often life threatening. Radiological changes may lag behind the clinical manifestations and serial chest X-rays are essential.

Hypotension, sinus tachycardia, arrhythmias and left ventricular failure may indicate associated myocardial injury. It is important not to ignore the abdomen as blast can cause disruption of the liver, spleen, kidneys and contusion or perforation of the intestines.

Primary blast injuries to the lung are rare in civilian casualties from terrorist bombings, although chest injuries from materials energized by the blast (secondary effects) or the individual being thrown against a solid object (tertiary effect) are not uncommon.

Blast injury is frequently observed in fatalities from explosions, particularly if the incidence of penetrating wounds is reduced by body armour (Mellor and Cooper, 1989).

MANAGEMENT

Patients who have been in close proximity to a bomb explosion and present with minimal injuries and show no obvious respiratory symptoms, should nevertheless be considered to be at risk of developing ARDS from the primary blast lung injury for up to 48 hours. During this period of observation particular attention should be paid to all aspects of respiratory function and the ECG.

The management approach is in general similar to that for the injured chest (see Chapter 10). Assisted ventilation is controversial in blast injury, in that it can increase pulmonary barotrauma in patients already at risk. Chest drains *must* be in place. Given that artificial ventilation should be avoided if possible, there remains a group of critically ill patients in which there is no other practical alternative if they are to survive. Positive pressure should be adjusted to keep airway pressure as low as possible because of the fragility of the alveoli. Prophylactic placement of chest drains has been advocated but one should bear in mind that

further alveolar rupture and the development of a tension pneumothorax can occur even with drains *in situ*. A right to left shunt requires high oxygen tensions in the inspired air, and if oxygen toxicity is to be avoided positive end expiratory pressure (PEEP) is mandatory (Coppel, 1979).

Some clinicians advocate pressure-controlled inverse ratio ventilation (PCIRV) to reduce barotrauma (Shuster *et al.*, 1991). There is no evidence to suggest that other novel techniques, such as high-frequency jet ventilation, reduce barotrauma. There may well be an indication for differential lung ventilation when the blast effect is unilateral (Geiger, 1983), but although there are reports of the use of this technique in other forms of lung trauma, none so far have been documented in primary blast injury.

Patients with blast injuries of the lung may have sustained other severe injuries which require large volumes of fluid and blood replacement. Wherever possible, care should be taken to use only the appropriate amount of crystalloid or colloid solutions, as there is every likelihood of enhancing the pulmonary oedema.

There is no doubt that in the past, patients survived the severe effects of blast lungs only to die at a later stage from infection and sepsis. The problem can now be, at least partially, controlled.

REFERENCES

Bebb A.H., Temperley H.N.V., Rawlins J.S.P. (1981). *Underwater blast: experiments and researches by British Investigators*. AMTE(E) R81 401 1981. UK Admiralty Marine Technology Establishment.

Benzinger T. (1950). Physiological effects of blast in air and water. In *German Aviation Medicine, World War II*, Vol. II. Washington, DC: US Government Printing Office, pp. 1225–59.

Blaisdell F.W., Lewis F.R. Jr. (1979). Respiratory distress syndrome of shock and trauma: post traumatic respiratory failure. In *Major Problems in Clinical Surgery*, Vol. XXI. Philadelphia: W.B. Saunders, pp. 1–9.

Brown R.E., Cooper G.J., Maynard R.L. (1993). The ultrastructure of rat lung following acute primary blast injury. *Int. J. Exp. Pathol.*, **74**, 151–62.

Buffe P., Cedenec Y.F., Baychelier J.L., Grateau P. (1987). Les lesions laryngees par explosion. (Blast laryngees). *Ann Otolaryngee*, **104**, 379–82.

Cameron G.R., Short R.H.D., Wakeley, C.P.G. (1943). Abdominal injuries due to underwater explosion. *Br. J. Surg.*, **31**, 51–66.

Cassen B., Kistler K. (1954). Effects of prior administration of various drugs on the acute pulmonary oedema produced by blast injury and the intravenous injection of epinephrine. *Am. J. Physiol.*, **178**, 53–7.

Chiffelle T.L. (1966). Pathology of direct air blast injury. In *Technical Progress Report on Contract DA-49–146-XZ-055*, Ref No DASA-1778. Albuquerque, New Mexico: Lovelace Foundation for Medical Education and Research.

Clemedson C-J. (1949). An experimental study on air blast injuries. *Acta Physiol. Scand.*, **18** Supp. LXI 7–200.

Clemedson C-J. (1956). Blast injury. *Physiol. Revs.*, **36**, 336–54.

Clemedson C-J., Hultman H.I. (1954). Air embolism and the cause of death in blast injury. *Milit. Surg.*, **114**, 424–37.

Cohen H., Biskind G.R. (1946). Pathological aspects of atmospheric blast injuries in man. *Arch. Pathol.*, **42**, 12–34.

Cooper G.J., Taylor D.E.M. (1989). Biophysics of impact injury to the chest and abdomen. *J.R. Army Med. Corps*, **135**, 58–67.

Cooper G.J., Maynard R.J., Cross N.L., Hill J.F. (1983). Casualties from terrorist bombings. *J. Trauma*, **23**, 955–67.

Cooper G.J., Townend D.J., Cater S.R., Pearce B.P. (1991). The role of stress waves in thoracic visceral injury from blast overloading: modification of stress transmission by foams and high density materials. *J. Biomechanics*, **24**, 273–85.

Coppel D.L. (1976). Blast injuries of the lungs. *Br. J. Surg.*, **63**, 735–7.

Damon E.G., Yelverton J.T., Luft U.V., Jones R.K. (1970). Recovery of the respiratory system following blast injury. In *Technical Progress Report DA-49–146-XZ-372. Ref. No. DASA 2580*. Albuquerque, New Mexico: Lovelace Foundation for Medical Education and Research.

Damon E.G., Yelverton J.T., Luft U.C., Mitchell K. Jr, Jones R.K. (1971). Acute effects of air blast on pulmonary function in dogs and sheep. *Aerospace Med.*, **42**, 1–9.

Falla S.T. (1940). Effect of explosion-blast on the lungs: report of a case. *Br. Med. J.*, **2**, 255–6.

Finlay W.E.I., McKee J.I. (1982). Serum cortisol levels in severely stressed patients. *Lancet*, **ii**, 1414–15.

Geiger K. (1983). Differential lung ventilation. *European Advances in intensive Care. Int. Anaesthesiol. Clin.*, **21**, 83–96.

Greaves F.C., Draeger R.H., Brines O.A. et al. (1943). An experimental study of underwater concussion. *US Naval Med. Bull.*, **41**, 339–52.

Hadfield G. (1941) Discussion of the problem of blast injuries. *Proc. R. Soc. Med.*, **34**, 189–91.

Haldane J.B.S. (1938). *A R P*. Toronto: Ryerson Press.

Hooker D.R. (1924). Physiological effects of air concussion. *Am. J. Physiol.*, **67**, 219–74.

Jonsson A. (1979). Experimental Investigations on the Mechanisms of Lung Injury in Blast and Impact Exposure. Linkoping, Sweden, Linkoping University Medical Dissertations No. 80.

Krohn P.L., Whitteridge D., Zuckerman S. (1942). Physiological effects of blast. *Lancet*, **i**, 252–8.

Latner A.L. (1942). The low pressure phase of blast. *Lancet*, **ii**, 303–4.

Logan D.B (1939). War wounds and air raid casualties. *Br. Med. J.*, **2**, 864–6.

Marshall T. (1977). In *Forensic Medicine*, Vol. 1 (Tedeschi C.G., Eckert W.G., Tedeschi L.G., eds) pp. 612–35. Philadelphia: Saunders.

Maynard R.L., Cooper G.J., Evans V.A., Kenward C.E. (1984). Histological study of the resolution of pulmonary contusions. Chemical Defence Establishment Porton Down UK, TP 360 1984.

Mellor S.G., Cooper G.J. (1989). An analysis of 828 servicemen killed or injured by explosions in Northern Ireland 1970–1984: the HACS statistics. *Br. J. Surg.*, **76**, 1006–10.

Moore F.D., Lyons J.H., Pierce E.C., Morgan A.P., Drinker P.A., MacArthur J.D., Dammin G.J. (1969). Post-traumatic pulmonary insufficiency. Philadelphia: W.B. Saunders.

Osborn G.R. (1941). Pulmonary concussion ('Blast'). *Br. Med. J.*, **1**, 506–10.

Richmond D.R., White C.S. (1966). Biological effects of blast and shock. In *Technical Progress Report on contract No. DA-49–146-XZ-055*, Ref No. DASA-1777. Albuquerque, New Mexico: Lovelace Foundation for Medical Education and Research.

Rossle R. (1950). Pathology of blast effects. In *German Aviation Medicine World War II*, Vol. II. Washington, DC: US Government Printing Office, pp. 1260–73.

Savage O. (1945). Pulmonary concussion ('Blast') in non-thoracic battle wounds. *Lancet*, **i**, 424–9.

Shuster S., Weilemann L.S., Kelbel C. et al. (1991). Inverse ratio ventilation improves pulmonary gas exchange and systemic oxygen transport in patients with congestive left heart failure. *Clin. Intens. Care*, **2**, 148–53.

Thomas A.R. (1941). Blast chest. The radiological aspect of the pulmonary changes following exposure to high pressure waves. *Br. J. Radiol.*, **14**, 403–6.

Topliff E.D.L. (1976). Mechanism of lung damage in explosive decompression. *Aviat. Space Environ. Med.*, **47**, 517–22.

Tunbridge R.E., Wilson J.V. (1943). The pathological and clinical findings in blast injury. *Q.J. Med.*, **12**, 169–84.

Williams E.R.P. (1942). Blast effects in warfare. *Br. J. Surg.*, **30**, 38–49.

Wilson J.V., Tunbridge R.E. (1943). Pathological findings in a series of blast injuries. *Lancet*, **i**, 257–61.

Zuckerman S. (1940). Experimental study of blast injuries to the lungs. *Lancet*, **ii**, 224–6.

Zuckerman S. (1941). Discussion of the problem of blast injuries. *Proc. R. Soc. Med.*, **34**, 171–88.

Zuckerman S. (1952). Vulnerability of human targets to fragmenting and blast weapons. In *Textbook of Air Armament*. Ref: TAA/2/12/52. Ministry of Supply.

18. Blast Injury of the Ear
R. J. N. Garth

INTRODUCTION

The ear is a particularly sensitive organ which has evolved to enable sound to be detected and interpreted over a wide range of sound pressure. As an air-containing organ, the ear is particularly susceptible to blast injury or barotrauma.

Blast injury is relatively uncommon during peacetime, with the notable exception of terrorist bombings. Few otolaryngologists see this type of problem frequently, although sporadic cases occasionally occur as a result of accidents. Otological injury is often of relatively minor importance during the early stages of management of the blast victim with multiple injuries and may easily be overlooked. Many tympanic membrane perforations heal spontaneously and minor cases of sensorineural hearing loss may go undiagnosed. In a review of 1535 consecutive terrorist explosion victims in Belfast (Hadden et al., 1978), only 15 patients were noted to have perforated tympanic membranes. Although the details of the explosions were not given, many of these are likely to have been unconfined free-field explosions which may account for the low incidence of perforations. It is also possible that some otological injuries went unrecorded.

The management of casualties from terrorist bombing campaigns have resulted in a number of published reports on otological injury. Kerr and Byrne (1975) reported the injuries resulting from a confined explosion when the Abercorne Restaurant in Belfast was bombed in 1972. This resulted in 60 perforated tympanic membranes. Pahor (1981) reported the otological findings in 41 survivors following the Birmingham pub bombings, in which 37% of patients had ENT problems. Half of these had suffered perforated tympanic membranes. Ruggles and Votypka (1973) reported the results of treating 11 tympanic membrane perforations resulting from the bombing of a police station at Shaka Heights in Ohio. There have also been a number of reports from military conflicts, Singh and Ahluwalia (1968) reported 79 cases from the Indo-Pakistan conflict and Sudderth (1974) 107 tympanic membrane ruptures from the Vietnam War. Apart from these large series, sporadic cases occur as the result of industrial accidents or military training – a military 'Thunderflash' used for training may generate a 200-dB sound pressure level (SPL) in a confined space. Such cases are rarely reported unless there is some unusual feature.

These reports are of clinical interest to the otolaryngologists involved in the management of such patients but the broad spectrum of injuries resulting from the uncontrolled conditions at the time of the explosion means that there is often little information of scientific value which can be obtained to add to our understanding of the mechanisms or criteria of injury. Laboratory investigations using animals, cadaver ears and models have added greatly to our knowledge of the biophysical interactions of pressure waves with the ear and form the basis of our understanding of the susceptibility of the ear.

Blast injuries are of particular relevance in a military environment, as modern warfare carries a significant risk of blast injury. The hazards presented to the ear depend on the type of conflict. During the Second World War, grenades and booby-traps were the cause of only 2–5% of all tympanic membrane perforations (Korkis, 1945) but in the Vietnam War they accounted for 68% (Sudderth, 1974). In armoured combat vehicles penetrated by shaped charges, the blast-wave may have multiple peaks (generally designated 'complex' waveforms) and the nature of the pressure/time profile may modify the susceptibility of the ear to blast compared to its susceptibility to unconfined free-field waveforms. Although the occupants of such a vehicle may be afforded considerable protection from the blast and fragments of an external explosion, a relatively small blast occurring within the confines of the vehicle or gaining access through defeated armour, may cause extensive injury due to the reflection and multiple shock loading and build up of pressure within the vehicle interior. The incapacitation caused by a blast injury to the ear is likely to be of greater significance in an age of high technology on the battlefield where the ability to use communication systems is vital.

ANATOMY AND PHYSIOLOGY

Figure 18.1 shows the structure of the human ear.

External ear

The external ear comprises the pinna and the external auditory canal. The pinna consists of a plate of elastic cartilage in a number of complex folds and has a covering of skin which is firmly bound to the cartilage on its anterolateral surface, becoming continuous with the skin of the external auditory canal.

The external auditory canal is approximately 24 mm in length, and in the outer one-third consists of a cartilaginous framework continuous with the cartilage of the pinna. The inner two-thirds has a bony wall which is narrower than the cartilaginous portion. There is a gentle curve to the canal, the outer third running slightly upwards and backwards. The inner two-thirds runs forwards and downwards. At the junction of the bony and

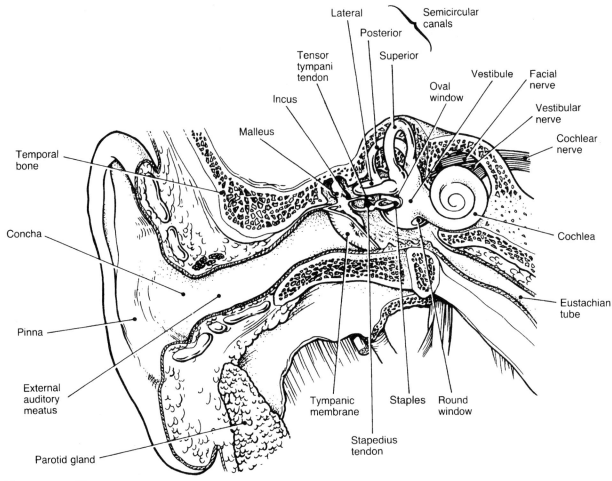

Figure 18.1 The human ear. (Reproduced from Kessel and Kardon, 1979.)

cartilaginous portions the canal narrows slightly. It also narrows at the isthmus, situated half-way along the bony canal.

Tympanic membrane

The tympanic membrane is slightly oval-shaped set at an angle of 55 degrees to the floor of the canal. The membrane forms a flattened cone with its apex directed medially into the middle ear.

The membrane is composed of three layers. The outer is stratified squamous epithelium, continuous with the skin of the external auditory canal. The inner is a mucous membrane continuous with the lining of the middle ear cleft. The middle, or lamina propria, is formed of elastic and collagen fibres and is responsible for the main mechanical characteristics of the tympanic membrane. These fibres radiate outwards from the umbo and handle of malleus towards the edge of the drum head, where they become incorporated into a fibrocartilaginous ring which lies in the bony tympanic sulcus. In addition to these radial fibres, there are also some inner circular fibres. Super-

iorly lies the pars flaccida in which the fibrous layer is usually said to be absent, though electron-microscope studies have shown some collagen and elastic fibres in this region (Lim, 1970). The main fibrous part of the tympanic membrane is known as the pars tensa.

Middle ear

The middle ear cleft consists of a tympanic or middle ear cavity which communicates anteriorly with the nasopharynx via the eustachian tube, and posteriorly with the mastoid antrum and air cells via the aditus. In the tympanic cavity lie the malleus, incus and stapes with their ligamentous attachments within the attic. The footplate of the stapes occupies the oval window between the vestibule and the middle ear and is held in place by the annular ligament. Below this, the round-window membrane sits in the medial wall of the middle ear and separates the middle ear from the scala tympani. The tendons of the tensa tympani and stapedius muscles are attached to the neck of the malleus and head of the stapes respectively.

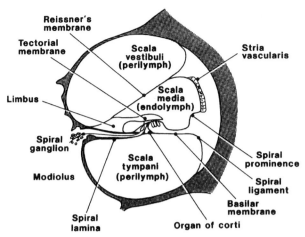

Figure 18.2 Cross-section of the cochlea. (Reproduced from Pickles, 1982.)

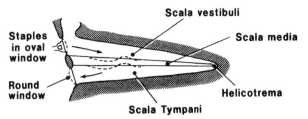

Figure 18.3 Schematic diagram depicting the unrolled membranes of the cochlea. (Reproduced from Pickles, 1982.)

Inner ear

The inner ear is situated in the dense bone of the otic capsule. It has a vestibule into which the semicircular canals of the vestibular labyrinth open, the scala vestibuli of the cochlea and the vestibular aqueduct. The bony cochlea is a snail-shaped structure which is divided into three components by the membranous cochlea. It contains the organ of Corti. This system is fluid filled – the scala media contains endolymph and perilymph fills the scala tympani and scala vestibuli (Figure 18.2).

Functional aspects of the ear

The transformer mechanism of the middle ear overcomes the impedance mismatch between air and perilymph and couples sound waves from the external auditory canal to the inner ear. Sound waves entering the external auditory canal initiate movements in the relatively low impedance tympanic membrane. These vibrations are transmitted to the malleus handle and through the malleo-incudal complex to the stapes. The malleo-incudal complex rotates about an axis which passes from the anterior process of the malleus to the short process of the incus. At low sound intensities, the movement of the long process of the incus results in a piston-like movement of the stapes. As sound levels increase, the movement of the footplate becomes more like a door with its hinge posteriorly. When sound is sufficiently loud to initiate the stapedius reflex, this changes to a rotating action along the longitudinal axis of the footplate. The action of the stapedius muscle attenuates the sound transmitted to the cochlea.

The area of the tympanic membrane is much greater than that of the footplate, with an effective surface area ratio of 14:1. In addition to this, the differing lengths of the malleus and long process of incus create a lever with a mechanical gain of 1.3.

The combined effect results in an 18-fold increase in pressure at the oval window.

Movement of the stapes footplate produces a displacement of perilymph in the scala vestibuli, resulting in movement of Reissner's membrane (Figure 18.2) and basilar membrane. Displacement of perilymph in the scala tympani is made possible by the bulging of the round-window membrane into the middle ear (Figure 18.3). Movement occurring in the basilar membrane is transmitted to the organ of Corti, and results in a shearing action on the stereocilia of the hair cells embedded in the tectorial membrane. This action changes current flowing through the hair cells and alters the endocochlear potential. This may initiate a cochlear nerve action potential.

INTERACTION OF BLAST WITH THE EAR

Acoustic trauma may be considered in terms of noise-induced hearing loss, impulse noise (which may be reverberant or repetitive) and blast trauma. The distinction between impulse noise and blast is arbitrary and can be classified both in terms of the source of the pressure and the characteristics of the waveform; there is no formal distinction. Weapons such as hand guns and rifles produce impulse noise, but the sound energy from the firing of larger weapons such as howitzers and anti-tank weapons is usually described as blast.

In general, differentiation of impulse noise and blast may be made using the following criteria:

1. The peak overpressures of impulsive noise are usually less than 1–2 kPa (160 dB). Large guns may produce SPLs of tens of kPa and are usually described as producing 'muzzle blast'.
2. Blast involves considerable movement of air and combustion products – impulsive noise does not.
3. The frequency content of impulsive noise may include low-frequency features such as mechanical clatter.

This chapter is primarily concerned with auditory injury from blast overpressure. Descriptions of the effects of impulsive noise, and occupational guidelines to limit exposure, are dealt with else-

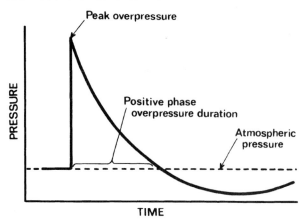

Figure 18.4 Idealized (Friedlander) free-field blast overpressure.

where (e.g. Powell and Forrest, 1988). The physics of detonations and blast-waves are described in Chapter 15 and will not be repeated here. However, there are some points that require emphasis in relation to the ear and these are discussed below.

The detonation wave coupling into air (shock-wave) and the massive increase in gas volume are collectively described as a blast-wave. The shock-wave is an effectively instantaneous overpressure, travelling through undisturbed air at a velocity greater than the speed of sound in ambient air. Behind the shock-wave is a region of gas flow of the combustion products. The motion of gas results in a lower pressure – the dynamic overpressure. These combined pressures decay during the short positive overpressure phase. There is then a longer sub-atmospheric pressure phase. In Figure 18.4, these features are shown on an idealized free-field (Friedlander) waveform.

The degree and type of damage to the ear is influenced by the peak overpressure, the positive impulse and the duration of the positive wave (James *et al.*, 1982). These factors will be determined by the size and type of explosion and the distance of the victim from the source.

In reality most blast victims are exposed to considerably more complex blast-waves resulting from interaction of the waves with the local environment. In a confined space, such as a building or an armoured combat vehicle, the overpressure comprises the initial shock and additional multiple loadings arising from surface reflections. In addition to this, heating of the gases within a vehicle may give a slowly rising pressure build up after 10–20 ms which may last for several hundred milliseconds (Phillips *et al.*, 1989). Therefore there are multiple short-duration, repetitive loadings superimposed on a long-duration increase in ambient pressure of long rise time (Figure 18.5).

With nuclear weapons, a much greater proportion of the energy is dissipated as heat. The positive

pressure duration of a nuclear blast may last for seconds and the peak overpressure are low at ranges where survival is conceivable. The dynamic overpressures are notable and displacement of personnel is the principal risk.

The tympanic membrane and ear are situated at the end of a slightly curved external auditory canal and the blast-wave is modified by reflections and refractions during its passage down the canal. The curve, the change in diameter, the elasticity of the tissues and the conical shape of the tympanic membrane may modify both the magnitude and shape of the incident blast-wave during its passage down the meatus.

The orientation of the canal in relation to the incident wave may also have a significant effect on pressure propagation (Figure 18.6). In comparison to the normal reflected overpressure from a surface, the peak overpressure measured at the eardrum is greater for a shock-wave with a normal incidence to the side of the head but reduced when the incidence is side-on (James *et al.*, 1982).

Stinson (1985) used scaled replicas of the human external auditory canal to investigate sound pressure distribution at the tympanic membrane. His results showed a considerable variation in sound pressure as a result of the shape of the ear canal. At 15 kHz the area near the top of the drum had 20 dB of attenuation compared to the centre of the drum, and in the lower part the sound pressure was increased by 4 dB. Although these findings were related to continuous sound and cannot be extrapolated directly to blast-waves, they do illustrate that the external auditory canal can modify a wave and that different parts of the tympanic membrane may be exposed to different pressure levels during a blast injury. This may explain in part the uneven

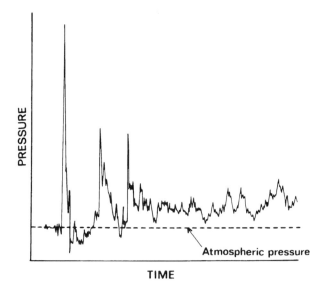

Figure 18.5 Complex waveform resulting from an explosion in a confined space.

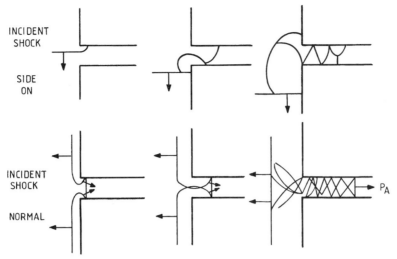

Figure 18.6 Diagrammatic representation of the entry of a blast-wave into a duct such as the external ear canal. In the upper diagram, the incident blast is side-on to the axis of the duct. The lower figure shows the reflection for a shock incident normal to the surface and transmission down the duct. (Reproduced from James *et al.*, 1982.)

distribution of injury to the tympanic membrane commonly found following explosions.

The pinna also has a role to play in modifying the initial peak pressure at the tympanic membrane. Although their data were limited, James *et al.* (1982) also found that the presence of a pinna reduced the impulse and pressure when the incidence was normal to the ear. The peak pressure increased with the side-on shock incidence; the impulse did not.

With such a large number of variable factors it is inevitable that in the event of an explosion, very few tympanic membranes would be exposed to the same blast magnitude or profile. When the normal biological variability of the eardrum is also considered, it is not surprising that there can be such a broad spectrum of injuries to the ear arising from an apparently identical blast.

THE EFFECTS OF BLAST ON THE EAR

The external ear

It is unlikely that injury will result as a primary effect of the blast-wave, but secondary injuries from flying debris may occur. In principle these will be much the same as any other soft tissue injury from penetrating projectiles and will not be further discussed.

The tympanic membrane and middle ear

The blast-wave may produce a wide spectrum of injury to the tympanic membrane and middle ear. If examined soon after a small explosion, only injection of the vessels lying along the malleus handle may be evident. With more severe blast loadings,

subepithelial haemorrhages may occur and the tympanic membrane may be perforated. These perforations occur in the pars tensa and are often small slit-like tears following the radial fibres of the lamina propria (Figure 18.7). Larger perforations may have smooth or ragged edges and there may

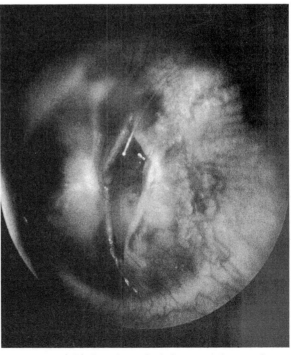

Figure 18.7 Perforation of a left tympanic membrane showing a defect following the radial fibres running from the centre of the drum to the annulus inferiorly.

TABLE 18.1
OSSICULAR INJURIES. (DATA FROM SUDDERTH, 1974)

Incudo-malleolar joint disruption	25%
Incudo-stapedial joint disruption	4%
Incudo-stapedial disruption + stapes superstructure fracture	2%
Incus dislocation	2%
Fractured stapes superstructure	1%

be flap-like tears with inversion or eversion of the flap. Although the perforations are usually single, multiple perforations of the drum can occur and severe blasts may result in subtotal or total perforations.

Pahor (1981) recorded the site of smaller perforations following the Birmingham pub bombing. Sixty per cent occurred in the central portion of the drum, 25% were anterior and 15% were posterosuperior. More severe injury may result in damage to the ossicular chain, although this is found in a small proportion only of surviving victims. There were no cases of ossicular damage in a combined total of 95 perforated tympanic membranes reported by Pahor (1981) and Kerr and Byrne (1975), though Singh and Ahluwalia (1968) reported ossicular damage in two of 52 ears with perforations. A much greater incidence of disruption was found by Sudderth (1974), who found ossicular damage in approximately 33% of ears undergoing tympanoplasty.

The reason for this great difference is not clear but may well lie in the selection criteria for the different populations studied rather than in the magnitude of the blast-wave. The ossicular damage reported in Sudderth's series is summarized in Table 18.1. Other reports of isolated cases of ossicular injury are found in the literature but the most prevalent injuries are as described, with the exception of dislocation and fracture of the stapes footplate (Singh and Ahluwalia, 1968).

When a tympanic membrane is ruptured by a blast-wave, small fragments including squamous keratinizing epithelium from the outer surface of the drum head may be blown into the middle-ear cleft. Small fragments in contact with the middle-ear mucosa may remain viable and keratin production may result in cholesteatoma formation. Whether this squamous epithelium is confined to the tympanic cavity at this early stage or whether it is also seeded throughout the mastoid system is not clear. Kronenberg et al. (1988) found an incidence of cholesteatoma formation of 7.6% in a series of 210 ears. Of these, six were cholesteatoma pearls and 10 were invasive cholesteatomas involving the middle ear and extending throughout the mastoid system. These more extensive cases could result from the wide dissemination of fragments of squamous epithelium throughout the middle ear and mastoid system, or alternatively represent the extension of an aggressive cholesteatoma starting in the middle-ear cavity. As most of these ears would have been normal before the blast, these patients would have well-pneumatized mastoid systems which would provide little in the way of a barrier to the cholesteatoma.

Laboratory studies have provided information on the susceptibility of the ear to blast that cannot be obtained from investigations of human blast

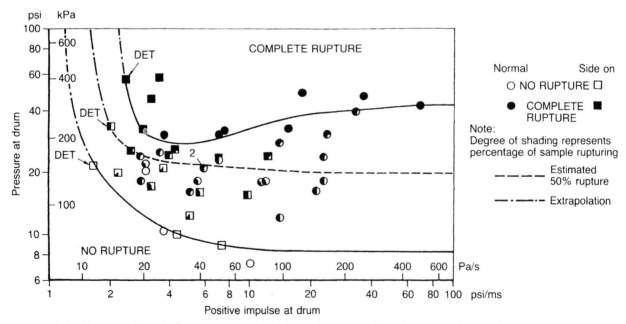

Figure 18.8 Pressure–impulse rupture criteria for bare human cadaveric tympanic membranes (no meatus or pinna). (Reproduced from James et al., 1982.)

victims. Animal studies have correlated blast-wave parameters and the incidence of tympanic membrane rupture. Other experiments have determined the peak overpressure required for a 50% incidence of rupture but there is poor consistency as a result of different species of animal employed and differing blast overpressure features. Nearly all investigation have failed to define the duration dependency of tympanic membrane rupture.

There have been few investigations on humans. In one of the earliest experiments, static overpressures were measured and the lowest pressure for tympanic membrane failure was found to be 37 kPa (5.4 psi), a figure that is frequently quoted in the literature (Zalewski, 1906).

James *et al.* (1982) gathered sufficient data using fresh cadaver temporal bones to draw up 50% rupture curves as a function of pressure and positive impulse (Figure 18.8). They concluded that for long-duration blasts (greater than 2 ms), a maximum peak pressure of 50–56 kPa was required for rupture. For shorter durations, a minimum impulse of about 8 kPa was required. The quoted

overpressures describe the susceptibility of the tympanic membrane alone and do not take into account modification of the incident overpressure by the pinna or meatus. The information has been used to construct a relationship predicting the incidence and nature of eardrum rupture *in situ* in terms of the maximum incident overpressure and the overpressure duration. Figure 18.9 shows the relationship for a person in free-field with the long axis of the front of the body facing the blast source (Richmond and Axelsson, 1990). Figures for the susceptibilities of the tympanic membrane with the body prone or close to a reflecting surface are given in the same reference.

It is clear that there are variations in susceptibility of a tympanic membrane to perforation from one individual to another. The drum head is an elastic structure and has slightly different physical characteristics as a result of normal biological variability. Furthermore, previous injury to the tympanic membrane and ageing may also increase the vulnerability of the drum. Animal studies have suggested differences in susceptibility to blast perforation

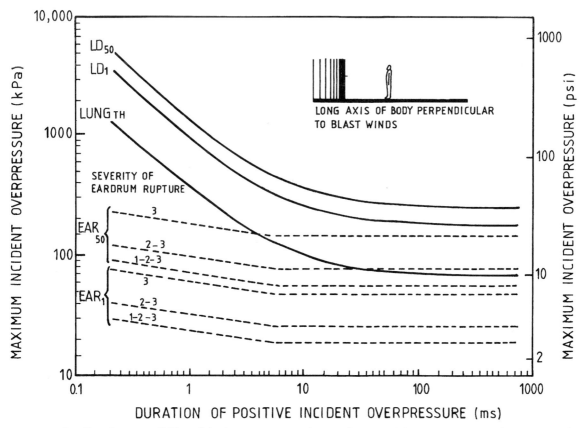

Figure 18.9 Predicted susceptibility of the human tympanic membrane to blast overpressure for a person facing the blast source (ears side-on to the blast). The data of Figure 18.8 was used to construct the relationship. EAR_{50} and EAR_1 are 50% and 1% probability of eardrum rupture respectively. The three categories of rupture are: 1 = minor: minor slits and linear disruptions; 2 = moderate: large tears; 3 = major: total disruption; large flaps. $LUNG_{TH}$, LD_1 and LD_{50} are threshold of primary blast injury to lung, 1% and 50% probability of death from blast lung respectively. (Reproduced from Richmond and Axelsson, 1990.)

from one species to another, although these conclusions were based on limited data (Roberto *et al.*, 1989).

The stress within the tympanic membrane during a blast is not uniformly distributed. Stuhmiller (1989) studied the tensile stress within different parts of the pars tensa using a model and he showed quite marked variation in stress maximal around the periphery of the tympanic membrane (Figure 18.10). The variation resulted from uniform static pressure loading which is not the case following a shock-wave but does demonstrate the degree to which stress may vary throughout the drum. Continuous acoustic stimulation is also associated with considerable variation in the sound pressure level over the surface of the tympanic membrane (Stinson, 1985). If a similar variation also applies to pressure loading from blast, the stress distribution within the tympanic membrane is further complicated by the uneven distribution of the pressure loading on the tympanic membrane.

Stress imposed on the drum which is well beyond normal physiological levels results in damage and alters its mechanical characteristics. Tympanometry on chinchillas exposed to repeated 166-dB impulse stimuli demonstrated an increased compliance immediately after exposure (Eames *et al.*, 1975). The tympanogram also became a little irregular, gradually returning to normal over the following 2 weeks. This is likely to be the result of rupture of some of the radial fibres of the lamina propria stretched beyond their limits of elasticity followed by gradual reorganization and repair.

As the tympanic membrane is displaced medially by the positive phase of the blast it is cushioned to some extent by the increase in pressure within the middle ear. The increase in pressure will depend upon the size of the middle-ear cleft and how quickly the air within the middle ear can be displaced into the mastoid system or down the eustachian tube. It is uncertain to what extent this cushioning protects the tympanic membrane from rupture but, if the effect is significant, an ear with a large mastoid system or patulous eustachian tube may be more vulnerable to blast injury.

White *et al.* (1970) proposed the theory that an elastic tympanic membrane may be displaced sufficiently to 'bottom out' on the promontory and ossicles, gaining extra support in these areas. This may explain the distribution of perforations – the anterior portion of the tympanic membrane near the eustachian tube opening is unlikely to be supported and is therefore a common site for perforation. Further, the fact that tympanic membranes often perforate more easily when exposed to a static negative canal pressure may reflect the lack of support from middle-ear structures with these forces.

There has been debate in the past about the relative contribution of the positive and negative phase of a blast-wave in relation to middle-ear injury. The presence of perforations with an inverted flap of drum, and cholesteatoma following perforation, suggests that many of these injuries are caused by the positive phase of the blast. The negative phase is probably of less importance, and it is likely that in some cases where an everted flap of drum is found, the perforation was caused by the positive phase, the negative phase merely everting the loose flap.

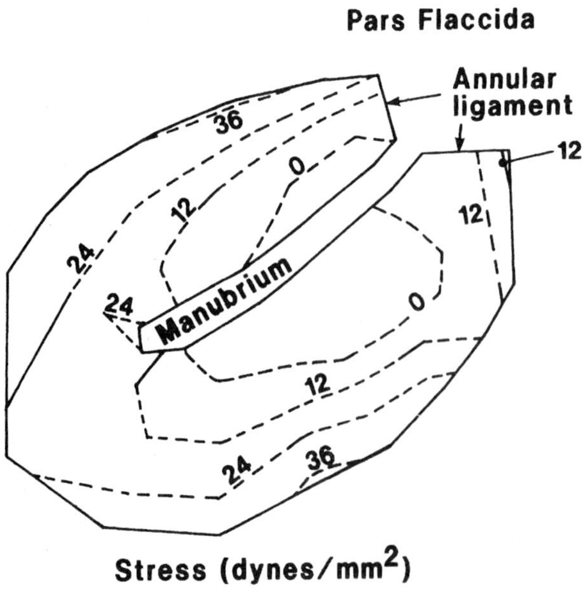

Figure 18.10 Stress loading occurring in a tympanic membrane model as a result of uniform pressure loading. (Reproduced from Stuhmiller, 1989.)

The inner ear

Clinical accounts of blast casualties report marked tinnitus and a temporary profound sensorineural hearing loss in many patients. This temporary threshold shift and tinnitus is often short lived and lasts only a few hours. In some patients, however, recovery may take months and a few are left with a permanent hearing loss (Kerr and Byrne, 1975). Many patients may be unaware of this because it is often in the high frequencies, and good speech discrimination is retained. Teter *et al.* (1970) described four different audiometric configurations in a retrospective study of blast injury but a wide variety of audiometric patterns have been reported, the most common being a predominantly high-tone sensorineural loss. The 4-kHz dip, usually found in noise-induced hearing loss, is not generally a feature of that resulting from blast and suggests a different mechanism of injury.

Vertigo is an uncommon problem following blast. Kerr and Byrne (1975) found that most patients suffering vertigo following the Belfast bombing had also had a significant head injury and the vertiginous problems were very similar to those often associated with a postconcussional state. A very small number who had not suffered head injury developed benign paroxysmal positional vertigo. Only two cases of the 111 victims of the Birmingham bombing suffered vertigo, and of these, one had an exacerbation of a previous vertiginous problem, and in the other it was considered that the question of litigation and compensation was of significance (Pahor, 1981).

Perilymph fistula following blast is rare but may occur as a result of disruption of the stapes footplate (Singh and Ahluwalia, 1968). It has also been demonstrated in animals (Yokoi and Yanagita, 1984).

The use of the scanning electron microscope in studies on laboratory animals has given considerable insight into the damage occurring within the cochlea (Hamernik *et al.*, 1984a, b; Yokoi and Yanagita, 1984). These changes may remain for a considerable time after the injury. The anatomical disruption is most easily studied and correlates with the permanent threshold shift following a blast. The temporary threshold shift is more difficult to explain in these terms but has been postulated as resulting from changes in the integrity of the tight cell junctions of the reticular lamina, local biochemical abnormalities from membrane permeability changes or holes in the reticular lamina. Such breaches may allow perilymph to mix with the endolymph of the scala media, which in turn interferes with electrophysiological events, or even leads to further degenerative changes within the organ of Corti because of the altered ionic environment. In addition to these metabolic changes, the physical damage to the cochlear may be quite extensive even to the extent that it changes the pattern of vibration in the basilar and tectorial membranes.

Hamernik *et al.* (1984a) described the changes occurring in the chinchilla exposed to multiple 160-dB impulsive noises. Many ears suffered limited cochlear damage consisting of loss of hair cells but the structural elements of organ of Corti remained intact. In ears which are more severely damaged, there may be more striking changes – detachment of the long segment of the organ of Corti may occur and this may float free in the scala media with other cellular debris. The outer hair cells may suffer damage similar to that caused by continuous noise exposure – cilia are bent, usually at the point where the hair is attached to the cuticular plate. Some cilia may fuse, others break and the occasional giant cilia is found. Similar changes are found in the inner hair cells though usually to a lesser degree. Holes appear in the reticular lamina, and in places cytoplasmic extrusions occur at the apex of the inner hair cells, principally at the site of maximal cochlear disruption. Perilymph may mix with endolymph through the holes and crevices, and damaged cells may leak cytoplasmic contents giving localized changes in endolymph composition. The stria vascularis and Reissner's membrane are not grossly damaged. The cells of the inner sulcus undergo changes with the development of numerous pseudopodia and microvilli and macrophages increase within the cochlear reaching a peak at 12–16 days after injury. Claudius cells appear to be able to spread their membranes over a considerable area to cover damaged portions of the organ of Corti. Phagocytic activity is still evident 30 days after exposure and there may still be some communication between perilymph and endolymph at this stage though many of these holes will have closed and there may be extensive scar formation.

Yokoi and Yanagita (1984) found rupture of the round window and nystagmus after blast exposure in 40% of animals studied. However, such an injury is not reported in most animal studies and vestibular problems are rare in humans following blast injury. The histological findings in this study are otherwise in keeping with those already described, with most of the damage at the basal turn of the cochlear. It is likely that the high incidence of round-window rupture in this series resulted from the extremely long overpressure duration employed (200 ms).

Kumagami (1992) observed endolymphatic hydrops in guinea-pigs after exposure to single fire cracker explosions. He noticed degeneration and fibrous changes in the rugose portion of the endolymphatic sac and some degree of endolymphatic hydrops in the cochlear, vestibule and semicircular canals 6 months after blast exposure. Whether such changes occur in humans is not clear, as the clinical features of endolymphatic hydrops are not generally associated with blast injury.

In an environment with high levels of ambient noise, the stapedius muscle contracts to reduce sound transmission to the cochlea. However, with blast-waves or impulse noise the peak overpressure is attained well before the stapedius reflex can take effect.

There is evidence to suggest that perforation of the tympanic membrane and disruption of the ossicular chain affords some protection to the cochlea. Guinea-pigs exposed to a single blast suffered less cochlear damage when exposed to larger blasts that resulted in disruption of the sound-conducting mechanism (Akiyoshi *et al.*, 1966). Similar findings have been reported in animals exposed to multiple shock-waves (Eames *et al.*, 1975; Hamernik *et al.*, 1984a). However in man evidence of cochlear protection from tympanic membrane rupture has not been found, though none of the victims studied were reported to have ossicular damage (Kerr and Byrne, 1975). It is likely that any protective effect will be much more significant in ears exposed to multiple shock-waves as the initial disruption to the conducting mechanism will reduce the transmission of subsequent pressure waves to the cochlea.

The central nervous system

There is evidence that degeneration of the central nervous system can occur following acoustic trauma from continuous noise. Cats and chinchillas show degenerative changes in the axonal endings and ascending pathways (including the superior olivary complex) following acoustic trauma (Morest, 1982). It was also suggested that some of the larger endings were more resistant to degeneration. It is uncertain whether such degeneration occurs to any significant extent in humans following blast exposure. Clinical reports usually comment on good speech discrimination when speech audiometry is performed on blast victims which suggests that axonal degeneration is not an important component of the hearing loss. Further evidence is provided by Pratt *et al.* (1985) on the failure to detect any abnormality in the auditory brain-stem-evoked potentials of 37 human blast survivors (Pratt *et al.*, 1985). Although central degeneration is unlikely to be of clinical significance, it may nevertheless occur to a degree that is not detected by the relatively crude techniques of speech audiometry and evoked potentials.

TREATMENT

Most clinicians involved in the management of blast injuries would agree that ears that have not suffered perforations do not require active treatment. There is little evidence that treating the immediate sensorineural hearing loss with vasodilators, steroids or vitamin supplements makes any difference to recovery. The spontaneous healing of 83% of perforations makes it difficult to justify grafting as a primary treatment.

Ears with perforations should be kept dry, and antibiotics or ear drops reserved for those that become infected. Perforations that do not heal spontaneously within 3–6 months may be grafted and any ossicular damage reconstructed. Should patients be troubled by persistent vertigo, the rare complication of a perilymph fistula must be considered and a tympanotomy performed if necessary to confirm the diagnosis and close the fistula.

Follow-up is important if the tympanic membrane has been perforated. If there is any suspicion of cholesteatoma, the middle ear and mastoid must be explored.

PREVENTION

In the military environment, the design of armoured vehicles may help protect the occupants from an external blast. The exposed individual must rely on ear muffs or plugs for protection. Jonsson (1990) has shown that the use of ear plugs during exposure to blasts with overpressures of 190 kPa gives sufficient protection to make perforation unlikely, with only 14 kPa recorded in the ear canal. Ear muffs provide much less protection, with pressures of 100 kPa recorded in the canal, and the muffs may be displaced by the blast. Protection against blast is covered in more detail in Chapter 21.

REFERENCES

Akiyoshi M., Amemiya A., Sato K. et al. (1966). On the pathogenesis of acoustic trauma in rabbits and guinea pigs due to explosion. *Int Audio.*, **5**, 270–1.

Eames B.L., Hamernik R.P., Henderson D., Feldman, A.S. (1975). The role of the middle ear in acoustic trauma from impulses. *Laryngoscope*, **85**, 1582–92.

Hadden W.A., Rutherford W.H., Merrett J.D. (1978). The injuries of terrorist bombing: a study of 1532 consecutive patients. *Br. J. Surg.*, **65**, 525–31.

Hamernik R.P., Turrentine G., Roberto M. et al. (1984a). Anatomical correlates of impulse noise-induced mechanical damage in the cochlea. *Hearing Res.*, **13**, 229–47.

Hamernik R.P., Turrentine G., White C.G. (1984b). Surface morphology of the inner sulcus and related epithelial cells of the cochlea following acoustic trauma. *Hearing Res.*, **16**, 143–60.

James D.J., Pickett V.C., Burdett K.J., Cheesman A. (1982). Part 1: The effect on the ear drum of a short duration, fast rising pressure wave. In *The Response of the Human Ear to Blast*. AWRE/CDE Report No. 04/82. AWRE Foulness/CDE Porton.

Jonsson A. (1990). Pressure measurement in the external auditory canal of a human head model exposed to air shock waves. National Defence Research Establishment (Stockholm) FOA Report, C20802–23.

Kerr A.G., and Byrne J.E.T. (1975). Concussive effects of bomb blast on the ear. *J. Laryngol. Otol.*, **89**, 131–43.

Kessel R.G., Kardon W.H. (1979). *Tissues and Organs*. New York: W.H. Freeman.

Korkis F.B. (1945). Rupture of blast origin. *J. Laryngol. Otol.*, **61**, 367–90.

Kronenberg J., Ben-Shoshan J., Madan M., Leventon G. (1988). Blast injury and cholesteatoma. *Am. J. Otol.*, **9**, 127–30.

Kumagami H. (1992). Endolymphatic hydrops induced by noise exposure. *Auris. Nasus. Larynx (Tokyo)*, **19**, 95–104.

Lim D.J. (1970). Human tympanic membrane. An ultrastructural observation. *Acta Otolaryngol. (Stockholm)*, **70**, 176–86.

Morest D.K. (1982). Degeneration in the brain following exposure to noise. In *New Perspectives in Noise Induced Hearing Loss* (Hamernik R.P., Henderson D., Salvi R., eds). New York: Raven Press, pp. 87–93.

Pahor A.L. (1981). The ENT problems following the Birmingham bombings. *J. Laryngol. Otol.*, **95**, 399–406.

Phillips Y.Y., Mundie T.G., Hoyt R., Dodd K.T. (1989). Middle ear injury in animals exposed to complex blast waves inside an armoured vehicle. *Ann. Otol. Rhinol. Laryngol.*, **98**, 17–22.

Pickles J.O. (1982). *An Introduction to the physiology of Hearing*. London: Academic Press.

Powell R.F., Forrest M.R. (1988). *Noise in the Military Environment*. Brassey's Defence Publishers Ltd.

Pratt H., Goldsher M., Netzer A., Shenhav R. (1985). Auditory brainstem evoked potentials in blast injury. *Audiology*, **24**, 297–304.

Richmond D.R., Axelsson H. (1990). Airblast and underwater blast studies with animals. *J. Trauma (China)*, **6**, (Suppl.), 229–34.

Roberto M., Hamernik R.P., Turrentine G.A. (1989). Damage of the auditory system associated with acute blast trauma. *Ann. Otol. Rhinol. Laryngol.*, **98**, 23–34.

Ruggles R.L., Votypka R. (1973). Blast injuries of the ear. *Laryngoscope*, **83**, 974–6.

Singh D., Ahluwalia K.J.S. (1968). Blast injuries of the ear. *J. Laryngol. Otol.*, **82**, 1017–28.

Stinson M.R. (1985). The spatial distribution of sound pressure within scaled replicas of the human ear canal. *J. Acoustic Soc. Am.*, **78**, 1596–602.

Stuhmiller J.H. (1989). Use of modelling in predicting tympanic membrane rupture. *Ann. Otol. Rhinol. Laryngol.*, **98**, 53–60.

Sudderth M.E. (1974). Tympanoplasty in blast-induced perforation. *Arch. Otolaryngol.*, **99**, 157–9.

Teter D.L., Newell R.C., Aspinall K.B. (1970). Audiometric configurations associated with blast trauma. *Laryngoscope*, **80**, 1122–32.

White C.S., Bowen I.G., Richmond D.R. (1970). The relation between eardrum failure and blast induced pressure variations. *Space Life Sci.*, **2**, 158–205.

Yokoi H., Yanagita N. (1984). Blast injury to sensory hairs: a study in the guinea pig using scanning electron microscopy. *Arch. Otorhinolaryngol.*, **240**, 263–70.

Zalewski T. (1906). Experimentelle Untersuchungen uber die Resistenzfahigkeit des Trommelfells. *Z. Ohrenheilkd.*, **52**, 109–28.

19. Terrorist Bombings: Pattern of Injury

S. G. Mellor

TERRORISM IN THE TWENTIETH CENTURY

It has been said that terrorism is a consequence of an affluent society. The century began at the height of the Anarchist movement in Great Britain and Europe. To some extent the First World War mitigated the effects of this movement which was replaced by the spread of communism: it appears that terrorist tactics are more the province of religious and nationalist fanatics than of idealogical political extremism. More grotesque and barbarous acts have been carried out in the name of religion (other than Buddhism) than any other cause (Clutterbuck, 1986). With the demise of the influence of communism and the dramatic improvement in living standards for some, the divisions in society are again becoming increasingly apparent and terrorism is again a significant problem. The situation at the end of the twentieth century seems not dissimilar to that at the end of the nineteenth. Few countries in the world are free from hostile pressure groups prepared to make their point by acts of aggression, whether their governments are democratic or totalitarian.

In modern society, the terrorist has many weapons. He/she can pollute water supplies, poison goods on the supermarket shelf, disrupt computer communications, or he/she may threaten to undertake these acts. However, the bomb and bullet are still his/her principal weapon. With sophisticated remote detonation, the bomber can keep well away from victims although deliberate suicide by the delivery of large quantities of explosive is not uncommon, particularly in the Middle and Far East.

Whilst attention to personal security is the mainstay of defence against the terrorist, vast resources in terms of police and military time and manpower are expended each year in the fight against terrorism. It is by the dislocation of normal life that the terrorist hopes to maintain his/her cause high on the agenda. Placing small bombs at railway stations, for example, can cause chaos. Although public sympathy may not follow, public outrage may be enough to move political change towards the wishes of the terrorist, simply because of the necessity to curtail personal freedom, within a democracy, in order to enhance security.

Over the past 20 years at least 10 000 people around the world have been killed by acts of terrorism, many with bombs of various types. Appalling though these figures may appear, they must be viewed in relation to other sources of injury. In Northern Ireland over the past 20 years, death and injury from terrorist incidents is less than half that caused by road traffic accidents (RTAs). It is even more salutary to note that over the same period the total numbers of dead and injured per head of population in Northern Ireland, caused by terrorist incidents and RTAs, is less than half that in Scotland caused by RTAs alone, though these estimates are not population adjusted.

EXPLOSIVE DEVICES AND TECHNIQUES USED BY TERRORISTS

Kill one; frighten ten thousand (Chinese proverb)

An explosion is a rapidly expanding sphere of the high temperature gaseous products of detonation. This process is much more rapid than combustion, consisting of a wave which propagates through the explosive at around 4000 m/s for commercial gelignite, and at about twice this value for military explosives.

The terrorists' armoury is dependent upon local laws pertaining to the possession of guns and high explosives. In the UK, both of these are strictly controlled and possession alone may be a criminal offence. There is a very large variation across different countries and states and even within these there may be adequate opportunity to avoid the law.

Explosives may be improvised from available commercial ingredients, but in small quantities produce little damage. In large quantities, as may be employed in large car bombs with a small detonating charge, home-made explosive can be devastating, as was demonstrated by the Shia Muslim fundamentalists in Lebanon in 1983–4. The Provisional IRA recently readopted this tactic in Northern Ireland by employing hostage drivers to deliver the car bomb to its destination (proxy bombing). This has been made even simpler by laser-operated triggering devices.

Whilst 'home-made' bomb making is possible, and does occur, most terrorist organizations rely on supply from some other country intent on destabilization.

Electronically timed and radio-controlled explosions are a more recent threat, an example being the attempt in 1985 on the life of the British Prime Minister of the day (Mrs Margaret Thatcher) at the Conservative Party Conference. This was thought to be the first attack of this type in mainland UK.

Specific targeting

Small bombs may be planted in places where a specific person or type of person can be targeted, possibly with few other casualties. The murders in the early 1980s of senior British politicians, Airey

Neave and Ian Gow, are examples of this method of terrorist attack. In both of these murders, car bombs were employed. These can be detonated in a variety of ways. If fixed to the car a trembler device can be employed to trigger when the car is started, or simply when the door is slammed. Wiring the device to the ignition is much more complex and time consuming. Whilst this will not guarantee that the owner of the car will be killed, this is the type of threat from which military and police personnel are most at risk. Radio-controlled detonators allow for greater target specificity.

If the bomb is fixed to the car, and particularly if a shaped charge is employed, the car and occupant will be disintegrated. On the other hand, a similar sized charge not fixed to the car may displace the vehicle and its occupant without such severe damage. If the car doors and windows are closed when the bomb is detonated, the occupant may be protected from the blast-wave by reflection off the car body. The victim may receive injuries from displacement, but these may not be fatal.

In Northern Ireland, 'culvert' bombs are used to attack military convoys and patrols, or military/ police personnel in unmarked cars. In such cases, very large quantities of home-made explosive are employed and can create very large craters. Vehicles may be destroyed completely or thrown into the air for considerable distances. Those strapped in are still at risk from impact with internal features of the vehicle, loose equipment and deceleration injuries on landing. Where open-backed Land Rovers or other military vehicles are used, the blast-wave from an explosion behind the vehicle may enter it and be reflected and reinforced within its rigid structure. Improvised 'Claymore mines', which propel a swathe of nails, steel balls and other large fragments, may also be used against military vehicles.

Indiscriminate bombing

In this context, indiscriminate bombing encompasses any bomb placed in or near public buildings or military and police installations. Passenger aircraft are also a frequent target, a recent example of this being the Lockerbie air disaster in the UK. Warnings may or may not be given allowing for evacuation of buildings, with all the inconvenience that that entails. Once such a bombing campaign starts, equal inconvenience can be engendered by hoax warnings. This puts a considerable strain on the police who are eventually obliged to make judgements on the nature of the warning (hoax or real), and therefore to ignore many of the warnings, with all the risk that that entails.

Many examples of such incidents over the last three decades may be quoted and have been extensively analysed. Incidents are related to political tension: Coventry was extensively bombed by the IRA in 1939 at the start of the Second World War, the bombing of London railway stations by the IRA and a mortar attack on the British Prime Minister coincided with the recent Gulf War.

PATTERNS OF INJURY

Patterns of injury resulting from terrorist bombings depend on:

1. Type of explosive.
2. Quantity of explosive.
3. Construction, in terms of inclusion of metal and other materials designed to produce penetrating injuries.
4. Position of the bomb in relation to walls, furniture and, in some cases, other explosive material.
5. Position of victims in relation to the bomb.
6. Environment in which the bomb is placed.

Every explosion has a lethal zone within which survival is not possible. Outside this area death and injury may be caused by secondary missiles, the blast winds (flow of the combustion products) and, under certain circumstances, the shock-wave.

Most injuries, both of a minor and serious nature, are caused by flying debris. Most victims of explosions will have multiple bruises and abrasions from flying debris with characteristic tattooing where small particles of dirt have been driven into the skin. The intense but short-lived heat of the explosion can cause burns to exposed skin, but these are generally superficial.

When a blast-wave impinges on a medium of different density, pressure is both reflected and coupled into the medium. When the shock-wave is reflected, reinforcement of the oncoming wave front may occur. Energy is lost when the differences in the density are most marked, such as the interface between air and fluid. Hence, the ear, lungs and bowel which contains air are most affected by the shock-wave which is coupled into the body.

Perforation of the eardrum can occur with relatively low increases in overpressure. Other tissues are less susceptible to the effect of the blast-wave – blast lung results from very large incident overpressures. Consequently, significant blast-induced primary lung and bowel damage are rare in survivors but require clinical attention.

Effect of location of the bomb on death and injury from explosion

The incidence of death and injury caused by an explosion will depend on the proximity of people to the explosion and on the environments within which the device detonates. The latter may conveniently be divided into explosions occurring in the open air, inside buildings and inside vehicles.

What follows is an analysis of recent occurrences and their significance.

Explosions in open air

The car bomb detonated outside the Old Bailey, London in 1973 was placed against an outside wall and although it caused 160 casualties, mainly from flying debris and collapsing masonry, there were no directly attributable deaths (Caro and Irving, 1973). This pattern is observed in large buildings, such as railway stations, which are uncrowded.

Explosions in buildings

In the Bologna Railway Station explosion in 1980, 73 out of 291 died at the scene of the explosion, the high incidence of fatalities undoubtedly arose from the crowding at the railway station, but there were several quite severe injuries at a considerable distance from the explosion due to flying glass and debris (Brismar and Bergenwald, 1982). The bombing of Beirut International Airport in 1983 resulted in 346 casualties, of whom 68% were killed (Frykberg and Tepas, 1988). It was an extremely large explosion, and collapse of the building contributed to many of the injuries.

The relationship between death/injury and the characteristics of the device and environment has been analysed (Cooper et al., 1983). In the 'Horse and Groom' public house incident in Guildford, UK, in 1974, a small explosive device had been placed in an alcove. Those close to the incident were killed or seriously injured (Figure 19.1). Of those admitted to hospital (n = 24), two were reported as having blast lung and nine had eardrum rupture. The latter were reported as far away from the explosion as 8 m, whilst some close in to the explosion had intact eardrums (Figure 19.2). Those sufficiently seriously injured to require hospital admission (Figure 19.3) had extensive soft tissue laceration (46%), burns (42%) and fractures (29%). Few others were seriously injured, with the notable exception of the barman directly opposite the opening of the alcove, and two people near the door who were also very seriously injured, and had ruptured eardrums.

In the 'Tavern in the Town' public house explosion in Birmingham, UK, the explosive device, of a similar size to that in the 'Horse and Groom' explosion, was again placed in an alcove. Death and injury occurred in the alcove where the explosion occurred, but also against the opposite wall, about 12 m away (Figure 19.4). In this case there were 21 fatalities and 119 casualties, of whom 42 were admitted to hospital. Of those admitted to hospital,

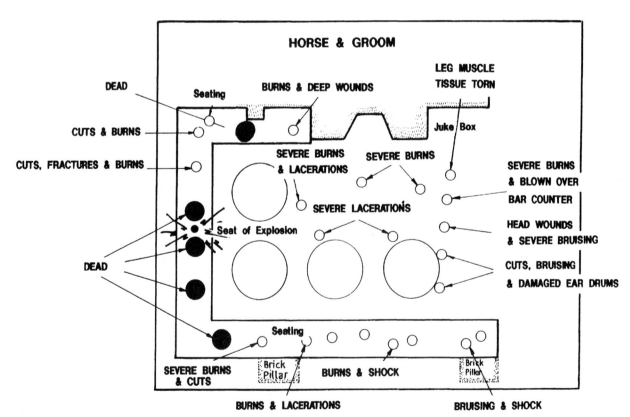

Figure 19.1 'Horse and Groom' Public House Bombing UK 1974: those close to the injury were killed or seriously injured.

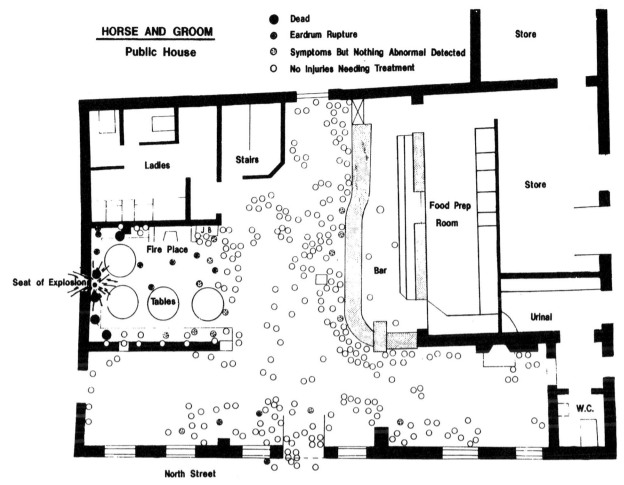

Figure 19.2 'Horse and Groom' Public House Bombing UK 1974: position of casualties sustaining eardrum rupture.

55% were burned, 52% had serious soft tissue damage and 35% had fractures. Forty-one per cent of the hospital admissions had ruptured eardrums (Figure 19.5).

Explosions in vehicles

In an incident in Israel, an explosive device equivalent to 6 kg of TNT was placed on a crowded city bus (Katz *et al.*, 1989). Several passengers immediately adjacent to the bomb were uninjured. Eight casualties sustained life-threatening multiple injuries, some of whom were some distance from the explosion. Twenty-nine casualties had primary blast injuries. Of these, 22 had ruptured tympanic membranes, 11 had blast lung and four had abdominal injuries which might be ascribed to the blast-wave. This incident was of particular significance because there were uninjured people next to the bomb, yet there were deaths from blast lung well away from the bomb, but against the side of the bus where the blast-wave would be reflected and reinforced to result in high local overpressures.

In 186 deaths from explosions in Northern Ireland, multiple rib fracture and lung contusion were significantly more common in victims in vehicles than in buildings (Hill, 1979). Major penetrating wounds of the chest were more common in fatalities in the open than in buildings. This illustrates the concept that in an enclosed space the lethal zone due to the blast-wave itself is not confined to the area immediately around the charge (as it would be in the open) but is reflected and reinforced by walls and debris generated other than at the point source of the charge. This is particularly well demonstrated by the large proportion of blast-wave-related injury seen in the bus bomb incident (Katz *et al.*, 1989), where almost half the passengers had ruptured eardrums. In addition, 11 patients had blast lung, which is rarely seen in survivors of civilian bombing incidents (Cooper *et al.*, 1983).

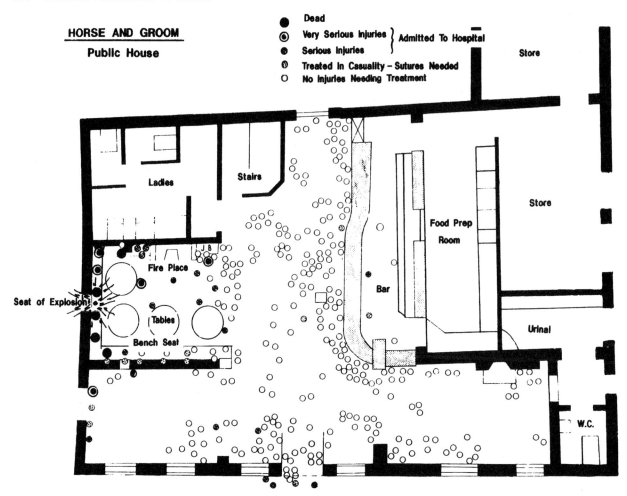

Figure 19.3 'Horse and Groom' Public House Bombing UK 1974: position of dead and seriously injured casualties.

Thus a small charge in an enclosed space may cause more deaths from the effect of the blast than would secondary missiles directly from the device area, and from a much smaller charge than would be necessary in the open to have the same effect. On the other hand, in the open, where the blast-wave is not contained and reflected, fatality is likely to be due to secondary missiles beyond the lethal zone for the particular charge, as in the Old Bailey incident described above.

Regional distribution of injury

The probability that any particular part of the body will be struck by flying debris is proportional to the area presented, which is largely constant for the various areas whatever the position of the body. The head and neck present about 12%, thorax 16%, abdomen 11%, upper limb 22% and lower limbs 39%.

In general, this finding is reflected in the distribution of injuries occurring, although is not helpful

for predicting outcome. For example, of 290 bomb-blast victims studied between 1971 and 1976, 38% sustained head injuries, of whom half died. Twenty-one per cent had chest and abdomen wounds of whom one-third died. In particular, head injuries feature prominently in those who have been more severely injured or killed by explosions (Hill, 1979). Frykberg and Tepas (1988) noted a 70% incidence of head injury in immediate fatalities in their large review. Clearly these findings do not reflect the number of hits on the area, more its inherent vulnerability.

Eye injuries have been noted in up to 40% of fatalities from explosions (Hill, 1979). This high number of injuries relative to the small presenting area reflects the sensitivity of the eye to very small fragments of debris which would not affect other parts of the body.

Half of all fatalities from explosions have penetrating injury to the chest and abdomen with consequent laceration of contained organs and vessels. Some of these injuries will be non-penetrat-

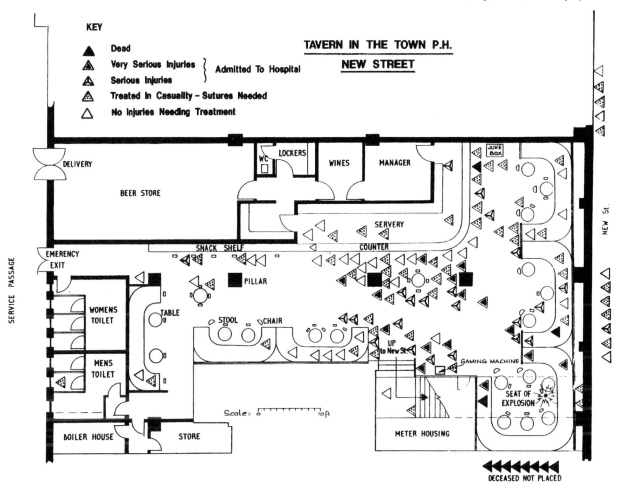

KEY

▲ Dead
⟁ Very Serious Injuries ⎫ Admitted To Hospital
△ Serious Injuries ⎭
⟁ Treated In Casualty – Sutures Needed
△ No Injuries Needing Treatment

TAVERN IN THE TOWN P.H.
NEW STREET

◀◀◀◀◀◀◀◀
DECEASED NOT PLACED

Figure 19.4 'Tavern in the Town' Public House Bombing UK 1974: position of dead and seriously injured casualties.

ing, from movement of the body by the blast wind, or from larger pieces of flying debris.

Those dying as a result of an explosion all have the characteristic triad of bruises, abrasions and tattooing due to the flying dust and debris (Marshall, 1977). In addition, soft tissue damage severe enough to warrant surgery is seen in those killed by explosions. Hill noted extensive lacerations and soft tissue loss around the head and neck in 60% of 186 deaths. Twenty-five per cent of fatalities had severe soft tissue damage in other areas.

Fractures and traumatic amputations are very common in those killed by explosion. Skull fracture is significantly more frequent in fatalities in the 18–30 age group than in the over 50 age group. This observation would suggest that fatalities occur in the older age group with less severe injuries. As might be expected, the older age group has a much higher incidence of rib fracture, due to the lower fracture threshold of the rib cage with age (Hill, 1979).

Cause of death following explosions

Those in the immediate vicinity of an explosion will usually be killed and are often blown to pieces. Very close to an explosion source, the peak over-pressure in air decays with the cube of the distance. Unless the explosion is very large and lasts for several milliseconds, those further away from the explosion will not be significantly injured by the blast-wave. They may, however, sustain fatal injuries from primary and secondary missiles. In between these two regions, there will be a group which receives fatal primary blast injuries and penetrating wounds/serious soft tissue injury without total body disruption.

There is little published information differentiating the causes of death from individual explosions, but a survey of servicemen killed in Northern Ireland by explosions (Mellor and Cooper, 1989) indicated that 14% were totally disrupted by the explosion, 39% died of multiple injuries and 21%

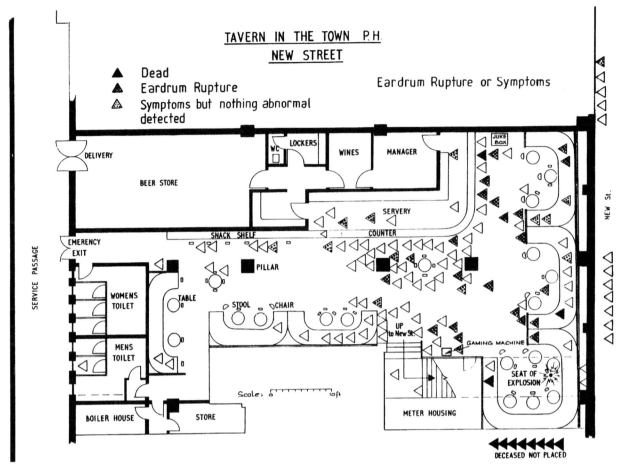

Figure 19.5 'Tavern in the Town' Public House Bombing UK 1974: position of casualties sustaining eardrum rupture.

died of head and chest injuries (blunt and penetrating). Eleven per cent died of chest injury alone, whilst 12% died of head injury alone. Apart from the last group, the evidence available suggested that all had primary blast lung as a contributory factor in their demise. Head injury alone is identified as a common cause of death in other series where this has been analysed (Hill, 1979; Cooper *et al.*, 1983; Frykberg and Tepas, 1988; Mellor and Cooper, 1989).

The group of servicemen in Northern Ireland who died of chest injury alone are a selected group, unrepresentative of the general population because they were wearing body armour. Body armour is remarkably effective against fragments, but offers no protection against shock-waves that may be coupled into the body and produce primary blast lung. Although the total number of dead will be reduced by body armour, the proportion of dead exhibiting primary blast injuries will increase.

Marshall (1977) points out that secondary missiles from explosions can cause fatal penetrating injuries at a considerable distance from the explosion.

The foregoing has dealt with immediate death from explosions. A small percentage die in hospital. Some die during resuscitation, some on the operating table and others several days later.

Early deaths in hospital are generally due to uncontrollable haemorrhage or to true blast lung which develops over a few hours and is often fatal, especially if combined with other injuries (Mellor and Cooper, 1989).

Traumatic amputation caused by the blast wind is rarely survivable as those near enough to an explosion to sustain such an injury invariably have some degree of blast lung and penetrating injury. Head injury will also account for some of these early deaths in hospital.

Late deaths (after several days) contributed to by adult respiratory distress syndrome (ARDS) should not be attributed solely to the effects of the blast. Sepsis, shock, repeated blood transfusion and prolonged artificial ventilation are far more likely to be the cause. Head injuries are also a cause of late death in hospital following explosions (Mellor and Cooper, 1989). It may be surmised that after explosions early deaths in hospital, despite early intense resuscitation, are not a reflection of poor management, but of the inherently very serious nature of the injury.

Damage to specific areas of the body by explosions

The ear

Virtually everyone injured by an explosion will have some auditory disturbance, even if it is only transient deafness or tinnitus. An already inflamed tympanic membrane will rupture with an overpressure as low as 15 kPa sustained for a few milliseconds. By contrast, 50% of humans with normal eardrums can expect to withstand overpressures of 100 kPa for as long as 10 ms.

It has been suggested that the presence of a ruptured eardrum following an explosion indicates exposure to a significant overpressure, and such patients warrant careful observation for the development of clinically significant blast lung. This is certainly true, but the absence of damage to the tympanic membrane does not exclude exposure to a high overpressure.

The propensity to rupture is critically dependent upon the orientation of the head to the incident blast. A direct overpressure of only a few kPa is required to rupture an exposed tympanic membrane, but the incident overpressure can be over 200 kPa before rupture of the tympanic membrane in a normal ear occurs. Some authors suggest that over 300 kPa may be tolerated, but do not specify the duration of the maximum overpressure (Blake et al., 1943). Individual tolerances of tympanic membrane to blast loading are wide.

Damage to the tympanic membrane varies from slight bruising to large defects, always located in the anterior inferior quadrant. Tears of the pars flaccida have not been reported.

Rupture of the tympanic membrane is the most obvious form of trauma to the ear in blast injury, but the shock-wave may be transmitted and cause dislocation of the ossicles in severe cases. Recent work demonstrates the damage done to the organ of Corti (Roberto et al., 1989). Damage to the labyrinth is also known to occur with rupture of the membrane of the round window. This probably heals spontaneously: it would be unwise to cite this as a frequent cause of dizziness following an explosion, as minor head injury is so common.

In the Old Bailey bombing, no eardrum ruptures were noted (Caro and Irving, 1973), but where the explosion is enclosed, as in the Guildford and Birmingham pub bombings, some 40% of survivors requiring admission to hospital had ruptured eardrums (Figures 19.2, 19.5) (Cooper et al., 1983). In the Israeli bus bombing, 76% of the 29 casualties had ruptured eardrums (Katz et al., 1989).

These figures suggest that, as expected, the degree of blast loading to which the victims are subjected is increased when they are enclosed. Clearly, in the Old Bailey bombing the blast loading declined rapidly in the open air. On the other hand, the overpressures must have been very high within the bombed Israeli bus due to shock-wave reflection and generation of the gaseous products of the explosive. In the survey of soldiers killed and injured by explosions in Northern Ireland, an attempt was made to correlate eardrum ruptures with blast loading sustained. When the fatalities were considered, none of those in the low blast loading group had ruptured eardrums, whereas this injury was seen in 96% of those fatalities thought to have been exposed to overpressures of more than 500 kPa (Mellor and Cooper, 1989). The survivors of such a high blast loading appeared to have a much lower incidence of perforation (38%). This observation may have been because the blast loading was lower than supposed in these cases, or due to the protective effect of the auditory meatus, or simply underreporting. About 50% of those surviving blast loading less than 500 kPa had perforated eardrums.

Blast injury to lung and gastrointestinal tract in survivors

Injury to the lung and gastrointestinal tract are frequently associated. Gut injury due to blast may occur in isolation in underwater explosions (Adler, 1981), but this is rather an unusual circumstance in terrorist bombings.

Clinically apparent blast injury to the lung is not common in survivors. Whilst it is clear that there is a wide variation in the damage that the blast-wave may do to the lungs, it must be appreciated that in less severe cases it rarely becomes evident, and that those with more severe blast lung die either of blast lung or the secondary injuries which are necessarily severe due to proximity to the explosion.

Twenty-seven servicemen supposedly exposed to severe blast loading in the early days of the Second World War were reviewed specifically for chest signs and symptoms (Dean et al., 1940). Six had abnormal radiological appearances, but since they had suffered burns and other injuries, this could not definitely be attributed solely to blast.

Body armour worn by security forces in Northern Ireland protects against potentially severe penetrating injury but not against blast. Two servicemen from Northern Ireland have required ventilation for blast lung, with no concurrent penetrating injury, and both were wearing body armour (Mellor and Cooper, 1989). One anecdotal incident from the Gulf War involved blast injury to a serviceman wearing body armour. A chest radiograph taken immediately had shown pulmonary contusion: this was no longer apparent 5 days later, and it could not be demonstrated on CT scanning, which would show pulmonary contusion not demonstrated by X-ray.

The lack of survivors with demonstrable pulmonary contusion suggests that if it does occur, the victim is probably close enough to be killed by penetrating missiles (hence its frequent incidence in those wearing body armour).

Contusion of bowel wall due to the blast-wave is seen experimentally in animal studies, but rarely appears clinically. The appearance of bruising in the caecal region is a common finding, and may reflect compression of gas against a competent ileocaecal valve. Perforation, or the colicky pain said to be due to submucosal haemorrhage, rarely appear because blast loading sufficient to cause symptomatic bowel damage is usually accompanied by blast lung which carries a high mortality.

Penetrating thoracic and abdominal injury

Penetrating injury of the abdomen resulting from explosions and involving intraperitoneal structures is rarely survivable. No survivors are recorded in data collected by the UK Royal Army Medical Corp's Hostile Action Casualty reporting System (HACS) from Northern Ireland. The same applies to injuries following explosion in which the thoracic wall is penetrated with resultant damage to intrathoracic structures. The combination of such injuries with the high blast loading is largely incompatible with survival. It should be stressed that these observations are on victims of terrorist devices which generate secondary fragments from debris: these fragments have poor aerodynamic qualities and would have insufficient energy for notable tissue penetration outside the lethal blast zone of the explosion. Although a percentage will reach hospital alive, they mostly die within a few hours of admission, either of uncontrollable haemorrhage or rapidly progressing ARDS.

These remarks do not apply to military munitions producing preformed fragments: these are projected much more widely resulting in severe secondary injuries well outside the lethal zone of the explosion, and indeed beyond the zone where any significant blast loading would be experienced.

Injury to solid viscera

Damage to solid organs, such as liver and spleen, is comparatively rare in survivors of explosions but may be seen in those wearing body armour which protects the chest. It is probably not the stress waves responsible for blast lung which cause tears of the solid organs, but transverse, low-frequency, shear waves. These cause tearing of organs with fixed mesenteries due to their differing inertial properties. Tears of the spleen occur near the hilum and can be reproduced experimentally. Lacerations of the liver will occur where it strikes the rib cage. If there is no evidence of blast lung then such injuries will have been caused by direct blows, as the body is displaced by the explosion or struck by flying objects. Only two survivors with closed abdominal injury following explosion have been recorded in HACS data from Northern Ireland. Waterworth and Carr (1975) record one patient with blast lung who required splenectomy, and survived. Other series report laparotomies for various abdominal injuries following explosions, but do not comment on the outcome (Scott et al., 1986; Frykberg and Tepas, 1988).

Head injury

This is an important source of morbidity and mortality in terrorist explosions. At least half of the late deaths from explosions are due to head injury (Frykberg and Tepas, 1988; Mellor and Cooper, 1989). In the Northern Ireland survey (Mellor and Cooper, 1989), 70% of those killed had significant head injuries. Of the survivors, 18% had significant head injuries (n = 113), but only seven of these had long-term sequelae. Hill's series of deaths from Northern Ireland bombings notes that 51% had skull fractures and 66% had evidence of brain damage. Subdural and subarachnoid vessels were the most common source of intracranial haemorrhage, but in 17% of cases were not associated with skull fracture. Major soft tissue loss around the head occurred in 61% of fatalities (Hill, 1979).

Head injury in survivors appears mainly restricted to concussion and cerebral contusion. Compound skull fractures requiring surgery were recorded in 10% of head injuries following the Bologna bombing (Brismar and Bergenwald, 1982).

Eyes

In spite of the small presented area of the eyes, injuries to the eye are common. Hill's data from Northern Ireland records 20% closed eye injury in fatalities and 18% perforating eye injury. Information gained from HACS data from Northern Ireland indicates 8% of all casualties sustained eye injury. Of these, 25% had penetrating injuries.

Burns

An explosion results in an intense but short-lived burst of thermal energy. Fires are caused, but the effect on the body is to cause rather superficial burns from the radiant heat, and from conduction from the hot explosive products (the flame front). Burns are usually only on exposed areas of skin, unless the casualty has been trapped by a secondary fire. Severe burns after explosions are uncommon. The head, neck and hands are the more frequently burned areas which simply reflects skin most commonly exposed.

Inhalation injuries

These are more likely to result from secondary fires than from the explosion itself, and may be another cause of ARDS which results in death more than 48 hours after the explosion.

Crush injuries

Crush injuries are an important source of morbidity and mortality when buildings collapse, but survivors of such injuries are unlikely to have sustained blast injury as well. The high mortality rate in the Beirut bombing was probably due in part to collapse of the building. The bombing of the Royal Marine Band depot at Deal in 1990 resulted in a large number of injuries due to collapse of the building.

Traumatic amputation of limbs

As already mentioned, traumatic amputation at any level is common in fatalities and survival is rare. In one series with 2934 immediate survivors, only 35 (1.2%) had such an injury, four of whom rapidly succumbed (Frykberg and Tepas, 1988). If the degree of blast loading is taken into account (Mellor and Cooper, 1989), half those surviving traumatic amputation will have sustained a blast

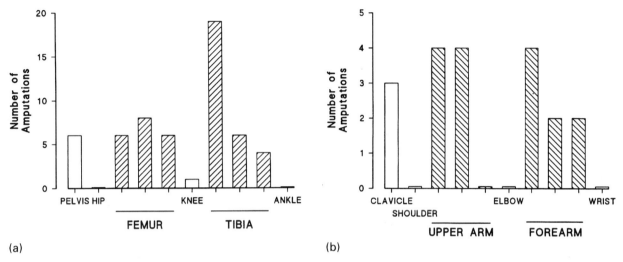

Figure 19.6 Sites of lower-limb (a) and upper-limb (b) amputations from bomb blast in fatalities from Northern Ireland.

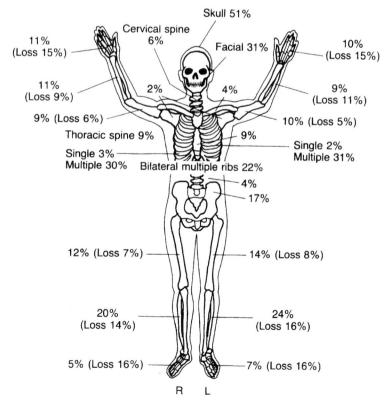

Figure 19.7 Distribution of skeletal fractures following explosions. (Taken from Hill, 1979.) Crown Copyright

loading of up to 500 kPa. However less than 10% will survive a blast loading greater than this, and it is in this group that most traumatic amputations occur. Those traumatic amputations that are survived are usually of digits alone. In the Paris bombings (Rignault and Deligny, 1989), resuscitation of victims with major traumatic amputations from the blast was attempted on the spot, but with no success.

Traumatic amputation from the blast is largely regarded as being due to forces arising from the motion of the combustion products (dynamic overpressure). This may produce limb-flailing, or bending forces on limbs. There is some evidence from a recent survey to suggest that flailing is not the principal mechanism; the primary interaction is probably the coupling of the very intense shock-wave into the limb, leading to bone failure.

A recent survey of amputations in fatalities from explosions in Northern Ireland, reviewed post-mortem reports and police photographs in Northern Ireland (Hull, 1994). A total of 73 amputations were observed in 100 consecutive deaths from bomb blast from 1987 to 1992. Specific note was made of the level of amputation. Very few of the amputations were through joints, the site likely to be described if flailing was the mechanism. Amputations caused by blast were commonest at the level of the upper third of the tibia for lower-limb injuries, and at the upper third of both the upper arm and the forearm (Figure 19.6).

Other limb injuries

When amputation because of blast is excluded, limb injuries severe enough to require surgery are seen in 20% of survivors (Mellor and Cooper, 1989). These injuries are caused by the violent displacement of the victim by the blast wind, blunt secondary missiles and collapse of buildings. In this series, 106 sustained lower-limb injuries, 89 upper-limb injuries and 103 both. Forty-five had residual lower-limb injuries, and two required amputation. Twenty-one had residual upper-limb injuries, and again two required amputation. These findings are similar to those described by Hadden *et al.* (1978). Frykberg and Tepas (1988) noted fractures in 10% of immediate survivors of explosions. The distribution of skeletal fracture as a result of such injuries is shown in Figure 19.7.

REFERENCES

Adler J. (1981). Underwater blast injury. *Med. Bull. US Army Europe*, **38**, 33–5.

Blake P.M., Douglas J.B.W., Krohn P.L., Zuckerman S. (1943). *Rupture of the Eardrums by Blast*. Ministry of Home Security Report BPC 43/169/WS21, Military Personnel Research Committee (Medical Research Council). Oxford: Department of Human Anatomy, Oxford University.

Brismar B., Bergenwald L. (1982). The terrorist bomb explosion in Bologna, Italy: an analysis of effects and injuries sustained. *J. Trauma*, **22**, 216–20.

Caro D., Irving M. (1973). The Old Bailey Bomb Explosion. *Lancet*, **i**, 1433–5.

Clutterbuck R. (ed.) (1986). *The Future of Political Violence*. New York: Royal United Services Institute, St Martins Press.

Cooper G.J., Maynard R.L., Cross N.L., Hill J.F. (1983). Casualties from terrorist bombings. *J. Trauma*, **23**, 955–67.

Dean D.M., Thomas A.R., Allison R.S. (1940). Effects of high explosive blast injury on the lungs. *Lancet*, **ii**, 224–6.

Frykberg E.R., Tepas J.J. (1988). Terrorist bombings. Lessons learned from Belfast to Beirut. *Ann. Surg.*, **208**(5), 569–76.

Hadden W.A., Rutherford W.H., Merritt J.D. (1978). The injuries of terrorist bombing: a study of 1532 consecutive patients. *Br. J. Surg.*, **65**, 525–31.

Hill J.F. (1979). Blast injury with particular reference to recent terrorist bombing incidents. *Ann. R. Coll. Engl.*, **61**, 4–11.

Hull J.B. (1994). Pattern of injury in those dying from traumatic amputation caused by bomb blast. *British Journal of Surgery*, **81**(8), 1132–5.

Katz E., Ofek B., Adler J. et al. (1989). Primary blast injury after a bomb explosion in a civilian bus. *Ann. Surg.*, **209**(4), 484–8.

Marshall T.K. (1977). Explosion injuries. In *Forensic Medicine*. (Tedeschi C.G., Eckert W.G., Tedeschi L.G., eds). Philadelphia: W.B. Saunders, pp. 612–35.

Mellor S.G., Cooper G.J. (1989). Analysis of 828 servicemen killed or injured by explosion in Northern Ireland 1970–1984. *Br. J. Surg.*, **76**, 1006–10.

Rignault D.P., Deligny M.C. (1989). The 1986 terrorist bombing experience in Paris. *Ann. Surg.*, **209**(3), 368–73.

Roberto M., Hamernik R.P., Turrentine G.A. (1989). Damage of the auditory system associated with acute blast trauma. *Ann. Otol. Rhinol. Laryngol*, **98**, 23–34.

Scott B., Fletcher R., Pulliam M. (1986). The Beirut terrorist bombing. *Neurosurgery*, **18**, 107–10.

Waterworth T.A., Carr M.J.T. (1975). Report on injuries sustained by patients treated at the Birmingham General Hospital following the recent bomb explosions. *Br. Med. J.*, **2**, 25–7.

20. Military Explosions*†

G. R. Ripple and Y. Phillips

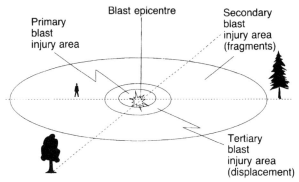

Figure 20.1 Blast injuries' distance of occurrence from the blast epicentre. The usual location of primary, secondary and tertiary blast injuries, in relation to an explosion regardless of blast intensity or distance, is shown.

BLAST-RELATED INJURIES IN THE MILITARY

Throughout modern military history, the majority of traumatic injuries occurring on the field of combat have been caused by exploding munitions. The wounding mechanisms associated with explosions are:

- Primary blast injury (PBI) due to the direct effects of the blast.
- Secondary ballistic injuries due to munition fragmentation and flying debris.
- Tertiary injuries, the outcome of the combatant being tumbled across the ground, thrown against a solid structure, or struck by a large object.

Fragmentation leading to penetrating wounds is the injury mechanism of most military ordnance with an anti-personnel role.

The three blast-related effects generate wounds according to the victim's distance from the centre of the explosion (Figure 20.1). Casualties close to the detonation are likely to show evidence of all three effects, while those who are farther away generally sustain only penetrating injury. Combined PBI ballistic and thermal injuries incurred close to an exploding munition are usually severely mutilating and survival is unlikely. Because the radius for ballistic injury is much larger than the corresponding radii for primary and tertiary blast effects, munitions designers capitalize on the ballistic effects by ensuring optimal fragmentation from each weapon, both in terms of fragment size and numbers. However, with the advance of the technology of fragment protection, both personal and within vehicles, and the improvement of blast weapons' performance, primary blast injury may become more significant in future combat.

PBI has received far less attention in military circles than secondary blast effects, largely because it is more difficult to recognize and diagnose, and because it is easily masked by more obvious ballistic wounds. Nevertheless, in certain military environments, PBI is now recognized as a distinct injury which requires specialized knowledge for optimal care.

MILITARY EXPERIENCE WITH PRIMARY BLAST INJURY

Primary blast injury is most likely to occur during conflicts in which powerful, sophisticated weapons are used. However in recent years, it has not been commonly reported in casualty statistics from military operations. This may be attributed to the low-intensity conflicts that have preoccupied Western nations during the second half of this century and which have employed relatively small ordnance on a limited scale. In contrast, however, wars in the Middle East during the same period have involved massed deployment of armour and powerful conventional weapons. Israeli writers have reported some primary blast injuries, though the accounts are limited by a lack of precision and autopsy data. Arab nations have not revealed any casualty information which may have been obtained from the Arab–Israeli conflicts, the Iran–Iraq War or Operation Desert Storm.

The earlier military medical literature contains remarkably little careful documentation of PBI. Either it occurs infrequently or it has gone unrecognized or unreported. American casualties from blast in Vietnam were probably few in number because the opposing forces utilized mostly light, hand-held infantry weapons. There were few large, special-purpose explosive munitions which might have generated large overpressures sufficient to produce primary blast injury. However, the opposing forces would have been more likely to suffer blast injuries from US weapons than vice versa, but no detailed medical data are available from Vietnamese sources.

Data collection

The US forces went to great lengths to compile accurate casualty data during the Vietnam conflict. The most ambitious data-collection effort was

* Portions of the text are taken from office of the Surgeon General, Department of the Army (1991). *Conventional Warfare: Ballistic, Blast and Burn Injuries (Textbook of Military Medicine*, Part I, Vol. 5). Washington, DC: US Government Printing Office.

† The opinions or assertions contained herein are the private views of the authors and are not to be construed as official policy or as reflecting the views of the Department of the Army, the Department of Defense or the United States Government.

conducted by the Wound Data and Munitions Effectiveness Team (WDMET), which accumulated detailed tactical and medical information on over 17 000 wounded or killed soldiers (Wound Data and Munitions Effectiveness Team, 1970).

In all the WDMET data, only two incidents were reported in which PBI was recognized and neither was the result of heavy enemy ordnance. In one case, a 500-lb (227-kg) conventional bomb dropped by US aircraft inadvertently fell on a US patrol. The fragments from the bomb caused many deaths and injuries but, in addition, two soldiers presented with haemoptysis and pulmonary contusion without external evidence of injury. Both clearly had blast-induced lung injury but neither required mechanical ventilation and both survived.

The second incident involved a rocket attack on an armoured vehicle which killed two soldiers. One was mutilated as he was blown through an open hatch. The other had only a scratch on his chin but was dead on the scene. Autopsy revealed that he had extensive blast injuries to his internal organs and fatal pulmonary haemorrhage. Air embolism was the probable cause of death; however, air emboli were not identified but it is unlikely that the tissues were carefully examined.

Data from other countries is also limited and difficult to interpret. According to Chinese experts, blast injuries accounted for only 0.3% of Chinese casualties during the Korean conflict (Wang, 1987). However, in the prevailing hardships of that time, data collection must have been very difficult. In China's more recent border conflict with Vietnam, 20% of the injuries that were caused by artillery or mines were said to include PBI (Wang, 1987). Unfortunately, details of PBI and concurrent injuries, including their morbidity and treatment, are not available.

Little precise documentation of the Israeli or Arab experiences in the 1980s is available on the incidence and consequence of PBI. Israeli Defense Force physicians reported that blast was responsible for 2.3% of the casualties in Lebanon in 1982 (Danon and Nili, 1984). Whether this refers only to PBI or includes the mutilating effects of mines and other explosives is not known. However, artillery explosions, which caused 53% of battle injuries, were identified separately as sources of injury which suggests that the 2.3% blast casualty rate may refer to PBI only. Injured personnel in armoured vehicles accounted for 14% of all casualties but the data do not indicate whether PBI was a significant cause or complication of injuries in tank crews. The collection of Israeli mortality data was also complicated by religious objections to autopsy so that the precise cause of death was not always determined.

The patterns of wounding described above would be more likely in a prolonged conflict against an enemy using sophisticated, conventional weapons. However, though PBI is a recognized result of explosive munitions, the actual incidence, morbidity and mortality of PBI remain unknown.

SPECIAL MILITARY BLAST HAZARDS

Future military conflicts will probably produce casualties with PBI, usually as an injury concurrent with other more obvious injuries in a severely wounded patient. PBI may become a significant injury mechanism for crews of modern armoured vehicles in which the other threats of fragments and fire have been reduced. Blast may also have serious effects on soldiers who wear body armour, who are exposed to enhanced-blast munitions or who are partially submerged during underwater denotations. Hearing loss and non-auditory injury from effects of either high-intensity blast or repeated low-intensity blast may also inhibit a combatant's ability to carry out military operations.

Exploding munitions are designed for anti-material effects, antipersonnel effects or both. Any munition may cause PBI and other blast-related injuries but the former is one of the antipersonnel effects most likely to be caused by specialized ordnance, such as armour-penetrating munitions, enhanced blast munitions and nuclear weapons. Underwater blast and repetitive low-level blasts are also injury-producing environments that are largely unique to the military environment.

Blast within penetrated armoured vehicles

In the past, fragments and fire have posed the greatest threat to crewmen when their armoured vehicle was penetrated by an antitank munition. However, design improvements in these vehicles and in personal protective clothing have significantly reduced the vulnerability of the crew to these injuries (Kennedy, 1983). The improvements include the use of: (a) spall-suppression linings; (b) compartmentalization of fuel and munitions; (c) flame resistant clothing and interior materials; and (d) automatic-fire suppression systems. As the threat of fragment and burn injuries lessens, those of blast and other ancillary effects may increase in significance.

Many Israeli armour casualties in the 1967 war occurred inside vehicles that were penetrated by antitank guided missiles (ATGMs) equipped with shaped-charge warheads. Some casualties suffered from respiratory failure and extensive (but superficial) burns. This combination of symptoms became known as the *ATGM syndrome* (Owen-Smith, 1977). The pulmonary component was attributed to a combination of PBI and toxic-fume inhalation.

Neither British nor US casualty data from armoured conflicts during the Second World War are particularly useful in determining the incidence of such primary blast injury. However, more recently, the introduction of aluminium armour for light vehicles has raised new concerns. Vaporific effect is a term introduced to describe a process in which aluminium, or any other component of armour, is vaporized and fragmented, mixed with atmospheric oxygen and is then rapidly oxidized to cause an explosive chemical reaction. Indeed, some arms manufacturers have proclaimed that new anti-tank rockets produce enhanced behind-armour blast effect because of this phenomenon. The biological significance and alleged increased incapacitating effects have not so far been sustained. Vaporific effect was studied in the mid 1980s by the US Army Medical Research and Developmental Command (USAMRDC). USAMRDC investigators conducted experiments using anaesthetized sheep and pigs inside armoured vehicles but outside the area of fragment injury. Two different armoured personnel carriers were penetrated by either small shoulder-fired antitank munitions or other larger calibre warheads (Phillips *et al.*, 1989a). These experiments revealed that, outside the fragment spall cone, significant primary blast injury to the lungs and gut did not occur.

A US Congress mandate in 1987 decreed that all US military weapons systems must be tested against realistic threats from munitions in simulated combat operating conditions. As a result, the US Army completed an extensive series of tests with the Bradley fighting vehicle (Figure 20.2), the M60A3 tank and the M1A1 Abrams tank (Phillips *et al.*, 1989b). Fragment injuries were assessed on ballistic mannequins positioned as the crew would be. USAMRDC investigators determined the risk of other non-fragment injury from data collected to evaluate: (a) heat; (b) acceleration/displacement; (c) primary blast and (d) inhalation of toxic fumes. Although the results of these tests were not published in the open literature, PBI was assessed as a probable casualty effect in only a few circumstances.

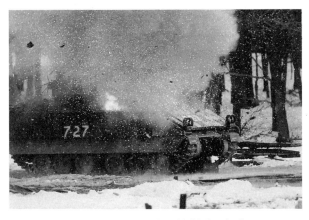

Figure 20.2 Bradley Fighting Vehicle during armour perforation.

The number of PBI casualties in a modern armour conflict is difficult to predict, but the incidence of crewmen injured by fragment wounds is still expected to exceed by far that of PBI injury. Based on the USAMRDC studies in which an armoured vehicle was penetrated by a large warhead, 1–20% of the survivors would be expected to have some degree of PBI in addition to their other wounds. Whether the blast effects would dominate or merely complicate the clinical course of these casualties is not known. Therefore, casualties who are injured in these circumstances should be observed closely for signs of PBI.

Enhanced blast munitions

Some modern weapons are specially designed to enhance blast effectiveness (enhanced-blast technology). Modern fragmentation munitions are one example but the weapon most capable of producing PBI is the fuel-air explosive (FAE). Munitions of this kind are designed to injure by their direct blast effects rather than by fragmentation. Most 'modern' military powers have these at their actual or potential disposal. Until recently, delivery of these bulky, heavy weapons and their associated explosion/fire hazards precluded their routine use in naval and land warfare. However, they have become more reliable and sophisticated, and hence more prevalent in modern arsenals.

A typical FAE munition is constructed with a bursting charge placed in the central long axis of a cylindrical container filled with a low-volatility liquid fuel such as ethylene oxide or propylene oxide. The walls of the container are scored so that it can break apart in a predictable way when the bursting charge explodes. A second, delayed, igniting charge then detonates the dispersed liquid. The weapon is usually delivered by aircraft as a gravity, sometimes 'steerable', bomb or by low-velocity guided missile. To allow efficient dispersal of the fuel-air cloud, the munition may be parachute-braked before impact. The bursting charge detonates and the container's contents are dispersed as a disc-shaped, fuel-aerosol cloud at low altitude (Figure 20.3(a)). The diameter may range from 15 m from a 36-kg FAE to 45 m with a 900-kg FAE (Bellamy and Zajtchuk, 1990). The second, 'trailing' charge ignites the fuel-air mixture, causing an explosion of high peak overpressure and duration (Figure 20.3(b)).

The cloud's characteristics allow it to disperse widely and to enter foxholes, fortifications, and other structures which are inaccessible to fragments. Thus, blast effects which are not possible through the use of any single conventional, solid, explosive munition can be created over a wide area and within protective structures. Given appropriate though complex conditions, the detonation creates an almost universally lethal blast pressure of

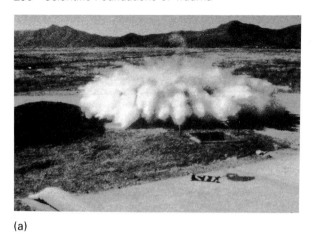

(a)

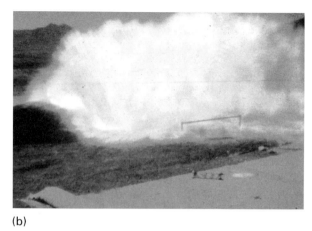

(b)

Figure 20.3 Fuel-air explosion sequence. (a) Fuel-air cloud dispersed by bursting charge. (b) Fuel-air explosion detonated by 'trailing', igniting charge.

1700–2000 kPa throughout the cloud (Bellamy and Zajtchuk, 1990). Lethal effects from a 900-kg FAE may encompass as much as 4500 m².

FAEs were utilized in the Vietnam War to clear mine fields and landing sites. In addition, they have probably been used against 'soft' military material, such as vans, radar antennae and other light, tall structures. The Egyptians reportedly used FAE munitions to knock down and disable Israeli radar antennae during the Yom Kippur War (Phillips and Richmond, 1990). FAE weapons could be used for other special-purpose missions such as clearing helicopter landing zones, destroying buildings, fuel depots and ammunition stacks and clearing dense foliage.

Although FAE should be effective against personnel in foxholes, bunkers and tunnels, the role of enhanced-blast munitions as antipersonnel weapons has not been established. FAE munitions were reportedly used by Soviet forces against Afghanistan emplacements and resulted in immense fires (Phillips and Richmond, 1990). Whether they were used as a primary blast weapon, as a 'terror' weapon or as an incendiary munition is unclear. More recently, in Operation Desert Storm, US Forces used FAE munitions against Iraqi bunkers and defense fortifications. The rationale for using FAE munitions in such instances can only be conjectured, and the resulting antipersonnel effects are undocumented.

Injuries produced by enhanced-blast munitions

Enhanced-blast weapons, which include FAE, generate all forms of blast-associated injuries. Personnel in the open can be thrown by an explosion and suffer impact injuries. The latter include skin lacerations and abrasions, muscular contusions, skeletal fractures and joint dislocations. Internal organ contusions and ruptures are also common impact injuries, and usually cause hypovolaemic shock from bleeding into a body cavity or muscle.

Sand, twigs and other objects can be propelled by a blast to cause penetrating injuries and a high incidence of eye damage. FAE munitions also cause significant burn injuries in victims caught within or just outside the area of cloud.

Blast effects are magnified in enclosed areas. Foxholes afford little, if any, protection from the blast and burn effects of an enhanced-blast munition. In fact, some foxholes may magnify blast effects because enclosures of certain dimensions produce reflected pressures which magnify the incident pressure and/or extend the pressure duration.

As enhanced-blast munitions are used more frequently in combat, PBI and ear injury will likely become more common. Because FAE produce long-duration blast-waves similar to a nuclear explosion, these effects are discussed below in the section 'Blasts from nuclear explosions'.

Blast from nuclear explosions

Nuclear weapons effects

The blast, thermal and radiation resulting from the detonation of a nuclear weapon are dependent on the total energy produced by a weapon – yield in kilotons (KT) of an equivalent conventional explosive – usually TNT. The intense heat radiating from a nuclear blast is the most immediate injury-producing mechanism to a soldier in the field. This burn threat dominates other injury effects for large-yield strategic weapons (Joint DNA–USANCA Study: Combined Injury from Nuclear-Weapons Effects, 1979). Nuclear radiation is not immediately incapacitating but may render troops ineffective in combat within hours. Blast effects are of little concern, except in special instances where the individual may be protected from the thermal and radiation effects (Bellamy and Zajtchuk, 1989).

The detonation of a nuclear device produces a blast (shock) wave which is a function of the weapon's yield. The blast-wave contains both high static pressures and intense dynamic pressures (nuclear wind) which can produce primary, secondary and tertiary injuries. The static pressures occur within an expanding envelope of compressed air which crushes soft objects. The dynamic pressure is produced by and is proportional to the difference between the expanding static pressure envelope and the ambient air pressure. In this discussion, the static and dynamic components are referred to as blast overpressure and blast wind, respectively.

Injuries induced by long-duration blast-waves

Both the blast overpressure and the blast wind can cause injury to unprotected individuals. The blast overpressure with its very short rise time and long duration produces primarily internal injuries in gas-containing organs. For example, rupture of the eardrum occurs at about 50 kPa, while a static, long-duration, free-field overpressure of 250 kPa produces serious intrathoracic injuries which include alveolar and pulmonary vascular rupture, interstitial haemorrhage, oedema and air emboli. Bowel injuries (contusion, perforation) occur at approximately the same levels which cause pulmonary injuries. Hepatic and splenic rupture may also occur with higher levels of blast overpressure because of violent compression of the abdomen or tertiary impact following displacement.

The blast winds that accompany the blast overpressure produce mainly secondary and tertiary blast injuries. Loose debris is hurled by the blast wind which, depending on the size, shape and mass of the fragments, can cause injuries ranging from lacerations and contusions to fractures, blunt trauma and dismemberment. Blast winds in excess of 160 kph can violently hurl a person and cause lacerations, contusions and fractures from tumbling across the terrain or from being thrown against a stationary object. Blast winds produce more significant injuries than the accompanying static component of the blast-wave.

Lethality from tumbling begins when blast winds move at speeds greater than 80 kph and the LD_{50} is when a human impacts the ground at about 32–40 kph (Bellamy and Zajtchuk, 1989). These blast winds are usually associated with static pressures of approximately 40 kPa. Therefore, the LD_{50} for a nuclear blast is calculated to occur at 40 kPa (Bellamy and Zajtchuk, 1989), but the primary wounding effects are secondary and tertiary blast effects, not PBI. For a small nuclear munition with a yield of 0.5 kiloton (KT), the LD_{50} range extends to approximately 0.5 km. Larger weapons with yields of 50 and 500 KT produce an LD_{50} which extends to just under 2 km and just under 4 km, respectively (Bellamy and Zajtchuk, 1989).

Records from Nagasaki and Hiroshima indicate that 5% of injuries were caused by blast injuries (probably secondary and tertiary effects), another 5% were attributed to combined blast and burn injury, and 20% were the outcome of burn, blast and radiation injuries combined. Approximately 70% of survivors from Nagasaki and Hiroshima suffered mechanical injuries from translation or flying debris (Joint DNA–USANCA Study: Combined Injury from Nuclear-Weapons Effects, 1979). Primary blast injury could compound these more serious injuries in multiple-injured patients. However, survival of those so close to 'ground zero' would be doubtful, due to the coincident extremes of thermal and radiation energy. As with enhanced-blast weapons, foxholes and surrounding barriers afford little protection from PBI and they may actually magnify the blast and the resulting injuries.

The best protection from a nuclear blast is within a blast-resistant shelter but some protection can be achieved behind an immovable object which offers protection from the radiant thermal pulse and the blast wind. In the absence of other protection to reduce the body's surface area that is exposed to wind-borne debris and to lessen the body's aerodynamic resistance to the blast wind, personnel should lie face down on the ground with the head pointed toward the explosion.

Underwater blast

Blast injuries in partially submerged individuals exposed to subsurface explosions are common in naval combat and are probably the most numerous and lethal of all primary blast injuries. During the Second World War, combatants in the water near a subsurface explosion are known to have suffered severe lung and abdominal injuries. Many casualties were reported by US and British authors; however, the exact number of those afflicted, which includes those who died, is not accurately recorded. Pugh (1943) identified 50 casualties with abdominal blast injuries who were evacuated to Pearl Harbor following the Battle of Midway in 1942. The British recorded an incident in which only 90 out of 125 sailors who had safely abandoned ship survived a nearby depth-charge explosion (Cope, 1953). In another incident, 24 sailors were rescued after having survived an underwater explosion in a North Sea combat action; however, 11 died within the first few days following the incident. Seven of the dead suffered intestinal perforations (Gordon-Taylor, 1953).

More recently, Huller and Bazini (1970) reported an action from the 1967 Arab–Israeli War in which an Egyptian missile struck and sank the Israeli destroyer Eilat. After the crew abandoned ship, another missile detonated nearby. The number who were in the water and the number of immediate deaths were not reported but 32 survivors were rescued within a few hours. PBI was documented in all but one. This individual suffered a fractured tibia before abandoning ship, and Huller raises the supposition that hypovolaemia may protect against PBI. Twenty-seven of the 32 survivors showed evidence of blast lung injury, and five of these required positive-pressure (mechanical) ventilation. Twenty-four underwent laparotomy for abdominal symptoms, and 22 were found to have bowel perforations. Nineteen sailors had concurrent thoracic and gastrointestinal injuries. Ultimately, four of the 27 died, and three of these expired during or shortly after general anaesthesia.

In another incident from the Middle East, 13 soldiers suffered injuries from an underwater detonation while they were swimming for recreation (Weiler-Ravell *et al.*, 1975). Although all quickly left the water, two sailors suffered cardiac arrest within the first minute. Within 10 minutes, two more died of unknown causes. By 30 minutes after the blast, two more died. The remaining seven survivors were flown by helicopter to a nearby medical facility. Despite intensive treatment all but three ultimately died. Air embolism to the heart and brain was assumed to be the cause of the early deaths.

Blast-waves are transmitted more efficiently in water – the peak impulse is transmitted farther with less energy dissipation. This expands the lethal radius by a factor of at least three over that for an explosion in air. The water–air interface reflects the shock-wave as a tension wave and this combines in a complex manner with the initial wave and effectively cancels some of the injurious effect near the surface (Fletcher *et al.*, 1976). The injurious effect of the blast increases with depth

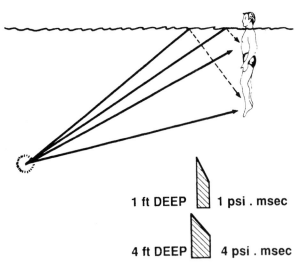

1 ft DEEP   **1 psi . msec**

4 ft DEEP   **4 psi . msec**

Figure 20.4 Underwater explosion. The reflective properties of the air–water interface disrupt a blast-wave near the surface and magnify its intensity at increasing depth.

(Figure 20.4), which is thought to be one of the reasons why abdominal injuries occur more frequently in water.

Body depth and orientation in the water is an important determinant of the severity of underwater blast injuries. Cope, a British naval surgeon in the Second World War, observed that if an individual was floating on his back, no serious injury was sustained from a nearby subsurface explosion (Mellor, 1988). Therefore, when exposure to underwater blast is expected, floating on the back as near to the water's surface as possible is probably the safest course of action.

Repetitive low-intensity blast

Weapon crews in training and combat are exposed to repetitive blasts. The auditory health hazard created by such exposures is well recognized by the military (see 'Hearing loss' below). However, other organs that contain gas are also susceptible to injury from repetitive blasts – the mechanical reasons are not known. With the development of more powerful weapons and better hearing protection, non-auditory injury induced by repetitive low-level blasts could become a significant occupational hazard for the military.

Investigators at the Walter Reed Army Institute of Research (WRAIR) determined the intensity and number of repetitive blast exposures which caused trivial submucosal punctate haemorrhages to appear in the trachea of sheep (Dodd *et al.*, 1990). As it is difficult to diagnose minor blast injuries (e.g. small asymptomatic pulmonary or gastrointestinal contusions) in man, and because sheep have proven to be a reasonable human surrogate model for studying blast overpressure injury, pressure limits slightly lower than these curves have been accepted by the US Army as the absolute upper limits of human exposure for free-field air blasts. These safety levels for 5, 25 and 100 sequential exposures are illustrated in Figure 20.5.

Using these human exposure limits, US Army Medical Research and Development Command initiated a study to determine the human auditory exposure limits for soldiers wearing single and double hearing protection while exposed to a repetitive blast overpressure. The study is complex and carefully designed to limit human risk. In brief, males wearing ear muffs, foam ear plugs, or both, are exposed to increasing numbers and blast intensities (Table 20.1), according to an exposure matrix (Figure 20.6) based upon the non-auditory limits. Audiometry is performed before and after the exposures to determine early hearing decrements as defined by a subject's temporary threshold shifts (TTS). Preliminary data has revealed no TTS or non-auditory physical injury in the first 94 subjects. All subjects left the study in good health and without medical complaints, which suggests

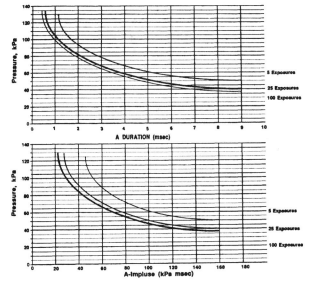

Figure 20.5 Human exposure limits to repetitive blast overpressure. These curves were experimentally derived from a large animal model and represent the blast intensity levels for 5, 25 and 100 blast exposures which cause trivial, small visceral submucosal haemorrhages (petechia). Each intensity is plotted by two parameters: (a) pressure versus the time of positive deflection, A-Duration; (b) pressure versus the integral of the initial positive deflection A-Impulse.

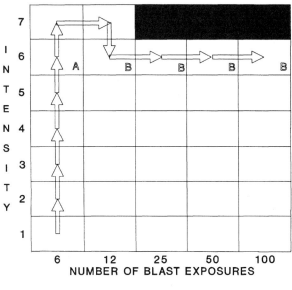

Figure 20.6 Human tolerance study: exposure matrix. This matrix shows the allowable exposures which were tested by the United States Army Medical and Development Command. The arrows show the exposure sequence for an individual who showed no auditory or non-auditory effects during the experiment. Intensity levels can be determined from Table 20.1.

TABLE 20.1

AVERAGE BLAST EXPOSURES: HUMAN TOLERANCE STUDY. VALUES ARE THE AVERAGE BLAST INTENSITIES STUDIED BY THE UNITED STATES ARMY MEDICAL RESEARCH AND DEVELOPMENT COMMAND IN THE FIRST PHASE OF A HUMAN TOLERANCE STUDY TO DETERMINE HUMAN SAFETY STANDARDS FOR REPETITIVE BLAST EXPOSURES

Intensity code	Peak (kPa)	Peak (dB)	A-duration (ms)	B-duration (ms)	A-impulse (kPa/ms)
1	9.0	172.1	2.2	21.9	9.2
2	13.7	176.7	2.4	22.3	14.2
3	18.6	179.4	2.5	20.2	19.8
4	25.9	182.2	2.8	22.2	27.7
5	34.9	184.4	2.9	21.5	38.0
6	50.3	187.9	2.9	22.6	55.9
6B	45.3	187.1	3.0	22.1	51.4
7	65.8	190.3	2.9	27.7	72.5

Note: Intensity 6B maintains a maximum exposure level below the non-auditory limits.

that cumulative blast effects did not occur at the levels tested.

These initial results suggest that humans can tolerate low-intensity, repetitive blast exposures without significant physical injury. However, the study also revealed that humans feel discomfort at the highest levels tested. Exposures above an unknown 'nuisance level' might produce discomfort which could adversely affect an individual's performance or willingness to serve in such a noisy environment.

Body armour

Although the effects of body armour are discussed elsewhere in this text, a brief discussion is included in this section because it has been shown to enhance PBI. Blast researchers have studied clothing effects during blast overpressure exposure to determine their effect on the injury mechanism and to determine if an individual can be protected by a practical body covering. Research to date has documented the enhancement of blast injury by certain outerwear.

Jönsson (1979) demonstrated that foam rubber covering a rabbit markedly increased primary blast lung injury and lethality. However, shielding the animal's chest in a steel pipe protected the animal from lung injury. A human volunteer study conducted by WRAIR showed that the US Army standard-issue Kevlar cloth ballistic vest caused an increase in intrathoracic pressures at the overpressure levels found in the crew areas during the firing of heavy weapons as compared to intra-thoracic pressure when the vest was not worn (Young *et al.*, 1988).

This study was followed by one using large animals and much higher levels of blast (Phillips *et al.*, 1985), which indicated that the ballistic vest significantly increased both lung haemorrhage and mortality compared to controls. At the highest overpressure level, five of the six animals wearing the vest died immediately from the blast compared to only two of six uncovered animals.

Combat records do not confirm – or refute – this enhancement of PBI by fragmentation rests. However, a British study of IRA bombings documents lethal pulmonary blast injuries in some soldiers wearing ballistic vests (Mellor and Cooper, 1989). PBI was the presumed cause of death in some casualties and had a higher incidence than that normally reported in civilians. Enhancement of PBI may be implicated, but the British authors suggest that the high incidence arises from a failure of fragmentation vests to decouple the shock-wave. The total number of dead due to fragments is reduced, and thus the apparent incidence of PBI increases. Although Israeli soldiers commonly wear body armour, the authors are unaware of any publication which documents the incidence of PBI in soldiers wearing ballistic vests and wounded in recent Middle-East conflicts.

The mechanism for this enhancement of PBI has not been satisfactorily determined, but two theories have been proposed (Phillips *et al.*, 1988; Cooper *et al.*, 1989). The vest may serve to increase the body's surface area thus increasing the total energy delivered to the chest, or it may alter the acoustic impedance of the air/body interface and transmit more of the blast overpressure into the chest (see p. 263). Both theories suggest that the chest wall is compressed more violently when a cloth ballistic vest is worn. Therefore, although ballistic vests are necessary to protect individuals from potentially lethal fragment injuries, some investigators believe they may do so at the cost of compounding PBI. This enhancement may not be as great when more rigid ballistic protection is used, such as overlapping metal plates (Z.G. Wang, 1991, personal communication).

This information that personal body armour may enhance PBI must not be seen as a recommendation to abandon its use. The ballistic vest is a proven lifesaver and the threat of injury by bullets or fragments is far greater that the threat of pure PBI on any battlefield that can currently be imagined. Instead, the data should be used by physicians when they make triage and treatment decisions; they must suspect PBI in individuals wearing ballistic vests who are exposed to blast overpressure even in the absence of significant ballistic wounds.

Hearing loss

The most sensitive organ to the primary effects of a blast-wave is the ear. Military personnel are at particular risk for hearing loss during training, not only from blast exposure but also from higher frequency impulse noise, such as rifle firing, and from continuous noise exposure during the operation of aircraft and tracked vehicles. Hearing loss is the largest category of medical disability for the US military, and in 1985 it resulted in the payment of more than $165 million in benefits (Phillips and Richmond, 1990).

Information on combat-related hearing loss is scanty. Brown (1985) reported 338 soldiers with hearing loss sustained during the campaign in the Falklands. The soldiers were divided into three groups according to their exposure: (a) support weapon operators, e.g. mortar crews; (b) infantrymen using small arms and (c) survivors of blast injuries sustained in an attack on a transport ship. Brown discovered that those using heavier weapons were at greater risk with the mean hearing loss when compared with preconflict hearing levels being 5.1 dB in the right ear and 5.5 dB in the left ear. Compliance in the use of hearing protection was so poor that no conclusion could be reached regarding its effectiveness. In a second study from the Falklands, 114 soldiers in the Royal Artillery were exposed to very high levels of impulse noise from the sustained firing of 105-mm artillery (Anderson, 1984). The data are summarized in Table 20.2.

Soldiers who fail to wear hearing protection and are inside an armoured vehicle during penetration are likely to suffer severe ear damage as the outcome of the complex reverberant blast environment. In one study, large animals were placed inside armoured vehicles that were penetrated by shaped-charge warheads (Phillips and Patterson, 1988). A 5-in. warhead penetration caused tympanic-membrane rupture in 71% of ears, compared to 36% during penetration of a 3-in. warhead.

TABLE 20.2
HEARING LOSS IN BRITISH COMBATANTS: FALKLAND ISLANDS CONFLICT. SUMMARY OF THE HEARING DECREMENTS FOUND IN BRITISH COMBATANTS FOLLOWING THE FALKLAND ISLAND CONFLICT (ANDERSON, 1984; BROWN, 1985)

Test group	No. studied	% of combatants whose hearing was affected
All infantry	338	13.3
Infantry using small arms	109	7.3
Infantry using 81-mm mortars	76	23.7
105-mm Howitzer gun crew	84	11.9

Prevention of hearing loss is possible. Conventional hearing protection plugs should greatly reduce or eliminate the risk of tympanic-membrane rupture and hearing loss.

PREDICTING BLAST-INDUCED INJURY SEVERITY

Human injury and performance decrements attributable to conventional or nuclear explosions cannot be studied experimentally. However, military planners must approximate injury incidence and human performance as a first step in estimating effective troop strength for combat operations. Predictive criteria have been suggested to estimate the incidence of PBIs and their resulting performance decrement.

Historically, performance decrement estimates have been based on a subjective linking of performance with lethality criteria. A consensus meeting of US investigators in 1983 (Phillips Y.Y. and Kokinakis W., 1983, personal communication) suggested that degrees of incapacitation should be assigned to the Bowen's injury/lethality curves (Bowen *et al.*, 1968; White *et al.*, 1971), which define the probability of lethality or injury for certain blast exposures, e.g. body prone head-on to blast or body against reflecting surface. These curves are shown in Chapter 16. The meeting participants recommended that incapacitation be extrapolated between three points:

1. Total incapacitation should be considered to occur at blast levels causing 50% mortality (LD_{50}).
2. Fifty per cent incapacitation should be considered to occur at LD_1.
3. One per cent incapacitation should be considered to occur at threshold lung injury levels.

Since the Second World War, physicians have recognized that exercise enhances the severity of blast injury (O'Reilly and Gloyne, 1941). It probably exacerbates a moderate blast injury into severe injury or death by extending the area of pulmonary haemorrhage, by enhancing pulmonary oedema or by increasing the frequency and size of air emboli (Yelverton *et al.*, 1971). The window of susceptibility for increased lethality due to exercise following blast injury probably lasts 4 hours; however, decrements in exercise performance may last 2–3 days (Yelverton *et al.*, 1971). Although the extent to which exercise increases PBI in humans has yet to be determined, the authors suggest that the injury or incapacitation prediction be doubled for individuals who may undergo severe exercise (e.g. that performed by a munitions handler or an infantryman).

These models cannot be directly applied to injury and performance for soldiers suffering PBI from a *complex* blast-wave, e.g. from an explosion inside a bunker or armoured vehicle. Such a wave is composed of multiple reflective spikes which do not allow easy comparison to the characteristic free-field blast waveforms on which the Bowen curves are based. Until the interaction of complex blast-waves and the human torso is more completely characterized, the injury potential of a complex wave will have to be extrapolated in some way from free-field criteria.

The above incapacitation criteria are based on limited scientific data and provide only rough estimates of PBI severity and its effect on human performance. The authors also recognize that other unmeasurable factors can greatly affect an individual's performance in combat; e.g., motivation from fear of death or from group cohesiveness can overcome pain and physical weakness. This method of determining blast injury/performance decrements is of limited use, except to military planners who seek a method to quantitate the human effects during expected combat operations.

SUMMARY

Although fragments and mechanical translation cause most of the injuries that result from explosive munitions on the field of combat, PBI has been found at autopsy in soldiers dying of other causes and it may be a contributor to early mortality in many instances. The actual incidence of PBI in military casualties has probably been clouded by the low-intensity nature of most Western combat operations since the Korean Conflict and a lack of blast-casualty data from Middle-East wars.

A small number of casualties who present to a medical care facility following traumatic injuries induced by an explosion will be likely to have PBI of varying severity. Pulmonary PBI is an immediate concern because it results in early respiratory failure and high mortality. Use of positive-pressure ventilation or general anaesthesia induces high levels of morbidity and mortality in PBI casualties. Abdominal PBI may not be obvious initially, but it may result in perforation of the bowel with subsequent peritonitis and death. Therefore, the triage physician must recognize the conditions which are associated with a higher likelihood of PBI. Medical officers should be particularly alert for PBI in casualties from armoured-vehicle penetration, enhanced-blast munitions (such as fuel-air explosives), nuclear explosions or underwater blasts.

Repeated exposure to blast overpressure is a unique occupational hazard of the military. Certain levels of blast overpressure, which are not dangerous if experienced once, can cause both auditory and non-auditory injuries if an individual is exposed to repetitive blasts. Although experimental work has determined levels of repeated blast which are safe, repeated exposures above a yet to be determined level probably would produce enough discomfort that an individual might be unwilling to remain and work in such a noxious environment.

Even in peacetime, hearing loss is a common occupational hazard for soldiers. The limited available data and common sense suggest that intense combat operations – even those that are as brief as the Falkland Islands War and Operation Desert Storm – can result in significant hearing loss for many combatants. Wearing standard-issue hearing protection should greatly ameliorate this acoustic injury.

Improved ballistic protection (e.g. armoured vehicles and body armour) for soldiers in modern conventional wars may increase a soldier's vulnerability to blast effects while providing better protection from fragments.

So long as wars are fought, military leaders and physicians must remain attentive to all effects of explosive munitions. As yet, primary blast injury has not been a major determinant of morbidity or mortality during military training or combat; however, changes in weaponry and war-fighting doctrine will probably increase the incidence of primary blast injury. Military physicians must be prepared during future conflicts to suspect, to recognize and to treat primary blast injury.

REFERENCES

Anderson J. (1984). An audiometric survey of royal artillery gun crews following 'Operation Corporate'. *J. R. Army Med. Corps*, **130**, 100–8.

Bellamy R.F., Zajtchuk R. (eds) (1989). The weapons of conventional land warfare. In *Textbook of Military Medicine, Part I, Vol. 2, Medical Consequences of Nuclear Warfare*. Washington, DC: US Government Printing Office, pp. 4–5.

Bellamy R.F., Zajtchuk R. (1990). The weapons of conventional land warfare. In *Textbook of Military Medicine, Part I, Vol. 1, Conventional Warfare: Ballistic, Blast, and Burn Injuries* (Bellamy R.F., Zajtchuk R., eds). Washington, DC: US Government Printing Office, pp. 35–6.

Bowen I.G., Fletcher E.R., Richmond D.R. (1968). *Estimates of Man's Tolerance to the Direct Effects of Air Blast*, Technical Report under contract No. DA-49–146-XZ-372 (DASA-2113). Government Printing Office.

Brown J.R. (1985). Noise-induced hearing loss sustained during land operations in the Falkland Islands campaign. *J. Soc. Occup. Med.*, **35**, 44–54.

Cooper G.J., Pearce B.P., Cater S.R. et al. (1989). Augmentation by foam materials of lung injury produced by blast waves; the role of stress waves in thoracic visceral injury at high rates of energy transfer. In *Proceedings of the International Research Council on the Biokinetics of Impacts*. Stockholm, Sweden: International Research Council on the Biokinetics of Impacts.

Cope Z. (1953). The general effects of blast. In *Surgery*, part 1 (Cope Z., ed.). London: HMSO, pp. 652–63.

Danon Y.L., Nili E. (1984). Triage, primary treatment and evacuation: the IDF experience in Lebanon. In Paper presented at the Second International Congress in Israel on Disaster Management, 16–19 September, at Israel Defense Force, Jerusalem.

Dodd K.T., Yelverton J.T., Richmond D.R et al. (1990). Nonauditory injury threshold for repeated intense freefield impulse noise. *J. Occup. Med.*, **32**, 260–6.

Fletcher E.R., Yelverton J.T., Richmond D.R. (1976). The thoraco-abdominal system's response to underwater blast. In *Final Report to Naval Research Contract N0014–75-C-1079*, Lovelace Foundation for Medical Education and Research. Springfield, VA: National Technical Information Service, US Department of Commerce.

Gordon-Taylor G. (1953). Abdominal effects of immersion blast. In *Surgery*, part 2 (Cope Z., ed.). London: HMSO, pp. 664–72.

Huller T., Bazini Y. (1970). Blast injuries of the chest and abdomen. *Arch. Surg.*, **10**, 24–30.

Joint Defence Nuclear Agency – United States Army Nuclear and Chemical Agency (DNA – US ANCA): Combined Injury from Nuclear-Weapons Effects (1 Jan. 1979), Washington DC, pp. 1–2.

Jönsson A. (1979). Experimental Investigations on the Mechanisms of Lung Injury in Blast and Impact Exposure. PhD Dissertation no. 80, Department of Surgery, Linköping University, Stockholm, Sweden.

Kennedy D.R. (1983). Improving combat crew Survivability. *Armor*, **9**, 16–22.

Mellor S.G. (1988). The pathogenesis of blast injury and its management. *Br. J. Hosp. Med.*, **39**, 536–9.

Mellor S.G., Cooper G.J. (1989). Analysis of 828 servicemen killed or injured by explosion in Northern Ireland 1970–84: The Hostile Action Casualty System. *Br. J. Surg.*, **76**, 1006–10.

O'Reilly J.N., Gloyne S.R. (1941). Blast injury of the lungs. *Lancet*, **ii**, 423.

Owen-Smith M.S. (1977). Armored fighting vehicle casualties. *J.R. Army Med. Corps*, **123**, 65–76.

Phillips Y.Y. III, Patterson J.H. (1988). Protection against noise and blast. *Med. Bull. U.S. Army Med. Dep.*, **PB8–88–2**, 17–20.

Phillips Y.Y. III, Mundie T.G., Yelverton J.T., Richmond D.R. (1988). Cloth ballistic vest alters response to blast. *J. Trauma*, **28**, S149–52.

Phillips Y.Y. III, Mundie T.G., Hoyt R., Dodd K.T. (1989a). Middle ear injury in animals exposed to complex blast waves inside an armored vehicle. *Ann. Otol. Rhinol. Laryngol.*, **98**, 17–22.

Phillips Y.Y. III, Ripple G.R., Dodd K.T., Mundie T.G. (1989b). Medical evaluation of live fire test injuries: predicting medical effects behind defeated armor. *Army RD A Bull.*, **89**, 16–18.

Phillips Y.Y. III, Richmond D.R. (1990). Primary blast injury and basic research: a brief history. In *Textbook of Military Medicine, Part I, Vol. 1, Conventional Warfare: Ballistic, Blast, and Burn Injuries* (Bellamy R.F., Zajtchuk R., eds). Washington, DC: US Government Printing Office, pp. 227–33.

Pugh H.L. (1943). Blast injuries. *Surg. Clin. North Am.*, **23**, 1589–602.

Rose T.F. (1944). Lung blast. *Med. J. Aust.*, **1**, 784.

Wang Z.G. (1987). Research on blast injury in China. *Chuang Shang Tsa Chih*, **6**, 222–8.

Weiler-Ravell D., Adatto R., Borman J.B. (1975). Blast

injury of the chest: a review of the problem and its treatment. *Isr. J. Med. Sci.*, **11**, 268–74.

White C.S., Jones R.K., Damon E.G. et al. (1971). *The Biodynamics of Airblast*, DNA 2738T under contract no. DASA 01–70-C-0075, 1 July. Government Printing Office.

Wound Data and Munitions Effectiveness Team (1970). *Evaluation of Wound Data and Munitions Effectiveness in Vietnam (Final Report)*. Alexandria, VA: Defense Documentation Center of the Defense Logistics Agency.

Yelverton J.T., Viney J.F., Jojola B., Jones R.K. (1971). *The Effects of Exhaustive Exercise on Rate at Various Times Following Blast Exposure*, DASA 2702, DNA Contract No. DA-49–146-XZ-359. Government Printing Office.

Young A.J., Jaeger J.J., Phillips Y.Y. III et al. (1988). The influence of clothing on intrathoracic pressure during airblast. *Aviat. Space Environ. Med.*, **89**, 49–53.

21. Protection Against Blast Injury

G. J. Cooper and A. Jönsson

INTRODUCTION

This chapter discusses the attenuation of air-blast and underwater blast, and presents the scientific basis for protection from the primary effects of blast, and from traumatic amputation. An understanding of the biophysical interactions of blast-waves with the body is central both to the development of personal protective materials and the identification of the risk of blast injury by the employment of mathematical models and anthropomorphic dummies.

The greatest threat to civilians or soldiers exposed to bombs is penetrating injury from primary and secondary fragments. The principles of ballistic protection are covered in Chapter 8 and will not be discussed here – this chapter is concerned solely with the interaction of fast-rising pressure waves with the body.

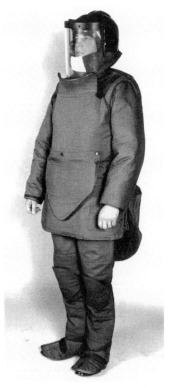

Figure 21.1 An explosive ordnance disposal (EOD) suit.

There are notable extremes in blast protection. At one end of the scale is equipment used by the Military and Police, such as the Explosive Ordnance Disposal suit (EOD), which is designed to withstand severe explosions at close range (Figure 21.1). At the other is ear protection from impulsive noise (very low level blast), commonly worn not only by the Services for protection from weapon noise, but also in widespread industrial use in the civilian sphere.

Blast protection will be considered in two principal areas:

1. The scientific basis for personal protection from impulsive noise, severe air-blast and blast underwater.
2. The use of model systems such as dummies and mathematical models to assess the threat from blast overpressures, the efficiency of protective measures and options for reducing personal exposure to blast.

The protection concepts which can reduce the incidence and severity of the following blast injuries are also outlined:

1. Primary blast injury to the lung and bowel.
2. Tympanic rupture and sensorineural hearing loss in air-blast.
3. Traumatic amputation of limbs.

During the Second World War, Desaga (1950) wrote: 'On the basis of my investigations, it can be asserted that it is impossible to design a practical protective suit for the individual'. This statement cannot be sustained today, largely because a more detailed understanding of the biophysical interactions that produce lung injury, knowledge that has allowed development of protective measures with an appropriate theoretical, rather than empirical, base.

There are four main approaches in reducing blast forces externally to the body, or within the body:

1. Increase the separation of the explosive charge from the body.
2. Reduce the loadings of incident overpressures, reflected overpressures and dynamic pressure by alteration in their shape, position and orientation. Shielding of the body or limiting the number of exposures will also reduce blast loading.
3. Attenuation of the power of an explosive at source by using added protection such as aqueous foams and bomb blankets.
4. Reduction of the inward acceleration and deflection of the body wall under blast loading, and thus diminishing both direct compression of underlying structures and the generation of waves in the body.

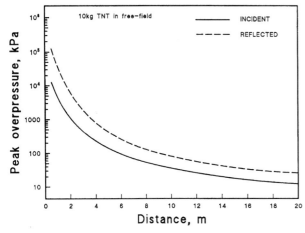

Figure 21.2 Peak overpressure from detonation of 10-kg TNT in free-field.

Increasing the distance of the body from the charge

The relationship between the peak overpressure and the distance from an explosive charge is shown in Figure 21.2 (Turnbull and Walter, 1982; Baker, 1983). In very close proximity to the charge, the overpressure declines very quickly with distance. This is the result of loss of energy through heating of the atmosphere by the progressing shock-wave and the rapidly increasing sphere surface area with increasing range. The latter predominates at medium to long ranges, the former within a few charge diameters. Close to the charge, peak overpressure is proportional to $1/r^3$ where r is the distance from the charge but the power to which r is raised declines with increasing range.

The overpressure at a particular distance from a charge is proportional to $W^{1/3}$, where W is the charge weight. It is more usual to express the overpressure/distance relationships for explosives as the scaled distance $(r/W^{1/3})$ (Turnbull and Walter, 1982). A log/log plot of peak overpressure against scaled distance will result in a straight line for a specific explosive. Explosives of different power result in parallel relationships.

In water, detonation initially produces a primary shock of very short duration. Subsequently, longer duration pulses (bubble pulses) are formed and result from the expansion and subsequent collapse of the bubble produced by the gaseous products of the explosion. Multiple reflections from the sea bed and sea surface may give rise to a complex pressure environment. Peak overpressure declines very rapidly with distance, and close to the charge it is proportional to $1/r^3$. By about five charge radii, the relationship is a simple inverse one with overpressure proportional to $1/r$.

Thus, for both air-blast and underwater blast, peak incident overpressure declines very rapidly

with distance, particular very close to the charge. It should be noted however that water is a more effective medium than air for transmitting shock-waves – safe distances from explosions in water are about three times the corresponding distances in air.

Separation of the body, or parts of the body, from the charge is an obvious but nevertheless very effective way of reducing blast forces.

Changes in geometry

The susceptibility of man to primary lung injury is dependent upon the peak overpressure, and positive-phase duration (Bowen *et al.*, 1968). The loading resulting from an incident overpressure is modified by:

1. The orientation of the thorax to the incident pressure.
2. The proximity of the man to large reflecting surfaces.

Figure 21.3 demonstrates that if the man is close to a reflecting surface a lower incident overpressure is required to produce 50% mortality from lung injury. Reflection of the incident wave at a barrier produces an overpressure that may be up to eight times the incident overpressure. A man close to the surface (say within 1 wavelength) is subjected to a higher pressure than if the barrier is absent.

Changing the orientation so that the transverse axis of the thorax is parallel to the incident blast significantly reduces susceptibility to blast by reducing the local overpressure at the thoracic wall.

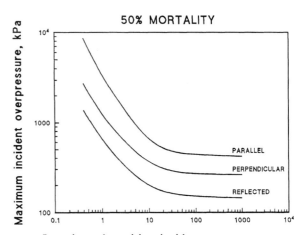

Figure 21.3 Predicted 50% mortality within 24 hours from primary blast lung injury for man in three orientations – axis of the body parallel or normal to the incident overpressure propagation axis (perpendicular); the response for man close to a large reflecting surface is also shown. (Derived from Bowen *et al.*, 1968.)

The principal loading is the incident pressure alone, with little reflected component or dynamic overpressure (Figure 21.3).

Changes in orientation and removal of the body from the reflecting surfaces is an effective way of reducing blast forces and thus decreasing the incidence of lung, ear and bowel injury. These procedures assume that the person is aware of an impending blast loading but there are scenarios such as 'Take Cover Drills' on board ships under attack by missiles or torpedos or in the design of underground shelters that can provide a reduced risk of lung injury.

The general principles of reducing blast loading by appropriate changes in the shape of protective equipment can be seen in some EOD suits, where the front breastplate may be shaped to divert the blast winds away from the neck and face and so reduce the dynamic pressure loadings to these regions (Figure 21.1). Similar principles have also been employed in footwear designed to protect the foot from mines (see below).

Repetitive loading to blast overpressures that are above an injury threshold will result in an increased severity of primary injury (Figure 21.4). Repeated subthreshold blast loadings do not create injury (Richmond, 1990). The time interval between the blasts determines the increased severity of the injury from multiple loadings – blasts given daily (or less frequently) have little effect on overall mortality when compared to single blasts. Rats exposed to a long-duration blast-wave (100 ms) of ~180 kPa had a 5% incidence of mortality at 24 hours. Three blasts at an interval of 15 minutes

resulted in 85% mortality. At 30 minute, 4-hour and 24-hour intervals of blast loading, mortality was 26%, 27% and 7% respectively (Richmond, 1990).

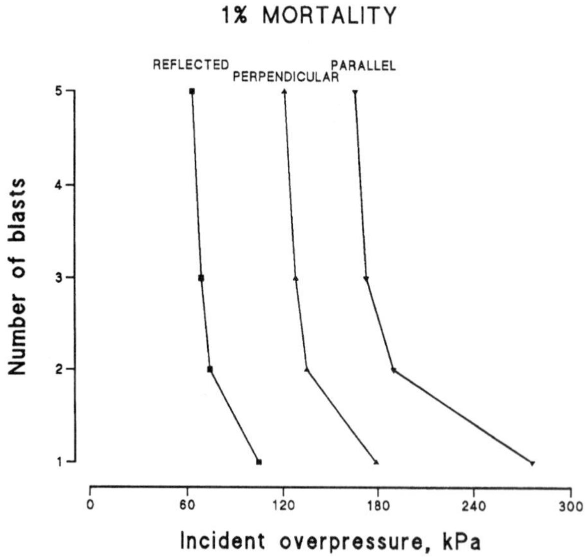

Attenuation of the power of an explosive

There are techniques for reducing the destructive ability of explosives by increasing the rise time and attenuating the peak overpressure. An aqueous foam around an explosive will attenuate blast by consuming some of the energy of the shock and converting the foam into minute droplets of water – energy is also used in the evaporation of the droplets (Aubert et al., 1986). Some police forces also use 'bomb blankets' to cover the device or employ mobile bomb containment units, but these facilities can only deal with small charges. The principal problem with this approach is that the forensic investigation of the device in situ is hampered. Filling a city street with aqueous foam reduces the options open to the bomb disposal officer and makes examination of the device and application of some techniques, such as disruption of the explosive device by high-velocity water jets, difficult to achieve.

Reducing the motion of the body wall

The body wall exposed to blast is very rapidly displaced inwards. The high initial accelerations may generate stress-waves particularly with short-duration blast-waves (Cooper et al., 1991), and these coupled waves will lose energy and perform work when they encounter regions of different density such as air/tissue interfaces (Bush and Challener, 1988). Motion of 'particles' at these internal boundaries is necessary for stress transmission and, although the accelerations are high, the actual motion of tissue is quite small. Lacerations are uncommon; contusion is the principal outcome – blast lung and blast damage to the gut.

If the blast-waves are of long duration, the gross compression of the body wall is severe and is probably of greater importance than stress-wave transmission. The velocity of the gross deformation may be correlated to the severity of injury (Jonsson et al., 1988); additionally, shear waves may be initiated by the deformation (Cooper and Taylor, 1989).

Protection from primary blast is aimed at reducing these deformations, whether they be small and fast from short-duration waves or larger but slower from long-duration loadings.

PROTECTION FROM AIR-BLAST

Primary blast injuries to the lung

It is important to emphasize that the tolerance of the body to blast is very dependent upon the duration of the overpressure (Bowen et al., 1968).

Figure 21.4 Predicted 1% mortality of man to blast lung injury from multiple, long-duration (10–15 ms) blast loading in three orientations. The time interval between blast loadings is 1 minute. (Reproduced from Richmond, 1990.)

Explosive charges range in weight from a few grams to an equivalent weight of megatons for nuclear devices. These charges can generate over-pressure durations in air ranging from less than 1 ms to hundreds of milliseconds or even seconds. An example serves to demonstrate the dependence of primary blast lung injury upon overpressure duration (t). A man, standing in the open and exposed to a blast-wave of approximately half a millisecond and peak incident overpressure (P_{max}) of ~680 kPa will receive a blast loading just on the limit of lung injury. He will experience the same risk when exposed for approximately fifty milliseconds at P_{max} = 80 kPa. Furthermore, when the incident shock-waves reflect on the body wall, the 680 kPa will theoretically rise by a factor of 3–4, and the 80 kPa will be doubled.

It is difficult to believe that the mechanical processes in the body are the same in the two cases, although the predicted risk of injury is the same. Rather, it would seem plausible that the higher overpressure of short duration may invoke wave phenomena such as direct stress coupling, while longer duration wave of lower overpressure produces greater gross deformation. It must not be assumed therefore that protective measures designed to combat exposure at one end of the range of time will necessarily be efficient at the other.

Most of the experimental work directed towards blast protection has addressed relatively short-duration, high-overpressure loadings – the principles discussed below – and the protective concepts developed have not been tested against very long duration blast. They are unlikely to be as effective.

Mechanism of injury
Although the features of an incident blast-wave that determine the severity of primary lung contusions have been empirically determined and scaled to man (Bowen *et al.*, 1968), the biophysical factors leading to the transfer of energy internally and the production of the lung injury following the interaction of the blast-wave with the thoracic wall are still unclear for both short-duration and long-duration waves. Work during the Second World War showed that pulmonary contusions arise from the interaction of the blast-wave with the chest wall, not from the passage of the blast-wave down the respiratory passages.

Any impact to the body will generate direct stress and shear waves (Cooper and Taylor, 1989; Taylor *et al.*, 1990; Cooper *et al.*, 1991). The body is a very complex structure in which to initiate the propagation of waves – there are marked differences in density, elastic modulus and propagation velocities within the various thoracic tissues and complex geometric configurations; any sort of impact, including blast, is likely to excite a broad spectrum of frequencies and stress concentration at multiple sites.

High-speed photography of the chest under blast or under impact loading shows that the thoracic cage undergoes considerable compressive strain and exhibits a damped, viscoelastic behaviour. The compressive strain may be considerable and it is tempting to ascribe the resultant visceral injury solely to local shear or compression underneath the advancing body wall or to shear waves producing strain at sites of fixation such as the hilar region of the lung.

Jonsson (1979) concluded that gross thoracic deformation with corresponding compression of the lungs and associated oscillation of pressure within them is the main origin of the pulmonary injuries, certainly for long-duration air-blast. Direct coupling of stress-waves into the thoracic cavity was not considered to be a primary cause of injury for long-duration waves. However, the evidence outlined below shows that for *short*-duration waves, the direct coupling of the blast-wave into the thorax is the principal injury mechanism.

The interrelationship of the two phenomena may be illustrated by the simple analogy of striking a cushion with the fist. A 'boom' and compression of the cushion occurs. The boom occurs during the initial stages on impact when the fist accelerates particles of cushion and propagates a weak stress-wave into the material which is reflected within the cushion to produce the sound. The motion of the cushion wall under the loading of the fist continues over a longer time scale and eventually results in gross compression of the body of the cushion – its contents may be subjected to shear and a slow, long-duration wave may propagate through them. The same phenomena are thought to occur with interaction of blast-waves with the body – stress coupling, followed by gross deformation and both local and indirect shear.

Experimental data and modelling studies (Bush and Challener, 1988; Cooper *et al.*, 1991) support the following sequence of events for *short*-duration waves:

1. The coupling of the incident shock-wave into the thorax is achieved by the initial rapid acceleration of the thoracic wall; the velocity and displacement associated with the very short duration acceleration are small in magnitude.
2. A pressure-wave is propagated into the lung, the magnitude of which is probably determined by the initial peak velocity of the body wall. The more important feature of the pressure pulse (in terms of lung injury) is the rate of pressure rise which is determined by the peak acceleration of the thoracic wall.
3. The pressure propagates through the lung and results in pressure differentials across the capillary/alveolar interface, the magnitude of which

is dependent upon the rate of pressure rise of the pulse. Failure at the interface and therefore haemorrhage will occur if the pressure differential reaches a critical failure level (of unknown magnitude).

4. The stress-wave will also reflect and reinforce within the thoracic cavity to result in stress concentration and injury at sites some distance from the lateral thoracic wall (such as the mediastinum and anteromedial pleural niche).

The interrelationship of these events in time is shown in Figure 21.5. The incident pressure-wave results in a short-duration acceleration of the thoracic wall in the same direction as the blast. After a slight delay, the shock loading reaches the rear accelerometer to result in a complex acceleration profile of relatively low magnitude. The relative velocity of the front and rear thoracic walls shows a two-phase response – an initial pulse arising from the high acceleration of the front wall

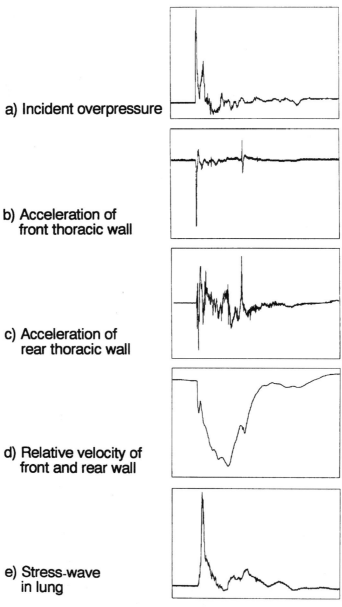

a) Incident overpressure

b) Acceleration of front thoracic wall

c) Acceleration of rear thoracic wall

d) Relative velocity of front and rear wall

e) Stress-wave in lung

Figure 21.5 The relationship in time from the detonation of the explosive (time 0) of the incident overpressure and the biomechanical response of the thorax. (a) Incident overpressure measured just below the front thoracic wall. (b) The acceleration of the front thoracic wall (negative-going is positive acceleration along the same axis as the advancing shock front). (c) The acceleration of the rear thoracic wall (output reversed from (b) above). (d) The relative velocity of the front and rear accelerometers estimated by integration and subtraction of (b) and (c). (e) The stress-wave within the right lung measured with a gauge in the medial part of the lung. The y-axes are arbitrary.

and a much slower acceleration to a higher velocity. The latter probably represents the later gross compression produced by the dynamic pressure loadings. The rise in intrathoracic (lung) pressure is associated with the initial peak acceleration and not with the slower gross compression

The pattern of injury in lungs subject to blast also suggests that stress-waves contribute to the injury. Contusions are generally most severe close to the inner surfaces of the lung adjacent to the mediastinum and liver and in acute angles within the parenchyma such as the anteromedial border where stress concentration occurs. The peripheral pleural surface and parenchyma directly compressed by the gross deflections of the thoracic wall are often less severely injured, suggesting that direct shear or compression may not necessarily be the principal injury mechanism.

Finite element modelling of the transmission of impact-induced stress-waves in pulmonary parenchyma support these empirical observations (Bush and Challener, 1988) and demonstrate that, because of reflection and reinforcement of the waves within the thoracic cage, the stress at internal sites may exceed the peak stresses close to the body wall. Modelling has also demonstrated that direct stress-waves may also steepen during transmission through the parenchyma because of increased wave velocities of the high-pressure components and consequently result in greater pressure differentials across the alveolar/capillary interface. These pressure differentials may lead to failure of capillary walls and produce haemorrhage into the alveoli.

Protective clothing

The relative contributions of *stress coupling* and *gross distortion* to lung injury, are of fundamental importance in the construction of protective clothing designed to attenuate primary blast effects.

If different fundamental mechanisms are responsible for lung injury with short- and long-duration waves, the appropriate methods of protecting the body may also be different. If stress-wave coupling dominates, then acoustic decoupling layers may be effective. To reduce gross deflection of the thoracic wall, its effective mass or stiffness must be increased by placing heavy plates against the chest. This is not likely to be a very effective option, as deflection of the combined mass of the chest and plate will undoubtedly still occur but to a lesser extent. Ideally, a rigid box should envelope the torso although the operational limitations of this are obvious.

The categories of 'short' and 'long'-duration blast-waves are somewhat arbitrary, but they are related to body size (for air-blast) and resonances within the body. Between these extremes, that may extend from about 1 ms to 100 ms for conventional explosives, is a spectrum of durations within which the relative roles of stress coupling and gross compression have not been determined.

Increased severity of injury with foam protection

Perhaps the most obvious way of protecting the thorax from a blast-wave would be to employ a foam material such as natural rubber or foamed polymer to attenuate the transferred energy, either by reducing the rate of rise time of the incident pressure or absorbing some of the energy of the wave by allowing the wave to perform work on the foam. This approach was investigated in the Second World War. Desaga (1950) experimented with rubber sponge and other elastic materials and concluded that the foam would have to be 150–200 mm thick and encompass the whole trunk.

Other investigators have also studied foams but Clemedson *et al.* (1971) published an observation that called in question such an approach. Rabbits were used to investigate the efficiency of rigid coverings of parts of the torso and soft foams as protection from long- (25-ms) and short- (3-ms) duration blast-waves. A rigid covering significantly reduced the severity of lung injury (Figure 21.6); in these circumstances, the intrathoracic pressure (an index of the thoracic compression) was only modestly reduced but greater reductions were seen in the *rate* of intrathoracic pressure rise (dP/dt_{max}). They concluded that any protective method should aim towards a reduction in the low-frequency oscillations and associated inward deflection of the

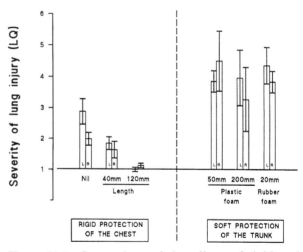

Figure 21.6 Comparison of the effects of rigid and soft materials upon the torso of rabbits exposed to long-duration blast-waves (~20 ms). With the rigid protection, steel coverings were applied to the thorax from the 1st to the 4th rib (40 mm), or to the whole thorax and part of the abdomen (120 mm). For the soft protection, 50-mm or 200-mm plastic foam, or 20-mm rubber foam, was applied to cover the whole animal. The lung quotient (LQ) is a gravimetric index of lung injury severity – the ratio of the actual lung weight to the predicted normal weight. L and R denote left and right lungs. Blast loadings were to the right thorax, and the animals were upon a reflecting surface. (Reproduced from Clemedson *et al.*, 1971.)

thoracic wall – it was surmised that the rigid covering was limiting the motion of the thoracic wall.

When plastic foam and rubber sponge of thickness from 20 to 200 mm covered the whole body, and the rabbit was exposed to long-duration blast-waves, *the severity of lung injury increased* (Figure 21.6).

The conclusions were that:

1. Protection was only afforded to weak shocks that were incapable of compressing the foam.
2. If the blast was severe enough to completely compress the foam, this increased the loading to the chest and thus would give rise to more severe injuries.

The exacerbation of blast injuries by the foams were explained as a result of a reduction in the time-scale of the incident blast within the foam because of the low wave propagation speed in foam which could lead to an increase in the forces applied to the body wall during the critical period between arrival of the shock at the surface and the peak intrathoracic pressure. Alternatively, as a result of the lower wave velocity and compressibility of the foam, a greater potential energy may possibly be stored within the compressed foam than would normally arise from the incident wave impinging upon the unprotected thorax. The higher initial velocity of the chest wall that could then occur may produce more serious injury.

The augmentation of blast injury by foams is rather more than a novel observation and holds the key to the investigation of the role of directly coupled stress-waves in the cause of lung injury for both short- and long-duration waves.

An alternative explanation of the augmentation of injury by foam materials can be formulated in terms of impedance matching (see below). The materials might act as acoustic couplers/transformers, resulting in an augmented transfer of direct stress-waves from the air into the tissues.

The observation by Clemedson *et al.* (1971) of augmented injury was confirmed by Cooper *et al.* (1991) and formed the basis of experimental and modelling work that clarified the important role of stress-waves in lungs exposed to shorter-duration waves and led to the development of effective personal protection from primary blast lung injury based on the principles of acoustic decoupling. These are important and as they form the backbone of much of the blast protection work to be reviewed later, they are now considered.

Theory of stress-wave decoupling Decoupling layers have applications in civilian and military spheres but it is in the military that surface coatings have been used widely. They are used to reduce radiated energy – anechoic claddings on submarines, or radar absorbing materials to reduce the

target strength of ships and aircraft. Laminated armours on armoured fighting vehicles are designed to reduce stress transmission from an impact or explosion on the outer surface, and thus reduce the incidence of spalling (secondary fragments, see below) and other effects at the internal surface of the vehicle.

An incident pressure-wave at an interface of materials with dissimilar properties will give rise to a wave reflected back in the opposite direction (for normal approach), and a wave transmitted on into the second material. The magnitude of the reflected and transmitted waves is dependent upon the relative characteristic acoustic impedances of the materials at the interface (Kirsler *et al.*, 1980). The characteristic acoustic impedance (Z) is the product of the speed of sound in the material (*c*) and its density (ρ).

Thus, for an acoustic wave (propagating in one dimension) of amplitude P_i travelling through material 1, incident upon a boundary with material 2, a reflected wave (P_r) and a transmitted wave (P_t) will be generated. The magnitudes of the incident and transmitted waves are related by the expression:

$$P_t/P_i = (2Z_2)/(Z_1 + Z_2). \qquad (21.1)$$

The wave reflected into material 1 (P_t) can be calculated from:

$$P_r = P_t - P_i. \qquad (21.2)$$

For conventional engineering materials, the characteristic acoustic impedance, Z, may also be expressed in terms of the Young's modulus, E. As:

$$c = \sqrt{(E/\rho)} \qquad (21.3)$$

Z in equation (21.1) may be substituted by $\sqrt{(E \times \rho)}$.

It can be seen from equation (21.1) that if material 2 has a much higher acoustic impedance than material 1 (such as a wave going from air into a metal), the wave is totally reflected (in the same phase) and the transmitted pressure is double the incident pressure. However, if the position is reversed, i.e. material 1 is steel and material 2 is air, the pressure is nearly totally reflected (in reverse phase – a rarefaction wave) and very little pressure is transmitted from the metal into air. The pressure has been 'decoupled'. If the pressure propagating through the steel is very high, the tensile forces at the steel/air interface due to the change in phase of the reflected wave may actually disrupt the steel to form scabs – this is spalling, and is the principle of High Explosive Squash Head (HESH) ammunition used to defeat tanks. It also accounts for the initial spray dome of water seen at the water surface in underwater explosions which results from the reflection of the shock-wave in water from the water/air interface.

Acoustic theory governing the coupling of acoustic waves through adjoining layers of materials is well described and straightforward. The transmission of stress-waves of very large amplitude (shockwaves) does not follow simple acoustic theory. In the transmission of shock fronts through multilayers, there are significant differences in the absolute pressures predicted at boundaries using acoustic and non-acoustic theory.

Nevertheless, predictions made from simple acoustic theory have been borne out qualitatively and often quantitatively in the evaluation of the performance of air-blast decoupling layers, both *in vivo* and in test models such as shock coupling into anechoic chambers (Cooper *et al.*, 1991).

Acoustic theory of stress transmission is founded on two assumptions:

1. The velocity of the pressure-wave in the material is equal to the speed of sound in the material and does not vary with the magnitude of the pressure.
2. The reflection of a wave at a boundary cannot result in a pressure at the boundary greater than twice the incident pressure.

Shock-waves or high-magnitude stress-waves do not satisfy these assumptions. The local properties in materials – such as density and stiffness – in which the shock-waves are propagating may be altered by the high pressures, and thus increase the speed of wave propagation. Thus the acoustic impedance ($\rho \times c$) may be markedly different for high-pressure waves. Reflected overpressures at interfaces exposed to shock fronts may be up to eight times the incident overpressure.

As an illustration of the principles of acoustic coupling and decoupling, equation (21.1) may be used to calculate the direct stress transferred into the lung after propagation of a compressive stress in the air through materials and into the body. For the reasons outlined above the calculation of these stresses can only be considered to be semiquantitative. The effects of oblique incidence and multiple internal reflections within each material are also not considered. Nevertheless, this simple one-dimensional model demonstrates the principle of acoustic decoupling.

The relative acoustic impedances of air/foam/body wall/lung is assumed to be 1/4.7/3700/23; the acoustic impedance of air at atmospheric pressure is 415 Pa/s/m.

Using the simple model above, the peak stress transmitted through the bare, uncovered chest wall into *lung* for an incident stress in air of 100 units is estimated to be 2.5 units. Interposition of a foam *increases* this stress to 4.2 units – the foam is acting as an acoustic coupler and more energy is coupled into the chest.

A dense material such as copper has a relative acoustic impedance of 7.7×10^4 compared to air. Putting the metal layer *on top* of the foam, i.e. facing the incident pressure, significantly reduces the

transmitted stress to 0.0006 units. This is a *decoupling layer* – the impedance difference at the metal/foam interface reflects the incident wave within the metal and very little energy is transmitted into the foam layer, and on through the chest wall into the body.

This simple example does not take into account the frequency components of the coupled pressure – any attempt to attenuate the energy coupled into a system should ideally be designed to decouple energy at the frequencies considered to result in damage to the system. The performance of such a simple decoupling system such as a metal backed by foam is not uniform across the frequency spectrum; indeed at some frequencies (the decoupling layer's resonant frequency) the decoupling layer may actually transmit *more* energy into the body and act as an acoustic coupler. This may be of little consequence if the frequencies responsible for injury are well separated from this resonance, but the effects could be disastrous if the frequencies coincided.

It is essential therefore that the design of primary blast protection considers the frequency domain and optimization of the layers and must be directed towards maximum decoupling performance *at the frequencies responsible for the injury*. The definition of these frequencies is a difficult but critical part of the design of protective measures and is discussed below.

In simple terms, a metal/foam decoupling layer may be thought of as a simple mass/spring system where the mass represents the metal, and the spring represents the foam (Figure 21.7). Consider the

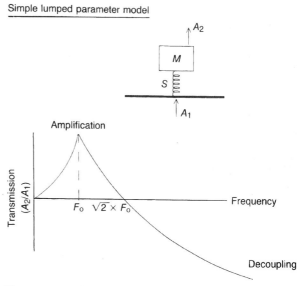

Simple lumped parameter model

Figure 21.7 A simple mass (M)/spring (S) model showing the transmission response of the system with respect to frequency. Decoupling is achieved when the acceleration of the mass (A_2) is less than the input acceleration (A_1). F_o is the resonant frequency of the system.

response of this simple system to acceleration (impact) at different frequencies – at very low frequency the incident and transmitted accelerations will be equal. As the frequency of excitation is increased, the system will resonate and at this resonant frequency (F_o), the transmitted acceleration is amplified. If there is no damping in the system, the incident and transmitted accelerations will again be equal at $\sqrt{2} \times F_o$. As the frequency is increased, the transmitted acceleration is much less than the incident, and the system is acting as a *decoupler*. This simple system makes no allowance for wave effects such as multiple reflections within layers which will be present in practical designs, and a more rigorous mathematical solution is required.

The material parameters required to optimize the performance of a decoupling ensemble can be determined using a mathematical approach based on transmission line theory. By entering appropriate frequencies and material properties into transmission line equations, the reflection and transmission coefficients for simple and complex multilayered systems may be computed. The effective bulk and shear moduli for common materials such as metals and glass-reinforced plastic are obtainable from reference texts. For air-filled polymers, these values may be calculated from the polymers' basic dynamic mechanical properties using Kerner's theory (Kerner, 1950). Thus, the complex wave velocity and hence impedance for each layer of a multilayer system may be calculated. The derivation of these equations will not be discussed here, but models employing them are used later.

Performance of simple decoupling layers In experiments with anaesthetized rats exposed to short-duration, reflected blast overpressures from a laboratory blast-wave generator, Cooper *et al.* (1991) confirmed the observation of Clemedson *et al.* (1971) that foams augment lung injury. Coverage of the right lateral thoracic wall with either a natural rubber foam or viscoelastic open-cell polyurethane-silicone foam significantly *increased* the severity of lung injury (Figure 21.8). The intensification of

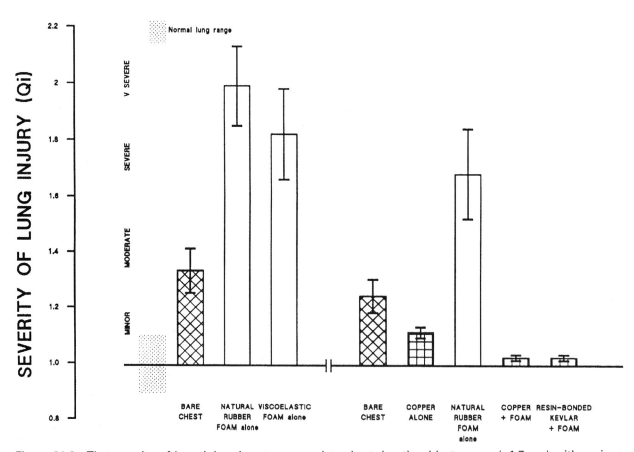

Figure 21.8 The severity of lung injury in rats exposed to short-duration blast-waves (~1.7 ms) with various materials covering the presented area of the right lateral thorax facing the blast. The severity of lung injury, *Qi* is the ratio of the actual lung weight to the predicted normal weight. A *Qi* of 1 denotes normal, uninjured lungs – the dotted area is ±1 s.d. of the normal *Qi*. The foams were 9.3–10.3 mm thick; the resin-bonded Kevlar and copper had an areal density 5.1 kg/m². For the two decoupling layers (copper + foam and resin-bonded Kevlar + foam) the foam was placed between the dense layer and the body.

primary blast effects evident with the rats placed upon a reflecting surface, could also be demonstrated in rats exposed in free-field conditions.

High-speed cine photography of the foam exposed to blast loading on an unyielding surface and upon the rat thoracic wall showed that rubber foam underwent considerable compression with subsequent recovery. However, viscoelastic foam failed to show any dynamic compression or distortion under identical loading. Both foams, of very different static and dynamic properties, produced exacerbation of primary blast lung injury. Augmentation of lung injury was also evident with a high-density cross-linked polyethylene closed cell foam and even 'bubble pack' packaging material used as thoracic coverings.

The application of a thin sheet of copper to the thorax failed to significantly reduce the severity of lung injury (Figure 21.8). However, placing the copper *on top* of the foams produced a substantial reduction in the severity of the lung injury, and with the natural rubber foam the injury was eliminated.

The elimination of primary blast lung injury was mirrored when other relatively dense armour materials such as resin-bonded Kevlar (at the same areal density as copper) was used as facing on the foams. Severe primary blast lung injury, produced with foams alone, was eliminated when the foam was faced with either copper or resin-bonded Kevlar (Figure 21.8).

These data support the assertion that for short-duration waves, direct stress coupling was producing the lung injury and facing the foam with a dense material such as copper or resin-bonded Kevlar provided a decoupling interface.

The augmentation and decoupling in the frequency domain achieved by the materials was established using an underwater anechoic chamber. The materials were floated on the water surface and air-blast directed at the air/material interface. The stress coupled through the layers into the water (representing the soft tissue of the body) was detected using a hydrophone. Logarithmic spectra of the measured pressures were produced in the frequency domain and the frequency content of the transmitted pressure profiles was compared to that of the waveforms transmitted *without* materials by subtracting logarithmic spectra, thus giving the ratio of coated to uncoated transmission in dB (the definition of dB and its use in decoupling studies is summarized in the Appendix at the end of this chapter).

Both types of bare foam significantly increased the power within certain frequency bands transmitted into the anechoic water chamber. The blast coupling produced by the rubber foam showed a 5–10 dB enhancement over the bandwidth 0.5–3.5 kHz (Figure 21.9). Copper or resin-bonded Kevlar alone did not significantly modify the severity of

injury in the rat model and this was mirrored in the comparative logarithmic spectra, with minor changes in the transmitted frequencies over the bandwidth 0.5–5 kHz (Figure 21.9).

Placing the resin-bonded Kevlar or copper as facings upon both types of foams achieved substantial decoupling over a wide frequency range. Copper upon foam resulted in a 10–20 dB reduction over a bandwidth of 2–6 kHz (Figure 21.9). Frequencies of less than 2 kHz were largely unaffected.

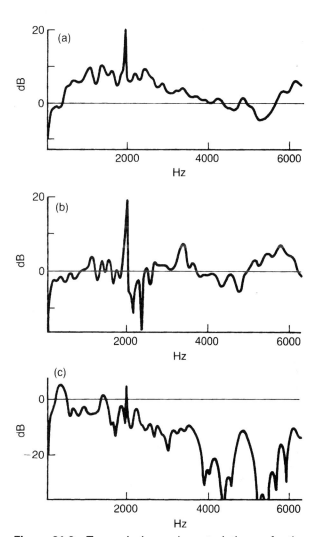

Figure 21.9 Transmission characteristics of the materials shown in Figure 21.8 acquired by subjecting the materials to air-blast loading at the air/water interface of an underwater anechoic chamber, and recording the pressures coupled into the water beneath the layers: 9.3-mm natural rubber foam alone on the water surface (a), 0.58-mm copper sheet alone (b) and 0.58-mm copper facing upon 9.3-mm natural rubber foam (c). The results of subtraction of the logarithmic spectrum in the frequency domain of the directly coupled waveform (acquired in the absence of any coverings) from the logarithmic spectrum of the waveforms transmitted with each type of covering is shown. (Reproduced from Cooper *et al.*, 1991.)

A very similar pattern was also seen with the resin-bonded Kevlar as a facing on foam.

In experimental work with rats, rigid heavy materials placed alone on the thoracic wall failed significantly to reduce the severity of lung injury; these materials doubled the effective mass of the body wall and would be expected to reduce the peak velocity and gross deflection of the body wall under the same blast loading. Their failure to diminish the injury is indirect evidence that the gross deflection is not a major determinant of the severity of injury with short-duration waves; frequency analysis of the transmitted waveforms demonstrated little loss in transmission over a wide frequency band (Figure 21.9) and thus corresponded to the lack of effect demonstrated *in vivo*.

The natural rubber foam alone without a facing resulted in an increased transmission of power within the bandwidth 0.5–3.5 kHz (Figure 21.9). The resonant frequency of the rat thoracic wall is around 0.35–0.8 kHz (Von Gierke, 1968) and it is conceivable that the foam was increasing the deflection of the chest because of resonance at this frequency. The elimination of thoracic injury with the high acoustic impedance materials placed upon the foams resulted from significant decoupling at frequencies much higher than these resonant frequencies (Figure 21.9), and would suggest that the primary lung injury is a high-frequency damage mechanism. Foams also produce exacerbation of injury in anaesthetized pigs; the thoracic wall resonances in this model are about 70–150 Hz and, in the anechoic chamber studies, the foams did not result in significant increases in transmission at these very low frequencies.

Studies were extended into pig models, with three aims:

1. To determine if the same general principles applied to larger animal models, with different body wall resonances.
2. To measure the intrathoracic stresses within the lungs and oesophagus in animals protected with different assemblies. Peak oesophageal pressure in the rats exposed to short-duration waves showed no correlation with the severity of lung injury. However, modelling of the pig thorax subjected to blunt impact had indicated that for short-duration impacts at high velocity, the *rate* of intrathoracic pressure rise was a more appropriate index of the potential for lung injury (Dodd *et al.*, 1989).
3. To measure the acceleration of the body wall beneath the various enhanced coupling and decoupling layers and to determine both the role of this variable in the stress transmission process and its correlation with both the stress transferred in to the lung and the severity of lung injury.

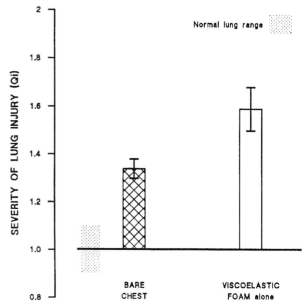

Figure 21.10 Augmentation of lung injury by 32 mm foam in anaesthetised pigs exposed to short-duration blast loading (~4 ms).

Anaesthetized pigs were exposed to short-duration (~5 ms) incident overpressures from an explosively driven shock tube; incident blast overpressures of either ~300 kPa or ~380 kPa were employed.

Coverage of the right lateral thoracic wall with a viscoelastic foam resulted in an augmentation of the severity of lung injury produced with moderate blast loading which mirrored the response observed in rats (Cooper *et al.*, 1991) (Figure 21.10).

The pigs with bare thoraces exposed to the severe loadings had a considerable lung injury. Coverage of the right thorax with a resin-bonded Kevlar plate failed significantly to reduce the severity of lung injury (Figure 21.11). However, providing acoustic decoupling by backing the plate with the viscoelastic foam virtually eliminated lung injury (Figure 21.11). Backing the resin-bonded Kevlar with natural rubber foam was not as successful, but still offered notable protection.

The peak accelerations (A_F) measured on the front thoracic wall along the same vector as the advancing shock front ranged from 2800 to 87 700 m/s/s depending on the particular materials placed upon the thorax and on the rear (A_R) 981 to 4510 m/s/s. An example of the acceleration waveform is shown in Figure 21.5. The A_F showed a positive correlation to the severity of lung injury (Figure 21.12). There was little variation in the mean intrathoracic pressure ($ITP_{(max)}$) within the lung and oesophagus beneath the various thoracic coverings, and no significant correlation with the peak acceleration of the thoracic wall.

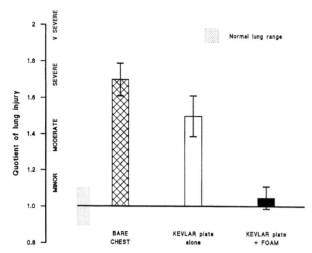

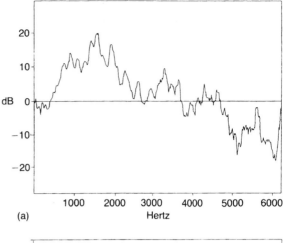

Figure 21.11 Protection from short-duration blasts achieved by a resin-bonded Kevlar plate (12 kg/m²) backed with 32-mm viscoleastic foam. The plate alone had no significant effect on the severity of injury.

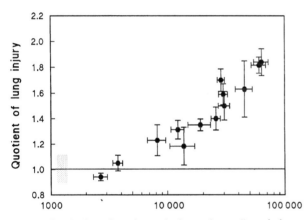

Figure 21.12 The correlation between the peak acceleration of the thoracic wall facing the blast (R), and the severity of lung injury, (Qi) for short-duration waves. Individual points are the means (±s.e.) of groups of anaesthetized pigs with different types of materials covering the right lateral thorax.

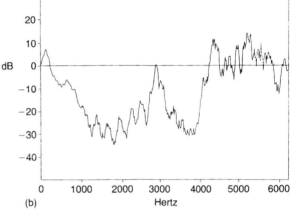

Figure 21.13 *In vivo* transmission characteristics of viscoelastic foam alone (a) and foam faced with resin-bonded Kevlar (b). The figures show the result of subtraction of logarithmic spectra in the frequency domain of the intrathoracic pressure in the lung in pigs without any coverings from the logarithmic spectrum of intrathoracic pressure coupled with the materials. Transforms were performed on the time-averaged pressures within the lung. Foam alone increased the power coupled over the frequency band 0.5–2.5 kHz and augmented the severity of lung injury; the Kevlar/foam configuration decoupled power over the same bandwidth and protected the lung from injury.

However, the *rate* of pressure rise did differ between the groups – both the rise time of $ITP_{(max)}$ in the lung and the average $ITP_{dP/dt}$ in the lung showed significant correlation to A_F – rapid rise in ITP in the lung (but not oesophagus) was associated with high peak acceleration levels and lung injury.

These observation support the concept of injury outlined above which is based on general physical principles and FE modelling: the rate of pressure rise within the lung is determined by the peak acceleration of the body wall during the coupling of the pressure wave in air into the thorax.

The frequency content of the stress-wave coupled into the lung beneath acoustic coupling and decoupling layers is shown in Figure 21.13. In the comparison of the frequency content of the averaged stress-wave in the lung of a group with coverage of the right thoracic wall with foam alone, to the stress in the pigs subjected to severe blast loadings with bare thoraces, the foam produced up to 10–20 dB amplification over the frequency band 0.5–2.5 kHz – this enhanced coupling was associated with an increase in the severity of lung injury. The decoupling layer significantly reduced the frequency content of the stress-wave in the lung and effectively eliminated the lung injury. Figure 21.13 shows up to a 30 dB decoupling over the same bandwidth.

In its simplest form, therefore, personal blast protection is best achieved by the use of a low-acoustic-impedance foam layer faced with a high-acoustic-impedance layer to decouple the blast and thus reduce the direct stress transferred into the body.

Work with long-duration waves (Clemedson *et al.*, 1971) demonstrated that gross deflection is the primary mechanical response of the body wall responsible for lung injury and that $ITP_{(max)}$ was correlated with the degree of lung injury. This is at odds with the observations of others (Cooper *et al.*, 1991) on short-duration waves, but it was noted that: 'a protective device which decreases the steepness of the pressure pulse may have a good protective effect, even if the reduction of the maximum pressure is only insignificant.'

The same studies demonstrated that any protective device must reduce the *low*-frequency oscillations of the thoracic wall. Rigid plates alone applied to the thorax reduced lung injury (Figure 21.6) and this was attributed to the rigid protection which prevented the shock acting on the chest wall and thus limited the inward deflection. Rigid materials closely applied to the thoracic wall in experiments with short-duration blast did not significantly reduce the severity of lung injury – a lack of effect that would be expected if direct stress coupling was the principal injury mechanism.

If direct stress coupling is involved in the cause of lung injuries from long-duration blast, the above observations are not incompatible with a stress-wave cause. The protection produced by rigid covering alone could be attributed to the air gap between the rigid protection and the thoracic wall (see figure 3 (lower) in Clemedson *et al.*, 1971).

Flexible body armour It is alleged that conventional textile 'fragmentation' vests may increase the susceptibility of the soldier to blast-waves (Young *et al.*, 1985; Dodd *et al.*, 1989). Young *et al.* exposed human volunteers to simulated artillery muzzle blast with a mean peak incident overpressure of 18.6 kPa and measured intraoesophageal pressure. They showed that a flexible ballistic vest increased the peak intrathoracic pressure when compared to thin clothing alone; the peak intrathoracic pressure was not affected by other clothing ensembles such as ceramic armour or ceramic armour and flexible Kevlar. $ITP_{dP/dt(max)}$ was not different between the clothing groups. The conclusion of the study was that ballistic vests offer no protection from blast and that further work was required to investigate if the increase in peak intrathoracic pressure was reflec-

ted in an increased severity of lung injury with more severe blast loadings.

Phillips *et al.* (1988) exposed sheep to one of four peak reflected overpressures: 115, 230, 295 or 420 kPa. In a comparison of the severity of lung injury between groups of sheep wearing or not wearing 'cloth ballistic vests' (CBV), a significant increase in lung weight could only be demonstrated in the 230 kPa group; a higher mortality was demonstrated at 420 kPa but this was not associated with a significant increase in lung weight. In a small number of sheep, intrathoracic pressure was measured but no significant differences between the CBV and non-CBV groups could be demonstrated.

A recent retrospective review of 828 soldiers in Northern Ireland killed or injured by explosions has described a higher incidence of primary blast lung injury in fatally injured soldiers when compared to the incidence in civilian casualties (Mellor and Cooper, 1989). Ninety per cent of the soldiers were wearing body armour. The predicted blast loadings to the soldiers were categorized into four levels, ranging from 'minor' to 'very severe'. The 'very severe' category was associated with a mortality of 50%. The majority of these victims died from multiple wounds but 17% of the dead had no external injury that could account for their death. It is probable that the majority died of primary lung injury.

The difference in the incidence of blast lung injury between military and civilian casualties does not necessarily imply that the body armour contributed to their deaths. Fatally injured soldiers may have been closer to the devices because wearing body armour effectively reduces the lethal radius of an explosive device – there would be a higher incidence of civilian deaths (from penetrating injuries) at longer ranges where blast overpressure levels would be significantly lower. Thus, body armour artificially increases the incidence of blast lung in the dead but the total number of deaths is reduced by the fragmentation protection afforded by the armour.

It has been shown that for short-duration loadings, textile body armour does not result in a significant increase in the severity of lung injury and, reflecting this, it did not significantly change the magnitude or rise time of $ITP_{(max)}$ in the lung or A_F (Cooper *et al.*, unpublished observations). Flexible textile armour, even if backed by foam, is also not an efficient decoupling layer against severe blast loads. The lack of effect probably arises from the relatively low areal density of most textile body armours.

The principal threats to soldiers and the police are antipersonnel fragments and bullets; it would be unacceptable to inhibit the wearing of body armour because of an alleged increase in blast injury which is of relatively low incidence.

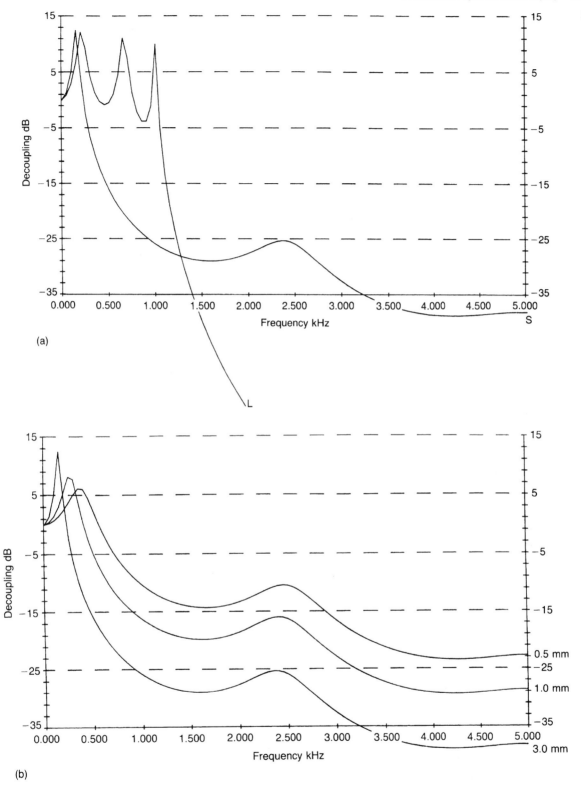

Figure 21.14 Decoupling predicted from an acoustic transmission model of an acoustic wave in air into an infinite water layer. (a) Decoupling achieved by a 3-mm GRP layer facing on a 9-mm foam layer (S), and the change in performance when the same thickness layers are split into three and laminated, i.e. GRP/foam/GRP/foam/GRP/foam (L). High-frequency performance is substantially increased, but additional resonance peaks due to added mass layers can degrade performance at lower frequencies. (b) Improved decoupling achieved by increasing the mass of the facing layer on 9-mm foam; 0.5-mm, 1-mm and 3-mm GRP shown.

Optimization of decoupling layers The change in frequency content of the direct stress-wave coupled into the thorax by acoustic couplers and decouplers mirrors the response predicted both by acoustic transmission models and anechoic chamber studies. Foam alone produced a 5 dB amplification over the bandwidth 0.5–2 kHz, and dense materials such as resin-bonded armours or metals placed on top of the foam achieved substantial decoupling, principally over the bandwidth 2–6 kHz.

The *in vivo* data (Figure 21.13) showed substantial amplification of the stress-wave in the lung behind a viscoelastic foam over the frequency range 0.5–2.5 kHz. Behind the resin-bonded/foam layers, the decoupling was also substantial over approximately the same frequency range (0.5–3 kHz). This suggests that the frequencies responsible for producing primary blast lung injury are within the frequency band 0.5–3 kHz, which is an important observation because it provides a window within which maximum decoupling must be achieved in the development of blast-protective clothing.

The most simple way to improve the blast protection of EOD suits is to place foam material behind the existing thoracic and pelvic plates present in nearly all designs. This ensemble may be optimized further in a number of ways, detailed below.

Laminating Splitting the mass and foam layers and interleaving them as a laminate will substantially increase the decoupling at high frequencies (Figure 21.14). However, each mass/foam layer will have a characteristic resonance and thus for a three-layer laminate, three resonance peaks will be present in the coupled energy and care must be taken to ensure that these do not extend into the frequency considered to be responsible for lung injury with short-duration blasts.

Experiments with bare charges in air showed that GRP plates backed with a closed-cell cross-linked polyethylene foam could eliminate lung injury resulting from an exposure to an incident overpressure of ~700 kPa (~2.5 ms duration) capable of producing very serious lung injury in the unprotected animal. However, attempts to optimize performance by laminating with a thin lead insert in the foam reduced performance due to the additional resonance (Figure 21.15). Care is therefore needed.

Mass layer Increasing the mass of the facing layer will increase decoupling across the frequency band and shift unwanted resonance peaks to lower frequencies (Figure 21.14(b)).

Foam properties and thickness The foam should ideally be highly compliant and have a large air content. It is essential however that during practical use in the field the foam is not compressed during

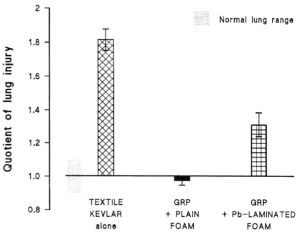

Figure 21.15 The protection achieved by a 20 kg/m² GRP plate backed with 20-mm foam against severe, short-duration blast loadings (~2.5 ms). Textile Kevlar is used for fragmentation protection and offers no protection from blast. An attempt to optimize the decoupling layer by adding an additional mass layer of 0.41-mm lead within the foam (GRP + Pb-LAMINATED FOAM) actually reduced performance due to an additional resonance from the extra mass layer encroaching into the frequency band responsible for lung injury. High-frequency performance was substantially increased (e.g. Figure 21.14).

bending; nor should it creep during storage. Air content must be maintained.

Increasing the thickness of a foam generally increases decoupling performance; however, across the frequency spectrum this enhancement of performance is not uniform and indeed at certain frequencies, performance can actually be decreased due to half-wave resonances.

All these means of optimizing necessitate a compromise between comfort, weight, bulk, possible degradation of personal performance and the degree of protection achievable. It is also very important to ensure that maximum coverage compatible with comfort of the thorax and abdomen is achieved.

Blast injury to bowel

Bowel contusions occur in most animals exposed to sufficient air-blast to produce lung injury. They are not commonly noted in human casualties, probably because of the lack of acute effects of bowel contusion but their presence is undoubtedly underreported. Abdominal injuries generally have a higher incidence in underwater explosions (Rawlins, 1974).

The dominance of both the acute and chronic effects of primary blast by injury to the lung in blast-injured casualties has directed most research effort addressing protection from air-blast to this organ, and little work has been undertaken on the protection of the bowel.

When examined at post-mortem, contusions to small bowel are usually associated with air-filled segments and this observation is compatible with a direct stress-coupling cause. Contusion to the colon and caecum do not show such association, and coincident injuries such as bruising around the peritoneal folds that bind the coils of the colon (in the pig model) and injury to small bowel mesentery indicate that shear arising from gross distortion of the abdominal wall is also implicated in the abdominal response to air-blast (shear and displacement injuries are very prevalent in underwater blast).

In a sequence of experiments on anaesthetized pigs designed to optimize thoracic protection, the same decoupling materials being used for thoracic protection were employed on the abdominal wall facing an explosive charge. The decoupling layer was GRP backed with a low-density closed-cell foam. The protected animals were in two groups – a group in which the decoupling plate was small and covered only about 60–70% of the presented area of the abdomen facing the charge, and a second group in which the coverage was optimized to envelop all the abdominal surface except the downstream side.

Small bowel injury was practically eliminated by the large coverage decoupling plates. Shock decoupling was remarkably effective and this observation supports the role of stress-waves in small bowel injury. However, the small decoupling plates were not effective against small bowel injury which emphasizes that extensive coverage of the body wall is essential for adequate performance of decoupling layers

For large bowel, neither the use of small nor large area coverage plates produced a significant difference in the contusion size and frequency when compared to the unprotected group, i.e. shock decoupling did not protect against large bowel injury, even in the pigs with maximal abdominal coverage.

The lack of effect on large bowel supports the observations on the nature of large bowel injuries that stress-waves may have a minor role in their causation but that abdominal compression and shear may predominate.

Clemedson *et al.* (1971) assessed the severity of abdominal injuries in their experiments on rabbits designed to attenuate blast lung with rigid shells around the torso. There was no clear relationship between the severity of the blast loading and the severity of abdominal injuries – undoubtedly resulting in part from variability in the gas content of the bowel. With a rigid shell covering the thorax and most of the abdomen, the incidence of injury to the intestines (large and small bowel not differentiated) was reduced from 85% to 17% for large rabbits, and from 80% to 50% for small ones.

Blast injury to the ear

The ear is the part of the body most sensitive to shock fronts and impulsive noise (e.g. from the firing of weapons). Injury to the ear has two implications

1. It may result in incapacitation of a soldier and reduce his operational effectiveness.
2. It may be an unacceptable consequence of weapon training in peacetime.

Eardrum rupture in a person close to a bomb is an injury whose significance is overshadowed by fragmentation and other wounds, and thus protection of the eardrum is not undertaken in combat soldiers.

Protection of the ear during training or for specialized personnel is a different matter. Although firing modern weapons will not result in eardrum rupture for single blasts, repeated exposure of the unprotected ear to weapon impulsive noise carries an unacceptable risk of permanent shift in auditory threshold. Most weapons produce hearing loss when the ear is not protected.

Exposure limits

An effective way of protecting the ear from impulsive noise is to limit exposure. There are a number of published guidelines and the principal limitations are on peak overpressure, impulse duration and the number of impulses permissible per day. Impulsive noise from the firing of weapons generally has a complicated pressure/time profile arising from reflections off adjacent objects and the ground and in some cases from secondary sources in the weapon such as venturi (Powell and Forrest, 1988). Firing weapons in reverberant rooms may result in an extremely complex envelope of pressure where the initial direct effect may be less of a hazard than the reflections. In these circumstances, the effective duration of the impulsive noise is defined as the time during which the envelope of the pressure fluctuations is within one-tenth of the peak overpressure (i.e. a 20 dB reduction in peak overpressure) – known as the B-duration.

Standards are published by many countries (e.g. MOD, 1986) that define, for the unprotected ear, maximum permissible combinations of peak overpressures and duration for a stated number of firings (100/day for the UK standard – corrections may be applied for greater or lower numbers of exposures ranging from +10 dB for 1 exposure to –10 dB for 1000). For the UK military standard, allowances of 20 dB (or exceptionally 25 dB) are permitted if hearing protection is used.

Hearing protection

Hearing protectors should be seen as the last resort in the conservation of hearing and should not be used as a substitute for other methods of noise reduction. They are widely used in civilian and military spheres but compromises have to be made in their design and use; the maximum protection available from hearing protectors is rarely achieved in practice.

There are two main types (Powell and Forrest, 1988):

1. Earplugs that fit into the external auditory meatus. These are often constructed from rubbery, malleable materials that can be shaped to fit closely the meatus of an individual – a good fit is essential for efficient performance.
2. Earmuffs that cover the pinna and meatus. They tend to be bulky and can interfere with military equipment such as helmets. Performance can be significantly degraded either by damage from careless handling or by poor adjustment and fit.

A noise-excluding helmet with an ear cup is also used in some military situations, such as within aircraft and tanks.

The same well-established principles employed in the protection of the ear from industrial noise are also used for impulsive noise (blast). An earmuff should consist of a rigid shell and a compliant cushion that seals it against the side of the head. The shell should be as heavy as can be compatible with comfort. The preferred acoustic characteristics of earmuffs can be gauged by an examination of the general principles of attenuation of noise with muffs (Zwislocki, 1955).

The forces on the side of the head and muff are shown schematically in Figure 21.16 (Zwislocki, 1955). The total force acting on the external surface S_o, F, is the sum of F_c, the reaction force due to the compression of the air volume V_c enclosed by the muff, and F_m, the reaction force due to the impedance of the muff and lining.

This relationship can be rewritten in terms of the impedances of the air and the muff/lining, and the velocity of displacement of the muff in the direction of F:

$$F = u(Z_m + Z_c) \qquad (21.4)$$

where u is the velocity of displacement, Z_m is the impedance of the muff and lining combined, and Z_c is the impedance of the air volume.

The pressure external to the muff is:

$$p_o = F/S_o$$

and internally:

$$p_i = F_c/S_i$$

The sound attenuation, A, is the ratio of these two pressures (p_o/P_i) and by using equation (21.4)

$$A = S_i/S_o \times |Z_m + Z_c|/|Z_c| \qquad (21.5)$$

The mechanical impedance of the enclosed air volume:

$$Z_c = -j((\rho_o c^2 S_i^2)/(\omega V_c))$$

If the average depth of the earmuff is d, the air volume enclosed by the earmuff, $V_c = S_i d$, thus:

$$Z_c = -j((\rho_o c^2 S_i)/(\omega d)) \qquad (21.6)$$

$$A = d/S_o(\omega |Z_m + Z_c|/\rho_o c^2) \qquad (21.7)$$

Equation (21.5) shows that if the impedance of the earmuff shell and associated lining (Z_m) is much greater than the impedance of the air volume (Z_c), then the attenuation will be large. Equation (21.7) shows that the ratio of the effective depth of the earmuff and the effective contact area (d/S_o) should be as great as possible compatible with comfort, i.e. a deep, narrow earmuff will produce superior attenuation than a broad shallow muff. Z_m is a function of the mass of the earmuff and, for optimal attenuation, the mass of the shell should be high.

For optimal performance, muffs should also have a sealing cushion that ideally is very compliant to provide an effective seal but conversely has high internal viscosity to reduce vibration of the muff and seal. As well as high mass, the shell should also be rigid to reduce sound conduction by shell deformation.

The sound attenuation provided by muffs is not uniform across the frequency range. Although this is an important consideration for protection from general environmental noise, the more usual solution for protection from impulsive noise is to

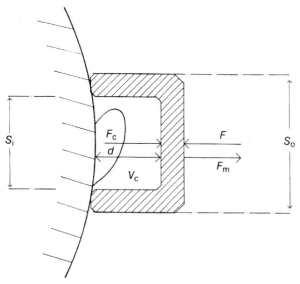

Figure 21.16 Earmuff model (Reproduced from Zwislocki, 1955.)

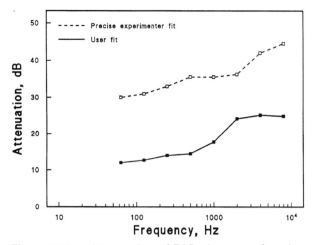

Figure 21.17 Attenuation of EAR plugs as a function of frequency when an experimenter gave each subject precise instructions on fitting and supervised the fitting procedure, and when the subject fitted the plug without guidance (user fit). (Reproduced from NATO, 1987.)

assume an attenuation of around 20 dB and apply this figure to the standards.

Expanded foam earplugs are particularly good for impulsive noise but the sound attenuation achieved by plugs (and muffs) is critically dependent on the quality of the fit – poorly fitted muffs or plugs provide poor attenuation. Figure 21.17 shows the attenuation as a function of frequency for a particular type of hearing plugs when fitted following precise instructions from an experimenter and under direct supervision, and when the subject fits the earplug without guidance. The change in performance is marked, amounting to a difference of around 20 dB.

An important aspect of hearing protection is education of the wearer about the benefits and limitations of hearing protection, and the importance of correct fit. The use of standard operating procedures to ensure implementation of protective measures is mandatory.

Traumatic amputation

Traumatic amputation by blast is associated with high mortality for lower-limb injury and in the upper limb when amputation occurs at a level above the hand. There has been no systematic survey of the nature of traumatic amputations that can be used as a basis for designing protective measures to reduce the incidence.

The delineation of mechanical injury from shock coupling into the limbs, direct effects of the blast winds (dynamic overpressure) on the tissues and avulsion of limbs at joints due to overextension or flailing is an important first step in combating this severe injury. A notable observation is that most traumatic amputations are not through the joints but usually occur through the shaft of the bone. In many cases, the bone injury is a cleaver-type break and is not severely comminuted. Soft tissue may also be stripped back from the bone, suggesting that for limbs in the same axis as the blast this may be the outcome of the dynamic overpressure.

Protective measures designed to reduce the forces of the gas flow over the tissues may have little effect on the direct coupling of the shock front into the tissues and, as with primary lung injury, bulky, strong materials that, on the face of it, suggest a degree of protection may not actually be effective. Nearly all bomb suits have no specific design aspects to address the risk of traumatic amputation – the layers of textile armour designed for fragmentation protection are merely assumed to offer a degree of protection against traumatic amputation. Steps can be taken to reduce the overextension of the arms under blast loading and to strengthen the joins between suit arms and the armour covering the torso. There is an inevitable compromise between comfort, manoeuvrability and the degree of protection: a suit that impairs the performance of an EOD operator may actually increase the risk of an inadvertent detonation. Few EOD operators wear heavy gloves for this reason and loss of hands or fingers is then inevitable.

The small amount of work on protection against traumatic amputation has been almost exclusively directed towards footwear designed to protect the lower limb from mines – there are few effective antimine boots and the more effective models tend to have limitations in movement, stability and general comfort.

There are two general approaches to the design of protective footwear:

1. Reduce the ground pressure (usually by increasing the contact area of the boot with the ground) to reduce the probability of mines detonating under the foot.
2. Try to maintain a boot that fulfils the requirement of comfort, stability and mobility and design the boot to withstand the detonation of the mine and so limit injuries to those that have low residual disability.

Other options tried in the Second World War were to remove the contact forces away from the foot by having extensions to the boot, forward and rear. The man walked on an elevated platform supported by a tubular frame, relying on a lower probability of activating a mine by point contacts, and separation of the foot from the ground to attenuate the blast loading should the mine detonate.

There are a number of operational considerations that direct designers towards the latter of the two main options. This is a difficult design problem – a conventional antipersonnel blast mine which contains 50–100 g high explosive is a severe threat, and rather more sophisticated mines using focused explosives and the shaped-charge effect escalate this to insurmountable levels. There are few effective antimine boots available and they fall into two general types – those designed for general combat use and those for specialized personnel involved in mine clearance.

The designs use one or all of three general principles:

1. Increase the stand-off of the foot from the mine.
2. Incorporate energy-absorbing materials such as metallic honeycombs or foam materials to reduce the peak overpressure loading to the boot. The materials may extend the duration of the loading, absorb some of the energy of the blast and employ decoupling principles to reduce the shock coupled through the boot to the foot.
3. Incorporate a wedge to reduce the dynamic pressure loading and effectively reduce the impulse to the lower limb.

The materials used in the construction of the boot must be strong, lightweight and, in some circumstances non-metallic, not only to reduce weight but also to reduce interference with mine detection equipment.

Stand-off is perhaps the most effective option but will inevitably result in instability to the wearer if carried to extreme. Elevation of the floor of the boot will permit incorporation of a wedge – and there is also a compromise between the small wedge angle required, the available height, and the reduction of impulse per unit area on the stiffened surface of the boot in contact with the foot.

In the 1960s a combat boot was developed in the USA that incorporated an aluminium honey comb, large angle wedge and a fairly small stand-off (Fujinaka and MacDonald, 1966). Tests on cadaver limbs attacked with a US Army M-14 mine containing about 1 ounce (~30 g) explosive, showed that in the evaluation of eight variants of a prototype design, 45% of the limbs protected by the variants had injuries that were 'probably salvageable'. The optimal design had a 'probable salvage' rate of 63%.

The Chinese FLX-1 mine-protective boot relies on a stand-off of 10 cm and also incorporates 'foamed plastic' to attenuate the shock loading (Liu Yin-Qiu *et al.*, 1990). It is very lightweight (1.1–1.5 kg) and has a sole shaped at the front and rear to provide comfort and stability during walking. Evaluation of the boot against 56 g TNT using pig and human cadaver limbs, showed that with a separation of 10 cm, 38% of injuries were linear lacerations with no tissue loss, 47% had loss of skin and soft tissues and bone fractures, 9% showed multiple comminuted fractures and severe tissue loss and 6% were

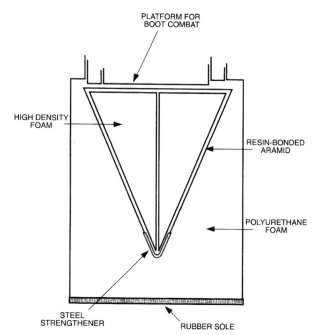

Figure 21.18 Section of a mine-protective overboot incorporating a wedge, and substantial stand-off.

assessed as beyond repair. The final design offered good protection – all injuries were repairable and would permit return to units after repair and recovery.

The antimine boot developed in the UK was designed for mine clearance. It is an overboot and is constructed largely from resin-bonded Kevlar (International Defence Review, 1988). Within the sole is a wedge fabricated from resin-bonded Kevlar with a 16-SWG steel-angled plate placed over the apex for additional strength (Figure 21.18). The inner part of the wedge is filled with a high-density polymethacrylamide foam and a polyurethane sole cast around the whole assembly. The contact with the ground is with a 5-mm microcellular rubber sole.

Tests on early prototypes suggested that compression fracture of the bones of the lower limb could result from the severe threat that the overboots were designed to defeat but the inclusion of energy-absorbing foams between the overboot and the combat boot significantly reduced the impulse transferred. Not only does the overboot effectively eliminate the risk of traumatic amputation but also the incidence of serious fracture to the bones of the foot and lower limb is likely to be low. The penalty for this efficient protection is a high sole but the limitations imposed by this can be overcome by training.

With all designs, injury is still largely inevitable – the aim of the protection is to reduce the incidence of traumatic and elective amputation, to limit the severity of the wounds and thus improve the long-term outlook for the casualty. Achievement of low residual disability is the priority. Total protection will never be achieved – most of the boots are designed to attenuate the effects of small blast mines. Unfortunately, it is a simple matter to design a mine to defeat the protection concepts.

PROTECTION FROM BLAST IN WATER

Prediction of the blast forces upon a man in water are difficult. Not only are the forces dependent upon charge weight and distance but also both the sea bed, sea surface and the location of the diver between these reflecting surfaces can result in a complex pressure environment (Rawlins, 1974).

The primary shock-wave from the charge propagates at around 1500 m/s and is reflected from the surface as a rarefaction wave (due to the impedance mismatch between the water and air) and, depending upon the distance of the diver from the surface, the rarefaction may actually reduce the total impulse. In shallow waters, there may also be reflection from the sea bed and these subsidiary pulses may reinforce the incident wave or produce double pulses.

The primary shock-wave is not the only load on the diver. There is a mass movement of water, the velocity of which is proportional to the shock-wave overpressure. An expanding bubble forms from the hot gases of the explosion, and this subsequently collapses to produce a pressure wave – the bubble wave. There may be several pulsations – the overpressures are less than the primary shock but the durations are longer resulting in approximately similar impulses for the primary shock and the bubble. There is also an after-flow of water associated with the bubble.

The diver is constrained by his environment and in most cases can achieve little even if he is prewarned of an explosion. The reduced impulse because of rarefaction of the reflected shock at the surface, is maximal close to the surface and some have advocated the opinion that divers close to the surface are subjected to less total impulse and therefore have a lower risk of injury. The safest place in underwater explosions is actually just out of the water – very little energy is coupled from the water into air and partial submersion of the body such that only the abdomen is in the water is preferred to total submersion when the chest is also exposed to the overpressures. It has also been stated that swimming on one's back offers a degree of protection.

The incident primary shock and multiple reflections between the sea bed and the surface may produce the same pattern of injury seen with air-blast – lung contusions, bowel contusions and perforations. It is important to recognize however that the bubble pulse, and the after-flow of water arising from the primary shock, are also capable of producing injury. The general pattern is very similar to those outlined above; additionally, intra-abdominal injuries such as subcapsular injury to the liver and tearing of the attachment of the gall bladder suggest that direct coupling of the shock front is not the only injury mechanism. The latter injuries probably result from shear arising from gross compression of the abdominal (and thoracic) wall undoubtedly from the after-flow of water. This is unlike the situation with air-blast – the momentum of the gross motion of water ('water-ram') is considerable and severe body wall distortions will occur.

The definition of 'safe' distances from charges is extremely difficult and it is unwise even to have confidence in the definition of a worst possible case. 'No damage' ranges are frequently expressed in terms of peak overpressure for structures of high natural frequency because the overpressure duration is long compared to the response of the object; if the natural oscillation is long compared to the wavelength, the displacement of the structure (and thus the propensity for injury) is related to the total impulse (the integral of the pressure/time profile).

The identification of both high frequency and low frequency injury mechanisms in man has led to a confused picture in which tolerance is expressed in terms of peak overpressure and impulse. The values of Christian and Gaspin (1973) for 'safe' ranges are frequently quoted – peak overpressure of 125 psi (about 900 kPa) and impulse 2 psi/ms (14 kPa/ms) but the caveats attached by the authors to the use of these figures suggests caution in their use.

Protection concepts must be directed not only to shock decoupling but also to reduce the gross compression of the body wall.

Shock-wave decoupling can be achieved by enveloping the torso in foam. Unlike air-blast, a decoupling facing of high acoustic impedance is not necessary underwater as water itself has high impedance and the decoupling interface is at the water/foam discontinuity. Research by Bebb in 1952 (MOD papers) showed that aerated rubber offered protection to rats but rigidity was of paramount importance for protection against bubble pulses and after-flow. A combination of a metal shield enclosing rubber foam prevented injury to the rats at lethal ranges from underwater charges.

Experiments with sheep showed that a steel jacket one-sixteenth-inch thick and a rigid diving helmet, both lined with foam rubber, ensured complete protection. Bebb noted that rubber foam alone appeared to increase the impulse in deep water and resulted in an increase in the severity of injuries. Rawlins (unpublished observations) considered that compression of the foam rubber by the hydrostatic pressure at depth may have negated the shock decoupling performance of the material.

Interaction of the bubble pulses and water after-flow could compress the foam to its limit and thereafter transmit an enhanced acceleration because of rebound expansion. The rubber foam (Rubazote) was more effective as an attenuator of shock pulses for small charges than for large in deep water. Close to the surface, it performed well for both small and large charges.

With our present knowledge of the cause of underwater blast injuries, effective protection can be achieved only by a rigid layer to attenuate the displacement of the body wall and an internal layer of foam to decouple the shock front.

USE OF DUMMIES IN BLAST PROTECTION AND ASSESSMENT OF THREAT LEVELS

After the Second World War, anthropomorphic models, colloquially called *dummies*, were used extensively both in the study of the impact of materials upon the body and in displacement of the body with subsequent impact upon solid objects (Fletcher *et al.*, 1970). These dummies often consisted of a strong metallic 'skeleton' covered with a foam-like material to simulate soft tissue. They were generally well modelled with respect to size and shape: the most important considerations were overall weight and weight distribution in that blast-induced motion of the dummy – and the velocity of the impact in particular – is often used to predict the risk of injury. The trajectory and velocity of the dummies was usually determined from high-speed photography; accelerometers placed in the head and chest provided additional information on forces involved.

Response characteristics required

It was not until the 1980s (Jonsson *et al*, 1983) that anthropomorphic dummies were used in experiments investigating the direct or primary effects of air-blast. The design criteria for these dummies was not in their behaviour during gross displacements but in fidelity to predict or replicate the response of the thoracic wall and the generation of pressure within the thorax.

It has been indicated above that, over the very wide range of overpressure durations, there is unlikely to be a common mechanical basis for lung injury. It is important therefore that any dummy developed to assess protective measures can address both direct stress transmission and gross compression. The latter has been achieved; the replication of the former has not yet been undertaken in detail.

Modelling of the torso requires a reasonable knowledge of the mechanism of injury in critical organs. It is essential therefore that a dummy should be able to replicate the motion of the body wall both on a gross scale to model long-duration impacts and, at a very different level, to model very transient small distortions of high acceleration with low overall velocity that couple direct stress-waves into the body. The dummy should also contain a lung simulant to provide an assessment of stress within the lung parenchyma, whether the rise time or the peak overpressure is taken as the index of injury potential.

Experiments performed in Sweden and the USA recording the intrathoracic pressure in lungs of animals exposed to long-duration shock-waves, showed that intrathoracic pressures could considerably exceed the external pressures acting on the thoracic wall (Clemedson *et al.*, 1969; White *et al.*, 1971). This indicated a large displacement of the thoracic wall and the motion of the wall was largely retarded by the build up of pressure in the lungs, and manifested as high intrathoracic peaks. Increasing the blast load accentuated the effect. A theoretical model describing the large displacements of the thoracic wall and associated intrathoracic pressure variations was developed in the USA (Bowen *et al.*, 1965).

If the blast loading was low or of short duration, the intrathoracic pressure was lower than the external pressure acting on the thoracic wall and, by implication, the gross deformation appeared to be less (Clemedson and Jonsson, 1961; White *et al.*, 1971). In other experiments (Clemedson and Jonsson, 1964) in which the motion of the body wall, exposed to small charges (short duration) was measured, maximal displacements of 5–10% of the relative chest diameter were recorded with chest wall velocities around 30 m/s. The acceleration of the body wall was estimated to be around 10^4G ($\sim 10^5$ m/s/s) – of the same order as the pig data outlined above. The maximum velocity of the body wall correlated with lung injury but the correlation with gross displacement was poor.

With large charges, deflections of up to 30–40% were recorded and in some experiments the deflections exceeded the lateral dimensions of the lungs – the peak velocities were low within the range 5–20 m/s (Clemedson *et al.*, 1969; Jonsson, 1979). An example of simultaneous recordings of chest wall motion and intrathoracic pressure is shown in Figure 21.19 – the maximal overpressure in the lung closest to the charge was three times the extra-thoracic pressure.

In summary, with long-duration waves, experimental evidence and modelling work suggest that gross deformations are the principal mechanism of injury, and that the severity of injury is also dependent upon the maximum velocity of the deformation (Clemedson *et al.*, 1968; Jonsson, 1979). The maximum intrathoracic pressure is an index of the injury potential and because of the dynamic overshooting of the thoracic wall, may be many times the external loading. Conversely for short-duration waves, gross compression is not severe

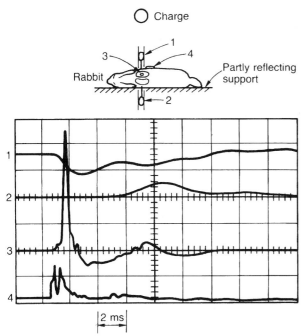

Figure 21.19 Example of simultaneous recordings of inward deflection of chest wall and intrathoracic pressure in rabbits exposed to air shock-waves produced by 'large' charges of TNT (8–32 kg). Animals lying on their left side on a rigid and partly reflecting support and the charge suspended above. Curve 1, Deflection of right chest wall facing the charge. Curve 2, Deflection of left chest wall. Curve 3, Intrathoracic pressure in right lung facing the charge. Curve 4, Extrathoracic pressure acting on the right chest wall. Intrathoracic pressure about three times the extrathoracic pressure. Time 2 ms between vertical lines (Reproduced from Clemedson *et al.*, 1969.)

but the acceleration of the thoracic wall generates a stress-wave whose rise time is the index of injury. Peak intrathoracic pressure is not relevant in this context.

Development of the dummy

Before the construction of the human dummy, a mechanical model of a rabbit was designed. The simplified lung model made of foam plastic was mounted in a water-filled rubber tube with closed ends (Jonsson, 1979). Pressure patterns recorded in the lung model were found to be very similar to intrathoracic patterns recorded in rabbits under nearly identical blast conditions and were considered to indicate a similarity in dynamic response. A factor that increased the risk of injury was reflected in a higher overpressure recorded in the lung model. Exposures to long-duration waves showed fast-rising waves in the water surrounding the lung but not in the parenchyma itself. The overpressures appeared to result from the gross compression and distortion of the mechanical

model by water being forced against the lung. High-speed photography revealed that the lung underwent a larger and more complicated deformation than could be anticipated from the external deformation of the model.

In exposure to short-duration blast-waves in water, signs of typical shock-waves were seen in the lungs; the maximal overpressure recorded seemed to have been produced mainly by mass motion in the surrounding water.

These experiments, and the difficulty of measuring body wall deformation and velocity reproducibly and accurately, led the Swedish investigators to define the intrathoracic pressure as the primary output of a model to predict the blast overpressure to *long*-duration waves which constituted a threat to man. The efficiency of protective measures, principally in terms of changes in geometry and location of the body in a complex blast environment and to a lesser extent in the development of personal protection, could be determined using this index. The subsequent work of Cooper *et al.* (1991) on *short*-duration waves suggests that the rise time of this pressure would be an acceptable index for injury potential but the acceleration of the thoracic wall would be even better.

The torso of the model was constructed from strong rubber tube closed at both ends with transparent material to facilitate inspection, The rubber tube was formed to approximate the exterior of the human thorax (Jonsson *et al.*, 1983, 1988) and simplified models of the human lung were mounted in it (Figure 21.20). The models were made of foamed plastic, formed as cylinders with a volume corresponding to the average of an adult human. At the central part of each, a pressure transducer was placed for the recording of pressure/time sequences used for predicting the risk of lung injury. The torso is filled with water before use and thereby attains basic dynamic properties similar to the human thorax. Studies to date have used the maximal overpressure recorded as the measure of blast severity.

Dummy validation

The dummy has been used principally with shock-waves of long duration. Experiments in the USA compared the response of the dummy and sheep to nearly identical shock-waves generated in a shock tube (Jonsson *et al.*, 1983). The severity of lung injury was correlated to the intrathoracic pressures recorded in the dummy 'lung'. From Figure 21.21 it can be seen that the maximal overpressure recorded in the animals and the dummy agreed fairly well over a range of injuries from threshold, to the lower probabilities of mortality. Over this range, the intrathoracic pressures in sheep and dummy varied from approximately 100 kPa to 1 MPa. Figure 21.21 also shows that the ratio of internal to external

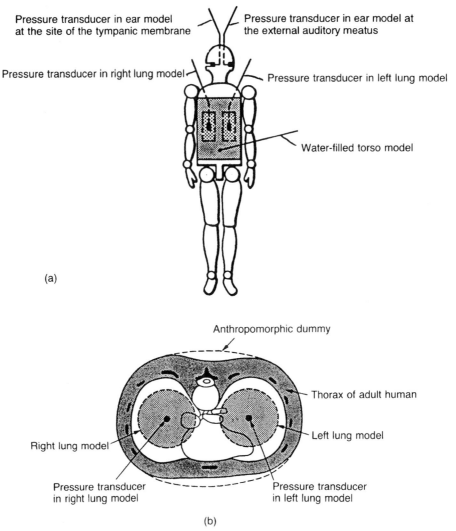

Pressure transducer in ear model at the site of the tympanic membrane

Pressure transducer in ear model at the external auditory meatus

Pressure transducer in right lung model

Pressure transducer in left lung model

Water-filled torso model

(a)

Anthropomorphic dummy

Thorax of adult human

Right lung model

Left lung model

Pressure transducer in right lung model

Pressure transducer in left lung model

(b)

Figure 21.20 (a) Anthropomorphic dummy for the study of direct or primary effects of air shock-waves. Transducers for recording of pressure in models of left and right lung, and left and right external auditory canal for predicting effects on lungs and ears, respectively. (Reproduced from Jonsson *et al.*, 1988.) (b) Schematic cross-section of adult human torso taken at the level of the heart, and of the corresponding part of the anthropomorphic dummy (dashed line). (Reproduced from Jonsson *et al.*, 1988.)

pressure increased significantly with increasing blast load.

Modification for underwater blast

The hydrostatic pressures experienced by the dummy underwater necessitate modification. As with divers using pressurized air, the dummy must be provided with a device for pressure/volume compensation of the lung models so that their volume can remain constant irrespective of the hydrostatic pressure. Plastic tubes simulating the upper respiratory airways were joined to the lung models and, via a shut-off valve, were connected with a demand valve of the type used by divers. Tubed air at pressure is used to manipulate the demand valve.

For an anthropomorphic dummy to be used in blast experiments, the shape and size of the torso and limbs are probably less important in water than in air. Surface properties however may be more important. The arms are made of water-filled rubber tubes fixed to the side of the dummy. Legs are replaced by simple supports to facilitate manipulation of the dummy and the head is replaced by a strong housing to protect the shut-off valve.

The dummy was initially evaluated in an underwater blast test facility in the USA (Yelverton *et al.*, 1973). Previous experiments on animal models designed to establish risk of injury criteria for divers had demonstrated that the impulse correlated well with the injury, better than the peak overpressure or energy in the same part of the waveforms.

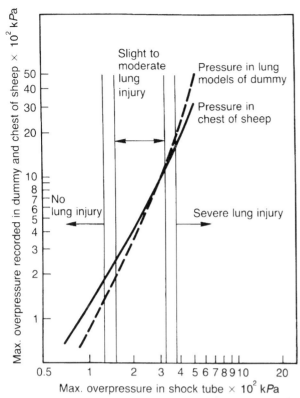

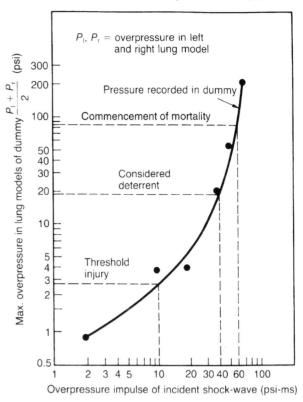

Figure 21.21 Validation of the anthropomorphic dummy for the study of air-blast effects. Dummy and sheep exposed to nearly identical shock-waves in a shock tube at the Biodynamics Laboratory, ITRI, Albuquerque, New Mexico, USA (Jonsson *et al.*, 1988). Duration of overpressure in the incident waves 10–20 ms. Criteria for predicting injury obtained from Dr Donald R. Richmond (Head of Biodynamics Laboratory, ITRI).

Figure 21.22 Validation of anthropomorphic dummy for the study of underwater blast effects on divers. Pressure recorded in the lung models of the dummy related to overpressure impulse of incident shock-wave. Experiments at a depth of 3 m performed in the pond (Lake Christian) at the Biodynamics Laboratory, ITRI, Albuquerque, New Mexico, USA. Criteria for predicting risk of injury derived from Yelverton *et al.* (1973), and from personal communication with Dr Donald R. Richmond (Head of the Biodynamics Laboratory, ITRI).

The dummy was exposed at a depth of 3 m. Figure 21.22 shows the correlation of the impulse with the maximum pressure measured in the dummy. The criteria demanded from the animal models are also shown in Figure 21.22 and it can be seen that the intrathoracic pressure in the dummy used for predicting the risk of injury varied from 10 to 700 kPa with a range of injuries from threshold of lung injury to mortality.

Experiments were also performed in the open sea at depths down to 20 m. Intrathoracic pressures (in the dummy) in experiments with small charges of TNT were characterized by a pronounced low-frequency oscillation. Typically, the dummy responded to underwater blast with a sequence of intrathoracic pressure oscillations divided into two distinct groups each containing at least one peak of relatively high overpressure. The leading group of each sequence was attributed to the shock-wave generated by the charge and the remainder to subsequent bubble pulses

with significant mass movement of water. The dummy showed that at 10 m depth the bubble pulses may produce higher intrathoracic overpressures than the shock-wave.

Acknowledgements

The unpublished writings and internal MOD reports of the following people have been consulted. On underwater blast: J.S.P. Rawlins, A.H. Bebb and H.N.V. Temperley. On stress analysis: I.S. Bush, S.A. Challener, A.R. Duffin and M.J. Hodson. Mr D.J. Townend has provided invaluable, practical advice on decoupling principles.

Dr D.R. Richmond and his colleagues at the Biodynamics Laboratory, formerly affiliated with the Inhalation Toxicology Research Institute (ITRI), Lovelace Biomedical and Environmental Research Institute, Albuquerque, New Mexico, USA, provided facilities and performed the experiments to validate the dummies for use in air and water.

REFERENCES

Aubert J.H., Kraynick A.M., Rand P.B. (1986). Aqueous foams. *Sci. Am.*, **254**, 58–68.

Baker W.E., *Explosions in Air*. San Antonio, TX: Wilfred Baker Engineering.

Bowen J.G., Holladay A., Fletcher E.R. et al. (1965). *A Fluid-Mechanical Model of the Thoraco-Abdominal System with Application to Blast Biology*. DASA-1675. Albuqurque, New Mexico: Lovelace Foundation for Medical Education and Research.

Bowen I.G., Fletcher E.R., Richmond D.R. (1968). Estimate of man's tolerance to the direct effects of air blast. In *Defence Atomic Support Agency Report DASA-2113*. Dept of Defense, Washington.

Bush I.S., Challener S.A. (1988). Finite element modelling of non-penetrating thoracic impact. In *Proceedings of the International Research Council Biokinetics Impacts (IRCOBI), Bergisch-Gladbach, FRG*.

Christian J., Gaspin J. (1973). Swimmer safe stand-offs from underwater explosions. In *US Navy Assistance Programme Report on Project PHP 11–73*. Dept of Defense, Washington.

Clemedson C-J., Jonsson A. (1961). Transmission of elastic disturbances caused by air shock waves in a living body. *J. Appl. Physiol.*, **16**, 424–36.

Clemedson C-J., Jonsson A. (1964). Dynamic response of chest wall and lung injuries in rabbits exposed to shock waves of short duration. *Acta Physiol. Scand.*, **62**, (Suppl.) 233.

Clemedson C-J., Hellstrom G., Lindgren S. (1968). The relative tolerance of the head, thorax and abdomen to blunt trauma. *Ann. N.Y. Acad. Sci.*, (152 Art.), **1**, 187.

Clemedson C-J., Frankenberg L., Jonsson A. et al. (1969). Dynamic response of the thorax and abdomen of rabbits in partial and whole-body blast exposure. *Am. J. Physiol.*, **216**, 615–20.

Clemedson C-J., Frankenberg L., Jonsson A. et al. (1971). Effects on extra and intrathoracic pressure pattern and lung injuries of rigid and soft protection of the thorax in blast exposed rabbits. *Forsvarmedicin*, **7**, 172–90.

Cooper G.J., Taylor D.E.M. (1989). Biophysics of impact injury to the chest and abdomen. *J. R. Army Med. Coll.*, **135**, 58–67.

Cooper G.J., Townend D.J., Cater S.R., Pearce B.P. (1991). The role of stress waves in thoracic visceral injury from blast loading: modification of stress transmission by foams and high-density materials. *J. Biomechanics*, **24**, 273–85.

Desaga H. (1950). Blast injuries. In *German Aviation Medicine, World War 2*, Vol. 2. US Department of the Air Force, pp. 1274–93. Dept of Defense, Washington.

Dodd K.T., Ripple G.R., Mundie T.G. (1989). Current injury assessment techniques for complex waves. In *Proceeding of the 6th International Symposium on Military Operational Research*. RMCS Shrivenham, UK.

Fletcher E.R., Richmond D.R., Jones R.K. (1970). *Blast Displacements of Prone Dummies*. Operation Prairie Flat. Project Officers Report – Project LN 402, Technical Report on contract no. DA-01-68-C-0118. Washington, DC: Defense Atomic Supply Agency, Department of Defense.

Fujinaka E.S., Macdonald J.L. (1966). *Research and Development of Blast Protective Footwear. Fabrication and Proof-testing*. Technical Report 67–5-CM. Natick: US Army Natick Laboratories.

Jonsson A. (1979). Experimental Investigations on the Mechanism of Lung Injury in Blast and Impact Exposure. Linkoping University Medical Dissertation No. 80.

Jonsson A., Clemedson C-J., Arvebo E. (1983). Experiments with an anthropomorphic dummy for blast research. In *Proceedings of the Eighth International Symposium on Military Application of Blast Simulation (MABS8), Spiez, Switzerland, 20–24 June 1983*. Spiez: Gruppe Fur Rustungsdienste, AC-Laboratorium.

Jonsson A., Arvebo E., Schantz B. (1988). Intrathoracic pressure variations in an anthropomorphic dummy exposed to air blast, blunt impact and missiles. *J. Trauma*, **28**, S125–31.

Kerner E.H. (1950). The elastic and thermo-elastic properties of composite media. *Proc. Phys. Soc.*, **B 63**, 2.

Kinsler L.E., Frey A.R., Coppens A.B., Sanders J.V. (1980). *Fundamentals of Acoustics*, 3rd edn. Chichester: John Wiley.

Liu Yin-Qiu, Wang Zheng-Guo, Chen Xie-Min et al. (1990). Development of Model FLX-1 mine protective footwear and its protective effectiveness. *J. Trauma (China)*, **6**, (Suppl.), 173–6.

Mellor S.G., Cooper G.J. (1989). An analysis of 828 servicemen killed or injured by explosions in Northern Ireland, 1970–1984. The HACS statistics. *Br. J. Surg.*, **76**, 1006–10.

Mine-resistant boots (1988). *Int. Defence Rev.*, **12**, 1661.

MOD (UK) (1988). Defence Standard 00–27/1 *Acceptable Limits for Exposure to Impulse Noise from Military Weapons, Explosives and Pyrotechnics*.

Phillips Y.Y., Mundie T.G., Yelverton J.T. et al. (1988). Cloth ballistic vest alters response to blast. *J. Trauma*, **28**, (Suppl.), S149–52.

Powell R.F., Forrest M.R. (1988). Noise in the military environment. In *Land Warfare: Brassey's New Battlefield Weapon Systems and Technology Series*, Vol. 3. London: Brassey's Defence Publishers.

Rawlins J.S.P. (1974). Physical and pathophysiological effects of blast. *Journal of the Royal Naval Medical Service*, **29**, 124–9.

Richmond D.R. (1990). Blast criteria for open spaces and enclosures. In 'Effects of noise and blasts.' (Borch-grevink, ed.). *Scand. Audiol.*, (Suppl.) **34**, 49–76.

Taylor D.E.M., Cooper G.J., Maynard R.L., Whammond J. (1985). Biomechanics of ribs and thoracic cage in relation to chest injury. In *Proceedings of the Conference on Material Properties and Stress Analysis in Biomechanics*. Bristol: Institute of Physics.

Turnbull J.H., Walter K. (1982). *Explosions in Air and Water*. Shrivenham: Department of Chemistry and Metallurgy, Royal Military College of Science.

von Gierke H.E. (1968). Response of the body to mechanical forces – an overview. *Ann. N. Y. Acad. Sci.*, **152**, 172–86.

White C.S., Jones R.K., Damon E.G. et al. (1971). *The Biodynamics of Air Blast*. DNA-2738T. Albuquerque, New Mexico: Lovelace Foundation for Medical Education and Research.

Yelverton J.T., Richmond D.R., Fletcher E.R., Jones R.K. (1973). *Safe Distances from Underwater Explosions for Mammals and Birds*. Technical Progress Report DNA 3114T. Washington DC: Department of Defense, Defense Nuclear Agency.

Young A.J., Jaeger J.J., Phillips Y.Y. et al. (1985). The influence of clothing on human intrathoracic pressure during airblast. *Aviat. Space Environ. Medi.*, **56**, 49–53.

Zwislocki J. (1955). Design and testing of ear muffs. *J. Acoust. Soc. Am.*, **27**, 1154–63.

APPENDIX: THE DECIBEL

The intensity of a sound is measured in terms of how many times more intense the sound is than a reference sound. A logarithmic scale is used to cover the large range of the human ear. The unit *bel* is used to measure the intensity of sound. A bel is defined as:

$$\text{Intensity in bels} = \log_{10}(I/I_o) \quad (21.A1)$$

Where I_o is a reference intensity of 10^{-12} W/m^2. Thus a sound of identical intensity as the reference sound will have an intensity of 0 bels ($\log_{10}$ of 1). A sound 10 times as intense will have an intensity of 1 bel, 100 times will be 2 bels.

Sound intensity is the rate of energy transmitted across a unit area normal to the propagation direction (J/s/m^2 or Watts/m^2). The relationship between intensity and the pressure generated is:

$$I = P^2/(2\rho c)$$

where ρ = density of the medium and c = speed of sound in the medium. Thus, $I \propto P^2$, and the equation above can be rewritten as:

$$\text{Intensity in bels} = \log_{10}(P^2/P_0^2)$$

where P_0 is a reference pressure at I_0 (2×10^{-5}Pa). This reference pressure is conveniently close to the pressure just detectable by the ear in its most sensitive frequency range.

The bel is actually a large unit, and sound intensities and pressures are more conveniently expressed as decibels. Thus:

$$\text{Intensity in decibels} = 10(\log_{10}(P^2/P_0^2)$$

As $\log_{10}x^2 = 2\log_{10}x$:

$$\text{sound pressure level in decibels} = 20 \log_{10}(P/P_0)$$

The attenuation in intensity (or power) achieved by acoustic decoupling or other attenuation techniques is generally expressed in terms of dB. From equation (21.A1) it can be seen that an attenuation of 10 dB (1 bel) is a 10-fold reduction in intensity. Pressure attenuation is also expressed in dB and as $P \propto I^2$, a 10 dB reduction in pressure is equal to a 3.16-fold ($\sqrt{10}$) reduction in pressure.

This is summarized below:

Attenuation (dB)	Reduction in intensity (power)	Reduction in pressure
10	10	3.16
20	100	10
30	1000	31.6
40	10000	100

22. Crush Injury
S. Burzstein and G. Carlson

INTRODUCTION

Crush injuries were first reported during the Messina earthquake in 1909 (Colmers, 1909), and the air raids of the First World War (Frankenthal, 1916). The first definitive description of the clinical syndrome associated with crush injuries to the limbs was provided by Bywaters and Beall (1941), during the 'Blitzkreig' of the Second World War. Bywaters and Beall noted that resuscitation of shocked patients, extricated from the rubble of bombed buildings, did not prevent death from acute renal failure. Moreover, post-mortem examination revealed the presence of numerous casts, predominantly in the distal renal tubules, a phenomenon referred to as 'lower nephron nephrosis'. Bywaters and his colleagues systematically explored the mechanisms responsible for the development of renal failure in patients subjected to crush injury, and demonstrated that in animal models of crush injury, extensive damage to skeletal muscle leads to haemoconcentration and shock (Bywaters and Popjak, 1942). Myoglobin was believed to be the major nephrotoxic factor responsible for acute renal failure after muscle injury, and Beall and Stead (1944) demonstrated that the nephrotoxicity of myoglobin could be attenuated by alkalinization of the urine. The demonstration of a causal link between muscle injury and the development of shock, haemoconcentration and acute renal failure subsequently led Bywaters to suggest that the term 'crush syndrome' should be abandoned in favour of 'ischaemic muscle necrosis' (Bywaters and Dible, 1942). While the relative contributions of vascular impairment and direct mechanical injury to muscle in the pathogenesis of crush injury are unclear (see later), the complications of this unique form of injury continue to cause considerable clinical problems, and crush injury is still recognized to be associated with a high mortality (Bentley and Jeffreys, 1968; Brown and Nichols, 1977), particularly if renal failure supervenes (Ward, 1988).

The fundamental mechanism underlying the pathogenesis of crush injury is limb compression. A combination of ischaemia, owing to the compression of the vascular supply to the limb, and direct injury leads to necrosis of skeletal muscle. Subsequent extrication of the injured limb may restore perfusion, but may also exacerbate the injury (see later), and provoke the release of intracellular muscle con-

stituents into the systemic circulation (rhabdomyolysis), resulting in a series of systemic disturbances including metabolic acidosis, myoglobinaemia, myoglobinuria, hypocalcaemia, hyperphosphataemia, hyperuricaemia and defects of coagulation (Honda, 1983; Better, 1989; Curry et al., 1989).

RHABDOMYOLYSIS AND THE LOCAL INJURY

Injury to skeletal muscle and leakage of the intracellular contents of myocytes into plasma may be provoked by a number of conditions, including excessive physical activity (Olerud et al., 1976), drugs and toxins (Berlin, 1948; Koffler et al., 1976), alcohol (Schneider, 1970), viral infection (Minow et al., 1974), severe potassium depletion (Campion et al., 1972) and hereditary disorders of muscle metabolism (Bank et al., 1975). Although other forms of physical injury, including electrical injury (Artz, 1967), the injudicious use of pneumatic antishock trousers (Bass et al., 1983) and acute arterial occlusion (Haimovici, 1979), have also been reported to cause rhabdomyolysis, compression of skeletal muscle is thought to be aetiologically important in up to 40% of patients with rhabdomyolysis (Odeh, 1991).

The mechanisms of local injury are complex and incompletely understood. It is now clear, however, that both local pressure and vascular changes may contribute, in an independent, though related manner, to the development of muscle necrosis. While the systemic manifestations of crush injury begin only after the patient has been extricated from the scene of injury, the local injury begins while the limb is trapped. The relative contributions of ischaemia and pressure to the development of local injury are difficult to separate. Although ischaemia alone may produce a similar spectrum of responses to crush injury (Haimovici, 1979), and muscle necrosis is known to occur after approximately 6 hours of total warm ischaemia (Whitesides et al., 1971) (the application of a limb tourniquet has, in fact, been used as an experimental model of crush injury (Bywaters and Popjak, 1942)), rhabdomyolysis may occur in cases where limbs have been compressed despite an adequate blood supply, with a warm limb and palpable distal pulses. Complete recovery from limb entrapment for periods of up to 28 hours suggests that total warm ischaemia of this duration is unlikely to have occurred (Ron et al., 1984). These observations imply that although ischaemia may play a role in the pathogenesis of the local injury, total ischaemia is not an essential prerequisite.

LIMB COMPRESSION

Sustained compression of skeletal muscle, together with complete immobilization, may lead to local muscle necrosis. Although skeletal muscle is sensitive to ischaemic injury, the 'warm ischaemia time' required to produce muscle necrosis, of approximately 6 hours (Whitesides et al., 1971), compares favourably with the time required for necrosis to occur as a result of mechanical compression. Significant pathological changes have been described within skeletal muscle subjected to sustained mechanical pressure over periods as short as 60 minutes (Better and Stein, 1990; Better et al., 1990). Skeletal muscle may therefore be much more sensitive to mechanical than ischaemic injury. Intramuscular pressures as high as 240 mmHg have been recorded in patients with compressed limbs, and have been associated with rhabdomyolysis, despite the presence of an intact vascular supply (Owen et al., 1979). The mechanism by which mechanical pressure leads to muscle injury is unclear. While high intramuscular pressures may compromise the microvasculature of skeletal muscle, irrespective of the state of major blood vessels, and intramuscular pressure has been shown to exceed arterial pressure within minutes of trauma (Awbrey et al., 1988), the relatively long duration of ischaemia, compared with pressure, required to produce muscle necrosis suggests that mechanisms other than ischaemia must be involved. Alterations in myocyte function, associated with the flux of calcium across the plasma and mitochondrial membranes of the myocyte, may be of importance in this respect. The permeability of the plasma membrane of the myocyte is altered by mechanical stretching. In particular, stretching has been shown to increase the permeability of the plasma membrane to calcium ions (Guharay and Sachs, 1984). The resulting flux of calcium into the muscle cell may have adverse consequences. An increase in cytosolic and mitochondrial calcium concentration may interfere with mitochondrial function, and inhibit oxidative metabolism and sodium-potassium ATPase activity, leading to a secondary flux of sodium and water into the muscle cell, and swelling (Better et al., 1990). In addition, calcium may lead to activation of a number of intracellular proteolytic enzyme systems, modulated by calmodulin and resulting in autolysis (Better et al., 1990), and also the conversion of xanthine dehydrogenase to xanthine oxidase within muscle. This process may play a role in the generation of oxygen-derived free radicals and tissue injury (Roy and McCord, 1983; McCord, 1985) (see later).

ISCHAEMIA AND REPERFUSION

The potential role of ischaemia in the pathogenesis of crush injury is exemplified by the fact that tourniquet ischaemia is recognized to be a useful model of muscle injury and rhabdomyolysis (Bywaters and Popjak, 1942). Ischaemic injury leads to muscle necrosis, and significant morbidity from both local and systemic complications, as does crush injury (Haimovici, 1979; Cambria and Abbott,

1984; Walker et al., 1987). In models of ischaemic injury, however, the damage to skeletal muscle appears to occur primarily during the period of reperfusion (Cambria and Abbott, 1984; Jennische, 1984; Walker et al., 1987). In fact, skeletal muscle is relatively resistant to ischaemic injury, compared with tissues such as brain, gut and cardiac muscle. The reintroduction of oxygen to ischaemic muscle appears to be the key factor responsible for this 'reperfusion injury' (Presta and Ragnotti, 1981; Korthuis et al., 1989). It is perhaps surprising that the reoxygenation of ischaemic tissues should produce a greater injury than ischaemia alone. This phenomenon has therefore been called the 'oxygen paradox' (Braunwald and Kloner, 1985). The reasons for the oxygen paradox are only recently becoming clear. As in the case of mechanical muscle injury, there is evidence to support the suggestion that calcium ions may play a role in the injury associated with ischaemia and reperfusion (see later). The fundamentally injurious agents appear, however, to be oxygen-derived free radicals, such as superoxide, hydrogen peroxide and hydroxyl ions (Freeman and Crapo, 1982). These agents are believed to play a major role in the parenchymal and microvascular injury associated with ischaemia and reperfusion in a number of tissues, including skeletal muscle (Presta and Ragnotti, 1981; Jackson and Veal, 1989; Korthuis et al., 1989). While ischaemia directly impairs oxidative metabolism, restoration of the supply of oxygen has been shown to increase the extent of skeletal muscle necrosis (Jennische, 1984; Perry et al., 1984; Korthuis et al., 1985; Walker et al., 1987; Korthius et al., 1989; McCutchen et al., 1990; Sexton et al., 1990). Administration of compounds which inhibit the production of, or neutralize oxygen-derived free radicals, such as superoxide dismutase (SOD) and catalase, have been shown to attenuate the injury to tissue and its microvasculature associated with ischaemia-reperfusion injury (Korthuis et al., 1985; Walker et al., 1987; Smith et al., 1988). Reperfusion of the ischaemic limb with hypoxaemic blood increases microvascular permeability and vascular resistance only slightly, and the muscle necrosis can be reduced substantially by the gradual restoration of oxygenation, combined with SOD, catalase and mannitol (Walker et al., 1987).

The production of oxygen-derived free radicals in reperfused tissues has been attributed to the actions of the enzyme xanthine oxidase (XOd) (McCord, 1985; Van Gilst, 1989; Linas et al., 1990), although polymorphonuclear leucocytes may also play a role (Freeman and Crapo, 1982). Most tissues within the body contain two related forms of XOd; XOd itself and xanthine dehydrogenase (XdH), with a preponderance of XdH (>90%). This is of importance, because XdH uses nicotinamide adenine dinucleotide (NAD) as an electron acceptor, rather than oxygen. Since the activity of XdH does not, therefore lead to the transfer of electrons to molecular oxygen, oxygen-derived free radicals are not generated. In contrast, XOd uses oxygen as an electron carrier, and activity of XOd *is* associated with the formation of free radicals (McCord, 1985). In many tissues (though not apparently in skeletal muscle), XdH is converted to XOd in conditions of ischaemia (McCord, 1985), the reaction being catalysed by an intracellular proteolytic enzyme, regulated by ionic calcium and calmodulin. In ischaemic tissue, the ability of the cell to maintain the extrusion of calcium is impaired, and activation of the protease results in the conversion of XdH to XOd (McCord, 1987). This finding is supported by the observation that conversion of XdH to XOd is significantly reduced in rats by the administration of trifluoperazine (an inhibitor of calmodulin) (Roy and McCord, 1983). Although XOd may play a role in the generation of free radicals, the mechanism by which XOd is produced from XdH in the crush-injured limb may be related less to ischaemia than to the effect of mechanical pressure on calcium flux. As indicated above, ischaemia may lead to the generation of XdH in many tissues, but this does not seem to occur in skeletal muscle (McCord, 1985). This has been suggested as a possible reason for the relative resistance of skeletal muscle to ischaemic injury (Labbe *et al.*, 1987). The production of XOd in the crush-injured limb may be a result of calcium influx occurring due to mechanical pressure rather than ischaemia, although the relative influences of the two pathways are difficult to separate. While calcium enters the cell subjected to mechanical pressure owing to a direct effect on membrane permeability to calcium (see above), the mechanism by which ischaemia leads to the influx of calcium is probably more complex. Relatively little calcium enters the cell during the period of ischaemia, the majority of calcium flux occurs during the process of reperfusion (Shen and Jennings, 1964; Watts *et al.*, 1980). In ischaemic tissue, a decline in the activity of sodium–potassium ATPase leads to the accumulation of sodium ions within the cell, and leakage of potassium into the extracellular fluid (Daly *et al.*, 1984). Sodium ions are then exchanged for calcium ions during reperfusion, due to the activity of a specific sodium–calcium exchange pump. The overloading of the cell with calcium not only results in the generation of XOd, but also impairs mitochondrial function, and thus ATP generation. Since ATP is vital for the activity of sodium–potassium ATPase, the influx of calcium leads to further accumulation of sodium within the cell, and these sodium ions are in turn exchanged for calcium. A vicious cycle therefore develops, promoting the generation of oxygen free radicals and cellular injury. Oxygen free radicals attack the lipid bilayer of the cell membranes (lipid peroxidation), leading to structural and functional disturbances, including further sodium influx, which

merely exacerbates the vicious cycle (Korthuis *et al.*, 1985; Walker *et al.*, 1987). The cellular injury is compounded by calcium-mediated impairment of cellular oxidative metabolism (Wrogemann and Pena, 1976), free radical production (Braughler, 1988) and activation of phospholipase A_2 which leads to the generation of lysophospholipids, leukotrienes and prostaglandins which also promote cell injury (Duncan and Jackson, 1987) and muscle contracture (Ogilvie *et al.*, 1988). These processes are believed to contribute significantly to progressive muscle necrosis (Lakatta *et al.*, 1979; Nayler *et al.*, 1979; Trump *et al.*, 1980; Poole-Wilson *et al.*, 1984).

In addition to calcium- and calmodulin-mediated generation of free radicals, polymorphonuclear leucocytes may also generate highly reactive oxygen metabolites, and have been implicated in ischaemia-reperfusion injury in several organ systems (Romson *et al.*, 1983; Jolly *et al.*, 1984; Grisham *et al.*, 1986; Klausner *et al.*, 1988b; Ciuffetti *et al.*, 1989; Suzuki *et al.*, 1989). Almost half the capillaries in skeletal muscle have been shown to contain trapped leucocytes (Bagge *et al.*, 1980), and this persists despite reperfusion (Korthuis *et al.*, 1988). Oxygen free radicals produced by these cells have been shown to damage the endothelium of the skeletal muscle microvascular bed (Korthuis *et al.*, 1970). The role of leucocytes is supported by the demonstration that depletion of polymorphonuclear cells reduces the pathological microvascular changes associated with reperfusion injury (Klausner *et al.*, 1988a; Korthuis *et al.*, 1988), and attenuates the increase in lymphatic flow and protein content associated with reperfusion (Belkin *et al.*, 1989). Polymorphonuclear cells have to establish a secure site of adherence to the endothelium prior to producing free radical-mediated injury, and prevention of adherence, by the administration of monoclonal antibodies to the CD11/CD18 adherence receptor, has been shown to attenuate microvascular injury (Carden *et al.*, 1990).

LOCAL INJURY – AN INTEGRATED HYPOTHESIS (Figure 22.1)

The mechanisms described above provide a means by which the combined effects of local pressure and ischaemia may lead to muscle injury. The increase in microvascular permeability leads to the sequestration of oedema fluid within the tissues of the injured limb (Korthuis *et al.*, 1985, 1989). As explained above, this fluid equilibrates with the cytosol of the injured muscle cells, to an extent determined by the disturbance of cell membrane function. Water penetrates the injured muscle, under a head of pressure which may exceed mean arterial pressure, even in a normotensive subject. This intra- and extracellular sequestration of fluid is

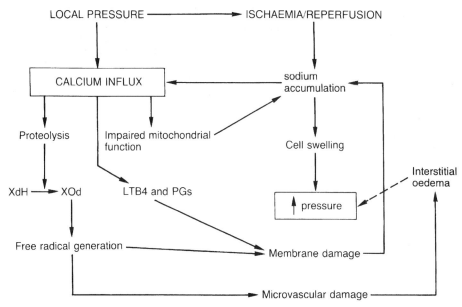

Figure 22.1 An integrated hypothesis for the pathogenesis of local crush injury.

made more significant by the anatomical arrangement of muscle groups within the limbs. Muscle groups tend to be confined within compartments bounded by bone and dense, unyielding fascial sheaths. The total volume of a muscular compartment is therefore limited, and the oedema fluid can only be accommodated at the expense of an increase in the hydrostatic pressure within the compartment. The clinical and structural consequences of this process, whatever the underlying cause, have been referred to as the 'compartmental syndrome' (Matsen, 1975; Mubarak et al., 1975; Whitesides et al., 1975; Matsen et al., 1980), and compartment syndromes have been described in a number of anatomical locations (Matsen et al., 1980; Bonutti and Bell, 1986; Tarlow et al., 1986; Schmalzreid et al., 1992). The mechanisms responsible for the maintenance of the intracompartmental hypertension are unclear. It might be expected that the development of increased hydrostatic pressure within the muscle compartment would rapidly oppose the movement of fluid into the compartment, since the increased tissue pressure would balance the Starling forces encouraging the movement out of capillaries, even in the presence of altered capillary permeability. Better (1990) has suggested that intracompartmental hypertension develops not only as a result of the accumulation of oedema fluid within the limb, but also as a result of the failure of the injured cells to maintain the extrusion of sodium and water, compounded by an increase in cytosolic osmotic or oncotic pressure, because of an increase in the number of 'idiogenic molecules', owing to the breakdown of larger molecules such as glycogen and protein within the

cytosol of the muscle cell. The increase in intracompartmental pressure may exceed arterial perfusion pressure, and the perfusion of the limb may therefore be secondarily compromised. This combination of pressure and ischaemia appears to be particularly injurious to both nerve and muscle (Sheridan et al., 1977). The metabolic and histological disturbances of skeletal muscle in the compartment syndrome significantly exceed those observed with ischaemia alone – hydrostatic pressure and ischaemia thus appear to act synergistically (Heppenstall et al., 1986). The time required to produce a complete failure of peripheral nerve conduction is inversely proportional to compartment pressure, and total conduction block occurs within 2 hours at pressures between 80 and 120 mmHg (Hargens et al., 1979).

The end result of the pathological processes described above, even after extricating the victim, and administering adequate resuscitation, is a limb in which vast amounts of fluid are sequestered, with a marked increase in intracompartmental pressure, progressive muscle injury and impairment of myoneural function.

Clinical aspects of the local injury

The clinical features of the local injury relate primarily to manifestations of the increased hydrostatic pressure within the affected muscle compartments. While cutaneous and bony injury may be readily apparent during routine clinical and radiological examination, the earliest evidence of a developing compartment syndrome is pain which may be of disproportionate severity for the external evidence of injury, and is characteristically exacerbated by passive stretching of the muscles involved (Matsen *et al.*, 1980). The pain may be accompanied by visible and palpable swelling of the affected muscle.

The presence of neural involvement is heralded by the development of paraesthesiae, progressing to complete anaesthesia, and weakness with depression of neuromuscular reflexes, progressing to complete paralysis of the injured limb. Vascular involvement is suggested by impairment of capillary return (increased time for cutaneous blanching to disappear after cutaneous pressure), and reduction of arterial pulse pressure or even complete disappearance of the arterial pulse distal to the injury. It is essential that a full neurological and vascular assessment be conducted early in the course of management, to distinguish neurological and vascular impairment secondary to a compartment syndrome from primary neurological and vascular injury, as the therapeutic consequences may be quite different.

The diagnosis of compartment syndrome may be confirmed by direct measurement of intramuscular pressure (Whitesides *et al.*, 1975; Matsen *et al.*, 1976, 1980). A critical pressure of 40 mmHg, or 30 mmHg less than systemic diastolic pressure has been defined (Owen *et al.*, 1979), with a critical time period for this pressure of 6–8 hours (Hargens *et al.*, 1979).

The management of the local injury has been the subject of some controversy. While some authors have advocated prompt operative decompression of all affected muscle groups (Jepson, 1926; Mubarak and Owens, 1977; Whitesides *et al.*, 1977; Matsen *et al.*, 1980), this view has not been supported by others (Better, 1990; Better and Stein, 1990). The principal argument in favour of early operative decompression is that this treatment may help in the preservation of limb function, particularly with respect to the avoidance of ischaemic muscle contracture, which has been recognized for more than a century (Volkmann, 1881). While fasciotomy allows oedematous muscle to bulge into the wound, and may be associated with an improvement in arterial pulse pressure (both of which might suggest a beneficial effect of therapy), fasciotomy is not without problems. Muscle necrosis may be extensive, even if fasciotomy is performed shortly after the signs of compartment syndrome have developed. Arguments against fasciotomy are as follows:

1. Provided the initial injury is 'closed', the contents of the muscle compartment remain sterile, even in the presence of substantial muscle necrosis. Fasciotomy therefore converts a clean closed injury to a potentially or actually contaminated 'open' one. Even if bruised, skin constitutes a highly effective barrier to the ingress of microorganisms (Reis and Michaelson, 1986). Fasciotomy exposes a considerable area of potentially necrotic muscle to infection, and, in particular, the possibility of infection with saprophytic organisms such as *Clostridium welchii*, leading to gas gangrene with potentially fatal consequences. While thorough debridement of necrotic muscle at the time of fasciotomy might be expected to reduce the risk of this complication, it may be extremely difficult for the surgeon to ascertain the exact extent of muscle necrosis. Bleeding from the cut edge of muscle is *not* a sign of viability, since the blood vessels to necrotic muscle may remain patent. Indeed, severe primary or secondary haemorrhage may develop as a complication of fasciotomy. Electrical or mechanical stimulation of muscle has been advocated to be a more useful guide to the extent of muscle necrosis (Reis and Michaelson, 1986). Since muscle necrosis might be expected to progress, even after an apparently successful fasciotomy, because of reperfusion injury (see above), it is important to recognize that a decision to perform fasciotomy may necessitate repeated trips to the operating theatre, with increasingly aggressive debridement, and a continuing risk of sepsis, which may ultimately necessitate amputation.

2. The evidence that fasciotomy is necessarily associated with a more favourable functional outcome is relatively poor. While Sheridan and Matsen (1976) reported that the timing of fasciotomy was critical to outcome, with a good functional result in only 8% of cases in which fasciotomy was delayed for greater than 12 hours, compared with 68% in those subjected to fasciotomy within 12 hours, these differences might equally have been attributable to the severity of primary injury in the delayed group. Conversely, Better (1990) has indicated that failure to perform fasciotomy is by no means associated with a poor functional outcome. While there is thus some evidence to suggest that the effect of fasciotomy may not be entirely predictable, the authors believe that the weight of evidence currently indicates an aggressive surgical approach to the crushed limb and prompt operative decompressions of affected muscle at the earliest opportunity is advocated.

Despite the experimental evidence to suggest a role for oxygen-derived free radicals and calcium ions in the pathogenesis, and the availability of free radical scavengers and antagonists of the sodium-calcium exchange pump, such as amiloride and benzamil (Odeh, 1991), there is no direct clinical evidence that such agents are useful in the management of the local injury.

SYSTEMIC MANIFESTATIONS OF THE CRUSH SYNDROME

Before the Second World War, patients with crush injuries frequently died as a result of uncontrollable sepsis or haemorrhage due to the local injury. With improvement in resuscitation and surgical techniques, the systemic manifestations of crush injury have assumed major importance. While the crushed patient lies trapped, the risk of systemic complications appears to be negligible. After the patient is extricated, however, a series of pathological disturbances occur as a result of a bidirectional flux of solute and water into and out of the injured muscles (Table 22.1). As indicated earlier, the massive fluid sequestration within the injured limbs may lead to marked hypovolaemia. Efflux of intracellular constituents from damaged muscles leads to a series of metabolic disturbances, including hyperkalaemia, acidosis, hyperuricaemia, hyperphosphataemia and an elevation of the plasma concentration of creatinine and creatine kinase. Myoglobin is released into the systemic circulation and filtered at the glomerulus, resulting in myoglobinuria. Hypocalcaemia has been recognized for many years and has been shown to result from a massive influx of calcium from the extracellular compartment into damaged muscle (Meroney et al., 1957). This hypocalcaemia cannot be corrected by intravenous calcium administration (Meroney et al., 1957). The magnitude of these metabolic alterations is hardly surprising, since muscle represents, by weight, the largest single organ system of the body, accounting for 40% of total body weight, and 75% of whole body potassium (De Franzo and Bia, 1985). While the metabolic disturbances described above may be associated with a host of systemic complications, the life-threatening complication encountered with the greatest frequency is acute renal failure (Ward, 1988), which is still associated with a high mortality. The mechanisms underlying the development of acute renal failure in the crush syndrome will therefore be discussed separately.

MECHANISMS OF RENAL FAILURE

Nephrotoxicity

A number of potentially 'toxic' factors have been implicated in the development of acute renal failure complicating crush injury, including hyperuricaemia (Honda, 1983; Better, 1989, 1990) and hyperphosphataemia (Better and Stein, 1990). The chief nephrotoxin, however, may be myoglobin (Beall and Stead, 1944; Braun et al., 1970; Blachar et al., 1981). Myoglobin is a haem pigment with a molecular weight of approximately 17 800 Daltons. It is readily filtered at the glomerulus and excreted in the urine at serum concentrations of less than 15 mg/dl (Finn, 1979). This appears to require

TABLE 22.1

BIDIRECTIONAL FLOW OF SOLUTES AND WATER ACROSS SKELETAL MUSCLE CELL MEMBRANES IN RHABDOMYOLYSIS (CRUSH SYNDROME). (ADAPTED FROM BETTER, 1990)

Efflux from damaged muscles	
Myoglobin	Nephrotoxicity, particularly on the background of oliguria, aciduria and uricosuria
Thromboplastin	Disseminated intravascular coagulation with thrombi in the glomeruli
Potassium	Hyperkalaemia and cardiotoxicity aggravated by hypocalcaemia and hypotension
Purines from the disintegration of cell nuclei	Increased urate load on the kidney and nephrotoxicity
Lactic and other organic acids	Metabolic acidosis and aciduria
Creatine phosphokinase (CPK)	Extreme elevation of serum CPK levels
Creatinine	Disproportionate rise in blood creatinine/blood urea nitrogen ratio
Phosphate	Hyperphosphataemia, aggravation of hypocalcaemia and metastatic calcification

Influx from extracellular compartment into muscle cells	
NaCl and water	Hypovolaemia, haemodynamic shock, prerenal and later acute renal failure
Calcium	Hypocalcaemia, aggravation of hyperkalaemic cardiotoxicity, activation of cytosolic proteases

damage to at least 200 g of muscle (Rowland and Penn, 1972). While the finding of red or brown pigmentation of the urine in cases of acute renal failure strongly suggests myoglobinuria, myoglobin must be distinguished from other haem pigments such as haemoglobin, which are also filtered and excreted in the urine. Myoglobinuria is likely if the plasma is not pigmented (pigmentation suggesting the presence of free haemoglobin and therefore haemoglobinuria). In addition, haemoglobin, unlike myoglobin, is bound to plasma haptoglobins and a normal plasma haptoglobin concentration in the presence of urinary haem pigment is suggestive of myoglobinuria (Finn, 1979). Simple bedside tests, such as a positive benzidine reaction in the presence of ammonium sulphate precipitation (Braun *et al.*, 1970), may also help to distinguish myoglobinuria from haemoglobinuria, although false-negative results have been reported (Barbanel, 1979). The optimum test for the identification of myoglobin in urine appears to be immunoassay (Kagen, 1970; Hibrawi and Blaker, 1975). The attention devoted to the detection of myoglobin in the urine of patients with crush injuries and acute renal failure implies a clear causal link between myoglobin and renal failure. Unfortunately, the evidence supporting such a link is by no means clear. Myoglobinaemia and myoglobinuria may certainly occur without renal failure (Kagen, 1971; Grunfeld *et al.*, 1972; Olerud *et al.*, 1976) and there is no clear relationship between the degree of myoglobinuria and the prevalence of anuria (Barbanel, 1979). Even the nephrotoxicity of myoglobin is questionable – myoglobin itself appears to be relatively inert, but may become nephrotoxic in the presence of dehydration and acidosis (Lalich, 1952; Perri and Gorini, 1952). Intravenous administration of myoglobin to animals has been shown to induce acute renal failure only in the presence of a metabolic acidosis and a urinary pH less than 6.0 (Perri and Gorini, 1952). This finding has implications for the potential mechanisms of myoglobin-induced renal damage. Myoglobin is converted to haematin (ferrihaemate) at a urinary pH of less than 5.6, and haematin is known to be toxic to the kidney, vascular and reticuloendothelial systems (Anderson *et al.*, 1942; Braun *et al.*, 1970). The iron moiety of myoglobin may stimulate the production of hydroxyl radicals, leading to lipid peroxidation and damage to the membranes of cells in the proximal convoluted tubule (Paller, 1988).

Hypotension

As indicated earlier, the flux of electrolytes from the systemic circulation into injured muscle may be considerable, and the associated movement of water from the extracellular to the intracellular compartment may lead to hypovolaemic shock and haemoconcentration. This may result in prerenal failure and oliguria, and, if volume replacement therapy is inadequate or delayed, acute tubular necrosis and established renal failure. While prompt resuscitation may reduce the risk of acute renal failure, renal impairment may still develop, despite the restoration of extracellular fluid volume, indicating that factors other than systemic haemodynamics may play a role in the pathogenesis of acute renal failure.

Reduction in glomerular filtration rate due to intrarenal haemodynamic changes, or changes in glomerular permeability

While reduced renal cortical blood flow and increased renal vascular resistance have been suggested as potential mechanisms for the reduction in glomerular filtration rate (Oken *et al.*, 1966; Ayer *et al.*, 1971; Chedru *et al.*, 1972; Flamenbaum *et al.*, 1972), it has been suggested that the significance of intrarenal haemodynamic alterations may depend upon the experimental model of acute renal failure adopted (Stein *et al.*, 1978). Although the relevance of the glycerol-induced myoglobinuric acute renal failure model to human crush injury is debatable, renal failure in this model is accompanied by a significant increase in renal vascular resistance and a fall in renal blood flow (Better, 1989), the latter associated with intrarenal shunting, and a redistribution of blood flow from the outer to the juxtamedullary cortex (Ayer *et al.*, 1971). This finding has been supported by the results of angiographic studies performed in a rabbit model of crush injury (Trueta *et al.*, 1948). The reduction in renal blood flow appears to be accompanied by both afferent and efferent glomerular vasoconstriction (Venkatachalam *et al.*, 1976), but may only play an early role in the reduction in glomerular filtration rate. Extracellular volume expansion attenuates the early reduction in glomerular filtration rate following glycerol administration, but this effect is not observed 18 hours later, when the reduction in glomerular filtration rate persists, despite volume expansion sufficient to restore renal blood flow (Reineck *et al.*, 1980). A variety of mechanisms have been postulated to account for the apparent renal vasoconstriction in myoglobinuric renal failure, including increased activity of the renin–angiotensin system and the sympathetic nervous system, abnormalities of renal prostaglandin metabolism, vasopressor substances such as antidiuretic hormone (ADH) and glomerular microthrombosis associated with disseminated intravascular coagulation (DIC).

Increased activity of the renin–angiotensin system

The role of the renin–angiotensin system in the pathogenesis of acute renal failure has been recognized, even if incompletely understood, for many years. Increased granularity of the cells of the juxtaglomerular apparatus was first reported in 1945, in patients with anuria associated with crush injury (Goormaghtigh, 1945). Goormaghtigh postulated that these granules might represent the accumulation of a vasopressor substance. Subsequently, elevated plasma renin concentrations have been demonstrated in animal models of acute renal failure (DiBona and Sawin, 1971; Grandchamp *et al.*, 1971; Brown *et al.*, 1972) and in patients with acute renal failure due to a number of causes (Tu, 1965; Clarkson *et al.*, 1970). Chronic sodium loading, which leads to intrarenal renin depletion, appears to protect animals from experimental acute renal failure (McDonald *et al.*, 1969; Flamenbaum, 1973). Renal renin levels may be of greater relevance than plasma renin levels, because an acute reduction in plasma renin activity without a corresponding fall in renal renin levels has not been shown to protect animals from acute renal failure (Flamenbaum *et al.*, 1973). Chronic potassium loading (which has a greater suppressive effect upon plasma renin activity than upon renal renin activity) appears to be less effective than chronic sodium loading in the prevention of glycerol-induced acute renal failure (Powell-Jackson *et al.*, 1972).

In patients with crush injuries, renin production may be stimulated by increased renal sympathetic nervous activity (see below). In addition, damage to the epithelium of the proximal convoluted tubule may lead to an increase in the sodium content of the filtrate entering the distal nephron. Tubuloglomerular feedback mechanisms, induced by this increased sodium load, have been proposed to increase renin production, causing afferent glomerular vasoconstriction and a fall in glomerular filtration rate (Thurau and Boylan, 1976).

Although the renin–angiotensin system may thus play a role in the persistent reduction in glomerular filtration rate in the face of the restoration of extracellular fluid volume, the evidence that the renin–angiotensin system is of pathological importance to the maintenance of renal functional impairment is not unequivocal. In some models of acute renal failure, the elevation of plasma renin levels is short-lived, and renin levels may return to normal without a measurable improvement in renal blood flow (Montoreano and Ruiz-Guinazu, 1972). As suggested above, however, renal renin levels may be of greater importance than plasma renin levels, and the two may correlate poorly (Mason, 1976). While this may indeed be the case, one would expect that pharmacological blockade of the actions of renin or angiotensin might prevent, or at least attenuate, acute renal failure, but active or passive immunization to renin or angiotensin has been ineffective (Flamenbaum *et al.*, 1972a; Oken *et al.*, 1975; Powell-Jackson *et al.*, 1978).

Activation of the sympathetic nervous system

Increased activity of the sympathetic nervous system characteristically accompanies injury (Wilmore *et al.*, 1974). The kidneys receive a dense sympathetic innervation, and stimulation of the renal sympathetic nerves has been shown to induce renal vasoconstriction and a reduction in glomerular filtration rate (Pomeranz *et al.*, 1968). If persistent activation of the sympathetic nervous supply to the kidneys explained the reduction in glomerular filtration rate, one might expect that pharmacological adrenergic blockade might modify the course of acute renal failure. Although α-blockade has been claimed to reduce renal impairment and histological changes, renal failure is not prevented (McLean and Thomson, 1970). Similar results have been reported for β-blockade (Eliahou *et al.*, 1973; Stein *et al.*, 1973; Takemura and Matsubara, 1975; Kokot and Kuska, 1976).

Abnormalities of renal prostaglandin metabolism

Abnormalities of renal prostaglandin metabolism have been implicated, at least in a permissive role, in the glomerular vasoconstriction associated with acute renal failure. Renal prostaglandin synthesis is known to be enhanced in conditions in which renal blood flow is reduced, including a reduction in renal perfusion pressure (Herbacynska-Cedro and Vane, 1973), renal sympathetic nerve stimulation and following the administration of vasoconstrictor substances (McGiff *et al.*, 1970; Needleman *et al.*, 1973). Prostaglandins may play a protective role – the renal vascular response to angiotensin and noradrenaline is augmented following the inhibition of prostaglandin synthesis (McGiff *et al.*, 1970; Aiken and Vane, 1973). Fine (1970) has postulated a central role for prostaglandins in the development of acute renal failure, with ischaemic damage to the tubules of the outer renal medulla resulting in a fall in renal prostaglandin synthesis, cortical ischaemia and a fall in glomerular filtration rate. Other studies have supported the suggestion that a fall in renal prostaglandin synthesis contributes to the development of acute renal failure (Oken, 1975; Torres *et al.*, 1975; Solez *et al.*, 1977). Indomethacin not only increases the incidence and severity of acute renal failure (Torres *et al.*, 1975; Solez *et al.*, 1977), but also abolishes the protective effect of plasma volume expansion in glycerol-treated rats (Papanicolau *et al.*, 1975).

Antidiuretic hormone

Antidiuretic hormone (ADH) may also play a role in the pathogenesis of acute renal failure. Although rats with diabetes insipidus still develop acute myoglobinuric renal failure after subcutaneous injection of glycerol, the severity of renal injury appears to be attenuated (Wilson *et al.*, 1969). Plasma ADH concentrations increase markedly after glycerol injection (Hofbauer *et al.*, 1977), and administration of exogenous ADH increases the severity of acute renal failure in animal models (Iaina *et al.*, 1980).

Disseminated intravascular coagulation

While the mechanisms discussed above relate to disturbances in the normal mechanisms for the control of renal blood flow, filtration fraction and solute handling, an alternative possibility for the development of acute renal failure pertains to the observation of disseminated intravascular coagulation (DIC) in the crush syndrome. Thromboplastins released from damaged muscle may activate the clotting cascade (Honda, 1983), provoking DIC (Clarkson *et al.*, 1970; Wardle, 1975; Schor *et al.*, 1981), and glomerular microthrombi have been demonstrated in rabbits infused with muscle extract (Blachar *et al.*, 1981). Although there is little direct evidence to support the suggestion that the perfusion of glomeruli with blood containing microthrombi is responsible for the development of acute renal failure in the patient with crush injury, it seems reasonable to expect that the effect of numerous microthrombi upon renal haemodynamics might be sufficiently marked to explain a reduction in glomerular filtration rate.

Changes in glomerular membrane permeability

The glomerular filtration rate is determined not only by the filtration pressure within the glomerular capillaries but also by the permeability of the glomerular membrane. While there is little evidence to support the hypothesis that a reduction in glomerular capillary permeability is responsible for the reduction in glomerular filtration rate observed in acute myoglobinuric renal failure, it is interesting to note that angiotensin II and ADH (which have both been implicated in the pathogenesis of acute renal failure) have been shown to reduce glomerular permeability, possibly by inducing the contraction of glomerular mesangial cells (Schor *et al.*, 1981). Swelling of mesangial cells has been observed for up to 16 hours after glycerol injection (Suzuki and Mostofi, 1970), although the relevance of these morphological changes to glomerular permeability are uncertain.

Tubular obstruction

Obstruction to the flow of filtrate represents a possible explanation for the persistence of oliguria, despite the restoration of renal perfusion. Cellular debris and pigmented casts are characteristically found in the renal tubules of patients with acute renal failure complicating crush injury (Bywaters and Beall, 1941; Finckh, 1957), the implication being that these abnormal constituents of urine might obstruct the flow of filtrate within the renal tubules. Proximal tubular pressures have not, however, been shown to rise consistently in experimental models of acute renal failure (Flanigan and Oken, 1965; Oken *et al.*, 1966). In the study reported by Oken *et al.* (1966), tubular flow ceased but tubules were collapsed and not dilated, contrary to what one might have expected if tubular obstruction was responsible for the cessation of flow. Micropuncture studies of rats with acute renal failure have shown that both single nephron glomerular filtration rate *and* intratubular pressure falls (Flanigan and Oken, 1965). In this study, tubular sodium absorption was preserved, indicating that the primary mechanism responsible for the reduction in tubular flow was the reduction in glomerular filtration rate.

The assumption that tubular obstruction is, of necessity, accompanied by an increase in tubular hydrostatic pressure is, however, simplistic. An increase in the resistance to tubular flow might be masked if filtration pressure also fell, or disruption of the tubular epithelium allowed 'passive backflow' of filtrate into the interstitium (see below). The former possibility has been strongly supported (Finn *et al.*, 1975). Even taking these possibilities into account, the evidence that tubular obstruction contributes to the development of acute renal failure remains equivocal. Arendshorst *et al.* (1975) have shown that in the early stages of acute ischaemic renal failure, filtration pressure remains normal, while proximal tubular pressure rises. Dye injected into the proximal convoluted tubule is retained, suggesting tubular obstruction. At a later stage in the development of acute renal failure, however, both filtration pressure and tubular pressure fall, and dye injected into the tubules appears to leak into the interstitium. Extracellular volume expansion at this stage leads to a rise in both glomerular capillary pressure and proximal tubular pressure. In contrast to these results, which appear to support the possibility of tubular obstruction in the early stages of acute renal failure, tubular pressures have been shown to be low in the early stages of acute myoglobinuric renal failure (Oken *et al.*, 1966), and other studies have reported normal tubular pressures, despite a fall in glomerular filtration rate (Stein *et al.*, 1978).

While haematin and urate both precipitate in acidic urine (Knochel, 1981b), the role of casts in tubular obstruction is also unclear. Tanner and Steinhausen have investigated the role of casts in the genesis of tubular obstruction (Tanner and Steinhausen, 1976). Early in the development of acute renal failure, tubular casts can easily be flushed out at low tubular pressures, suggesting that casts do not contribute to tubular obstruction. Subsequently, however, relatively high pressures are required to flush out casts from the tubules. The authors concluded that casts may contribute to the development of acute renal failure, but that tubular obstruction as a result of the deposition of casts was unlikely to be the primary factor responsible for the development of acute renal failure.

Passive backflow

Oliver *et al.* (1951) suggested that breaks in the renal tubular epithelium might allow leakage of tubular fluid into the renal interstitium, allowing filtrate to equilibrate with blood, and an associated rise in renal interstitial pressure might also contribute to the obstruction of renal tubules. While some studies have demonstrated tubular leakage occurs (Arendshorst *et al.*, 1975), others have not (Oken *et al.*, 1966), and the recovery of the majority of tracer substances injected into the proximal tubule, in the distal nephron (Olbricht *et al.*, 1977) suggests that leakage of filtrate is unlikely to be of sufficient magnitude to play a significant role in the pathogenesis of acute renal failure.

MANAGEMENT OF THE SYSTEMIC COMPLICATIONS OF CRUSH INJURY

The most important aspect of the management of the systemic complications of crush injury is prophylaxis. The value of the prophylactic approach in the prevention of acute renal failure has been summarized by Better (1990). Awareness of the risk of hypovolaemia, and the role of hypovolaemia in the development of renal failure, necessitates vigorous resuscitation of the patient, if possible even before extricating the victim from the scene of the accident. Normal saline or Ringer's lactate should be infused (for a 75-kg adult) at 1.5 l/h. It may take over an hour for the complete extrication of the patient and subsequent transfer to an intensive care unit. While the orthopaedic surgeon may be involved in the management of the local injury, the aim of systemic treatment is to prevent the development of the systemic complications which are associated with a poor outcome, and, in particular, acute renal failure (Ward, 1988). Vigorous resuscitation should be continued, with colloid or crystalloid, and central venous pressure and urine output monitored carefully. Despite the conflicting evidence for the nephrotoxicity of myoglobin (see above), the evidence demonstrating that acute renal impairment is particularly likely in the presence of a concentrated acidic urine is sufficiently strong to make the establishment of a forced alkaline diuresis desirable (Eneas *et al.*, 1979; Ron *et al.*, 1984). The suggested regimen is an intravenous infusion of hypotonic saline and sodium bicarbonate (NaCl 70 mmol/l in 5% dextrose, $NaHCO_3$ 50 mmol/l), together with 120 g of mannitol per day. This fluid regimen is appropriate to a 75-kg adult, and is administered at a rate of approximately 12 l/day, to produce a target urine output of 8 l/day, with a

urinary pH above 6.5. The urine should be tested 6 hourly for evidence of myoglobinuria (see above), which generally subsides within 3 days of admission. Serum electrolytes, and, in particular, serum potassium concentration should be monitored closely, because of the risk of hyperkalaemic cardiotoxicity. The suggested fluid regimen should, however, correct hyperkalaemia and acidosis adequately. The use of mannitol is supported by its well-recognized protective effect with respect to the development of acute renal failure (Better, 1989, 1990). This may relate to its diuretic action, in that potentially nephrotoxic substances are diluted and flushed out of the renal tubules. In addition, mannitol may protect the cells of the renal tubule by inhibiting sodium reabsorption, thus reducing the oxygen requirements of the tubular epithelium, and therefore increasing their capacity to withstand the metabolic insult associated with nephrotoxic damage (Knochel, 1981b). Finally, as indicated above, mannitol is an effective scavenger of oxygen-derived free radicals (Freeman and Crapo, 1982). Loop diuretics are not indicated in the management of the patient with crush syndrome, and may compound the nephrotoxicity of the injury, acidify the urine and aggravate hypovolaemia. While amiloride and its analogues appear attractive, because their effects upon the sodium-calcium exchange pump might be expected to reduce the extent of muscle injury (see above), concern has been expressed at the potentially serious hypovolaemia (Odeh, 1991), and hyperkalaemia (Screaton *et al.*, 1991) that might result from their use.

Significant metabolic alkalosis (arterial blood pH over 7.45) occasionally presents problems because alkalosis tends to increase the amount of calcium bound to albumin. This may result, on a background of hypocalcaemia related to muscle injury, in hypocalcaemic tetany. Alkalosis should be treated with acetazolamide, an inhibitor of carbonic anhydrase, because urinary alkalinization is further enhanced.

Calcium infusion is not indicated, except when the hypocalcaemia presents a serious risk of hyperkalaemic cardiac arrhythmias, or tetany (Knochel, 1981a). Calcium infusion will only partly correct the hypocalcaemia of crush injury, because of the magnitude of the calcium flux into injured muscle, and the effects are temporary, hypocalcaemia recurring shortly after calcium infusion has ceased. In addition, the majority of infused calcium appears to be deposited in injured muscles, aggravating metastatic calcification (Meroney *et al.*, 1957).

SUMMARY

The aetiology of crush injury is undoubtedly complex. This century has seen the recognition of the systemic complications of crush injury, the development of effective renal replacement therapy in the management of the acute renal failure complicating crush injury, and the emergence of a prophylactic approach to the management of the systemic complications. Controversy still exists regarding the optimum management for the crushed limb. In the future, our emerging understanding of the cellular and biochemical mechanisms responsible for muscle and renal injury may allow the development of effective medical therapy for both the local and the systemic complications of this unique clinical condition.

REFERENCES

Aiken J.W., Vane J.R., (1973). Intra-renal prostaglandin release attenuates the renal vasoconstrictor activity of angiotensin I. *J. Pharmacol. Exp. Ther.*, **184**, 678–87.

Anderson W.A.D., Morrison D.B., Williams E.F. Jr (1942). Pathological changes following injections of ferrihemate (hematin) in dogs. *Arch. Pathol.*, **33**, 589–602.

Arendshorst W.J., Finn W.F., Gottschalk C.W. (1975). Pathogenesis of acute renal failure following temporary renal ischemia in the rat. *Circ. Res.*, **37**, 558–68.

Artz C.P. (1967). Electrical injury simulates crush injury. *Surg. Gynecol. Obstet.*, **125**, 1316–17.

Awbrey B.J., Sienkiewicz P.S., Mankin H.J. (1988). Chronic exercise-induced compartment pressure elevation measured with a minituarised fluid pressure monitor: a laboratory and clinical study. *Am. J. Sports Med.*, **16**, 610–15.

Ayer G., Grandchamp A., Wyler T., Truniger B. (1971). Intrarenal hemodynamics in glycerol-induced myohemoglobinuric acute renal failure in the rat. *Circ. Res.*, **29**, 128–35.

Bagge U., Amundson B., Lauritzen C. (1980). White blood cell deformability and plugging of skeletal muscle capillaries in hemorrhagic shock. *Acta Physiol. Scand.*, **108**, 159–63.

Bank W.J., Dimauro S., Bonilla E. et al. (1975). A disorder of muscle lipid metabolism and myoglobinuria: absence of carntinine palmityl transferase. *N. Engl. J. Med.*, **292**, 443–9.

Barbanel C. (1979). Hemoglobinuria and myoglobinuria. In *Nephrology* (Hamburger J., Crosnier J., Grunfeld J.P., eds). New York: Wiley, p. 185.

Bass R.R., Allison E.J., Reines H.D. et al. (1983). Thigh compartment syndrome without lower extremity trauma following application of pneumatic antishock trousers. *Ann. Emerg. Med.*, **12**, 382–4.

Beall D., Stead J.K. (1944). The production of renal failure following injection of solutions containing myohaemoglobin. *Q. J. Exp. Physiol.*, **33**, 53–79.

Belkin M., Lamorte W.L., Wright J.G., Hobson R.W. II (1989). The role of leukocytes in the pathophysiology of skeletal muscle ischemic injury. *J. Vasc. Surg.*, **10**, 14–19.

Bentley G., Jeffreys T.E. (1968). The crush syndrome in coal miners. *J. Bone Joint Surg.*, **50B**, 588–94.

Berlin R. (1948). Haff disease in Sweden. *Acta Med. Scand.*, **129**, 560–72.

Better O.S. (1989). Traumatic rhabdomyolysis ('crush syndrome') – updated 1989. *Isr. J. Med. Sci.*, **25**, 69–72.

Better O.S. (1990). The crush syndrome revisited (1940–1990). *Nephron*, **55**, 97–103.

Better O.S., Stein J.H. (1990). Early management of shock and prophylaxis of acute renal failure in traumatic rhabdomyolysis. *N. Engl. J. Med.*, **322**, 825–9.

Better O.S., Abassi Z., Rubinstein I. et al. (1990). The mechanism of muscle injury in the crush syndrome: ischemic versus pressure-stretch myopathy. *Minerva Electrolyte Metab*, **16**, 181–4.

Blachar Y., Fong J.S.C., De Chadarévian J-P., Drummond K.N. (1981). Muscle extract infusion in rabbits. A new experimental model of the crush syndrome. *Circ. Res.*, **49**, 114–24.

Bonutti P.M., Bell G.R. (1986). Compartment syndrome of the foot. *J. Bone Joint Surg.*, **68A**, 1449–51.

Braughler J.M. (1988). Calcium and lipid peroxidation. In *Oxygen Radicals and Tissue Injury* (Halliwell B., ed.). Bethesda, MD: Federation of the American Society of Experimental Biology, p. 99.

Braun S.R., Weiss F.R., Keller A.I. et al. (1970). Evaluation of the renal toxicity of heme proteins and their derivatives. A role in the genesis of acute tubular necrosis. *J. Exp. Med.*, **131**, 443–60.

Braunwald E., Kloner R.A. (1985). Myocardial reperfusion: a double-edged sword? *J. Clin. Invest.*, **76**, 1713–19.

Brown A.A., Nichols R.R. (1977). Crush syndrome; a report of 2 cases and a review of the literature. *Br. J. Surg.*, **64**, 397–402.

Brown W.C.B., Brown J.J., Gavras H. et al. (1972). Renin and acute circulatory renal failure in the rabbit. *Circ. Res.*, **30**, 114–22.

Bunn H.F., Jandl J.H. (1966). Exchange of heme among hemoglobin molecules. *Proc. Natl. Acad. Sci. USA*, **56**, 974–8.

Bywaters E.G.L., Beall D. (1941). Crush injuries with impairment of renal function. *Br. Med. J.*, **1**, 427–32.

Bywaters E.G.L., Dible J.H. (1942). The renal lesion in traumatic anuria. *J. Pathol. Bacteriol.*, **54**, 111–20.

Bywaters E.G.L., Popjak G. (1942). Experimental crushing injury. *Surg. Gynecol. Obstet.*, **75**, 612–27.

Cambria R.P., Abbott W.M. (1984). Acute arterial thrombosis of the lower extremity: its natural history contrasted with arterial embolism. *Arch. Surg.*, **119**, 784–7.

Campion D.S., Arias J.M., Carter N.W. (1972). Rhabdomyolysis and myoglobinuria associated with hypokalaemia of renal tubular acidosis. *JAMA*, **220**, 967–9.

Carden D.L., Smith J.K., Korthuis R.J. (1990). Neutrophil-mediated microvascular dysfunction in post-ischemic canine skeletal muscle: role of granulocyte adherence. *Circ. Res.*, **66**, 1436–44.

Chedru M.F., Baethke R., Oken D.E. (1972). Renal cortical blood flow and glomerular filtration in myohemoglobinuric acute renal failure. *Kidney Int.*, **1**, 232–9.

Ciuffetti G., Balendra R., Lennie S.E. et al. (1989). Impaired filterability of white cells in acute cerebral infarction. *Br. Med. J.*, **298**, 930–1.

Clarkson A.R., MacDonald M.K., Fuster V. et al. (1970). Glomerular coagulation in acute ischaemic renal failure. *Q.J. Med.*, **39**, 585–99.

Colmers (1909). Ueber die durch das Erdbehen in Messian am 28 Dec. 1908 verursachten Verletzungen. *Arch. Klin. Chir.*, **90**, 701–5.

Curry S.C., Chang D., Connor D. (1989). Drug and toxin-induced rhabdomyolysis. *Ann. Emerg. Med.*, **18**, 1068–84.

Daly M.J., Elz J.S., Nayler W.G. (1984). Sarcolemmal enzymes and Na$^+$:Ca^{2+} exchange in hypoxic, ischemic and reperfused rat hearts. *Am. J. Physiol.*, **247**, H237–43.

DeFronzo R.A., Bia M.B. (1985). Extrarenal potassium homeostasis. In *The Kidney: physiology and pathophysiology* (Seldin D.W., Giebisch G., eds). New York: Raven, p.1179.

DiBona G.F., Sawin L.L. (1971). The renin–angiotensin system in acute renal failure in the rat. *Lab. Invest.*, **25**, 528–32.

Duncan C.J., Jackson M.J. (1987). Different mechanisms modulate structural changes and intracellular enzyme efflux following damage to skeletal muscle. *J. Cell Sci.*, **87**, 183–8.

Eliahou H.E., Brodman R.R., Friedman E.A. (1973). Adrenergic blockers in ischemic acute renal failure in the rat. In *Proceeding of the Conference on Acute Renal Failure* (Friedman E.A., Eliahou H.E., eds). Publ. No. (NIH) 74–608. Washington: DHEW.

Eneas J.F., Schoenfeld P.Y., Humphreys M.H. (1979). The effect of infusion of mannitol-sodium bicarbonate on the clinical course of myoglobinuria. *Arch. Intern. Med.*, **139**, 801–5.

Finckh E.S. (1957). Experimental acute tubular nephrosis following subcutaneous injection of glycerol. *J. Pathol. Bacteriol.*, **73**, 69–85.

Fine L.G. (1970). Acquired prostaglandin E2 (medullin) deficiency as the cause of oliguria in acute tubular necrosis. A hypothesis. *Isr. J. Med. Sci.*, **6**, 346–50.

Finn W.F. (1979). Acute renal failure. In *Strauss and Welt's Diseases of the Kidney*, 3rd. edn. (Earley L.E., Gottschalk C.W., eds). Boston: Little, Brown, pp. 167–210.

Finn W.F., Arendshorst W.J., Gottschalk C.W. (1975). Pathogenesis of oliguria in acute renal failure. *Circ. Res.*, **36**, 675–81.

Flamenbaum W. (1973). Pathophysiology of acute renal failure. *Arch. Intern. Med.*, **131**, 911–28.

Flamenbaum W., Kotchen T.A., Oken D.E. (1972a). Effect of renin immunisation on mercuric chloride and glycerol-induced renal failure. *Kidney Int.*, **1**, 406–12.

Flamenbaum W., McNeil J.S., Kotchen T.A., Saladino A.J. (1972b). Experimental acute renal failure induced by uranyl nitrate in the dog. *Circ. Res.*, **31**, 682–98.

Flamenbaum W., Kotchen T.A., Nagle R., McNeil J.S. (1973). Effect of potassium on the renin–angiotensin system and HgCl-induced acute renal failure. *Am. J. Physiol.*, **224**, 305.

Flanigan W.J., Oken D.E. (1965). Renal micropuncture study of the development of anuria in the rat with mercury-induced acute renal failure. *J. Clin. Invest.*, **44**, 449–57.

Frankenthal L. (1916). Ueber Verschuttungen. *Virchows Arch.* [A], **222**, 332–7.

Freeman B.A., Crapo J.D. (1982). Biology of disease. Free radicals and tissue injury. *Lab. Invest.*, **47**, 412–26.

Goormaghtigh N. (1945). Vascular and circulatory changes in the renal cortex in the anuric crush syndrome. *Proc. Soc. Exp. Biol. Med.*, **59**, 303–5.

Grandchamp A., Veyrat R., Rosset E. et al. (1971). Relationship between renin and intrarenal hemodynamics in hemorrhagic hypotension. *J. Clin. Invest.*, **50**, 970–8.

Grisham M.B., Hernandez L.A., Granger D.N. (1986). Xanthine oxidase and neutrophil infiltration in intestinal ischemia. *Am. J. Physiol.*, **251**, G567–74.

Grunfeld J.P., Ganeval D., Chanard J. et al. (1972). Acute renal failure in McArdle's disease. *N. Engl. J. Med.*, **286**, 1237–41.

Guharay F., Sachs F. (1984). Stretch activated single ion channels currents in tissue cultured embryonic chick skeletal muscle. *J. Physiol. (Lond.)*, **352**, 685–701.

Haimovici H. (1979). Metabolic complications of acute arterial occlusions. *J. Cardiovasc. Surg. (Torino)*, **20**, 349–57.

Hargens A.R., Romine J.S., Sipe J.C. et al. (1979). Peripheral nerve-conduction block by high muscle-compartment pressure. *J. Bone Joint Surg.*, **61A**, 192–200.

Heppenstall R.B., Scott R., Sapega A. et al. (1986). A comparative study of the tolerance of skeletal muscle to ischemia. *J. Bone Joint Surg.*, **68A**, 820–8.

Herbacynska-Cedro K., Vane J.R. (1973). Contribution of intrarenal generation of prostaglandins to autoregulation of renal blood flow in the dog. *Circ. Res.*, **33**, 428–36.

Hibrawi H., Blaker R.C. (1975). Improved estimation of urinary myoglobin by counterimmunoelectrophoresis, as compared with the double immunodiffusion technique. *Clin. Chem.*, **21**, 765–8.

Hofbauer K.G., Konrads A., Bauereiss K. et al. (1977). Vasopressin and renin in glycerol-induced acute renal failure. *Circ. Res.*, **41**, 424–35.

Honda N. (1983). Acute renal failure and rhabdomyolysis. *Kidney Int.*, **23**, 888–98.

Iaina A., Orndorff M., Gavendo S., Solomon S. (1980). ADH effects on development of ischemic acute renal failure. *Proc. Soc. Exp. Biol. Med.*, **163**, 206–11.

Jackson R.M., Veal C.F. (1989). Re-expansion, re-oxygenation and rethinking. *Am. J. Med. Sci.*, **298**, 44–50.

Jennische E. (1984). Post-ischemic calcification in skeletal muscle: a light microscopic study in the rat. *Acta Pathol. Microbiol. Immunol. Scand.*, **92**, 139–45.

Jepson P.N. (1926). Ischemic contracture. Experimental study. *Ann. Surg.*, **84**, 785–95.

Jolly S.R., Kane W.J., Bailie M.B. et al. (1984). Canine myocardial reperfusion injury: its reduction by the combined administration of superoxide dismutase and catalase. *Circ. Res.*, **54**, 277–85.

Kagen L.J. (1970). Immunofluorescent demonstration of myoglobin in the kidney: case report and review of forty three cases of myoglobinemia and myoglobinuria identified immunologically. *Am. J. Med.*, **48**, 649–53.

Kagen L.J. (1971). Myoglobinemia and myoglobinuria in patients with myositis. *Arthritis Rheum.*, **14**, 457–64.

Klausner J.M., Paterson I.S., Valeri C.R. et al. (1988a). Limb-ischemia-induced increase in permeability is mediated by leukocytes and leukotrienes. *Ann. Surg.*, **208**, 755–60.

Klausner J.M., Anner H., Paterson I.S. et al. (1988b). Lower torso ischemia-induced lung injury is leukocyte dependent. *Ann. Surg.*, **208**, 761–7.

Knochel J.P. (1981a). Serum calcium derangement in rhabdomyolysis (editorial). *N. Engl. J. Med.*, **305**, 161–2.

Knochel J.P. (1981b). Rhabdomyolysis and myoglobinuria. In *The Kidney in Systemic Disease* (Suki N.N., Eknoyan G., eds). New York: Wiley, p. 263.

Koffler A., Friedler R.M., Massry S.G. (1976). Acute renal failure due to non-traumatic rhabdomyolysis. *Ann. Intern. Med.*, **85**, 23–8.

Kokot F., Kuska J. (1976). Influence of extracorporeal

dialysis on parathyroid hormone secretion in patients with acute renal failure. *Nephron*, **16**, 302.

Korthuis R.J., Granger D.N., Townsley M.I., Taylor A.E. (1985). The role of oxygen-derived free radicals in the ischemia-induced increases in canine skeletal muscle vascular permeability. *Circ. Res.*, **57**, 599–609.

Korthuis R.J., Grisham M.B., Granger D.N. (1988). Leukocyte depletion attenuates vascular injury in post ischemic skeletal muscle. *Am. J. Physiol.*, **254**, H823–7.

Korthuis R.J., Smith J.K., Carden D.L. (1989). Hypoxic reperfusion attenuates post ischemic microvascular injury. *Am. J. Physiol.*, **256**, H315–19.

Labbe R., Lindsay T., Walker P.M. (1987). The extent and distribution of skeletal muscle necrosis after graded periods of complete ischemia. *J. Vasc. Surg.*, **6**, 152–7.

Lakatta E.G., Nayler W.G., Poole-Wilson P.A. (1979). Calcium overload and mechanical function in post hypoxic myocardium: biphasic effect of pH during hypoxia. *Eur. J. Cardiol.*, **10**, 77–87.

Lalich J.J. (1952). The influence of in vitro hemoglobin modification on hemoglobinuric nephrosis in rabbits. *J. Lab. Clin. Med.*, **40**, 102–10.

Linas S.L., Whittenberg D., Repine J.E. (1990). Role of xanthine oxidase in ischemia-reperfusion injury. *Am. J. Physiol.*, **258**, F711–16.

Mason J. (1976). Tubuloglomerular feedback in the early stages of experimental acute renal failure. *Kidney Int.*, **10**, S106–14.

Matsen F.A. (1975). Compartmental syndrome. A unified concept. *Clin. Orthoped.*, **113**, 8–14.

Matsen F.A., Mayo K.A., Sheridan G.W., Krugmire R.B. (1976). Monitoring of intramuscular pressure. *Surgery*, **79**, 702–9.

Matsen F.A., Winquist R.A., Krugmire R.B. (1980). Diagnosis and management of compartmental syndromes. *J. Bone Joint Surg.*, **62A**, 286–91.

McCord J.M. (1985). Oxygen-derived free radicals in post-ischemic tissue injury. *N. Engl. J. Med.*, **312**, 159–63.

McCord J.M. (1987). Oxygen-derived radicals: a link between reperfusion injury and inflammation. *Fed. Proc.*, **46**, 2402–6.

McCutchen H.J., Schwappach J.R., Enquist E.G. et al. (1990). Xanthine oxidase-derived H_2O_2 contributes to reperfusion injury of ischemic skeletal muscle. *Am. J. Physiol.*, **258**, H1415–19.

McDonald F.D., Thiel G., Wilson D.R. et al. (1969). The prevention of acute renal failure in the rat by long-term saline loading: a possible role for the renin-angiotensin axis. *Proc. Soc. Exp. Biol. Med.*, **131**, 610–14.

McGiff J.C., Crowshaw K., Terragno N.A., Lonigro A.J. (1970). Release of prostaglandin-like substance into renal venous blood in response to angiotensin II. *Circ. Res.*, **27**, (suppl. 1), 121–30.

McLean D., Thomson A.E. (1970). Effect of phenoxybenzamine on glycerol-induced acute renal failure in the rat. *Fed. Proc.*, **29**, 478.

Meroney W.H., Arney G.K., Segar W.E., Balch H.H. (1957). The acute calcification of traumatised muscle, with particular reference to acute post-traumatic renal insufficiency. *J. Clin. Invest.*, **36**, 825–32.

Minow R.A., Gorbach S., Johnson B.L., Dornfeld L. (1974). Myoglobinuria associated with influenza A infection. *Ann. Intern. Med.*, **80**, 359–61.

Montoreano R., Ruiz-Guinazu A. (1972). Renin content of the kidneys during the course of methemoglobin-induced acute renal insufficiency in the rat. *Medicina (B Aires)*, **32**, 209–14.

Mubarak S.J., Owens C.A. (1975). Compartmental syndrome and its relation to crush syndrome: a spectrum of disease. A review of 11 cases of prolonged limb compression. *Clin. Orthoped.*, **113**, 81–9.

Mubarak S.J., Owens C.A. (1977). Double-incision fasciotomy of the leg for decompression in compartment syndromes. *J. Bone Joint Surg.*, **59A**, 184–7.

Nayler W.G., Poole-Wilson P.A., Williams A. (1979). Hypoxia and calcium. *J. Mol. Cell Cardiol.*, **11**, 683–706.

Needleman P., Kaufman A.H., Douglas J.R. et al. (1973). Specific stimulation and inhibition of renal prostaglandin release by angiotensin analogs. *Am. J. Physiol.*, **224**, 1415–19.

Odeh M. (1991). The role of reperfusion injury in the pathogenesis of the crush syndrome. *N. Engl. J. Med.*, **324**, 1417–22.

Ogilvie R.W., Armstrong R.B., Baird K.E., Bottoms C.L. (1988). Lesions in the rat soleus muscle following eccentrically biased exercise. *Am. J. Anat.*, **182**, 335–46.

Oken D.E. (1975). Role of prostaglandins in the pathogenesis of acute renal failure. *Lancet*, **i**, 1319–22.

Oken D.E., Arce M.L., Wilson D.R. (1966). Glycerol-induced hemoglobinuric acute renal failure in the rat. Micropuncture study of the development of oliguria. *J. Clin. Invest.*, **45**, 724–35.

Oken D.E., Cotes S.C., Flamenbaum W. et al. (1975). Active and passive immunisation to angiotensin in experimental acute renal failure. *Kidney Int.*, **7**, 12–18.

Olbricht C., Mason J., Takabatake T. et al. (1977). The early phase of experimental acute renal failure II. Tubular leakage and the reliability of glomerular markers. *Pflug. Archiv.*, **372**, 257–8.

Olerud J.E., Homer L.D., Carroll H.W. (1976). Incidence of acute exertional rhabdomyolysis. *Arch. Intern. Med.*, **136**, 692.

Oliver J., MacDowell M., Tracy A. (1951). The pathogenesis of acute renal failure associated with traumatic and toxic injury: renal ischemia, nephrotoxic damage and the ischemuric episode. *J. Clin. Invest.*, **30**, 1305–51.

Owen C.A., Mubarak S.J., Hargens A.R. et al. (1979). Intramuscular pressures with limb compression: clarification of the pathogenesis of the drug-induced muscle compartment syndrome. *N. Engl. J. Med.*, **300**, 1169–72.

Paller M.S. (1988). Hemoglobin and myoglobin acute renal failure in rats: role of iron in nephrotoxicity. *Am. J. Physiol.*, **255**, F539–44.

Papanicolau N., Callard P., Bariety L., Milliez P. (1975). The effect of indomethacin and prostaglandin (PGE_2) on renal failure due to glycerol in saline-loaded rats. *Clin. Sci. Mol. Med.*, **49**, 507–10.

Perri G.C., Gorini P. (1952). Uraemia in the rabbit after injection of crystalline myoglobin. *Br. J. Exp. Pathol.*, **33**, 440–1.

Perry M.O., Shires G.T., Albert S.A. (1984). Cellular changes with graded limb ischemia and reperfusion. *J. Vasc. Surg.*, **1**, 536–40.

Pierce G.N., Maddafard T.G., Kroeger E.A., Cragoe E.J. (1990). Protection by benzamil against dysfunction and damage in rat myocardium after calcium depletion and repletion. *Am. J. Physiol.*, **258**, H17–23.

Pomeranz B.H., Birtch A.G., Barger A.C. (1968). Neural

control of intra-renal blood flow. *Am. J. Physiol.*, **215**, 1067–81.

Poole-Wilson P.A., Harding D.P., Bourdillon P.D.V., Tones M.A. (1984). Calcium out of control. *J. Mol. Cell Cardiol*, **16**, 175–87.

Powell-Jackson J.D., Brown J.J., Lever A.F. et al. (1972). Protection against acute renal failure in rats by passive immunisation against angiotensin II. *Lancet*, **i**, 774–6.

Powell-Jackson J.D., MacGregor J., Brown J.J. et al. (1978). The effect of angiotensin II antisera and systemic inhibitors of the renin-angiotensin system on glycerol-induced acute renal failure in the rat. In *Proceedings of the Conference on Acute Renal Failure* (Friedman E.A., Eliahou H.E., eds) Publ. No. (NIH) 74–608. Washington: DHEW.

Presta M., Ragnotti G. (1981). Quantification of damage to striated muscle after normothermic or hypothermic ischemia. *Clin. Chem.*, **27**, 297–302.

Reineck H.J., O'Connor G.J., Lifschitz M.D., Stein J.H. (1980). Sequential studies on the pathophysiology of glycerol-induced acute renal failure. *J. Lab. Clin. Med.*, **96**, 356–62.

Reis N.D., Michaelson M. (1986). Crush injury to the lower limbs: treatment of the local injury. *J. Bone Joint Surg.*, **68A**, 414–18.

Romson J.L., Hook B.G., Kunkel S.L. et al. (1983). Reduction of the extent of ischemic myocardial injury by neutrophil depletion in the dog. *Circulation*, **67**, 1016–23.

Ron D., Taitelman U., Michaelson M. et al. (1984). Prevention of acute renal failure in traumatic rhabdomyolysis. *Arch. Intern. Med.*, **144**, 277–80.

Rowland L.P., Penn A.S. (1972). Myoglobinuria. *Med. Clin. North Am.*, **56**, 1233–56.

Roy R.S., McCord J.M. (1983). Superoxide and ischemia: conversion of xanthine dehydrogenase to xanthine oxidase. In *Oxygen Radicals and their Scavenger Systems*, Vol. 2. *Cellular and Medical Aspects* (Greenwald R., Cohen, G., eds). New York: Elsevier Science, p. 145.

Schmalzreid T.P., Neal W.C., Eckardt J.J. (1992). Gluteal compartment and crush syndromes. Report of three cases and review of the literature. *Clin. Orthoped.*, **277**, 161–5.

Schneider R. (1970). Acute alcoholic myopathy with myoglobinuria. *South. Med. J.*, **63**, 485–7.

Schor N., Ichikawa I., Renke H.R. et al. (1981). Pathophysiology of altered glomerular function in aminoglycoside-treated rats. *Kidney Int.*, **19**, 288–96.

Screaton G.R., Cairns H.S., Cohen S.L. (1991). The role of reperfusion-induced injury in the pathogenesis of the crush syndrome (letter). *N. Engl. J. Med.*, **325**, 1383.

Sexton W.L., Korthuis R.J., Laughlin M.H. (1990). Ischemia-reperfusion injury in isolated rat hindquarters. *J. Appl. Physiol.*, **68**, 387–92.

Shen A.C., Jennings R.B. (1964). Kinetics of calcium accumulation in acute myocardial ischemic injury. *Circ. Res.*, **14**, 260–9.

Sheridan G.W., Matsen F. (1976). Fasciotomy in the treatment of acute compartment syndrome. *J. Bone Joint Surg.*, **58A**, 112–14.

Sheridan G.W., Matsen F.A. III, Krugmire R.B. (1977). Further investigations on the pathophysiology of the compartmental syndrome. *Clin. Orthoped.*, **123**, 266–70.

Smith J.K., Carden D.L., Grisham M.B. et al. (1988). Role of iron in ischemia-reperfusion injury to skeletal muscle microvasculature. *Physiologist*, **31**, A31.

Solez K., Altman J., Rienhoff H.Y. et al. (1977). Early angiographic and renal blood flow changes after HgCl$_2$ or glycerol administration. *Kidney Int.*, **10**, S153–9.

Stein J.H., Boonjarern S., Mauk R.C., Ferris T.F. (1973). Mechanism of the redistribution of renal cortical blood flow during hemorrhagic hypotension in the dog. *J. Clin. Invest.*, **52**, 39–47.

Stein J.H., Lifschitz M.D., Barnes L.D. (1978). Current concepts on the pathophysiology of acute renal failure. *Am. J. Physiol.*, **234**, F171–81.

Suzuki T., Mostofi F.K. (1970). Electron microscopic studies of acute tubular necrosis. Early changes in the rat kidney after subcutaneous injection of glycerin. *Lab. Invest.*, **23**, 8–14.

Suzuki M., Inauen W., Kvietys P.R. et al. (1989). Superoxide mediates reperfusion-induced leukocyte–endothelial cell interactions. *Am. J. Physiol.*, **257**, H1740–5.

Takemura T., Matsubara O. (1975). Renal microvasculature in acute renal failure. *Bull. Tokyo Med. Dent. Univ.*, **22**, 9–14.

Tani M., Neely J.R. (1989). Role of intracellular Na$^+$ in Ca^{2+} overload and depressed recovery of reticular function of reperfused rat hearts: possible involvement of H$^+$–Na$^+$ and Na$^+$–Ca^{2+} exchange. *Circ. Res.*, **65**, 1045–56.

Tanner G.A., Steinhausen M. (1976). Tubular obstruction in ischemic-induced acute renal failure in the rat. *Kidney Int.*, **10**, S65–73.

Tarlow S.D., Achterman C.A., Hayhurst J., Ovadia D.N. (1986). Acute compartment syndrome in the thigh complicating fracture of the femur. *J. Bone Joint Surg.*, **68A**, 1439–43.

Thurau K., Boylan J.W. (1976). Acute renal success. The unexpected logic of oliguria in acute renal failure. *Am. J. Med.*, **61**, 308–15.

Torres V.E., Strong C.G., Romero J.C., Wilson D.M. (1975). Indomethacin enhancement of glycerol-induced acute renal failure in rabbits. *Kidney Int.*, **7**, 170–8.

Trueta J., Barclay A.E., Daniel P.M. et al. (1948). *Studies of the Renal Circulation.* Oxford: Blackwell.

Trump B.F., Berezesky I.K., Laiho K.W. et al. (1980). The role of calcium in cell injury. *Scanning Electron. Microsc.*, **2**, 437–62.

Tu W.H. (1965). Plasma renin activity in acute tubular necrosis and other renal diseases associated with hypertension. *Circulation*, **31**, 686–95.

van Gilst W.H. (1989). Protection of the myocardium against post ischemic reperfusion damage. *J. Cardiovasc. Pharmacol.*, **14**, (suppl. 9), S49–54.

Venkatachalam M.A., Rennke H.G., Sandstrom D.I. (1976). The vascular basis for acute renal failure in the rat. Preglomerular and postglomerular vasoconstriction. *Circ. Res.*, **38**, 267–79.

Volkmann R. (1881). Die ischaemischen muskellahmungen und kontrakturen. *Centrabl. Chir*, 51.

Walker P.M., Lindsay T.F., Labbe R. et al. (1987). Salvage of skeletal muscle with free radical scavengers. *J. Vasc. Surg.*, **5**, 68–75.

Ward M.M. (1988). Factors predictive of acute renal failure in rhabdomyolysis. *Arch. Intern. Med.*, **148**, 1553–7.

Wardle E.N. (1975). Endotoxinaemia and the pathogenesis of acute renal failure. *Q. J. Med.*, **44**, 389–98.

Watts J.A., Koch C.D., LaNoue K.F. (1980). Effects of Ca^{2+} antagonism on energy metabolism: Ca^{2+} and heart function after ischemia. *Am. J. Physiol.*, **238**, H909–16.

Whitesides T.E. Jr, Harada H., Morimoto K. (1971). The response of skeletal muscle to temporary ischemia: an experimental study. *J. Bone Joint Surg.*, **53A**, 1027.

Whitesides T.E., Haney T.C., Murimoto K., Harada H. (1975). Tissue pressure measurements as a determinant for the need of fasciotomy. *Clin. Orthoped.*, **113**, 43–51.

Whitesides T.E., Harada H., Morimoto K. (1977). Compartment syndromes and the role of fasciotomy. Its parameters and techniques. In *Instructional Course Lectures, the American Academy of Orthopedic Surgeons*. St Louis: Mosby, p. 179.

Wilmore D.W., Long J.M., Mason A.D. Jr et al. (1974). Catecholamines: mediators of the hypermetabolic response to thermal injury. *Ann. Surg.*, **180**, 653–69.

Wilson D.R., Thiel G., Arce M.L., Oken D.E. (1969). The role of the concentration mechanism in the development of acute renal failure: micropuncture studies using diabetes insipidus rats. *Nephron*, **6**, 128–39.

Wrogemann K., Pena S.D.J. (1976). Mitochondrial calcium overload: a general mechanism for cell-necrosis in muscle diseases. *Lancet*, **i**, 672–4.

23. Barotrauma

Z. Török

INTRODUCTION

Barotrauma embraces the circumstances when increased pressure within the airway and across tissue–air interfaces causes pathological effects. The 'design pressure' of the human body is 1 bar and, apart from the few who live at high altitude, this is not often departed from (Figure 23.1). Nevertheless, function is possible without injury at pressures from 0.5 to 70 bar (Paton *et al.*, 1984). Applied pressure is well tolerated; it is *change* of pressure that leads to barotrauma.

All the important forms of barotrauma man suffers from will be discussed in the following pages. The clinical picture is always more grave when the lungs are affected. This is essentially due to the continuous, uninterruptable nature of lung function in supporting life. Lung function cannot yet be suspended for a convenient period of time whilst repair takes place. In addition, air often gains entry to arteries such as the carotid, via a damaged lung. Once the carotid artery is embolized, most of the therapeutic effort will be directed at the resulting hypoxic brain. For this reason some aspects of carotid gas embolism, especially those with direct impact on therapy, are also included.

A modicum of common sense of the mechanical engineering kind, aids understanding of the pathogenesis described in the second half of the chapter. Quantitative aspects of the volume changes and forces involved aid the construction of a dynamic picture. Similarly, simple concepts like squeeze and reverse squeeze are of value and will be outlined.

Barotrauma is conspicuously a man-made problem. Apart from a few cases of spontaneous pneumothorax, most cases of barotrauma follow the use of the mechanical ventilator or the endeavour of man, a terrestrial form of life, to penetrate the sea, the atmosphere and beyond. Ideas bearing on prevention are therefore important and will be presented.

Nowadays barotrauma is most frequently encountered in two different circumstances. First in clinical practice it may occur spontaneously but is more often seen when respiration is assisted by the use of positive pressure ventilators. Pulmonary barotrauma and its sequelae, such as respiratory distress, pneumothorax or carotid arterial gas embolism, are well-recognized complications. In published series the incidence of barotrauma ranges from around 8% when peak airway pressure is below 70 cmH$_2$O, to 43% with higher pressures (Petersen and Baier, 1983). If pulmonary interstitial emphysema on X-ray is accepted as the criterion of barotrauma, the incidence in a small group of patients with adult respiratory distress syndrome was 88% (Woodring, 1985). Amongst patients with barotrauma which resulted from mechanical ventilation and complicated further therapy, mortality rates in excess of 50% have been reported (Fleming and Bowen, 1972; de Latorre *et al.*, 1977; Cullen and Caldera, 1979). Though these improve with a high index of suspicion and early diagnosis (Steir *et al.*, 1974), iatrogenic barotrauma remains a frequent and serious complication of intensive care.

Second, barotrauma due to changes in environmental pressure is a hazard of activities such as diving and aviation. It affects the potentially closed air-filled cavities of the body, most often the middle ear, but also the facial sinuses and the lungs. It is one of the dysbaric illnesses. Barotrauma of the lung is rare in aviation, even after sudden failure of the pressure cabin at high altitudes (Fryer, 1965).

Barotrauma is eminently preventable. In practice, whenever it is seen, an excessive rate of change of pressure coupled with some loss of control, such as breath holding, panic or an unchecked buoyant fast ascent in water, plays a dominant part. Viewed simply, the key feature is stretch with overdistension of some part of the human body, caused either by a trapped volume of air expanding according to Boyle's law as pressure is reduced, or by the positive pressure ventilator, when 'breath-stacking' occurs. The alternative term 'expansion rupture' focuses attention on this aspect (Lenaghan *et al.*, 1969).

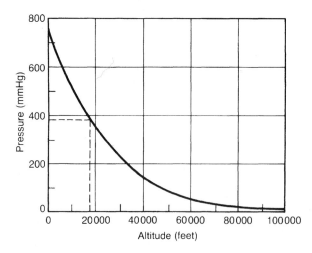

Figure 23.1 Atmospheric pressure is an exponential function of altitude, it is halved at 13 000 ft (4000 m). In contrast, pressure increases linearly with sea water depth.

Related forms of injury

In primary blast injury, a wave or front of pressure is responsible for damage. This lasts but a few tens of milliseconds; the resulting clinical picture (Mellor, 1988) is quite different from barotrauma proper which is considered in other sections of this text (Chapters 16 and 17). Noise-induced hearing loss is caused by peak sound pressure levels at audible frequencies and is cumulative over a relatively long period of time. Because sound energy propagates by longitudinal waves, that is by a periodic compaction and rarefaction of the conducting medium, the damage to the cochlea so caused could be regarded as barotrauma. However it falls outside the scope of this chapter.

PULMONARY BAROTRAUMA

Reports of spontaneous pulmonary barotrauma of a clinically relevant degree at normal atmospheric pressures have been more common in the past. The first substantial analysis of its mechanisms was provided in this context by Macklin and Macklin (1944). The end result of many respiratory diseases was death following respiratory failure, with or without a pneumothorax. Post-mortem the lungs appeared to splint the rib cage, were stiff, light and would not collapse when squeezed: this being the description of pulmonary interstitial emphysema. Alveolar rupture was established as the cause. The non-partitional or marginal alveoli are vulnerable because they are adjacent to blood vessels, with walls subject to a pressure gradient which is the transpulmonary pressure (defined as intratracheal minus pleural pressure). On rupture, gas is discharged into the perivascular sheaths, and then tracks towards the hilum of the lung.

Further tearing of connective tissue may result in pneumomediastinum, pneumothorax, pneumopericardium, pneumoprecordium (with its accompanying Hamman's sign – squelchy sounds in phase with the heart beat) and, following gradients of pressure, gas may find its way out of the thorax and present as subcutaneous emphysema, often in the neck (Boetger, 1983). Rupture into the peritoneal cavity is rare, even in the more dramatic cases which result from uncontrolled buoyant ascent in diving where large volumes of expanding gas force their way through the tissues (Schriger *et al.*, 1987). A similarly rare event in divers is rupture of the visceral pleura without involving the hilum of the lung. When pneumothorax is caused in this way, pre-existing bullae or other local pathological conditions are often responsible. Subpleural air cysts are common in ventilator-induced pulmonary barotrauma. They were originally recognized in children with hyaline membrane disease when their appearance often heralded the development of tension pneumothorax (Johnson and Altan, 1979; Albelda *et al.*, 1983).

Pathogenesis

A large proportion of our present understanding of the fundamental mechanics of pulmonary barotrauma stems from military research. Escape of survivors from a damaged submarine lying on the sea bed requires rapid increase of pressure upon the crew to equal sea-water pressure prevailing outside the boat and then buoyant ascent to the surface whilst continuously exhaling (Crocker, 1955). In-water training for this procedure involves a risk of 1 in 2300 ascents of producing pulmonary barotrauma (Greene, 1978). The correct diagnosis was often missed in the early US training casualties (Polak and Adams, 1932) and this experience led to quantitative work to determine the forces and the strength of the intrathoracic structures involved. In England such work followed the loss of HMS *Truculent* in 1950.

High intrathoracic pressure produced by the expiratory muscles was excluded as the causative mechanism of pulmonary barotrauma. The average expiratory peak pressure in 419 trainees was 114 mmHg, the maximum 350 mmHg, which agrees well with other series (Shilling, 1933). The crucial point is that muscular force to produce these pressures is applied evenly to all the contents of the thorax and stretch, hence tearing of pulmonary tissues, cannot take place. Macklin and Macklin (1944), amongst their causes of interstitial emphysema where intrapulmonary pressure is prominent, described events such as blowing against obstruction, violent cough, violent straining and parturition. Others of their examples, such as hiccough, illustrate the role of negative pressure and stretch as during forced inspiration. Some important aspects of the causative mechanisms of pulmonary barotrauma await clarification.

The magnitude of transpulmonary pressure necessary to cause barotrauma of the human lung has been measured in cadavers (Malhotra and Wright, 1954). Rupture of alveoli at 80–95 mmHg accord well with results of more recent work on cadavers, dogs and rabbits (Malhotra and Wright, 1960; Calder, 1985). These experiments have also shown the protective effect of uniformly reducing the compliance of the whole thorax by binding of the thorax and abdomen to prevent expansion as intratracheal pressure is applied. Threshold pressure to cause trauma rose to 133–190 mmHg and 85–210 mmHg in cadavers, and to more than 180 mmHg in dogs. Volumetric air expansion in closed trachea experiments, where decompression in a pressure chamber is used to achieve over-inflation and stretch, is exponential following Boyle's law, and the starting volume of trapped air is much less in bound animals (Malhotra and Wright, 1960; Schaefer *et al.*, 1960). Care must be exercised when comparing these results to the more controlled experiments performed at one atmosphere with linear expansion rates (Malhotra and Wright, 1954).

A given transpulmonary pressure produces more expansion in a compliant than in a stiff lung; thus, everything else being equal, the former is more vulnerable. However the opposite was reported in a study of six divers who suffered pulmonary barotrauma on ascent, compared to ten normal controls (Colebatch *et al.*, 1976). Larger regional differences in stiffness of the lung in the barotrauma group could explain this result. Thus the stiff regions would be protected, resulting in less local expansion and increased overall transpulmonary pressure. This in turn would lead to increased distension of regions of the lung with higher compliance than would be the case in lungs with evenly distributed mechanical properties. Most evidence for this concept comes from retrospective clinical studies, correlating high vulnerability with pre-existing regional lung disease (Kumar *et al.*, 1973; Steir *et al.*, 1974; Woodring, 1985). Cases with unilateral distribution are particularly convincing (Graziano *et al.*, 1978; Siegel *et al.*, 1985).

A similar conceptual model assumes the outflow from a lobule of lung to become obstructed, once filled with air at increased pressure such as at depth in diving. Unable to escape, air in such a lobule would cause rupture after maximal local distension, even though the rest of the lung was functioning normally. Though this is an attractive concept, its relative importance in the pathogenesis of barotrauma remains unclear.

If regional idiosyncracies are disregarded, a number of simple and instructive calculations can be made using Boyle's law and the following figures: maximum tolerable transpulmonary pressure 70 mmHg; total lung capacity 6.5 litres; pulmonary compliance (the slope of the pressure–volume curve at this lung capacity) 17 ml added lung volume per cmH_2O pressure; and the elastic recoil pressure of the thorax and contents 50 cmH_2O. Starting with a voluntarily fully inflated lung, the pressure and stretching of the tissues generated by an additional 800 ml or so of air will cause barotrauma. Should a trainee diver breathe from the 'SCUBA' gear at the bottom of a 3-m swimming pool and hold breath at maximum lung volume, there will be potentially disastrous barotrauma about a metre below the surface. Starting with a fully inflated lung at 20-m depth, the diver will suffer the same fate at around 2 m below the surface. The effect of Boyle's law is clearly illustrated: per metre ascent, the expansion of gas and the accompanying risk of barotrauma is greater near the surface. A given volume of gas will double during a 20-m ascent from 30 m to 10 m, and double again during half that amount (10 m) of ascent from 10 m depth to the surface.

Pulmonary interstitial emphysema

Pulmonary interstitial emphysema in mechanically ventilated patients may be regarded as an intermediate stage in a sequence of events set in motion by barotrauma. The process will continue unless the positive-pressure ventilation can be stopped. Its characteristic early radiological signs are therefore particularly important. Apart from the subpleural air cysts referred to above, perivascular air halos and linear air streaks radiating from the hilum may be seen. Pneumatoceles and subpleural air may represent a somewhat later stage (Johnson and Altan, 1979; Woodring, 1985). The lung fields may be unusually translucent, and with some measure of splinting of the rib cage the diaphragm will appear low and flat, moving poorly with respiration.

Pneumothorax

Pneumothorax is a serious sequel of pulmonary barotrauma. It occurs in up to 15% of mechanically ventilated patients depending on the underlying pathological process (de Latorre *et al.*, 1977), and on the technique and duration of the positive-pressure ventilation used (Zwillich *et al.*, 1974; Zimmerman *et al.*, 1975; Siegel *et al.* 1985). Tension pneumothorax – an acute medical emergency – is the usual form encountered as opposed to the closed and the open varieties, where the mean pleural pressures are respectively negative and atmospheric. The positive mean pleural pressure results from a valvular mechanism in the path of escape of air from the lung. Rise in pressure often leads to mediastinal shift towards the unaffected side, causing both respiratory and circulatory embarrassment and cyanosis. As prognosis worsens markedly with delay in diagnosis on a timescale of minutes or hours, the early clinical signs must be borne in mind: hyperresonance with regionally diminished breath sounds, and tachycardia with a systolic blood pressure below 90 mmHg (Steir *et al.*, 1974).

Pneumothorax may occasionally present weeks after withdrawal of ventilatory support (Cooper *et al.*, 1989). The mechanism has been shown to be the earlier development of subpleural and parenchymal cysts. Once formed, these may expand and eventually rupture into the pleural cavity.

Arterial gas embolism

From studies of the various routes extra-alveolar gas may take (Macklin and Macklin, 1944), it seems surprising that, in mechanically ventilated adults, pulmonary barotrauma only rarely leads to arterial gas embolism. Gas escaping the non-partitional alveoli may follow the transatrial pressure gradient and enter the pulmonary veins and, via the left heart, the systemic circulation. This course of events is well known in diving (see below), and also in ventilated infants (Brown *et al.*, 1977; Kogutt, 1978). In adults it causes focal cerebral infarction, myocardial injury with ECG signs and characteristic patchy dermal venodilation – *livedo reticularis* – that is known to develop following arteriolar occlusion (Marini and Culvert, 1989). Some authors consider such marbling of the skin as pathognomonic (Durant *et al.*, 1949). Though systemic gas embolism as the causative agent has not been proven conclusively, the case is convincing. Indeed, it seems likely that the diagnosis is sometimes missed because of the extreme difficulty of obtaining firm confirmatory evidence. Massive embolization of the pulmonary artery and right heart has been described at post-mortem in ventilated patients (Tremonti and Halka, 1972). However, minor degrees of this condition may go unrecognized in that large volumes of air in the pulmonary circulation can remain asymptomatic (Moore and Braselton, 1940).

It appears from first principles that high transpulmonary pressure is the likeliest damaging factor and results from excessive peak airways pressure. Thus, given that satisfactory gas exchange can be maintained, reduction of the ventilated tidal volume to around 10 ml/kg body weight or lower, and reduction of peak flow rates, should result in increased safety (Boetger, 1983). Adequate sedation prevents patients 'fighting the ventilator', and thus causing extra respiratory muscle force to increase the airway pressure or cause breath stacking.

Conversely, to use the ventilator in patient-triggered mode may be an effective means of avoiding man–machine conflict. Clearly, a tolerable degree of controlled hypoventilation is preferable to barotrauma. Such underventilation may be unavoidable in patients where lung tissue compliance is non-uniform, as in status asthmaticus, necrotizing pneumonitis or pre-existing regional pathological conditions (Menitove and Goldring, 1983; Carioli and Perret, 1984). Though high-frequency jet ventilators offer a number of theoretical advantages, these have not been apparent in every series of patients assembled to assess their utility (Carlon *et al.*, 1983).

Pulmonary barotrauma in aviation

In aviation medicine, the main interest in pulmonary barotrauma has always been vested in events following the structural failure of a pressure cabin at altitudes of up to 45 000 ft (approx 14 000 m) where the atmospheric pressure is about 0.15 bar. The duration of the sudden steep decrease in pressure is of prime prognostic interest, 'explosive decompression' being defined to occur in less than 1 second. The final value of cabin pressure at the end of such a step change is not necessarily that ambient at the aircraft's altitude, since it may be increased by ram effects or lowered by venturi suction effects depending on the location, size and nature of the rupture. Much of the work describing quantitatively the physics of explosive decompression has been aimed at determining the duration of the step change and the ensuing effects on the occupants of the aircraft (Lovelace and Gagge, 1946; Violette, 1954).

Very few instances of pulmonary barotrauma consequent upon cabin failure at altitude have been reported. Some of the early cases were the result of deliberate breath-holding, leading to systemic arterial gas embolism (Bentzinger, 1950; Luft, 1954). Decompression from an equivalent pressure of 8000 ft (2500 m) to 31 000 ft (13 000 m) in 0.5 seconds caused pneumomediastinum in two cases, whilst unexplained syncope, pneumothorax and subcutaneous emphysema of the neck followed decompression in 2.0 seconds from 8000 ft (2500 m) to 22 000 ft (9200 m) (Holmstrom, 1958). It is conspicuous that in all the above cases there was some reason to believe that there was breath-holding. Overall the low incidence of pulmonary barotrauma is thus seen to follow the small probability of the glottis being closed with the thorax in maximum inspiration at the unpredictable instance of explosive decompression.

The few reports of explosive decompression from the hyperbaric state describe disasters with numerous casualties (Richter and Loeblich, 1978; Giertsen *et al.*, 1988). These include all the occupants of the chamber, even at comparatively low pressures such as 3 bar. The post-mortem appearances depend on the state of saturation of the body, which is in turn a function of both, pressure and the length of exposure. Gas bubbles may form in every tissue with gross mechanical disruption.

Pulmonary barotrauma in diving

A large proportion of cases of uncomplicated pulmonary barotrauma leading only to extra-alveolar air during diving must remain unreported and may not require specific treatment; the true incidence is thus unknown. Its most feared complication, carotid arterial gas embolism, is an important cause of diving fatalities, second only to drowning. The overall risk is nevertheless small. The number of sports divers in Britain is about 60 000, each diving on average about 20 times per year. Assuming that about 350 cases of dysbaric disease were treated in the dozen or so available hyperbaric chambers in the 1989 diving season at a ratio of decompression sickness to arterial gas embolism of about 10 : 1, the estimated death rate is very roughly about 1 in 30 000 dives. Annual statistics available from sources such as the US National Diver Alert Network and the British Sub Aqua Club present a similar but equally uncertain picture. British records of military diving show 35 cases of arterial gas embolism over 20 years, an incidence of 1 in 20 000 dives (Dickson *et al.*, 1947) and in the US Navy the incidence was 1 in 15 000 dives (US Navy Diving Statistics, 1978). It is conspicuously an injury of the novice diver, who is more easily stampeded into some form of uncontrolled ascent whilst not exhaling properly.

Differential diagnosis between decompression sickness and arterial gas embolism is difficult. The chain of events leading to decompression sickness is started by bubbles of gas arising afresh in the blood or other tissues, after an excess of inert gas has been previously dissolved. Diagnostic problems occur when divers present with neurological symptoms after short, shallow dives not capable of generating enough supersaturation for gas bubbles to form on decompression. It is possible that minor degrees of pulmonary barotrauma which admit small volumes of gas into the systemic circulation are very much more frequent than hitherto thought (Francis and Smith, 1991). This fundamental uncertainty in the diagnosis of dysbaric illnesses is acknowledged but the following section describes the classical presentation of arterial gas embolism – a major event by any standard.

Arterial gas embolism in diving

Classical cases of pulmonary barotrauma which originate during ascent present with evidence of cerebral involvement within 10 minutes of breaking surface. Loss of consciousness, possibly with epileptiform convulsions, accounts for up to half of the highly symptomatic cases. Altered consciousness with weakness or deranged coordination affecting the motor system, sensory or visual loss together is seen in two-thirds of the remainder. Vertigo, amnesia, deafness and a characteristic loss of rapport with the surroundings characterize the rest. A few patients go into cardiorespiratory arrest early and some of these die in spite of energetic therapy. Myocardial or brainstem emboli are the likely causes in such cases (Evans *et al.*, 1977).

In a retrospective review of 140 divers with pulmonary barotrauma of ascent, only 23 were uncomplicated (Leitch and Green, 1986). Presenting features were chest or abdominal pain, dyspnoea with or without pneumothorax and cough with haemoptysis. The patient may remain asymptomatic in spite of marked degrees of subcutaneous emphysema, and the main complaint may be a change in the pitch of the voice. Direct X-ray evidence of lung damage in divers with arterial gas emboli is rarely found (Gorman, 1984; Kizer, 1987).

Once gas enters the pulmonary vein, the left heart and the aorta, it will be distributed in the systemic circulation according to the haemodynamic factors that prevail. In that the forward flow velocity of blood in the aorta is only a few cm/second, gravity, and hence the position of the patient, plays an important role. However a detailed experimental study on dogs illustrated that *any* position of the body at the time of embolization endangers a vital organ, either the heart or the brain (Van Allen *et al.*, 1929).

The optimal body position during transport is an exercise in applied physiology and its determination is further complicated by the way gravity is expected to affect cerebral blood flow and intracranial pressure, given that the state of autoregulation of cerebral blood vessels is in most cases an unknown variable. With deranged autoregulation, the head-down position will probably result in increased carotid and cerebral venous pressures, hence in increased blood flow and volume. A small drop in systemic blood pressure and increased intracranial pressure would also result. With intact autoregulation the cerebral perfusion rate may fall in the head-down position. Advantageous redirection of further emboli away from the carotid arteries in the head-down position only ensues in cases where further emboli form during transport.

Nevertheless, in the absence of conclusive evidence some physicians still prefer the head-down position (Gorman, 1989). Controversy over the best position for transport must not be allowed to delay the treatment of the patient in a pressure chamber and, all things considered, the horizontal recovery position may be a good choice. Patients must never be transported head up.

Once gaseous emboli become lodged in cerebral arterioles, a number of pathological changes occur. Some are mentioned here to provide the rationale for the treatment of the majority of divers with pulmonary barotrauma where the clinical picture is dominated by cerebral features. The main feature is focal neuronal ischaemia proceeding to oedema, infarction and haemorrhage. Endothelial damage is shown by local swelling, platelet deposition, polymorphonuclear infiltration and disruption of the blood–brain barrier (Catron *et al.*, 1984). The autoregulation of cerebral perfusion may be deranged. Some cerebral oedema must be expected in every case, with a subsequent rise in intracranial pressure and a drop in blood flow which can lead to further ischaemic damage and, if gross, herniation of cortex with further local and generalized effects.

The primary lesion in arterial gas embolism involves elements of both cytotoxic and vasogenic oedema, with an unknown relative contribution of each to a given clinical case (Klatzo, 1967). Cytotoxic oedema follows the ischaemic disruption of intracellular energy management, and is commonly seen after cardiac arrest. The sodium pump fails, followed by an ingress of water. The blood–brain barrier remains intact and in most cases there is no rise in intracranial pressure. Steroids are ineffective.

Vasogenic oedema is essentially extracellular and extravascular and follows injury to the capillary endothelium. The blood–brain barrier is disrupted, the intracranial pressure is raised with a decreased rate of blood flow. Steroids are of proven benefit. Steroids can thus only be expected to help by opposing the pathological chain of events set in motion by direct mechanical injury of blood vessels, and then only after a time lag of some hours after administration. Nevertheless, large dose steroid therapy is a routine adjunct in the management of serious cerebral arterial gas embolism.

A further pathophysiological model which aids understanding of the clinical course and response in time and to therapy is the concept of the 'ischaemic penumbra' (Astrup *et al.*, 1977). Clear electrophysiological evidence exists to show that quantitative measures of neuronal function depend linearly on blood perfusion at flow rates of 12–16 ml/min/100 g brain tissue. Below about 12 ml/min neuronal function is not detectable, yet until a much lower perfusion rate was reached, the neurones remained viable (Heiss *et al.*, 1976). Thus, absence of neuronal function is not synonymous with cell death. As the blood supply improves, function can return after an absence of hours or longer.

Treatment of arterial gas embolism

The generally accepted treatment of arterial gas embolism is described in the *Royal Navy Diving Manual* (1991). It consists of immediate compression of the diver to 6.0 bar on air. In most cases symptoms will resolve in 30 minutes when chamber pressure is lowered to 2.8 bar following the pressure–time profile of Treatment Table 63. The patient is given 100% oxygen to breathe for the following 4 hours 45 minutes as chamber pressure is lowered returning to surface pressure. If symptoms persist at 6.0 bar pressure, then up to 2 hours may be spent there; however, the patient and attendants will be committed to a stay of 2 days in the chamber. The option of follow-on hyperbaric oxygen treatments on a daily basis is available for patients with residual neurological deficit. For this purpose oxygen is given in a pressure chamber at 2.0–2.8 bar for 1 hour, interrupted after 25 minutes with 5 minutes air breathing to lessen oxygen toxicity effects.

On the basis of the pathophysiology outlined above, the shorter the time delay between the onset of the neurological features and the hyperbaric therapy, the more meaningful it is to apply the 6.0 bar pressure during the initial half-hour. In practice, a delay up to about 2 hours is compatible with good prognosis, and beyond 5 hours the patient is likely to obtain all the benefit he/she can be given from 2.8 bar maximum pressure on oxygen (Peirce, 1980).

The treatment pressures of 6.0 bar and 2.8 bar were chosen as a compromise between the therapeutic objective of decreasing the linear diameter of the offending gas bubble, thus enabling it to pass downstream, and the toxicity (dose) limits of oxygen in terms of both its partial pressure and exposure time. After many years experimentation, there is considerable agreement on both sides of the Atlantic about the use of these tables (Kindwall, 1973; Catron *et al.*, 1984; Gorman, 1989). The efficacy of an initial 6.0-bar pressure has been confirmed by the direct observation of air emboli in the dog (Fries *et al.*, 1957; Waite *et al.*, 1967; Mader and Hulet, 1979).

General intensive care measures are used during and after re-compression. Mechanical ventilation of lungs already damaged by barotrauma must only be given if unavoidable. The hazards of fire in a high oxygen atmosphere make special equipment necessary for this and for defibrillation.

Without a pressure chamber being available there is little justification to use the word 'therapy' to describe the management of a victim of dysbaric arterial gas embolism. Such cases illustrate the natural history of the disorder. A few die almost instantly of cardiac arrest. About two-thirds show significant improvement in the first hour but most of these will deteriorate later. In only 10–20% is the initial improvement maintained and few recover completely. In one-third the initial neurological deficit is maintained and will only improve with hyperbaric therapy.

Deterioration is commonly seen on a timescale of hours even after successful hyperbaric therapy (Gorman, 1984). It is possible only to speculate about the cause. Redistribution or coalescence of gas bubbles, re-embolization on postural change, formation of thrombi on the damaged endothelium, focal haemorrhage and oedema, interactions involving the von Willebrand factor protein and the prostaglandin system have, amongst many other mechanisms, been suggested. Interestingly, in one retrospective study of 140 divers, no secondary deterioration was seen in any of the 33 patients where early steroid administration was prescribed, against 20% relapse rate without steroids (Leitch and Green, 1986). All cases of dysbaric arterial gas embolism should be treated in a pressure chamber, as early improvement or its extent were poor predictors of the final outcome.

In practical terms, prevention amounts to identification of susceptible individuals and their exclusion from diving, good training practices, and dealing with the problem of recurrent pulmonary barotrauma once more in the context of return to diving. Fitness of dive is determined during an annual medical examination mandatory for all professional divers. Chronic lung disease, any disorder which causes altered general or local lung compliance, obstructive airways disease and penetrating chest injuries are excluded. Silent structural abnormalities of the lung, such as bullae and old tuberculous scars, are excluded on the basis of full plate X-rays taken both in inspiration and expiration. Proper training and selection based on aptitude also plays a vital role.

BAROTRAUMA OF BODY CAVITIES

When gas contained in a closed cavity within or on the surface of the body is subjected to a change in pressure, a volume change occurs according to Boyle's law, so that for constant temperature the product of pressure and volume remains constant. On increasing ambient pressure, the chain of ensuing events depends on the physical properties of the walls of the cavity, with special reference to the weakest area. Were the walls infinitely compliant, the intracavity volume would follow perfectly Boyle's law with the transmural pressure staying at zero. In reality, beyond a critical point of volume expansion, the wall will start to stretch, exhibiting a tendency to recoil under the forces of elasticity, so generating an increased pressure within. When measured against the outside ambient pressure, this pressure difference across the cavity wall is the transmural pressure and the cause of barotrauma. When stretching forces exceed the elastic limit of the wall, rupture occurs. Table 23.1 gives some figures relevant to these general observations.

Squeeze and reverse squeeze (Table 23.2)

Squeeze is a mechanism of barotrauma that follows failure of air to enter a body cavity, such as a paranasal sinus. It occurs on descent (compression) as the ambient pressure is rising. The resultant negative transmural pressure causes oedema, transudation and haemorrhage from vascular structures such as the mucosa. Such fluid shifts tend to decrease the transmural pressure. Rupture, when it occurs, is implosive in nature and it is then that significant pain is caused instantly, and remains intractable.

In *reverse squeeze*, gas cannot get out of a cavity on ascent or decompression. The transmural pressure is positive, and stretches the walls. As the capillary perfusion pressure is exceeded, ischaemia ensues. There is a time lag even without further increase of transmural pressure, before pain is felt. Symptoms other than pain and variable pathological signs may result when blood flow in the vasa nervosum is prevented by positive transmural pressure. Recovery is prompt on reperfusion, which usually follows a remarkably small change in pressure applied in a compression chamber. Trauma due to reverse squeeze occurs less frequently than that from squeeze.

An understanding of the above principles is crucial to the interpretation of symptoms and signs and subsequent management.

Barotrauma of the middle ear

Air contained in the middle ear changes volume as the environmental pressure varies and some portion of the wall of the cavity has to change shape and yield to the transmural pressure gradient. The tympanic membrane is most affected and clinically most prominent: stretch gives rise to pain; bulging and injury is visible through the otoscope; rupture

TABLE 23.1

CHANGES IN ALTITUDE AND IN SEA WATER DEPTH TO CAUSE A DOUBLING OF PRESSURE. THE THIRD COLUMN SHOWS CORRESPONDING CHANGES IN VOLUME OBEYING BOYLE'S LAW, AND THE LAST INDICATES HOW THE DIAMETER OF A GAS BUBBLE, CHOSEN TO BE UNITY AT SEA LEVEL, CHANGES. A FORCE TO CAUSE BAROTRAUMA TO A GAS-FILLED, RIGID-WALLED CAVITY VARIES LINEARLY WITH THE QUANTITIES IN THE LAST COLUMN

Pressure		Altitude or depth		Volume factors	Diameter factors
Bar	mmHg	metres	feet		
0.25	190	10 360	34 000	4.00	1.61
0.50	380	5486	18 000	2.00	1.26
1.00	760	0.0	0.0	1.00	1.00
2.00		10.0	30.0	0.50	0.80
4.00		30.0	91.4	0.25	0.63

TABLE 23.2

MECHANISMS AND PROPERTIES OF SQUEEZE AND REVERSED SQUEEZE

	Squeeze	Reverse squeeze
Direction of positive pressure	From outside, inwards	From the inside, excess gas
Transmural pressure	Negative	Positive
Failure of air to	Enter	Exit
Pathology	Transudation and haemorrhage	Ischaemia, haemorrhage later
Pain	On compression at higher pressures	On decompression, after delay caused by low (80 mmHg) pressure
Leading to	Implosion	Explosion
Relative frequency of occurrence	3	1

affects hearing. A decrease in environmental pressure will normally result in automatic venting through the Eustachian canal but the process does not normally happen in reverse without some voluntary intervention. Thus, otic barotrauma is most common on descent in both diving and aviation, when the eardrum is bulging inwards. Its incidence is between 25 and 33% in trainees on first exposure to pressure, but declines rapidly with experience. Seventy-five per cent of dives stopped by ear pain are shallower than 10 m, with monaural pain being twice as common as bilateral presentation (Bayliss, 1968). It is a significant cause of novice divers failing to complete their training course and the most common diving-related malady. Though the pressure gradients involved are more severe in diving, a proportion of airline passengers may also be considered at risk.

Without a transmural pressure difference, the impedance of both the tympanic membrane and oval window at the inner end of the ossicular chain is optimal for sound transmission. As the diver descends with the Eustachian canals closed, these membranes begin to bulge into the middle ear cavity, hearing appearing muffled (hence the phrase 'ear clearing' used for the process of equilibrating middle ear pressure). At a depth of less than 1 metre, when the transmural pressure is about 60 mmHg, stretch of the thin skin of the eardrum is sufficiently pronounced to cause pain. The temporary conductive hearing loss is marked, and rarely vertigo is noticeable (alternobaric vertigo). At 1.2 m depth, with 90 mmHg transmural pressure, the nasopharyngeal ostium of the Eustachian canal is locked in the sense that ear clearing becomes much more difficult. Petechial bleeding and congestion will have occurred into the substance of the drum and pain is considerable. On continued descent to depths of about 3–6 m producing transmural pressures of 100–500 mmHg, rupture of the tympanic membrane occurs with relief of pain.

Experimental work on cats has confirmed the vascular origin of middle ear congestion (Dickson *et al.*, 1947). Oedema is followed by seromucinous effusion, haemorrhagic bullae and polymorphonuclear infiltration of the affected membranes.

There are two different widely used grading schemes of the degree of trauma to the drum as seen through the otoscope (Teed, 1944; MacFie, 1964). In the Teed scheme, Grade 1 denotes patchy congestion and erythema over the malleus; Grade 2 the same appearances over the whole drum; Grade 3 signifies haemorrhage into the drum; and Grade 4 refers to rupture of the drum with fluid-containing bubbles visible behind it. Gross damage is rated Grade 5, with copious amounts of dark blood in the middle ear cavity. The MacFie classification is probably simpler to use: erythema, slight haemorrhage, gross haemorrhage, free blood behind, and rupture of drum define five stages of increasing severity.

Though these formal classifications are of value in epidemiological work, a clear verbal description is simpler to use and less ambiguous.

Rupture of the drum occurs at widely varying transmural pressures (100–500 mmHg). In one series of 897 aviators' ears with otic barotrauma, the incidence of tear was 4.2% (King, 1975). The commonest site in a healthy drum is the anteroinferior quadrant. Scars formed on previous rupture, or thin vascular areas are preferentially affected. Rarely, with rapid large pressure changes a circular tear may develop around the handle of the malleus.

Normal function of the Eustachian tube is the key to prevention of otic barotrauma (Aschan, 1955). Gases, especially oxygen, are continuously being absorbed in the middle ear cavity and the necessary extra volume of air enters along the tube. This function is assisted by the contraction of nearby muscles, such as the tensor palati, the levator palati, the salpingopharyngeus and the superior constrictor. Normally the tube begins to open from above with closure starting at the nasopharynx. Both are easier in the upright position when the neck veins are empty.

Experienced divers and aviators usually make up middle ear volume by voluntary contraction of pharyngeal muscles only. Nose-clips are provided so this process can be aided by a slight blow against the clip, the procedure being widely known as the Valsalva manoeuvre. It is not instantaneous; a slight pressure of 33 mmHg generated by the blow is sufficient, provided it is maintained for a time whilst pressure progressively separates the moist walls of the normally closed tube. Toynbee's method consists of swallowing whilst the nose is closed. Frenzel's manoeuvre is more efficient than any other, in that it requires only a mean of 6 mmHg for opening pressure, but it requires some training. The nose, mouth and glottis are closed voluntarily whilst muscles of the floor of the mouth and the superior pharyngeal constrictors are also contracted.

Eustachian tube function may fail for many reasons. Coryza, nasal infections, allergic rhinitis and hypertrophy of lymphatic tissue may narrow the canal, or increase the viscosity or the rate of production of mucus. Failure of a more permanent nature may result from the presence of a tumour, defective mucosal lymphatic drainage or loss of integrity of the tube-opening mechanism. Flying or diving may permanently be denied to such individuals. In a series of 37 deserving cases, submucous resection of the nasal septum was carried out, excising the vomer and perpendicular plates with the vomero-ethmoid suture (McNicoll, 1982). Thirty-four patients had their Eustachian canal function restored, as established by an exposure to 2.0 bar. The high success rate in this group of keen volunteers is conspicuous. Apart from proper training, avoidance of predisposing factors such as the above goes a long way towards prevention of middle ear barotrauma.

Delayed-onset otic barotrauma may constitute a diagnostic problem. Typically, it occurs after breathing 100% oxygen in flight. The pilot, perhaps suffering from coryza, seeks medical help for some unilateral hearing loss and ear pain first presenting the following morning. The combination of an oxygen-filled poorly venting middle ear and the insidious development of negative pressure, perhaps during sleep by the absorption of oxygen, may provide the explanation (Comroe *et al.*, 1945).

The transmural diffusion into the middle ear cavity of another gas, nitrous oxide, can increase the middle ear pressure during general anaesthesia and rupture of the tympanic membrane has been attributed to this cause (Owens *et al.*, 1978; Bailie and Restal, 1988). Nitrous oxide is some 30 times more soluble in blood than nitrogen. When it is first added after induction of general anaesthesia, it is rapidly absorbed into the tissues in large quantities. On reaching any surface of the body, some of the newly acquired nitrous oxide is lost by diffusion into the gas space concerned. The rate of diffusion in the reverse direction across such surfaces is initially negligible, because of a low partial pressure of the gas in that space. Thus, diffusion predominates until equilibrium is reached. In the interim, as a transient effect, the total ambient pressure will be increased if the gas space concerned is closed. Increases in transmural pressure of 15 mmHg within 5 minutes of the start of nitrous oxide breathing have been recorded (Mann *et al.*, 1985). This isobaric transient gas transport effect has several practical consequences. Nitrous oxide should not be used during surgical repair of tears in the tympanic membrane. First aid analgesia using nitrous oxide (in the form of Entonox, commonly available in ambulances) is absolutely contraindicated in arterial gas embolism, decompression sickness and related conditions, as its 'bubble amplifier' effect is counter-therapeutic.

Isobaric decompression sickness is a term used to explain skin lesions and severe vestibular damage in deep saturation diving experiments using more than one inert gas (Lambertsen and Idicula, 1975). It is classified as decompression sickness, in that gas bubbles emerge out of solution at tissue boundary layers not normally delineating gas from fluid. Were this criterion abandoned, decompression sickness would properly be regarded as barotrauma, the agent of trauma being gas, its mechanism hypoxic or mechanical.

Facial baroparesis

Compressive ischaemia in the bony canal of the facial nerve is taken as the causative mechanism of Bell's palsy in normobaric clinical practice; it is not surprising that an analogous condition has been described in divers and aviators, though it is uncommon, less than 20 cases having been reported (Eidsvick and Molvaer, 1985). There is little doubt that the dysbaric chain of events starts in a very few individuals only in whom middle ear pressure can be transmitted to the facial nerve. On failure to vent during ascent, the excess middle ear pressure can exceed the capillary perfusion pressure of the nerve trunk and, if sustained, after about 20–30 minutes, a sudden unilateral facial lower motor neurone lesion results.

As with all ischaemic lesions of the nervous system, therapeutic relief is urgent. It may follow successful venting of overpressure using the Toynbee manoeuvre or, in the recompression chamber, an overpressure equivalent to only a few metres of water.

Perilymph fistula

Rupture of the oval or round window membrane with subsequent perilymph fistula was first suggested in 1968 as a possible mechanism to explain sudden profound unilateral hearing loss. In the same year three patients were described after head injury with surgically verified and repaired oval window membrane perilymph fistulas (Fee, 1968). Five years earlier experimental work on cats had shown that perilymph pressures were almost identical to cerebrospinal fluid pressures (Kerth and Allen, 1963). After a number of reported case histories, it became clear that brief but violent events with straining, coughing and sneezing were frequently responsible for rupturing the fenestral membrane of the oval or round windows.

The oval window receives the sound energy from the footplate of the stapes; the round window is believed to increase the compliance of the fluid-filled, and therefore incompressible, transducer system to sound waves whilst damping out irrelevant low frequencies. Rupture of the oval window is less common than that of the round one.

Two different mechanisms of rupture can be distinguished. Intralabyrinth pressure follows ambient pressure with little delay or damping. Should the middle ear pressure fall below ambient because of inadequate ear clearing, both windows and the eardrum will bulge into the middle ear cavity. In such a prestretched state the window membranes, especially of the round window, are vulnerable to the effects of an explosive impulse such as straining, the mechanism of injury being called explosive (Goodhill, 1971). By contrast, implosive injury occurs when a forceful sudden increase in middle ear pressure pushes the stapes as a piston into the labyrinth (Figure 23.2).

The clinical features of perilymph fistula are somewhat varied. Perhaps the most significant feature is profound, usually complete unilateral hearing loss (dead ear). There is a characteristic delay, perhaps overnight, before it develops fully.

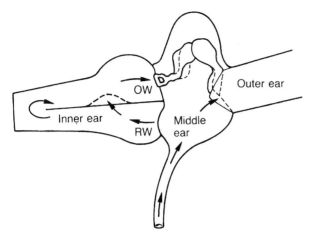

Figure 23.2 A diagram of the air-filled outer and middle ear, and the fluid-filled inner ear. The direction of forces causing perilymph fistula in one of the mechanisms of barotrauma is shown by the arrows. OW = oval window; RW = round window.

The causative event may be accompanied by a 'pop' and 'bubbling' sounds which the subject perceives in the affected ear, followed closely by tinnitus, violent vertigo, disorientation, nausea and vomiting, which lasts for 1–2 hours. In some patients these features persist.

It is the sudden onset of vertigo and disorientation, perhaps in the pilot of a high-performance aircraft, which gives this form of barotrauma its significance in aviation. In diving, the usual cause is an unduly forceful and sudden, impulse-like Valsalva manoeuvre at a point during descent when the Eustachian tube has blocked due to middle ear pressures in excess of 90 mmHg a few metres below the surface. Snorkelling, with its repeated ascents and descents near the surface, seems particularly risky. Correct training goes a long way towards prevention.

Perilymph fistula must be regarded as an acute surgical emergency which requires immediate tympanotomy. No doubt most fistulas heal spontaneously; the objective is to restore normal intracochlear pressure and fluid circulation within days before neurociliary function deteriorates irredeemably. There is probably no longer any justification for conservative expectant management of a unilateral dead ear of sudden onset preceded by a typical history; such a patient has very little to lose on exploratory tympanotomy.

In a diver, differentiating from a (Type II) neurological decompression sickness is difficult and important, since recompression in the case of perilymph fistula would result in further damage. Trial recompression or diagnosis by therapy must be avoided here. Useful diagnostic pointers may emerge on taking a detailed history: type of diving, time and mode of onset of symptoms and the range of symptoms (and findings on examination).

Gastrointestinal barotrauma

In its mild form, this condition is caused by expansion during ascent of gas contained in the intestinal tract, usually the stomach and colon. It rarely amounts to more than discomfort. Occasionally forcible distension of a viscus has been advanced as explanation for syncope immediately on surfacing from a dive.

In all cases of reported rupture, swallowing of air, usually by frightened novices, is involved (Margreiter *et al.*, 1977; Cramer and Heimbach, 1982). The Valsalva manoeuvre performed in the head-down position forces air up the oesophagus, and may be a contributory factor. The stomach is the viscus most at risk, and rupture can occur along the lesser curvature. Radial rupture of the mucosa around the cardia may create a one-way valve mechanism. Experimental work confirms the preferential location of rupture, indicating that overpressure of 96–146 mmHg is required at a filling volume of 1.7–2.0 litres (Margreiter *et al.*, 1977).

It is important to realize that free air in the peritoneal cavity, for example after diving, may not indicate a ruptured viscus, and is not an indication for exploratory laparotomy (Rose and Jarczyk, 1978; Rashleigh-Belcher and Ballham, 1984). Air which has caused pulmonary interstitial emphysema may have tracked along tissue planes to find its way into the abdomen. Occasionally, the time and cause of rupture of the stomach after energetically performed resuscitation of a diver shortly after surfacing is difficult to determine (Halpern *et al.*, 1986).

Barotrauma of the facial sinuses

The paranasal sinuses, though vulnerable, are not affected quite as frequently in diving and aviation as is the middle ear. The frontal sinuses are more frequently involved than the maxillary in a ratio of 2:1, probably because of the narrowness of the nasofrontal duct which is the single ostium of each sinus. Both squeeze and reverse squeeze may lead to barotrauma, squeeze being more frequent.

The pathogenesis is readily understood. On descent either in water or from altitude, if the ostium of a sinus becomes blocked, air will not enter as it should. The resulting negative pressure inside the cavity leads to engorgement of mucous membranes and other vascular structures, transudation and haemorrhage. Pain is a relatively inconspicuous feature. On ascent, ischaemia predominates once the capillary perfusion pressure is exceeded in a blocked rigid-walled cavity. Experiments with intra-antral balloons have shown that about 2–3 hours at an overpressure of 80 mmHg is required to produce pain. Direct pressure within that period of time was well tolerated, which emphasizes the importance of the ischaemic mechanism in pain production.

In practice, the pressure cycle during a conventional bounce dive or a flight lasting 1 or 2 hours in a subject with a partially blocked sinus can cause both negative and positive barotrauma. Painless haemorrhagic transudation may occur first, the mucinous transudate partially filling the sinus and compensating for some of the pressure change. On ascent the initially compressed gas re-expands and the positive pressure so generated may force the obstructed ostium open and eject the offending fluid. In a unique and well-documented case (Leitch, 1969), the weakest point in the wall of the frontal sinus was a recent fracture line in the roof of the orbit. The previous contents of the sinus, including air, had to be evacuated from the orbit. Normally nothing more than a sense of facial fullness is left as a reminder of the haemorrhagic discharge on ascent. When the rate of change of pressure is large and the ascent of an aircraft at, say, 6000 ft/min (1830 m/min) is not readily interrupted, barotrauma may lead to the mucosa being stripped off the wall of a sinus and the cavity filling with blood (Weisman *et al.*, 1972; Fagan *et al.*, 1976).

The severity of sinus barotrauma is graded into three. Class I: mild symptoms which last for a few hours only, slight mucosal swelling and normal X-rays. Class II: symptoms present for more than 24 hours, mucosal thickening is demonstrated on the X-ray film and blood-stained transudate is obtained on aspiration or on spontaneous discharge. Class III: a rare squeeze type with sudden severe pain on descent; a haematoma may completely fill the affected sinus, causing pain for several days (Weisman *et al.*, 1972). Surgical evacuation and repair may be indicated.

Pain and a history of epistaxis are the usual presenting features. Frontal pain is much more common than that over the ethmoid or maxilla. Tenderness on percussing the involved sinuses was only present in 33% of the cases in a series of barotrauma of sufficient severity to show X-ray changes in 80% (Fagan *et al.*, 1976). Neurological clinical features may occur. Pain may be accompanied by unilateral numbness and rarely paraesthesia in the face, upper lip and lower eyelid (Wright and Boyd, 1945).

Their significance is the need to avoid misdiagnosis of neurological (Type II) decompression sickness which should lead to therapeutic compression. Such therapy in sinus barotrauma has the potential to cause significant further injury.

The common cold and other short-lasting pathological processes which cause mucosal swelling are responsible for most barotrauma in the paranasal sinuses. The ball valve action of a pedunculated tumour, usually a polyp, may cause reverse squeeze. A history of chronic sinusitis and rhinitis should eliminate candidates from diving and flying. In a typical series of 50 divers, over half had chronic respiratory problems such as sinusitis, infections or hay fever. In a quarter deviated septa or nasal polyps were present (Fagan *et al.*, 1976).

Lung squeeze

As the breath-hold diver descends with full lungs, the contained gas is compressed and the geometry of the thorax approaches that of the functional residual lung volume. Elastic recoil tends to expand the rib cage passively and generates a transthoracic pressure of approximately 40 cmH$_2$O at functional residual volume. Below this the negative pressure increases rapidly because of the low compliance of the chest wall. Intrathoracic blood volume rises, the governing factor being the distensibility of the great veins and the pulmonary vascular bed. Interstitial and intra-alveolar oedema follows, then petechial and pronounced pulmonary haemorrhage. Consciousness is rapidly lost due to circulatory changes. Once correctly diagnosed, therapy follows the standard principles of intensive care. In hard hat diving, the same sequence may occur if depth is increased without a follow on of supply pressure or if the hose breaks with a concurrent failure of the nonreturn valve.

There are three distinct types of air diving. Free descent and ascent without equipment but holding the breath – breath-hold diving. A metal helmet with a supply of compressed air from the surface by hose with the pressure adjusted so that excess air overflows from the hard hat whatever the depth. Demand valve diving where the valve automatically adjusts to supply the breathing gas at ambient pressure. In the last, lung squeeze cannot occur but in the first two it is a recognized but extremely rare form of barotrauma.

Barotrauma caused by man-made external cavities

A number of divers' ailments can be brought together under this heading. Their common feature is a cavity usually enclosed by an item of the diver's equipment on the surface of the body. Change in ambient pressure may cause painful barotrauma by squeeze or reverse squeeze.

Royal Navy divers in the 1950s equipped with a rubber hood fitting particularly closely around the external auditory meatus noticed a sense of fullness with some bleeding around the ears on surfacing. The divers coined the phrase 'reversed ear', in the mistaken belief that outward bulging of the drum was causative. This incorrect ascription may still be encountered today. Careful inspection through the otoscope shows oedematous skin in the meatus, with petechial haemorrhages and blood-filled bullae, some of which may have ruptured. Experiment indicates that about 100–200 mmHg negative pressure in the auditory meatus is required to reproduce the condition (Jarrett, 1961a). Fourteen cases were collected in the Royal Navy in 4 months of 1960 (Jarrett, 1961b). It is clear that the reserved ear syndrome is caused by external ear squeeze. This type of diver's hood was withdrawn and the condition is rarely seen today.

Face-mask squeeze occurs when the diver fails to exhale into his face-mask during descent; negative pressure develops because the rubber is relatively non-compliant. Capillary dilatation in the conjunctival membranes and nasal mucosa is then followed by petechial haemorrhages. If goggles are worn which do not cover the nose, they must have a small reservoir of air attached in a floppy rubber balloon to prevent conjunctival barotrauma.

Dry suits can never fit perfectly to the diver's torso and, as the air contained between it and the skin is compressed, some of the suit can be thrown into folds. Negative transmural pressure beneath them causes painful red skin lesions in branching lines. Petechial haemorrhages are common, occasionally the skin surface is broken by extravasated blood. The remedy is correct use of compressed air from the suit inflation bottle. This manoeuvre is also a useful means of adjusting the diver's buoyancy when a dry suit is worn.

Painful teeth (aerodontalgia) can be the outcome of raised transmural pressure in the maxillary sinus (see above). A more frequent cause, which may affect mandibular teeth as well, is a small volume of gas trapped underneath a filling. During decompression, such fillings can be lifted, or the tooth shattered. Occasionally a crown is lifted off its stump.

Negative pressure (i.e. squeeze mechanisms during compression) is three times more frequent as a cause of dental pain than is decompression (Shiller, 1965). Aerodontalgia may also be produced in a different way, though the mechanism is unclear. Teeth with damaged pulp or damaged nearby structures may become painful and sensitive to minor stimuli at altered ambient pressure, though asymptomatic under normobaric conditions.

REFERENCES

Albelda S.M., Gefter W.B., Kelley M.A. et al. (1983). Ventilator induced subpleural air cysts: clinical, radiographic and pathologic significance. *Am. Rev. Resp. Dis.*, **127**, 360–5.

Aschan G. (1955). The anatomy of the Eustachian tube with regard to its function. *Acta Soc. Med. Upsalien*, **60**, 131–49.

Astrup J., Symon L., Branston N.M., Lassen N.A. (1977). Cortical evoked potential and extracellular K^+ and H^+ at critical levels of brain ischaemia. *Stroke*, **8**, 51–7.

Bailie R., Restal J. (1988). Otic barotrauma due to nitrous oxide. *Anaesthesia*, **43**, 888–9.

Bayliss G.J.A. (1968). Aural barotrauma in naval divers. *Arch Otolaryngol*, **88**, 49–55.

Bentzinger T. (1950). *German Aviation Medicine in World War II*. Washington: US Govt Printing Office, pp. 404–8.

Boetger M.L. (1983). Scuba diving emergencies: pulmonary overpressure accidents and decompression sickness. *Ann. Emerg. Med.*, **19**, 563–7.

Brown Z.A., Clark J.M., Jung A.L. (1977). Systemic gas embolus. *Am. J. Dis. Child.*, **131**, 984–5.

Calder I.M. (1985). Autopsy and experimental observations on factors leading to barotrauma in man. *Undersea Biomed. Res.*, **12**, 165–82.

Carioli E., Perret C. (1984). Mechanically controlled hypoventilation in status asthmaticus. *Am. Rev. Resp. Dis.*, **129**, 385–7.

Carlon G.C., Howland W.S., Ray C. et al. (1983). High frequency jet ventilation: a prospective randomised evaluation. *Chest*, **84**, 551–9.

Catron P.W., Hallenbeck J.M., Flynn E.T. et al. (1984). Pathogenesis and treatment of cerebral air embolism and associated disorders. *US Naval Med. Res. Inst. Rep.*, 84–20.

Colebatch H.J.H., Smith M.M., NG C.K.Y. (1976). Increased elastic recoil as a determinant of pulmonary barotrauma in divers. *Res. Physiol.*, **26**, 55–64.

Comroe J.H., Dripps R.D., Dumke R.R., Deming M. (1945). Oxygen toxicity. *Jama*, **128**, 710–17.

Cooper M., Mackeen A.D., Janigan D.T., MacGregor J.H. (1989). Delayed sequelae of pulmonary barotrauma. *J. Canad. Assoc. Radiol.*, **40**, 232–3.

Cramer F.S., Heimbach R.D. (1982). Stomach rupture as a result of gastrointestinal barotrauma in a scuba diver. *J. Trauma*, **22**, 238–40.

Crocker W.E. (1955). Principles and techniques of free ascent in submarine escape. *J. R. Naval Med. Serv.*, **16**, 133–40.

Cullen D.J., Caldera D.L. (1979). The incidence of ventilator induced pulmonary barotrauma in critically ill patients. *Anaesthesiology*, **50**, 185–90.

de Latorre F.J., Thomas A., Klamburg J. et al. (1977). Incidence of pneumothorax and pneumomediastinum in patients with aspiration pneumonia requiring ventilatory support. *Chest*, **72**, 141–4.

Dickson E.D.D., McGibbon J.E.G., Campbell A.C.P. (1947). Acute otitic barotrauma. In *Contributions to Aviation Otolaryngology* (Dickson E.D.D., ed.). London: Headley Bros, p. 60.

Durant T.M., Oppenheimer M.J., Webster M.R. (1949). Arterial air embolism. *Am. Heart J.*, **38**, 481–500.

Eidsvick S., Molvaer O.I. (1985). Facial baroparesis: a report of 5 cases. *Undersea Biomed. Res.*, **12**, 459–63.

Evans D.E., Hardenberg H.E., Hallenbeck J.M. (1977). Cardiovascular effects of arterial air embolism. In *Undersea Med Soc 'Workshop' on Arterial Air Embolism and Stroke*. UMS Report No 11–15–17. Washington: Undersea Medical Society.

Fagan P., Mckenzie B., Edmonds C. (1976). Sinus barotrauma in divers. *Ann. Otol. Rhinol. Laryngol.*, **85**, 61–4.

Fee G.A. (1968) Traumatic perilymph fistulas. *Arch. Otolaryngol.*, **88**, 477–80.

Fleming W.H., Bowen J.C. (1972). Early complications of long-term respiratory support. *J. Thorac Cardiovasc. Surg.*, **64**, 729–37.

Francis T.J.R., Smith D.J. (eds) (1991). In *Proceedings: Decompression Illness 'Workshop' at INM*. Bethesda, MD: Alverstoke Undersea Biomed Soc.

Fries C.C., Levowitz B., Adler S. et al. (1957). Experimental cerebral gas embolism. *Ann. Surg.*, **145**, 461–70.

Fryer D.I. (1965). Failure of the pressure cabin. In *A Textbook of Aviation Physiology* (Gillies J.A., ed.). Oxford: Pergamon, pp. 187–206.

Giertsen J.C., Sandstad E., Morild I. et al. (1988). An explosive decompression accident. *Am. J. Foren. Med. Pathol.*, **9**, 94–101.

Goodhill V. (1971). Sudden deafness and round window rupture. *Laryngoscope*, **81**, 1462–74.

Gorman D.F. (1984). Arterial gas embolism as a consequence of pulmonary barotrauma. In *Diving and Hyperbaric Medicine IX. Proceedings of the International Symposium. European Undersea Biomed Soc in Barcelona* (Desola J., ed.). pp. 348–68. Barcelona: CRIS ISBN 84-398-2285-5.

Gorman D.F. (1989). Decompression sickness and arterial gas embolism in sports scuba divers. *Sports Med.*, **8**, 32–42.

Graziano C.C., Kahn R., Howland W.S. et al. (1978). Acute life threatening ventilation-perfusion inequality: an indication for independent lung ventilation. *Crit. Care Med.*, **6**, 380–3.

Greene K.M. (1978). *Causes of Death in Submarine Escape Training Casualties.* Admiralty Marine Technology Establishment Report (E) R78–402. Alverstoke: AMTE.

Halpern P., Sorkine P., Leykin Y., Geller E. (1986). Rupture of the stomach in a diving accident with attempted resuscitation – a case report. *Br. J. Anaesth.*, **58**, 1059–61.

Heiss W.D., Haykawa T., Waltz A.G. (1976). Cortical neuronal function during ischaemia: effects of occlusion of one middle cerebral artery on single unit activity in cats. *Arch. Neurol.*, **33**, 813–20.

Holmstrom F.M.G. (1958). Collapse during rapid decompression. *J. Aviat. Med.*, **29**, 91–6.

Jarrett A. (1961a). Reversed ear syndrome and the mechanism of barotrauma. *Br. Med. J.*, 483–4.

Jarrett A. (1961b). Ear injuries in divers. *J. R. Nav. Med. Serv.*, **47**, 13–19.

Johnson T.H., Altan A.R. (1979). Pulmonary interstitial gas: first sign of barotrauma due to positive end-expiratory pressure therapy. *Crit. Care Med.*, **7**, 532–5.

Kerth J.D., Allen G.W. (1963). Comparison of the perilymphatic and cerebrospinal pressures. *Arch. Otolaryngol.*, **77**, 581–5.

Kindwall E.P. (1973). Massive surgical air embolism treated with brief recompression to 6.0 Atm followed by hyperbaric oxygen. *Aerospace Med.*, **44**, 663–6.

King P.F. (1975). Otic barotrauma and related conditions. *Proc R Soc. Med.*, **68**, 817.

Kizer K.W. (1987). Dycbaric cerebral air embolism in Hawaii. *Ann. Emerg. Med.*, **16**, 535–41.

Klatzo I. (1967). Neuropathological aspects of brain oedema. *J. Neuropathol. Exp. Neurol.*, **26**, 1–14.

Kogutt M.S. (1978). Systemic air embolism secondary to respiratory therapy in the neonate: nine cases including one survivor. *AJR*, **131**, 425–9.

Kumar A., Pontoppiadan H., Falke K.J. et al. (1973). Pulmonary barotrauma during mechanical ventilation. *Crit. Care Med.*, **1**, 181–6.

Lambertsen C.J., Idicula J. (1975). A new gas exchange lesion syndrome in man induced by isobaric gas counterdiffusion. *J. Appl. Physiol.*, **39**, 434–43.

Leitch D.R. (1969). Unusual case of emphysema. *Br. Med. J.*, **383**, 8.

Leitch D.R., Green R.D. (1986). Pulmonary barotrauma in divers, and the treatment of cerebral arterial gas embolism. *Aviat. Space Environ: Med.*, **57**, 931–8.

Lenaghan R., Silva Y.J., Walt A.J. (1969). Haemodynamic alterations associated with expansion rupture of the lung. *Arch. Surg.*, **99**, 339–43.

Lovelace W.R., Gagge A.P. (1946). Aeromedical aspects of cabin pressurisation for military and commercial aircraft. *J. Aero Sci.*, **13**, 143–50.

Luft U.C. (1954). *Handbook of Respiratory Physiology.* USAF School of Aviation Medicine, pp. 134–5. Randolph Field, TX: USAF.

MacFie D.D. (1964). ENT problems of diving. *Med. Ser. J. Can.*, **20**, 845–61.

Macklin M.T., Macklin C.C. (1944). Malignant interstitial emphysema of the lungs and mediastinum. *Medicine*, **23**, 281–358.

McNicoll W.D. (1982). Remediable Eustachian tube dysfunction in diving recruits: assessment, investigation and management. *Undersea Biomed. Res.*, **9**, 37–43.

Mader J.T., Hulet W.H. (1979). Delayed hyperbaric treatment of cerebral embolism. *Arch. Neurol.*, **36**, 504–5.

Malhotra M.S., Wright H.C. (1954). The effect of a raised intrapulmonary pressure on the lungs of fresh unchilled bound and unbound cadavers. *J. Pathol Bacteriol*, **82**, 198–202.

Malhotra M.S., Wright H.C. (1960). Arterial air embolism during recompression, and its prevention. *Proc. R. Soc. B.*, **154**, 418–27.

Mann M.S., Woodsford P.V., Jones R.M. (1985). Anaesthetic carrier gases: their effect on middle ear pressure peri-operatively. *Anaesthesia*, **40**, 8–11.

Margreiter R., Unterdorfer H., Margreiter D. (1977). Positive barotrauma of the stomach. *Zbl Chir (Germany)*, **102**, 226–30.

Marini J.J., Culvert B.H. (1989). Systemic gas embolism complicating mechanical ventilation in the Adult Respiratory Distress Syndrome. *Ann. Intern. Med.*, **110**, 699–703.

Mellor S.G. (1988). The pathogenesis of blast injury and its management. *Br. J. Hosp. Med.*, **39**, 532–9.

Menitove S.M., Goldring R.M. (1983). Combined ventilator and bicarbonate strategy in the management of status asthmaticus. *Am. J. Med.*, **94**, 898–901.

Moore R.M., Braselton C.W. (1940). Injections of air and carbon dioxide into a pulmonary vein. *Ann. Surg.*, **112**, 212–18.

Owens W.D., Gustav E., Scarloff A. (1978). Tympanic membrane rupture with nitrous oxide anaesthesia. *Anaesth. Analg.*, **57**, 283–6.

Paton W., Elliott D.H., Smith E.B. (1984). Diving and life at high pressures. In *Proceedings of the Royal Society Discussion Meeting, Royal Society (London)*, p. 200.

Peirce E.C. (1980). Cerebral gas embolism (arterial), with special reference to iatrogenic accidents. *HBO Rev.*, **1**, 161–84.

Petersen G.W., Baier H. (1983). Incidence of pulmonary barotrauma in a medical ICU. *Crit. Care Med.*, **13**, 67–9.

Polak B., Adams H. (1932). Traumatic air embolism in submarine escape training. *US Navy Med. Bull.*, **30**, 165–77.

Rashleigh-Belcher H.J.C., Ballham A. (1984). Pneumo peritoneum in a sports diver. *Injury*, **16**, 47.

Richter K., Loeblich H.J. (1978). Fatal decompression sickness. *Z. Rechtsmed.*, **81**, 45–61.

Rose D.M., Jarczyk P.A. (1978). Spontaneous pneumo peritoneum after scuba diving. *JAMA*, **239**, 223.

The Royal Navy Diving Manual (1991). BR 2806. London: HMSO/MOD.

Schaefer K.E., McNulti W.P., Carey C., Liebow A.A. (1958). Mechanisms in development of interstitial emphysema and air embolism on decompression from depth. *J. Appl. Physiol.*, **31**, 15–29.

Schriger D.L., Rosenberg G., Wilder R.J. (1987). Shoulder pain and pneumoperitoneum following a diving accident. *Ann. Emerg. Med.*, **16**, 1281–4.

Shilling C.W. (1933). Expiratory force as related to submarine escape training. *US Nav. Med. Bull.*, **31**, 1–7.

Shiller W.R. (1965). Aerodontalgia under hyperbaric conditions. *Oral Surg.*, **20**, 694–7.

Siegel J.H., Stoklosa J.C., Borg U. et al. (1985). Quantification of asymmetric lung pathophysiology as a guide to the use of simultaneous independent lung ventilation. *Ann. Surg.*, **202**, 425–39.

Steir M., Ching N., Roberts E.B., Nealon T.F. (1974). Pneumothorax complicating continuous ventilatory support. *J. Thorac. Cardiovasc. Surg.*, **67**, 17–23.

Teed R.W. (1944). Factors producing obstruction of the auditory tube in submarine personnel. *US Nav. Med. Bull.*, **44**, 293–306.

Tremonti L.P., Halka J. (1972). Death due to pulmonary air embolism in bronchial asthma: case report. *Military Med.*, **137**, 194–5.

US Navy Diving Statistics Jan – Dec (1977). Norfolk, VA: Navy Safety Center.

Van Allen C.M., Hrdina L.S., Clark J. (1929). Air embolism from the pulmonary vein: a clinical and experimental study. *Arch. Surg.*, **19**, 567–99.

Violette F. (1954). Physiological effect of explosive decompression and its mechanisms. *Med. Aeron.*, **9**, 223–71.

Waite C.L., Mazzone W.F., Greenwood M.E., Larsen R.T. (1967). Dysbaric cerebral air embolism. In *Proceedings of the 3rd Symposium on Underwater Physiology* (Lambersen C.J., ed.). Baltimore: Williams and Wilkins, pp. 205–15.

Weisman B., Green R.S., Roberts P.T. (1972). Frontal sinus barotrauma. *Laryngoscope*, **82**, 2160–8.

Woodring J.H. (1985). Pulmonary interstitial emphysema in the adult respiratory distress syndrome. *Crit. Care Med.*, **13**, 786–91.

Wright R.W., Boyd H.M.E. (1945). Aerosinusitis. *Arch. Otolaryngol.*, **41**, 193–203.

Zimmerman J.E., Dunbar B.S., Klingenmaier C.H. (1975). Management of subcutaneous emphysema, pneumo-mediastinum and pneumothorax during respirator therapy. *Crit. Care Med.*, **3**, 69–73.

Zwillich C.W., Pierson D.J., Creagh C.E. et al. (1974). Complications of assisted ventilation: a prospective study of 354 consecutive episodes. *Am. J. Med.*, **57**, 161–70.

24. Acceleration Injury

D. Glaister

With the exception of chemical and thermal insults, most injuries result from the application of excessive forces to the body as a whole, or to specific areas of the body. Since force is numerically equal to mass multiplied by acceleration, and the mass involved will usually be constant, trauma can generally be characterized in terms of the resulting acceleration. Thus, a blow from a hammer will cause the underlying tissues to be displaced over a given period and undergo measurable and predictable accelerations. However, the displacements, forces and accelerations will vary over a very wide range with distance from the impact point. The concept of acceleration tolerance is usually restricted to instances in which the whole body moves effectively as a single mass (a rearward-facing passenger in an aircraft crash, for example), or to head impacts in which the head can be considered as a mass freely mobile about the neck. This chapter will concentrate, therefore, upon these two aspects of acceleration injury and, since the injuries can largely be prevented by appropriate protective measures, it will also discuss methods of protection.

WHOLE-BODY IMPACT

Mechanical principles

Acceleration is the rate of change in velocity and so can be simply calculated from a known (or estimated) stopping distance in any accident in which an overall velocity change has occurred. Thus in a car crash, for example, the stopping distance can usually be estimated from the measured deformation of the vehicle structures or from the deformation of another vehicle, pavement furniture, trees or other objects. If the velocity before impact is known or can be assumed, then the average deceleration is given by the relationship

$$V^2 = 2as$$

where V is the pre-impact velocity (in m/s); a, the acceleration (in m/s/s); and s, the stopping distance (in metres). Accelerations are usually expressed in units of G, the ratio of the measured acceleration to that of normal gravity ($g = 9.81 \, \text{m/s/s}$). So, by rearranging and taking $g \simeq 10$, the average acceleration

$$G = \frac{V^2}{20s}$$

and may be easily calculated and applied to known human tolerance limits. It is important to stress that

this is the average acceleration and implies a rectangular acceleration/time pulse, most unlikely to be seen in practice. Usually, the acceleration pulse is very irregular with several peaks and troughs and a tendency to increase terminally as any energy-absorbing structures 'bottom out'. If one assumes a triangular pulse, the peak acceleration is twice the average value as calculated above and this probably gives the best rough estimate of the forces involved in a vehicle collision (or head impact). Any traumatic effect of acceleration on the body will be proportional to the magnitude of the force.

Other factors affecting human tolerance to impact

Velocity is a vector quantity, having direction as well as magnitude. It follows that acceleration, the rate of change in velocity, is also a vector quantity. Thus, in determining the effects of acceleration on the body, its orientation relative to the force vector becomes a second important determinant of human tolerance. Note that it is the inertial reaction (equal and opposite to the acceleration vector, as propounded in Newton's third law of motion) that determines the pathophysiological response. Thus, a headwards acceleration ($+G_z$) tends to displace body organs and blood towards the feet and evokes quite a different physiological response to that of $-G_z$ (footwards) acceleration or from forces acting in the front to back ($\pm G_x$), or lateral axes ($\pm G_y$). This three-coordinate system of acceleration terminology was standardized by Gell (1961) and is illustrated in Figure 24.1. Needless to say, forces are not restricted to these three orthogonal axes but can occur in any direction or rotate about the body during the accident sequence. However, at any one instant all forces acting on the body can be resolved into a single vector having a measurable magnitude and direction.

A third factor which affects human tolerance to acceleration is the length of time for which the force acts. It is intuitively apparent that a very short-lasting acceleration will have less effect than if the same force is applied for a long time. The product of acceleration and time is velocity, and the kinetic energy which must be dissipated by bringing the body to rest is equal to its mass (a constant) multiplied by the square of the initial velocity. The SI unit of energy is the Joule and is the unit commonly used in references to energy dissipation in head impacts and head impact protection (1 Joule (J) is the energy acquired when a mass of 1 kg is accelerated at $1 \, \text{m}^{-2}$ through a distance of 1 m and is equal to 1.36 ft 1bf. Consequently, a mass of 1 kg, raised 1 m against the Earth's gravitational acceleration, acquires a potential energy of 9.81 J).

The above relationships would be adequate descriptions of acceleration events were the human

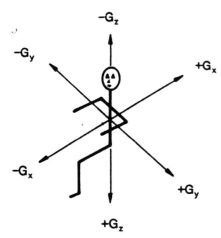

Figure 24.1 Definition of inertial force vectors using the three coordinate system proposed by Gell (1961).

body a rigid mass. In mechanical terms however, it consists of very many masses coupled together by springs and dampers and its dynamic response to impact forces is complex. One very simple model has proven useful in assessing aircraft ejection forces in relation to their potential to produce compression fractures of the spine. As illustrated in Figure 24.2, this treats the body as a system with a single degree of freedom and a single lumped mass, spring stiffness and damping coefficient (Payne, 1962). In such a model the output (spring compression, or peak compressive force in the spine) is related to the acceleration input in a manner determined by the ratio between the acceleration pulse length and the natural period of oscillation of the mass/spring system (about 8 Hz for the average seated adult male). For very long pulses, the system

reaches equilibrium and output and input acceleration are identical. However, for very brief short pulses (pulse length ≪ natural period), the spring will still be compressing up to the end of the input pulse and the output force will be attenuated. Under these conditions the response becomes proportional to the induced velocity change and is a further reason for using this parameter in describing human tolerance to impact forces.

A critical situation occurs when the pulse length approximates to the natural period. Then the spring will start to rebound and its stored energy will be returned coincident with the peak input force – termed 'dynamic overshoot'. Without damping, an amplification factor of × 2 can be induced in this way.

These relationships are illustrated in Figure 24.3 which plots the peak acceleration needed to produce unit output against the pulse length/natural period ratio. Note that the left-hand portion of the relationship has a 45 degrees slope since any point gives the same product of acceleration and time, or velocity change. To the right, the line becomes horizontal (response simply dependent upon peak acceleration), while the intermediate dip represents the dynamic overshoot. This curve has been calculated for a triangular acceleration pulse, but exactly the same considerations apply when a plateau level of acceleration is attained at differing rates of onset. Onset rate, the rate of change of acceleration (termed 'jolt'), is measured in G per sec (m/s/s/s) and is a critical factor in the design of aircraft ejection seats in which the sustained rocket thrust must be reached as rapidly as possible to maximize clearance from the aircraft structure, using explosive cartridges and telescopic gun tubes. Ideally, the dynamic overshoot should be constrained to occur during the rising phase of the acceleration profile so

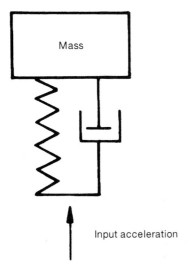

Figure 24.2 A simple lumped parameter model for spinal compression as developed by Payne (1962).

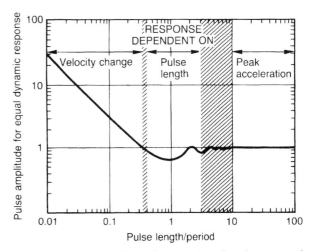

Figure 24.3 The effect of pulse duration (expressed as a proportion of the natural period) on the amplitude of the triangular acceleration pulse needed to give an equal dynamic response in a simple dynamic system. (After von Gierke, 1964.)

that the required plateau level of acceleration is not amplified and the risk of spinal fracture kept to a minimum.

Two further factors which determine the response of the body to acceleration are the site of application of the force and the use of restraint systems. A localized application of force is obviously going to produce local deformation and even penetrating injury, without necessarily accelerating the body as a whole, while restraint systems can be utilized to spread the forces over body strong points and so reduce local pressure effects. A fundamental concept of crashworthy design as applied to any passenger vehicle is the requirement to spread impact forces over as large an area of the body as possible, by use of restraint systems, air bags, deformable panels and, best of all, a rearward-facing seat with adequate head restraint. In this way contact forces are kept as low as possible and the flailing of limbs or head, with further risk of injury, prevented. In his studies to define pure acceleration tolerance, Stapp (1951) used head, arm, upper torso and leg restraints in addition to a conventional full aircraft harness (Figure 24.4).

Most data on human acceleration tolerance have been obtained from healthy young adult male volunteers and relatively little is known about other groups, though females and the elderly of either sex would be expected to have a weaker bone structure. A curious feature of much accident data has been the apparently high tolerance to impact forces of the inebriated (Snyder, 1963). Though possibly anecdotal, this could be related to a lack of muscle activity producing a more yielding body response.

Tolerance criteria

There are two major sources of data on human tolerance to impact forces. First, impact devices

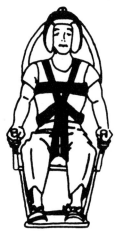

Figure 24.4 The full torso, limb and head restraint system used by Stapp (1951) in human impact studies.

(accelerators or decelerators, drop towers and ejection rigs) in which impact levels are gradually increased until the volunteer withdraws, either because of the onset of unacceptable symptoms suggesting an underlying soft tissue injury or because of belief that a further increment will indeed produce such symptoms. The measurement of physiological variables – pulse rate, blood pressure, hormone levels – is unlikely to be helpful as their critical 'pathophysiological' levels are also poorly defined. Obviously, motivation has much to do with the tolerance levels achieved in such experiments and ethical considerations make it even harder to approach true thresholds for injury.

The second source is the investigation of accidental exposures to whole-body impacts in which survival, injury or fatality can be related to estimates of the forces involved. In most of these, however, injury will be due to localized forces, particularly to the head or limbs and the criterion of uniformly applied force is rarely met. Free falls into water, or soft snow, are possible exceptions.

The definition of tolerance also depends upon the situation. A compression injury to the spine is acceptable if the alternative is failure to escape from a crashing aircraft while, at the other end of the scale, a moving walkway would be considered to produce unacceptable accelerations upon boarding were any passengers to fall.

Pathophysiology of inertial forces

It is not intended to go into details of the pathological changes likely to be seen if impact tolerance levels are exceeded, since these are covered elsewhere. A wide spectrum of injuries is likely from muscle and ligament strains and tears, through injuries of the bony skeleton, to ruptures of abdominal and thoracic viscera. Most of these injuries could be prevented by proper immobilization and/or restraint during the impact sequence but, because the heart is a massive organ surrounded by low-density and yielding lung tissue, it will be displaced by inertial forces and fatal injury will result if the elastic limits of the major blood vessels are exceeded. Similarly, the diaphragm offers inadequate support to abdominal viscera, a further major site of damage from excessive inertial forces.

Sustained acceleration exerts its major effect through hydrostatic pressure gradients in the vasculature, and inertial displacement of the circulating blood. Excessive $+G_z$ forces ($+5G_z$, or more) lead to cerebral ischaemia and, 5 or 6 seconds later, to loss of consciousness. Ethical considerations have prevented acceleration studies from being prolonged beyond this endpoint, though loss of consciousness appears to be a protective mechanism, aimed at ensuring a horizontal posture and improved cerebral circulation, rather than the first symptom of irreversible brain damage (Glaister and Miller, 1990). Voluntary exposures to sustained accelerations – either on centrifuges or in aircraft – have produced no significant short-term, nor any documented long-term, disorders. Presumably, were the acceleration stress to be continued and the posture maintained, the persistent cerebral ischaemia would lead to permanent brain damage and death.

Lower levels of sustained $+G_z$ acceleration lead to dimming of vision or 'greyout', as the intraocular pressure of some 20 mm Hg impedes retinal artery inflow. Cerebral blood flow may remain unimpeded or even be somewhat assisted by a subatmospheric pressure developed in the jugular venous outflow – the so-called jugular siphon (Henry et al., 1951). Symptoms first appear in the peripheral parts of the visual fields as the more distant branches of the retinal artery have reduced perfusion pressures. Then, with increasing acceleration, visual loss spreads centrally with coning and tunnelling of the visual fields, until blackout supervenes. Note that this is still a retinal perfusion problem and full cerebral function is maintained for a further $+1G_z$ increment until cerebral blood flow becomes compromised and unconsciousness (G-induced loss of consciousness, or G-LOC) ensues. For an unprotected subject, peripheral vision is lost on average at $+3.6G_z$, blackout occurs at $+4.0G_z$ and G-LOC at $+5.0G_z$, though there is considerable subject variation with a standard deviation around these figures of about $\pm0.8G$.

A further factor affecting tolerance is the rate at which the acceleration level is reached. Thus, a slow onset, say 0.1G/s, allows baroreceptor reflex mechanisms to be activated with an increase in tolerance of about 1G. Sustained acceleration also leads to an exaggeration of the normal gravitational inequalities in blood and gas distributions within the lung. This leads to significant falls in arterial oxygen saturation, closure of dependent airways with gas trapping and to acceleration atelectasis, a condition in which soluble trapped gas is absorbed to cause collapse of dependent lung zones. Needless to say there are measures which can be used to increase tolerance to sustained $+G_z$ acceleration such as anti-G straining manoeuvres, anti-G trousers, positive-pressure breathing and appropriate body positioning. For a full description of the physiology of sustained acceleration and counter-measures, the reader is referred to a specialist textbook such as Ernsting and King's *Aviation Medicine* (1988).

Human tolerance to impact forces

From the earlier discussion it can be predicted that human tolerance curves should have the general form shown in Figure 24.3 but exhibit wide variations depending upon the degree of body restraint, G vector and selected tolerance criterion. For any particular impact condition, it should be possible to state two threshold values, a maximum acceptable velocity change (for short-duration impacts) and a maximum acceptable plateau acceleration level (for longer-lasting events). The trough caused by dynamic overshoot has, however, only been satisfactorily demonstrated for the particular case of aircraft ejection (see Chapter 14). A similar trough would be expected for each specific injury mechanism but the paucity of experimental data and scatter of human response has precluded identification of any other example.

In that it has become customary to express human impact tolerance in terms of plots of acceleration versus time, the form of presentation used in Figure 24.3 has been adhered to though additional figures are included in Figures 24.5 and 24.6 for the velocity change and plateau G thresholds. In order to simplify the presentations, impacts are divided into two categories: those such as falls which normally occur vertically (Figure 24.5); those such as vehicle collisions which normally occur horizontally (Figure 24.6). This is an arbitrary classification because the critical vector is not Earth's gravity – which has only a very minor influence – but the alignment of the body in relation to the resultant impact vector.

Vertical impacts

Figure 24.5 illustrates impact tolerance curves for lying, seated and standing subjects exposed to a vertical force vector. The logarithm of acceleration is plotted against the logarithm of time and points of equal velocity change lie on a 45 degrees slope from top left to bottom right. The data given are for

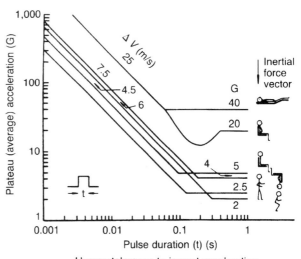

Human tolerance to impact acceleration

Figure 24.5 Tolerance to whole-body impacts in the attitudes and restraints indicated in the inset diagram, for a perpendicular inertial force vector. For a body brought to rest by the impact, the initial motion would have been in the same direction.

idealized rectangular pulses but, as pointed out earlier, irregular-shaped pulses are more likely to be seen in practice. A more representative triangular pulse would have a peak value twice that seen here for the same pulse width but the quoted velocity changes would be the same and provide a more meaningful tolerance criterion.

Figure 24.5 also demonstrates that the highest tolerances are seen when the impact forces are uniformly distributed and the lowest are found for a standing, unrestrained subject. Thus, the uppermost curve represents an impact applied through a form fitting couch or a fall onto a conforming surface such as deep soft snow with the force vector in the $+G_x$ direction. Under these conditions a velocity change of the order of 30 m/s can be tolerated without injury, and there have been spectacular cases of survival following falls from great heights such as those reported by Snyder (1963). Given such a uniform load distribution, comparable tolerances would be expected for $-G_x$ and $\pm G_y$ impacts, though difficulties in supporting the anterior chest wall and face, and the greater potential displacement of the heart within the thoracic cavity, suggest that tolerance levels may be lower for these vectors (Figure 24.6). The right-hand portion of the $+G_x$ line in Figure 24.5 shows that 40G can be tolerated for up to 1 second but this horizontal line cannot be extrapolated beyond a few seconds as physiological endpoints similar to those discussed earlier take over from structural ones and become limiting.

The other curves in Figure 24.5 all refer to $+G_z$ impacts with differing restraints and postures, as indicated by the stick figures. The seated figure with torso restraint represents aircraft ejection and illustrates the trough in tolerance for impacts lasting around 200 ms (Figure 24.3). Without restraint, tolerance for a seated subject falls dramatically, as might be expected because, depending upon the precise force vector in relation to the centres of mass of head and thorax, the body will tend to slump forwards. Tolerance figures of 5 m/s and 5G are relevant for a seated subject.

Studies on the feasibility of escaping from large military aircraft by downwards ejection gave tolerances of 8 m/s, but only 4G, the crossover relative to the other curves being the consequence of the fact that though reasonable load distribution could be provided by lap and shoulder harness, haemodynamic effects within the circulation produced unacceptable symptoms at head level.

Data on unrestrained subjects come from three main sources: centrifuge studies on locomotion; drop rigs; and cages which can be accelerated vertically by precisely controlled hydraulic rams to simulate the heave of a ship's deck which can follow the nearby detonation of a mine. Again, the two curves exhibit a crossover because flexed legs can absorb a greater velocity change without injury

by acting as energy absorbers (as in jumping, or parachute landing) but are less able to support an increased body weight. Voluntary tolerance in these tests tends to be limited by leg pain but in military situations (such as deck heave) it is the secondary impacts which can occur following upward projection or falls which cause injury, most commonly to the head (Glaister, 1974).

Horizontal impacts

Figure 24.6 illustrates, in the same format, human tolerance curves for impacts in which the force vector is generally horizontal to the Earth's surface. The uppermost curve represents a forwards-facing impact ($-G_x$) for a seated subject with a full body restraint system similar to that illustrated in Figure 24.3. It also applies to a rearwards-facing impact ($+G_x$) provided that there is an adequate head support and that a lap belt is in place to prevent the subject rebounding out of the seat. The tolerance levels are the same for the upper curve of Figure 24.5, as are the force vectors. The second curve shows that a simple torso restraint reduces $-G_x$ tolerance significantly, as the head is now free to be thrown forward to sustain high angular accelerations with the potential for brain injury and sternal fracture from chin contact. This curve is also applicable to $\pm G_y$ impacts with the body fully supported (Weis *et al.*, 1963). Simple lap belt restraint permits a comparable velocity change (10 m/s) but a lower sustained G with all the forces being taken on the small area supported by the belt around which the body is free to flex, or 'jack-knife' (Ryan, 1962).

The addition of a head support is patently of no benefit in a $-G_x$ impact though the head may rebound from the chest to cause overextension of

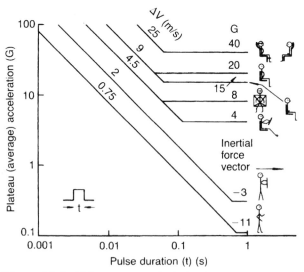

Figure 24.6 Tolerance to whole-body impacts in the attitudes and restraints indicated in the inset diagrams, for a horizontal inertial force vector.

the neck and 'whiplash'. Comparison of the curve of $-G_x$ and a lap belt only with the uppermost, $+G_x$, curve demonstrates the enormous gain in tolerance potentially achieved by simply turning the seat around to face rearwards (see p. 318).

Tolerance to lateral ($\pm G_y$) impacts decreases dramatically if the head is free to move sideways. Voluntary exposures are limited by neck pain and, presumably, soft tissue injury at levels of about $\pm 8G_y$. With only a steering wheel and foot pedals for support, a car driver can sustain the same 5 m/s velocity change but if this is sustained for more than 100 ms, arm strength becomes insufficient to prevent forwards displacement of the torso at forces greater than about $-4G_x$.

The data for the lower two curves of Figure 24.6 are from studies on passenger conveyers (Browning, 1974). The tolerance criterion is based on public acceptance of a transport system which even an elderly person, encumbered with shopping or a suitcase, must be able to use without injury or discomfort. This is obviously far more stringent than in other studies using highly motivated fit young volunteers and often militarily acceptable pass/fail criteria where some risk of injury may be acceptable provided that the subject can still perform his allotted task. The lower tolerance of about 1 m/s and 0.1G was obtained for a free standing subject while the addition of a grab handle (as on the platform of a double-decker bus) increases these figures to 2 m/s and 0.3G respectively.

Protection against impact forces

The data summarized in Figures 24.5 and 24.6 were mostly obtained in experimental exposures of volunteer subjects in which the inertial load distributions were clearly determined by the configuration of the couches or seats and by the restraint system used. In all circumstances adequate space was available around the subject to permit free movement of the head and limbs and to preclude secondary contact injuries. In real accidents these ideals are rarely achieved, though the concept of a 'safety capsule' has been applied to the design of racing cars with the obvious benefit of often negligible injury in what would otherwise have been fatal collisions. More usually, relatively rigid objects intrude into the potential strike envelope of the head and limbs and serious contact injuries can result. Any such injury mechanisms are excluded from Figures 24.5 and 24.6 but must be borne in mind. Also excluded is any indication of the scatter of experimental results for this would have concealed the apparently clear influences of restraint and posture on human impact tolerance. Needless to say, there is a very great variation in response and the published tolerance curves should be used with caution in the design of any impact protection system.

Figure 24.6 shows that appropriate body positioning and restraint can be applied to achieve a 30-fold increase in acceptable velocity change and an even greater 400-fold increase in plateau G tolerance while the benefit of simply turning a seat around, providing that the impact vector is known, has already been mentioned. The reader need only spare a glance at Figure 24.5 to know what to do in a lift in the event of a cable failure (and if he can persuade any other occupants to lie down first, so much the better).

Vehicle designers must of course consider all aspects of crashworthiness, but one which derives from the shape of the tolerance curves is of great importance. It is noted for example that, with appropriate restraint, a velocity change as great as 30 m/s can be sustained without significant injury. However, 40G for up to 1 s is also acceptable and this represents a velocity change of 400 m/s. Thus, if the duration of the impact can be extended beyond the inflexion points in the curves, greater velocity changes become tolerable. This is the principle behind crush zones, energy-absorbing seats, deformable panels and protective padding and is illustrated in Figure 24.7. Unfortunately, the limit to the protection available is given quite simply by the increased stopping distance which must be provided. To come to rest from 400 m/s in 1 s at a constant 40G requires some 200 m and an energy absorber which will deform uniformly and inelastically over this whole distance. Though this may appear not very practical, good results have been obtained by applying this principle to aircraft and car components and even to aircraft seats, particularly those of helicopters.

Of the potential secondary impacts, those to the head are the most important because of the great risk of fatal injury or permanent brain damage. If

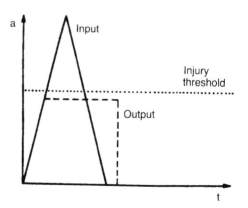

Figure 24.7 By placing an 'ideal' energy absorbing system between the input force and the body, the peak force experienced (the output of the system) can be kept below the injury threshold. The crush properties of the system must be carefully controlled and it must provide sufficient stopping distance to preclude its 'bottoming out'.

contact injuries cannot be avoided by design, then the addition of specific head protection is an acceptable alternative. The tolerance of the head to impact and the mechanisms of head protection provide the subject matter for the following section.

HEAD IMPACT

Tolerance

Two mechanisms for brain injury are discussed here, neither of which need involve deformation of the skull. The first is excessive linear acceleration with the production of diffuse axonal injury due to cavitation effects (Ward *et al.*, 1948), while the second is caused by excessive angular acceleration with the production of surface contusions and disruption of bridging veins (Löwenhielm, 1977; Voigt *et al.*, 1977). In that protective helmets are used to mitigate the effects of penetrating and non-penetrating blunt injuries but inevitably permit the application of controlled levels of linear forces, the mechanics of head protection also merit discussion.

Linear forces

Ward *et al.* (1948) proposed that concussion, or even greater levels of brain injury, might result from excessive linear acceleration of the head in the absence of any local deformation of the skull. They suggested that, because of its inertia, brain tissue would be subjected to brief hydrostatic pressure effects, positive pressures occurring beneath the site of application of force and negative pressures developing at distant sites as the skull accelerated away. If tissue pressures fell low enough, even transiently, then bubbles of water vapour would form (cavitation) which would subsequently collapse implosively as pressures returned to normal, so causing intense local shear forces and tissue damage. A comparable effect may be seen in ship's propellors where the bronze is in time eaten away by imploding cavitation bubbles on the low-pressure face of the blades.

Subsequently, Lissner and Gurdjian (1960) produced concussion in experimental animals by the application of negative pressure pulses through burr holes, and Lindgren (1966) recorded similar negative pressure waves in experimental impacts (Figure 24.8). Some doubt has been cast on much of the early work, in that in experimental impacts designated as 'linear', the heads of the animal subjects were not prevented from undergoing secondary rotation. Thus, Genarelli *et al.* (1972) found it very difficult to induce concussion in squirrel monkeys when the head was constrained to move only linearly, so supporting Holbourne's (1943) thesis that 'shear strains are the cause of (brain) injury, whereas compression and rarefaction strains are not'.

Research work at Wayne State University, Detroit, culminated in the publication of the 'Wayne State Concussion Curve' – an attempt to relate human tolerance to the linear acceleration level and duration (Figure 24.9). It must, however, be noted that three regions of this curve refer respectively to: the fracture tolerance of cadaveric skulls; experimental concussion in dogs (burr hole studies); and human voluntary (whole-body) tolerance to acceleration. The joining of these disparate data by a single curve is to say the least of doubtful validity. Nevertheless, the curve has filled a requirement, especially among engineers, for a single numerical index for tolerance of human head to impact. Mathematical derivatives from it – the Gadd Severity Index (GSI) and, particularly, the Head Injury Criterion (HIC) – have become widely used in crash analysis and vehicle safety standards. However, to

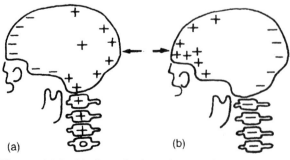

Figure 24.8 Lindgren's (1966) experiment on the intracranial pressure changes produced by head impact. (a) Occipital impact. (b) Frontal impact.

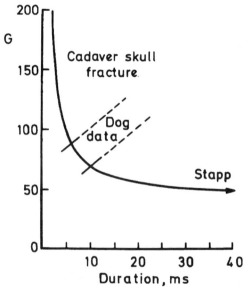

Figure 24.9 Human tolerance to concussion as defined by the Wayne State curve, a plot of peak acceleration (G) against impact duration in milliseconds.

quote from Newman (1982): 'It does not appear at this time, that there is any great validity in those particular criteria'.

Swearingen (1971) reviewed the literature and concluded that, in the absence of deformation of the skull, the brain can withstand forces in the region of 300–400G without concussion. Realistically, these forces must be very transient, since they are far above tolerance levels for the body as a whole (Figures 24.5, 24.6), to which the head must remain attached and share a common overall velocity change.

Angular forces

The mechanism by which brain damage can result from exposures of the head to excessive angular acceleration is easy to appreciate. Inertia of the brain mass and its relative lack of fixation implies that its rotation will lag behind that of the skull. Then, as the cranium rotates relative to the brain, surface bruising (gliding contusions) can result from friction between brain and dura and, if the relative displacement becomes excessive, parasagittal bridging veins will be overstretched and rupture, leading to subdural haematoma. Other damage can occur whenever the brain's motion is resisted by local irregularities in the internal shape of the skull or by the falx cerebri and, in particular, where the brain stem and cord are relatively fixed at the foramen magnum.

Löwenhielm (1977) developed mathematical models based upon the anatomy, and has also used mechanical models and accident analysis to assess the tolerance of the human brain to angular accelerations. He showed that both a critical angular acceleration and a critical angular velocity must be exceeded for injury to be produced. In other words, the excessive angular acceleration must be applied for long enough to attain a critical angular velocity and excessive displacement between brain and skull. His values for tolerance for both bridging vein disruption and gliding contusions are illustrated in Figure 24.10 as shaded areas on a plot of angular velocity against angular acceleration. It may be noted that no axis of rotation is specified, but it is obvious from the complex anatomy of the brain and its non-isotropic 'restraint' within the cranium, that differences in sites of injury, as well as in tolerance levels, will be expected depending upon the axis about which the skull is rotated. Ljung *et al.* (1983) have pointed out that families of tolerance curves would be expected for the three axes of rotation as well as for three major axes of linear acceleration, and indeed for each different injury mechanism. The data presented in Figure 24.10 (and in Figure 24.9) must be considered as approximations and used only as a rough guide in assessing potentials for brain injury.

Unfortunately, research into the effects of rotational forces has, until recently, been hampered by

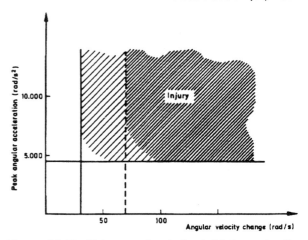

Figure 24.10 Tolerance levels for bridging vein disruption (solid lines) and for gliding contusions (dashed line). Note that critical values for peak angular acceleration and angular velocity must both be exceeded for injury to result. (Reproduced from Löwenhielm, 1977.)

the lack of a simple angular acceleration transducer. Assemblies of 9, or even 11, linear accelerometers have had to be employed with appropriate computation to derive the three-axis rotational data. The development of an oblique impact test for the British Standard specification for protective helmets for vehicle users (BS 6658:1985) was based on the work of Aldman *et al.* (1976) using such linear accelerometer arrays, but could be loosely correlated with Löwenhielm's tolerance data (Glaister, 1986).

Recent studies at the Transport Research Laboratory, Crowthorne (Chinn, personal communication), have used a 9 accelerometer array mounted in a Hybrid II dummy headform in tests based on the BS oblique impact procedure. These have led to the recommendations of maximum pass criteria of 6600 or 9950 rad s^{-2} and 30 or 46 rad s^{-1} (depending upon anvil configuration), values in good agreement with Löwenhielm's human tolerance data, and so providing confidence in the earlier BS specification.

Principles of head protection

Helmets can be designed to protect against the two injury mechanisms discussed above as well as against penetrating and non-penetrating head injuries. A shell, manufactured normally from either a glass-reinforced or thermoplastic material, resists penetration and, together with a buffer layer of foam liner (or space maintained by a suspension system), can prevent a sharp object from reaching the skull. Under these conditions the energy of the impact is absorbed by the liner and transmitted to a large area of the skull at a tolerably low level of linear acceleration (Figure 24.11). Similarly, by resisting deformation, the shell and liner will

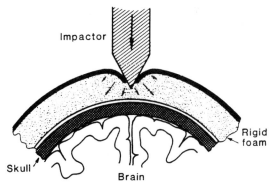

Figure 24.11 The helmet shell and rigid foam liner resist penetration, absorb energy and spread the impact load over a large area of skull surface.

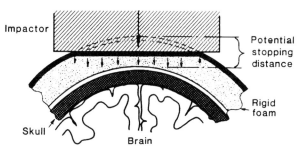

Figure 24.12 The rigid foam crushes at a predetermined pressure to absorb energy over a finite stopping distance and to spread the impact load over a larger area of skull surface.

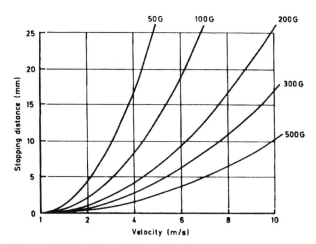

Figure 24.13 The relationship between stopping distance, velocity on impact and resultant acceleration for idealized rectangular pulses.

increase the area over which the impact force is distributed to the head, even for an impact against a flat surface (Figure 24.12). The force per unit area (pressure) transmitted to the skull will be decreased proportionately and deformation of the skull and the potential for skull fracture will be thereby reduced.

For any given velocity change (i.e. the head coming to rest upon striking a solid object), the average acceleration will be inversely proportional to the stopping distance. Thus, an increase in this allows the helmet liner to attenuate the force applied to the head. For reasons of weight and mobility, the maximum liner thickness is restricted to some 25 mm, and Figure 24.13 shows that, under ideal conditions, a velocity change of about 12 m/s could be sustained without exceeding a 300G tolerance level. However, there are no materials available which crush at a uniform 300G (especially as the area being crushed is likely to increase over the course of the impact (Figure 24.12)); most materials, such as the expanded polystyrene foam in general use, 'bottom out' and become stiffer after 70% or so of compression. A considerably reduced velocity change is, therefore, achievable and the

7.5 m/s demanded by the current British Standard (BS 6658: 1985) for an impact of a Type A helmet against a flat anvil comes close to the practicable limit of helmet design.

The limited stopping distance available within the confines of the shell of a practicable helmet contrasts with the far greater crush zones which can be designed into vehicles, or crash barriers. Within any vehicle, therefore, a helmet should be considered only as a last resort in head protection once design and restraint of the occupant can no longer preclude the possibility of a head strike.

An off-axis impact will induce helmet (and head) rotation depending upon friction between the struck object (i.e. road surface) and the helmet shell. Protrusions such as visor mounts can exacerbate this effect and a good helmet is designed to be as smooth and 'slippery' as possible. The potential for actively protecting against rotational forces exists either by letting the helmet surface abrade readily or by introducing controlled slippage between the shell and head (or between concentric layers of liner). A recently introduced 'oblique impact test' measures the reaction induced in an anvil as the helmet shell or any protrusion slides down it (BS 6658:1985). The anvil is faced either with a standard abrasive material or with a series of horizontal steel slats to reproduce potential accidents. The peak tangential force is recorded and used as an index of angular acceleration while the integral of force against time (impulse) is used as an index of the angular velocity achieved during the impact. The application of this test has already led to 'smoother' helmets and freed manufacturers from many preexisting design restraints. The potential exists, by tightening the pass/fail criteria, to force the introduction of active protection in future helmet design.

REFERENCES

Aldman B., Lundell, B., Thorngren L. (1976). Non-perpendicular impacts – an experimental study on crash helmets. In *Proceedings of the IRCOBI 1st International Meeting on Biomechanics of Injuries to Pedestrians, Cyclists and Motorcyclists*, Amsterdam, September, p. 322.

British Standards (1985). BS 6658:1985. Protective Helmets for Vehicle Users. London: British Standards Institution.

Browning A.C. (1974). *The Tolerance of the General Public to a Speed Differential between Adjacent Floors, with Special Reference to Pedestrian Conveyors. Exploratory and preliminary experiments*. Technical Report 74076. Farnborough: Royal Aircraft Establishment.

Ernsting J., King P. (eds) (1988). *Aviation Medicine*, 2nd edn. London: Butterworths, chaps 10, 11.

Gell C.F. (1961). Table of equivalents for acceleration terminology. *Aerosp. Med.*, **32**, 1109–11.

Gennarelli T.A., Thibault L.E., Ommaya A.K. (1972). Pathophysiologic responses to rotational and translational accelerations of the head. In *16th Stapp Car Crash Conference*. SAE Paper No. 720970. November 1972.

Glaister D.H. (1974). *Human response to +G_z ship-shock Acceleration*. Scientific Memorandum No. 109. Farnborough: Royal Air Force Institute of Aviation Medicine.

Glaister D.H. (1978). Human tolerance to impact acceleration. *Injury*, **9**, 191–8.

Glaister D.H. (1986). Protective helmets for motorcyclists – a new British Standard (BS 6658). *Injury*, **17**, 376–9.

Glaister D.H., Miller N.L. (1990). Cerebral tissue oxygen status and psychomotor performance during lower body negative pressure (LBNP). *Aviat. Space Environ. Med.*, **61**, 99–105.

Henry J.P., Gauer O.H., Kety S.S., Kramer K. (1951). Factors maintaining cerebral circulation during gravitational stress. *J. Clin. Invest*, **30**, 292–300.

Holbourne A.H.S. (1943). Mechanics of head injuries. *Lancet*, **245**, 438–41.

Lindgren, S.O. (1966). Experimental studies of mechanical effects in head injury. *Acta Chir. Scand. Suppl.*, 360.

Lissner H.R., Gurdjian E.S. (1960). Experimental cerebral concussion. Paper No. 60-WA-273. In *Proceedings of the Winter Annual Meeting of the American Society of Mechanical Engineers*. New York, November/December.

Ljung C., Lindgren S. and Aldman. B. (1981). On the analytical approach to head injury criteria. In *Head and Neck Injury Criteria. A Consensus Workshop*. Washington, DC: Department of Transportation, Highway Safety.

Löwenhielm, C.G.P. (1977). *On Bridging Vein Disruption and Rotational Cerebral Injuries due to Head Impact*. Department of Forensic Medicine and Division of Solid Mechanics, University of Lund, Sweden.

Newman J.A. (1982). Biomechanics of brain injury – a brief overview. In *Head Protection: The State of the Art. Proceedings of University of Birmingham Symposium, September 1982* (Pedder J.B. and Mills N.J. eds), pp. 31–41. Department of Metallurgy and Materials, The University of Birmingham.

Payne P.R. (1962). An analog computer which determines human tolerance to acceleration. In *Impact Acceleration Stress*. Publication No. 977. Washington: National Academy of Sciences–National Research Council.

Ryan J.J. (1962). Human crash deceleration tests on seat belts. *Aerosp. Med.*, **33**, 167–74.

Snyder R.G. (1963). *Human Survivability of Extreme Impacts in Free-fall*. Report No. 63–15. Oklahoma: Federal Aviation Agency Civil Aeromedical Research Institute.

Stapp J.P. (1951). *Human Exposures to Linear Deceleration, Part 2. The forward-facing position and the development of a crash harness*. AF Technical Report No. 5915. Wright Air Development Centre, Ohio.

Swearingen J.J. (1971). *Tolerances of the Human Brain to Concussion*. Federal Aviation Administration Report No. FAA-AM-71–13. Washington, DC: Department of Transportation.

Voigt G.E., Löwenhielm, C.G.P., Ljung C.B.A. (1977). Rotational cerebral injuries near the superior margin of the brain. *Acta Neuropathol.*, **39**, 201.

Von Gierke H. (1964). Transient acceleration, vibration and noise problems in space flight. In *Bioastronautics* (Schaefer K.E., ed.). New York: Macmillan, pp. 27–75.

Ward J.W., Montgomery L.H., Clark. S.L. (1948). A mechanism of concussion: a theory. *Science*, **107**, 349.

Weis E.B., Clarke N.P., Brinkley J.W. (1963). Human response to several impact acceleration orientations and patterns. *Aerosp. Med.*, **34**, 1122–9.

25. Injury from Falls
G. W. Bowyer

INTRODUCTION

The essence of a fall is that potential energy due to height is converted to kinetic energy under the influence of gravity. At impact some of this energy is imparted to the body and may result in injury.

The *Oxford English Dictionary* defines a fall as a dropping down from a height or relatively high position, by the force of gravity. This fits with the concept above but begs the question 'how high is "high or relatively high"?' A broad definition of the height allows for a wide range of injuries. The International Classification of Diseases (ICD9) gives a range of heights in its definition of falls, including slipping or stumbling, through to falls from scaffolding or cliffs. This chapter attempts to resolve the problem of what constitutes 'falls', by considering the *mode* of injury involved.

I will develop the concept of two major modes of injury. Direct injury is immediately anatomically related to the point of impact; indirect injury is more distant. The latter results from forces transmitted through the body or from its deceleration. Using this concept falls can usefully be divided into:

1. Falls resulting in direct injury.
2. Falls resulting in direct *and* indirect injury.

A scientific foundation on which to build an understanding of injury from falls requires consideration of the physics and biomechanics involved. The former is not complex but there are misunderstandings which have found their way into the medical literature and which may be avoided if the subject is approached from first principles. The biomechanics, particularly of deceleration and transmission of forces within the body, may be unfamiliar to many medical readers, so a theoretical and experimental background is provided in this chapter.

The few medical publications dealing specifically with falls tend to concentrate on heights causing death or serious injury, such as falls from buildings or bridges. However, there are lessons to be learnt from these papers, as they give an indication of indirect injury patterns. Thus, falls from buildings and bridges may be used as a paradigm for falls which produce both direct and indirect injury.

Direct trauma principally involves the musculoskeletal system and its soft tissue covering. Injuries depend on the part which impacts, and are therefore diverse. To avoid producing a catalogue of orthopaedic injuries, I will concentrate on the skeletal injuries resulting from a single cause – military parachuting. The literature on parachuting offers information on injury which results from falls in a narrow range of velocities, almost exclusively to the musculoskeletal system and largely by direct trauma. Parachuting injury will therefore serve as a paradigm for direct injury.

Reviews of the relevant literature offer an insight into the type of injuries which result from each mode of injury. The injury patterns from direct and indirect trauma will therefore be discussed, along with the factors which determine the likely injuries. The trauma will be considered from a mechanistic perspective. Particular attention will be paid to those injuries which may be difficult to diagnose if not suspected and actively sought. Thus, management will be discussed from the viewpoint of potential pitfalls in diagnosis and treatment and the effect of optimum management on outcome. The importance of appreciating the potential effects of indirect trauma will be emphasized.

PHYSICS OF FALLS

Velocity of fall – basic equations

For a fall to earth from a height it is appropriate to assume that the acceleration due to gravity is constant during the fall and, for a free-fall, is the only acceleration which the body experiences.

It is accepted that the force of gravity varies slightly from place to place on the earth's surface, by a factor of about 0.3%. There is also variation with distance from the earth's centre of mass, but by a negligible amount for falls which are in the order of metres rather than kilometres. Hence for a body a distance x from the Earth's centre of gravity, where time is t:

$$\mathrm{d}^2x/\mathrm{d}t^2 = \text{Constant} \qquad (25.1)$$

This constant is commonly referred to as 'gravity' or g, and is about $9.8\,\mathrm{m/s^2}$. Integrating both sides of equation (25.1) with respect to time:

$$\mathrm{d}x/\mathrm{d}t = gt + k \qquad (25.2)$$

where k is $\mathrm{d}x/\mathrm{d}t$ at $t = 0$, the initial velocity, which for a body falling from rest, is zero. Integrating equation (25.2) with respect to time:

$$x = kt + 0.5\,(gt^2) + \mathrm{h}$$

where h is a constant, representing the height of the body at $t = 0$, i.e. the height from which the body fell. Rearranging for t, and putting in the initial conditions for initial velocity (0) and height of the fall (h):

$$t^2 = 2\mathrm{h}/g$$

Substituting into equation (25.2):

$$\mathrm{d}x/\mathrm{d}t = g_{\backslash}(2\mathrm{h}/g)$$
$$(\mathrm{d}x/\mathrm{d}t)^2 = 2gh$$

Velocity, v, after a fall from rest from height h, is given by:

$$v = \sqrt{(2gh)} \qquad (25.3)$$

Velocity of fall – correction factors

The equations above are true for a fall in a vacuum; however, during a fall in the earth's atmosphere the body experiences drag or air resistance, which is itself a function of the body's velocity, presented area and the air density.

Work by Cotner and Early in the 1960s, referred to by Snyder (1965b), calculates velocity using a constant drag factor based on a standardized body surface area, standardized clothing and a constant orientation (horizontal). This predicts a terminal velocity of 120 mph (53.6 m/s) for the body in this orientation and clothing. In a head-down vertical position the terminal velocity is about 185 mph (82.7 m/s).

No allowance is made in these solutions for changes in orientation during the fall. This factor is of particular importance in extreme falls, since the human body's flexibility and non-homogeneous mass distribution makes it inherently unstable in free-fall. The tendency is towards a head-down falling position but other meta-stable positions may be maintained by voluntary efforts. The effect of this instability, and perturbations in presented area, is to reduce further the velocity but in a manner which is non-linear and difficult to predict.

These calculations also make no allowance for differences in clothing, which may act to increase drag and hence slow a fall. However, reports which suggest that skirts act as a parachute (Lukas et al.,

1981; Harvey and Solomons, 1983) are entirely anecdotal and improbable.

The solution for velocity at impact produced by Snyder (1965b) has been utilized in several subsequent reports (Lukas et al., 1981; Harvey and Solomons, 1983; Fortner et al., 1983), to give a more realistic prediction of velocity at impact than that produced by equation (25.3). However, Lewis et al. (1965) misrepresented the situation by simply calculating the height which would allow 120 mph (53.6 m/s) (terminal velocity) to be reached, using equation (25.3), and stated that terminal velocity is reached in a fall from 482 ft. (147 m). This is of course incorrect, as it effectively implies that the drag forces which limit velocity suddenly act at terminal velocity. In reality the retardation acts throughout the fall, as a function of the velocity reached, so a more accurate figure for the height required to reach terminal velocity is around 570 m. The error made by Lewis et al. (1965) has persisted in subsequent work, which quotes them as the authority (Isbister and Roberts, 1992).

Other authors prefer to use the simple equation (25.3), which gives an error of less than 5% for jumps of up to 23 m. This error is probably less than that made in estimating the height of the jump: several publications convert a reported height to an equivalent number of 'floors', or vice versa, but the conversion factor varies from 3.7 m (Isbister and Roberts, 1992) to 4.5 m per floor (Steedman, 1989).

An approximation for velocity reached after a fall of known distance, and for two orientations, is given in Figure 25.1. It must be emphasized however that this assumes air conditions to be uniform and of standard sea-level density. Thus the terminal velocities are for 'low-level' free-fall.

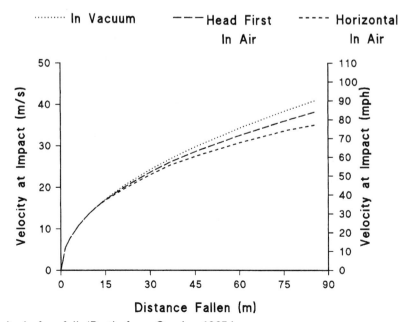

Figure 25.1 Velocity in free-fall. (Partly from Snyder, 1965.)

For falls at very high altitudes this assumption does not hold. The fastest velocity achieved in free-fall was 625 mph (279.4 m/s) attained by Captain J.T. Kittinger in 1960, when he jumped from a test balloon at 31 333 m, reaching his greatest velocity at an altitude of 27 430 m, before landing safely by parachute (*Guinness Book of Records*, 1991).

A parachute acts to increase the drag of a falling body, to the extent that terminal velocity is then low enough to make the descent relatively safe. Actual descent speed will vary with the type of parachute, the weight of man and equipment and meteorological conditions. For a typical military parachute the vertical descent rate is 5.6–6.5 m/s (Pirson and Verbeist, 1985). This is equivalent to jumping from a height of 1.6–2.2 m. However, an important factor to consider is the ground speed – the velocity relative to the ground, due to the wind blowing the body and the canopy; this may be reduced by the inherent drive in certain steerable parachutes. Parachuting is usually restricted to conditions where the wind is below 16 knots (8.23 m/s), since the ground speed generated has a clear effect on injury rates (Essex Lopresti, 1946; Pirson and Verbeist, 1985; Lillywhite, 1990).

Deceleration on impact

Changes in velocity result when a falling body impacts a surface. The body is decelerated, and the unit of measurement conventionally used in considering the deceleration acting is gravity, or *G* forces (actually only strictly speaking a force when the mass is taken into consideration but mass is assumed to remain constant). As noted in equation (25.1) above, the acceleration due to gravity, *g*, is 9.8 m/s^2.

As an example of deceleration forces, if a body of mass 50 kg falls at 19.6 m/s, and is brought to rest in 0.1 s, then it experiences a deceleration of 196 m/s^2, or 20*g*. The force of the ground reacting on it as it comes to a halt is 50 kg × 20*g* = 1000 Newtons, or 20 times the force when it is standing at rest on the ground – its weight is effectively increased 20-fold.

From the preceding example, it is apparent that the quicker a body is brought to rest, the greater will be the forces acting on it. The rate at which it gives up its kinetic energy, as it decelerates, depends on the surface on which it impacts. On a relatively yielding surface, such as a safety net, the energy is given up slowly, but on a relatively unyielding surface, such as concrete, the time period of deceleration is much shorter, and hence the forces on the body are much greater.

It should be appreciated that from the point of view of forces acting in deceleration, it does not matter if the body bounces back up, in that it has been brought to zero velocity momentarily between falling and bouncing (i.e. deceleration has been complete). Of course from the viewpoint of energy dissipation, the bounce is of great importance, representing kinetic energy which has not been dissipated within the body or impacted surface at the point of impact. Bouncing will also lead to a secondary impact, and repeated deceleration, with the potential for further injury.

Duration of deceleration

Some confusion has arisen in the literature when deceleration analysis has been applied to the human body falling from a height onto a hard surface such as concrete. Snyder (1963) reported the minimal deformation in a concrete slab which results when a man falls onto it (maximum deflection without cracking of the order of 0.2 mm or less); it may be inferred that the duration of deceleration must therefore be extremely short, in the order of tenths of a millisecond. This type of calculation has been taken up by others (Lewis *et al.*, 1965; Isbister and Roberts, 1992). The calculations are themselves correct but an error arises in assuming that the human body acts as a homogeneous rigid structure during this deceleration.

The analysis of the forces acting in this brief period as a human body comes to a halt is complex; the body is of course non-homogeneous and the whole body is not brought to rest in the same manner. Snyder himself makes the point that the body is heterogeneous and viscoelastic: that is, its resistance to a force varies with the rate at which the force is applied.

The G forces at the point of impact will indeed be very great, but the deformation brought about in the body tissues and structures act to damp the deceleration and greatly reduce the deceleration force at other, distant, parts of the body. Experimental studies of rapid human deceleration have shown this phenomenon of differential rates of deceleration very clearly (Stapp, 1951; Evans *et al.*, 1958; Swearingen *et al.*, 1960). These results are considered in detail below in the section on experimental deceleration. They allow an insight into the injuries which may result from deceleration and the factors contributing to human tolerance of deceleration forces. The differential rates of deceleration lead to tension in tissues, and inertia becomes a mechanism of injury (von Gierke, 1967).

Rate of change of deceleration

An important factor in determining the human tolerance to deceleration is the rate of onset or change in the deceleration (the third derivative of distance with respect to time, d^3x/dt^3). When gravity is the only force acting, then the rate of change is zero, but when a body impacts after falling, it experiences deceleration which may change rapidly, depending in great part on the material which it impacts. Hence a fall onto concrete results in a very rapid onset of deceleration, or a high 'jolt' factor. It is this factor, or rate of change of deceleration, which distinguishes the response in this situation from a G force of similar magnitude applied gradually in an experimental centrifuge or in a rocket at lift-off.

There is considerable evidence that the rate of deceleration – as well as its magnitude – are of importance in determining the body's responses and injuries (Rushmer *et al.*, 1946; Stapp, 1951, 1957; Cook and Mosely, 1960; Swearingen *et al.*, 1960) and these will be discussed below.

Kinetic energy dissipation

The falling body converts its potential energy (due to its height) into kinetic energy due to its motion. In the consideration of velocity attained in a fall, it was observed that some energy is expended in travelling through the air at a given velocity and orientation.

At impact a body comes to a halt (even if only momentarily before rebounding). In doing this it must give up its kinetic energy. The magnitude of the kinetic energy, and the way in which it is dissipated determines the changes to the body's tissues. If certain tolerance limits are exceeded, then injury results.

The body may transfer energy to the surface with which it impacts, deforming it either temporarily or permanently. The reactive force of impact on the body is either absorbed by the tissues underlying the impact (which may result in direct injury), or is transmitted to distant structures (which may result in indirect injury).

If the surface impacted or the body, undergoes temporary elastic deformation, then it contains potential energy which is released as it reverts towards its original state; this may cause the body to rebound (i.e. kinetic energy is again imparted to the body). The rebound will be to a lesser height than the initial fall, since some energy has been expended at the first impact but the subsequent secondary impact may still be sufficiently energetic to produce further, secondary, injury.

Falls into water

Deceleration by falling into water is an interesting case, and appropriate to consider because it is not uncommon in falls and jumps from bridges (Snyder, 1965a,b; Snyder and Snow, 1967; Lukas *et al.*, 1981; Fortner *et al.*, 1983; Harvey and Solomons, 1983). The more extreme survived falls are usually into water (Steedman, 1989; Isbister and Roberts, 1992).

Falls into water offer the chance of a longer deceleration period, hence lower direct forces of

deceleration, and smaller deceleration differentials in different tissues. Hence a fall into water is likely to be better tolerated than a fall from the same height on to a relatively non-yielding surface.

Hydrodynamics

The manner in which the body is slowed as it enters water was considered by Stewart *et al.* (1955). They discussed the hydrodynamics of a sphere falling into water which effectively carries with it a mass of water equal to a hemisphere of water based on the wetted perimeter of the partially immersed sphere. They applied the principle of conservation of momentum at impact to derive a formula for the resulting velocity of that wetted part of the body plus its associated 'load' of water, and derived an equation for the relative inward velocity of the immersed front. They applied these mathematics to an approximate model of the chest wall at immersion, to show the inward velocity of the chest wall at a given velocity of impact with water. Their subsequent animal experimental work supported the approximations inherent in the mathematical model.

It seems reasonable to apply this model to a body falling into water, with the mass of water effectively associated with the immersed part being related to the cube of the wetted circumference, $f(c^3)$. This gives some insight into the way such a body is decelerated, since the deceleration is related to the associated water volume, hence is related to the third power of the wetted circumference. The presented cross-sectional area is a function of the square of the wetted circumference (since $C = 2\pi r$, and area $= \pi r^2$), hence the deceleration will be a function of the presented cross-sectional area to the power of $\frac{3}{2}$. Consideration of this statement confirms that a smaller presented cross-section will lead to a smaller deceleration and hence lower deceleration forces on the body.

This helps to resolve an apparent inconsistency which was highlighted by Maull (1981), who discussed how force spread over a greater impact area will result in a lower pressure on that area, which may be expected to cause less damage. This is simply resolved if one considers that the pressure (force per unit area) is related to the inverse of the area but that the force itself is related to the $\frac{3}{2}$ power of the area:

$$\text{Pressure} = \text{force}/\text{area}, \quad \text{if area} = a, \text{ then}$$
$$\text{Pressure} = \text{force} \times f(a^{-1})$$
$$\text{Force} = f(a^{3/2})$$
$$\text{Pressure} = f(a^{1/2})$$

Hence the pressure is directly related to the presented cross-sectional area to the power of $\frac{1}{2}$ (that is the square root of the presented cross-sectional area). As the area presented to the water increases, so the pressure increases as well, because deceleration is increased by more than the cross-sectional area is increased.

The deceleration force due to hydrodynamics is related to the circumference of the presented area. If the circumference gradually increases as the body is immersed, then the deceleration applied also changes; hence a conical solid entering apex first, or a man diving, will experience progressively greater retardation through increased hydrodynamic effects as well as the gradually increasing upthrust due to the volume of water displaced. Hence both hydrodynamic and hydrostatic forces produce a lower jolt factor (d^3x/dt^3) as well as lower deceleration (d^2x/dt^2) for a tapered shape than they do for a body of near uniform cross-sectional circumference making the same plunge (as in a belly-flop dive).

Hydrostatics

The other force acting to decelerate a body falling into water is the upthrust due to the weight of water displaced on the Archimedean principle. As more of the body is immersed, so the deceleration force increases, proportional to the volume of the body which is immersed.

There are theoretical reasons derived from stagnation theory for expecting the G forces associated with a fall into water to be five to seven times greater in the prone, supine or lateral orientation than in the head-first or feet-first position (Snyder, 1965b).

BIOMECHANICS INVOLVED IN INDIRECT INJURY

It is important to consider two factors acting at impact which may produce indirect injury. The first is deceleration of the body, and the second is the transmission of the local loads applied to the limbs or body wall. These forces will be considered in turn. Because of the importance of the experimental work on deceleration, and its direct homology with forces acting at impact from a fall, some outline of the experiments is given.

Experimental work on deceleration

From the late 1940s onward, with the development of the jet and rocket engines, much attention has been focused on the effects of deceleration. This was in response to the demand for improved pilot and passenger restraint in aircraft seating and ejection systems in military aircraft. Further impetus was provided by the developing space programme, with its requirement for astronaut safety during the acceleration of take-off and deceleration at re-entry and splash-down.

Experimental work has involved the use of drop-platform systems for inflicting rapid vertical deceleration (Rushmer *et al.*, 1946; Swearingen *et al.*, 1960), or a sled-on-track arrangement (Stapp, 1957; Cook and Mosely, 1960; Becding, 1961).

Rushmer *et al.* (1946) exposed cats in various orientations to abrupt deceleration of between 140 and 1045G peak for durations of 0.002–0.012 seconds. They found the lungs, liver and spleen to be frequently injured, regardless of orientation. They also found that the rate of change of deceleration (d^3x/dt^3) was more important than the total deceleration applied.

The importance of the former factor (d^3x/dt^3) in determining tolerance limits was confirmed by experimental work on pigs, chimpanzees and human volunteers (Stapp, 1957). The important finding was that decelerations of less than 0.2 seconds duration produce no fluid displacements within the tissues or systems and hence did not alter hydrostatic pressures within the body. The latent period for displacement of body fluids is about 0.2 second and their hydrostatic effects become evident by 0.4 second; this is beyond the duration of deceleration experience in impacts from falls.

Von Gierke (1967) has described how the body's natural frequency of oscillation determines its sensitivity to linear impact acceleration. This applies provided that impact duration is less than a value designated τ_{crit}. This value depends on the steady state natural frequency of the system, its damping coefficient and the shape of the impulse. This tolerance changes as the duration of the acceleration varies, and is shown in Figure 25.2. For durations longer than 0.2 second the tolerable acceleration level is constant, at about 20g. These findings for τ_{crit} and tolerance of acceleration/

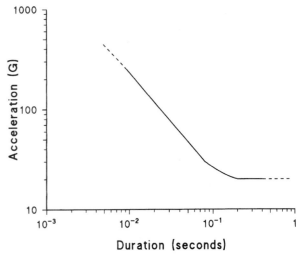

Figure 25.2 Human tolerance to vertical acceleration. (Redrawn from von Gierke, 1967.)

deceleration are consistent with the experimental findings of Rushmer *et al.* (1946) and Stapp (1957).

Cook and Mosely (1960) studied black bears subjected to deceleration (25–125*g* at 1000–9400*g*/s) in a variety of orientations. The most important information was obtained at post-mortem, which showed lesions of viscera and their attachments, many of which were potentially reversible. Lesions around the diaphragm included haemorrhage around the phrenic vessels, the coronary and falciform ligaments of the liver and within the muscular portion of the diaphragm. Other injuries included hepatic damage without rib fractures, contusion of the attachments of the gallbladder to the liver, perirenal bleeds, tears of the gastric mucosa, full-thickness contusions of the gastric wall and contusions of the lower portions of the lung which abut the diaphragm. The mechanism proposed was the upward displacement of the abdominal contents against the relatively yielding diaphragm, or downward traction of the liver on its suspension from the diaphragm; both may occur in the same impact, as the viscera oscillate. Many of these injuries correlate with the subjective complaints of human volunteers undergoing deceleration trials and with sporadic operative findings.

Swearingen *et al.* (1960) investigated human voluntary tolerance to sudden vertical impacts. Tolerances were established by progressively increasing loads until the subject complained of severe pain. Impact loads were measured at the point of contact and at remote sites on the body. The most important finding was the body's ability to effectively damp the transmitted deceleration forces, by landing with feet first and allowing the knees to flex on impact. The deceleration (as measured at shoulder level) which produced severe pain was about 10*g* at 600+*g*/s; however, the magnitude of impact deceleration to produce such symptoms varied more than four-fold, depending on whether knees were locked or allowed to flex on impact. This is illustrated in Figure 25.3; those experiments in which the knees and hips were allowed to flex on impact show a later and more gradual onset of deceleration at shoulder level, with a lower but more sustained plateau, around 5*g*.

The vertical axial orientation may not be optimum for experiencing deceleration (tolerance to *g* is about twice as much in the transverse plane) but the lower limbs are capable of acting as effective shock absorbers. This greatly reduces the level of deceleration experienced by other body structures if impact is taken feet first and the lower limbs flex.

These deceleration experiments were not without risk to volunteers: Beeding (1961) reported the termination of one series of experiments when a man suffered three vertebral fractures (40*g* at 500–1000*g*/s, forward facing).

Transmission of local loads

The transmission of force to the tissues is complex, and involves a variety of mechanisms, depending on the way in which the force is imparted. Both magnitude and rate of application are important in determining the injury pattern. For example: the effects of explosive blast on the body, a cricket ball striking the chest, or a fall from 3 m onto concrete all impart energy to the body. The magnitude of the force is different in each but, in addition, because of the differences in velocity of impact and the momentum involved, there will also be different mechanisms of force transmission within the body. The predominant mechanisms involved in each example are shock-waves, stress-waves and shear waves respectively.

In most falls the impact is relatively slow (tens of milliseconds or more) but of great momentum and the mechanism which predominates are the shear waves. These are transverse waves of low velocity and long duration which produce gross distortion of the tissues (Cooper and Taylor, 1989). The motion may be imparted by distortion of the body wall or transmitted through a limb, and injury is typified by contusion and laceration. The injuries arise from:

1. Asynchronous motion of connected structures of differing inertia.
2. Stress at sites of attachment of viscera set in motion.
3. Collision of viscera with other structures.
4. Compression of a body cavity by pressure from adjacent viscera set in motion.

Each of these mechanisms can be shown to act in various ways in the trauma which result from falls and will be mentioned as injuries are described (see below).

Body's response to forces

The effects of the application of force to body tissues, by either deceleration or transmission of local force, was investigated by von Gierke (1967). He has described the Breaking Index for various human tissues. This is derived from the breaking strength of the tissue, divided by Young's modulus of elasticity (stress required to produce unit increase in length), and is expressed as the fractional increase in length required to break the tissue. Some typical values are 0.3 for the diaphragm, 0.5 for the thoracic aorta under longitudinal stretch, 0.3 for the lower oesophagus under longitudinal stretch and 0.45 for the stomach. These all have a bearing on the injuries seen in extreme falls.

The response of bone and the skeletal system to forces, both direct and indirect, is considered in Chapters 4 and 6.

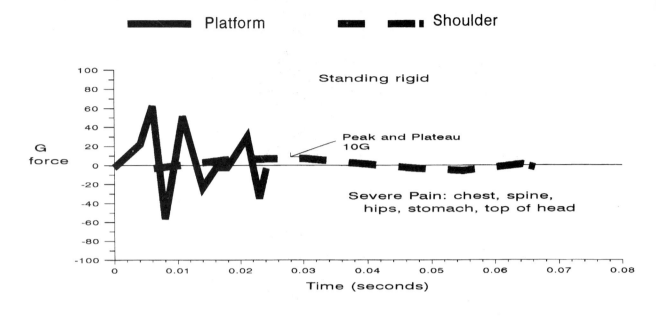

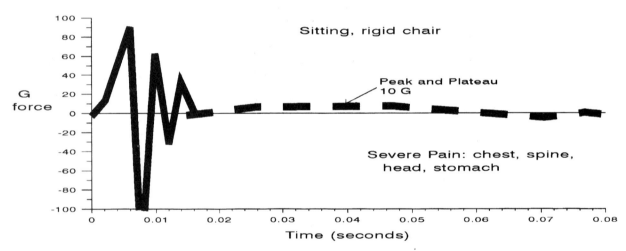

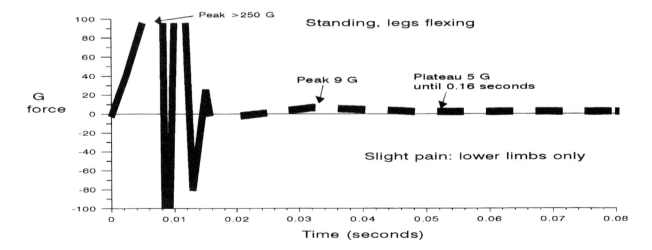

Figure 25.3 Effects of deceleration in various postures. (Reproduced from Swearingen *et al.*, 1960.)

EPIDEMIOLOGY OF FALLS

Incidence

In 1990 there were 3400 deaths from accidental falls in England and Wales (Office of Health Economics, personal communication), a figure based on the broad definition of falls given in ICD9. However, given the current system of reporting, it is not possible to ascertain the morbidity or data on hospital admission as a result of falls. Details of injury resulting from a non-fatal fall will often not have a circumstance or mechanism of injury recorded, and cannot be abstracted from the official statistics. It is also likely that many patients – particularly the elderly – die from complications initiated by the fall but this mechanism is not recorded or reported (Baker *et al.*, 1984).

Age and sex

The population which experiences falls depends on the type of fall being considered, and clearly the possibilities are manifold. The range extends from children falling from cots through to the elderly slipping on the ice or falling at home.

Falls in the elderly may have many contributing factors. The intrinsic factors include neurological, cerebrovascular and cardiovascular disease. In addition, both age and medication may adversely affect their gait, stability and coordination.

Osteoporosis is a major factor in fractures in the elderly, particularly in women aged over 65 years. The condition is morphologically heterogeneous (Lane and Vigorita, 1983) but affects especially the proximal femur, distal radius and vertebrae. Indeed, the commonly used index for osteoporosis involves a grading of the trabecular pattern of the proximal femur (Singh *et al.*, 1970). Fractures at these sites in the elderly often involve abnormal bone.

Extrinsic or environmental factors which may predispose the elderly to falls, include steep or uneven steps and floors, loose carpets, inappropriate footwear and poorly used walking aids.

The causes of fractures in the elderly are clearly multifactorial. There is also evidence that the incidence, particularly of proximal femoral fractures, is increasing. This rise is not simply due to demographic change (Boyce and Vessey, 1985). The problem is such that 20% of orthopaedic beds in the UK are occupied by patients with femoral neck fractures.

At the lower energy end of the range, fracture of the distal radius resulting from a fall has an estimated incidence approaching 0.2% of the population per year (Allfram and Bauer, 1962), with two clear peaks of incidence: in mid-childhood (6–10 years) and in those between 60 and 69 years of age. However, at the more extreme limit of trauma from falling, a study of fatalities shows a different age and sex distribution (Goonetilleke, 1980). The group of accidental falls can be divided into those related to a trade or work, those occurring whilst engaged in 'Do It Yourself' (DIY) type activity and accidents unrelated to work, such as from trees, windows or down flights of stairs. The suicidal falls make a sizeable group, and a further group are those coroner's cases in which an open verdict is returned. Variation in age and sex depending on the circumstances of the fall are demonstrated in Figure 25.4. Others (Lewis *et al.*, 1965; Rozycki and Maull, 1991) also noted this variation in population age and sex, which reflect the circumstances surrounding the fall.

Seasonal trends have been identified, with children frequently sustaining accidental falls in the summer months; adult violence and crime followed a similar pattern (Lewis *et al.*, 1965). A review of falls from Seattle's Aurora bridge – the great majority being suicide attempts – also shows a peak in the late spring and summer months (Fortner *et al.*, 1983).

Geography

There are marked differences in the numerical patterns of falls depending on the geographical location. This is particularly so near certain high bridges, which have become a favoured venue for suicide attempts. This has led to interesting reports on the traumatic effects of falls into water at the Golden Gate Bridge, San Francisco (Snyder and Snow, 1967; Lukas *et al.*, 1983), the Aurora bridge, Seattle (Fortner *et al.*, 1983) and Sydney Harbour bridge (Harvey and Solomons, 1983). Although some victims in these studies were workmen who fell accidently, the majority were suicide attempts, many having travelled considerable distances to their chosen site.

The preponderance of high-rise buildings in a particular area will also influence the demographics of the population suffering falls, a point made by Lewis *et al.* (1965) in their report of fatal falls in Harlem. Pounder (1985) made a similar observation when commenting on the higher frequency of suicide by leaping from high buildings in New South Wales compared to the rest of Australia.

Coexisting psychiatric conditions

Jumping from a height is a relatively uncommon form of suicide – about 5% of all successes. In England and Wales in 1990 there were 143 suicidal deaths from falls/jumps (Office of Health Economics, personal communication). However, there are certain regions, mentioned above, where suicidal jumping makes up a considerable proportion of those who die from falls; in this group psychiatric conditions are common. Goonetilleke's (1980) report of 146 fatal falls in the London area found

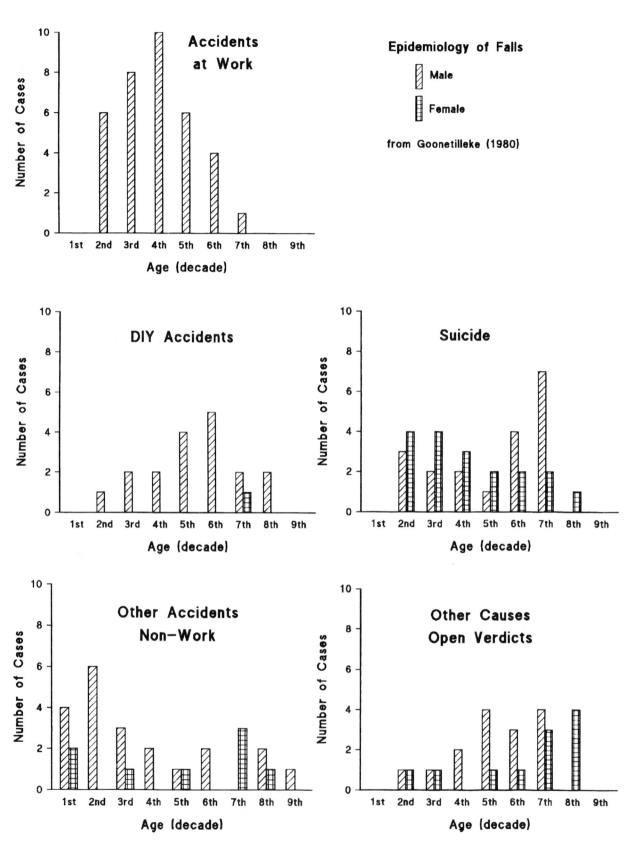

Figure 25.4 Epidemiology of falls. (Reproduced from Goonetilleke, 1980.)

that 25% were suicides, more than 50% of these having a previous psychiatric condition or having previously taken an overdose.

A recent study in Glasgow looked at 60 instances of intentional self-harm by jumping, an important source of multiple injury in that city, with a markedly rising incidence (Isbister and Roberts, 1992). A common pattern was of a young, single, unemployed man. In 72% there was a known psychiatric diagnosis, with psychotic illness in 36% and depression and anxiety in 55%. Drugs or alcohol had been taken before the jump in 32%. Only 15% had neither psychiatric history nor evidence of drug or alcohol abuse; of these nine, five had serious medical conditions which may have precipitated their falls (see remarks on coexisting physical illness below). In Pounder's (1985) review of the increasing incidence of suicidal leaping in Adelaide, he discussed the possibility of media reports prompting copy-cat suicides shortly thereafter. He concluded that media reporting tended to follow rather than precede the deaths and in only two cases was copy-cat behaviour implicated. However, it may be that reporting popularized the method and particular venues (multistorey car parks), possibly increasing suicide attempts by that method at a considerably later date.

A review of psychiatric inpatients who died by jumping, showed that 21 of the 22 fatalities were psychotic, most commonly schizophrenic (Sims and O'Brien, 1979). However, this probably reflects the population in a psychiatric hospital rather more than it does the population of deliberate jumpers at large. The Glasgow figures show 15 with psychosis out of 58 individuals attempting suicide by jumping from a height (26%) (Isbister and Roberts, 1992), and this is close to the Adelaide finding of eight psychotics out of 29 suicides (27.6%) (Pounder, 1985).

Coexisting medical conditions

In patients aged over 55 years, fatalities from falls are most commonly related to pre-existing medical conditions (Rozycki and Maull, 1991). Surprisingly few falls considered here were directly *caused* by a medical condition. Goonetilleke (1980) mentions four in his series of 146 fatal falls: one an epileptic, two with a history of dizzy spells and one asthmatic who fell from a first-floor open window. However, when managing casualties who have suffered a fall, it is important to consider whether there is a medical condition which caused the fall or may complicate the response to injury, such as a seizure, syncopal attack, cardiac arrhythmia or ischaemic heart disease. Rozycki and Maull (1991) identified many pre-existing medical risk factors in those aged over 55 years.

The effects of alcohol and drugs, both prescribed and 'recreational', also require consideration. Alcohol, either acutely or in the context of chronic alcoholism, figures large in several reports of those injured or killed by falls (Lewis *et al.*, 1965; Reynolds *et al.*, 1971; Goonetilleke, 1980). An interesting, and sad, subgroup can be identified in the suicides reported in the series of Goonetilleke (1980) and Isbister and Roberts (1992) – patients under medical investigation or with a serious medical, often neoplastic, condition such as myelomatosis, Hodgkin's disease or other malignancies.

INJURIES

Reports on direct and indirect injury in falls

The medical literature which describes the injuries caused by falls is rather limited, with few accounts dealing specifically with circumstances. As we have seen, series are often selected by the venue of the fall such as a bridge or a specific urban area. The injuries also tend to be at the more severe end of the spectrum, often concentrating on fatal falls, because these are readily identified as a group. However, half a dozen papers have been identified in which the authors have given considerable detail on the injuries sustained by the victims. This allows a picture to be built up of the relative frequency of injuries, qualified by the fact that these represent a very selected subpopulation. Altogether more than 500 cases are included in this collated analysis. It is worth reiterating that these results cannot be pooled to give a figure for the incidence of any particular injury or lesion in a fall; rather they may give an indication of the type of trauma which occurs in patients whose mechanism of injury is labelled as 'a fall' and serve as a paradigm for trauma from direct and indirect mechanisms.

The Tables 25.1–25.4 below indicate the injuries reported for head trauma (Table 25.1), thoracic trauma (Table 25.2), abdominal trauma (Table 25.3) and skeletal trauma (Table 25.4); the reports used are the same in each. Where possible the injuries have been divided into those in survivors and those in fatalities. Where the information is insufficient to allow this, then the overall survival rate for the study group as a whole is given. The data are arranged in the tables such that the group with the lowest mean fall is to the left, highest to the right. For brevity the source papers are indicated only by first authors' name. Further details about the particular studies are provided below:

- *Steedman* (1989) Review of 28 patients injured in falls, between 1981 and 1986, to which the Edinburgh Accident Flying Squad was called. Mean fall was 8.5 m, with two falls into water. Survival rate was 71%.

TABLE 25.1
HEAD INJURES REPORTED

Injury	Steedman (28 falls, mean ht 8.5 m) 71% survived	Reynolds (200 falls, 83% survived)	Lewis (53 falls, > 10m fall)		Goonetilleke 146 falls 100% fatal	Lukas (106 falls, approx 75 m)		Synder (169 falls, approx 75 m) 100% fatal
			22 survived	31 fatal		100 fatal	6 survived	
Skull fracture	7	44[a]	3	16	87	7[b]		40
Facial bone fracture						5		
Brain damage[c]			1	12	105			62[a]
Subarachnoid haemorrhage	2				65	24		
Cerebral contusion	4[d]				15	13		
Subdural haematoma	3				10	5		
Cerebral laceration					10			
Extradural haemorrhage					4			
Concussion	1		16	0				
Fracture, no brain damage[e]					3			14[f]
Brain damage, no fracture[e]					23			31[f]

[a] 14 in survivors, 30 in fatalities.
[b] All basal skull fractures in this series.
[c] No more specific detail available.
[d] Laceration and contusion not distinguished in this series.
[e] Brain damage detected at autopsy, including subarachnoid haemhorrhage, contusions, lacerations and subdural bleeds.
[f] Insufficient data to determine this in most series.

TABLE 25.2
THORACIC INJURIES REPORTED

Injury	Steedman (28 falls, mean ht 8.5 m) 71% survived	Reynolds (200 falls, 83% survived)	Lewis (53 falls, > 10m fall)		Goonetilleke 146 falls 100% fatal	Lukas (106 falls, approx 75 m)		Synder (169 falls, approx 75 m) 100% fatal
			22 survived	31 fatal		100 fatal	6 survived	
Rib fractures	8		3	11	77	71	1	144
Pulmonary contusion	4	3	1[a]	10[a]	19	87[a]	2	
Pulmonary laceration		4			17			129
Pneumothorax	3	7			2	34	3	
Haemothorax	1	3				82		
Bronchial rupture	1							
Haemomediastinum	1							
Myocardial laceration						13		42
Myocardial contusion	1		0	3[b]	13[b]	6		10
Diaphragmatic tear	1							
Atelectasis		2						
Sternal fracture			1	1	17	7		
Hilar laceration					6			
Haemopericardium						21		
Pericardial tear					6	10		
Pericardial bruise					4			
Aortic tear [c]					8	23		38
Vena cava tear						4		11
Pulmonary vessel tear						2		18

[a] Lacerations and contusions of lung not distinguished in this series.
[b] Lacerations and contusions of heart not distinguished in this series.
[c] Anatomy of aortic tears considered further in text.

TABLE 25.3
ABDOMINAL INJURIES REPORTED

Injury	Steedman (28 falls, mean ht 8.5 m) 71% survived	Reynolds (200 falls, 83% survived)	Lewis (53 falls, > 10 m fall)		Goonetilleke 146 falls 100% fatal	Lukas (106 falls, approx 75 m)		Synder (169 falls, approx 75 m) 100% fatal
			22 survived	31 fatal		100 fatal	6 survived	
Splenic laceration	3	4	0	5	2	50	3	a
Liver laceration	2	4	2	10	16	80	2	91
Perinephric haematoma	1					4		13
Retroperitoneal haematoma	1					12	1	32
Mesenteric laceration	2					1		
Mesenteric contusion					8	1		
Pancreatic laceration	1							
Bladder rupture		6	1	1		4		1
Stomach rupture		2						2
Kidney rupture laceration		1			3			4
Kidney contusion					7	1		4
Gallbladder performation		1						
Ileal contusion							1	
Bowel perforation					2[b]			5
Haemoperitoneum						84		
Adrenal haemorrhage						1		5

[a] Not possible to abstract figures for splenic injury from this series.
[b] One case of ileal perforation by a wooden railing.

TABLE 25.4
SKELETAL INJURIES REPORTED

Injury	Steedman (28 falls, mean ht 8.5 m) 71% survived	Reynolds (200 falls, 83% survived)	Lewis (53 falls, > 10 m fall)		Goonetilleke 146 falls 100% fatal	Lukas (106 falls, approx 75 m)		Synder (169 falls, approx 75 m) 100% fatal
			22 survived	31 fatal		100 fatal	6 survived	
Clavicle	1				14	9	2	18[a]
Scapula					4			a
Shoulder dislocation	1		4	0		2		
Humerus	1		2	3	14	14		25[b]
Elbow joint					8			
Radius	2	42[c]	7	1	9	1		b
Ulna	d	18	d	d	d	2		b
Wrist					6			b
Cervical spine	2	1			14	3	2	13
Thoracic spine	2				28	5	4	8
Lumbar spine	5	39[e]	5[f]	7[f]	6	1	2	1
Pelvis	9	35	7	9	31	11		20
Sacroiliac joint					16			
Sacrum					2	1		3
Hip dislocation						1		
Femur	4	13	6	10	17	13		24[g]
Knee joint					3			
Tibia	3	35[h]	5[d]	5[d]	11[d]	11[d]	1	g
Fibula	d	26	d	d	d	d		g
Ankle	1		4	0	4			g
Os calcis	1	22	5	0				g
Tarsal metatarsal		10	3	0				

[a] Clavicle and scapula not distinguished in this series.
[b] Bones of upper limb not distinguished in this series.
[c] Radius and ulna both fractured in 12 cases.
[d] Tibia and fibula and radius and ulna not reported separately in this series.
[e] 85% of vertebral fractures were thoracolumbar in this series.
[f] Vertebral level not distinguished in this series.
[g] Bones of lower limb not distinguished in this series.
[h] Tibia and fibula both fractured in 15 cases.

- *Reynolds et al.* (1971) Review of 200 patients falling in New York City, from 1965–1969, admitted alive to a municipal hospital. Mean fall approximately 13 m, where height was known, all on to ground. Survival rate was 83%.
- *Lewis et al.* (1965) Review of 53 casualties who fell or jumped from three or more storeys (>12 m) in Harlem, New York City in 1964. All on to ground, with a survival rate of 42%.
- *Goonetilleke* (1980) Review of 146 autopsies on victims of falls in London from 1958 to 1978. Falls were all on to ground. All were fatal but 24% were admitted to hospital alive.
- *Lukas et al.* (1981) Review of 100 consecutive autopsies on victims who jumped into water from the Golden Gate Bridge, San Francisco (75 m), from 1972 to 1978. Also a record of injuries to six others who survived the leap in that period.
- *Snyder and Snow* (1967) Review of 169 autopsies on victims who jumped into water from the Golden Gate Bridge, San Francisco (75 m), from 1937 to 1966. All were fatalities.

Difficulties in analysis of reports

There are many difficulties inherent in assessing the data, both within the individual review and across the six series brought together here. They are heterogeneous in many respects, and subject to three of the types of bias which Rudicel and Esdaile (1985) identified in their critique of orthopaedic trials: susceptibility, performance and detection.

Susceptibility bias arises when prognostically dissimilar groups are compared. The degree of trauma to which the casualties had been submitted varied from falls of less than a metre to falls from 75 m. The surface on to which they fell also varied, as did other factors such as body orientation at impact, age and pre-existing disease. The effects of these factors are considered below.

Performance bias is that attributable to different techniques used in treatment. The delay in the casualties receiving medical help varied greatly and the quality of medical care spanning 50 years would also be expected to have changed. The effects of delay and the quality of immediate and subsequent care are discussed below in the section on management.

Detection bias arises when injuries are sought in different ways. Many of the fatalities were subjected to a full and thorough autopsy but others, often within the same series, had only an 'examination and incision' or merely an 'inspection' (Lewis *et al.*, 1965). There are also differences in reporting injuries both in the original post-mortem reports and within the published papers. An example is haemoperitoneum, which would be expected in many of the cases but was only recorded in one of the papers (Lukas *et al.*, 1981). This must not, of course, be taken to imply that it was not more frequently present. Other problems which arise from the grouping together of certain injuries have been highlighted in the tables and accompanying notes.

Further difficulties arise in comparing the findings in the survivors with those who have had an autopsy. Of course many of the more subtle lesions, such as mesenteric contusion, detected at post-mortem examination would not be expected to be diagnosed in the surviving casualty. The clinical problems associated with missed diagnoses in the severely injured are discussed in the section on management.

Injury patterns from direct and indirect trauma

Not withstanding the reservations expressed above, the findings, as tabulated, do give some important information about the injuries caused by both direct and indirect mechanisms in falls. Those highlighted below are the particularly frequent injuries, those of major clinical importance or injuries which may be missed if not carefully sought:

Head
  Skull fracture
  Intracranial haemorrhage
  Brain or brain stem injury
Thorax
  Multiple rib fractures
  Pulmonary laceration or contusion
  Pneumo/haemothorax
  Myocardial laceration or contusion
  Diaphragmatic tear
  Aortic and other great vessel rupture
Abdomen
  Hepatic laceration
  Splenic laceration
  Renal laceration or contusion
  Rupture of a hollow viscus
Skeleton
  Fractures of pelvis/sacrum
  Fractures of vertebras
  Fractures about the ankle
  Fractures of bones of the foot

These injuries, and the mechanisms producing them, are considered in greater depth below.

Direct trauma – parachuting injury

Useful information about skeletal injury may be gained from a study of the injuries caused by military parachuting. Provided that the parachute has not malfunctioned, the rate of descent is roughly equivalent to a jump from a 1.5–2.5 m wall, with the addition of speed along the ground: forward, backward or sideways.

Several papers have reported military parachuting injuries and the injury rate is remarkably

TABLE 25.5

SKELETAL INJURIES IN PARACHUTING (NUMBER OF JUMPS IN SERIES INDICATED IN PARENTHESES)

Injury	Ciccone (600 000)	Neel (174 220)	Kirby (208 000)	Hallel (83 718)	Petras (90 000)
Clavicle	35	1	3		
Scapula	6	4	2		
Shoulder dislocation	39	28	45		
Humerus	38	7		18[a]	6[a]
Elbow dislocation	9				
Radius	16	1	4		
Ulna	5	1			
Wrist	36				
Cervical spine		1	2		
Thoracic spine	129[b]	19	10	23	12
Lumbar spine		76	23		
Pelvis	22	16	4	3	3
Sacroiliac joint					
Sacrum		5	1		
Symphysis pubis separation	8				
Hip dislocation	1	2			
Femur	36	27	9	8	1
Knee joint[c]	93	2	33	7	
Patella	11	2			
Tibia	173	31	18	12	6
Fibula	78[d]	46			
Ankle	1462	56	119	94	41
Os calcis	40		3		
Tarsal/metatarsal	339[e]	16	21	4	2

[a] All upper limb fractures and dislocations grouped together in this paper.
[b] Cases of vertebral disruption, levels not distinguished; two-thirds were single vertebra.
[c] Major knee ligament disruption or dislocation.
[d] Fibula alone – 125 cases of tibia plus fibula.
[e] Phalanges, metatarsals (cases, not fractures) and tarsals excluding os calcis.

consistent, at about 0.5–1% in British, US, Belgian and Israeli forces (Lillywhite, 1990). The injury rate has been at or about this level since shortly after the Second World War (Neel, 1951; Kiel, 1965). The findings from five major reviews of injuries are presented in Table 25.5; taken together these represent the moderate to severe skeletal injuries (excluding skull fracture) resulting from more than 1 million military parachute jumps. For brevity, the source papers are indicated only by first author's name in the table. Further details about the particular studies are given below:

- *Ciccone and Richman* (1948)   Review of 3000 fractures and major soft tissue injuries resulting from more than 600 000 military parachute descents. Series from Fort Benning, USA after the Second World War.
- *Neel* (1951)   Review of injuries from 174 220 jumps at Fort Bragg, USA from 1946 to 1949. Approximately 36% of all injuries reported were fractures or dislocations.

- *Kirby* (1974)   Review of 520 injuries in British soldiers, requiring admission to hospital, from more than 200 000 jumps over a 5-year period, in the early 1970s.
- *Hallel and Naggan* (1975)   Injuries from 83 718 Israeli Army parachute jumps. Approximately 35% of recorded injuries were fractures or moderate or severe soft tissue injuries.
- *Petras and Hoffman* (1983)   Injuries from 90 000 jumps at Fort Bragg in 1981. Only fractures were recorded in detail in this paper.

The results in these series are subject to much less susceptibility variation than those in more extreme civilian jumping injuries. The vast majority descended in a narrow velocity range (5.6–6.5 m/s), and with an upper limit on ground speed due to wind of about 15 knots. The factors which influence injury rate have been analysed by Lillywhite (1990) and others (Essex Lopresti, 1946; Pirson and Verbeist, 1985). Although there are circumstances, such as operational jumps at night with heavy equipment, which will increase the risk of injury, the range of probabilities of injury is much smaller than that in the more extreme injury group.

The injuries highlighted are the direct ones of impact, usually involving the ankle. Indirect injuries to the thoracolumbar spine are also relatively common. Both these patterns of injury are discussed further below.

Indirect injuries in parachute accidents

The fatality rate from military parachute jumps, generally caused by a failure of the parachute to deploy properly, is about 1 in 50 000 descents. The more severe injuries in the parachute group tend to be the result of a parachute malfunction or a mishap in mid-air which leads to a very rapid descent comparable to a fall from a much greater height than 2 m. This type of malfunction accounts for the overlap between the parachuting injuries and injuries from falls from bridges or buildings. The skeletal injuries then include pelvic fractures; visceral injuries of the deceleration and indirect type may occur. These have been reported in fatalities from parachuting (Kiel, 1965), and include pulmonary laceration, cardiac injury and aortic rupture.

Factors influencing the injury pattern

The discussion of the physics of falls (above) has already highlighted factors which may be expected to influence injury. These are:

- Height.
- Orientation of the body, and impacting part.
- Surface impacted.
- Other factors such as meteorology and environment.

The importance of subsequent medical attention in determining the outcome which results from injury is discussed in the section on management.

Height
Several reports have shown a direct relationship between the height fallen and survival (Lewis *et al.*, 1965; Reynolds *et al.*, 1971), illustrated in Figure 25.5. The height fallen also correlates with the extent of injury as measured by the Injury Severity Score (Steedman, 1989).

Visceral injuries have been shown to be common in falls of more than 6.1 m (Steedman, 1989). Hepatic injury has been demonstrated in 43% of falls over 15 m but in only 4.7% of lower falls (Goonetilleke, 1980). Other reports have given the mean height for pelvic fracture as 11 m and for multiple rib fractures as 12 m (Steedman, 1989).

However, the relationship between height fallen and injury sustained is not simple, being confounded by the other factors already discussed.

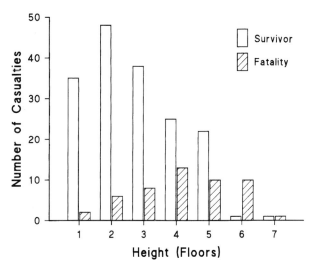

Figure 25.5 Outcome related to height fallen. (Reproduced from Lewis *et al.* (1965) and Reynolds *et al.* (1971).)

Snyder (1963) was unable to show a clear height/trauma relationship for falls to the ground nor for falls into water (Snyder, 1965a). Goonetilleke (1980) also found the relationship between severity of brain injury and height fallen was non-linear.

Orientation
Body orientation at the point of impact is of importance in determining both injury pattern and mortality.

Snyder (1963) popularized a standard notation for direction of force at impact which has been adopted by subsequent authors. It is based on the direction that a body organ would be displaced by the acceleration (deceleration at impact is a negative acceleration). The z axis is the longitudinal axis of the body, the x axis runs antero-posteriorly from umbilicus to small of back and the y axis transversly from flank to flank. In Snyder's 1963 series the majority of falls were $+G_z$: that is vertical landing, feet first. The next most common was $-G_z$, that is head first; a buttocks-first landing is a special case of $+G_z$.

Goonetilleke (1980), in the fatal falls he reported, carried out a thorough analysis of the injuries sustained in each orientation. The findings for skeletal injury are largely as would be intuitively expected: lower limbs injured almost exclusively in $+G_z$ falls, upper limbs mainly in side impacts but also common in feet-first falls, because of secondary impact. The incidence of deceleration-type indirect injury (discussed further below) was highest with feet and buttock impact.

Snyder (1965b) investigated the critical velocity for survival of a fall into water (the velocity above which 'few' survive). He reported this as just over 30 m/s, corresponding to a fall of about 50 m, but emphasized the importance of body orientation in determining survival. He reported the highest survived impacts in his series as: 26.5 m/s in the lateral position ($-G_y$), 26.8 m/s when prone ($-G_x$), 28.3 m/s supine ($+G_x$) and 29.6 m/s head-first ($-G_z$). One individual survived at each of these velocities, whereas five survived at more than 30.5 m/s in the feet-first orientation. The assertion that the most survivable body orientation for impact with water is the feet-first position seems valid from the clinical findings (Snyder 1965a; Snyder and Snow, 1967) and the consideration of forces (above). Snyder (1965b) proposed an increased safety factor of five to seven times for the $+G_z$ orientation, which seems to have been based on calculations of G forces rather than on actual observations: there were only small numbers in the groups other than $+G_z$ (five or fewer in each other orientation).

Isbister and Roberts (1992) related approximate height fallen and orientation at impact to the approximate 50% chance of survival; this is about one floor for head-first, three to four floors for side-first and four to five floors for feet-first.

Surface impacted

As discussed at the beginning of this chapter, the surface onto which a body falls determines the pattern of deceleration and energy exchange. Cummins and Potter (1970) suggested that in head injury the contact surface may be even more important than the height fallen. Water is obviously a special case, which has also been discussed at some length. In addition, water alters the pattern of limb injuries, with more fractures occurring midshaft, in a configuration suggesting angulation as a mechanism rather than rotation. Foot or ankle fractures were not found with falls into water (Snyder, 1965a). The visceral injuries sustained by those who fell from the Aurora Bridge differ depending on whether impact was on land or water: cardiac, major vessel, CNS and musculoskeletal injuries were all less common in those hitting the water (Fortner *et al.*, 1983).

Other factors

Meteorological factors may play a part in determining injury. Wind may affect the velocity of the body in the same plane as the ground, i.e. forward, backward or laterally, although this effect will be much less marked in free-falls than beneath a parachute canopy. Weather conditions may also have a bearing on the surface, disturbing water surface into waves, or covering the ground with snow or ice.

The effect of water as an *environment* must also be remembered. There are several reports of falls into water where the primary cause of death is recorded as drowning (Snyder and Snow, 1967; Harvey and Solomons, 1983). This may be related to inability to swim, incapacity due to injury or lack of volition. Other hazards presented by the water environment include sharks, with one case in the series reported by Lukas *et al.* (1981) having suffered severe mutilation whilst in the water. The hypothermic effects of cold water may also influence the outcome and need to be borne in mind when managing these patients.

'Miraculous' escapes

There are cases where the height of fall seems to produce disproportionate injury or lack thereof. The record height for a survived free-fall is more than 10 000 m, when Vesna Vulovic survived the disintegration of a DC9 aircraft over Czechoslovakia (*Guinness Book of Records*, 1991). By contrast a fall from less than 1 m has proved fatal (Goonetilleke, 1980).

Numerous reports testify to 'miraculous' survival of what should be considered extreme falls. These have sometimes served to confuse the relationship between height fallen and injury sustained, so it is worth considering some examples:

A man fell from 13.5 m on to granite (Snyder, 1963), survived without loss of consciousness, and walked away though he sustained a fracture of a cervical vertebra and a pubic ramus. These injuries are entirely consistent with such a fall and could easily have had more severe consequences. The case represents someone whose outcome is of lower probability than most but is in keeping with the degree of energy imparted.

A suicide attempt from 21.9 m resulted in cuts alone, sustained when the casualty fell through a skylight (Snyder, 1963). However, it must be appreciated that in breaking the glass of the skylight there would have been considerable deceleration, before striking the ground. Again, the injuries may be at the lower end of the expected range but need not be considered miraculous, other than in the journalistic use of the word.

A soldier parachuting in Alaska fell 374 m when his parachute failed completely to deploy. He landed 'like a mortar round exploding in the snow', creating a 1-m crater, and sustained only a clavicular fracture, a chip fracture of a lumbar vertebra and contusions (Kiel, 1965). The light injuries can be attributed to his relatively slow and gradual deceleration by the thick snow which was composed of alternating layers of soft snow and frozen crust.

It must be remembered that a fall from a given height will result in a narrow range of kinetic energies but that this may be dissipated in a wide range of ways at impact. The energy exchanged at impact will lead to a *probability* of injury but this will be subject to a statistical distribution which, if normal, would lead to half suffering less than the median injury.

INJURY – PATTERN AND PATHOGENESIS

Skull fracture

The pattern of skull fracture in fatalities was classified by Goonetilleke (1980) into five groups. These are:

1. Fractures of the vault, including depressed fractures.
2. Fractures at the level of the brim of a hat.
3. Fractures of the base only.
4. Extensive fractures of both vault and base.
5. Ring fracture separating the rim of the foramen magnum from the remainder of the base.

Lissner and Evans (1956) showed the fracture patterns that may be produced with various impacts, and demonstrated basal fractures following occipital impact (pattern 3 above). They reported that only a small increase in energy beyond that needed to produce a linear fracture would cause extensive destruction of the skull (pattern 4 above). They also demonstrated the considerable shock-absorbing capacity of the scalp, usually of 20 J or more. They found that the energy needed to produce a fracture on the intact cadaveric adult skull (in situations where the skull impacts a virtually unyielding surface) was about 18–55 J and varied between specimens and with the site of impact. Furthermore, Evans *et al.* (1958) showed that the rate of application or absorption of the energy was of great importance in determining the mechanism of skull fracture.

The first four patterns of skull fracture above are attributable to direct head impact, either primary or secondary. However, the ring fractures form an interesting group, associated with feet-first or buttocks-first landing, and are attributable to indirect fracture, the deceleration force being transmitted up the spine to the atlanto-occipital joint. Indirect fracture of the base of skull, as in a ring fracture, occurred only in cases of $+G_z$ impact. Skull fracture is particularly uncommon following falls into water, those which were reported (Lukas *et al.*, 1981) being basal fractures, possibly arising from an indirect mechanism of injury.

Brain injury

A wide variety of brain injury has been reported, and is the commonest cause of death in falls on to land. Brain injury is present in most of those who die and, as would be expected, is present in almost all who die following head-first impacts. However, brain damage is also prominent in more than 50% of those whose impact is in another orientation (Goonetilleke, 1980). A range of intracranial injury has been reported, from extradural, subdural and subarachnoid bleeds to brain laceration or contusion. Four cases of bruising or laceration of the corpus callosum were reported following falls onto the occiput (Goonetilleke, 1980).

It is clear from many reports that brain injury may be present without skull fracture, and vice versa. Brain and skull injury offer the poorest correlation with the height fallen but the severity of brain injury correlates well with probability of mortality.

Gurdjian *et al.* (1961) described the manner in which intracranial pressure may be generated as the head decelerates and the cranium is distorted at impact so that pressure may reach nearly 1.5 atm (152 kPa) for 6 to 12 ms. Shear waves are created at impact which tend to disrupt the mid-brain and the brain stem at the level of the foramen magnum.

Multiple rib fractures

Severe disruption of the bony thorax is a frequent finding in many series of extreme falls; thoracic trauma is the most common cause of death in falls into water (Snyder and Snow, 1967).

The ribs are prone to fracture through direct force and break at the point of impact. Anterior impact – such as a blow to the sternum – produces indirect stress concentration at the posterolateral angle of the rib, and laterally because of the posterior curvature and caudal angulation of the ribs (Cooper and Taylor, 1989). Fractures may occur at these points in several ribs and, with anterior compression, may also be found in the mid-clavicular line.

Viano (1978a) has shown a relationship between thoracic deflection (normalized by dividing the distance deflected inward by thoracic diameter, P/D) and the overall degree of thoracic trauma. However, he also demonstrated that life-threatening thoracic injuries were generated when P/D exceeded 0.32. He postulated that this degree of deflection corresponds to a deformation limit to the thorax. Beyond P/D of 0.32, there is a high likelihood of collapse of the rib cage, with a subsequent avalanche effect, resulting in multiple rib fractures which allow even greater deformation of the thorax. Deformation in the structurally unstable thorax may reach P/D of 0.4, at which point the sternum comes virtually into direct contact with the vertebral column.

Cardiac and pulmonary contusion and laceration

Cardiac contusion and laceration are frequently reported in extreme falls (Snyder and Snow, 1967; Goonetilleke, 1980). Any chamber may be affected, the atria more often than ventricles, but with no preponderance of a particular side when all series are considered. The pericardium may be contused anteriorly or posteriorly, or split open. These injuries are commonly found without rib fractures.

Lung contusion and laceration is a common finding in the more extreme falls with several reports of these injuries in the absence of rib fractures. Laceration and contusion is also noted at the hila of the lungs.

The organs within the thorax are susceptible to indirect injury mediated by shear waves resulting from thoracic indentation at impact. This would explain the contusions at sites remote from direct impact (such as the hilum). The mechanism also accounts for the lacerations which occur in the absence of rib fractures or with contralateral injuries to the chest wall.

Beyond the structural stability limit of the thorax, multiple rib fractures will result allowing direct compression of the heart and lungs between the sternum and spine. Furthermore, jagged ends of broken ribs or the sternum may contribute to the lacerations to these organs.

The heart is susceptible to damage through asynchronous motion and inertial injury and from upward compression by the abdominal contents displaced against the diaphragm. This upward movement may also account for the pulmonary contusions seen at the bases of the lungs (Cook and Mosely, 1960), as these are 'pinched' between the diaphragm and thoracic wall.

Aortic damage

Injury to the aorta and other great vessels occurs in more extreme falls. The force to rupture the aorta probably requires a fall of more than 12 m; no aortic ruptures were present in Steedman's (1989) series, almost all of these falls being of less than 12 m.

The sites of aortic rupture have been carefully studied, as they give a clue to the mechanisms involved. Those recorded in falls (Snyder and Snow, 1967; Lukas et al., 1981) correspond broadly to the pattern reported by Sevitt (1977) from road traffic accidents. The majority occur at the aortic isthmus, at or near the origin of the left subclavian artery but with the ascending aorta – at its root – also a common site.

The possible mechanisms are the subject of debate but the evidence has been summarized by Sevitt (1977) and Viano (1978b). Anatomical factors play an important part: in falls tension is induced by relative displacement of the heart, contributing to rupture at the sites where the aorta is partially fixed. This occurs at the isthmus, just distal to the origin of the left subclavian artery, as the arch undergoes transition to the descending aorta which is firmly held on the posterior wall of the thorax. Other sites of relative fixation include the aortic root and the diaphragmatic hiatus and at these rupture is also common. The ligamentum arteriosum is thought by some (Sevitt, 1977) to exert a pull on the anterior wall of the isthmus, to cause anterior tears but others

doubt its significance (Viano, 1978b). The hilum of the lung passes beneath the aortic arch, and may act as a fulcrum for motion of the heart on the aorta, concentrating stresses at the root or the isthmus.

Movement leading to stresses at these points of fixation may arise from impacts to the chest or deceleration of the body. Blows to the sternum and even laterally on the chest can be shown to displace the heart and aorta (Viano, 1978b; Cooper and Taylor, 1989). In addition, the heart may be displaced relative to the thorax during deceleration. The heart has relatively high inertia, compared to the rest of the thorax, and would tend to continue in downward motion in feet-first falls, stressing its attachments to the aorta (root) and the aorta itself at the transition from isthmus to descending portions. This longitudinal tension would account for the commonly described circumferential tears at the sites where stress is concentrated.

An alternative view is that hydrodynamic forces associated with a sudden rise in aortic blood pressure cause the tears; however, tears due to increased internal pressure would be expected to be longitudinal, whereas those found in falls are circumferential or transverse – consistent with a deceleration or shear mediated mechanism of injury (Sevitt, 1977).

Aortic ruptures are primarily internal, involving the intima and media. The initial false aneurysm is contained by the adventitia and mediastinum and, in consequence, it may be concealed clinically, manifesting later as delayed rupture or a chronic aneurysm. Less commonly the adventitia is also torn, resulting in mediastinal haemorrhage. A complete tear will usually lead to exsanguination and death at the scene of accident; however, some 20% survive hours or even days. This is long enough for operative intervention and repair to be undertaken if the diagnosis is made. The overall survival rate from thoracic aortic rupture is about 15% but paraplegia is a common and severe postoperative complication is a consequence of poor distal aortic perfusion and inadequate flow through the anterior spinal artery supplying the cord (Jamous et al., 1992). The relative roles of the injury and reparative surgery in causing this underperfusion remain controversial.

Chronic aneurysms may result if the lesion is self-limiting and undetected. A fascinating case of a man who jumped from the Aurora bridge on *two* occasions showed that in the second fall he died from rupture of an old false aneurysm of the aortic arch, presumably sustained on his first fall (Fortner et al., 1983).

Many other great vessel injuries are associated with overlying bony injury; it seems likely that in these circumstances direct tearing by bony fragments causes the damage.

Pneumothorax and haemothorax

These injuries occur commonly in association with thoracic trauma. Several of the injuries described above lead to haemothorax or haemomediastinum. Pneumothorax in the presence of rib fractures is explained by rupture of the visceral pleura. However, pneumothorax also occurs without rib fractures for which the explanation is advanced that air leaks from parenchymal tears, induced by shear forces, tracks to the hilum and finally distends the ruptured mediastinal pleura (Harvey and Solomons, 1983).

Diaphragmatic injury

Diaphragmatic injury is infrequently recorded in falls but evidence from deceleration experiments suggests that subtle injuries to and around the diaphragm may be quite common. This is a potentially serious complication of non-penetrating trauma, and may be present in 3–8% of patients who have sustained blunt trauma to the trunk sufficient to require surgical intervention for visceral injury (Johnson, 1988). The mechanism involved is the relative upward movement of the abdominal contents, forced up against the diaphragm, as a result of impact to the abdomen or deceleration (feet first or head first), as the abdominal contents oscillate up and down on impact.

If a tear is neglected or undetected, then diaphragmatic herniation of some abdominal contents is almost inevitable, because of the pressure differential between abdomen and thorax. Hence early diagnosis and repair are essential if late complications are to be avoided.

Abdominal viscera

Damage to the solid viscera, the liver and spleen, were common findings in the group suffering higher falls, particularly those in excess of 12–15 m (Goonetilleke, 1980; Steedman, 1989). The liver seems to be more at risk than the spleen, often with extensive laceration or 'pulpification' (Lukas et al., 1981). These injuries were usually coincident with severe overlying trauma to the bony thorax; direct injury to the organ by rib fractures may contribute to the lacerations but in most cases a further indirect shearing mechanism was also likely.

Contusion and laceration of the kidney was occasionally related to overlying lower thoracic fractures; however, the indirect mode of injury, particularly shear stresses, seems to be implicated in the majority.

The hollow viscera seem less vulnerable than the solid ones. Bladder lacerations and contusions were almost always related to fractures of the pubic rami, their injury pattern being consistent with direct injury by bone ends. Rupture of the gallbladder and avulsion of the gallbladder from its hepatic attachments are compatible with indirect injury through deceleration or shear forces.

Pelvic fractures

The pelvis is fractured in many of the more extreme falls; in parachuting it is usually related to a parachute malfunction or mishap resulting in a faster landing than normal. The pelvis is susceptible to both direct and indirect trauma. In a buttocks-first impact, pelvic fracture was a common finding in Goonetilleke's (1980) series; indirect fracture may result from force being transmitted up the lower limbs, affecting the bony pelvis, hips or sacroiliac joints. Such an indirect mechanism has been investigated by Roy-Camille et al. (1985), in sacral fractures. By comparing clinical and cadaveric findings they demonstrated that the fracture pattern was determined by the position of the lumbar spine in kyphosis or lordosis at impact.

Lissner and Evans (1956) carried out a detailed analysis of the tension induced in the pelvis by static and dynamic loading. It is notable that loading of the ischial tuberosities produces tensile stresses in the ischium, acetabulum, iliac fossae and both pubic rami. Hence direct loading of the ischium (in a buttocks-first fall) could lead to failure of the pubic rami from tensile stress and stressing of the sacroiliac joints. This accords with the reported fracture patterns in a clinical series (Goonetilleke, 1980).

Sacral fracture is easily overlooked in multiple trauma patients (Roy-Camille et al., 1985). There is little indication of the fracture on the standard anteroposterior pelvic radiograph; lateral views and tomography are indicated when the lesion is suspected. There should be a high index of suspicion when the history suggests the mechanism and the casualty has altered perineal sensation.

Spinal fractures

The vast majority of vertebral fractures are about the thoracolumbar junction, affecting either T_{11}, T_{12}, L_1, L_2 alone or in combination with an adjacent vertebra. This pattern holds true in all series, including military parachuting. The commonest pattern is of anterior compression wedge fracture, usually without neurological involvement. A review of thoracolumbar fractures in vertical plunges (Smith et al., 1977) found that the extent of bony injury was directly related to the height fallen and that all patients with neurological involvement had fractures involving the posterior vertebral elements as well as the vertebral bodies.

Flexion forces tend to produce a wedge fracture of the vertebral body, the compression being anterior. However, if there is additional rotation at impact, the pattern is changed, with lateral wedging and an increased risk of posterior element fracture. Direct compression produces end plate disruption but in the majority the pattern suggests forward flexion as the mechanism of injury in the thoracolumbar spine.

Stapp (1957) showed that the human spine has a low failure limit, being particularly vulnerable in vertical deceleration due to its cervical and lumbar lordotic curves (animals such as the chimpanzee without these primary curves are more tolerant of axial G forces). In optimal alignment the human spine can withstand 35G at rates <500G/s, but in hyperflexion this falls to less than 15G at the same rate of onset. Vertebral fractures result from this indirect application of force as the spine undergoes forward flexion and longitudinal compression.

The sequelae of thoracolumbar wedge fractures are generally mild and several reports suggest that they may pass unnoticed. A review of the spine in veteran parachutists showed radiological evidence of wedge fracture (most commonly L1) in 10 out of 46 subjects (Murray-Leslie et al., 1977), but eight of these were unaware of any injury having occurred.

The more extreme trauma in fatalities in falls to the ground (Goonetilleke, 1980) or into water (Snyder and Snow, 1967) results in a greater number of fractures in the cervical and thoracic spine, often associated with contusion, laceration or transection of the spinal cord. In those falling a mean of 6.4 m, spinal injury was present in four out of nine (Steedman, 1989).

Cervical fractures tend to predominate in head-first impacts, and neurological involvement is more common in these than in the thoracolumbar wedge fractures. However, cervical compression fractures may also be clinically silent, as was shown in a study of high-divers in Acapulco (Schneider et al., 1962), which demonstrated old compression fractures in the radiographs of three, each of whom had made the 41-m dive on more than 8000 occasions. None had any abnormal neurological symptoms or signs. It is of interest that the diving technique of those with old fractures involved entering the water with the hands apart, hence taking some of the impact directly on the head; the other three divers locked their hands over the head, and no evidence of cervical spine injury was noted on their radiographs.

Ankle fractures

The common injury pattern arises from torsion, and mostly affects the lateral malleolus. The torsional force arises through the combination of descent and speed along the ground, resulting in inversion plus internal rotation, or eversion with external rotation. Fracture of the posterior malleolus occurs if the talus is forced back up and backwards as the plantarflexed foot contacts the ground. This fracture of the posterior malleolus was labelled a 'paratrooper fracture' by Tobin (1943). During training for parachuting much emphasis is placed on keeping the feet and knees tightly together, to offer mutual splintage (Essex Lopresti, 1946), a technique which altered the rate and pattern of lower limb injuries in the US parachute training schools when it was adopted in 1943 (Lord and Coutts, 1944). In the British Parachute Training School the emphasis is also on a flat-footed landing but the posterior malleolar fracture does still occur if a parachutist reverts to the more instinctive landing with toes pointing down, or 'ballet dancer' position.

Strain of the superior tibiofibular joint was described by Essex Lopresti as a typical parachuting injury, arising as the fibular head springs sideways during a roll on landing. Petras and Hoffman (1983) found that 10% of ankle fractures from parachuting involve a fracture of the proximal fibula, often arising from a long torsional mechanism with disruption of the deltoid ligament and tibiofibular syndesmosis (Maissoneuve pattern). This emphasizes the need to include the joint above when examining ankle injuries clinically and radiologically.

Foot injuries

Fractures of the os calcis are regarded by many as a typical injury from a vertical fall and are relatively common. The mechanism of fracture and a classification of the patterns has been described by Essex Lopresti (1952). The intra-articular fractures may be divided into two major groups depending on the manner in which the posterior facet of the subtalar joint is displaced. In the 'tongue' pattern the posterosuperior part of the calcaneum and the joint facet are rotated, the posterior part going up and the facet going down, as the talus forces down between the facets of the subtalar joint. In the 'joint depression' pattern the force of the talus is directed more posteriorly, as though the impact of landing has been taken towards the back of the heel, on the tuberosity of the calcaneum; the posterior facet of the subtalar joint is forced into the substance of the cancellous bone of the calcaneum. Variations on this classification exist but the fractures involving the subtalar joint remain a challenging clinical problem (Giachino and Uhthoff, 1989).

It is commonly believed that os calcis fracture is often associated with fractures of the lumbar spine; in the series reviewed in this account there were coexisting vertebral fractures in 20–40% of calcaneal fractures (Lewis et al., 1965; Reynolds et al., 1971).

MANAGEMENT

Direct injury to the soft tissues and bony skeleton may present challenging problems and advances in care with improved restoration of function are being made. The diagnostic problems have been mentioned, and a more detailed discussion of management can be found in standard orthopaedic works. The problems associated with indirect injuries are less well defined, so this section will focus on that area, highlighting problems in management and steps which might be taken to improve care.

Problems in diagnosis

A major problem in managing falls is a failure to appreciate fully the nature and extent of indirect injury. The Royal College of Surgeons Working Party on the management of major injury listed the 18 commonest missed diagnoses in a study of 1000 trauma deaths (Anderson *et al.*, 1988). The most frequent were:

- Ruptured liver – 22
- Lung laceration – 18 (4 hilar)
- Ruptured spleen – 12
- Subdural haematoma – 12
- Haemo- or pneumothorax – 9

Other injuries featuring high on the list of missed diagnoses included ruptured kidney (five), perforated bladder (three) and ruptured diaphragm (two). Around 33% of trauma deaths were considered preventable, the majority of preventable deaths being in those without central nervous system injury. These are precisely the injuries which have been highlighted in this chapter, and often result from the indirect mode of injury.

Improving immediate care

Much can be achieved through early skilled intervention in trauma casualties. The effects of pre-hospital care in Seattle have been reported (Fortner *et al.*, 1983), looking specifically at the consequences for casualties falling from the Aurora bridge (50 m). The 'Medic I' programme ensures that paramedics go to the scene and commence care, usually within 15 minutes of the fall. Attention is given to airway control, with 55% of survivors being intubated at the scene. Oxygen is administered, and ventilatory support given when needed, and an intravenous infusion is commenced, with blood being drawn for cross-matching. The paramedics are also able to insert chest drains, and immobilize extremity and spinal fractures. This has been shown to improve the casualties' haemodynamic status and arterial oxygen tension on arrival at the hospital. The result has been an increased overall survival of three-fold when compared with casualties having made the same jump before the introduction of the pre-hospital treatment programme. In addition the injury severity of the patients surviving has increased.

Transfer to appropriate hospital

The report of the Royal College of Surgeons of England on care of the severely injured recommends that patients with life-threatening injury should be treated at a regional trauma centre (Royal College of Surgeons of England, 1988). Studies in the USA have shown markedly improved survival rates when operating such a policy and the philosophy has been summarized by Trunkey (1985).

In order for transport to an appropriate hospital to take place, the casualty needs to be adequately assessed at the scene. It is accepted that assessment of abdominal and thoracic injuries, particularly those arising from indirect trauma, is difficult; there are therefore guidelines in the USA that direct any casualty from a fall of more than 6.1 m to a Level I trauma centre (Champion and Sacco, 1986). The data reviewed in this chapter supports this recommendation, since significant injury to abdominal or thoracic viscera has been shown to be uncommon in lesser falls but to increase in incidence and severity above this height. There may of course be other reasons for transfer to a trauma centre, such as neurological injury or severe skeletal injury, which can result from a lower fall.

Management in hospital

Appropriate hospital management will ensure that the patient is promptly resuscitated and assessed, using the principles of Advanced Trauma Life Support (American College of Surgeons, 1989). A thorough assessment will reveal the injuries listed above. An appropriate trauma centre has the expertise available not only to make these diagnoses but also to act on them operatively where indicated. The majority of preventable deaths are a result of failure to stop bleeding and prevent hypoxia; hence the problem does not extend far beyond the essential ABC – airway, breathing and circulation.

The pulmonary trauma highlighted in falls is, for the most part, potentially reversible. The American and Australian groups reporting extreme falls from bridges have each advocated prompt ventilatory support for those suffering pulmonary contusion (Lukas *et al.*, 1981; Harvey and Solomons, 1983). It is also appropriate to insert chest drains prophylactically in those exhibiting radiographic evidence of pulmonary contusion before instituting mechanical ventilatory support.

Evaluation of the liver and spleen should be a priority in the haemodynamically unstable patient who has suffered a fall. This often proves to be the source of continued bleeding and surgery is generally required. Assessment of the kidneys with an intravenous pyelogram and the bladder by cystogram may be indicated; the former when there is macroscopic haematuria, the latter in pelvic fracture.

Rupture of the aorta is not easy to diagnose; the cardinal radiological sign is widening of the superior mediastinum, but this may not be present, particularly when there is concomitant pneumothorax, haemothorax or surgical emphysema (Bryan and Angelini, 1989). Widening is an indication for aortography.

Neurosurgical and orthopaedic opinion and intervention is often required in those with multiple injuries from falls; there are circumstances, such as intracranial bleeding or pelvic fracture, where this may be life-saving. The medical problems associated with drug or alcohol dependency and withdrawal need to be considered, and coexisting disease also taken into account when planning management.

Some specific considerations peculiar to falls into water are the possibility of hypothermia – manifest by core temperature and by J waves on the ECG – and electrolyte imbalance resulting from near drowning and fresh-water aspiration.

Many problems in the management of multiple trauma patients, such as those suffering high falls, arise from difficulty in diagnosis of the injuries. This is particularly true in those injuries resulting from deceleration or non-penetrating trauma. By considering the scientific basis for these indirect injuries it is hoped that a greater appreciation of the mechanisms will be gained, and the potential for injury recognized.

REFERENCES

Allfram P.-A., Bauer G.C.H. (1962). Epidemiology of fractures of the forearm. A biomechanical investigation of bone strength. *J. Bone Joint Surg.*, **44A**, 105–14.

American College of Surgeons (1989). *Advanced Trauma Life Support Course*. Chicago, Illinois: American College of Surgeons.

Anderson I.D., Woodford M., de Dombal T., Irving M. (1988). Retrospective study of 1000 deaths from injury in England and Wales. *Br. Med. J.*, **296**, 1305–8.

Baker S.P., O'Neill B., Karpf R.S. (1984). *The injury fact book*. Lexington, MA, USA: D.C. Heath & Company.

Beeding E.L. (1961). Human forward facing impact tolerance. *Aerospace Med.*, **32**, 220–30.

Boyce W.J., Vessey M.P. (1985). Rising incidence of fracture of the proximal femur. *Lancet*, **331**, 150–1.

Bryan A.J., Angelini G.D. (1989). Traumatic rupture of the aorta. *Br. J. Hosp. Med.*, **41**, 320–5.

Champion H.R., Sacco W.J. (1986). Triage of trauma victims. *Curr. Ther. Trauma*, **2**, 5–8.

Ciccone R., Richman R.M. (1948). Mechanisms of injury and distribution of 3000 fractures and dislocations caused by parachute jumping. *J. Bone Joint Surg.*, **30A**, 77–97.

Cook J.E., Mosely J.D. (1960). Visceral displacement in black bears subjected to abrupt deceleration. *Aerospace Med.*, **31**, 1–8.

Cooper G.J., Taylor D.E.M. (1989). Biophysics of impact injury to the chest and abdomen. *J. R. Army Med. Corp.*, **135**, 58–67.

Cummins B.H., Potter J.M. (1970). Head injury due to falls from heights. *Injury*, **2**, 61–4.

Essex Lopresti P. (1946). The hazards of parachuting. *Br. J. Surg.*, **34**, 1–13.

Essex Lopresti P. (1952). The mechanism, reduction technique and results in fractures of the os calcis. *Br. J. Surg.*, **39**, 395–419.

Evans F.G., Lissner H.R., Lebow M. (1958). The relation of energy, velocity, and acceleration to skull deformation and fracture. *Surg. Gynecol. Obstet.*, **107**, 593–601.

Fortner G.S., Oreskovich M.R., Copass M.K., Carrico C.J. (1983). The effects of prehospital trauma care on survival from a 50-meter fall. *J. Trauma*, **23**, 976–81.

Giachino A.A., Uhthoff H.K. (1989). Current concepts review: intra-articular fractures of the calcaneus. *J. Bone Joint Surg.*, **71A**, 784–7.

Goonetilleke U.K.D.A. (1980). Injuries caused by falls from heights. *Med. Sci. Law*, **20**, 262–75.

Guinness Book of Records 1992 (1991). London: Guinness Publishing.

Gurdjian E.S., Lissner H.R., Evans E.G., Patrick L.M., Hardy W.G. (1961). Intracranial pressure and acceleration accompanying head impacts in human cadavers. *Surg. Gynecol. Obstet.*, **113**, 185–90.

Hallel T., Naggan L. (1975). Parachuting injuries: a retrospective study of 83 718 jumps. *J. Trauma*, **15**, 14–19.

Harvey P.M., Solomons B.J. (1983). Survival after free falls of 59 metres into water from the Sydney Harbour Bridge, 1930–1982. *Med. J. Aust.*, **1**, 504–11.

Isbister E.S., Roberts J.A. (1992). Autokabalesis: a study of intentional vertical deceleration injuries. *Injury*, **23**, 119–22.

Jamous M.A., Silver J.R., Baker J.H.E. (1992). Paraplegia and traumatic rupture of the aorta: a disease process or surgical complication? *Injury*, **23**, 475–8.

Johnson C.D. (1988). Blunt injuries of the diaphragm. *Br. J. Surg.*, **75**, 226–30.

Kiel F.W. (1965). Hazards of military parachuting. *Milit. Med.*, **130**, 512–21.

Kirby N.G. (1974). Parachuting injuries. *Proc. R. Soc. Med.*, **67**, 17–21.

Lane J.M., Vigorita V.J. (1983). Current concepts review: osteoporosis. *J. Bone Joint Surg.*, **65A**, 274–8.

Lewis W.S., Lee A.B., Grantham S.A. (1965). Jumpers syndrome: the trauma of high free fall as seen at Harlem Hospital. *J. Trauma*, **5**, 812–18.

Lillywhite L.P. (1991). Analysis of extrinsic factors associated with 379 injuries occurring during 34 236 military parachute descents. *J. R. Army Med. Corp.*, **137**, 115–21.

Lissner H.R., Evans F.G. (1956). Engineering aspects of fractures. *Clin. Orthop.*, **8**, 310–22.

Lord C.D., Coutts J.W. (1944). Typical parachuting injuries. *JAMA*, **125**, 1182–7.

Lukas G.M., Hutton J.E., Lim R.C. (1981). Injuries sustained from high velocity impact with water: an experience from the Golden Gate Bridge. *J. Trauma*, **21**, 612–18.

Maull K.I. (1981). Discussion following injuries sustained from high velocity impact with water: an experience from the Golden Gate Bridge. *J. Trauma*, **21**, 617–18.

Murray-Leslie C.F., Lintott D.J., Wright V. (1977). The spine in sport and veteran military parachutists. *Ann. Rheum. Dis.*, **36**, 332–42.

Neel S.H. (1951). Medical aspects of military parachuting. *Milit. Surg.*, **108**, 91–105.

Petras A.F., Hoffman E.P. (1983). Roentgenographic skeletal injury patterns in parachute jumping. *Am. J. Sports Med.*, **11**, 325–8.

Pirson J., Verbeist E. (1985). A study of some factors influencing military parachute landing injuries. *Aviation Space Environ. Med.*, **56**, 564–7.

Pounder D.J. (1985). Suicide by leaping from multistorey car parks. *Med. Sci. Law*, **25**, 179–88.

Reynolds B.M., Balsano N.A., Reynolds F.X. (1971). Falls from heights: a surgical experience of 200 consecutive cases. *Ann. Surg.*, **174**, 304–8.

Roy-Camille R., Saillant G., Gagna G., Mazel C. (1985). Transverse fracture of the upper sacrum: suicidal jumpers fracture. *Spine*, **10**, 838–45.

Royal College of Surgeons of England (1988). Commission on the Provision of Surgical Services. Report of the Working Party on the Management of Patients with Major Injury. London: Royal College of Surgeons of England.

Rozycki G.S., Maull K.I. (1991). Injuries sustained by falls. *Arch. Emerg. Med.*, **8**, 245–52.

Rudicel S., Esdaile J. (1985). The randomized clinical trial in orthopaedics. Obligation or option? *J. Bone Joint Surg.*, **67A**, 1284–93.

Rushmer R.F., Green E.L., Kingsley H.D. (1946). Internal injuries produced by abrupt decleration of experimental animals. *Aviation Med.*, **17**, 511–25, 89.

Schneider R.C., Papo M., Alvarez C.S. (1962). The effects of chronic recurrent spinal trauma in high diving. *J. Bone Joint Surg.*, **44A**, 648–56.

Sevitt S. (1977). The mechanisms of traumatic rupture of the thoracic aorta. *Br. J. Surg.*, **64**, 166–73.

Sims A., O'Brien K. (1979). Autokabalesis: an account of mentally ill people who jump from buildings. *Med. Sci. Law*, **19**, 195–8.

Singh M., Nagrath A.R., Maini P.S. (1970). Changes in the trabecular pattern of the upper end of the femur as an index of osteoporosis. *J. Bone Joint Surg.*, **52A**, 457–67.

Smith G.R., Northrop C.H., Loop J.W. (1977). Jumpers fractures: patterns of thoracolumbar spine injuries associated with vertical plunges. *Radiology*, **122**, 657–63.

Snyder R.G. (1963). Human tolerances to extreme impacts in free-fall. *Aerospace Med.*, **38**, 695–709.

Snyder R.G. (1965a). *Survival of High-velocity Free-falls in Water*. Report no. AM 65–12. Oklahoma City, OK: Federal Aviation Agency, Office of Aviation Medicine.

Snyder R.G. (1965b). Human tolerance limits in water impact. *Aerospace Med.*, **36**, 940–7.

Snyder R.G., Snow C.C. (1967). Fatal injuries resulting from extreme water impact. *Aerospace Med.*, **38**, 779–83.

Stapp J.P. (1951). Human tolerance to deceleration: summary of 166 runs. *Aviation Med.*, **22**, 42–5, 85.

Stapp J.P. (1957). Human tolerance to deceleration. *Am. J. Surg.*, **93**, 734–40.

Steedman D.J. (1989). Severity of free-fall injury. *Injury*, **20**, 259–61.

Stewart W.K., Spells K.E., Armstrong J.A. (1955). Lung injury by impact with a water surface. *Nature*, **175**, 504–5.

Swearingen J.J., McFadden E.B., Gardner J.D., Blethrow J.G. (1960). Human tolerance to vertical impact. *Aerospace Med.*, **31**, 989–98.

Tobin W.J. (1943). Paratrooper fracture. *Arch. Surg.*, **46**, 780–3.

Trunkey D.D. (1985). Towards optimal trauma care. *Arch. Emerg. Med.*, **2**, 181–95.

Viano D.C. (1978a). *Thoracic Injury Potential*. General Motors Research Laboratories, Report GMR-2683. Warren, Michigan: GMRL.

Viano D.C. (1978b). *Traumatic Aortic Ruptures*. General Motors Research Laboratories, Report GMR-2712. Warren, Michigan: GMRL.

Von Gierke H.E. (1967). Response of the body to mechanical forces – an overview. *Ann. NY. Acad. Sci.*, **152**, 172–86.

26. Injury from Bites
T. R. Mokoena and G. Cliff

INTRODUCTION

Man is not a natural prey of any other animal. Rarely, humans have been reportedly preyed upon by predators under extraordinary circumstances such as by a wounded or otherwise physically compromised animal. Human wounding by animals therefore is either: by accident; defence of territory or self under anticipated, mistaken or real human aggression; or by a rogue or otherwise unhealthy animal such as a rabid animal.

The extent of the problem is difficult to assess accurately because most of the injuries are minor and probably heal with self treatment, or without any treatment. This is particularly true for most rural and underdeveloped communities with limited medical facilities who are the very people most apt to be victims of animal bites. Furthermore, the circumstances in which some bites occur are socially or legally censured, such as human or guard dog attacks, thus discouraging the victim from seeking medical attention willingly and timeously unless complications set in. It is estimated that there are up to 2 million animal bites per year in the USA alone.

Dog bites constitute the vast majority of reported animal bites, up to 90% (Table 26.1), and cats trail a poor second. Because of the social stigma surrounding human bites their true extent is grossly under-recorded. Sporadic cases of animal bites from other varieties of both domestic and wild animals have been reported. An account on terrestial animal bites is therefore based largely on experience with dog bites.

Most reported bites are from pet dogs (McDonough *et al.*, 1987). However, our experience and that reported by others shows a different pattern (Nguyen, 1988). The majority of bites in our community result from police dogs (80%) followed by guard-dog bites. Pet-dog bites form a small proportion (6%). This partly reflects the relatively high frequency of use of dogs in policing in South Africa, especially during crowd control, coupled with the fact that the largely poor African population served by our hospital would not seek medical advice for minor injuries especially from domestic pets. More than 90% of bites involve the limbs, with the lower limbs the predominant site to be attacked. Most pet-dog bites are usually single, but bites from police or guard dogs tend to be multiple and to involve the upper limbs – probably as the victim attempts to ward off the attack – and the head and neck. However children tend to sustain upper limb and neck domestic dog bites probably because of their height as well as attack while kneeling or seated during play. Although most dog bites are not usually fatal, attacks from fighting breeds such as Pit Bull Terriers and Rottweilers or cross-breeds can be fatal (Sacks *et al.*, 1989). Sporadic cases continue to be reported in the lay press where children have been mauled by these types of dogs. Most wounds involve the skin and subcutaneous tissue, although deep wounds into the muscles also occur. Wounds into the joints and bones or those involving vital structures such as the nerves and vessels take place from time to time.

The seriousness of the bite is determined by the size and natural aggressiveness of the attacking animal, the circumstances in which the attack is taking place, the age and physical state of the victim. Children are the most common victims of domestic animal bites some of which prove fatal especially if no adult help is readily available. Large predator attacks happen both in the wild and in captivity and are often fatal while most bites by domestic pets or rodents are minor but none the less serious because of their potential to become septic. Transfer of specific diseases which are harboured by animals are a further area of grave medical concern and rabies is the preeminent example. Victims may sometimes sustain various degrees of serious or even fatal secondary injuries such as drowning during aquatic attacks, crush injury from hooves of animals or a fall during attempted escape and tears from claws or horns.

TABLE 26.1
PROPORTION OF MAJOR ANIMAL BITES.
(ADAPTED FROM WILEY, 1990)

Type of animal	% of bites
Dog	80–90
Cat	5–10
Human	2–3
Other*	2–3

* Every animal that man has come across has attacked him on occasion, including wild terrestial and marine inhabitants.

FACTORS THAT INFLUENCE WOUNDING AND SIZE OF WOUND

Circumstances and factors that influence the nature and extent of animal bite wounds are listed in Table 26.2 and further discussed below.

TABLE 26.2
FACTORS THAT INFLUENCE
NATURE AND EXTENT OF ANIMAL
BITE

Animal factors
    Size and power
    Number
    Natural aggressiveness
    Defence of territory or kind
    Socialization; poor
    Predation
    Dentition
    Feeding
    Mating

Victim factors
    Size
    Loner
    Provocation
    Misadventure
    Socialization; poor
    Hunting
    Leisure activity
    Hand feeding
    Clothing

Environmental factors
    Terrain
    Pollution

Factors concerning the attacking animal

Dentition

The setting of an animal's teeth determines the type of wound it can inflict. Animals with well-developed incisor teeth such as herbivours like horses and donkeys can inflict large cutting wounds if the bite is fully executed, those with large flat molars like ruminants result in crush injuries, while carnivores with well-developed canine teeth wound by tearing into flesh.

Power of the animal

The larger and more powerful the animal the more extensive is the resulting damage. A large Pit Bull Terrier can exert a force of up to 1800 psi (12 420 kPa) (Baack *et al.*, 1989) which is enough to pierce a light metal sheet. Likewise because predators are built for and are well atuned to killing, they impart more severe injuries than herbivores of the same size.

Natural aggressiveness of the animal (aggression)

The extent of wounding also depends on the natural aggression of the animal. Carnivores, especially predators, have evolved special biting apparatus and biting forms part of their primary fighting apparatus. They use their limbs as secondary fighting weapons and therefore tend to claw and pin their victim down resulting in secondary injuries. Generally carnivores tend to be naturally proactively aggressive and, although man may not be their primary prey, a mauling attack from a carnivore tends to be very severe. It is probably because of their ancestral trait in part that domesticated canine and feline classes account for most reported human bites. The practice of cross-breeding these domestic animals with their wild cousins creates a potential for tragedy which should be strongly discouraged. An attack from most large herbivores is usually by hooves or horns and biting is only secondary or incidental. Herbivore bites usually result during feeding, patting or activity related to their use for labour, and as such are relatively minor and rare. Bites from wild animals in captivity can be severe. The public should refrain from feeding and patting such wild animals. Starving, wounded or otherwise incapacitated animals tend to be more aggressive and less selective of prey than usual and if predator, may attack a human for food.

Predation on man

A deliberate proactive aggression for mistaken or displaced prey or by a rogue animal may result in severe if not fatal wounds.

Defensive attack

Active defence of self, litter, pack or territory against real, as during a hunt, or apparent threat from humans can result in an attack.

Habitual group hunting by domestic animals

Dogs that are accustomed to hunting in a pack for human sport or for feeding purposes are more likely to attack humans as a pack and inflict severe injuries. Hunting canids immobilize victims by biting the legs and begin feeding while the victim is still alive (Borchelt *et al.*, 1983). A simultaneous attack by a number of animals such as by a pack of dogs increases the number and ferocity of the bites sustained by the victim.

Mating activity

Virile males tend to be more aggressive especially in the presence of a receptive or oestrus female. Furthermore, an oestrus female attracts a larger number of males each jostling for a position to mate. This increases the chances of an attack on an intruding human.

Social interaction with humans

Animals that have been trained to relate socially to people are less likely to bite than untrained ones. Guard dogs and police dogs are trained especially to attack on command or in the presence of an erratic stranger.

Hunger and feeding

The likelihood of an attack on a human as a displaced or mistaken prey has already been alluded to. In addition feeding animals tend to defend their food by attacking competitors and intruders including humans.

Incidental bite

Incidental and warning bites such as many inflicted by domestic animals during 'forced' play, labour or some other disturbance tend to be minor. Likewise wounds sustained during active play or hand to mouth feeding tend to be less extensive although partial loss of digits, and tears to the lip from a jumping dog are not uncommon. These circumstances are some of the most common that occur during domestic animal bites experienced by children.

Victim-related factors

Size

Children are by far the most frequent victims of animal bites, not only because of their higher exposure and relative lack of experience in relating to animals in general but primarily because their size makes them less formidable in the eyes of a potential attacking animal. Clearly children and small individuals or otherwise handicapped people would fare less well against an attack of comparable ferocity than an able-bodied adult man. It is mainly in this group of victims that most severe dog bites have occurred (Jaffe, 1983; Wright, 1985).

Provocative behaviour

A number of attacks from domestic animals result from provocative behaviour often in a form of taunting usually by children. Hunting is the extreme form of provocation although most victims of the hunted animal end up being hounds and horses. Fox-bites of humans by hounded animals have been recorded. All animals, including humans, tend to guard their young jealously and to protect them with utmost ferocity. An erratic approach, however well intended it might be, is often met with an unprecedented attack from an otherwise hitherto friendly bitch or mother especially during nursing. Children should be warned against playing with fresh puppies lest they be attacked by the mother. Likewise a nursing wild animal and her young ones should be given a wide berth.

Labour activity

Man has harnessed other animals for his labour and leisure activities. Even the most domesticated beast sometimes revolts especially when treatment is not altogether humane and bites may result (Al-Boukai *et al.*, 1989).

Leisure and pleasure activity

Pranks and acts with captive wild animals still remain the mainstay of circus shows. Tragically some of these come to a fatal ending.

Mating activity in humans

Human lovers often express their pleasure during sexual activity by biting which may be severe enough to breach the skin including the amputation of nipples (Al Fallouji, 1990).

Misadventure

Some tribal young men demonstrate their valour by hunting and fighting wild animals, including lions, while wearing rudimentary armour (Burge *et al.*, 1985). Some urban youths likewise aim to impress by disregarding warnings at zoos, e.g. one youth reportedly took a tiger by its tail and sustained a bite for his efforts (Woolfrey *et al.*, 1985).

Animal husbandry activity

Humans often demonstrate their affection for their pets and domestic animals by letting them feed directly out of their palms. Unfortunately this not infrequently results in accidental bites. Extension of this practice to wild animals in captivity is very hazardous since these animals are more likely to bite than are domestic ones.

Occupational

Zoo and game keepers, circus and laboratory animal attendants are continually exposed to wild animals. Great care should be taken to avoid provocative or otherwise threatening behaviour that might excite the animals' aggression. Those who have to feed and transport captive animals should take extra precautions. Feeding animals manually should be avoided, as should lone interaction with them. A second attendant suitably armed or otherwise equipped to intervene and assist in the event of an attack should always be present.

Incidental bite

Incidental bites sometimes occur when no biting activity was intended by either party. The most common example is injury to the ungloved hand during a punch that lands on the teeth. This usually leads to extensor tendon expansion injury with or without associated phalangeal fractures and is frequently followed by infection with organisms that originated in the mouth of attacked individual.

Clothing

Clothing helps in preventing or minimizing wounding during a bite. The stronger the material the more protective it is (Figure 26.1). Those who tend captive animals, especially research laboratory attendants, should take the extra precautions of

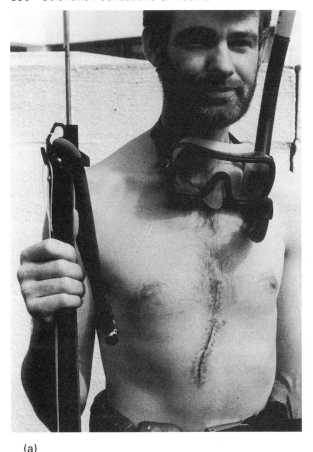

(a)

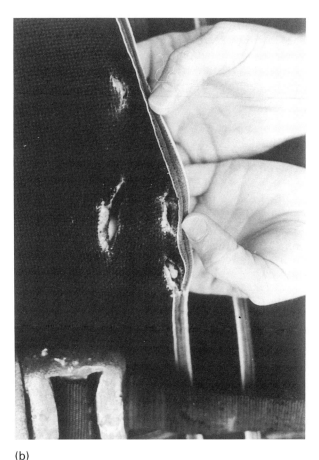

(b)

Figure 26.1 A spear fisherman escaped a shark attack with only superficial laceration (a), having been protected by his Neoprene suit and a metal weight on his belt which took the brunt of the bite (b). (Courtesy Mr George Askew.)

being suitably and fully clad which mean protective gloves, head wear and masks if necessary.

Environment-related factors

Terrain
A victim in an open terrain is potentially more vulnerable than someone in a wooded environment where evasive action can be taken in the event of an attack. By contrast, secondary injuries may result from collision with obstacles. An attack in water is more dangerous because of the threat of drowning posed even to an otherwise competent swimmer. Lone adventure or straying into potentially dangerous game parks or waters should be avoided. Indeed hunting or hiking expeditions should be organized as a group with a clearly laid down set of safety guidelines, appropriate medical first aid preparation and a leader to monitor the group whose members should keep within sight at all times.

Contamination
All animals inject saliva which includes mouth flora during the process of biting. Tables 26.3 and 26.4

show some of the organisms that have been recovered from wounds as well as mouths of the types of animals that have bitten people. Except under surgical experimental conditions, animal bites occur in natural surroundings where there is environmental dirt or water which harbour microorganisms. The extent of contamination of the wound depends on the ferocity of the attack, the size of the wound, the presence and type of clothing and the topography of the terrain where sandy, dusty, muddy surrounds are more likely to result in more soiling than on hard earth or slate. The nature of microorganisms that gain access into the wound from the environment is influenced by the extent of pollution present. Thus pathogenic enteric organisms such as *Salmonella spp.* are more likely to be found in areas of sewage disposal. Attending physicians should always bear this factor in mind, especially if the attack occurred in or near rivers and oceans which receive sewage effluent.

A victim or lay colleagues may unwittingly introduce secondary contamination directly into the wound during efforts at self-medication. Lay people, e.g. rural Africans, often help secure hae-

TABLE 26.3
ORGANISMS CULTURED FROM ANIMAL BITE WOUNDS OR
ANIMAL MOUTHS. (DERIVED FROM AUTHORS' EXPERIENCE AND
REVIEW OF THE LITERATURE)

Pasteurella multicida
Bacteroides spp.
Streptococcus spp.
Actinobacter spp.
Staphylococcus aureus
Staphylococcus epidermidis
Corynebacterium spp.
Enterobacter spp.
Enterobacter agglomeratus
Enterobacter cloacae
Enterococcus
Eikenella corrodens
Peptostreptococcus spp.
Pseudomonas aeruginosa
Fusobacterium spp.
Dysgonic Fermenter 2 (DF2)
(*Capnocytophaga canimorsus* sp. nov. and *C. cynodegmi* sp.
  nov.)
Actinomycosis
Blastomycosis
Streptococcus faecalis
Staphylococcus intermedius
Pasteurella pneumotropia
Actinobacillis lignieresii
Proteus mirabilis
Clostridium spp.
Citrobacter
Group EF-4
Acinetobacter amitradi
Escherichia coli
Non-haemolytic streptococcus
Aeromonas hydrophilia
Serratia marcescens
Klebsiella oxytoca

TABLE 26.4
ORGANISMS CULTURED FROM HUMAN BITE WOUNDS OR
HUMAN MOUTHS.

Bacteroides spp.
Streptococcus spp.
Staphylococcus aureus
Staphylococcus epidermidis
Corynebacterium spp.
Enterobacter spp.
Eikenella corrodens
Peptostreptococcus spp.
Fusobacterium spp.
Actinomycosis
Blastomycosis
Tuberculosis
Streptococcus faecalis
Hepatitis B and C
Clostridium spp.
Escherichia coli
Non-haemolytic streptococcus
Haemolytic streptococcus
Enterobacter cloacae
Klebsiella pneumoniae
Haemophilus parainfluenza
Neisseria spp.

mostasis by putting soil or dirt into the wound which nearly always succeeds in promoting clot formation but also introduce environmental micro-organisms. Often people wash off blood stains or soiling with water obtained directly from a nearby source including stagnant puddles, rivers or beach and thus introduce secondary contamination.

THE WOUND

The primary wound

The nature and extent of the wound depends on:

1. *Energy transfer* – the higher the energy transferred from the attacking animal to the victim the more severe the wound. The amount of energy to be transferred is related to the size and attitude of the attacking animal; an attack from a fighting dog such as a Pit Bull Terrier can exert up to 1800 psi (12 420 kPa) and is more severe than that from a rat. Given a certain amount of energy at impact, the quantity transferred depends on the angle of impact (e.g. a glazing bite is less severe than a full frontal attack) and on the size, attitude and clothing of the victim. If the victim is in the process of taking evasive action, energy transfer is less than in a passive or pinned-down position or in a counter-attacking charge. Likewise clothing absorbs some of the energy and, depending on the type of clothing, wounding might be obviated altogether from some bite attacks.

2. *Wounding apparatus* – the size, shape and nature of the wound depend on that of the wounding teeth. Animals with big flat teeth designed for chewing of vegetable matter, such as ruminants, tend to produce crushing injury with ragged edges. Carnivores with well-developed canine teeth inflict deep, punctured wounds or tears. Those animals with razor sharp teeth such as some sharks tend to produce incised wounds. Worrying or shaking also modify the damage profile.

3. *Additional injuries* – incidental wounding may be occasioned by an attack with claws, horns, hooves, thorns (porcupine) or by coming into contact with scales. Secondary injury may also occur from drowning or near drowning when an attack happens in or near large collections of water. Crush injuries occur when an attacking animal falls or tramples over the victim. The victim may also sustain injuries from falling objects disturbed during the fracas or might fall or jump steps, cliffs, banks or walls or run into obstacles while attempting to escape.

TABLE 26.5
ANATOMICAL SITE OF ANIMAL BITE WOUND. (DERIVED FROM
OUR OWN EXPERIENCE AND WILEY, 1990)

	General* (%)	Children (%)
Lower extremities	57	25
Upper extremities	34	38
Head and neck	4	30
Trunk	4	7

*Includes children

Site of the wound

The most frequently bitten parts of the human anatomy are limbs (Table 26.5), partly because they are more accessible and partly during attempts to fend off the attack. The head and neck area, more common in children, is of particular concern because the wound may involve the respiratory apparatus directly or indirectly by secondary swelling. Bites to the trunk other than buttocks are relatively infrequent. Injuries may not only involve skin and related muscles but may also affect vessels and nerves sometimes with loss of function of the part. Bones and joints are often implicated in crushing injuries. Human and other animal incisor teeth and razor sharp shark's teeth have been recovered from fractured bones (Figure 26.2).

Complications

Infection
Primary infection of the wound may be established by colonization by contaminating microbial flora of the attacking animal's mouth or microbes from the environment (Tables 26.3 and 26.4, see also Table 26.8). Tetanus, gas gangrene and necrotizing fasciitis are a real danger. Secondary infection may result from colonization by the victim's own microbial flora or microorganisms from clinical attendants, other patients, hospital or domestic environment.

Allergies
A number of atopic and some apparently normal individual have clinical or subclinical allergy to animal fur, saliva and other products. An animal bite may precipitate an allergic reaction in a susceptible person (Teasdale and Davies, 1983; Wong et al., 1984).

Loss of function
Apart from haemorrhage or interruption of respiratory apparatus which are life threatening, injury to vital structures may result in loss of function with vascular injuries leading to ischaemia, nerve injuries to paresis and/or hypoaesthesia or anaesthesia leading to contractures or dystrophic changes.

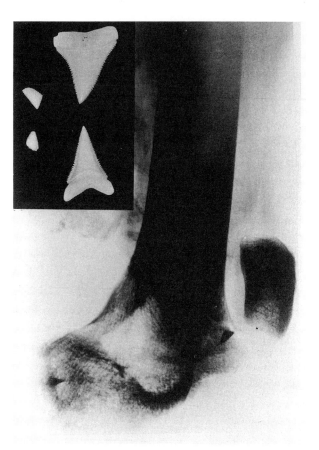

Figure 26.2 A radiograph of the lower limb of a victim of shark attack showing fragments of shark teeth which were removed at operation. Comparison with intact great white shark teeth (insert) suggest this was the culprit. (Courtesy Oceanographic Research Institute, Durban).

Transmission of specific diseases

Animals harbour microorganisms which may not be pathogenic to them but may be so to man. Furthermore wild animals form a reservoir of diseases which may be transmitted to man with devastating results. Table 26.6 shows the diseases that have been or may be transmitted to man during a bite. Transmission of syphilis (Fiumar and Exnor, 1981) and hepatitis B (Cancio-Bello et al., 1982) have been recorded. However, there is as yet no documented case of transmission of HIV though the risk is clearly present (Shirley and Ross, 1988).

MANAGEMENT

Management of an animal bite victim follows established lines of management of injuries in general, with first aid at the point of injury and as rapid as possible evacuation to an institution where formal trauma care can be undertaken.

Those who treat bites should remember that foreign bodies are common and include complete

TABLE 26.6
DISEASES TRANSMISSIBLE TO HUMANS DURING AN ANIMAL BITE

Diseases	Microbial agent	Animal source
Rabies	Rabies virus (Rhabdovidae)	Dogs, cats, variety of wild canids and other mammalian spp.
Viral hepatitis	Hepatitis B and C viruses	Humans
Simian hepatitis B	Simian hepatitis B virus	Non-human primates
Adult immune deficiency syndrome*	Human immunodeficiency virus	Humans
Cat scratch disease	?Chlamydia-like	Cats, dogs, monkey
Tularaemia	*Francisella tularensis*	Cats, coyotes, squirrels
Rat-bite fever	*Streptobacillus moniliformis* or spirillum minor	Rats, mice and other small rodents
Syphilis	*Treponema pallidum*	Humans
Leptospirosis	*Leptospira* spp.	Many wild and domestic mammals.

Notes:
Most of the bacterial diseases are amenable to penicillin therapy.
General reference: Mandell *et al.* (1985).

* There is no conclusive evidence of transmission of AIDS by biting.

teeth or fragments from the attacking animal. Radiography is therefore essential.

Treatment

A summary of guidelines to management of different special risk areas and circumstances is presented in Table 26.7. Some authors advocate thorough debridement and primary closure of all animal bite wounds (Callaham, 1980). This practice relies on unconventional use of local and systemic antimicrobial agents to suppress infection. Primary closure of face and neck wounds is more widely practised with early reconstructive surgery in order to ensure better cosmetic results. Primary repair following human bite wounds of the face has been less frequently undertaken because of the fear of an increased sepsis rate (Early and Bardley, 1984; Srivasta, 1989). Except for the most minor incidents the victim should be observed in hospital at least overnight especially with injuries of the face and limbs where secondary swelling may compromise function.

Prophylaxis

Against general wound infection

Systemic antimicrobial agents are used empirically depending on the animal and circumstances of the bite. Broad-spectrum antibiotics to cover gram-positive and gram-negative, aerobic and anaerobic bacteria should be used for 24–48 hours especially if the wound is extensive and contamination severe.

If sewage-bearing water formed part of contamination, coliforms and *Salmonella* spp. must be covered. Tables 26.3, 26.4 and 26.8 show a possible spectrum of reported organisms grown from bite wounds or mouths of different animals which attack humans. Of note is the dysgonic fermenter (DF2) which has not only produced morbidity and mortality in immunocompromised victims but also in healthy ones (Job *et al.*, 1989). *Pasteurella multicida* which is present in most animal mouth flora can lead to a rapidly spreading local infection which if unchecked may progress to septicaemia. It is for this reason as well that recommendation of in-hospital observation for 24 hours or more is made as cases of rapidly spreading cellulitis have been reported to occur within this time period. A rare but interesting complication of animal bites is reabsorption of bone. The cause is as yet unsettled but could be due to the direct effect of the colonizing organism or due to hyperaemia from chronic infection (Al-Boukai *et al.*, 1989). Antimicrobial therapy should supplement rather than replace sound use of local antiseptic measures.

Against specific infections

Tetanus: *Clostridium tetani*, the causal microbe of tetanus, is ubiquitous being abundant in dirt and animal excrement including that of humans. Extensive contamination is not necessary for colonization. Indeed small scratches have been known to provide a portal of entry with subsequent colonization by *Cl. tetani* and the development of tetanus. Prophylaxis against tetanus should form part of

TABLE 26.7

SUMMARY OF MANAGEMENT APPROACH TO SPECIAL RISK SITES OR CIRCUMSTANCES IN ANIMAL BITES

Head and neck	Healing good and cosmesis important, therefore debridement and primary suture recommended. Proximity to CNS creates special danger in rabid dog bite or *Cl. tetani* contamination, therefore prophylaxis more aggressive
Eyes	These communicate directly with CNS therefore managed aggressively with enucleation if function and/or viability doubtful
Nose/ears	Cartilage heals poorly so amputations better managed by reconstructive flaps than primary regrafting
Mouth	Liable to self-contamination from victim's mouth flora but successful acute reconstructive procedures reported
Hand foot and digits	The pulp spaces and the palmar/solar tendon sheaths allow infection to spread widely because of relative avascularity and the communication of the entire palmar or tarsal space. Primary closure should not be done. If infection sets in, management should allow all the spaces to be drained and the palmar incision placed such that contractures do not interfere with function. Immobilization should be avoided and early supervised exercise encouraged
Joints and bones	When joints or bones are involved the skin should be left open after thorough debridement of the joint or bone and its appropriate management. However, prosthesis placement should be used sparingly. Established septic arthritis or osteitis is managed on merit
Genitalia including nipples	Scrotal tears can be managed by absorbable suture repair, especially when the testis is exposed. Split-skin graft will be necessary in few patients where primary suture has not effected complete cover of the testis. Testes have been occasionally irretrievably lost during animal bites (Donovan and Kaplan, 1989). Lacerations of the foreskin may be managed by primary suture or by circumcision if severe. Partial amputation of the penile shaft may require split-skin graft. Nipple amputation following sexual/love bites are managed by refashioning of the areolar into a neo-nipple
Delayed and excessive devitalized tissues	All patients who present late (more than 12 hours) for attention to animal bites should be presumed infected and appropriate measures, including prophylactic antimicrobial therapy and open wound treatment, should be undertaken. Where there is excessive tissue devitalization extensive surgical debridement should be undertaken before closure of the wound.

TABLE 26.8

MICROBIAL ORGANISMS CULTURED FROM SHARK ATTACK WOUNDS OR SHARK MOUTHS (DAVIS AND CAMPBELL, 1962; WHITE, 1975; EDMONDS ET AL., 1981; BUCK ET AL., 1984; PARIA ET AL., 1989)

Vibrio alginolyticus
V. parahaemolyticus
V. fluvialis
V. carchariae
Pseudomonas putrefaciens
Staphylococcus aureus
Citrobacter
Micrococcus
Pseudomonas spp.
C. tetanus
C. welchii
Paracolon
Bacillus coli

every childhood immunization schedule. Once established, immunity is long lasting. However it is prudent to give a booster every 10 years or sooner if the patient receives a wound (Adams *et al.*, 1969; Veronesi, 1981).

In acute injury tetanus prophylaxis takes the form of thorough cleansing of the wound with debridement of all dead tissues. Most practitioners, including the authors, give a prophylactic antibiotic cover against clostridia while a few believe that wound cleansing alone should suffice. A tetanus toxoid booster or initial immunizing dose is started in nearly all cases except those adjudged to be candidates for antitetanus antibody therapy who should have tetanus toxoid delayed until the exogenous antibodies have substantially decreased. Indications for antitetanus antibody prophylaxis in bites, as well as other circumstances, remain controversial. The authors do not practise prophylactic antibody therapy but reserve this for treatment of established tetanus. Although the danger of serum sickness (anaphylactic shock) associated with horse serum is less with human-derived antibodies the risk of transmission of viral hepatitis and the human immunodeficiency virus make it difficult to justify its prophylactic use.

Rabies: Human infection by the rabies virus is nearly always fatal. This makes prophylaxis against it extremely important. Although the rhabdovirus is neurotropic it is secreted abundantly in the saliva of a rabid animal whence it is transferred during a bite.

Prophylactic active immunization of humans with an attenuated brain-tissue-passaged virus has not been as successful as hoped (Lancet, 1988). Side-effects of the preparation make its use justifiable only in victims of rabid animal bites but not in the general population or even high-risk individuals such as veterinary clinic/hospital attendants. The newer chick embryo cell and human diploid cell-derived inactivated virus vaccines have less side-effects. Apparently immune response develops rapidly enough to arrest the relatively slow growing virus.

Prophylactic passive immunization with antiserum is indicated in cases of proven rabid animal bites. Human hyperimmune gamma globulin is preferable to the equine product but fears of viral infection transfer exists. In this regard a more purified equine immune globulin (Wilde *et al.*, 1989) and experimental use of monoclonal antibodies (Schumaker *et al.*, 1989) are being pursued.

In practice most prophylaxis has been directed at controlling the virus spread in domestic animals, principally dogs, by mandatory immunization and strict quarantine of imported animals until it has been ascertained that they do not harbour the virus. Recently, efforts have been directed at controlling the virus within its wild animal reservoir. The recent vaccinia-based genetically engineered live vaccine used in foxes and other wild animals carriers in Europe and elsewhere promises the eradication of this disease if enough resources are devoted to it (Anderson, 1991). If the vaccine proves safe in animals it could be an ideal prophylactic measure in high-risk humans.

Management of special complications and infections

Septicaemia and toxic shock syndrome

Bites may provide a portal of entry for organisms which spread systemically to produce bacteraemia or septicaemia. Although this is more likely to occur in immunocompromised victims including those who have undergone splenectomy, hitherto healthy people have developed septicaemia from a number of organisms including *Pasteurella multicida* and DF2.

Staphylococcal toxic shock syndrome, which usually occurs in young menstruating women infected vaginally with a specific toxic-producing *Staphylococcus aureus*, has recently been identified in victims of human bite wounds of the hand (Karody *et al.*, 1988; Long *et al.*, 1988).

Gas gangrene and necrotizing fasciitis

Gas gangrene results from colonization of devitalized tissue by *Clostridium* spp. which are ubiquitous, especially *Cl. welchii* and *Cl. perfringes*. Necrotizing fasciitis is the consequence of infection with multiple organisms often working in synergy. Most of these are derived from the colon and are therefore present in sewage-bearing waters and dirt contaminated with excreta. *Pasteurella multicida* which has been isolated from the mouth flora of most domestic and wild animals results in a rapidly spreading infection like necrotizing fasciitis. *Vibrio* spp. from sharks and other marine animals also result in necrotizing fasciitis. Repeated debridement is often necessary.

Tetanus

Tetanus is managed along conventional lines (Adams *et al.*, 1969; Veronesi, 1981).

Rabies

Details of management can be found in Chutivongse *et al.* (1990), Kaplan *et al.* (1986) and Baer (1975).

PREVENTION OF ANIMAL BITES

Most prevention measures against animal bites and consequent reduction in morbidity and mortality entails the use of commonsense strategies:

1. Avoid solitary hiking, surfing or bathing, especially where wild game or sharks abound.
2. Members of the public must avoid provocative behaviour or behaviour that might give rise to bites from animals. People should not feed animals out of their hands, and should obey notices at zoo or game parks *not* to feed animals. The public should avoid dumping carcasses, blood or other edible material anywhere near sea/ocean waters that are frequented by humans for fear of attracting sharks. Bathers and surfers should restrict themselves to shark-protected areas.
3. Breeders of domestic animals should avoid cross-breeding large and aggressive dog breeds, as the behaviour of the cross-breeds is often unpredictable. The habit of breeding domestic animals with their wild cousins is to be deplored and even preferably outlawed worldwide.
4. Avoid keeping wild animals as pets.

SHARK-INFLICTED INJURIES

Introduction

No human injuries have aroused as much interest, concern or fear as those inflicted by sharks. Man has successfully minimized the threat posed by lions and tigers, the land's great predators, but he has not been able to overcome that posed by sharks. The result is an almost irrational fear of sharks, which has been fuelled by box office spectaculars, such as *Jaws* and its sequels. Here, sharks have been portrayed as monsters, tracking down and devouring unsuspecting bathers almost in a vengeful manner.

Throughout the world vast sums of money have been spent and scientists have given much attention to reducing the incidence of shark attack (Gilbert, 1963). Since they were first installed in Sydney in 1937, shark nets have been successfully used in parts of Australia and South Africa to protect popular bathing beaches. During the Second World War the United States Navy funded extensive research to find a repellent which would protect airmen and sailors who become vulnerable to shark attack following a disaster at sea. At a meeting of the American Institute of Biological Sciences in 1958, a scientific programme was formulated to deal with the shark hazard problem and included the formation of an International Shark Attack File to document shark attacks around the world whose analysis of more than 1650 incidents has been published (Baldridge, 1973).

Each year about 100 attacks are reported worldwide though no more than 30 prove fatal. South Africa has long been regarded as a country with a shark attack problem although since 1960 only an average of three such injuries have been recorded annually. The findings of Baldridge and of other subsequent studies show that sharks are man biters, but there are few cases of man eating. Given the appropriate treatment, victims can generally survive shark attack.

The shark's sensory apparatus

Sharks respond to internal drives (motivations) as well as external stimuli received by their sensory apparatuses and transmitted to the brain. An understanding of the nature and sensitivity of each of these senses (Hodgson and Mathewson, 1978) may assist in interpreting many of the circumstances surrounding shark attack.

Vision

Despite their reputation of having poor eyesight, sharks have a highly developed visual system. The eye has both rod, which are sensitive to movement in poor light, and cone photoreceptors, which detect colours in bright light. Sharks probably cannot distinguish shapes and colours nearly as well as they can detect contrasts and movements in poor light. This correlates with the nocturnal activity patterns of many sharks. Vision is probably only important in detecting prey at distances of less than 20 m, but some sharks such as the bull shark, *Carcharhinus leucas*, are able to feed in extremely turbid water, suggesting that in these circumstances vision is not particularly important in the capture of prey.

Smell and taste

On the underside of the snout there is a pair of nostrils which direct a continual stream of water over the sensory cells as the shark swims. Experiments have shown that sharks may detect one part of tuna extract in over a million parts of water, enabling them to track food several hundred metres downcurrent from its source. In many countries abattoirs pump their offal and other wastes directly in the sea. This has attracted sharks into the area, resulting in a high incidence of shark attack. Taste buds are located in the mouth and pharynx and sharks apparently reject unpalatable items after tasting them.

Sound and vibration

Sharks have a pair of well-developed inner ears which are highly sensitive to low-frequency sounds. They can therefore detect low-frequency vibrations several hundreds of metres from their source. They also possess a lateral line system extending along the sides of the head and body which comprises a series of fluid-filled canals with hair-like receptors which are stimulated by vibrations and pressure waves. These together with the ears are important in balance and orientation.

Electroreception

The ability to detect electrical fields is the least understood of all the senses. In the head region there are hundreds of tiny pores, known as the ampullae of Lorenzini, which house electro-magnetic receptor cells. Their sensitivity is probably the greatest in the animal kingdom, for sharks can establish the presence of potential prey by simply detecting the prey's electrical field without relying on sight or smell. Sharks may also use the earth's magnetic field to orientate and to carry out long-distance migrations. The great white shark, *Carcharodon carcharias*, is well known for attacking outboard motors and shark cages. It is possible that the shark is aroused by the electrical fields associated with these metallic objects.

Skin

The skin of a shark is covered with denticles, which are similar in origin and structure to teeth, comprising a dentine core covered by a hard layer of enamel. The denticles not only enhance the hydrodynamics of the faster moving sharks, but also protect the skin. The denticles make the skin abrasive, akin to coarse sandpaper, and can inflict considerable damage to human skin.

Dentition

Variation in dentition of sharks reflects the diverse nature of their diet. Three basic types of teeth are generally found:

1. Narrow, sharply pointed teeth have considerable piercing ability but limited cutting. These teeth are used by sharks to impale smaller prey, such as small fish and cephalopods, which are swallowed whole.
2. Teeth flattened to form a pavement are found in sharks which live on or feed on the bottom; they crush the hard exoskeletons of molluscs and crustaceans.
3. Triangular serrated teeth have considerable cutting ability and enable sharks to remove chunks from fairly large prey, such as marine mammals and other large sharks. Some species may be equipped with more than one type of teeth. The

bullshark and several other carcharhinid sharks have triangular, cutting teeth in the top jaw and narrower, grasping teeth in the lower jaw.

Teeth occur in multiple rows in the jaws (Figure 26.3). They are neither set in sockets, nor are they cemented to the underlying jaw cartilage, but are bedded in a collagenous membrane. The teeth are formed on the inside of the jaw and the outer, functional teeth, which are often broken or lost during feeding, are continually replaced by teeth from the row behind. In most sharks the teeth are not visible in the inferior positioned mouth. The jaw complex comprises a number of cartilages loosely connected to each other and to the chondrocranium. As a shark approaches its prey, it lifts its head and snout. Muscular contraction pulls the jaw complex forward; the lower jaw drops, the upper jaw protrudes and both jaws rotate outward to expose the teeth. Contrary to popular belief the shark does not have to turn on its side to bite.

In sharks which feed on prey too large to swallow whole the prey is impaled on the narrower, lower jaw teeth while serrated upper teeth cut out a chunk, aided by the violent side-to-side swings of the shark's head. The biting force of a 2-m shark has been calculated as being 3 metric tons per cm^2 at the tip of a tooth. Although this is little more than that measured in humans, the bite of a shark is far more damaging because a shark's teeth are razor sharp, there are more of them and a shark has the ability to project its jaws.

Sharks responsible for attacks

There are over 350 species of shark currently known to man (Compagno, 1984). They range in size from the dwarf shark *Squaliolus laticaudus*, which reaches a maximum of 27 cm, to the giant whale shark, *Rhiniodon typus*, the largest living fish, which may attain 13 m, but poses little threat to humans because it has minute teeth and is a filter feeder. About 27 species of sharks have been known to attack humans or boats. In a number of cases the identity of the species responsible is tenuous. Descriptions of the sharks by victims and eyewitnesses are of limited value, unless the shark has conspicious features such as the head of a hammerhead *Sphyrna sp*. A diver usually has the best opportunity to observe an attacking shark because he or she is wearing a face mask, however many divers did not see the shark prior to an attack. Bite patterns are used for identification, but the most positive information is provided by tooth fragments which are often found lodged against the victim's bones (Figure 26.2) or inside the surfboard. Three species have together been responsible for most of the attacks in coastal waters (Baldridge, 1973). Each of the three discussed, in more detail below, shares these attributes – a high level of

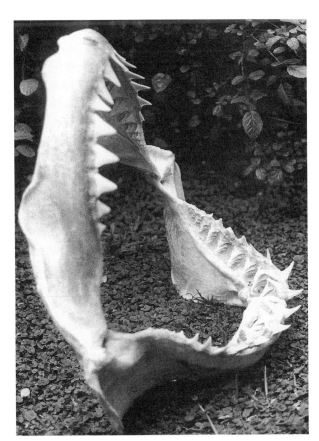

Figure 26.3 Great white shark jaw illustrating the wedge-shaped serrated teeth set in multiple rows.

aggression, serrated cutting teeth and wide mouth – which enable them to tackle prey too large to swallow whole.

The great white shark (*Carcharodon carcharias*)

This species has been implicated in more attacks than any other species. The main character in the motion picture, *Jaws*, it has a torpedo-shaped body, large gill slits and conical snout. The mouth is armed with large, triangular, serrated teeth. Although widely distributed in coastal waters, most attacks have occurred off California, Southern Australia, New Zealand and South Africa. This species is often concentrated near the rookeries of seals and sea lions, which are favoured prey for larger sharks. Smaller, agile members have a more varied diet, feeding on large fish and small sharks. There are several unconfirmed claims of great white sharks larger than 7 m and heavier than 3000 kg.

Little is known of its status and reproductive biology and, despite localized abundance, particularly around rookeries, there is growing concern of overexploitation by big game anglers and others who receive high prices for the jaws. In 1991 the species was granted protected status in South Africa to halt further exploitation while biologists assessed stock sizes.

The tiger shark (*Galeocerdo cuvier*)

This species has a blunt snout and vertical stripes along the length of the body which fade with age. The cockscomb-shaped teeth in both the upper and lower jaws are unique and function as a double bladed guillotine. In contrast to *C. carcharias*, this species has a more tropical distribution, favouring warmer waters. It is a solitary species. The largest accurately measured specimen was a 5.5-m shark caught off Cuba; however there is a photograph of a 7.4-m (3110 kg) female landed in Indo-China. It is well known for its indiscriminate eating habits with inedible items ingested which include gumboots, tin cans, a wide variety of plastics, a wallet and a vehicle registration plate having been recorded. Natural prey, much of which is scavenged, include turtles, sea birds, a wide variety of bony and cartilaginous fish, cephalopods and marine mammals. The species, like many other sharks, moves inshore to feed at night and retreats to deeper water during the day.

The bull shark (*Carcharhinus leucas*)

This species is a stout-bodied shark, with a rounded snout and triangular, serrated teeth in the upper jaw and narrower teeth in the lower jaw. Like *G. cuvier*, it is tropical and subtropical in its distribution. It is reknowned for spending long periods in freshwater. It is common in Lake Nicaragua and has been recorded 760 km up the Zambezi river, hence its common name – Zambezi shark – in southern Africa. It attains a length of up to 3 m.

Motivation behind shark attack

Some sharks have large brain mass–body mass ratios, close to those of birds and mammals (Northcutt, 1977) which exhibit complex behaviour. It is therefore not surprising that sharks do not necessarily behave predictably. In the presence of humans, attacks are not always the result of a feeding response. Despite being voracious predators, many sharks do not appear very aggressive. Given a shark's dentition and the powerful jaws, many of the wounds inflicted are not always consistent with an intention of eating the victim. There are at least five factors which may motivate a shark to attack.

Reproduction (species preservation)

During courtship many male sharks repeatedly nip the females as a prelude to copulation. Due to the shark's tough skin, these contacts leave superficial scars which soon heal. Similar contact with a human will cause more severe damage, although it seems unlikely that a human would generate visual or chemical signals that would result in that person being mistaken for a potential mate. It is conceivable, but not proven, that, during the mating season, sharks may become more aggressive.

Fear (self-defence)

Aggression shown by many animals is often greatest when they are threatened. The grey reef shark *Carcharhinus amblyrhynchos* only attains 1.8 m but has been known to attack divers and small manned submersibles. Johnson and Nelson (1973) showed that when the sharks were approached, they demonstrated agonostic behaviour consisting of exaggerated and jerky swimming patterns. The sharks lifted their snouts, depressed their pectoral fins and arched their backs and sometimes swam in figure-of-eight loops. This aggressive behaviour was regarded as a strategy to discourage a potential predator.

Shark attacks are often divided into provoked and unprovoked incidents. While the distinction may be unclear when a shark bites a spear fisherman handling a struggling fish, there are several cases of provocation, in which sharks, which have either been caught on hooks or in nets, have lashed out and injured their captors. The motive in such cases is fear or self defence.

Aggression (territoriality)

Baldridge (1973) concluded that 50–75% of cases in the International Shark Attack File may have been motivated by aggressive behaviour, indicative of fighting rather than feeding, termed by the author as 'non-foraging aggression'. Even the most docile of sharks, when provoked, may attack. Short fin mako sharks, *Isurus oxyrinchus*, are well known for ramming or even leaping into boats while they are being 'subdued' by anglers.

There is little evidence that sharks defend geographically defined territories, but a shark may repel any intruder which violates or intrudes its space. The agonostic behaviour described above may also be the response of a shark trying to evict a potential competitor from its territory or space.

Gregarious species tolerate conspecifics and a dominance hierarchy, usually based on size, may be established. Myrberg and Gruber (1974) found that bonnethead sharks, *Sphyrna tiburo*, kept in captivity were never seen to actively fight. When newcomers were added, some sharks bit others, suggesting that a hierarchy was being established, whereby smaller specimens would give way to avoid a collision with larger ones.

Large *Carcharodon carcharias* will chase away smaller conspecifics, particularly at a feeding session, and in so doing may resort to biting. Scars, clearly inflicted by other great white sharks, are found regularly on specimens examined at the Natal Sharks Board. The shark's rough skin reduces the severity of the wounds, but should a human be bitten in this way, the damage may be considerable.

Even in cases where the injuries are serious or subsequently fatal, rescuers may take considerable time (of the order of minutes) to assist the victim from the water, during which time the shark has ample opportunity to make a second attack. There are few cases in which a shark has made a second attack and even fewer in which the rescuer was attacked. Again this suggests that the aggressive response may not have been motivated by feeding.

Curiosity (investigation)

There are many incidents, including those involving large, powerful sharks such as the great white, in which the injuries were not only minor, but the contact made by the shark could be described as almost gentle. Many attacks may be motivated by curiosity, with the shark merely making an investigatory approach. Miller and Collier (1981) in an analysis of great white shark attacks off the California and Oregon coast concluded that many of the incidents 'were apparently slow, deliberate movements which could be described as an investigatory interaction of the shark with the object'.

Hunger (feeding)

Man is not a natural prey of sharks and in comparison to the total number of recorded shark-inflicted injuries there are few in which the shark devoured the victim. In South Africa between 1960 and 1991 there were only two cases of a shark or sharks repeatedly attacking a human, but there were at least six cases where victims of drowning had been partially eaten by sharks.

Another reason for an attack is mistaken identity, where a shark mistakes a human for its natural prey. The silhouette of a surfer on a surfboard, or a diver in a dark wetsuit and wearing fins, could easily be mistaken for a seal, dolphin or turtle (McCosker, 1985). Sharks often seize and shake a human and then immediately let him go, suggesting that the shark may have mistaken the victim for a natural prey.

There are instances of several attacks occurring over a short period and in a small area. In 1944, before shark nets were installed, there were five attacks in Durban within 81 days and again in 1946, four attacks in 23 days. In December 1957 there were three fatal attacks in 11 days at two adjacent holiday resorts on the east coast of South Africa which crippled the local tourist industry. These and other groups of incidents gave support to the hypothesis that a rogue shark, which had developed a taste for human flesh, was responsible (Coppleson, 1962). While that concept has been refuted by many scientists, recent research suggests that the highly dangerous *Carcharhinus leucas* may be otherwise relatively sedentary (Cliff and Dudley, 1991). Should a shark move into an area which is in close proximity to a popular swimming beach, it will come into contact with many bathers and several attacks could result.

Stimuli such as excessive blood and the vibrations of struggling fish can trigger off a feeding frenzy among a group of sharks. Individuals within the group swim more and more erratically and at increasing speeds, biting at anything in their path, including other sharks. A shark injured in this way may be attacked by the other sharks and devoured. Such strikes are most likely to be misplaced feeding responses of overstimulated sharks.

People exposed to shark attack

Victims of air and sea disasters

There have been a number of air and sea disasters, with sharks being attracted from vast distances by explosions. Both blood from injuries and the frantic struggling of the victims in the water arouse sharks, and where they occur in packs, feeding frenzies may result. In 1942 the British steamship *Nova Scotia* was torpedoed by a German U boat 50 km off the South African coast. Most of the life rafts were burned and hundreds of survivors were forced to cling to rafts and floating wreckage. Packs of sharks, possibly the oceanic white tip *Carcharhinus longimanus*, repeatedly attacked the men. Of the 765 prisoners-of-war and 134 soldiers on board, only 192 survived the ordeal of torpedoing, drowning and shark attack (Davies, 1964).

Recreational users of the sea

Historically more swimmers have been injured than any other recreational user of the sea. Recently in both Australia and South Africa more victims have been surfers and divers. This change can be attributed to the development of the wetsuit, with its thermo-insulatory properties, which has resulted in the increased popularity of these and a variety of other water sports. Surfers and divers stay in the water longer and venture further offshore than swimmers, which would increase their exposure to sharks. Among the divers many victims have been spear fishermen, whose quarry, when struggling and bleeding on the end of a spear, is highly attractive to sharks.

Harbour and other maritime workers
Of those working in the marine environment, commercial fishermen are exposed to the greatest risks. They may incur provoked attacks by sharks which are often trapped in nets or caught on hooks which are targeted for other fish. Commercial and naval divers are often called upon to work in waters which are known to be inhabited by dangerous sharks.

Factors favouring shark attack

Water temperature
The theory proposed by Coppleson (1962) that attacks will only occur in water warmer than 70°F (20°C) has been disproved by the many attacks in the colder waters of the Cape Province of South Africa and California and Oregon. The victims have primarily been wetsuit-clad divers and surfers, who have been able to tolerate the cold far better than an unprotected swimmer. Attack and feeding are not necessarily inhibited by cold water, but the cold water does restrict swimmers to short periods in the water, and hence limited exposure to sharks.

Turbidity
Attacks have taken place in clear as well as turbid water. Certain sharks, such as *Carcharhinus leucas*, do favour the shallow, turbid waters found close inshore. An ability to feed under these conditions would favour these sharks at the expense of predators which rely on clear water to locate their prey. *Carcharhinus leucas* often scavenges on terrestrial animals and freshwater fish flushed out of rivers in flood. On the east coast of South Africa over 70% of incidents have occurred in turbid water, highlighting the danger of entering the sea under these conditions. It is possible that in turbid waters a human is more easily mistaken for a natural prey than in clear water.

Beach profiles
Steeply sloping beaches often have a deep longshore channel immediately seaward of the shoreline and inshore of a variable sandbar, on which the main surf breaks. This deep channel allows large sharks to come very close to the shore. Wallett (1983) found that a high incidence of attacks at beaches on the east coast of South Africa occurred in the presence of a longshore channel.

Human activities
Dumping of fish and abbatoir offal is likely to attract sharks. Up until 1976 whales were brought into Durban harbour, attracting large sharks close inshore. These sharks were actively sought by anglers based on one of the two piers demarcating the entrance to the harbour, who used chunks of whale meat as bait. Many sharks weighing over 454 kg (1000 lb) were hooked, but only a few anglers gained membership of the elite '1000 Club' by landing one of these. Once whaling ceased very few of these large sharks were caught. Intense fishing may attract sharks to an area and sharks may become conditioned to the noise of fishing boats and the firing of spearguns by divers.

The discharge of blood and other fluids through an injury may put a person at risk. There is no evidence that sharks are attracted by urine or sweat. The colour and pattern of garments worn by the victim may be attractive to sharks. The yellow bright-coloured rescue vest is thought to be attractive to sharks but this is outweighed by the

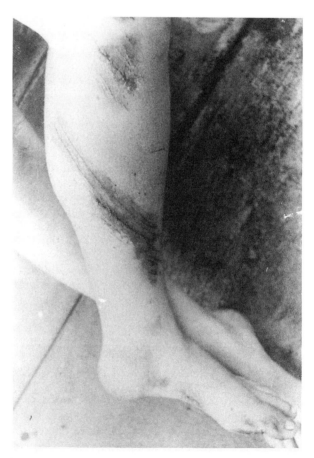

Figure 26.4 A bump attack producing abrasion whose denticle marks suggest a black tip shark.

advantages of being easily spotted by other rescuers.

Shark activities

In Natal, South Africa, more attacks have taken place in the seventeenth hour (16.00–16.59) than during any other hour of the day. This is not in keeping with numbers of beach users, which usually peak around noon, but is probably related to the activity patterns of sharks. Research has shown that most sharks are active at night when they move inshore to feed. As dawn approaches sharks move offshore and into deeper water.

Injuries inflicted

There are several ways in which a shark may make contact with its victim. This, when coupled with the dentition of the shark, may result in a wide variety of injuries.

Bump

This is usually caused by the shark's snout and results in an abrasion and bruising (Figure 26.4).

The victim, although conscious of being bumped, is often unaware that a shark was responsible.

Slash

This form of injury is caused by the teeth, but, as there is no associated biting action, it results in a series of parallel lacerations. Unserrated, needle-shaped teeth have virtually no cutting ability. A shark with such teeth, even if it were to bite, produces a tearing wound characterized by narrow, parallel lacerations.

Active bite

This is the most common, shark-inflicted injury in which a shark closes or partly closes its jaws on the victim. The bite is typically crescent shaped, reflecting the animal's jawline with separate incisions from each tooth (Figure 26.5). There are however major differences between the damage inflicted to a surfboard and to a living human victim. The former has a hard, rigid external coating of resin, while the latter is covered by a layer of soft, elastic skin and muscle. As a result the surfboard shows crushing around each incision which is not evident

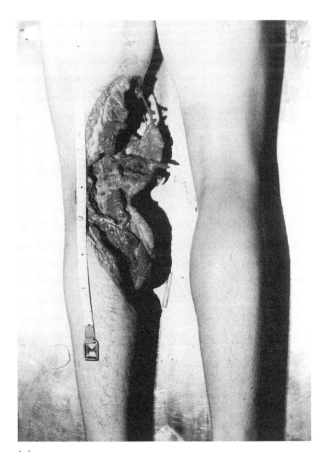

(a)

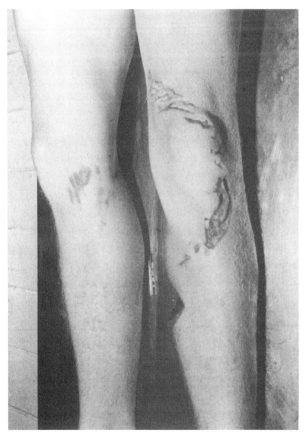

(b)

Figure 26.5 Fatal great white shark attack, illustrating the crescentic form of the bite as well as the possible mechanism of how it was executed where the deeper clean laceration was produced by cutting action of the upper jaw (a), while the more jagged and incomplete double-row lacerations on the anterior aspect of the knee suggest a steadying mechanism from the lower jaw (b). (Courtesy Dr M. D. Greyling, Mossel Bay).

on the skin. More important, the impression left by a shark on any inanimate object, such as a surfboard, or even a corpse, is determined largely by the action of the shark. When a living human being is seized, the victim instinctively responds by pulling away. This may result in a series of incisions running parallel or at a slight angle to the long axis of the shark.

The shark does not simply close its jaws with a clamp-like force, but may initiate a sawing action powered by the side-to-side swings of its head and upper body.

Crushing effect of the bite

While all bites confirm the cutting ability of shark teeth, there is also the crushing component. In an incident in which a shark severed both femora, the degree of comminution was similar to that of a severe motor vehicle accident. In this particular case two fragments of the shark's teeth were lodged in the bone and enabled the shark concerned to be identified (see also Figure 26.2).

Repeated mauling

Although sharks are well known as man biters, they seldom appear to be man eaters. A swimmer was repeatedly attacked by a great white shark. Two surfers came to assist the struggling victim thinking that he was in danger of drowning. When they realised that he was being attacked by a shark, they abandoned him. The shark attacked the body repeatedly and remained in the area for at least 20 minutes. Shots were fired at the shark with both a revolver and a shotgun. The corpse was later recovered with major injuries to the abdomen, left leg, left arm and right shoulder and minor injuries to the right lower leg, right forearm and right hand.

Incidental wounds

Incidental wounds may result from the victim's efforts to repel an attacking shark. In an effort to release a shark's grip on his right leg, the victim kicked out with his left foot and groped at the shark's snout with his hands. In addition to a heavily lacerated right leg which was subsequently amputated below the knee, the victim also suffered severe lacerations to the left foot and to both hands.

Scavenging

A corpse of a victim of drowning may be scavenged upon by a variety of marine organisms, including sharks. One such victim was last seen jumping into a heavily flowing river to perform a rescue. His corpse was recovered 2 days later on a beach 3 km north of the river mouth after having been heavily scavenged by sharks. An initial head injury was thought to have caused drowning.

Parts of the body injured

Most shark bites on humans are inflicted on the limbs, in particular the legs. Statistics from the International Shark Attack File (Baldridge, 1973) indicate that the vast majority occur below the knee followed by the thighs. Truncal injuries are less frequent. This is not surprising for several reasons:

1. Many attacks take place in waist-deep water.
2. The movement of the limbs may attract sharks.
3. It may be instinctive of sharks to immobilize their prey by seizing the tail which the legs of a swimmer might be mistaken for.

Management of shark attack

Though the handling of an incident of shark attack follows the same lines as for all trauma, the special circumstances of injury offshore and often in circumstances far from a trauma centre have lead to the development of special techniques which are beyond the scope of this account. They include special training facilities for emergency treatment on site such as the Feinberg Shark Attack Pack, a predetermined route for evacuation and an agreed antibiotic policy based on an understanding of the likely infecting organisms (Davis and Campbell, 1962). Application of these principles has led in South Africa to a decline in mortality from 21% in the 1960s to 6% in the 1980s.

Protection against shark attack

This may take one of two forms; either protection provided for an individual or that designed to protect a group.

Chemical protection

The Shark Chaser was supplied to United States airmen and sailors during the Second World War. It resembled a cake of soap and consisted of copper acetate, which smelt like putrefying shark and was intended to repel an approaching shark, and nigrosine dye which produced a cloud of black dye. Water currents rapidly dissipated both chemicals. The benefits of the Shark Chaser lay in the psychological reassurance it gave those who carried it.

Other toxins such as that derived from the Moses sole (*Pardachirus marmoratus*), which causes an instant but reversible paralysis and lockjaw if bitten into by a shark, have been investigated. This substance somewhat resembles some household detergents and these are now being studied.

Acoustic repellents

Low-frequency, irregularly pulsed sounds have been used to attract sharks. Less success has been achieved in using similar sounds, including the call of a killer whale, a known predator of sharks, to repel sharks.

In 1960 the bubble curtain or bubble fence was developed in Australia. It consisted of a perforated garden hose attached to an air compressor. When the hose was laid on the sea bed the air created a curtain or fence of bubbles. However testing has shown that only the most timid of sharks refuse to penetrate the fence.

Physical protection

The Shark Screen consists of a large cylindrical bag sealed at the bottom and supported at the top by three inflatable collars. The user climbs inside the bag which is filled with water. The Screen is made of an insulating material that prevents the transmission of any electrical fields which may be attractive to sharks, and it also prevents any blood from escaping into the surrounding water.

Divers have tried a variety of protective garments, including chain-mail and Kevlar suits, none of which have proved both practical and effective against shark attack.

Simple physical barriers consisting of iron and wooden poles and wire and nylon mesh have been erected at many swimming beaches. These structures did not survive long in areas with considerable wave action but have proved successful in sheltered conditions of lagoons and embayments such as Sydney harbour.

Shark netting Shark netting has proved the most successful form of protecting people frequenting popular swimming beaches against shark attack. The concept originated in Sydney, Australia, in 1937 and many beaches in Australia and South Africa are now protected. Their success is attributed to their achieving a substantial reduction in the number of sharks inhabiting a particular area, thereby diminishing the probability of a shark coming into contact with a bather.

Electrical repellents A number of efforts have been made to use electrical current to repel sharks. One of these was the Shark Shield, which was originally designed to protect the cod ends of shrimp fishermen's trawl nets from damage by sharks. A smaller version of this device is worn on a diver's belt; it emits 120-V pulses of electrical current into the water around the diver. Evaluation of efficacy is difficult but is being attempted*.

INJURIES CAUSED BY OTHER MARINE FISHES

In general these tend to be superficial as no other large fish has the dentition of a shark. Moray eels of

the family *Muraenidae* and barracuda *Sphyrna* sp. have sharp teeth, little more than 5 mm in length, which are capable of inflicting lacerations but with little tissue removal. Eels reside in holes on the reef and will only bite when their domain is threatened. Scuba divers have found that these fish are easily 'tamed' by frequent feeding, but the eels have also bitten divers who have approached them without food or who have panicked at the sight of an eel swimming toward them. Barracuda are attracted by bright-coloured objects and lights; they possibly regard such items as prey.

Groupers of the family Serranidae have numerous rows of small, brush-like teeth. Larger specimens, such as the brindle bass *Epinephalus lanceolatus*, which attains 250 kg, may inflict abrasions with associated contusion. Stingrays have one or two retroserrate, dentinal spines at the base of the tail, which are used in defence. The spines, being serrated, are not only difficult to remove, but they have an associated venom gland. Sawfishes (*Pristis* spp.) have saw-like, elongated snouts with a row of strong lateral teeth on each side. They are bottom dwellers which use their snouts to either stun small fish or to forage for shellfish in the sand or mud. Like the stingrays they are only dangerous when cornered or restrained.

REFERENCES

Adams E.B., Laurence D.R., Smith J.W.G. (1969). *Tetanus*. Oxford: Blackwell Science. U.K.

Al-Boukai A.A., Hawass Nour E-D., Patel P.J., Kolawole T.M. (1989). Camel bites: report of severe osteolysis as late bone complications. *Postgard. Med. J.*, **65**, 900–4.

Al Fallouji M. (1990). Traumatic love bites. *Br. J. Surg.*, **77**, 100–1.

Anderson R.M. (1991). Immunization in the field. *Nature*, **354**, 502–3.

Baack B.R., Kucan J.O., Demarest, Smoot E.C. (1989). Mauling by Pit Bull Terriers: case report. *J. Trauma*, **29**, 517–20.

Baer G.M. (ed.) (1975). *The Natural History of Rabies*. New York: Academic.

Baldridge H.D. (1973). *Shark Attack Against Man, A Program of Data Reduction and Analysis*. Sarasota, FL: Mote Marine Laboratory, 66 pp.

Borchelt P.L., Lockwood R., Beck A.M., Vaith V.L. (1983). Attacks by packs of dogs involving predation on human beings. *Pub. Health Rep.*, **98**, 57–66.

Buck J.D., Spotte S., Gadbaw J.J. Jr. (1984). Bacteriology of the teeth from a great white shark: potential medical implications for a shark bite victim. *J. Clin. Microbiol.*, **20**, 849–51.

Burge D.R., Scheifele, Speert D.P. (1985). Serious *Pasturella multicida* infections from lion and tiger bites. *JAMA*, **253**, 3296–7.

Callaham M. (1980). Dog bite wounds. *JAMA*, **244**, 2327–8.

Cancio-Bello T.P., deMedina M., Shorey J. et al. (1982). An institutional outbreak of hepatitis B related to a human biting earlier. *J. Infect. Dis.*, **146**, 652–6.

---

*The Natal Sharks Board has successfully tested a device which can protect scuba divers by repelling shark, *Carcharodon carcharias*.

Chutivongse S., Wilde H., Supich C. et al. (1990). Post-exposure prophylaxis for rabies with antiserum and intradermal vaccination. *Lancet*, **335**, 896–8.

Cliff G., Dudley S.F.J. (1991). Sharks caught in the protective gill nets off Natal, South Africa. 4. The bull shark *Carcharhinus leucas* (Valenciennes). *J. Mar. Sci.*, **10**, 253–70.

Compagno L.J.V. (1984). FAO Species Catalogue. Vol. 4. Sharks of the World. An annotated and illustrated catalogue of shark species known to date. Parts 1 and 2. *FAO Fish. Synop.*, **4**, (125).

Coppleson V.M. (1962). *Shark Attack*, 2nd edn. Sydney: Angus & Robertson.

Davies D.H. (1964). *About Sharks and Shark Attack*. Pietermaritzburg: Shuter and Shooter.

Davies D.H., Campbell G.D. (1962). The aetiology, clinical pathology and treatment of shark attack (based on observations in Natal, South Africa). *J.R. Nav. Med. Serv.*, **68**, 1–27.

Donovan J.F., Kaplan W.E. (1989). The therapy of genital trauma by dog bite. *J. Urol.*, **141**, 1163–5.

Earley M.J., Bardley (1984). Human bites: a review. *Br. J. Plast. Surg.*, **37**, 458–62.

Edmonds C., Lowry, C. and Pennefather, J. (1981). *Diving and Subaquatic Medicine*. Australia: Diving Medical Centre.

Fiumara N.J., Exnor J.H. (1981). Primary syphilis following a human bite. *J. Sex Transm. Dis*, **8**, 21–2.

Gilbert P.W. (ed.) (1963). *Sharks and Survival*. Boston: D.C. Health.

Hodgson E.S., Mathewson R.F. (eds) (1978). *Sensory Biology of Sharks, Skates, and Rays*. Arlington, VA: Office of Naval Research.

Jaffe A.C. (1983). Animal bites. *Pediatr. Clin. North Am.*, **30**, 405–13.

Job L., Horman J.T., Grigor J.K., Israel E. (1989). Dysgonic fermenter – 2: a clinico epidemiologic. *J. Emerg. Med.*, **7**, 185–92.

Johnson R.H., Nelson D.R. (1973). Agonistic display in the gray reef shark, *Carcharhinus menisorrah*, and its relationship to attacks on man. *Copeia*, **1**, 76–84.

Kaplan C., Turner G.S., Warrell D.A. (1986). *Rabies the Facts*, 2nd edn. Oxford: Oxford University Press.

Karody R., Nash N., Bhasin V., Balasubramanian (1988). Toxic shock syndrome due to an infected human bite. *Ann. Emerg. Med.*, **17**, 83–7.

Lancet (1988). Editorial: Rabies vaccine failures. *Lancet*, **331**, 917–18.

Long W.T., Filler B.C., Cox E.II, Stark H.H. (1988). Toxic shock syndrome after a human bite to the hand. *J. Hand Surg.*, **13A**, 957–9.

Mandell G.L., Douglas R.G., Jr, Bennett J.E. (eds) (1985). *Principle and Practice of Infectious Diseases*, 2nd edn. New York: John Wiley and Sons.

McCosker J.E. (1985). White shark attack behavior: observations of and speculations about predator and prey strategies. *Mem. South. Calif. Acad. Sci.*, **9**, 123–35.

McDonough J.J., Stern P.J., Alexander J.W. (1987). Management of animal and human bites and resulting human infections. *Curr. Clin. Top. Infect. Dis.*, **8**, 11–36.

Miller D.J., Collier R.S. (1981). Shark attacks in California and Oregon, 1926–1979. *Calif. Fish Game*, **67**, 76–104.

Myrberg A., Gruber S. (1974). The behaviour of the bonnethead shark, *Sphyrna tiburo*. *Copeia*, **2**, 358–74.

Nguyen D. (1988). Epidemiology of animal bites among American military personnel in central Germany. *Milit. Med.*, **153**, 307–8.

Northcutt R.G. (1977). Elasmobranch central nervous system organization and its possible evolutionary significance. *Am. Zool.*, **17**, 411–29.

Paria A.T., Bryan J.A., Maher K.L. et al. (1989). *Vibrio carchariae* infection after a shark bite. *Ann. Intern. Med.*, **111**, 85–6.

Sacks J.J., Sattin R.W., Bonzo S.E. (1989) Dog bite-related fatalities from 1979 through 1988. *JAMA*, **262**, 1489–92.

Schumaker C.L., Dietzchold B., Ertl H.C.L. et al. (1989). Use of mouse anti-rabies monoclonal antibodies in post-exposure treatment of rabies. *J. Clin. Invest.*, **84**, 971–5.

Shirley L.R., Ross S.A. (1989). Risk of transmission of human immunodeficiency virus by bite of an infected toddler. *J. Pediatr.*, **114**, 425–7.

Srivasta S. (1989). Reconstruction of traumatic loss of vermillion and mucocutaneous junction of the lips. *Br. J. Plast. Surg.*, **42**, 526–9.

Teasdale E.L., Davies G.E. (1983). Anaphylaxis after bites by rodents. *Br. Med. J.*, **286**, 1480.

Veronesi R. (ed.) (1981). *Tetanus Importat New Concepts*. Amsterdam: Excerpta Medica.

Wallett T. (1983). *Shark Attack in Southern African Waters and Treatment of Victims*. Cape Town: Struik.

White J.A.M. (1975). Shark attack in Natal. *Injury*, **6**, 187–94.

Wilde H., Chomchey P., Punyaratabandhu P. et al. (1989). Rabies immune globulin a safe and affordable alternative to human rabies immune globulin.

Wiley J.F. II (1990). Mammalian bites: review of evaluation and management. *Clin. Pediat.*, **29**, 283–7.

Wong A.K., Huang S.W., Burnett J.W. (1984). Hypersensitivity to rat saliva. *J. Am. Head Dermatol.*, **11**, 606–8.

Woolfrey B.F., Quall C.O., Lally R.T. (1985). *Pasturella multocida* in an infected tiger bite. *Arch Pathol. Lab. Med.*, **1109**, 744–6.

Wright J.C. (1985). Severe attacks by dogs. Characteristics of the dog, the victims and the attack settings. *Pub. Health Rep.*, **100**, 55–61.

27. Heat Transfer to Tissues

B. Lawton

INTRODUCTION TO HEAT TRANSFER

Temperature is usually thought of as the degree of hotness of a material. When a spatial temperature difference occurs, heat flows from the hot region to the cold region until the temperature difference is eliminated. The hot region loses energy and the cooler region gains energy so it is sometimes useful to think of heat transfer as energy transfer by virtue of temperature difference. This process does not occur instantly but requires a certain time and so heat transfer is the study of the relationships between energy, temperature, spatial coordinates, time and the properties of the materials involved.

Three modes of heat transfer are recognized, namely, *conduction*, *convection* and *radiation*:

In *conduction*, energy is transferred from molecule to molecule without the need for macroscopic movement of the material. This is the only way in which heat can be transferred through opaque solids, where the molecules are fixed and cannot easily move on a large scale. Conduction also occurs in fluids but is less vigorous because the molecules are farther apart. Heat transfer through the solid walls of a stove, or through skin, is by conduction.

In *convection*, energy is transferred by the macroscopic motion of the molecules themselves and it is, therefore, only possible in liquids and gases. *Natural convection* occurs if the fluid is nominally still and its motion is caused simply because a hot fluid, being less dense than the surrounding cold fluid, rises in a gravitational field. *Forced convection*, on the other hand, occurs when a heated fluid is moved by external means, such as a pump or a fan. Convection is commonly the mechanism of heat transfer between the surface of a solid and a surrounding fluid. For example, it is the way in which air is heated near the hot surface of stove. Warm blood pumped by the heart into cold extremities is another example of forced convection.

In *radiation*, energy is emitted, as infrared waves (part of the electromagnetic spectrum) and is emitted by all matter at absolute temperature greater than zero. Radiation exchange between matter does not depend on the existence of intervening material and it is the only method of heat transfer across a vacuum. It is only weakly absorbed by gases and liquids and it passes through some solids, such as glass. When radiation impinges on a solid surface it may by reflected, absorbed or transmitted. Absorption means that radiant energy is converted to a temperature rise in the solid. This usually occurs very close to the surface of opaque materials but in skin, for example, the sun's radiation may penetrate a few millimetres before being absorbed.

The laws of conduction

Heat transfer through a solid is governed by *Fourier's law*. It is based on the observation of one-dimensional steady-state conditions. A surface at a constant temperature is called an *isothermal* surface and the normal to such a surface is the direction of greatest temperature gradient. It is observed that heat flows in the direction of greatest temperature gradient and the rate of flow is directly proportional to that temperature gradient. Thus Fourier's law is:

$$q_x = -k \, \partial T/\partial x \qquad (27.1)$$

The negative sign is necessary because heat flux is considered to be positive in the direction of negative temperature gradient, i.e. heat flows from hot to cold. The constant of proportionality, k, is the thermal conductivity and is a property of the material through which the heat flows. The heat flux q_x is the rate of energy flow per unit area of the isothermal surface and has units of W/m^2. The temperature gradient in the x-direction has units of K/m and so the units of conductivity are W/mK. Typical values of thermal conductivity for good conductors, usually metals, are in the range 20–400 W/mK. Poor conductors of heat include gases, most liquids, and common insulating materials such as brick or cork; the conductivity of such materials varies from 0.01 to 1 W/mK. The conductivity of skin is about 0.5 W/mK and so it is a thermal insulator.

The net heat flowing into a region is stored as a temperature rise. The one-dimensional energy equation expressing this idea is:

$$C \, \partial T/\partial t = R - \partial q_x/\partial x \qquad (27.2)$$

C is the volumetric specific heat of the material, J/m^3K, and R is the volumetric rate of heat absorption, W/m^3. Heat absorption may be caused, for example, by partially transmitted radiation, by the passage of electrical current or by chemical reaction. Quite often its value is zero.

Differentiating Fourier's law and substituting into the energy equation gives the equation of heat diffusion:

$$\partial T/\partial t = R/C + \alpha \, \partial^2 T/\partial x^2 \qquad (27.3)$$

where $\alpha = k/C$ is the thermal diffusivity of the material and has units of m^2/s. Typical values lie in the range 5×10^{-6} to $100 \times 10^{-6}\,m^2/s$ for metals and gases and less than $1 \times 10^{-6}\,m^2/s$ for solid insulators and liquids. The thermal diffusivity of skin is about $0.14 \times 10^{-6}\,m^2/s$.

Equation (27.3) is particularly useful in determining the temperature distribution in a conductor at any instant. It can be solved by a variety of methods if the initial temperature distribution and two boundary conditions are known. Many solutions are given by Carslaw and Jaeger (1947).

Example 1 Skin has a thickness of 3 mm and a conductivity of 0.5 W/mK. Determine the temperature difference across the thickness if a body's metabolic rate is 120 W and the surface area is 1.8 m^2.

By Fourier's law: $q = Q/A = k\,\Delta T/\Delta x$

$$120/1.8 = 0.5 \times \Delta T/0.003$$

therefore $\Delta T = 0.4°C$.

This is the normal temperature difference through a 3 mm depth of skin. The surface temperature of skin is usually about 33°C and blood temperature is usually 37°C, so even deep layers of the dermis and subcutaneous fat are significantly cooler than the blood supply. Heat transfer between the dermis and the blood supply is by convection.

The laws of convection

When a hot fluid is in contact with a cold surface heat flows from the fluid to the surface. The fluid actually touching the surface is at the same temperature as the surface and a few millimetres from the surface the fluid is at its bulk temperature. This distance of a few millimetres in which the fluid temperature changes is called the boundary layer. If the temperature gradient is linear then Fourier's equation suggests:

$$q_x = -k\,(T_s - T_f)/\delta \qquad (27.4)$$

T_f is the bulk fluid temperature. T_s is the surface temperature and δ is the thickness of the boundary layer. Small-scale velocity oscillations in the fluid, known as turbulence, increase the fluid's effective conductivity by as much as 100 times. Moreover, the thickness of the boundary layer is not a fluid property but depends on many variables such as fluid velocity. It is usually convenient to simplify equation (27.4) to the form known as Newton's law:

$$q_x = h\,(T_f - T_s) \qquad (27.5)$$

the constant h is called the surface heat transfer coefficient or surface conductance and it has units of W/m^{2}K. For surfaces in contact with gases similar to air the surface conductance is often about 2–100 W/m^{2}K. Surface conductance is usually higher in forced convection than in natural convection where velocities are low. For surfaces in contact

with a liquid such as water the surface conductance may be in the range 500–20 000 W/m^{2}K.

Calculation, from first principles, of surface conductance is very complex and requires powerful computers. Before such computers were available simpler, semi-empirical, methods were used. These methods relied on non-dimensional numbers and it has been shown, by Chapman (1969), for example, that for natural convection the heat conductance may be determined from an equation of the form:

$$Nu = a\,(Gr)^b\,(Pr)^c \qquad (27.6)$$

where, Nu is the Nusselt number, hd/k
Gr is the Grashof number, $\beta g\,(T_f - T_s)\rho^2 d^3/\mu^2$
Pr is the Prandtl number, $C_p\mu/k$

and a, b, c are constants that depend on the level of turbulence and on the application, i.e. they are different for a vertical wall than for a horizontal cylinder. The values of a, b, c are usually determined by experiment and values may be found in textbooks on heat transfer and in published papers.

For forced convection the Grashof number is replaced by the Reynolds number:

$$Nu = a\,(Re)^b(Pr)^c \qquad (27.7)$$

where Re is the Reynolds number, $\rho c d/\mu$.

Again, the values of a, b, c must be determined by experiment or may be found in published material.

For the purposes of convective heat transfer most parts of the human body may be treated as a long cylinder of diameter d and thus the values of a, b, c in equations (27.6) and (27.7) are well established and are summarized in Table 27.1.

The requisite properties of air and water for these equations are given in Table 27.2. Substituting the values of a, b, c and the properties of air or water into equations (27.6 and 27.7) gives the following simple equations.

Natural convection in air:

$$h = 1.36\,(\Delta T/d)^{0.25} \text{ or } h = 1.54\,\Delta T^{0.333} \; (27.8)$$

The two equations are valid for their relevant range of Grashof numbers but it is often easier to work out both surface conductances and use the one with

TABLE 27.1

VALUES OF a, b, c FOR HORIZONTAL CYLINDERS IN NATURAL CONVECTION AND IN FORCED CONVECTION (CROSS-FLOW)

	a	b	c	
Grashof Number				
10^4 to 10^9	0.525	0.25	0.25	equation (27.6)
10^9 to 10^{12}	0.129	0.333	0.333	equation (27.6)
Reynolds Number				
4000 to 40 000	0.196	0.618	0.333	equation (27.7)
40 000 to 250 000	0.027	0.805	0.333	equation (27.7)

TABLE 27.2
RELEVANT PROPERTIES OF AIR AND WATER AT 20°C

	Air	Water	Units
Coefficient of cubical expansion, β	0.0034	0.00043	K⁻¹
Specific heat at constant pressure, Cp	1005	4183	J/kgK
Viscosity, μ	18.5	1002	μNs/m²
Thermal conductivity, k	0.0262	0.603	W/mK
Density, ρ	1.18	998.2	kg/m³
Prandtl number, Pr	0.71	6.95	–
Diffusivity, α = k/ C	22.1	0.144	μm²/s

Local gravity, g, is usually 9.81 m/s².

the larger value. The equations require the temperature difference, ΔT, to be in °C and the cylinder diameter, d, to be in metres for the surface conductance to be in W/m²K.

Natural convection in water:

$$h = 130 \, (\Delta T/d)^{0.25} \text{ or } h = 237 \, \Delta T^{0.333} \quad (27.9)$$

Forced convection of air:

$$h = 4.26 \, (c \, d)^{0.618}/d \quad \text{or} \quad h = 4.65 \, (c \, d)^{0.805}/d \quad (27.10)$$

The two equations are valid for their relevant range of Reynolds numbers but it is usually easier to work out both values of h and use the larger value. The air velocity over the cylinder should be in. m/s and the cylinder diameter should be in metres if the surface conductance is to be in W/m²K.

For forced convection of water:

$$h = 1150 \, (c \, d)^{0.618}/d \quad \text{or} \quad h = 2090 \, (c \, d)^{0.805}/d \quad (27.11)$$

Example 2 If a human finger of 10 mm diameter and 30°C surface temperature is placed into still water at 50°C, determine the heat flux into the finger.

For natural convection in water use equation (27.9):

$$h = 130 \times \{(50 - 30)/0.01\}^{0.25} = 876 \text{ W/m}^2\text{K or}$$

$$h = 237 \times (50 - 30)^{0.333} = 643 \text{ W/m}^2\text{K}$$

We use the larger of these values so:

$$q = h \, \Delta T = 876 \times (50 - 30) = 17\,520 \text{ W/m}^2$$

This is, of course, a heat flow into the skin; it is about 260 times greater than the normal heat flow out of the skin. Clearly, with such a large heat input the skin surface temperature increases very quickly. This reduces the temperature difference between the skin and the water and so reduces the heat input. After a few seconds the skin temperature will be very close to the water temperature and heat

flow will be much reduced. Immersion in still water at 50°C for 5 minutes normally produces a partial-thickness (second-degree) burn.

The laws of radiation

Infrared radiation is the name given to that part of the electromagnetic spectrum having wavelengths between about 1 and 100 μm. All matter at temperatures above absolute zero emits radiation, which travels in straight lines and passes through a vacuum and most gases with ease. When this radiation strikes a surface a proportion (ρ) is reflected, a proportion (α) is absorbed, producing a temperature rise in the material, and the remainder (τ) is transmitted through the material. Therefore:

$$\rho + \alpha + \tau = 1 \quad (27.12)$$

For most materials absorption takes place at the surface but some materials, skin is an example, allow the radiation to penetrate before it is absorbed. For most gases the absorptivity and reflectivity is very low and so the transmissivity, τ, is nearly unity. For most solids the transmissivity is zero and so:

$$\rho + \alpha = 1 \quad (27.13)$$

A perfectly white surface reflects all incident radiation, so $\rho = 1$ and $\alpha = 0$. A perfectly black surface absorbs all incident radiation and reflects none, so $\rho = 0$ and $\alpha = 1$. Surfaces are said to be grey if the absorptivity and reflectivity are greater than zero and less than unity and is independent of wavelength.

All these quantities may vary with the wavelength of the impinging radiation and this can lead to interesting phenomena such as the Greenhouse Effect. Glass has the ability to transmit short-wavelength radiation emitted by hot surfaces, such as sunlight, but is a poor transmitter of long-wavelength radiation emitted from cool surfaces. Thus sunlight passes through glass and is absorbed by surfaces behind the glass but the radiation emitted by these surfaces cannot be transmitted by the glass and so the sunlight is trapped. Similarly, materials such as steel are able to absorb sunlight but are poor emitters of radiation and so sunlight is trapped and the surface becomes very hot. This is the reason for motor cars made of steel becoming very hot, when left in bright sunlight.

It is found that a perfect black surface is the best emitter of radiation and the energy emitted per unit area per unit time is proportional to the fourth power of the absolute temperature:

$$q_b = \sigma T^4 \qquad (27.14)$$

This is the Stefan–Boltzmann law and the constant, σ, is the Stefan–Boltzmann constant and has a value of 5.67×10^{-8} W/m^2 K^4 (the number sequence 5,6,7,8 makes it very easy to remember).

For grey surfaces the energy emitted is less than that given by equation (27.14) and so a surface emissivity, $\epsilon < 1$, is introduced:

$$q = \epsilon \sigma T^4 \qquad (27.15)$$

By, Kirchoff's law the emissivity of a surface 1 at temperature T_1 is equal to its absorptivity for radiation received from a surface 2 at temperature $T_2 = T_1$. Thus:

$$\epsilon = \alpha = 1 - \rho \qquad (27.16)$$

Because of the possibility of confusion between α, meaning the absorptivity and α meaning the thermal diffusivity, the emissivity ϵ will be used when absorptivity is intended; this is justified by Kirchoff's law.

The net radiation exchange between two surfaces is usually expressed as:

$$Q = F_{1-2} A_1 \sigma (T_2^4 - T_1^4) \qquad (27.17)$$

where F_{1-2} is a form factor, having a value between 0 and 1, which takes account of the geometrical shape and emissivities of the two surfaces. The determination of form factors is usually very complex but values have been worked out for many configurations and may be found in textbooks on the subject.

The radiation from a surface is not emitted with equal intensity in all directions. The intensity of radiation in direction ø measured from the normal to a surface is given by Lambert's Law:

$$i = i_n \cos \phi \qquad (27.18)$$

where i_n is the intensity of radiation normal to the surface ($\sigma T^4/\pi$). The intensity of radiation emitted parallel to a surface ($\phi = 90$ degrees) is zero.

Similarly, the radiation emitted from a surface is not of a constant wavelength. If we define the energy emitted at wavelength λ as:

$$q_{b\lambda} = \partial q_b / \partial \lambda \qquad (27.19)$$

then by Plank's law:

$$q_{b\lambda} = \frac{c_1 \lambda^{-5}}{\exp(c_2/\lambda T) - 1} \qquad (27.20)$$

where $c_1 = 3.74 \times 10^{-14}$ Wm^2 and $c_2 = 0.01439$ mK

$q_{b\lambda}$ is called the monochromatic emissive power and, for a given temperature, it has a maximum value at a certain wavelength, λ_{max}. This is found by differentiating equation (27.20) with respect to λ and equating to zero to give the simple result known as Wien's displacement law:

$$\lambda_{max} T = 0.0029 \text{ m K} \qquad (27.21)$$

Thus the wavelength of sunlight ($T = 6000$ K) is $0.5 \, \mu$m and of low-temperature radiation ($T = 300$ K) is $10 \, \mu$m.

Example 3 A flame at a temperature of 2000 K exchanges heat with surface at (a) 30°C and (b) 500°C. If the form function is 0.8, determine the net heat flux in each case.

Use equation (27.17). Temperatures in °C are converted to K by adding 273.

(a) $q = 0.8 \times 5.67 \times 10^{-8} [2000^4 - (30 + 273)^4]$
    $q = 725.4$ kW/m^2

(b) $q = 0.8 \times 5.67 \times 10^{-8} [2000^4 - (500 + 273)^4]$
    $q = 709.6$ kW/m^2

In this case even a quite large change in the temperature of the cool surface (from 30°C to 500°C) makes only a 2% change in the radiant heat transfer. If the temperature ratio between the two surfaces is greater than two then the heat flux may be considered to be independent of the temperature of the cool surface.

APPLICATIONS

In this section some well-known solutions to the diffusion equation, equation (27.3), are described but not derived. Rigorous derivations may be found elsewhere (e.g. Carslaw and Jaeger, 1990). The solutions presented are chosen because of their usefulness in relation to skin burns. Experimenters normally carry out their measurements under well-defined and repeatable conditions that are amenable to mathematical analysis. Such analysis gives considerable insight into the conditions under which a burn occurs and also gives the experimenter confidence in the accuracy of the measurements.

The analytical solutions described all assume that the skin temperature is uniform immediately before the start of heat transfer ($T = T_i$ at $t = 0$ for all $x > 0$). This is nearly true as Example 1, above, has shown. It is also assumed that the temperature at great depths (i.e. about 5 mm) from the surface remains unchanged during the period of heat transfer ($T = T_i$ at $x = \infty$ for all $t > 0$). This is usually true for about 10 seconds after the start of heat transfer. Thus the analytical solutions are not useful for burns requiring exposure times greater than about 10 seconds. For longer times a numerical method, suitable for programming in a digital computer, is preferred.

A further assumption is that the thermal properties of skin remain unchanged during the period of heat transfer. This is approximately true but for long exposures to heat vasodilatation may occur which alters the skin's conductance. Finally, it is assumed that heat absorption (R) is zero. This means that the solutions cannot be used for cases of penetrating radiation such as sunlight.

For most cases in which simple boundary conditions are not valid, and this includes most real burns, analytical solutions are not possible. Under these more difficult conditions numerical solutions using a digital computer are necessary and so a simple numerical method for solving the diffusion equations is also described together with a suitable programming algorithm. Six solutions are considered to be particularly useful.

Step change in surface temperature

This boundary condition approximates the contact of skin with a dense fluid such as water where the skin surface temperature rises to the water temperature in a very short period of time. It is assumed that the surface temperature rises from $T = T_i$ to $T = T_0$ when $t = 0$ and remains at this temperature for all $t > 0$. The solution of the diffusion equation is:

$$\frac{T - T_i}{T_o - T_i} = 1 - erf(\theta) = erfc(\theta) \qquad (27.22)$$

where θ = dimensionless depth = $x/\sqrt{(4 \alpha t)}$

Alternatively the solution can be written in terms of dimensionless time as:

$$\frac{T - T_i}{T_o - T_i} = 1 - erf[1/\sqrt{\tau}] = erfc[1/\sqrt{\tau}] \qquad (27.23)$$

where τ = dimensionless time = $4 \alpha t/x^2$

The error function, erf, frequently arises in diffusion processes and is defined in terms of the integral:

$$erf(x) = \frac{2}{\sqrt{\pi}} \int_0^x \exp(-t^2) \, dt \qquad (27.24)$$

Values of the error function vary between 0 and 1 and are commonly tabulated in mathematical tables. The complementary error function, $erfc$, is defined such that $erf + erfc = 1$.

Equations (27.22) and (27.23) are plotted in Figure 27.1 in dimensionless format. The upper graph

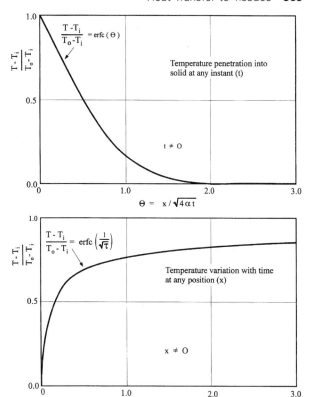

Figure 27.1 Response of a semi-infinite solid to a step change in surface temperature.

shows how the temperature varies with depth at any given instant of time, t. The lower graph shows how the temperature varies with time at any given point, x.

The depth of penetration into the surface of the temperature rise is given by $\theta = 2$; beyond this point the temperature rise is insignificant. Thus:

$$\theta = x/\sqrt{(4 \alpha t)} = 2 \text{ and so } x = 4\sqrt{(\alpha t)} \qquad (27.25)$$

This is a useful equation because it is very simple and gives a good indication of how far heat penetrates in a given time. For skin, $\alpha = 0.14 \times 10^{-6}\,m^2/s$, and so heat penetrates 1.5 mm in 1 second, 3 mm in 4 seconds and 6 mm in 16 seconds.

The surface heat flux, if the surface temperature is constant, is:

$$q_0 = k(T_0 - T_i)/\sqrt{(\pi \alpha t)} \qquad (27.26)$$

and the heat transferred (heat dose) is:

$$H = \int_0^t q_0 \, dt = k(T_0 - T_i)\sqrt{(4t/\pi \alpha)} \qquad (27.27)$$

Example 4 Determine the heat dose required to produce a partial-thickness burn by immersion in water at 56°C for 16 seconds. Conductivity is 0.5 W/mK and diffusivity is $0.14 \times 10^{-6}\,m^2/s$ and the skin's initial temperature is 37°C. Use equation (27.27):

$$H = 0.5 \times (56 - 37) \sqrt{(4 \times 16/3.142/0.14 \times 10^{-6}}$$

$$H = 0.115 \text{ MJ/m}^2$$

The equation used is in error for times greater than about 10 seconds and so the calculated heat dose is only approximate. The heat dose actually required to produce a partial-thickness burn in 16 seconds by immersion in water at 56°C is 0.1 MJ/m².

Contact between solids

An interesting and useful application of the theory for step changes in surface temperatures occurs when two solid surfaces touch. If the two surfaces are initially at temperatures T_a and T_b then the temperature at the point of contact changes to T_0, and remains at T_0, whilst the surfaces are in contact. The heat lost from material a is gained by material b and so, from equation (27.26), we may write:

$$q_0 = k_a (T_a - T_0)/\sqrt{(\pi \alpha_a t)}$$

$$= k_b (T_0 - T_b)/\sqrt{(\pi \alpha_b t)}$$

and the interface temperature T_0 is a constant given by:

$$\frac{T_0 - T_b}{T_a - T_b} = \frac{1}{1 + \lambda} \text{ where } \lambda = \frac{k_b}{k_a}\sqrt{\frac{\alpha_a}{\alpha_b}} \quad (27.28)$$

If the touching surfaces have the same thermal properties then $\lambda = 1$ and the interface temperature T_0 is the average of the two initial temperatures $(T_a + T_b)/2$. If the hot surface is a much better conductor than the cool surface then $\lambda = 0$ and the interface temperature is the same as the hot surface $(T_0 = T_a)$. By contrast, if the hot surface is a much worse conductor than the cool surface then $\lambda = \infty$ and the interface temperature is the same as the cool surface $(T_0 = T_b)$.

Equation (27.28) may be used in determining the thermal properties of skin. If the thermal properties of a hot probe are known together with the initial surface temperatures of the probe and the skin then, if the interface temperature is measured when the hot probe contacts the skin, the thermal properties of skin may be determined. Probe temperatures between 0°C and 55°C may be used without damage to the skin and the probe need only contact the skin for about 10 or 20 seconds to ensure that a constant temperature is attained. The method is good for low-conductivity materials but for high-conductivity materials, where the heat flow is large, the contact resistance at the interface becomes important and leads to errors if the simple theory is used.

Example 5 Skin at 35°C touches a plastic surface having a temperature of 140°C. Determine the temperature at the interface if the conductivity of plastic is 0.1 W/mK and the thermal diffusivity is 9 × 10⁻⁸ m²/s. For skin take the conductivity as 0.5 W/mK and the diffusivity as 0.14 × 10⁻⁶ m²/s.

From equation (27.28)

$$\lambda = 0.5/0.1 \times \sqrt{(9 \times 10^{-8}/14 \times 10^{-8})} = 4.01$$

and

$$\frac{T_0 - 35}{140 - 35} = 1/(1 + 4.01)$$

hence $T_0 = 56°C$

Clearly, contact with a low-conductivity material at 140°C is the equivalent of contact with water at 56°C and, as in Example 4, will produce a partial-thickness burn in 16 seconds.

Step change in surface heat flux

The heat flux at the surface is assumed to rise from zero to q_0 at $t = 0$ and remains at this value for all $t > 0$. This approximates radiant heating from a constant temperature source that is at least twice as hot as the irradiated surface; heating by the sun's rays or radiation from an electric fire or furnace are examples.

The solution of the diffusion equation is:

$$\frac{(T - T_i)k}{q_0 \sqrt{(\alpha t)}} = \frac{2}{\sqrt{\pi}} \exp(-\theta^2) - 2\theta \, erfc \, (\theta) \quad (27.29)$$

where θ = dimensionless depth = $x/\sqrt{(4\alpha t)}$ and the complimentary error function $erfc$ is defined as:

$$erfc \, (\theta) = 1 - erf(\theta) \quad (27.30)$$

Alternatively the solution may be written in terms of dimensionless time:

$$\frac{(T - T_i)k}{q_0 x} = \sqrt{(\tau/\pi)} \exp(-1/\tau) - erfc \, (1/\sqrt{\tau}) \quad (27.31)$$

where τ = dimensionless time = $4\alpha t/x^2$

At the surface $\theta = 0$ and thus equation (27.29) simplifies to:

$$T_0 - T_i = q_0 \sqrt{(4\alpha t/\pi)}/k \quad (27.32)$$

and so temperature rises as the square root of time if the surface heat flux is constant.

Equations (27.29) and (27.31) are plotted in Figure 27.2 in dimensionless format. The upper graph shows how temperature varies with depth at any given instant of time whereas the lower shows how temperature varies with time at any given point beneath the surface. As in the case of a step change in temperature the penetration of heat into the

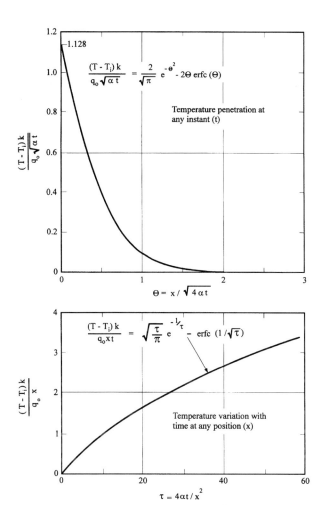

Figure 27.2 Response of a semi-infinite solid to a step change in heat flux.

surface is given by $\theta = 2$ and so equation (27.25) is also valid for the present case.

Since the surface heat flux is constant, the heat dose is determined from:

$$H = \int_0^t q_0 \, dt = q_0 t \qquad (27.33)$$

Example 6 If a heat dose of 0.28 MJ/m^2 is received at a constant rate in a time of 300 seconds, determine the maximum skin temperature. Assume that skin has the properties as in Example 4 and the initial temperature is 37°C.

From equation (27.33):

$$q_0 = 0.28 \times 10^6 / 300 = 933 \, W/m^2$$

From equation (27.32):

$$T_0 - 37 = 933/0.5 \times \sqrt{(4 \times 1.4 \times 10^{-7} \times 300/3.142)}$$

$$T_0 = 50.6°C.$$

Natural or Forced Convection

In this case it is assumed that the surface heat flux is given by the natural or forced convection equation $q_0 = h \, (T_f - T_0)$, where h, is the surface conductance and T_f is the bulk temperature of the fluid adjacent to the surface. The solution to the diffusion equation with this boundary condition is:

$$\frac{T - T_i}{T_f - T_i} = erfc \, \theta - \exp(2\theta\sqrt{\tau + \tau}) \, erfc \, (\theta + \sqrt{\tau}) \qquad (27.34)$$

where

$$\theta = x/\sqrt{4\alpha\tau} \text{ and } \tau = h^2\alpha t/k^2$$

and the complimentary error function is defined as:

$$erfc \, (x) = 1 - erf \, (x)$$

At the surface $\theta = 0$ and so equation (27.34) reduces to

$$\frac{T_0 - T_i}{T_f - T_i} = 1 - \exp(\tau) \, erfc \, \sqrt{\tau} \qquad (27.35)$$

The surface heat flux is given by $q_0 = h \, (T_f - T_0)$ and so the heat dose, H, is given by:

$$\frac{Hh\alpha}{(T_f - T_i) \, k^2} = 2 \, \sqrt{(\tau/\pi)} - \frac{T_0 - T_i}{T_f - T_i} \qquad (27.36)$$

Equations (27.35) and (27.36) are plotted in Figure 27.3.

Example 7 Skin at 37°C comes into contact with hot water at 56°C. If the surface conductance between skin and moving water is 6000 W/m^{2}K and the thermal properties of skin are as in Example 4,

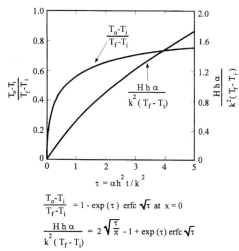

$$\frac{T_0 - T_i}{T_f - T_i} = 1 - \exp(\tau) \, erfc \, \sqrt{\tau} \text{ at } x = 0$$

$$\frac{Hh\alpha}{k^2 \, (T_f - T_i)} = 2\sqrt{\frac{\tau}{\pi}} - 1 + \exp(\tau) \, erfc \, \sqrt{\tau}$$

Figure 27.3 Transient response of a semi-infinite solid to a convective health flux $q = h \, (T_f - T_0)$.

determine the skin surface temperature after 10 seconds. What is the heat dose after 16 seconds. Use equation (27.34):

$$\tau = 6000^2 \times 1.4 \times 10^{-7} \times 10/0.5^2 = 201.6$$

$$T_0 - 37 = (56 - 37) \times [1 - \exp(201.6) \, erfc \, (14.2)]$$

$$T_0 = 56°C$$

Thus, after only 10 seconds the skin surface temperature has reached the same temperature as the water.

For the heat dose use equation (27.35). At $t = 16$ seconds the value of τ is 322.6 so:

$$\frac{Hh\alpha}{(T_f - T_i)\,k^2} = 2\sqrt{(322.6/\pi) - 1]} = 19.26$$

$$H = 19.26 \times (56 - 37) \times 0.5^2/(6000 \times 0.14 \times 10^{-6})$$

$$H = 0.109 \text{ MJ/m}^2$$

This is very close to heat dose calculated by a simpler method in Example 4 and it is subject to the same restrictions.

Exponentially decaying heat flux

In this case the surface heat flux, for $t > 0$, is defined by an exponential relationship of the form $q_0 = H/t_0 \exp(-t/t_0)$, where H is the heat dose and t_0 is a time constant. This form of heat transfer is typical of explosive events.

The solution of the diffusion equation with this boundary condition is most easily expressed as an integral or as an infinite series. The surface temperature is:

$$\frac{(T_0 - T_i)}{H}\sqrt{\frac{\pi k^2 t_0}{\alpha}}$$

$$= \exp(-u)\int_0^u \frac{1}{v}\exp(v)\,dv \tag{27.37}$$

where $u = t/t_0$ and v is the variable of integration between limits 0 and u. This has a series solution:

$$\frac{(T_0 - T_i)}{H}\sqrt{\frac{\pi k^2 t_0}{\alpha}}$$

$$= 2\sqrt{u}\exp(-u)\left[1 + \frac{u}{3} + \frac{u^2}{5.2!} + \frac{u^3}{7.3!} - - -\right] \tag{27.38}$$

Figure 27.4 shows equation (27.38) plotted in dimensionless format. The maximum surface temperature occurs when $t = 0.85\,t_0$ and has a value of:

$$T_{max} - T_i = 1.082\,H\sqrt{\alpha/(\pi k^2 t_0)} \tag{27.39}$$

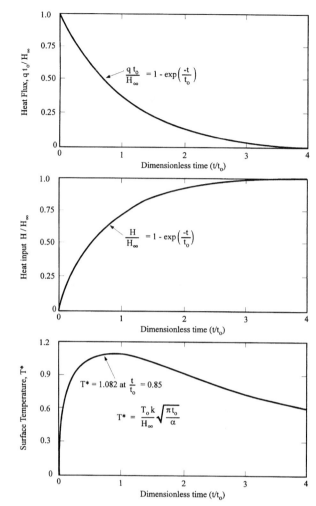

Figure 27.4 Heat flux, total heat input and surface temperature variation in time.

Example 8 In an explosion 0.1 MJ/m² of energy is transferred to skin at 35°C and having the thermal properties specified in Example 4. If the time constant is 0.05 s determine maximum skin temperature.

Use equation (27.39).

$$T_{max} = 35 + 1.082$$

$$\times 100\,000\sqrt{[0.14 \times 10^{-6}/(3.142 \times 0.5^2 \times 0.05)]}$$

$$T_{max} = 239°C$$

Although this is a very high skin temperature it lasts for only a short time and so the thermal damage inflicted is only just sufficient to produce a partial-thickness (second-degree) burn.

Nuclear explosions

The heat pulse from a nuclear explosion is due to radiation from the intensely hot fireball which lasts for several seconds depending on the size of the bomb (kT). It is usually assumed that 1 kT yields 4.2 $\times 10^{12}$ J of energy and that a third of this is converted into thermal radiation. Thus the heat per unit area, the heat dose, arriving at a surface depends on the size of the bomb and its distance from the surface (R):

$$H = \frac{1}{3} \frac{4.2 \times 10^{12} \times kT}{4\pi R^2}$$

$$= 0.1114 \times 10^{12}\, kT/R^2 \qquad (27.40)$$

The pulse shape is given by:

$$\frac{q}{q_{max}} = \frac{2.2u^2}{1 + 1.69u^{3.6}}$$

$$+ \frac{0.206\, \exp\,[-3.6\,(u-1.18)^2]}{1 + (u/1.6)^{10}} \qquad (27.41)$$

where $u = t/t_{max}$ and t_{max} is the time taken for the radiant flux to reach a maximum; it is usually estimated from $t_{max} = 0.042\, kT^{0.44}$. The maximum radiant heat flux is q_{max} and it has a value of $q_{max} = 0.38\, H/t_{max} = kT^{0.56}/R^2$.

The pulse shape, heat dose and surface temperature are plotted in Figure 27.5 in dimensionless format. The maximum temperature rise is given by:

$$T_{max} - T_i = 1.655\, q_{max}\, \sqrt{[t_{max}/(\pi\alpha)]}/C$$

$$T_{max} - T_i = 0.355\, \epsilon H/\sqrt{kCt_{max}} \qquad (27.42)$$

Of the heat dose H impinging on the skin, αH is absorbed and by Kirchoff's law this may be written as ϵH. Both equation (27.42) and Figure 27.5 assume that the material is opaque and so, while they are valid for many materials, they are not valid for human skin.

Example 9 Determine the maximum temperature of skin exposed to the radiation from a 1-MT nuclear bomb at a distance of 5 km. The thermal conductivity of skin is 0.5 W/mK, the volumetric specific heat is 3.57 MJ/m³K, the absorptivity of skin is 0.9 and the initial skin temperature is 35°C.

Use equation (27.40). 1 MT is 1000 kT.

$$H = 0.1114 \times 10^{12} \times 1000/5000^2 = 4.46\ \text{MJ/m}^2$$

This will produce very severe burns in excess of 3 mm deep. The temperature may be estimated from equation (27.42) but will be in error because radiation from a high-temperature source penetrates the skin to a considerable depth before being absorbed; equation (27.42) is valid for opaque materials where the radiation is absorbed at the surface. Nevertheless, equation (27.42) gives an approximation of the temperature rise.

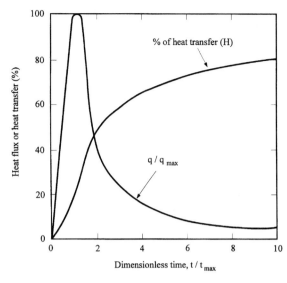

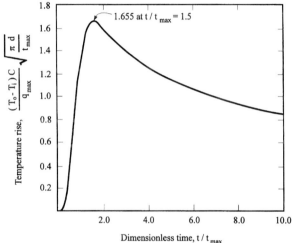

Figure 27.5 Heat flux, heat dose and surface temperature variation for radiation from a nuclear explosion.

$$t_0 = 0.042 \times 1000^{0.44} = 0.8775\ \text{s}$$
$$T_{max} = 35 + 0.355 \times 4.46 \times 10^6$$
$$\times\, 0.9/\sqrt{[0.5 \times 3.57 \times 10^6 \times 0.8775]}$$
$$T_{max} = 1174°C.$$

Numerical methods

The diffusion equation may be reduced to a set of simple finite difference equations and in this form is particularly suitable for digital computers. Also, many of the restrictions necessary for analytical solutions are removed without additional complication. For example, radiation and non-linear convective boundaries, heat absorption and finite wall thickness may be included in the calculation without increasing the complexity of the problem by a significant amount.

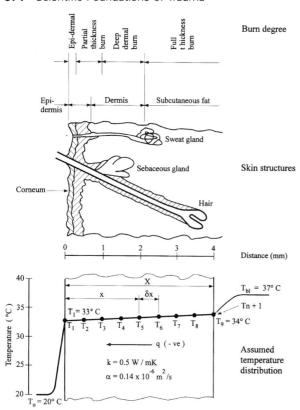

Figure 27.6 Assumed temperature distribution, skin structures and burn depths.

Figure 27.6 shows the position of imaginary nodes, distance δx apart, through the dermis. The temperature of the surface node is T_1 and there are n sections, hence the temperature at the inner surface is T_{n+1}. The temperature at any arbitrary node at time t is T_i and at δt seconds later the temperature is F_i. Using the usual finite difference approximations we may write:

$$\partial T / \partial t = (F_i - T_i)/\delta t$$

and

$$\partial^2 T / \partial x^2 = (T_{i+1} - 2T_i + T_{i-1})/\delta x^2$$

Substituting these into the diffusion equation, equation (27.3) gives:

$$(F_i - T_i)/\delta t = \alpha\,(T_{i+1} - 2T_i + T_{i-1})/\delta x^2 + R_i/C$$

which may be re-arranged to the more convenient form:

$$F_i = (1 - 2p)\,T_i + p\,(T_{i+1} + T_{i-1}) + u\,R_i \quad (27.43)$$

where $p = \alpha\,\delta t/\delta x^2 < 0.5$ for stability and $u = \delta t/C$.

This is the simple explicit finite difference form of the diffusion equation. The value of p is a constant and is fixed, by a suitable choice of δx and δt, to be less than 0.5. If the initial temperatures (T_i) are known then the temperature δt seconds later (F_i)

may be calculated. This is done for each of the nodes to give the new temperature distribution. The process is continued in this way for as long as is necessary.

At the surfaces ($i = 1$ and $i = n + 1$) equation (27.43) is invalid because the temperatures T_0 and T_{n+2} are required for the equation but are not defined. To define values for these *dummy* temperatures two boundary conditions must be specified.

If the heat flow into the skin, q, is known then, from Fourier's law:

$$q = -k\,\partial T / \partial x = k\,(T_0 - T_2)/(2\delta x) \text{ and so:}$$

$$T_0 = T_2 + 2\,\delta x q / k \quad (27.44)$$

Thus the dummy temperature T_0 is defined. The heat flux need not be constant but may be due to convection and radiation, so in general:

$$q = q_s + h\,(T_f - T_1) + \epsilon\sigma\,(T_f^4 - T_1^4) \quad (27.45)$$

Similarly at the inner surface:

$$T_{n+2} = T_n - 2\,\delta x q / k \quad (27.46)$$

At the inner surface the heat flux is caused by convection between the blood and the skin, so the heat flux is:

$$q = h_c\,(T_{n+1} - T_{bl}) \quad (27.47)$$

Equations (27.43) to (27.47) represent the most simple numerical approximation of the diffusion equation and its associated boundary and initial conditions. These equations are sometimes unstable but can be made to work for most problems. More advanced numerical methods are often used in order to improve accuracy, avoid instability or reduce computing time.

Example 10 Skin is subjected to a constant heat flux of 2000 W/m² for a period of 5 seconds. Determine the temperature distribution using a numerical method with $p = 0.25$, $\alpha = 0.14 \times 10^{-6}$ m²/s and $k = 0.5$ W/mK. The initial temperature is 30°C and the time step is 1 second.

Equation (27.43) is:

$$F_i = 0.5\,T_i + 0.25\,(T_{i+1} + T_{i-1}) \quad (27.48)$$

and

$$\delta x = \sqrt{(0.14 \times 10^{-6} \text{ x } 1/0.25)} = 7.5 \times 10^{-4} \text{ m}$$

Thus equation (27.44) is:

$$T_0 = T_2 + 2 \times 7.5 \times 10^{-4} \times 2000/0.5$$

$$T_0 = T_2 + 6 \quad (27.49)$$

The first line in Table 27.3, time = 0, has temperatures of 30°C and the dummy temperature is 36°C, equation (27.49). In the second line the temperatures T_1 to T_6 are calculated from equation (27.48). The dummy temperature is again $T_2 + 6$, equation (27.49), and so the process is repeated, line

TABLE 27.3
COMPUTATION OF SKIN TEMPERATURE

Time (s)	Dummy (T_0)	Surface					
		T_1	T_2	T_3	T_4	T_5	T_6
0	36	30	30	30	30	30	30
1	36	31.5	30	30	30	30	30
2	36.38	32.25	30.38	30	30	30	30
3	36.75	32.82	30.75	30.1	30	30	30
4	36.11	33.29	31.11	30.24	30.03	30	30
5	37.44	33.45	31.44	30.41	30.08	30.01	30
x(mm)		0.0	0.75	1.5	2.25	3.0	3.75

by line, until the 5 seconds are completed. This numerical analysis shows very clearly how the heat diffuses into the surface; after 5 seconds the heat has just penetrated to 2.25 or 3 mm.

The surface temperature after 5 seconds may be compared with the analytical solution, equation (27.32):

$$T_0 = T_i + q_0/k \sqrt{(4 \alpha t/\pi)}$$
$$T_0 = 30 + 2000/0.5 \times \sqrt{(4 \times 1.4 \times 10^{-7} \times 5/3.142)}$$
$$T_0 = 33.78°C$$

Thus there is an error of 9% in the change of surface temperature. This is quite large but it may be reduced to a very small value by choosing a smaller time step, δt. If the problem were programmed in a digital computer then a time step of 0.1 seconds gives a skin temperature of 33.69°C and a time step of 0.01 seconds gives the correct temperature of 33.78°C. The computing times are a few seconds.

THERMAL AND RELATED PROPERTIES OF HUMAN SKIN

The pertinent properties of human skin include thermal conductivity, density, specific heat, and thermal diffusivity. In order to model heat transfer through skin it is also necessary to know the skin's conductance, which is a combined measure of skin thickness, conductivity and the effectiveness of the blood supply (vasodilatation).

Optical properties are also important if the heat source is radiation. The reflectivity and emissivity of skin varies with the wavelength of incident radiation and with the skin's pigmentation. Also, skin is not perfectly opaque but allows short-wavelength radiation, e.g. sunlight, to penetrate a considerable distance before being absorbed. This has a marked effect in reducing the temperature rise and in protecting the skin against burns.

Geometrical and thermal properties

Roth *et al.* (1968) give the following geometrical properties for the average male weighing 70 kg and 1.7 m height.

Skin mass	4 kg
Surface area	1.8 m²
Volume	3.6 litre
Thickness (dermis)	0.5 mm (eyelids)
	5.0 mm (back)
	2.0 mm (average)
Epidermal thickness	80–300 μm
Density	1100 kg/m³
Water content	70–75%

With a water content as high as 70 or 75%, it is to be expected that the properties of skin are similar to those of water specified in Table 27.2.

A cross-section of human skin with some indication of the normal temperature distribution is shown in Figure 27.6.

Henriques found that pig skin produces very similar burns to human skin and, indeed, has very similar thermal properties (Henriques, 1947). The *in vitro* thermal properties of pig skin are given in Table 27.4.

Henriques reported that *in vivo* experiments confirm these values and suggested that increased blood flow could increase conductivity by about 15%. The influence of blood flow was also noted, in relation to human skin, by Buettner, and to allow for this he suggested that conductivity should increase with distance from the surface:

$$k = 0.293 (1 + 0.3x) \text{ W/mK} \text{ (when } x \text{ is in mm)}$$

Thus an average value ($x = 2$ mm) for human skin is 0.469 W/mK which is somewhat similar to Henriques' measurements.

Buettner (1952) also showed that conductivity apparently increased with temperature. However, he determined that this was due to radiant heat penetrating the skin to some depth rather than

TABLE 27.4

THERMAL PROPERTIES OF PIG SKIN (*IN VITRO*)

	Epidermis	Dermis	Fat	Muscle	Units
Specific heat	3600	3224	2300	3810	J/kgK
Conductivity	0.209	0.370	0.160	0.460	W/mK

being converted to a temperature rise at the surface as his analysis assumed.

Many researchers find it more convenient to measure the product $k/\sqrt{\alpha}$ which naturally occurs in heat transfer theory, as for example in equations (27.26), (27.27), (27.28), (27.32), (27.36), (27.39) and (27.42). It is easily shown that

$$k/\sqrt{\alpha} = \sqrt{(kC)} = \sqrt{(k\rho C_v)}$$

and the product kC or $k\rho C_v$ is called the *thermal inertia*. Thus any of the simple situations described in the previous section may be used to give a direct measure of the product kC and, from independent measurements of the volumetric specific heat, the conductivity and diffusivity is readily computed. The method lends itself to the measurement *in vivo* of thermal properties in humans (Perkins *et al.*, 1952). Some results are shown in Table 27.5.

Lipkin and Hardy (1954) also measured thermal inertia in human skin and found it to vary depending on the state of vasodilatation (Table 27.6).

Thermal inertia of skin increases with surface heat flux (Stoll and Greene, 1959), and it seems likely that this too is attributable to vasodilatation. In these tests the volumetric specific heat is taken to be 4.187 MJ/m^3 and some results are shown in Table 27.7.

Many measurements made by earlier workers have been summarized by Roth (1968), as shown in Table 27.8.

Other workers also take the volumetric specific heat to be 4.187 MJ/m^{3}K, and from measured temperature–time curves they used a computer to determine the variation of conductivity with temperature (Weaver and Stoll, 1969). Alas, the computer model ignored the penetration of radiation into the skin before being absorbed and their measurements are greatly in error at low temperatures. However, for much of this work average values are used. Conductivity is greater when heating than when cooling (some results are shown in Table 27.9).

These measurements have been much used in the USA, for example by Takata (1974) and by Kilminster (1974).

TABLE 27.7

INFLUENCE OF HEAT FLUX ON SKIN THERMAL PROPERTIES
(FROM STOLL AND GREENE, 1959)

q	4187	6280	8374	12 560	16 750	W/m^2
kC	1.68	1.93	2.22	2.46	2.78	× 10^{6}J^2/m^{4}K^{2}s
k	0.40	0.46	0.53	0.59	0.66	W/mK

TABLE 27.5

IN VIVO THERMAL PROPERTIES OF HUMAN SKIN

kC	2.58 × 10^6	J^2/m^{4}K^{2}s
C	3.35 × 10^6	J/m^3 K
k	0.77	W/$_2$mK
α	0.23 × 10^{-6}	m^2/s

TABLE 27.8

ROTH'S SUMMARY OF SKIN THERMAL PROPERTIES

k	0.63	W/mK	±20%
α	0.17 × 10^{-6}	m^2/s	surface layer 0.26 mm
kC	1.58 to 7 × 10^6	J^2/m^{4}K^{2}s	
C_v	3350	J/kgK	
ρ	1100	kg/m^3	
C	3.69 × 10^6	J/m^{3}K	

TABLE 27.6

INFLUENCE OF BLOOD SUPPLY ON THERMAL/PROPERTIES

kC	1.6 × 10^6	J^2/m^{4}K^{2}s	Vasoconstricted
kC	7.0 × 10^6	J^2/m^{4}K^{2}s	Vasodilated
k	0.48 to 2.1	W/mK	

TABLE 27.9

CONDUCTIVITY ON HEATING AND COOLING (FROM WEAVER AND STOLL, 1969)

k	0.586	W/mK	heating
k	0.523	W/mK	cooling
C	4.187	MJ/m^{3}K	

In vivo measurement of thermal properties

A simple method of measuring the thermal inertia of human skin is to bring a warm probe into contact with the skin and record the temperature change of the probe and the initial temperature difference between the probe and the skin. If the thermal inertia of the probe is known then the thermal inertia of skin may be determined using the theory set out in equation (27.28).

If the skin is given suffix a and the probe suffix b, then:

$$(T_0 - T_b)/(T_a - T_b) = 1/(1+ \lambda)$$

$$\text{where } \lambda = \sqrt{[k_b C_b/k_a C_a]}$$

The probe used at the Royal Military College of Science is a fast-response (1 μs) surface thermocouple and is a good conductor having a thermal inertia of $k_b C_b = 78.8 \times 10^6$; a typical set of results is shown in Figure 27.7. The linearity of Figure 27.7 confirms that the thermal inertia of skin is independent of temperature in the range 5°C to 55°C. The dwell time of the probe when these results were taken is about 20 seconds; 10 seconds to reach a steady state and 10 seconds to confirm that it remained steady. From Figure 27.7 it appears that:

$$(T_0 - T_b)/(T_a - T_b) = 1/(1 + \lambda) = 0.133$$

$$\text{hence } \lambda = 6.52$$

and

$$K_a C_a = 78.8 \times 10^6/6.52^2 = 1.85 \times 10^6 \text{ J}^2\text{s/m}^4\text{K}^2$$

If Roth's value of volumetric specific heat is accepted (3.69 MJ/m³K), then the conductivity is 0.50 W/mK and the diffusivity is 0.14×10^{-6} m²/s. Both these values correspond to the normal vasoconstricted condition.

Skin conductance

Skin conductance is a particularly useful measurement. Although it is a property of skin it is not strictly a thermal property. A simple model of the initial, steady conditions for heat flow through skin are shown in Figure 27.6. The outer surface is well defined as a smooth surface with convective or radiant heat supply. The inner surface, however, is ill defined and consists of an irregular dermis/fat interface perfused with a variable blood supply. This inner surface may be approximated by an idealized surface at which there is a sharp distinction between conduction and convection. Such an approximation greatly simplifies the analysis without introducing too much error at the outer surface.

The terms usually used to describe such a situation are: conductance, conductivity and heat transfer coefficient. They are defined as follows.

Conductance

A useful quantity because it is easily measured. It is the heat loss per unit area of skin divided by the difference between the blood temperature and the skin surface temperature.

$$U = q/(T_1 - T_{b1}) \text{ W/m}^2\text{K} \qquad (27.50)$$

where q is the heat flux (W/m²), T_1 is the skin surface temperature and T_{b1} is the blood temperature (310 K or 37°C). In equation (27.50) the sign convention adopted is that heat loss from the skin is negative. Conductance is not a thermal property of skin because its value depends on the closeness of the blood supply to the surface.

Conductivity

This is, as we have seen, a thermal property of skin and is defined in the usual way as the heat loss per unit area divided by the temperature gradient in the skin:

$$k = - q/[\partial T/\partial x] \text{ W/mK} \qquad (27.51)$$

The negative sign implies that heat flows in the direction of the negative temperature gradient, i.e.

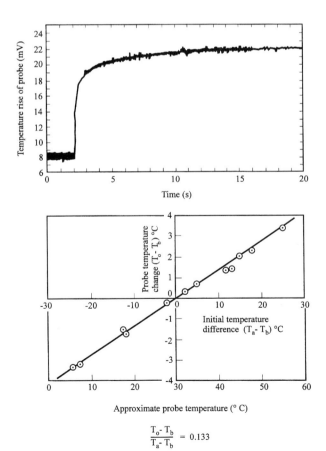

$$\frac{T_0 - T_b}{T_a - T_b} = 0.133$$

Figure 27.7 (a) Typical rise in contact probe temperature. (b) Change in probe temperature when a hot (or cool) probe is brought into contact with skin.

from hot regions to cold regions. If the temperature gradient is constant and the inner temperature is taken to be the blood temperature ($T_9 = T_{b1}$), then:

$$k = -qX/[T_{b1} - T_0] \qquad (27.52)$$

where X is a notional skin thickness. Eliminating q from equations (27.50) and 27.52 gives the simple result:

$$k = UX \text{ or } U = k/X \qquad (27.53)$$

and so conductance may be thought of as skin conductivity divided by skin thickness. Because of the difficulty in measuring skin thickness *in vivo* the conductance is usually easier to determine than the conductivity. If the conductivity is 0.5 W/mK and the skin thickness is 0.002 m, then the conductance is 250 W/m²K. This value is about 10 times greater than is usually observed and so equation (27.53) needs to be changed in some way.

Conductance of inner surface

In the above analysis it was assumed that the inner surface of the skin was at blood temperature. But clearly this cannot be true in general. If heat is lost from the blood to the skin then there must be a temperature difference between them. Denoting the inner temperature of the skin as T_9 (Figure 27.6), then the heat flow between the skin and the blood supply may be written as:

$$q = h (T_9 - T_{b1}) \text{ W/m}^2 \qquad (27.54)$$

where h is the conductance of the inner surface and may be thought of as the conductance of the blood in contact with the skin.

Heat conduction through the skin is, more correctly:

$$q = -k (T_1 - T_9)/X \qquad (27.55)$$

Writing equation (27.50) as:

$$q = U (T_1 - T_{b1}) = U [(T_1 - T_9) + (T_9 - T_{b1})]$$

and substituting from equations (27.54) and (27.55) gives:

$$q = U [qX/k + q/h]$$

and so

$$1/U = X/k + 1/h \qquad (27.56)$$

Conductance is thus made up of two parts that may be identified as the conductance of skin (k/X) and the conductance of the blood in contact with the skin (h).

If $X = 3$ mm, $k = 0.5$ W/mK and $h = 20$ W/m²K then $U = 17.9$ W/m²K and is typical of what is measured.

However, the inner surface conductance h is not usually known but many measurements of skin conductance, U, have been made and may be used to compute the inner surface conductance. Roth

TABLE 27.10
SKIN CONDUCTANCE OF VARIOUS PARTS OF THE BODY

Region	Preferred Temp. (°C)	Heat Loss (W)	Area (m²)	Conductance (W/m²K)
Head	34.7	4.66	0.20	9.1
Chest	34.7	9.55	0.17	22.0
Abdomen	34.7	5.25	0.12	17.1
Back	34.7	14.4	0.23	24.5
Buttocks	34.7	9.67	0.18	21.0
Thighs	34.7	14.0	0.33	10.0
Calves	30.8	17.0	0.20	13.3
Feet	28.6	11.6	0.12	11.2
Arms	33.0	9.8	0.10	23.3
Forearms	30.8	10.0	0.08	19.6
Hands	28.6	18.6	0.07	30.9
Total or mean		124.6	1.80	17.0

(1968) gives the data in Table 27.10 for the skin conductance of various parts of the body.

These variations are caused partly by differences in skin thickness and partly by differing blood supply. The values shown in Table 27.10 are minimum values and correspond to a metabolic rate of about 125 W. Increased activity increases metabolic rate and increases the skin conductance by increasing blood supply to the skin. The increased metabolic rate may also be dissipated by lowering skin surface temperature, equation (27.50), by the evaporation of sweat which lowers skin temperature towards the dew point temperature of the atmosphere. The influence of operative temperature on skin conductance is shown in Figure 27.8 (adapted from Roth, 1968).

Skin conductance and sweating is only important in burns caused by low heat flux over long periods of time. For the more usual burns of short duration and high heat flux, the influence of skin conductance and sweating is slight.

Radiation and optical properties

When radiation strikes a surface it may be reflected, transmitted or absorbed. The transmitted radiation may be partially or totally absorbed as it passes through the material. Only the absorbed radiation produces a temperature rise in the material. The reflectivity, ρ, the absorptivity, α, and the transmissivity, τ, are related by:

$$\rho + \alpha + \tau = 1 \qquad (27.57)$$

These quantities vary with the wavelength of the radiation, that is, with the temperature of the source. For black-body radiation the relationship between wavelength (for maximum monochro-

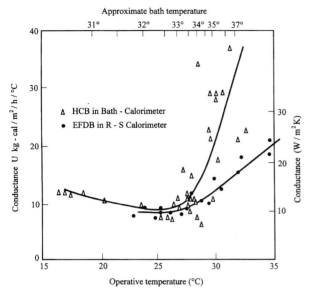

Figure 27.8 Relationship between conductance (a measure of peripheral blood flow) and operative temperature for a subject in two different calorimeters (Roth *et al.*, 1968).

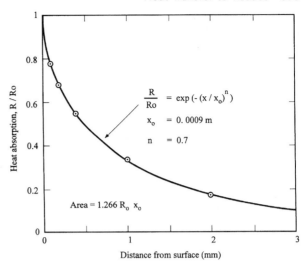

Figure 27.9 Absorption of penetrating radiation in white skin (Buettner, 1952).

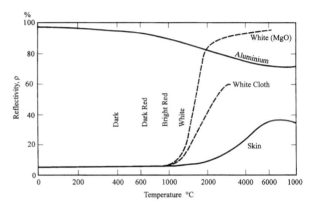

Figure 27.10 Total reflection by various 'white' surfaces and bright aluminium, as related to the temperature of the radiating body. It can be seen that if the radiator is cooler than 1000°C the whitest surfaces absorb entirely; i.e. they can be considered as 'black'. The appearance of the radiator to the eye is indicated by the words written vertically (Buettner, 1952).

matic emission) and source temperature is given by Wien's law:

$$\lambda T = 0.0029 \text{ mK} \qquad (27.58)$$

Buettner (1952) has examined all the available measurements of skin reflectivity and transmissivity. For solar radiation (source temperature 6000 K, wavelength 0.5 µm) he concluded that white skin reflected 42% of incoming radiation and absorbed 58%. He found that:

45.0% passed 0.1 mm depth
39.6% passed 0.2 mm depth
32.0% passed 0.4 mm depth
19.0% passed 1.0 mm depth
10.2% passed 2.0 mm depth

From these data it is possible to determine the rate of heat absorption at various depths (Figure 27.9). An approximate equation that fits this data is:

$$R = R_0 \exp\left[-(x/x_0)^{0.7}\right] \text{ W/m}^3 \qquad (27.59)$$

R is the heat absorption per unit volume, R_0 is the value of R at the skin surface $x = 0$, and x_0 is a constant that may be called the penetration depth. The total area under this curve is the total heat absorbed by the skin:

$$q_a = (1-\rho) \, q_r = \int_0^\infty R \, dx = 1.266 R_0 x_0 \qquad (27.60)$$

and so

$$R = (1-\rho) \, q_r / (1.266 \, x_0) \exp\left[-(x/x_0)^{0.7}\right] \qquad (27.61)$$

For sunlight the reflectivity is 0.42 and the penetration depth (Figure 27.9) is 0.9 mm. Both

these quantities change with the wavelength of radiation. The variation of reflectivity with source temperature for various white materials is shown in Figure 27.10. These white materials stay cool in sunlight, not only because they are good reflectors but also because they are good emitters (poor reflectors) of low-temperature infrared radiation. Other materials, such as stainless steel, show the opposite effect and become very hot when exposed to sunlight.

A simple polynomial equation may be used to fit the skin data shown in Figure 27.10:

$$\rho = 0.0621 - 4.335 \times 10^{-5} T + 3.546 \times 10^{-8} T^2$$
$$- 4.315 \times 10^{-12} T^3 + 1.49 \times 10^{-16} T^4 \qquad (27.62)$$
$$300 \text{ K} < T < 10\,000 \text{ K}$$

The other constant needed for equation (27.61) is the penetration depth x_0. This has a value of 0.9 mm for sunlight and zero for low-temperature radiation. Clearly, the penetration of radiation is related to its wavelength.

Infrared radiation
$$T = 300K \qquad \lambda = 10 \ \mu m \qquad x_0 = 0$$

Sunlight
$$T = 6000K \qquad \lambda = 0.5 \ \mu m \qquad x_0 = 0.9mm$$

X-rays, of course, have very short wavelengths, about 10^{-10}m, and very large penetration. It seems reasonable to take the penetration depth to be inversely proportional to the wavelength and, by Wien's law, to be proportional to the source temperature. Thus for the above data:

$$x_0 = 0.15 \times 10^{-6}T \qquad (27.63)$$

where x_0 is in m and T is in K.

The above equations apply only to white skin. For very black skin 10% of sunlight is reflected and 90% is absorbed. Eighty per cent passes a depth of 0.1 mm, about 40% is absorbed in the melanin layer at the base of the epidermis, and 35% passes 0.2 mm depth. Thus black skin burns more readily when subjected to high-temperature radiation.

THEORY OF SKIN BURNS

Classification of skin burns

Figure 27.6 shows a cross-section of the microstructure of skin. Healthy skin consists of two layers: the epidermis and the dermis. The epidermis is about 100–150 μm thick and has an outer layer of dead cells and a thin layer of epithelial cells containing the pigment melanin. The dermis makes up most of the skin thickness and varies in depth from about 0.5 mm on the eyelids to about 5 mm in the centre of the back. An average thickness is about 2 mm. The dermis is variably perfused by blood and contains skin structures such as hair follicles and the sweat and sebaceous glands.

Hair follicles are particularly important in burn healing because they are lined with epithelial cells from which a new epidermis can grow to cover an open wound. Consequently if the burn depth is greater than the depth of hair follicles, then the wound will not heal without a scar and a skin graft is necessary.

In the past it has been common to classify burns, in order of increasing severity, as first, second or third degree. Such classification depends on the appearance of the wound and corresponds to redness (first degree), blistering (second degree) and charring (third degree). This classification is being replaced because the numbering system can cause confusion. Afromowitz et al., 1987; Muir et al., 1987). A first-degree burn is sometimes erroneously considered to be more serious than a second or third-degree burn. Thus it is now increasingly common to use a classification that refers directly to the depth of burn:

shallow or superficial partial thickness   first degree
partial thickness,   second degree
full thickness   third degree.

Partial-thickness burns are sometimes referred to as deep dermal burns if it is suspected that most of the dermis has been destroyed to the level of the hair follicles, making healing unlikely or slow. These burn depths are indicated in Figure 27.6. Over the years many attempts have been made to devise a burn depth indicator, but so far with only limited success. (Dingwall, 1943; Patney and Scarfe, 1944; Godina et al., 1978; Afromowitz et al., 1987).

From a computational point of view burn depths may be taken as:

shallow   less than 100 μm
partial thickness   100 μm to 500 μm
full thickness   500 to 2000 μm depending on location.

This is, perhaps, a rather simple classification of burn depth but it is commonly used. More complex classifications are sometimes used. For example, Knox et al. (1978) used 11 grades (0–10).

Henriques' theory of skin burns

The action of heat on a surface usually causes some physical change in that surface. For example, a metal surface subjected to high heat flow usually softens (loses hardness and strength) and may melt. Many organic materials undergo chemical changes such as discoloration, scorching and charring. Sometimes vaporization occurs and, if the vapour is inflammable, a surface flame may occur. In 1947, Henriques assumed that skin cell destruction is an irreversible thermally activated process, similar to a chemical reaction, and can be described, as are many chemical reactions, by an Arrhenius equation of the form:

$$d\omega/dt = A \exp \left[-\Delta E / R_o T\right] \qquad (27.64)$$

where ω is a function of burn injury such that $\omega = 1$ for complete cell destruction and $\omega = 0.53$ for the onset of a partial-thickness burn. A is a rate constant, ΔE is an activation energy and R_o is the universal gas constant (8315 J/kg-mol). T is the temperature at any point, x, from the skin surface and when $\omega = 1$ at this point the skin is burned to this depth. Originally Henriques proposed this equation for a specific depth of 80 μm so it would give a prediction of a partial-thickness burn, but later workers have used it to predict burns at any depth.

The constants were determined by *in vivo* experimental scalds on pig skin and on human volunteers. Hot water at a constant temperature was applied to the skin to produce shallow burns or partial-thickness burns. After a few seconds' contact, the skin temperature is substantially the same as the water temperature and so equation (27.64) may be integrated to give:

$$t = \exp\left[\Delta E/(R_o T) - \ln A\right] \quad t > 100 \text{ s} \quad (27.65)$$

Henriques found that this equation fitted his experimental results very well and determined that the rate constant is $A = 3.1 \times 10^{98}$ and the activation energy is $\Delta E = 624$ MJ/kg-mol and so equation (27.65) may be written as:

$$t = \exp\left[75\,000/T - 226.78\right] \quad t > 100 \text{ s} \quad (27.66)$$

The time restriction on equation (27.66) is because it takes about 10 seconds for the skin temperature to rise to the same value as the water temperature, and so the skin temperature may be treated as a constant only if $t > 100$s.

Henriques noted that the theories advanced to explain thermal injury fall into three general groups:

1. *Thermal alteration of proteins.* Even minor increases in temperature, may result in irreversible change in protein structure and function. Examples are: increased permeability of the nuclear and/or the cell wall, structural alteration of the nucleus, disintegration of protein mitochondria present in the cytoplasm and inactivation of enzymes. Many of these processes have activation energies in excess of 200 MJ/kg-mol and some as high as 790 MJ/kg-mol. Thus Henriques concluded that skin burns may cause cell death due to the thermal alterations of as yet unknown proteins in epidermal cells. He based this conclusion on the fact that activation energies for proteins are of the same order as the activation energy required to produce skin burns.
2. *Other possible alterations in metabolic rate.* Since temperature affects the kinetics and thermodynamics of all chemical and physical phenomena, it may cause changes in metabolism irrespective of its affects on proteins. For example, temperature-induced changes in diffusion rates and the formation or degradation of chemical reactants may lead to abnormal functioning; certain normal metabolites may disappear and others of a toxic character may appear to cause cell death. However most of the possible metabolic reactions have activation energies between 40 and 80 MJ/kg-mol and none were found to exceed 200 MJ/kg-mol. Henriques concluded that this type of reaction was unlikely to lead to activation energies large enough to produce cell death in skin burns.
3. *Non-protein-induced changes in the physical characteristics of cells.* This group contains all physical phenomena characteristic of protoplasm but not primarily affected by thermal changes to the proteins. For example, diffusion of metabolites through a cell wall that has not undergone chemical change are included but diffusion rates affected by degradation of protein are excluded. All the biophysical rate processes were examined, such as diffusion through liquids and membranes, changes in viscosity, rigidity, tensile strength, liquefaction, and in every case the activation energy was less than 60 MJ/kg-mol. Many fat-like substances melt at temperatures in the range 45–48°C and this is sometimes considered as an instigator of thermal injury; however, the activation energy of the rate of melting is essentially zero and so it could not explain the observed relationship between skin temperature and time of exposure. Although all these processes are capable of producing cell death they are not the cause of cell death in skin burns.

Henriques concluded that the only known biokinetic phenomena that could account for cell death during skin burn are thermally induced changes in protein structure having an activation energy of about 600 MJ/kg-mol.

In general, therefore, cell destruction occurs to a depth x from the surface when:

$$\omega = 1 = \int_0^t \exp\left[226.78 - 75\,000/T\right] \, dt \quad (27.67)$$

where T is the temperature at depth x and, in general, is a function of time. This equation is quite difficult to integrate, except, for the special case when T is constant when it integrates to give equation (27.66). However, if a numerical computation of skin temperature distribution is made then it is perfectly easy to perform a numerical integration of equation (27.67) to give a prediction of burn depth.

Henriques' theory of skin burns has been much used by later workers, for example Kilminster (1974), Knox *et al.* (1978), Weaver and Stoll (1969), and Takata (1974). However, when this theory is applied to flash burns from a very hot radiation source the rate constant and activation energy are usually modified to fit the observed results. For example, Weaver and Stoll recommend:

For 44°C < T < 50°C

$$d\omega/dt = 2.185 \times 10^{24} \exp\left[-93\,535/T\right] \quad (27.68)$$

For T > 50°C

$$d\omega/dt = 1.823 \times 10^{51} \exp\left[-39\,110/T\right] \quad (27.69)$$

These changes to Henriques' theory are necessary because the heat transfer calculations used did not allow for the penetrating nature of short-wavelength radiation (Figure 27.9). Such calculations are difficult to perform unless numerical methods are used, so it is understandable that simple methods should be sought even when such methods cannot be justified.

However, when computer programs are adapted to allow for penetration of radiation before absorption then the constants originally measured by Henriques give perfectly accurate predictions of skin temperature, heat transfer and burn damage regardless of the nature of the heat source. An algorithm for such a computation is given below. A computer program based on this algorithm is then used to compute the heat dose required to produce skin burns from variety of heat sources and these computations are compared with measured data.

Computer program for predicting skin burns

The computer program solves the following equations using the explicit finite difference method. The equations to be solved are:

$$\partial T/\partial t = R/C + \alpha\, \partial^2 T/\partial x^2$$

where:

$$R = (1-\rho)\, q_r/(1.266\, x_0)\, \exp\left[-(x/x_0)^{0.7}\right]$$

$$\rho = 0.0621 - 4.335 \times 10^{-5}\, T_g + 3.546 \times 10^{-8}\, T_g^2$$

$$- 4.315 \times 10^{-12}\, T_g^3 + 1.49 \times 10^{-16}\, T_g^4$$

$$300\ K < T_g < 10\,000\ K$$

The value of R is determined only if there is radiation from a high-temperature source at temperature T_g otherwise its value is zero.

The initial condition is $T = 310$ K at $t = 0$, all x. The boundary condition at the outer surface is:

$$q = q_s + h\,(T_f - T_1) + \epsilon\sigma\,(T_f^4 - T_1^4) + F\,\epsilon\,\sigma\,(T_g^4 - T_1^4)$$

$$\text{at } x = 0, \text{all } t.$$

Thus the surface heat flux may be specified as a constant flux, a convective flux, a low-temperature radiant flux or a high-temperature radiant flux or any combination of these.

The boundary condition at the inner surface is:

$$q = h_c\,(T_{n+1} - T_{bl})$$

where the inner surface conductance, h_c, is determined from the skin conductance, U, by:

$$1/h_c = 1/U - X/k$$

The burn damage at any specified depth, b, is determined from:

$$\omega = \int_0^t \exp\left[226.78 - 75\,000/T_b\right]\, dt$$

and a superficial (first degree) burn occurs when $\omega = 0.53$ and complete cell destruction occurs when $\omega = 1$.

The heat dose is determined as the integral of the outer surface heat flux. Table 27.11 provides an algorithm for computing skin temperature, heat flows and burn damage.

TABLE 27.11

A SUITABLE ALGORITHM FOR COMPUTING SKIN TEMPERATURE, HEAT FLOWS AND BURN DAMAGE

Set initial conditions for:
skin properties k, α, ϵ
surface heat input, q_s, h, T_f

infra-red radiation, ϵ
high temperature radiation source, T_g, F

heat loss by sweating
skin conductance and skin thickness, U, X
burn depth, b
Run time of programme

Print the input data

Set the time increment δt and node spacing δx
ensure that $p = \alpha\, \delta t/\,\delta x^2 < 0.5$

Set initial conditions for
number of nodes $N = X/\delta x$
inner surface heat conductance, h_2

solar emissivity ϵ
internal heat absorption due to high temperature radiation, R
initial skin temperature

Print headings and initial temperature and heat flux values

Start of Main Loop
Calculate:
dummy temperatures at inner and outer surface and temperature at time $t + \delta t$ at each node (i.e. F_i)

Print current temperature T_i, heat dose H and burn damage ω if required

Replace current temperature by F_i

Calculate:
increment in heat dose and current heat dose, H
increment in burn function and current burn function, ω

If $w = 1$ or $t =$ run time
then exit Main Loop
else repeat Main Loop

Print end of program messages

End

Typical skin burns

The above algorithm and equations form the basis of a computer program to model the transient distribution of skin temperature, to predict the onset of pain and to determine the degree of burning at any depth from the skin surface. The temperature distribution calculated by the program was checked for accuracy against standard analytical solutions for opaque thick slabs (Carslaw and

Jaeger, 1990), and for semi-transparent slabs. These checks included:

a. constant heat flux at one surface and constant temperature at the other surface,
b. constant heat flux at one surface and zero heat flux at the other,
c. constant radiation into a semi-infinite, semi-transparent slab with a constant absorption coefficient.

In each case the error between the computed and analytical value was less than 0.3% and was usually less than 0.1%.

The program was then used to compute skin burns for various conditions of heat input, and the length of time required for superficial, partial thickness and deep dermal burns was determined. The program was tested against a wide range of experimental data for skin burns and found to predict the burn time with good accuracy. But before comparing the computed and clinical data, it is useful to examine the computed results in some detail.

For example, Figure 27.11a shows the skin temperature, heat dose, and burn damage during and after a 1.96 s exposure to hot water. In Figure 27.11a the calculation is made for a depth of 1 mm. The temperature at this depth rises by about 20°C after 4.5 s and then declines whereas the heat dose rises to

about 150 kJ/m² at 1.96 s and then remains constant. The burn damage function 1 mm from the surface does not begin to rise until 2.5 s, that is, until about 0.5 s after exposure has ended. This is because it takes a finite time for heat to diffuse from the surface. The burn function rises to 1.0 after 24 s. The burn damage caused after exposure to the hot source may be called *after-burning*. The after-burning period can be quite long, several minutes in some cases, and justifies the advice given to first aid workers, namely, that burn severity may be reduced by immersion in cold water immediately after exposure. In Figure 27.11a the exposure period is about 2 s whereas the after-burning period, during which burn severity could be reduced, is about 22 s.

It is a matter of trial and error, when using the computer program, to adjust the heat input to give zero slope at $\omega = 1$. A slightly smaller heat dose causes a very large increase in burn time whereas a slightly larger heat dose gives a non-zero slope when the burn function is 1.0 and so the heat dose required to produce a burn is well defined.

Figure 27.11b shows a similar set of results calculated for a burn depth of 0.1 mm. In this case the exposure time remains the same, 1.96 s, but the water temperature is decreased to produce a second-degree burn. The temperature at 0.1 mm rises quickly by about 20°C and then declines. At times greater than the exposure time the heat dose remains constant at about 52 kJ/m², the skin temperature falls and the burn function continues to rise, reaching 1.0 at 2.95 s. In this case the after-burning period is quite short, about 1 s. Once again a small decrease in heat dose makes it impossible for the burn function to reach 1.0 whereas a slight increase in heat dose gives non-zero slope when the burn function is 1.0 and, as before, the heat dose required to produce a burn is well defined.

When calculating the heat dose for skin burns it is important to include the after-burning period. Very misleading results may be obtained if the calculation is stopped when the exposure to heat ends. This is particularly important for short exposure times, intense heat transfer rates, and for deep dermal burns.

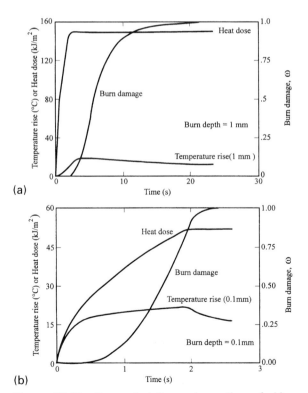

(a)

(b)

Figure 27.11 Computed thermal reaction of skin on exposure to flowing hot water. Exposure time is 1.96 s. Note the afterburning period. (a) third degree (1 mm) burn. (b) Second degree (0.1 mm) burn.

Comparison of computed and observed heat dose

Approximate analytical solutions for partial thickness burns are possible for certain cases over limited period of time. An example is the case in which the skin may be treated as a semi-infinite solid subjected to a constant surface temperature. This commonly occurs, for a limited time, when the skin touches a solid surface or is immersed in a dense fluid such as water. For time less than about 2 seconds the skin temperature, 100 µm from the surface, is unlikely to be constant if it touches a solid surface and may not be constant if time is less than 20 s if immersed in water and for a time greater than about 10 seconds skin can no longer be treated as semi-infinite. However, Equ.27.26 and 27.66 may be combined to give the solution:

$$H = k\sqrt{\frac{4t}{\pi\alpha}}\left[\frac{75\,000}{\ln(t) + 226.78} - T_i\right]$$

(27.70)

$$H = 1549\sqrt{t}\left[\frac{75\,000}{\ln(t) + 226.78} - 310\right]\,J/m^2$$

$$2 < t < 100\,s$$

where the thermal properties of skin have been taken as: $\alpha = 0.138 \times 10^{-6}\,m^2/s$, $k = 0.51\,W/mK$ and the initial skin temperature is taken to be 310 K. This equation is useful in its own right and gives satisfactory results for $2 < t < 100$ seconds. A simple approximation of Equ. 27.70 is:

$$H = 32\,000\,t^{0.42}$$

$$2 < t < 100\,s$$

(27.71)

where H is the heat dose in J/m^2 and t is the exposure time in seconds.

In general, numerical solutions are more accurate and flexible than analytical ones which, necessarily, are restricted to rather few cases if great complexity is to be avoided. All subsequent analysis of skin burns in this section is based on numerical, computer solutions using the algorithm of Table 27.11.

The observed and computed burn times for skin in contact with hot, flowing water at various temperatures are compared in Figure 27.12. The clinical data are those of Henriques (1947) and the computed curves assume the surface heat transfer coefficient is $10\,kW/m^2K$, skin thickness is 2 mm and conductance is $17\,W/m^2K$. The skin surface temperature rises to a constant value for $t > 100\,s$ and so Equ. 27.65 fits the observed results, but for

$t < 100\,s$ the skin temperature varies to some degree and must be computed numerically; the resulting burn times are then in good agreement with Henriques' observations.

It is more usual to plot the heat dose required for a given burn against the exposure time and so Figure 27.12 also shows the computed heat dose for these conditions. An advantage of this plot is that it is only slightly sensitive to changes in exposure time. For example, a one second exposure time requires about $0.04\,MJ/m^2$ for a partial thickness burn; this corresponds to a heat flux of $40\,kW/m^2$. For an exposure time of 1000 s the required heat dose is $0.4\,MJ/m^2$; this corresponds to a heat flux of only $0.4\,kW/m^2$. When the exposure time increases by three orders of magnitude, the heat flux decreases by two orders of magnitude and the heat dose increases by one order of magnitude. The heat dose is, therefore, the least variable quantity and is the preferred way of quantifying burn injuries. The numerical computation shown in Figure 27.12 compares quite well with the analytical solution, Equ. 27.70, over the relevant exposure times.

It also turns out that the required heat dose is almost independent of fluctuations in the heat flux during the exposure time. It is found that the computed heat dose for constant surface temperature, constant surface heat flux, convection, or non-penetrating radiation, all lie close to the same curve and give similar predictions for partial thickness burns.

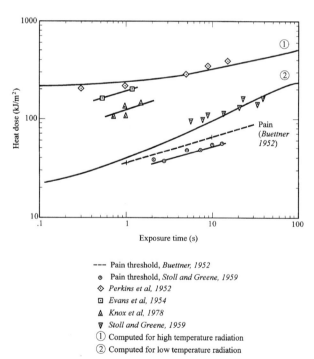

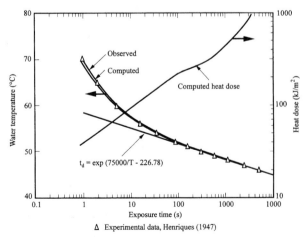

Figure 27.12 Comparison of computed and observed exposure time to produce second-degree skin burns by contact with hot flowing water.

Figure 27.13 Computed and observed heat dose for partial thickness (0.1 mm) skin burns due to low-temperature radiation and high-temperature radiation and data for the onset of pain.

The computer program also gives good predictions of partial thickness burns caused by radiation from low-temperature sources having temperatures less than about 1000°C. Up to this temperature the reflectivity of white skin is constant at about 5%. Thus the skin absorbs almost all the incident radiation and this absorption occurs at the skin surface, that is, it does not penetrate the skin before absorption. In running the program it is assumed that skin emissivity is 95% (reflectivity is 5%), incident heat flux varies from 0.3 to 25 kW/m², skin conductance is 25 W/m²K, skin thickness is 5 mm, diffusivity is 0.138×10^{-6} m²/s and burn depth is 100 μm.

The computed results are plotted in Figure 27.13 where they compare favourably with the clinical data of Stoll and Greene (1959). A satisfactory correlation is obtained without the need to change the constants in Henriques' thermal damage function, as suggested by Weaver and Stoll (1969). Note that the line for low temperature, non-penetrating radiation burns in Figure 27.13 is almost identical to that calculated for convection burns in Figure 27.12.

However, clinical results obtained by Evans *et al.* (1955), Knox *et al.* (1978) and by Perkins *et al.* (1952), show that, under different conditions, much greater heat doses are required for partial thickness burns. The reason for this is that these workers used high temperature radiation sources having temperatures in excess of 2000°C and as high as 6000 K. As we have seen, 42% of such incident radiation is reflected and the remaining 58% must penetrate the skin for 2 mm or so before it is absorbed. The incident energy is spread through a larger mass of material and produces a smaller temperature rise. Such short wavelength radiation is much less damaging than long wavelength radiation from a low temperature source from which only 5% is reflected and penetration is less than 0.2 mm. As can be seen in Figure 27.13, the computer models this behaviour with good accuracy and without having to change the constants in the Henriques equation. The computed curve for high temperature radiation is for the extreme case where 42% of incident radiation is reflected and the remainder is absorbed at various depths as specified by Equ. 27.61; all other data remain unchanged. The required heat dose is between 1.5 times and 9 times greater for penetrating radiation than for non-penetrating radiation. The computed results show very good agreement with the measurements of Perkins *et al.* (1952). The heat doses measured by Evans *et al.* (1954) and by Knox *et al.* (1978) are smaller because these workers used cooler, less penetrating, radiation sources.

For completeness, Figure 27.13 also shows clinical data for the onset of pain which, sensibly, occurs at low levels of heat dose. The data are those of Stoll and Greene (1959) and Buettner (1952).

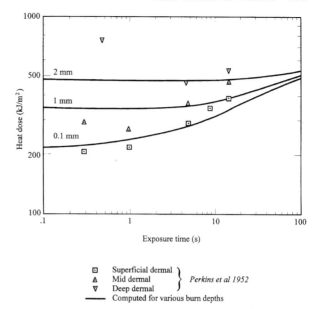

Figure 27.14 Comparison of computed and observed partial thickness (0.1 mm) and deep dermal (1 mm and 2 mm) burns from a high-temperature radiation source.

Figure 27.14 compares the heat doses required for deep dermal (third degree) burns from penetrating radiation. The computed curves are for 0.1 mm (partial thickness), and 1 mm or 2 mm (deep dermal) burns and the clinical observations are those of Perkins *et al.* (1952). For short duration burns there are marked differences between the heat doses required for different burn depths but for long exposures the required heat doses are almost the same. During long exposures the heat input is low and there is adequate time for conduction, thus the skin temperature is nearly uniform and the heat required to produce a burn on the surface is nearly the same as that required to produce a skin burn at 2 mm depth.

Perkins *et al.* have attempted to assess burn depth by classifying their results as superficial dermal, mid dermal or deep dermal; but they do not specify burn depth numerically. It appears, from Figure 27.14, that mid dermal burns are about 1.5 mm deep whereas deep dermal burns are in excess of 2 mm deep. Such burns are associated with very long afterburning periods so it is usually possible to reduce burn damage by surface cooling in cold water.

Heat flux variation

In experimental burns trials, the surface heat flux is often generated by radiation from a hot source and may be considered to be constant. Under these conditions the surface temperature rises as the square root of time. If the heat flux is generated by contact with a solid surface at a uniform temperature or by contact with hot water, then the

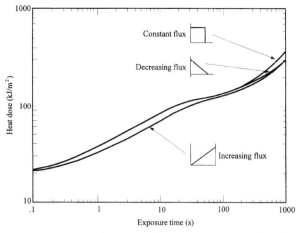

Figure 27.15 Influence of a constant, a linearly increasing, and a linearly decreasing heat flux on the heat dose for partial thickness burns from a low-temperature radiation source.

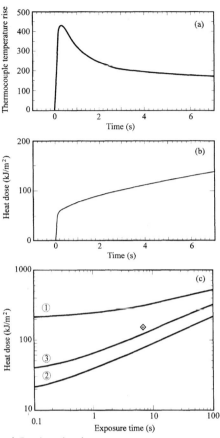

◇ Experimental result
① Computed curve for high temperature penetrating radiation
② Computed curve for low temperature non-penetrating radiation
③ Computed curve for 50% high temperature and 50% low temperature radiation

Figure 27.16 Interpretation of mixed convection and high-temperature radiation burns for a thermal pulse behind defeated armour. (a) Measured air temperature. (b) Measured heat dose (radiation and convection). (c) Allowable heat dose for partial thickness burns.

surface temperature quickly rises to a constant value and the surface heat flux decreases with time. Experimental burns are usually produced by one or other of these methods. But real burns are produced in more diverse circumstances and the surface heat flux may fluctuate in many different ways. Figure 27.15 demonstrates, numerically, the sensitivity of burns to such fluctuations in surface heat flux. Three cases are considered, namely, a constant heat flux, a linearly increasing heat flux and a linearly decreasing heat flux. The heat dose for partial thickness burns is calculated for each case. For short exposure the heat dose is nearly independent of the exposure time but for exposures between 1 s and 100 s the heat dose increases with exposure time to the power 0.375. There is very little difference between the constant heat flux and the declining heat flux cases but the linearly increasing heat flux produces burns at significantly lower doses; for an exposure time of about 20 s the required dose is reduced by about 18%. These variations may not be considered to be too serious and, as a reasonable approximation, we may assume that the heat dose for a given degree of burn is independent of heat flux variations.

The shape of the heat dose curve is governed by the skin geometry. In these calculations the skin thickness was taken to be 2 mm so for t < 10 s the skin wall behaves as a semi-infinite solid but for 10 < t < 100 s the temperature at the inner surface increases and the skin behaves as a slab of finite thickness. For t > 100 s the temperature difference across the skin thickness is small and constant and heat input causes a more or less uniform temperature rise throughout the skin thickness. As already mentioned, under these conditions the heat dose for partial thickness burns is almost the same as for deep dermal burns.

Mixed penetrating and non-penetrating radiation

One of the great advantages of a computer based theory of skin burns is that it allows us to interpret heat dose measurements without having to use live or anaesthetized animals (pigs). The main difficulty is when a burn is produced by a mixture of penetrating and non-penetrating radiation. In practical applications it sometimes happens that a burn is produced by more than one heat source. For example, Figure 27.16(a) and (b) show the air temperature and heat dose, measured using fast response gauges, when a shaped charge jet defeats (pierces) the armour plating of a military vehicle (Lawton and Laird, 1993). Immediately after the plasma jet perforates the armour the interior of the vehicle is filled with a short burst of intense penetrating radiation and the occupants receive an immediate heat dose. This is followed by a comparatively long period during which the air temperature rises by a few hundred degrees and the heat dose increases by convection and low temperature radiation. For the example shown, both the penetrating radiation dose and the convection dose are about $70\,kJ/m^2$ giving a total heat dose of about $140\,kJ/m^2$; the exposure time is 7 s. This result is plotted in Figure 27.16(c). Clearly, the measured heat dose is greater than that required to give a partial thickness burn by convection, which is $73\,kJ/m^2$ but is less than that required to give a partial thickness burn by penetrating radiation, which is $285\,kJ/m^2$.

We need to know the severity of the mixed radiation and convection burn and whether or not it produces a skin burn. This may be determined by using the measured heat doses as input to a computer program and calculating the skin temperatures and burn damage function with due allowance for after-burning. The resulting curve for the case where penetrating radiation and convection are equal, is shown in Figure 27.16(c). As might be expected, the combined curve lies between the curves for penetrating radiation and convection; but it does not lie exactly at the mid-way position between these curves. It may be shown that the heat dose required to produce a second-degree burn from a mixed penetrating radiation and convective heat source is

$$\frac{H}{G_E} = \frac{H_R + H_C}{G_E} = \frac{H_R}{G_R} + \frac{H_C}{G_C} \qquad (27.72)$$

where H is the heat dose, G is the allowed heat dose, suffix C refers to conduction or low temperature radiation, suffix R refers to high temperature radiation, and G_E is the equivalent heat dose allowed for mixed radiation and convection.

For pure convection the equivalent heat dose is $G_E = G_C$, whereas for pure penetrating radiation the equivalent heat dose is $G_E = G_R$. For the case shown in Figure 27.16 we have $H_R = 70$, $H_C = 70$, $G_C = 73$, and $G_R = 285\,kJ/m^2$. The convective heat dose is insufficient to cause a convection burn and the radiation dose is insufficient to cause a radiation burn. The total heat dose is insufficient to cause a radiation burn but it is sufficient to cause a convection burn. The interpretation of this burn data is not immediately obvious but from Equ. 27.72 the equivalent dose for a partial thickness burn is $G_E = 116\,kJ/m^2$. Because the actual heat dose is $140\,kJ/m^2$ the resulting burn is significantly more severe than partial thickness and burn depth will exceed $100\,\mu m$.

Conclusions

Henriques' theory of skin burns may be used to predict superficial, partial thickness, and deep dermal burns regardless of the heat source if due allowance is made for the penetrating nature of short wavelength radiation from hot radiation sources. The theory predicts conductive, convective and low temperature radiation burns and the heat dose required for such burns depends mainly on the burn time and is almost independent of transient variations in the surface heat flux. The only special case concerns radiation from high temperature sources (3000 K to 6000 K), emitted, for example, by the Sun or by nuclear explosions. Contrary to popular opinion, this type of radiation is much less damaging (typically 4 times less damaging) than either low temperature radiation or convection. This is because human skin is adapted to deal with high temperature radiation from sunlight. High temperature radiation is less damaging because it is reflected from the skin to a greater degree and also because such radiation that is not reflected must penetrate the skin to a depth of about 2 mm before being absorbed; as a smaller quantity of heat is absorbed by a larger mass of skin the temperature rise is smaller and the thermal damage is less.

Simple computer programs are able to model this behaviour using Henriques' original theory and the modifications proposed by Weaver and Stoll, and used by subsequent workers, are unnecessary. Such computer programs are able to include non-linear and time varying thermal and optical properties but such refinements do not seem to be necessary. Mixed conditions of penetrating and non-penetrating radiation may be assessed by a simple method which has been shown to agree with more rigorous computations.

Notation

a,b,c	constants
A	rate constant, s^{-1}
A_1	area of surface 1, m^2
c	velocity, m/s
C	volumetric specific heat, J/m^3K
C_p	specific heat at constant pressure, J/kgK
d	characteristic length (diameter), m
F_i	temperature at node i at time $t + \delta t$
F_{1-2}	radiation form factor between surfaces 1 and 2
g	local gravitation acceleration, 9.81 m/s^2
Gr	Grashof number, $\beta g(T_f-T_s)\rho^2d^3/\mu^2$
h	heat transfer coefficient, W/m^2K
H	heat transfer per unit area, J/m^2
i	radiation intensity, W/st
k	thermal conductivity, W/mK
k_a, k_b	thermal conductivity of a or b, W/mK
k_f	thermal conductivity of fluid, W/mK
kT	size of nuclear weapon in kilotonnes, kT
Nu	Nusselt number, hd/k_f

Pr	Prandtl number, $C_p \mu / k$
$q_{b\lambda}$	black-body radiance at wavelength λ, W/m^3
q_{max}	maximum radiation, W/m^2
q_x	heat flux in x direction, W/m^2
q_0	heat flux at $x = 0$, W/m^2
Q	heat transfer rate, W
R	volumetric rate of heat absorption, W/m^3 or radial distance, m
Re	Reynolds number, $\rho cd / \mu$
R_0	volumetric rate of heat absorption at $x = 0$, W/m^3 or universal gas constant, 8314 J/kg-molK
t	time, s
t_{max}	time at which radiation is maximum, s
t_0	time constant, s
T	temperature, K
T_a, T_b	initial temperature of a or b, K
T_{bl}	normal blood temperature, 310 K
T_f	temperature of fluid, K
T_i	initial temperature, K or temperature at node i at time t, K
T_{max}	maximum temperature, K
T_s	surface temperature, K
T_0	temperature at $x = 0$, K
T_1, T_2	temperatures of surfaces 1 or 2, K
u	dimensionless time, t/t_0
U	conductance, W/m^2K
x,y,z	coordinates, m
x_0	penetration depth, m
X	skin thickness, m
α	thermal diffusivity, k/C, m^2/s, or absorptivity
β	coefficient of cubical expansion, K^{-1}
δ	thermal boundary layer thickness, m
δt	time increment, s
δx	distance between nodes, m
ΔE	activation energy, J/kg-mol
ΔT	temperature difference, $T_f - T_s$, K
ϵ	emissivity
θ	dimensionless distance, $x/(4\alpha t)^{0.5}$
λ	wavelength, m or a constant
μ	viscosity, Ns/m^2
ρ	density, kg/m^3 or reflectivity
σ	Stefan-Boltzmann constant, 5.67×10^{-8}, W/m^2K^4
τ	transmissivity or dimensionless time, $4\alpha t/x^2$ or $h^2\alpha t/k^2$
ω	Henriques' burn damage function

REFERENCES

Afromowitz M.A., Van Liew G., Heimbach D.M. (1987). 'Clinical evaluation of burn injuries using an optical reflectance technique'. *IEE Trans. Biomed. Engin.*, **BME-34**, (2), 114–27.

Buettner K. (1952). Effects of extreme heat and cold on human skin. *Journal of Applied Physiology*, **5**, 207–20.

Carslaw H.S., Jaeger J.C. (1990). *Conduction of Heat in Solids.* Oxford: Oxford University Press.

Chapman A.J. (1969). *Heat Transfer*, 2nd edn. New York: Macmillan.

Davies J.W.L. (1982). *Physiological Response in Burning Injury.* New York: Academic.

Dingwall A.R. (1943). A clinical test for separating second from third degree burns. *Ann. Surg.*, **149**, 68–75.

Godina M. et al. (1978). The reliability of clinical assessment of the depth of burns. *Burns*, **4**, 92–6.

Henriques F.C. (1947). Studies of thermal injury: the predictability and the significance of thermally induced rate processes leading to irreversible epidermal injury. *Arch. Pathol.*, **43**, 489–502.

Kilminster D.T. (1974). *A Model to predict human skin burns.* BRL Report AD/A-003 918 Maryland: Aberdeen Proving Ground.

Knox F.S., Watchel T.L., Knapp S.C. (1978). *Mathematical Models of Skin Burns Induced by Simulated Postcrash Fires as Aids to Thermal Protective Clothing Design and Selection.* USAARL Report No 78–15. Fort Rucker, AL: US Army Medical Research Lab.

Lipkin M., Hardy J.D. (1954). Measurement of some thermal properties of human tissues. *J. Appl. Physiol.*, **7**, (2), 212–17.

Muir I.F.K., Barclay T.L., Settle, J.A.D. (1987). *Burns and their Treatment.* Oxford: Butterworth-Heinemann.

Odland G.F. (1983). Structure of skin. In *Biochemistry and Physiology of Skin* (Goldsmith L.A., ed.). Oxford: Oxford University Press.

Patney H., Scarfe R.W. (1944). The diagnosis of the depth of skin destruction in burning and its bearing on treatment. *Br. J. Surg.*, **32**, 32–49.

Perkins J.B., Pearse H.E., Kingsley H.D. (1957). *Studies on flash burns: the relation of time and intensity of applied thermal radiation to the severity of burns.* Atomic Energy Report UR 217. Rochester, NY: University of Rochester.

Roth E.M. (ed.) (1968). *Compendium of Human Responses of the Aerospace Environment*, Vol. 1, Section 6 (prepared by Bottomely, T.A., Roth E.M.), NASA-CR 1205. Washington, DC: National Aeronautics and Space Administration.

Stoll A.M., Greene L.C. (1959). Relationship between pain and tissue damage due to thermal radiation. *J. Appl. Physiol.*, **14**, (3), 373–82.

Takata A. (1974). Development of criterion for skin burns. *Aerospace Med.*, **45**, 634–7.

Weaver J.A., Stoll A.M. (1969). Mathematical model of skin exposed to thermal radiation. *Aerospace Med.*, **40**, 24–31.

28. Interactions of Heat with Tissues

J. W. L. Davies

In the UK it has been estimated that 17 000 people are admitted to hospital each year with thermal injuries and that about half this number have injuries severe enough to require surgical repair of the wounds. This review surveys the interactions between the thermal energy which produces the injury and the tissue changes which develop during the subsequent minutes and hours.

An account has been given in Chapter 27 of the modes of transfer of thermal energy onto the skin (by radiation and convection) and onto and into the skin by conduction. The severity of the injury to the skin and the subcutaneous tissues depends on the duration of exposure, the temperature, the efficiency with which the energy is transferred to the skin and the thermal conductivity of the tissues beneath the skin. The special situation where thermal energy is generated within the tissues by the passage of electrical energy, including microwaves, is discussed below.

Since the magnitude of the interactions between incident thermal energy and the responses of the tissues is dependent on both the temperature to which the tissues are exposed and the duration of the exposure, it is necessary here to summarize the studies which have defined this relationship. With very high temperatures (1000–3000°C) and brief exposures (200 ms), it was found by Evans *et al.* (1955) that:

- 8.4–13.4 J/cm^2 produced erythema of the skin in some subjects.
- 13.4–16.0 J/cm^2 produced both erythema and superficial/partial skin thickness damage.
- 16.4–19.7 J/cm^2 produced deep dermal skin thickness damage.
- Over 20.2 J/cm^2 produced full skin thickness damage.

About 90% of patients with scalds or burns treated in civilian hospitals are injured, in the domestic situation, following contact with hot liquids (scalds) or flames and very hot surfaces or electricity, which produce burns. The remaining 10% of thermal injuries follow industrial accidents. With domestic injuries the injuring temperatures are between 65 and 100°C for scalds and between 100 and about 500°C for flame and very hot surface contacts. Electrical injuries vary in temperature depending on whether the electricity passes *through* the tissues or the tissues are only very close to a very high temperature arc flash (see below).

The experimental studies in animals which have defined the tissue responses to heat have usually been conducted with incident (contact) temperatures of between 50 and 100°C applied for periods of time between 1 and 1000 seconds. Studies using heated metal blocks at temperatures up to 100°C applied to the skin surface show a very rapid, in less than 1 second, doubling of the temperature of the epidermis (which is between 100 and 500 μm in depth) and a ten times slower rate of rise in the temperature of the lower boundary of the dermis (which is many times thicker than the epidermis). Subdermal tissues do not reach the temperature of the applied block within 1000 seconds, partly due to the poor thermal conductivity of the tissue between the surface heat and the measuring thermistor probe and partly due to the removal of heat from the tissues by conduction to lateral and deeper tissues and by the flow of blood and lymph. A more recent computer modelling technique (Diller *et al.*, 1983) has explored the temperature gradients (portrayed as isotherms) within skin tissues of differing compositions and thickness during and subsequent to exposure to a circular disc heated to 90°C and applied to the skin for 15 seconds. The computed isotherms compared favourably with those reported 35 years earlier by Moritz and Henriques (1947).

There do not appear to be any studies of thermal gradients and subcutaneous tissue temperatures following higher temperature flame burns affecting the skin. Burning fabrics (clothing) produce temperatures around 500°C and inflict skin burns which are at least full skin thickness in depth and commonly also involve subcutaneous fat, findings which suggest that these tissues attained temperatures high enough to destroy deep tissues well within the 1000 seconds mentioned above.

The temperature–time relationship causing thermal damage is modified by applying pressure to a heat source in contact with the skin. In experimental animal studies (Suzuki *et al.*, 1991), applying a 400-g weight, and thus a total pressure on the skin of 49 mmHg to a disc at 50°C, produces a more severe thermal injury. Similarly, as for example when an unconscious person falls against the surface of a hot water heating radiator, the observed injury is more severe than would be expected from prolonged exposure to water at the same temperature. This enhanced severity of injury is attributed to the reduction of blood flow by pressure which impairs dispersion of heat to deeper and more distant sites.

INDICATORS OF THE SEVERITY OF THERMAL INJURY

The degree of tissue damage induced by radiative, convective and conductive heat transfer has been assessed by comparing the morphological,

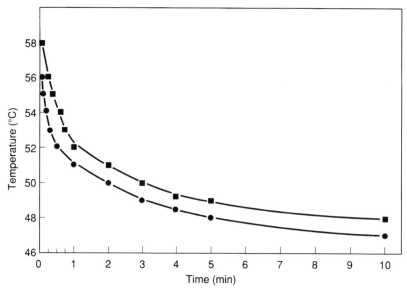

Figure 28.1 Minimal contact temperatures and periods of application which just produce an increase in permeability of the dermal capillaries of guinea-pig skin. There is an increase in permeability above line (■–■) and erythema without increased permeability below line (●–●).

histological and biochemical changes following application of different quantities of heat for differing periods of time to the skin of various animals. Time–temperature relationships ranging from 40°C for up to 48 hours to over 1000°C for only 50–60 milliseconds have been utilized. A wide range of techniques has indicated the macroscopic, microscopic and molecular changes associated with different degrees of injury inflicted on the epidermis, the dermis, the subcutaneous fat and muscle tissues and occasionally bone and nerve tissue.

When the skin of small animals, mainly rodents, is subjected to temperatures between 47 and 58°C for periods up to 600 seconds (Figure 28.1), erythema develops after short exposures to the lower temperatures, which becomes more intense and is associated with increased permeability of the dermal capillaries at the higher temperatures. For any given time of exposure a change in temperature of only about 1°C is required for progression from erythema to the induction of significant damage to the endothelial cells lining the capillaries which leads to virtually uncontrolled outward passage of a plasma-like fluid. Such altered capillary permeability is the typical response to scalding by water at temperatures between 60 and 100°C. In contrast, flame burns with temperatures ranging between 200 and 1000°C produce rapid coagulation of the tissues and blood vessels with minimal subsequent leakage of fluid. The combinations of time and temperature which induce erythema, kill epidermal cells and kill dermal cells and the skin adnexa contained within the dermis are shown in Figure 28.2. These changes in the tissues have been

intensively studied in an attempt to produce criteria where the conditions producing the injury are well defined, which will aid the assessment of the severity of injury in a burned/scalded patient where neither the duration of exposure to heat nor its temperature are known. The following subjective assessments and objective measurements have been used to indicate the extent and depth of a thermal injury.

Visual appearance

Accurate descriptions of the visual appearance of a burn wound have been available in the literature for over 300 years. In recent times Jackson (1953) described the appearance of human burn wounds with three recognizable zones following flame or boiling water injuries. He also stressed that the burn wound is three dimensional, the zones having depth as well as two surface dimensions. The three recognizable zones are:

1. A central zone of coagulated tissue where the incident heat has caused almost instantaneous destruction of tissue structure, cells and their contents.
2. An intermediate zone characterized by early stasis of blood flow in injured tissues which is maximal within 2 or 3 hours of injury and associated with gross swelling of the tissues, particularly following scalds.
3. An outer zone of least damaged tissue where hyperaemia is present initially although the early enhanced blood flow may subsequently return to normal or subnormal values.

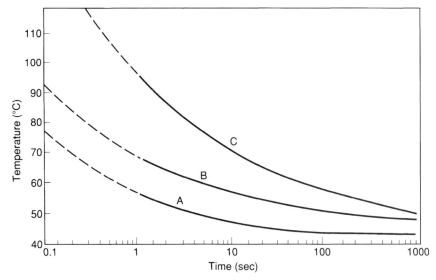

Figure 28.2 Relationships between time and temperature to cause discomfort in normal human volunteers (A), partial skin thickness burns (B) or full skin thickness burns (C). Values less than 1 second are extrapolations.

Histological examination of biopsy samples of skin and subcutaneous tissues taken within these three zones from rodents, primates and occasional burned patients have been reported by very many authors. On optical and scanning or transmission electron microscopy, the findings are summarized by Sevitt (1957) and Panke and McLeod (1985). A recent study (Suzuki *et al.*, 1991) has extended this outline by reporting, from numerous biopsies, the nature and anatomical levels of structural damage following *in vivo* exposure of rat tissues to temperatures between 37 and 60°C for between 3 minutes and 48 hours. The time/temperature exposures yielded the following five degrees of severity:

1. Vasodilatation with sparse perivascular infiltrations (erythema).
2. Epidermal necrosis with dense perivascular infiltration (partial skin thickness (partial-thickness) burn).
3. Collagen degeneration confined to the upper dermis (dermal depth burn).
4. Collagen degeneration affecting the lower zones of the dermis (deep dermal burn).
5. Collagen degeneration over the full depth of the dermis and into the tissues below it (full skin thickness (full-thickness) injury). For rat skin the critical temperatures producing superficial, partial-thickness and full-thickness injuries are 37.8, 41.9 and 47.9°C.

Nervous sensation

The nerve endings in skin responsible for the sensation of touch and the appreciation of pain are damaged by thermal injury to the extent that the nerve endings in the central zone of coagulated tissue are destroyed, leaving the tissue insensate. In the intermediate zone of stasis there is diminished, but still extant, nervous sensation whereas in the zone of hyperaemia nervous sensation is usually supranormal. The pin-prick test has been used to define the depth of injury. When a patient does not react to (i.e. feel) the pin prick, the burn is a full thickness injury; if the reaction is a feeling of touch rather than a sharp prick, the wound tissue is in the zone of stasis and therefore of superficial dermal depth. In the zone of hyperaemia it is not necessary to use the pin-prick test since the areas are subjectively very painful, even at complete rest. Analgesia is usually required for procedures involving movement, cleansing or the application of dressings. Of course these pin-prick assessments of burn depth will be of little or no value in babies, small children and in adults who are unconscious or analgesic due to the effects of ethanol or other drugs.

Visual appearance aided by dyes, stains, fluorescent compounds and differential reflectance photometry

Recent reviews by Heimbach *et al.* (1992) and Shakespeare (1992) have explored the usefulness of these guides to burn depth. A combination of Masson's trichrome stain and visual appearance can indicate the depth of thermal injury since normal collagen in tissue slices stains blue whereas heat-denatured collagen, with a loss of crystallinity and or parallel alignment of the collagen fibres, stains red. The depth of the abnormal staining of the skin is proportional to the time and temperature of the heat exposure. Other blue dyes, including methylene blue, are known to stain dead tissue blue and to be chemically reduced to a colourless or leuco form by the enzymes in living cells. In theory flooding a burn wound with the dye followed by washing the tissues should differentiate blue-coloured dead tissue from unstained viable tissue. In practice, however, Heimbach *et al.* (1992) found that the demarcation is too imprecise for guiding the surgical excision of non-viable tissue. Such imprecision has also nullified the usefulness of Patent blue V and tetracyclines for the differentiation of viable and non-viable tissues in wounds.

Almost 40 years before the use of the trichrome stain and blue dyes it was found that irradiation with ultra violet light after the intravenous injection of sodium fluorescein could differentiate between living tissues with an active blood flow and necrotic tissue which in consequence contained no fluorescein-labelled blood. This ability to distinguish qualitatively between partial- and full-thickness burns was rediscovered by Gatti *et al.* (1983), who were able to make quantitative measurements of the intensity of the fluorescence using a fibreoptic perfusion fluorimeter. Permanent records of the distribution and intensity of the fluorescence could be made using high-speed Polaroid photography (Grossman and Zuckerman, 1984), thereby permitting an investigation of possible changes in tissue viability with time. As is discussed in more detail below, partial-thickness zone of stasis burns may change to full-thickness zone of necrosis burns if the wound surface is treated unkindly (i.e. allowed to dry) (Zawacki, 1974). More recent assessments of the value of the fluorescein technique have provided contradictory evidence. Black *et al.* (1986) concluded from both experimental animal and burned patient studies that the use of fluorescein could not differentiate between partial- and full-thickness burns, though the clinical experience of Heimbach *et al.* (1992) confirms that very deep and very shallow burns can indeed be separated.

Differential reflectance photometry extends the visual capabilities of the eye in terms of the differing transmission and reflectance characteristics of incident light after the reflected portion has been split into bands for the infrared, red and green wavelength (Heimbach *et al.*, 1984; Afromowitz *et al.*, 1988). These original ideas were correct (Anselmo and Zawacki, 1977). The more recent simpler device requires pre-standardization which involves recording the spectral characteristics of wounds which are known to be shallow (which heal within 14–21 days), of partial-thickness depth (and require more than 21 days to heal) and those which are of full-thickness depth and will only heal after autografting. Once these results have been built into an 'instrument algorithm', the instrument may be used to predict the depth of a clinical injury (upon which the timing and degree of surgery may be chosen). The output was found to be con-

siderably more accurate than visual assessments made by experienced surgeons: the percentage accuracies were 86 vs. 71 for burns that healed by 21 days and 79 vs. 48 for burn wounds that only healed more than 21 days after injury.

This seeming ability to differentiate between shallow and deep dermal burns encouraged the development of other instruments based on the abnormal physiology of the burn, particularly those that attempted to quantify blood flow within thermally damaged tissue, since zone of stasis burns (with transient or permanent impairment of blood flow) are the clinical problem with respect to the timing of surgical repair.

Laser Doppler flowmetry

This technique measures blood flow using the Doppler shift in frequency of incident monochromatic light induced by movement of blood cells away from the light source. A comparison of the frequencies of the light reflected back from the bulk of motionless tissues, particularly the collagen in the dermis, and that from moving blood cells in a whole tissue sample of approximately $1 \, mm^3$, shows a very small change in frequency (about 1 part in 10^{12}) induced by the cell movement. When the two frequencies are mixed, the optical interference recorded by the detector results in a beat frequency (in the audible range of 2–3 KHz), the pitch of which is a direct measure of cell movement (Shakespeare, 1992).

This technique was first validated in rats with burns of varying severity, ranging from superficial epidermal to complete dermal depth. Helium neon laser light was used to measure the blood flow and tissue biopsies to confirm the depth of injury. A graded increase in the severity of injury produced by increasing time exposures to radiant heat from an incandescent light source (3100°C) was associated with graded reductions in capillary blood flow. In clinical studies normal or supranormal blood flows have been found with shallow burns affecting only the epidermis, whereas in deep burns involving most or all of the dermis blood flow was almost or completely absent. In patients with burns of intermediate depth (assessed clinically on admission), the Doppler flow measurements gave variable blood flows. When the blood flow measured soon after injury was compared with the subsequent pattern of wound healing or non-healing (Green *et al.*, 1988), it was found that wounds that healed without grafting always showed normal or elevated blood flows whereas in wounds that eventually required grafting flow was consistently reduced. At all times during the period of study there were statistically significant differences between the average levels of blood flow and whether the burns healed or did not heal.

The apparently variable Doppler blood flows in burns of intermediate depth may have other causes than changes in actual cell movement (Shakespeare, 1992). A degree of uncertainty has been introduced into the interpretation of Doppler flow measurements because of changes in the physical nature of the skin which govern the amount of light that reaches the blood cells. If the scattering characteristics of the skin are reduced, by for example the loss of the epidermis, then a higher proportion of the incident light will reach the remaining blood vessels. Such a change may produce a higher signal from the detector where the blood flow is reduced but more light reaches the vessels than from an area of high blood flow but which is masked by scattering structures above the blood vessels. These uncertainties arose following the simple experiment of placing a very thin slice of avascular epidermis over normal or burned tissue (between laser light source and detector) and showing an immediate decrease in detectable blood flow.

Thermography

Another characteristic of tissue with varying degrees of blood flow is that it has a variable temperature, which can be measured with a thermometer, thermocouples or with a thermographic camera. All warm objects emit radiation: the human body with a surface temperature of about 32°C emits infrared radiation with a wavelength of about 9.5 μm, it behaves as a perfect radiator, with high emissivity – a 'black body'. These criteria permit the mapping of isotherms using an infrared thermographic camera. Thermography has been used to study the depth of burning injury for over 25 years (see review by Shakespeare, 1992). Major interpretational problems which appeared during the thermographic measurements concerned the need to standardize the room temperature in which the measurements were made and to correct for changes in temperature of the burned tissue consequent upon the heat requirements for evaporative water loss. The evaporative water loss from a partial-thickness burn is approximately 20 times that from normal skin (Davies *et al.*, 1974) and requires approximately 580 Kcal for the evaporation of 1 litre of water. The early attempts to standardize the surface conditions of the wound by saturation with water have been superseded by covering the wound for the duration of the thermographic measurements with a water-impermeable film made of either polyethylene or polyvinyl chloride (Clingfilm) (Shakespeare, 1992). Currently the depth of a thermal injury is calculated from the differences in temperature between selected areas of the burn and adjacent areas of unburned skin. The consensus results of thermography are that, compared with adjacent normal skin temperatures, hyperaemic tissue has a higher temperature, zone

of stasis skin has a temperature between 0 and 1°C lower than normal and necrotic tissue may be cooler by 0.5–3°C. Simpler cheaper measurements using thermocouples or thermometers have provided similar temperature differences.

Diagnostic ultrasound measurements

These measurements basically indicate the distances between the sound transmitted at the skin surface and through tissue, until there is a change in the characteristics of the tissue which induces a reflection of the sound waves back towards the transmitter. The time taken between the transmitted pulse and the return of an echo indicates the depth of an echo-inducing interface.

Early observations in burned patients and pigs and in isolated pig skin, all burned to either partial-thickness or full-thickness depth, indicated that ultrasound pulses could differentiate boundaries between partial- and full-thickness injuries and subinjury normal tissues.

Contrary evidence in human burn patients has been presented by Wachtel *et al.* (1986), who made measurements of burn depth 24 and 72 hours after injury using a B mode 10-MHz scanning device. The data were found to be of no practical value to a burn surgeon for defining the difference in depth between partial-thickness and full-thickness burns. The explanation for this failure has been provided by Bauer and Sauer (1989), who made measurements with the same device between 1 and 6 hours after injury (but no later) and found a satisfactory relationship between the depth from the skin surface of the interface between heat-damaged and normal tissue and the time to healing.

INJURIES INDUCED BY ELECTRICITY

There are two methods by which electricity can cause thermal injury and one non-thermal mode of injury.

Arc injury

Arc injury occurs when a person approaches near enough to, but does not come in contact with, a conductor carrying electricity at a potential of 10 000 V AC or more. A very high temperature (c. 4000°C), short-duration (c. 100ms) pulse of electricity jumps between the electrical conductor and the person who is at 'earth' (ground) potential. Arcs can jump across a 10-cm gap with voltages of about 25 000 and across more than 40 cm when the voltage is about 100 000. These distances can increase dramatically if the air surrounding the conductor has a high water content.

The high temperatures of arc flashes cause radiant heat burns of exposed skin and will produce air temperatures at the surface of clothes sufficient for ignition if they are combustible.

Ignition is almost inevitably followed by deep skin burns. With this form of injury current rarely passes through the body to earth. The extreme example is when lightning strikes the ground or a tree close to where a person (or animal) is standing. The electrical potential of a lightning strike can range between 10 and 1000 million volts and can run into earth within 1–10 ms. An arc flash may extend for many metres around the strike. Clothing ignition is almost inevitable and some current from the ionized air around the flash may pass through the body inducing cardiac and respiratory arrests and muscle tissue and organ damage. Lightning strikes occur in two forms, discrete and continuing strikes. Discrete strikes are the more common: the current flows into the ground with a front waveform lasting about 1 μs, a tail waveform lasting about 40 μs and a peak current of about 20 000 A. Continuing strikes form a significant component of lightning strikes in about 50% of multistrike flashes where the current flow is only about 100 A but lasts for 40–300 ms. Some people survive discrete strikes whereas nobody survives the 1000 times longer continuing strikes, the current flow through the body always having lethal effects. Specific lightning injuries have also been described, including keraunoparalysis (Charcot's paralysis) – a transient paralysis associated with extreme vasoconstriction and sensory disturbances of one or more limbs and 'arborescent' flower or fern-like injuries affecting the skin (ten Duis *et al.*, 1987). The latter injuries appear to be associated with electrically positive discharges, in contrast to the former heat-induced injuries which result from electrically negative discharges.

Direct contact injury
Direct contact injury occurs when a person or animal at 'earth' potential makes physical contact with a conductor carrying electricity. Severe injury has been reported to follow contact with voltages as low as 250, where the electricity follows the paths of least tissue electrical resistance (the relative resistances to current flow from lowest to highest are nerve, blood, muscle, skin, tendon, fat and bone); and with powerlines carrying between 1100 and 500 000 V where the current flows along the shortest path to 'earth'.

Heat is the principal cause of tissue damage because the electrical resistances of many tissues are relatively small consequent on their high electrolyte contents. The body then acts as a volume conductor and heat is generated as a function of voltage drop and current flow per unit cross-sectional area – that is current density.

Simulation studies have been reported by Lee and Kolodney (1987) using an axisymmetric unidimensional model containing bone, skeletal muscle, fat and skin in a coaxial cylindrical geometry (as in a patient's upper or lower limb). After assigning appropriate thermal and electrical properties to each tissue the overall response to Joule heating was determined by a finite element numerical technique. The results indicated that when the tissues were electrically in parallel, skeletal muscle sustained the largest temperature rise, which then heated adjacent tissues. In the situation when bone was not in series with the other tissues, heating of bone was unlikely to be responsible for thermal damage to adjacent tissues. The simulation model also indicated that tissue perfusion (with blood and lymph) had a dramatic and direct effect on the rate of cooling of centrally located tissues.

These model-simulation studies used an electrical input spread uniformly over the end of the coaxial limb; in practice however patients injured by electricity usually receive the electrical input over a small area of the surface of the cylinder (i.e. on the skin). In this situation the current flow is markedly affected by the electrical resistance of the skin at the point of contact and with 'earth'; it will be relatively high in dry conditions and low when the humidity is high, particularly when there is sweating – induced by high ambient temperatures. Maximal current density at the skin surface continues until the tissue chars and the electrical resistance rises sharply to limit further passage of current and thus heating. The heated tissues then cool, the deeper zones cooling more slowly than the superficial. Since thermal damage of tissues is dependent upon both the achieved temperature and the duration of exposure, the deeper tissues are more liable to severe injury. Clinically such effects produce non-viable muscle near the centrally located bone of an extremity overlaid by more superficial viable or less damaged muscle. The extent of skin injury at the points of electrical contact with the conductor and with 'earth' may thus offer little indication of the extent of tissue damage.

The model simulation studies also explored the non-thermal modes of injury caused by the passage of electricity through tissues. Such current flows generate electrical fields which are capable of causing the breakdown of cell membranes and thus adjacent cell lysis. Large muscle and nerve cells have been found to be the most vulnerable. These studies have been reported in great detail in two recent multi-author books edited by Lee and his colleagues in 1992 and 1994.

Electricity-induced skin, other tissue and organ damage

Vascular damage
This is evident by 15 minutes after the passage of electricity and with some thromboembolic progression continuing for up to 48 hours. The blood flow in large distributive arteries is usually sufficient to dissipate the heat generated during the passage of

current, whereas smaller vessels such as muscular nutrient branches suffer significant damage manifest as endothelial cell membrane perforation or bursting and leucocyte margination. A special form of blood vessel damage follows the flow of current through bone marrow, there is then evidence of aplasia, leucocyte/granulocyte disintegration, a gross fall in the number of platelets and a failure of myelopoiesis.

Nerve damage

Because nerves convey more current per unit area they may become damaged before necrosis occurs in surrounding tissues. The injury to the nervous system may manifest itself immediately by loss of consciousness and respiratory and motor paralyses. Peripheral nerves may suffer direct injury at the entrance or exit sites of the electricity where there is commonly charring of all tissues down to fascia, or as a polyneuritic syndrome involving nerves far removed from the site of injury, which normally recover after a phase of reduced or lost function. When deep nerves are heated by direct current flow or by conduction of heat from adjacent heated muscle, recovery of nerve conduction is rare.

If the spinal cord is heat injured by current flows the response is either early death or a delayed neurological deficit manifest as hemiplegia or quadriplegia depending on the location of the entrance site. Recovery from the paralysis is unusual although not unknown. Perivascular haemorrhage, demyelinization, reactive gliosis and neuronal death have been observed in experimental animal studies of spinal cord heating by electricity.

Muscle tissue damage

Heat production by high current flows also damages muscle tissue with increased permeability of the intensely vascular tissue leading to impaired or stagnant blood flows, oedema formation, denaturation of the erythrocytes in the blood-rich tissue and the liberation of free haemoglobin, myoglobin and the creatine kinase isoenzymes, particularly the MM type. The latter materials are subsequently excreted in the urine, often aided by forced diuresis to limit the likelihood of renal impairment. Heat-affected muscle has a modified blood flow, changed tissue resistivity and an altered metabolic activity. Angiographic techniques (Hunt et al., 1974) have identified major blood vessel occlusions but are unable to visualize the small nutrient muscle branches which are commonly affected by sludged erythrocytes or microthrombi. [133]Xenon washout studies (Clayton et al., 1977) indicated areas of decreased muscle blood flow but could not provide accurate enough locations. Currently the most accurate measurements have been with pyrophosphate labelled with Technetium-99m ([99]Tc[m]-PYP), and indicate muscle necrosis – no uptake of [99]Tc[m]-

PYP – ischaemia where there is limited uptake of label and hyperaemic injury where there are areas of supranormal uptake.

Tissue resistivity and impedance measured by electrical frequency sweeping (Chilbert et al., 1985), and tissue metabolic activity measured by nuclear magnetic resonance spectroscopy (^{31}P) (Chilbert et al., 1990), have also provided evidence of the degree of injury affecting tissues hidden under the skin. Compared with the resistivity and metabolic activity of normal muscle, severe necrosis reduced both assessments by 70%, minimal necrosis plus oedema formation reduced them by 20–40% and oedema only reduced them by 10–30%.

In the absence of these sophisticated analytical measuring devices, satisfactory intraoperative identification of the degree of viability of muscle tissue suspected of being damaged by electrical heating has been reported using the nitro blue tetrazolium test (Hunt and Heck, 1984). Colourless nitro blue tetrazolium is normally reduced to a blue formazin by dehydrogenases in metabolically active or viable muscle fibres, but ischaemic or necrotic tissue has lost this enzyme reaction. Therefore during surgery blue-coloured muscle can be left *in situ*, very pale blue or uncoloured tissue can be excised.

Further studies of the increased dehydrogenase activity in heat-damaged muscle (Robson et al., 1984) explored the histochemical changes in tissue cross-sections of the hind limbs of rats which had been injured by the passage of 250 V AC for 10 seconds. The peroxidase-antiperoxidase method indicated an increased rate of production of arachidonic acid metabolites (see below), particularly the thromboxanes, at sites near the entrance point of the current and in periosseous tissue – areas likely to have been heated most intensely because of their high electrical resistance. The levels of these vasoactive substances (the thromboxanes) remained high during the development of necrosis which was apparent, microscopically, as intense vasoconstriction and its natural sequence of thrombus formation in the microcirculation. The role of the thromboxanes in this sequence of events was established by the administration of agents capable of blocking thromboxane production (imidazole, methyl prednisolone and aloa vera cream) which resulted in significantly less tissue destruction.

Ocular effects

It is uncertain whether thermal or electrostatic/ magnetic effects associated with the passage of high-voltage electricity induces the ocular effects seen in patients who show an electrical entry point on the head. The most common ocular effect is developing opacity of the lens which usually requires subsequent extraction (Boozalis et al., 1991).

Cardiac effects

When contact with high-voltage electricity conductors is by the head or hand(s), and with an exit to 'earth' by the contralateral hand or the feet, the flow of electricity is likely to cross the heart. Rhythm and conduction disturbances follow but usually resolve spontaneously. The most common electrocardiographic abnormalities are sinus tachycardia, non-specific ST-T segment alterations, which may be persistent (Hartford and Ziffren, 1971), and atrial fibrillation. Biochemical indications of cardiac injury following current flows are the tissue release and subsequent urinary excretion of the conduction-specific creatine kinase MB isoenzyme (Hammond and Ward, 1986). However, studies in electrically-injured patients have reported high levels of CK-MB isoenzyme in patients with presumed or known skeletal muscle damage and only transient or non-existent evidence of cardiac muscle damage (Ahrenholz et al., 1988). It has therefore been suggested that skeletal muscle contains both the MM and MB isoenzymes of creatine kinase. Both Housinger et al. (1985) and Ahrenholz et al. (1988) indicate that myocardial damage following electrical injury is rare.

Another rare manifestation of electricity induced cardiac injury is the pulmonary oedema which is a sequel to ventricular fibrillation (Schein et al., 1990). The haemodynamic findings and the ratios of the colloid osmotic pressures of the serum and the oedema fluid confirmed the cardiac origin of the oedema.

Not unexpectedly, when large quantities of electricity traverse the abdomen the heating effects damage a variety of internal tissues and organs. Nausea and vomiting are common symptoms and may reflect damage to the stomach. Stress ulceration, adynamic ileus, gallbladder necrosis, intestinal and colonic perforations also occur. When high-voltage electricity has an entrance point on the abdominal wall, the wall itself may be perforated leading to hepatic and pancreatic damage and single or multiple necrotic perforations of the small and large intestine, the caecum, bladder, sigmoid colon and terminal ileum. The nature and treatment of this wide variety of abdominal injuries has been recently reviewed by Nichter et al. (1984).

When high-voltage electricity enters the body near or via bony structures the high electrical resistance of bone leads to very high localized temperatures. Such temperatures may produce chemical fusion of the calcium phosphate matrix and more distant periosteal necrosis. As the limits of such necrosis may be difficult to define clinically, preoperative bone scans using ^{99m}Tc-labelled methylene diphosphonate have been found to be useful (Chang and Yang, 1991). The correlation between the results of scanning and the clinical findings was almost 89%.

MICROWAVE INJURIES

The now common domestic microwave oven uses a microwave frequency of 2.45 GHz to provide up to about 800 W of power. Foodstuffs, commonly meats and vegetables, are fully cooked within a few minutes by a mechanism which involves the violent movement of water molecules, the polarity of which changes from positive to negative or the reverse 2450 million times per second. The friction opposing this molecular movement appears as heat. The extent of microwave absorption and subsequent heat generation is determined by the relative dielectric constants of the materials being exposed. The higher the value of the dielectric constant the greater the amount of heat generated and vice versa. Animal and vegetable tissues with a high water content have high dielectric constants, whereas glass, plastics, porcelain, paper and fat all have low values. These properties account for the cooking of foodstuffs at 100°C in glass or porcelain containers which, on removal from the oven, are at a much lower temperature until conduction of heat from the contents raises the temperature of the container. A distressing example of this effect is seen when a baby's glass bottle of milk is warmed in a microwave oven for too long. On removal of the bottle from the oven the glass feels only warm whereas the milk may have a temperature above 75°C. Oral cavity scalds have been reported on a number of occasions.

The prospect that human extremities could be exposed to high doses of microwaves stimulated the studies reported by Surrell et al. (1987). Small deeply anaesthetized piglets were exposed to 750 W of microwaves for exposure periods of 90, 105 and 120 seconds and then were maintained in an anaesthetized state for 14 hours with appropriate fluid resuscitation before sacrifice. The macroscopic changes of the skin wound were studied as well as the autopsy collection of biopsies from all tissues that had been beneath the microwave-emitting device.

The animals showed very well demarcated full-thickness burns with severities that correlated well with the times of exposure to the microwaves. Macroscopic and microscopic inspection of the tissue samples showed destruction of the epidermis and dermis, relative sparing of the subcutaneous fat and a depth-related injury to the viscera – the viscera nearer the skin surface and microwave emitter being injured and the deepest tissues being uninjured. Electron microscopy of the tissues revealed oedema and acantholysis of the cells of the strata basale and spinosum and blisters located above the basement membrane. The relative layered tissue sparing (of relatively water-free fat) is a unique feature of thermal injury by microwaves. Furthermore, the microscopic nuclear streaming sometimes seen in burns caused by electricity having a low frequency (Hz or KHz) is not seen in burns caused by microwaves.

Isolated case reports of human hands being exposed to varying doses of microwaves (summarized by Surrell *et al.*, 1987) provided a spectrum of time exposure dependent injuries that ranged from full-thickness burns which ultimately led to amputation, through partial-thickness burns that healed spontaneously but with persistent neurological symptoms, to only a transient paraesthesia which completely resolved within 1 hour.

It is presumed, but does not appear to have been reported, that the heat-damaged tissue generated by microwave exposure shows the same biochemical abnormalities associated with, or induced by, oxygen free radicals, cytokines and inflammatory mediator cascades as described later in this chapter for flame burns and scalds.

LASER LIGHT INJURIES

Monochromatic coherent light produced by a number of laser systems also appears to be converted into heat when applied to the surface of samples of animal skin. This conclusion, reported by Lawrence (1967), followed metabolic studies where albino guinea-pig tissue samples composed mainly of epidermis and dermis were exposed to ruby laser light (λ = 694.3 nm) before *in vitro* microrespirometer measurements of oxygen consumption and the anabolic incorporation of ^{35}Sulphate into skin mucopolysaccharides. The response to the incident laser power given in graded doses produced the same tissue responses as found following exposure of the tissue samples to water at temperatures which produced graded epidermal, superficial dermal and deep dermal degrees of damage (44–54°C). Dose response curves indicated that 50% lethality occurred with an applied energy of 2 J/mm^2 of tissue. Histologically the ruby light did not appear to destroy, selectively, any particular zone of the skin. Attempts to induce complete necrosis of all layers of the skin samples failed because energy densities expected to do this induced explosive disintegration of the tissue, presumably due to the formation of steam.

ULTRASOUND-INDUCED INJURIES

Thermal injuries induced by accidental exposure to high-power levels of ultrasound appear to be rare, in contrast to the relatively frequent therapeutic use of ultrasound for thermal ablation of malignant tissues in the brain and eye, which have been reviewed in detail by Lizzi and Ostromogilsky (1987). As an example of the deep tissue temperatures that can be achieved, a 2-second exposure with 2.7 MHz ultrasound produced a brain tissue temperature in anaesthetized animals of 55°C.

When skin samples from albino guinea-pig ear were exposed by Carney *et al.* (1972) to 3 MHz ultrasound for 30 seconds at various power densities, heat damage occurred which had identical metabolic effects to those observed when the same tissues were exposed to water at a range of temperatures between 44 and 54°C. The rate of incorporation of ^{32}phosphate and ^{35}Sulphate into macromolecules, the rate of oxygen consumption and the activity of tissue dehydrogenases were impaired by energy inputs of between 11 and 13 W/cm^2 over a period of 30 seconds.

The ultrasound power densities and frequencies which induce tissue damage are very different from those used for estimating the depth of tissue necrosis induced by fire flames or hot water described earlier in this chapter.

BIOCHEMICAL EFFECTS OF THERMAL INJURY

The quantities of heat described earlier in this chapter which produce the three zones of graded damage to tissues are associated with the production of, and appearance in plasma, tissue fluid or wound exudate of a wide variety of substances with very diverse molecular sizes and chemical composition. Some of these substances are polymers of natural materials, others are degradation products and the remainder are normal intracellular compounds which are liberated from heat-activated cells or cells that have been ruptured by heat or by hydrostatic or osmotic pressures. A very wide range of biochemical, metabolic and physiological disturbances have been attributed to the formation and liberation of these substances into the lymph and blood streams.

The zone of stasis seems to be both the source of many of these compounds and to be most susceptible to their actions. Within minutes of injury it shows at least three visible changes: small blood vessels become more evident; the wound surface becomes wet with a clear fluid; and the tissues swell. *In vivo* microscopic examination of zone of stasis burns inflicted by scalding the hairless mouse ear have shown a pattern of changes that relates these events (Boykin *et al.*, 1981). Within 30 seconds of injury arterioles greater than about 12 μm in diameter undergo an immediate intense vasoconstriction down to 20% of preburn diameter, followed by dilatation up to 30% greater than preburn diameter, with return to preburn diameter about 30 minutes later. During this time, arterioles less than about 12 μm in diameter showed no appreciable change in diameter. In contrast, venular dilatation up to 42% greater than preburn diameter occurred promptly after injury. Commonly this persisted with erythrocyte sludging and aggregation, leucocyte clumping and margination along the vessel walls, platelet aggregation and the production of microthrombi.

Coincident with these blood vessel changes, full skin thickness punch biopsies from control ears, scalded ears and contralateral unburned ears showed (by comparison of wet and dry weights of the biopsies) that there was an early increase in the water content of the tissues, i.e. oedema formation. Scalded ears in another study became thicker, as measured with a micrometer screw gauge, and showed a wet surface (exudate). Observations in scalded patients admitted to hospital promptly (within an hour of injury) confirmed the developing wet surface, the tissue swelling and the blood vessel engorgement. When these observations are extended for 24–48 hours there is a rapid decrease in the number of circulating platelets, evidence of a much increased conversion of fibrinogen to fibrin and a sequence of other coagulation disorders (e.g. see Bartlett et al., 1981).

A number of reports (e.g. Massiha and Monafo, 1974) have shown that these induced changes in the capillary network within the zone of stasis tissues are progressive, ultimately leading to tissue ischaemia consequent upon the slowing and then cessation of blood flow and thus the supply of oxygen and tissue nutrients. Pharmacological treatment of the developing ischaemia with heparin to decrease coagulation effects and to increase blood flow has not been successful (e.g. see Robson et al., 1979). Further prolonged studies in scalded guinea-pigs defined the development and extent of vascular coagulation and oedema formation. By 4 hours after scalding oedema in the surrounding tissues had rapidly progressed to its maximal value, whereas capillary stasis had only involved about one-third of the thickness of the skin. Twelve hours later capillary stasis had progressed deeper, almost to the level of the panniculus carnosis, while the early oedema gradually diminished. Early oedema occurring within minutes of injury is considered to be a consequence of the direct effect of heat on the small blood vessels whereas the oedema that developed later is attributed to vascular occlusion. The vascular occlusion with sludged/aggregated red cells and marginated leucocytes leading to ischaemia is compounded by oedema formation since the volume of fluid escaping into the tissues through membranes having increased permeability exceeds that which can be removed by the lymphatic system. The net increase in extracellular water exerts a degree of hydrostatic compression on the blood vessels.

The necrotic effect of tissue ischaemia is exacerbated by evaporative water loss from the surface of the burn (Zawacki, 1974). The extent and depth of necrosis in a zone of stasis scald increases if the wound is left exposed to dry air whereas it either diminishes (if covered with a waterproof material after a few hours) or does not develop if the wound is covered within a few minutes of injury with xenografts, homografts, autograft or even a water-impermeable tape or plastic film. In scalded patients where zone of stasis burns are covered by blisters, leaving them intact as a wound covering ensures more rapid wound healing than if the blisters are removed (e.g. see Moserova et al., 1983).

In contrast to these relatively shallow burns with extensive oedema formation, it has been found that the necrotic tissue in the zone of coagulation produces relatively little oedema since the blood vessels and blood flow are completely destroyed by the incident heat (e.g. see Arturson and Jakobsson, 1985). The leathery texture of necrotic skin limits the evaporative water loss to low values and, as would be expected, covering the tissue has no beneficial effect on healing. In fact a cover enhances the rate of proliferation of any microorganisms that may have lodged on the surface of the wound subsequent to the injury though boiling water scalds and flame burns usually sterilize the skin.

Mechanisms of oedema formation

The early oedema occurring within minutes in injuries of the severity of the zone of stasis is attributed to the direct effect of heat on the smaller blood vessels which respond with an increased permeability of the damaged tissues to an outward leakage of water and ions, carbohydrates, fatty acids, peptides and proteins (see review by Arturson, 1985). Several endogenous compounds have been implicated in the mechanisms governing the increased permeabilities. The temporal sequence of appearance is oxygen and hydroxyl free radicals and hydrogen peroxide, the release of histamine and the activation of the kallikrein–kinin systems.

Free radical-induced mechanisms

Some types of microvascular endothelial cells are known to contain xanthine dehydrogenase and xanthine oxidase (Till et al., 1989), and that heat injury triggers the conversion of the former to the latter. The xanthine oxidase then leaks through the more porous cell membranes into the plasma, producing peak levels of xanthine oxidase activity (measured as the superoxide (O_2^-) anion or oxygen free radical) within 15 minutes of injury. Relative ischaemia affecting tissues distal, in terms of capillary blood flow (which may be less than 25% of control values), to the thermal injury also seems able to induce the conversion of xanthine dehydrogenase to xanthine oxidase.

It is also known that both ischaemia and heat injury cause the breakdown of adenosine triphosphate (ATP) to degradation products which include hypoxanthine, that are susceptible to enzymatic conversion to xanthine oxidase (in the presence of oxygen), xanthine, uric acid and the superoxide anion. This chain of events is strongly supported by the observed increases in the plasma levels of xanthine oxidase, xanthine, uric acid, allantoin and purine degradation products in burned rats. Of particular importance is the production of the superoxide anion during the conversion of hypoxanthine to uric acid, which is xanthine oxidase dependent, and which can be prevented by, pre-burn treatment with inhibitors of xanthine oxidase production or activity such as lodoxamide, allopurinol and oxypurinol.

This production of the super oxide anion within minutes of injury causes both fragmentation of the interstitial lattice of hyaluronic acid and oxidative degradation of cell membranes. Both these effects increase the permeability of the microvascular capillaries to water and macromolecules. This early superoxide anion effect is different from that involving neutrophils and other macrophages which produce toxic oxygen species (O_2^-, H_2O_2 and perhaps OH^-) via the myeloperoxidase enzyme. The cells are activated by a variety of compounds in plasma, including the complement degradation product C_{5a}, bacterial exo- and endo-toxins and, with respect to alveolar macrophages, the toxic chemicals in inhaled fire smoke (patients with flame burns usually inhale a certain amount of smoke from the fabrics burning on their skin).

The superoxide anions are normally short lived (milliseconds only) and their effects are limited to a radius of a few microns. However by reaction with polyunsaturated fatty acids in adjacent cell membranes, more stable but still highly reactive (oxidative) lipid peroxides are generated which may exert a damaging effect on more distant cell membranes. In addition, polyunsaturated fatty acids and their phospholipid esters are readily oxidized to lipid peroxides by a chain reaction involving arachidonic acid and subsequently the prostaglandins (see below). Once an initiating lipid radical has been generated, it attacks another cell membrane lipid to form a second lipid radical, thereby ensuring that the lipid peroxidation cycle is propagated; one initiating lipid radical induces oxidation of about 90 molecules of methyl linoleate.

The lipid peroxides with a relatively long biological half-life also have the ability to induce a systemic response. Following their distribution around the body in plasma and lymph they can cause tissue damage in remote organs and tissues such as the lungs, liver, kidney, muscles and skin (Sasaki *et al.* 1987; Demling and LaLonde, 1990). This damage may not cause immediate organ dysfunction but may sensitize the tissues to respond to a second insult, for example by various cytokines (see below) in a more serious way.

The chain of biochemical reactions leading to the reduction of oxygen to water not only involves the production of the superoxide anion but also that of hydrogen peroxide (Figure 28.3). Superoxide dismutase (a superoxide anion scavenger) inhibits the production of hydrogen peroxide and the administration of catalase (or activation of that already present in the tissues) destroys all pre-existing hydrogen peroxide. This scavenging action is of critical importance since, in its absence, hydrogen peroxide is able to activate complement with the formation of many degradation products, particularly C_{3a} and C_{5a}. These two peptides are important, since C_{3a} can induce the release of histamine from mast cells in rats and C_{5a} is a very potent endogenous chemotactic agent.

Histamine-related mechanisms

The delay of approximately 15 minutes between thermal injury and obvious oedema formation (although microscopically/histologically there is only a delay of a minute or so) has been attributed to the stages of complement activation, particularly the formation of C_{3a} from C_3 and C_{5a} from C_5. Both peptides are capable of initiating the release of histamine from basophils and mast cells in rats leading to a rapid rise in plasma histamine levels within 15 minutes of heat injury (Friedl *et al.*, 1989). It must be noted however that the temperature of the tissue must exceed 55°C before this happens. Concomitantly there is a further increase in the catalytic activity of xanthine oxidase. A vicious circle ensues (Figure 28.3) when the release of histamine and many of its metabolic derivatives stimulates xanthine oxidase to produce the superoxide anion, hydrogen peroxide and hydroxyl radicals which in turn stimulate further histamine release via C_{3a} and C_{5a} formation.

The histamine produced in this vicious circle does not appear to be directly responsible for the increased microvascular permeability because

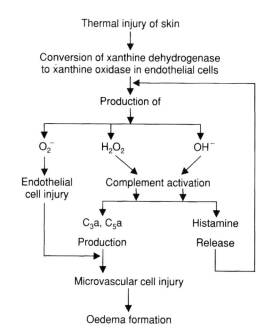

Figure 28.3 Events occurring within about 20 minutes of injury.

administration of mepyramine and diphenhydramine (H_1 histamine receptor antagonists) do not prevent it. However cimetidine (an H_2 histamine receptor antagonist) does inhibit the onset of increased microvascular capillary permeability, which can be attributed to its effectiveness as an hydroxyl radical scavenger. The sympatholytic drugs phenoxybenzamine and dibenamine also reduce oedema formation, which may be the result of their antihistaminic and antibradykin effects. In contrast to these 'antihistamines', the inhibitors of xanthine oxidase activity are highly protective, strongly suggesting that the reactive radicals O_2^- and OH^- and H_2O_2 derived from xanthine oxidase are the prime causes of the altered capillary permeability.

Aspects of complement activation Exploration of the mechanisms by which H_2O_2 initiates the appearance of C_{5a} suggests that the hydroxyl radical is critical. Hydrogen peroxide dissociates into OH^+ and OH^- in an iron-dependent reaction wherein Fe^{2+} changes to Fe^{3+}. Chemical scavengers of the hydroxyl radical dimethylthiourea (DMTU), dimethylsulphoxide (DMSO) and cimetidine are effective in preventing the appearance of C_{5a} following thermal injury. In an *in vitro* test system, the removal of iron has been shown to protect isolated pieces of tissue against injury by hydroxyl radicals. C_{5a} production in plasma is prevented by the addition of the iron chelating agent deferoxamine, an effect which can be partially reversed by the addition of ferric iron. Deferoxamine can also be complexed with the resuscitation fluid hetastarch to provide an *in vivo* form of therapy which decreases both systemic tissue oxidation changes and the volume of fluid required for effective resuscitation (implying reduced oedema formation).

The appearance of C_3 and C_5 is only part of the complement activation process induced by thermal injury and leading to the depletion of complement (and therefore opsonic activity) from plasma. The total haemolytic complement activity (CH_{50}) and other complement components (C_1, C_2, C_4, C_8) all show dramatic falls in concentration within hours of injury (Davies, 1982). Apart from the histamine releasing function of C_{3a} and the potent chemotactic activity of C_{5a}, both factors and C_{3b}, C_{3c}, C_{3d} and C_1 split products have a marked ability to induce an immunosuppressive state (Alexander, 1990).

The activation of complement following thermal injury may proceed by either the classical or the alternative pathways. The alternative pathway activation occurs with remarkable speed after significant injury, with a 75% depletion by 15 minutes and zero activity remaining by 60 minutes after scalds covering 25% of the body surface area (Gelfand, 1984). In contrast, the activation of the classical pathway caused only about a one-third depletion over the same time-scale.

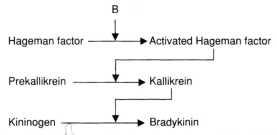

Figure 28.4 Stages in the formation of bradykinin from the Hageman factor. B = burn-induced liberation of proteolytic enzymes and exposure of the Hageman factor to collagen.

Hageman factor, kallikrein, kinin mechanisms
A second mechanism involved in the process, whereby endothelial cell membranes become more permeable to water and macromolecules, involves the activation of the Hageman factor. This factor is normally present in tissues and is activated by heat probably because of cell rupture, which allows the factor to come into contact with a mixture of intracellular proteases and with normal or heat-modified collagen. Activated Hageman factor (AHF) converts pre-kallikrein to kallikrein, which in turn converts kininogen into bradykinin (Figure 28.4).

Bradykinin has been shown to have a number of potentially pathogenic activities including the ability to dilate blood vessels, induce pain, initiate or enhance leucocyte migration and increase capillary permeability. Recent studies in burned guinea-pigs and patients with burns have strongly implicated bradykinin as another significant factor which increases microvascular capillary permeability (Holder and Neely, 1990). However there appears to be some delay (up to 2 hours) after injury before this mechanism makes a significant contribution to the volume of oedema and initially the free radical mechanisms appear to be dominant.

Bradykinin can also stimulate the production of the various prostaglandins through its ability to convert inactive phospholipase to active phospholipase (Figure 28.5), with the subsequent conversion of phospholipids to arachidonic acid, the precursor of first cyclic endoperoxide and then prostaglandin E_2 (PGE_2), prostaglandin I_2 (PGI_2) and thromboxane A_2 (TxA_2). One of these arachidonic acid metabolites, PGE_2, is further converted to $PGF_{2\alpha}$ by the enzymatic action of bradykinin. Further discussion of the actions of these arachidonic acid metabolites is given below.

Apart from initiating bradykinin formation, activated Hageman factor also appears to be involved in two aspects of the coagulation/fibrinolysis system. As may be seen (Figure 28.6), the enzymatic activity of AHF converts factor XI to factor XIa, which in turn leads to the conversion of factor IX to an active form which initiates the coagulation

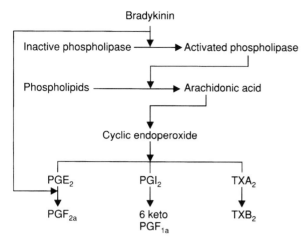

Figure 28.5 Mechanisms by which various prostaglandins are formed.

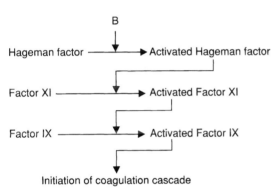

Figure 28.6 Stages in the initiation of the coagulation cascade. B as in Figure 28.4.

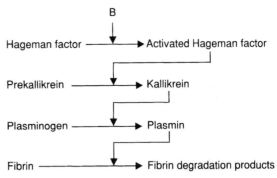

Figure 28.7 Stages in the formation of fibrin degradation products. B as in Figure 28.4.

cascade. The hypercoagulability of lymph and plasma during the early hours after scalding and burning is well known (Davies, 1982).

The AHF-induced production of kallikrein from pre-kallikrein also provides the enzyme action which converts plasminogen into plasmin (Figure 28.7), which is responsible for the degradation of insoluble fibrin into a sequence of soluble degradation products.

Metabolically active derivatives of arachidonic acid

These metabolites have a significant involvement in both the early and later responses to thermal injury (Harms *et al.*, 1981; Jin *et al.*, 1986). Two groups have been identified depending on the pathways involved in their production: the prostaglandins produced by the cyclo-oxygenase pathway and the leukotrienes produced by the lipo-oxygenase pathway.

Prostaglandins

The prostaglandins (prostanoids) are released in considerable amounts soon after thermal injury involving significant areas of the body surface (>10%). Two prostaglandins with different actions appear in both plasma and tissue fluid: one has a vasoconstricting activity (TxA_2) and the other a vasodilatory activity (Prostacyclin or PGI_2) (Harms *et al.*, 1981; Jin *et al.*, 1986). The persistent reduction in blood flow in the zone of stasis injury is most likely to be due to the effects of TxA_2 (DelBeccaro *et al.*, 1980) which also increases platelet aggregation and neutrophil margination and release in the burn microcirculation, which exacerbates the formation of oedema. The attribution of these effects to thromboxane A_2 has followed the use of specific TxA_2 inhibitors (imidazole, dipyridamole and methimazole) blended into a cream and applied topically to the burn wound (DelBeccaro *et al.*, 1980). In both burned animals and patients with burns there was an improved blood flow within the zone of stasis tissues and a decrease in the area of the wound that subsequently became necrotic. In addition, the intravenous administration of these TxA_2 inhibitors has been shown to decrease systemic vascular resistance.

The vasodilatory effect of prostacyclin (PGI_2) with increases in local blood flow probably accentuates the vascular permeability and oedema formation associated with free radical-induced cell membrane damage. Again the attribution of these effects to PGI_2 has followed the use of a known antagonist of prostacyclin activity (ibuprofen). When incorporated in a cream for topical application to the burn wound this agent induces a reduction in the volume of oedema (Demling and LaLonde, 1987), which may also follow, in part, the known antioxidant effects of ibuprofen (Demling and LaLonde, 1990).

Other prostaglandins have significant effects soon after thermal injury. PGE and PGE_2 are probably responsible for much of the erythema and pain found in the zone of hyperaemia. PGE_2 also appears to be a significant cause of the cell-mediated immunity which follows severe thermal injury as a consequence of its role as a mediator of the production of interleukin 2 (IL-2) (Hansbrough et al., 1984).

Leukotrienes

The leukotrienes originate in macrophages, mast cells, neutrophils and vascular tissues that have been activated by heat or the oxidizing effect of free radicals. Leukotriene B_4 is a potent chemoattractant that is associated with increased microvascular permeability (Lewis et al., 1990). It is found within a few hours of burn injury in the oedema fluid adjacent to the injured tissue and in the lymph draining from this tissue but not in plasma. Leukotriene C_4 and D_4 are potent vasoconstrictors of smooth muscle and have been detected in the fluid within burn blisters but not in plasma. It has been suggested, but not proven, that the C_4 and D_4 leukotrienes accentuate early post burn tissue ischaemia by mechanisms similar to those reported above for TxA_2.

In summary the biochemical studies discussed thus far indicate that skin burns induce the release of mediators that act both locally and systemically. These, including the very reactive oxidant radicals and the metabolites of arachidonic acid, both initiate and influence the formation of oedema by mechanisms which have been reviewed in detail by Youn et al. (1992). The heat injury also generates a number of factors which activate complement, stimulate further release of arachidonic acid and the production of a group of cytokines, particularly tumour necrosis factor, interleukins 1, 2 and 6, interferon γ and the colony stimulating factors.

Tumour necrosis factor (TNF)

TNF is produced primarily by macrophages but also by endothelial cells, neutrophils and lymphocytes, all of which would have been present in the tissues at the time of scalding or burning. A wide variety of cells, particularly those in the reticuloendothelial system, have specific receptors for TNF (Marano et al., 1990). There is a rapid production (within minutes) of TNF from heat-injured/activated cells. Although the burst of TNF production is short lived, with a plasma half-life of about 15 minutes, the response it produces is perpetuated through the initiation of secondary cascades. Lesser degrees of TNF activation produce stimulation of cell receptors with a delayed detrimental reaction.

Tumour necrosis factor generates a wide spectrum of activities, including the early release of neutrophils from the bone marrow, activation and margination of neutrophils in the injured area with the release of proteases and oxidants, and activation of macrophages which also release oxidants, the various metabolic degradation products of arachidonic acid and the production of inter-

leukins 1 and 6. These responses have both detrimental and beneficial effects – the potentiation of self-destructive inflammation coincides with stimulation of antibacterial defences.

Metabolic activity is also stimulated by TNF. There is an increased rate of catabolism of skeletal muscle in conjunction with secondary hormone release, stimulation of the hepatic production of acute phase proteins and peripheral lipolysis and hepatic lipogenesis. When the catabolic process is prolonged there will be significant weight loss through muscle wasting. Increased endothelial cell permeability and procoagulant activity have also been attributed to TNF; again these are activities which have both detrimental and beneficial effects, the localized inflammatory responses activating the cells required for initiating wound healing.

In patients with very severe thermal injuries there is an early acute, exaggerated secretion of TNF into the plasma with the increased likelihood of rapid cardiovascular collapse and death. Studies with ibuprofen can attenuate this, suggesting that the systemic response is caused by ibuprofen-sensitive secondary mediators released by TNF.

Interleukin 1 (IL-1)

IL-1 is produced primarily by heat-injured or activated blood monocytes and tissue macrophages and secondarily by keratinocytes and other cell types (Fong et al., 1990). This cytokine commonly remains bound to the cell membrane. T-cell proliferation follows contact with IL-1-activated macrophages. Other activities attributable to IL-1 include the production of IL-2, increasing the number of IL-2 receptors and enhancing the release of neutrophils from the bone marrow, the latter in collaboration with the granulocyte macrophage colony stimulating factor GM-CSF (see below).

A variety of metabolic events are induced by a mixture of IL-1 and IL-2, including: heat production associated with various prostanoids secreted by the central nervous system; the synthesis of IL-6 which, together with IL-1 and IL-2, stimulates the hepatic production of the acute phase plasma proteins; reductions in the plasma levels of iron and zinc; increased catabolism of skeletal muscle; anaemia as a consequence of erythrocyte stem cells being altered so that they form leucocytes and influence wound healing and connective tissue remodelling. In this sequence of metabolic events where TNF induces IL-1 production (and IL-1 increases TNF activity) and IL-1 also stimulates the production of IL-2, it is uncertain which factors are primarily involved with which changes. Considering the relationships between IL-1 and IL-2 it is not unexpected that early forms of treatment which reduce the production of IL-1 also decreases the levels of IL-2.

Interleukin 2 (IL-2)

IL-2 is produced by T lymphocytes and stimulates cell-mediated immunity and cytotoxic T-cell function. As stated above IL-2 production is dependent upon macrophage production of IL-1. Following severe thermal injury both the production and activity of IL-2 are depressed (Teodorczyk-Injeyan et al., 1986) attributable, in part, to a number of serum suppressive factors particularly PGE_2 (Wood et al., 1984). This decreased production and activity of IL-2 correlates well with increased mortality after a septic challenge in burned animals (Rodrick et al., 1989), which can be reversed by treatment with ibuprofen or the infusion of exogenous IL-2 (Gough et al., 1988). These studies, involving the close relationship between infection and IL-2 levels, underline the importance of this cytokine and the problems that depleted levels produce. The infusion of exogenous IL-2 however is not without hazard since organ dysfunction and hypermetabolism develop (Michie et al., 1988), which has been attributed to IL-2 induction of an enhanced release of TNF and interferon gamma.

Interleukin 6 (IL-6)

IL-6, which used to be called hepatocyte stimulating factor or interferon B_2, is a monocyte-derived human B-cell growth factor and is the general term for a family of phosphorylated glycoprotein cytokines produced following IL-1 stimulus (Bauer, 1989) by endothelial cells, macrophages, neutrophils and fibroblasts. They appear in the circulation very rapidly following thermal and other forms of injury and persist at high levels for many weeks. Their effects are immunological and metabolic: they stimulate acute phase protein synthesis by hepatocytes, immunoglobulin synthesis by B lymphocytes, the growth of megakaryocytes and also have pyrogenic properties (Nijsten et al., 1991).

Natural interferon gamma (IFNγ)

IFNγ is mainly derived from human helper T cells. Some macrophage populations also appear to produce this cytokine which has a significant role as a priming agent for macrophage function, which then leads to activation of other cytokines, particularly TNF.

Colony stimulating factors (CSF)

CSF are a family of glycoproteins produced by macrophages, activated T cells and endothelial cells following stimulation by interleukin-1. They stimulate the bone marrow to increase production of various cell lines, particularly neutrophils.

Heat-induced changes in erythrocytes

Subepidermal temperatures of 65°C and subdermal temperatures of 50°C cause almost immediate lysis (at about 65°C) or morphological and physiological changes (at about 50°C) of erythrocytes. In addition, microcytes, spherocytes and crenated erythrocytes are formed which may not undergo lysis or removal from the blood stream until some hours later.

Serum obtained within 30 minutes of burning may contain at least 300 mg haemoglobin/dl (Loegering, 1981), reflecting the early lysis of erythrocytes. In exceptional very extensive charring burns in patients greater serum haemoglobin levels have been observed (1040–2470 mg/dl serum, Muir, 1961), corresponding with the destruction of up to 10% of the circulating erythrocyte volume. In plasma, concentrations of haemoglobin such as these do not persist when renal function is relatively normal, since the renal threshold for haemoglobin excretion is 130–140 mg/dl. Haemoglobin may then accumulate in urine to levels of 500–1000 mg/dl, possibly accompanied in some patients by methaemalbumin.

Coincident with this early extensive haemolysis is the presence of erythrocyte membrane debris which is cleared from the circulation by the reticuloendothelial system. This system is thereby partially blocked with depressed phagocytic function and possibly impaired host defence against other particulate matter (e.g. microorganisms) which may enter the circulation. Contained within the debris of erythrocyte membranes will be the outer cell membranes (consisting of phosphatidylcholine and phosphatidylinositol) and at least two aminophospholipids (phosphatidylethanolamine and phosphatidylserine) which normally reside on the cytoplasmic side of the red cell membrane. Though the phospholipids of the outer cell membranes of erythrocytes have minimal toxicity in vitro and none in vivo, the inner red cell membrane aminophospholipids have numerous toxic properties depending upon their concentration in plasma. The nature of these toxic effects has been examined using either a suspension of murine peritoneal macrophages exposed in vitro to varying amounts of the aminophospholipids or following intravenous injections into rabbits (Feola et al., 1989).

The in vitro macrophage studies showed: that 0.5 μg/ml of the two aminophospholipids stimulated the production of hydrogen peroxide, complement factor C_{3a}, prostacyclin and TxB_2; that 50 μg/ml produced cell injury manifest by the release of lipid peroxides and lactic dehydrogenase, and by morphological changes observed using phase contrast and electron microscopy; and that 100 μg/ml caused the death of 50–66% of the macrophages.

The in vivo studies indicated; that 0.05 mg/kg body weight caused only transient hypotension; that 0.1 mg/kg caused significant hypotension, cardiac arrhythmias, bronchospasm, activation of intravenous coagulation, complement, platelets and leucocytes, which released histamine, serotonin and thromboxane; and that 0.3 mg/kg caused cardiac arrest and death. Many of these effects are observed in patients with extensive thermal injury.

Morphological and physical changes

When the ambient temperature around the erythrocytes during and for about 5 minutes after the thermal injury does not reach more than about 55°C, the cells are altered morphologically, structurally and biochemically. The sequence of structural changes has been determined *in vitro* by exposure of the cells in plasma or isotonic saline to various temperatures and for varying periods of time. At temperatures between 47 and 55°C the first alteration is the formation of buds which split off from the erythrocytes to form microcytes (about 3 µm in diameter). The cells then become crenated or spheroidal or fragmented. Spherocytes are osmotically very fragile. Such cellular species are also observed in blood films taken from patients within an hour or so of extensive burns. When these contain about 1% of microcytes among the apparently undamaged erythrocytes the patients usually have burned areas which cover between 20 and 45% of body surface area. More microcytes are seen in blood from patients with more extensive burns, who subsequently show clinically significant losses of red cell volume

Red cells from severely burned patients have an abnormal osmotic behaviour. Within a few hours after burning the erythrocytes have an increased osmotic fragility, which returns to normal by 12–24 hours after injury, but is then followed by a period of increased osmotic resistance, presumably due to the early loss of the most fragile (senescent) cells which results in a more resistant population of relatively young cells. Specific studies of this population of most thermally resistant cells has shown that they also retained their ability to change shape and recover. This ability to deform is an essential feature of normal erythrocytes if they are to pass through capillaries with diameters similar to or smaller than that of their usual biconcave shape. In contrast heat-injured cells that become spherocytes have an increased resistance to packing by centrifugation, increase the viscosity of the blood and have an increased mean cellular volume (a raised water content). If numerous, these spherical cells tend to block considerable volumes of the capillary network (another aspect of a zone of stasis thermal injury).

Although heat can directly cause the formation of rigid spherocytes (as when washed red cells are heated in isotonic saline), many of the heat-induced tissue cell changes involving free radicals, proteases, mediators and cytokines can lead to the production of various lipids, and some pharmacologically active materials (such as the catecholamines and prostaglandins) can also increase erythrocyte membrane rigidity by binding to receptor sites on the cell membrane. The lipid-coated cells become spiculated (echinocytes), are lysolecithin fragile and are found early in large numbers of patients with burns covering more than about one-third of the body surface area. Coincident with the echinocyte formation there are reductions in the plasma contents of alpha lipoproteins, cholesterol and phospholipids and an increase in the fatty acids associated with lysolecithin.

Biochemical changes

These spherocytes show increased rates of potassium transport and glycolysis, a variable rate of depletion of cellular adenosine triphosphate (ATP), a decreased response to stimulation with ascorbate, lowered activity of glucose-6-phosphate dehydrogenase, increased activity of methaemoglobin reductase and low concentrations of reduced glutathione. It appears that erythrocytes subject to an oxidative stress do not undergo acute haemolysis (Baar, 1978).

An alternative or additional abnormality found in some heat-damaged erythrocytes is the presence of heat-damaged haemoglobin. Normal haemoglobin is very sensitive to denaturation by alkali whereas erythrocytes from patients and experimental animals with extensive burns contain considerable amounts of alkali-resistant haemoglobin, which has an increased affinity for oxygen and may therefore reduce the efficiency with which oxygen is delivered to hypoxic tissues. Cells containing such altered haemoglobin may have an irreversible inactivation of either glucose-6-phosphate dehydrogenase or phosphoglyceraldehyde dehydrogenase or both enzymes and will be recognized by the reticuloendothelial system as abnormal cells. If such cells also have an altered cell membrane they may be removed from the active circulation. Sequestration of these cells occurs not only in spleen and liver but also in skin.

Measurements of the degree of hydration of the various types of erythrocyte induced by a thermal insult showed that

1. The cellular hydration of all sizes of cells increased when the temperatures exceeded 45°C.
2. The cellular hydration was maximal at 50°C.
3. Temperatures of 55°C and above caused lysis of all sizes of cells.
4. The oldest, most dense cells showed the greatest uptake of water since many of them were spheres rather than biconcave discs.

These changes in cellular hydration were usually accompanied by a gain in cellular sodium from 11.2 to 16.4 mmol/l and an equivalent loss of potassium from 87.8 to 80.5 mmol/l (Curreri *et al.*, 1974). Such a change in the partition of cations stimulates the ion-sensitive membrane ATPase with an early exhaustion of cellular ATP which, if not replaced, accelerates the death of the cell. Estimates of the activity of the ATPase enzyme show that red cell ghosts isolated from the blood of burned patients during the first few hours after injury had, on average, only 43% of the activity found in those prepared from normal blood. The ion-activated ATPase in red cell membranes is extremely sensitive to the concentration of calcium ions, where an increase from 0.0300 to 0.0317 mmol/l inhibited the activity of the membrane responsible for the transport of sodium and potassium against the concentration gradients which normally exist either side of the membrane. The pump which maintains the different Na to K ratio (normally 0.13 but rising to 0.20 in heat-damaged erythrocytes) within the cells compared with that outside requires energy. Glucose turnover in red cells from rats with scalds covering 20% of the body surface area increased moderately from 32 to 42 µg per ml red cells per minute, probably, as a result of a rise in the rate of glycolysis, as a normal consequence of an increased red cell glucose concentration. There is thus no evidence for a depressed rate of red cell glucose transport or metabolism during the first 5 hours after thermal injury.

BIOPHYSICAL EFFECTS OF THERMAL INJURY

It is well known that the increased permeability of the endothelial cells of the vascular system induced by direct heat injury and the variety of heat liberated mediators discussed above, leads to the loss of plasma-like fluid from within the capillaries into the interstitial tissues. The water content of these tissues may increase to twice that found in health and develops when the rate at which fluid is filtered out of the microvascular vessels exceeds the flow in the lymph vessels draining the same mass of tissue. At least two mechanisms are involved: a moderate increase in hydrostatic pressure inside the perfusing microvessels; and the development of a substantial negative (suction) pressure in the adjacent heat-injured tissues. This fluid transfer occurs within minutes of injury and is greater in extent following scalds than flame burns. The extravasated fluid mainly expands the extracellular compartment, although there is some intracellular fluid expansion.

Such expansion of the extracellular fluid volume is not confined to areas adjacent to the injury. When the burned area covers more than about one-quarter of the body surface area the oedema is generalized (determined from wet minus dry weights of tissue biopsies taken from unburned tissues before and after remote thermal injury), implying a systemic rather than just a localized disorder (Arturson, 1985). The inflammatory mediators discussed above, that enter the lymphatic and blood streams, appear to reach all distant organs and tissues and there induce an increase in vascular permeability.

TABLE 28.1
VARIABLES ASSOCIATED WITH THE MICROVASCULAR EXCHANGE OF FLUID AND PROTEIN IN NORMAL TISSUES AND FOLLOWING THERMAL INJURY (MODIFIED FROM LUND ET AL., 1992)

Variables	Postburn	Normal
CFC (ml/mmHg/min/100 g)	0.1	0.04
σ	0.4	0.85
P_c (mmHg)	48	24
P_{if} (mmHg)	−150	−1
COP_p (mmHg)	10	26
COP_{if} (mmHg)	10–15	15

Note: Explanation of abbreviations is given in the text.

σ = range of permeabilities of the vessel walls to macromolecules on a scale of 0–1 (where 0 = completely permeable and 1 = completely impermeable).

Vascular hypoproteinaemia and a raised extravascular tissue content of protein may also be causes of this remote oedema formation.

Extremely detailed accounts of the physiological changes which govern the microvascular exchanges of fluid and macromolecular proteins have been published and are reviewed by Lund *et al.* (1992). Calculations have provided details of the net increase in interstitial fluid volumes per unit time. Table 28.1 gives the range of numerical values for factors which contribute to this oedema formation; these include the capillary filtration coefficient (CFC), the capillary reflection coefficient (σ), the capillary hydrostatic pressure (P_c), the interstitial fluid hydrostatic pressure (P_{if}), the plasma colloid osmotic pressure (COP_p) and the interstitial fluid colloid osmotic pressure (COP_{if}).

Lymphatic fluid drainage

Lymphatic fluid drainage from tissues subjected to thermal injury commonly increases 20-fold in volume within an hour of injury and usually contains a much higher than normal concentration of the smaller molecular weight proteins (up to 100 000 daltons) normally present in plasma. In addition there is a moderate increase in lymph flow draining remote uninjured tissues, which is in part induced by mediators derived from heat-damaged cells circulating in the blood stream rather than directly heat induced and, in part, by the development of hypoproteinaemia (commonly exacerbated by early fluid resuscitation with crystalloid solutions) and subsequent increased capillary filtration.

Transcapillary protein exchange (Table 28.1)

The finding of significant levels of the smaller plasma proteins in blister and oedema fluids generated the term 'capillary leakage'. While commonly found in scald-induced blisters and scald- and burn-induced oedema, the capillary leakage also occurs following suction- and friction-induced blisters. The extravasation of plasma proteins into heat-damaged tissues, and to a lesser extent in uninjured tissues, that show evidence of oedema formation has been repeatedly demonstrated with radioactively labelled plasma proteins over the 50 years since it was first described using blue dyed proteins (see review by Davies, 1982). The amount of protein transferred from the plasma may increase by 100-fold the extravascular plasma protein content of tissues adjacent to the thermal injury (Arturson, 1985). There is a much smaller increase (about four-fold) in the extravascular plasma protein content in tissues remote from a relatively extensive thermal injury (greater than 30% TBSA).

The hypothesis that small pores in the endothelial cell membranes, which allow the normal, very limited leakage of small plasma proteins into the tissues, followed by lymphatic removal (σ = 0.85–0.90, Table 28.1), increase in size in thermally injured tissue to give σ values of 0.40 (Table 28.1), has been explored by Harms et al. (1982) and Pitt et al. (1987). In the earlier studies it was concluded that only proteins with a diameter of less than 1080 nm, corresponding to molecules of the size of immunoglobulin G, can pass through heat-damaged cell membranes. More recently Pitt and colleagues used a two-pore model and found that normal small pores 500 nm increase to 700 nm and large pores normally 3000 nm in diameter increase to 4000 nm following thermal injury.

MATHEMATICAL MODELS

Virtually all the factors discussed above which lead to the formation of oedema have been measured either in experimental animals with thermal injuries of varying severity or occasionally in scalded or burned patients. However there are a number of unmeasurable factors (e.g. cell membrane permeabilities and pressure differences across these altered membranes which govern the exchange of water and macromolecules between the intra-and extracellular compartments), the magnitudes of which are required for a complete understanding of the mechanisms involved in the transcapillary transport of fluid and protein.

Computer-derived or -assisted mathematical models have provided simulations of the physiological changes which are considered to take place during the formation of oedema following thermal injury. Such models have been reported by Arturson et al. (1984, 1989); Roa et al. (1988); Roa-Romero and Gomez-Cia (1986); Bush et al. (1986); Bert et al. (1989); Bowen et al. (1989); Diller et al. (1991) and Onarheim and Reed (1991). They have explored in detail the responses to variations in a wide range of

factors in unresuscitated burned animals and in burned animals and patients receiving various volumes of fluid therapy containing either crystalloids alone or admixtures with different amounts of colloidal carbohydrates or proteins with a wide range of molecular weights. Simulated predictions of the clinical responses to varying forms of fluid therapy have shown high correlations with the actual responses, implying that the numerical values accorded to the unmeasurable factors were realistic.

BURN TISSUE DERIVED 'TOXIC' MATERIALS

In the foregoing discussion the tissue effects of thermal injury have been presented in terms of a wide variety of stimulators and mediators which react with local fixed and wandering cells. One characteristic of these stimulators and mediators is that they are relatively small molecules ($\leq$1000 Da). In contrast over the past 50 years there have been periodic reports of the isolation of larger molecules (c. 5000–200 000 Da) that have adverse effects on cells, tissues and organs both in the vicinity of the injury and at remote cites (see review in Davies, 1982).

The most well characterized of these 'toxic' materials is the 'cutaneous burn toxin' (CBT) produced by high-temperature (250°C) flame injury of skin (Allgöwer et al., 1973; Schoenenberger, 1975). Recently and following closer examination of its chemical structure, this material has been renamed a burn-induced lipid-protein complex (LPC). It appears to be a trimerization product of a conglomerate of six naturally occurring proteins with lipid components derived from epidermal and dermal cell membranes. The molecular weights of the various components range between 40 000 and 160 000 Da. It is probable that four of the six monomer proteins are derived from epidermal T cells, keratinocytes and Langerhans cells. The complex, the activities of which have been reviewed by Sparkes et al. (1990a), appears in the circulation within hours of burning, with plasma concentrations of up to 40 µg/ml. It has been shown to induce a wide variety of effects including alterations in the permeability of parenchymal cells in all organs, to impair host immune defence response in a dose-related manner, to inhibit the mitogenic response of lymphocytes, the production of colony stimulating factor and to blockade the IL-2 dependent growth of cells. Thermal injury or an equivalent dose of LPC induces the same effects in whole mice, perfused rat livers and isolated hepatocytes. There were also the same degrees of membrane damage, mitochondrial destruction, inhibition of the electron transport system and the generation of ATP. A detailed interpretation of the interrelated responses associated with LPC has been provided by Allgöwer *et al.* (1995).

Some of these toxic effects of the LPC have been attributed to lipid peroxides (Hiramatsu *et al.*, 1984) but this mechanism has been eliminated by the detailed comparative studies reported by Sparkes *et al.* (1990a) who showed that pure LPC, which produced the above effects, contained no measurable lipid peroxide. Similarly, although impaired host immune defence mechanisms could have been due to the presence of endotoxins of bacterial origin, it has been found that on a molar basis the LPC was 1000 times more immunosuppressive than the most inhibitory endotoxin. The blockade of the interleukin-2-dependent growth of cells is directly related to the presence of LPC, it is not modified at all by endotoxin (Sparkes *et al.*, 1990b).

As described earlier, IL-1 production is an essential feature of the cytokine response to thermally induced tissue injury. The recent studies by Monge *et al.* (1991) indicate that LPC is a very potent stimulus for the production of IL-1 by monocytes.

A second relatively well characterized 'toxic' material has been isolated from serum taken from burned patients within a few hours of injury, and before any form of treatment other than fluid resuscitation with crystalloid solutions, or the possibility of the toxic material having a bacterial origin (Ozkan *et al.*, 1986). This material is a lipid-containing glycopeptide with a molecular weight of about 5000 Da; it has a profoundly suppressive effect, at concentrations of about 0.1 μg per ml of solution, on lymphocyte blastogenesis, it inhibits polymorphonuclear neutrophil chemotaxis and induces haemolysis of erythrocytes. Its discoverers believe that the suppressor active peptide (SAP) is produced by proteolytic degradation of normal tissue components. Amino acid analyses of the peptide showed the presence of hydroxylysine and hydroxyproline suggesting a firm link with collagen as the tissue precursor. SAP also contains carbohydrate and lipid components which, when removed from the peptide complex, abolish the suppressive activity. *In vitro* assessments of the mode of action of SAP indicate the obligatory requirement for the presence of some of the metabolites of arachidonic acid (most probably PGE_2) before the immunosuppressive activity is significant.

Comparison of the known biochemical structure and the biophysical characteristics of SAP, and the nature of the suppressive activity it induces, suggests that this 'toxic' compound may be similar to those described by Hakim (1977) and Garner *et al.* (1981). It remains to be proven whether this SAP is related to the myocardial depressant factors postulated by Baxter *et al.* (1966) and to those isolated by Hakim (1973), Moati *et al.* (1979) and Rosenthal (1982).

REFERENCES

Afromowitz M.A., Callis J.B., Heimbach D.M. et al. (1988). Multispectral imaging of burn wounds: a new clinical instrument for evaluation of burn depth. *IEEE Trans. Biomed. Eng.*, **35**, 842–50.

Ahrenholz D.H., Schubert W. and Solem L.D. (1988). Creatine kinase as a prognostic indicator in electrical injury. *Surgery*, **104**, 741–7.

Alexander J.W. (1990). Mechanism of immunologic suppression in burn injury. *J. Trauma*, **30**, (suppl.), S70–5.

Allgöwer M., Cueni L.B., Stadtler K. et al. (1973). Burn toxin in mouse skin. *J. Trauma*, **13**, 95–111.

Allgöwer M., Schoenenberger G.A., Sparkes B.G. (1995). Burning the largest immune organ. *Buns*, **21**,(suppl.1), S7–47.

Anselmo V.J., Zawacki B.E. (1977). Effect of evaporative surface cooling on thermographic assessment of burn depth. *Radiology*, **123**, 331–2.

Arturson M.G. (1985). The pathophysiology of severe thermal injury. *J. Burn Care Rehabil.*, **6**, 129–46.

Arturson G., Jakobsson O.P. (1985). Oedema measurements in a standard burn model. *Burns*, **12**, 1–7.

Arturson G., Groth T., Hedlund A. et al. (1984). Potential use of computer simulation in treatment of burns with special regard to oedema formation. *Scand. J. Plast. Reconstr. Surg.*, **18**, 39–48.

Arturson G., Groth T., Hedlund A. et al. (1989). Computer simulation of fluid resuscitation in trauma. First pragmatic validation in thermal injury. *J. Burn Care Rehabil.*, **10**, 292–9.

Baar S. (1978). The red cell enzyme response to thermal injury. *Burns*, **4**, 207–15.

Bartlett R.H., Fong, S.W., Marrujo G. et al. (1981). Coagulation and platelet changes after thermal injury in man. *Burns*, **7**, 370–7.

Bauer J. (1989). Interleukin-6 and its receptor during homeostasis, inflammation and tumour growth. *Klin. Wochenschr.*, **67**, 679–706.

Bauer J.A., Sauer T. (1989). Cutaneous 10 MHz ultrasound B scan allows the quantitative assessment of burn depth. *Burns*, **15**, 49–51.

Baxter C.R., Cook W.A., Shires G.T. (1966). Serum myocardial depressant factor of burn shock. *Surg. Forum*, **17**, 1–2.

Bert J.L., Bowen B.D., Gu X. et al. (1989). Microvascular exchange during burn injury. II. Formulation and validation of a mathematical model. *Circ. Shock*, **28**, 199–219.

Black K.S., Hewitt C.W., Miller D.M. et al. (1986). Burn depth evaluation with fluorometry: is it really definitive? *J. Burn Care Rehabil.*, **7**, 313–17.

Boozalis G.T., Purdue G.F., Hunt J.L. et al. (1991). Ocular changes from electrical burn injuries. A literature review and report of cases. *J. Burn Care Rehabil.*, **12**, 458–62.

Bowen B.D., Bert J.L., Gu X. et al. (1989). Microvascular exchange during burn injury. III. Implications of the model. *Circ. Shock*, **28**, 221–33.

Boykin J.V., Eriksson E., Pittman R.N. (1981). Microcirculation of a scald burn: an *in vivo* experimental study of the hairless mouse ear. *Burns*, **7**, 335–8.

Bush J.W., Schneider A.M., Wachtel T.L. et al. (1986). A simulation analysis of plasma water dynamics and treatment in acute burn resuscitation. *J. Burn Care Rehabil.*, **7**, 86–95.

Carney S.A., Lawrence J.C., Ricketts C.R. (1972). Some effects of ultrasound on guinea pig ear skin. *Br. J. Indust. Med.*, **29**, 214–20.

Chang L.Y., Yang J.Y. (1991). The role of bone scans in electric burns. *Burns*, **17**, 250–3.

Chilbert M., Maiman D., Sances A. et al. (1985). Measure of tissue resistivity in experimental electrical burns. *J. Trauma*, **25**, 209–15.

Chilbert M., Maiman D.J., Ackmann J.J. et al. (1990). Determination of tissue viability in experimental electrical injuries. *J. Burn Care Rehabil.*, **11**, 516–25.

Clayton J.M., Russell H.E., Hartford C.E. et al. (1977). Sequential circulatory changes in the circumferentially burned limb. *Ann. Surg.*, **185**, 391–6.

Curreri P.W., Hicks J.E., Aronoff R.J. et al. (1974). Inhibition of active sodium transport in erythrocytes from burned patients. *Surg. Gynecol. Obstet.*, **139**, 538–40.

Davies J.W.L. (1982). Effects of burning tissues. In *Physiological Responses to Burning Injury.* London: Academic, chaps 2, 3.

Davies J.W.L., Lamke L.O., Liljedahl S.O. (1974). A guide to the rate of non renal water loss from patients with burns. *Br. J. Plast. Surg.*, **27**, 325–9.

DelBeccaro E.J., Robson M.C., Heggers J.P. et al. (1980). Use of specific thromboxane inhibitors to preserve the dermal microcirculation after burning. *Surgery*, **87**, 137–41.

Demling R., LaLonde C. (1987). Topical ibuprofen decreases early post burn oedema. *Surgery*, **102**, 857–61.

Demling R., LaLonde C. (1990). Early post burn lipid peroxidation: effect of ibuprofen and allopurinol. *Surgery*, **107**, 85–93.

Diller K.R., Hayes L.J., Baxter C.R. (1983). A mathematical model for the thermal efficacy of cooling therapy for burns. *J. Burn Care Rehabil.*, **4**, 81–9.

Diller K.R., Hayes L.J., Blake G.K. (1991). Analysis of alternate models for simulating thermal burns. *J. Burn Care Rehabil.*, **12**, 177–89.

Evans E.I., Brooks J.W., Schmidt F.H. et al. (1955). Flash burn studies on human volunteers. *Surgery*, **37**, 280–97.

Feola M., Simoni J., Tran R. et al. (1989). Toxic factors in the red blood cell membrane. *J. Trauma*, **29**, 1065–75.

Fong Y., Moldawer L.L., Shires G.T. (1990). The biologic characteristics of cytokines and their implication in surgical injury. *Surg. Gynecol. Obstet.*, **170**, 363–78.

Friedl H.P., Till G.O., Trentz O. et al. (1989). Roles of histamine, complement and xanthine oxidase in thermal injury of skin. *Am. J. Pathol.*, **135**, 203–18.

Garner W.D., Proger M.D., Baxter C.R. (1981). Multiple inhibitors of lymphocyte transformation in serum from burn patients. *J. Burn Care Rehabil.*, **2**, 97–105.

Gatti J.E., La Rossa D., Silverman D.G. et al. (1983). Evaluation of the burn wound with perfusion fluorometry. *J. Trauma*, **23**, 202–6.

Gelfand J.A. (1984). How do complement components and fragments affect cellular immunological function? *J. Trauma*, **24**, (suppl.), S118–24.

Gough D.B., Moss N.M., Jordan A. et al. (1988). Recombinant interleukin-2 improves immune response and host resistance to septic challenge in thermally injured mice. *Surgery*, **104**, 292–300.

Green M., Holloway G.A., Heimbach D.M. (1988). Laser Doppler monitoring of microcirculatory changes in acute burn wounds. *J. Burn Care Rehabil.*, **9**, 57–62.

Grossman A.R., Zuckerman A. (1984). Intravenous fluorescein photography in burns. *J. Burn Care Rehabil.*, **5**, 65–8.

Hakim A.A. (1973). Thermal injury: release of a cytotoxic factor. *Experientia*, **29**, 865–7.

Hakim A.A. (1977). An immunosuppressive factor from serum of thermally traumatized patients. *J. Trauma*, **17**, 908–19.

Hammond J., Ward C.G. (1986). Myocardial damage and electrical injuries: significance of early elevation of CPK-MB isoenzymes. *South. Med. J.*, **79**, 414–16.

Hansbrough J., Peterson V., Zapata-Sirvent R. et al. (1984). Post burn immunosuppression in an animal model. II. Restoration of cell mediated immunity by immunomodulating drugs. *Surgery*, **95**, 290–6.

Harms B., Bodai B., Demling R. (1981). Prostaglandin release and altered microvascular integrity after burn injury. *J. Surg. Res.*, **31**, 274–80.

Harms B.A., Bodai B.I., Kramer G.C. et al. (1982). Microvascular fluid and protein flux in pulmonary and systemic circulations after thermal injury. *Microvasc. Res.*, **23**, 77–83.

Hartford C.E., Ziffren S.E. (1971). Electrical injury. *J. Trauma*, **11**, 331–6.

Heimbach D.M., Afromowitz M.A., Engrav L.H. et al. (1984). Burn depth estimation: man or machine? *J. Trauma*, **24**, 373–8.

Heimbach D.M., Engrav L., Grube B. et al. (1992). Burn depth: a review. *World J. Surg.*, **16**, 10–15.

Hiramatsu M., Izawa Y., Hagihara M. et al. (1984). Serum lipid peroxide levels of patients suffering from thermal injury. *Burns*, **11**, 111–16.

Holder I.A., Neely A.N. (1990). Hageman factor-dependent kinin activation in burns and its theoretical relationship to post burn immunosuppression syndrome and infection. *J. Burn Care Rehabil.*, **11**, 496–503.

Housinger T.A., Green L., Shahangian S. et al. (1985). A prospective study of myocardial damage in electrical injuries. *J. Trauma*, **25**, 122–4.

Hunt J.L., Heck E.L. (1984). Identification of non viable muscle in electric burns with nitro blue tetrazolium. *J. Surg. Res.*, **37**, 369–75.

Hunt J.L., McManus W.F., Haney W.P. et al. (1974). Vascular lesions in acute electrical injuries. *J. Trauma*, **14**, 461–70.

Jackson D.M. (1953). The diagnosis of depth of burning. *Br. J. Surg.*, **40**, 588–96.

Jin L., LaLonde C., Demling R. (1986). Lung dysfunction after thermal injury in relation to prostanoid and oxygen radical release. *J. Appl. Physiol.*, **61**, 103–12.

Lawrence J.C. (1967). *In vitro* studies of skin after irradiation by a ruby laser. *Br. J. Plast. Surg.*, **20**, 257–62.

Lee R.C., Cravalho E.G., Burke J.F. (eds) (1992). *Electrical Trauma – the pathophysiology, manifestations and clinical management.* Cambridge University Press, U.K. pp. 3–434.

Lee R.C., Capelli-Schellpfeffer M., Kelley K.M. (eds) (1994). Electrical injury. A multidisciplinary approach to therapy, prevention and rehabilitation. *Ann N.Y. Acad. Sci.*, **720**, 1–298.

Lee R.C., Kolodney M.S. (1987). Electrical injury mechanisms – dynamics of the thermal response. *Plast. Reconstr. Surg.*, **80**, 663–71.

Lewis R.A., Austen K.F., Soberman R.J. (1990), Leukotrienes and other products of the 5-lipoxygenase pathway. *N. Engl. J. Med.*, **323**, 645–55.

Lizzi F.L., Ostromogilsky M. (1987). Analytical modelling of ultrasonically induced tissue heating. *Ultrasound. Med. Biol.*, **13**, 607–18.

Loegering D.J. (1981). Hemolysis following thermal injury and depression of reticulo endothelial system phagocytic function. *J. Trauma*, **21**, 130–4.

Lund T., Onarheim H., Reed R.K. (1992). Pathogenesis of edema formation in burn injuries. *World J. Surg.*, **16**, 2–9.

Marano M.A., Fong Y., Moldawer L.L. et al. (1990). Serum cachectin/tumour necrosis factor in critically ill patients with burns correlates with infection and mortality. *Surg. Gynecol. Obstet.*, **170**, 32–8.

Massiha H., Monafo W.W. (1974). Dermal ischaemia in thermal injury: the importance of venous occlusion. *J. Trauma*, **14**, 705–11.

Michie H.R., Spriggs D.R., Manogue K.R. et al. (1988). Tumour necrosis factor and endotoxin induce similar metabolic responses in human beings. *Surgery*, **104**, 280–6.

Moati F., Sepulchre C., Miskulin M. et al. (1979). Biochemical and pharmacological properties of a cardiotoxic factor isolated from the blood serum of burned patients. *J. Pathol.*, **127**, 147–56.

Monge G., Sparkes B.G., Allgöwer M. et al. (1991). Influence of burn-induced lipid-protein complex on IL 1 secretion by PBMC in vitro. *Burns*, **17**, 269–75.

Moritz A.R., Henriques F.C. (1947). Studies of thermal injury. II. The relative importance of time and surface temperature in the causation of cutaneous burns. *Am. J. Pathol.*, **23**, 695–720.

Moserova J., Runtova M., Broz L. (1983). The possible role of blisters in dermal burns. *Acta. Chir. Plast.*, **25**, 51–4.

Muir I.F.K. (1961). Red cell destruction in burns with particular reference to the shock period. *Br. J. Plast. Surg.*, **14**, 273–302.

Nichter L.S., Bryant C.A., Kenney J.C. et al. (1984). Injuries due to commercial electric current. *J. Burn Care Rehabil.*, **5**, 124–37.

Nijsten M.W.N., Hack C.E., Helle M. et al. (1991). Interleukin-6 and its relation to the humoral immune response and clinical parameters in burned patients. *Surgery*, **109**, 761–7.

Onarheim H., Reed R.K. (1991). Thermal skin injury: effect of fluid therapy on the transcapillary colloid osmotic gradient. *J. Surg. Res.*, **50**, 272–8.

Ozkan A.N., Ninnemann J.L., Sullivan J.J. (1986). Progress in the characterisation of an immunosuppressive glycopeptide (SAP) from patients with major thermal injuries. *J. Burn Care Rehabil.*, **7**, 388–97.

Panke T.W., McLeod C.G. (1985). *Pathology of Thermal Injury: a practical approach*. Orlando, FL: Grune and Stratton.

Pitt R.M., Parker J.C., Jurkovich G.J. et al. (1987). Analysis of altered capillary pressure and permeability after thermal injury. *J. Surg. Res.*, **42**, 693–7.

Roa L.M., Gomez-Cia T., Cantero A. (1988). Analysis of burn injury by digital simulation. *Burns*, **14**, 201–9.

Roa-Romero L., Gomez-Cia. T. (1986). Analysis of the extracellular protein and fluid shifts in burned patients. *Burns*, **12**, 337–42.

Robson M.C., DelBeccaro E.J., Heggers J.P. (1979). The effect of prostaglandins on the dermal microcirculation after burning, and the inhibition of the effect by specific pharmocological agents. *Plast. Reconstr. Surg.*, **63**, 781–7.

Robson M.C., Murphy R.C., Heggers J.P. (1984). A new explanation for the progressive tissue loss in electrical injuries. *Plast. Reconstr. Surg.*, **73**, 431–7.

Rodrick M., Saporoschetz I., Wood J. et al. (1989). Serum suppression of interleukin-2 (IL-2) production and IL-2 action in thermal injury. *Surg. Forum*, **40**, 98–100.

Rosenthal S.R. (1982). Burn toxin and its competitin. *Burns*, **8**, 215–19.

Sasaki J., Cottam G., Baxter C.R. (1987). Lipid peroxidation following thermal injury. *J. Burn Care Rehabil.*, **4**, 251–4.

Schein R.M., Kett D.H., de Marchena E.J. et al. (1990). Pulmonary edema associated with electrical injury. *Chest*, **97**, 1248–50.

Schoenenberger G.A. (1975). Burn toxins isolated from mouse and human skin. *Monogr. Allergy*, **9**, 72–139.

Sevitt S. (1957). *Burns: pathology and therapeutic applications*. London: Butterworths, Chaps 1–3.

Shakespeare P. G. (1992). Looking at burn wounds. The A.B. Wallace Memorial Lecture 1991. *Burns*, **18**.

Sparkes B.G., Monge G., Marshall S.L. et al. (1990a). Plasma levels of cutaneous burn toxin and lipid peroxides in thermal injury. *Burns*, **16**, 118–22.

Sparkes B.G., Gyorkos J.W., Gorczynski R.M. et al. (1990b). Comparison of endotoxins and cutaneous burn toxin as immunosuppressants. *Burns*, **16**, 123–7.

Surrell J.A., Alexander R.C., Cohle S. D. et al. (1987). Effects of microwave radiation on living tissues. *J. Trauma*, **27**, 935–9.

Suzuki T., Hirayama T., Aihara K. et al. (1991). Experimental studies of moderate temperature burns. *Burns*, **17**, 443–51.

ten Duis H.J., Klasen H.J., Nijsten M.W.N. et al. (1987). Superficial lightning injuries – their 'fractal' shape and origin. *Burns*, **13**, 141–6.

Teodorczyk-Injeyan J., Sparkes B.G., Mills G. et al. (1986). Impairment of T cell activation in burn patients. A possible mechanism of thermal injury induced immunosuppression. *Clin. Exp. Immunol.*, **65**, 570–81.

Till G.O., Guilds L.S., Mahrougui M. et al. (1989). Role of xanthine oxidase in thermal injury of skin. *Am. J. Pathol.*, **135**, 195–202.

Wachtel T.L., Leopold G.R., Frank H.A. et al. (1986). B-mode ultrasonic echo determination of depth of thermal injury. *Burns*, **12**, 432–7.

Wood J.J., Rodrick M.L., O'Mahony J.B. et al. (1984). Inadequate interleukin-2 production. A fundamental immunological deficiency in patients with major burns. *Ann. Surg.*, **200**, 311–20.

Youn Y.K., LaLonde C., Demling R. (1992). The role of mediators in the response to thermal injury. *World J. Surg.*, **16**, 30–6.

Zawacki B.E. (1974) The natural history of reversible burn injury. *Surg. Gynecol. Obstet.*, **139**, 867–72.

Zimmerman T.J., Krizek T.J. (1984). Thermally induced dermal injury. A review of pathophysiological events and therapeutic intervention. *J. Burn Care Rehabil.*, **5**, 193–201.

29. Management of Burn Injury

L. W. Rue III, W. G. Cioffi, Jr., W. F. McManus and B. A. Pruitt, Jr.

The views of the authors do not purport to reflect the positions of the Department of the Army and the Department of Defense

From the US Army Institute of Surgical Research, Fort Sam Houston, San Antonio, Texas 78234–5012

INTRODUCTION

The exact incidence of thermal injury is unknown, but it has been estimated that over two million people in the USA are affected annually. The vast majority are managed as outpatients or in local hospitals, since over 80% of thermal injuries involve less than 20% of the body surface area (Mason and Pruitt, 1978). Approximately 300 burn patients per million population/year will require in-hospital care and 82 per million population per year are best cared for in a designated burn-care facility as a consequence of the extent or anatomical location of the burn, associated injury or illness, or extremes of age.

PATHOPHYSIOLOGY

Every organ system is involved in the pathophysiological response to burn injury. The magnitude of the physiological derangement is proportional to the extent of cutaneous injury, plateauing at approximately 60% BSA burn. Local cutaneous effects are influenced by the temperature of the wounding agent and the duration of contact. Temperatures below 45°C are not associated with burn injury regardless of contact duration (Sevett, 1957); with increases in temperature, the duration of contact required to produce a burn injury diminishes (Evans et al., 1955).

The area of protein coagulation and cell death associated with a burn injury has been referred to as the zone of necrosis (Jackson, 1969). This process involves the entire dermis in a full-thickness injury or a variable depth of dermis in a partial-thickness wound. Areas of lesser cellular damage have been designated the zones of stasis and hyperaemia. The zone of stasis, characterized by attenuated blood flow which is ultimately restored with successful resuscitation, extends to a variable distance around the zone of necrosis. The zone of hyperaemia usually manifested in superficial injuries is characterized by increased blood flow and an immediate inflammatory response following injury. Depending upon the extent of injury, these zones are seen as concentric tissue masses surrounding the point of contact (see also Chapter 28).

Thermal injury is also marked by increased capillary hydrostatic pressures in the early post-injury phase and later by increased capillary permeability which contributes to oedema formation. Cellular enzymes are released from damaged tissue following thermal injury. These include histamine, serotonin and various inflammatory mediators, such as prostaglandins, leukotrienes, complement and interleukins which impart local and systemic effects (Shea et al., 1973; Alexander et al., 1984; Herndon et al., 1984; Bjornson et al., 1986; Kupper et al., 1986). Oedema is also noted in unburned tissue following extensive thermal injury. This observation is most likely a consequence of combined osmotic and volume effects associated with burn resuscitation using large volumes of crystalloids (Mason, 1980; Demling et al., 1984). However, some investigators have attributed this to a generalized increase in capillary permeability (Arturson, 1961).

The initial cardiovascular response to burn injury is one of decreased cardiac output and increased peripheral vascular resistance as a consequence of the neurohormonal response associated with the stress of trauma (Pruitt et al., 1971). Fluid losses are promoted by alterations in vascular permeability, leading to hypovolaemia which further impairs cardiac output and reduces vital organ perfusion. Studies have attributed the subnormal cardiac output seen in this early period to decreased left ventricular end-diastolic volume, consistent with a hypovolaemic state (Dorethy et al., 1977), and improved cardiac performance can be achieved with fluid resuscitation (Cioffi et al., 1986). A proposed myocardial depressant factor, which adversely affects cardiac performance in the early postburn period (Baxter et al., 1966), has not been identified. As further repletion of plasma volume occurs during the second 24 hours, the cardiac output increases to supranormal levels. This correlates with the postburn hypermetabolic response which continues until the majority of the burn wound is closed.

Burn trauma, even in the absence of associated inhalation injury, induces physiological changes in the pulmonary system. Increases in pulmonary vascular resistance are noted postburn and are of a more prolonged duration than the increases in peripheral vascular resistance (Asch et al., 1973). The increase may be the result of the release of vasoactive amines and may have a protective effect in preventing pulmonary oedema during resuscitation. Lung lymph flow studies have demonstrated no change in pulmonary capillary permeability with simple thermal injury (Demling *et al.*, 1985). In the initial phase postburn, usually in association with modest hypovolaemia, minute ventilation is unchanged or perhaps even slightly decreased. With fluid resuscitation, minute ventilation progressively increases as a consequence of increased respiratory rate and increased tidal volume (Pruitt *et al.*, 1975). The extent of this increase is proportional to burn size and is thought to be a manifestation of postburn hypermetabolism. Additionally, decreased static and dynamic lung compliance cause a modest increase in the work of breathing.

The early gastrointestinal manifestations of extensive thermal injury are ileus requiring the use of nasogastric decompression to prevent emesis and possible aspiration (Pruitt, 1979a). Studies have demonstrated a significant decrease in gastric mucosal blood flow associated with shock (Levine *et al.*, 1978). This ischaemic phenomenon results in focal gastric mucosal cell injury. Superficial erosions in the stomach and duodenum may develop (Czaja *et al.*, 1974), and without protective measures such as H_2 blockers and antacid titration of gastric pH above 4 (McElwee *et al.*, 1979), frank ulcerations and gastrointestinal haemorrhage may occur. Following resuscitation, gastrointestinal motility returns and enteral nutrition can be initiated. Broad-spectrum antibiotic administration for septic complications can aggravate gastrointestinal dysfunction by allowing bacterial overgrowth which may cause diarrhoea and even pseudomembranous enterocolitis.

The renal response to burn injury parallels the cardiovascular changes. In the early postburn period, decreases in renal blood flow and glomerular filtration rate have been documented (O'Neill *et al.*, 1971). Markedly delayed or inadequate fluid resuscitation may lead to acute tubular necrosis and renal failure. Following resuscitation, the increased cardiac output and resorption of burn-associated oedema promote an increase in renal blood flow. The postburn diuretic response is modified by the large evaporative loss of fluids through the wound surface and the slow rate of oedema resorption. As a consequence of increased renal blood flow, the dose of drugs in use and excreted by the kidney may need adjustment (Aulick *et al.*, 1981). Excessive delivery of carbohydrate or protein for nutritional management may promote an osmotic diuresis, which further influences the physiological response.

Thermally injured patients typify the metabolic response to injury. In the immediate postburn period, a transient decrease in metabolic rate occurs. However, as resuscitation progresses, a catabolic hormonal pattern emerges. Increases in serum levels of catecholamines, glucagon and cortisol take place whereas insulin and triodothyrinine levels are decreased (Pruitt and Goodwin, 1983). The increase in metabolic rate is proportional to burn size and is mediated by catecholamine excess that is associated with negative nitrogen balance and increased glucose flux (Wilmore *et al.*, 1976b), which require a high level of nutritional supplementation. As the burn wounds are closed, the hormonal levels return toward normal and restoration of lean body mass ensues. Early sepsis exaggerates the hypermetabolic response normally encountered in the burn patient, while late sepsis is characterized by hypometabolism (Wilmore *et al.*, 1976a).

A generalized impairment of the immune system occurs following burn injury. Consequently, burn patients are more susceptible to infections. In addition to the obvious destruction of the cutaneous barrier to infection, thermal injuries are associated with decreased immunoglobulin levels. Initially burn patients manifest a leukopenia which is superseded by leukocytosis (McManus, 1983). Neutrophil chemotaxis, phagocytosis and bactericidal actions are adversely influenced postburn (Alexander and Wixson, 1970; Warden *et al.*, 1974; Allen and Pruitt, 1982). Alterations in lymphocyte subpopulations are also seen. Various investigators have demonstrated either a total decrease in T-cell number, with maintenance of the normal ratio of T-helper to T-suppressor cells, or a decrease in this ratio leading to impaired macrophage antigen presentation (Kupper *et al.*, 1985; Burleson *et al.*, 1988). Increased susceptibility to infection has also been attributed to decreased lymphocyte production of interleukin 2 and the magnitude of this suppression is related to the extent of burn (Wood *et al.*, 1986). The function of the reticuloendothelial system is also suppressed following burn injury and may be related to the diminished opsonic capability of the serum secondary to decreased fibronection levels (Hanback and Rittenbury, 1965).

Destruction of cellular elements of the haematopoetic system occurs to an extent directly proportional to burn size. Full-thickness burn injuries cause immediate red cell destruction in the involved microvasculature. Reticuloendothelial system clearance of damaged red cells and frequent blood sampling account for an 8–12% loss of circulating red cell mass per day during the first week postburn. Following successful resuscitation, increases in fibrin split products and decreases in platelet counts and fibrinogen levels are seen. Later, serum levels of fibrinogen, factors V and VIII, and platelet counts increase to supranormal levels (Curreri *et al.*, 1970, 1975).

INITIAL ASSESSMENT

A similar method is used as in all trauma patients. Table 29.1 shows the matters which should be considered.

TABLE 29.1
MATTERS TO BE CONSIDERED IN INITIAL ASSESSMENT OF
BURNED PATIENT

Airway integrity and supplementary oxygen

Complete history and physical examination

Tetanus status

Routine laboratory studies for serum electrolyte and glucose concentrations, liver function tests and full blood counts

Screening for hepatitis, syphilis, HIV if permitted, glucose-6-phosphate dehydrogenase deficiency and sickle cell disease

Surveillance bacterial colonization, especially in those already managed elsewhere

Chest radiography

Check on position and function of tubes and catheters

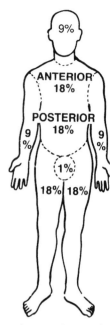

Figure 29.2 The 'Rule of Nines' can be used to make a quick and reasonably accurate assessment of extent of burn.

BURN DEPTH

This can be classified as first, second or third degree injury, with first degree representing the most superficial injury. A first degree wound, the best example being a sunburn, is dry, erythematous, painful and without bullae. Healing typically occurs within 3–6 days, often associated with a slough of the non-viable superficial epidermis. Second degree burn wounds, or partial-thickness burns, are either as superficial or deep dermal (Figure 29.1). Superficial partial-thickness wounds are erythematous or have a mottled appearance, moist and extremely sensitive and typically heal within 10–21 days. Deep dermal burns are characterized by a cherry-red or yellow-white appearance.

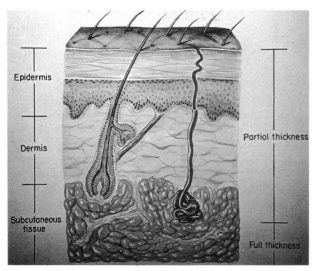

Figure 29.1 Diagram illustrating the depth of partial-thickness and full-thickness burns.

As a consequence of the depth of injury, pinpoint sensation is diminished but deep pressure sensation remains intact. These wounds require over 3 weeks to heal and often do so with significant hypertrophic scarring. Full-thickness burns or third degree injuries are pearly white or charred in appearance and often have thrombosed superficial veins visible. These wounds are insensitive and grafting is required for definitive wound closure.

The severity of burn injury is influenced by the extent and depth of the wound. Accurate assessment of the extent of the body surface injured is fundamental to the calculation of resuscitation fluid requirements. The 'Rule of Nines' provides a quick and reasonably accurate estimate of the percentage of body surface injured (Figure 29.2). The head and neck of the child account for a greater percentage of the body area and the lower extremities a lower percentage so that must be modified in children. More precise estimates of the extent of burn wound can be made by using a Lund–Browder chart, which provides estimates of the percentage of body surface area for various body parts at differing ages (Figure 29.3). A rough estimate of burn extent for irregular areas may be obtained by virtue of the fact that 1% of the total body surface area is equal to the area of the patient's palm.

RESUSCITATION

Many formulas have been proposed by various investigators as the ideal approach to burn resuscitation (Table 29.2) and they vary in the quantities

BURN ESTIMATE AND DIAGRAM
AGE vs AREA

Area	Birth 1 yr	1-4 yr	5-9 yr	10-14 yr	15 yr	Adult	2°	3°	Total	Donor Areas
Head	19	17	13	11	9	7				
Neck	2	2	2	2	2	2				
Ant Trunk	13	13	13	13	13	13				
Post Trunk	13	13	13	13	13	13				
R Buttock	2½	2½	2½	2½	2½	2½				
L. Buttock	2½	2½	2½	2½	2½	2½				
Genitalia	1	1	1	1	1	1				
R U Arm	4	4	4	4	4	4				
L. U. Arm	4	4	4	4	4	4				
R L Arm	3	3	3	3	3	3				
L L Arm	3	3	3	3	3	3				
R Hand	2½	2½	2½	2½	2½	2½				
L Hand	2½	2½	2½	2½	2½	2½				
R Thigh	5½	6½	8	8½	9	9½				
L. Thigh	5½	6½	8	8½	9	9½				
R Leg	5	5	5½	6	6½	7				
L Leg	5	5	5½	6	6½	7				
R. Foot	3½	3½	3½	3½	3½	3½				
L Foot	3½	3½	3½	3½	3½	3½				
						TOTAL				

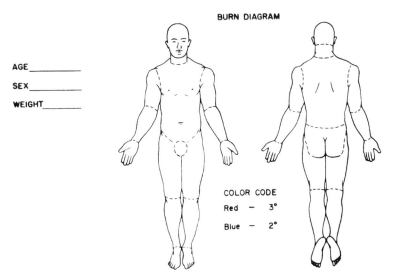

BURN DIAGRAM

AGE_____

SEX_____

WEIGHT_____

COLOR CODE

Red — 3°

Blue — 2°

Figure 29.3 The Lund–Browder chart enables an estimation of the extent of burn, on the basis of the relationship between the body surface area of various body parts and the age of the patient.

and composition of fluids employed. The predominant theme that the volume of fluids required is dependent upon the extent of burn and the patient's weight. Typically, one-half of he calculated 24-hour requirement is delivered in the first 8 hours postburn when capillary permeability is maximal. The remainder of the resuscitation volume is provided over the ensuing 16 hours. It is important to recognize that these formulas serve only as guides to volume resuscitation and the actual fluid requirements are dependent upon the individual physiological response of the patient. Fluid needs may deviate markedly from the calculated resuscitation volumes in patients with ethanol toxicity, inhalation injury and delayed onset of fluid resuscitation. High-voltage electrical injuries may also require more resuscitation fluid than that calculated on the basis of cutaneous injury.

Laboratory and clinical studies of transcapillary fluid movement during the first 24 hours postburn have found no advantage in the use of colloid-containing fluids in this phase of resuscitation. As functional capillary permeability returns to normal during the latter half of the first 24 hours (Pruitt and Mason, 1971), the fluid requirements begin to decrease. When capillary integrity is re-established,

TABLE 29.2

FORMULAS COMMONLY USED TO ESTIMATE RESUSCITATION FLUID NEEDS OF ADULT BURN PATIENTS

Formula	First 24 hours			Second 24 hours		
	Electrolyte-containing solution	Colloid-containing fluid equivalent to plasma	Glucose in water	Electrolyte-containing solution	Colloid-containing fluid equivalent to plasma	Glucose in water
Burn budget of F. D. Moore	Lactated Ringer's 1000–4000 ml 0.45 normal saline 1200 ml	7.5% of body weight	1500–5000 ml	Lactated Ringer's 1000–4000 ml 0.45 normal saline 1200 ml	2.5% of body weight	1500–5000 ml
Evans	Normal saline 1.0 ml/kg/% burn	1.0 ml/kg/% burn	2000 ml	One-half of first 24-hour requirement	One-half of first 24-hour requirement	2000 ml
Brooke	Lactated Ringer's 1.5 ml/kg/% burn	0.5 ml/kg/% burn	2000 ml	One-half to three-quarters of first 24-hour requirement	One-half to three-quarters of first 24-hour requirement	2000 ml
Parkland	Lactated Ringer's 4.0% ml/kg/% burn	–	–	–	20–60% of calculated plasma volume	As necessary to maintain urinary output
Hypertonic sodium solution	Volume of fluid containing 250 mEq of sodium per litre to maintain hourly urinary output of 30 ml hr	–	–	One-third isotonic salt solution orally up to 3500 ml limit	–	–
Modified Brooke	Lactated Ringer's 2.0 ml/kg/% burn	–	–	–	0.3–0.5 ml/kg/% burn	As necessary to maintain urinary output

the use of colloid-containing fluids repletes the intravascular volume more efficiently and with less volume than crystalloid fluids.

General use of the various burn resuscitation formulas has reduced the occurrence of shock and organ function impairment due to inadequate resuscitation. On the contrary, over-resuscitation of burn patients is now frequently encountered. Pulmonary, cerebral and exaggerated burn wound oedema often result. These complications are seen most often on the third to sixth postburn days when capillary integrity is restored, pulmonary vascular resistance is normal, and wound oedema is being reabsorbed.

Hypertonic saline has been proposed as a resuscitation fluid that will minimize early volume requirements, particularly in elderly or volume-sensitive patients. Additional claims of decreased fractional retention of sodium, decreased need for escharotomy and decreased ileus have not been supported by prospective studies (Moylan et al., 1973). Adverse consequences include hypernatraemia, often of sufficient magnitude to require infusion of hypotonic solutions, thereby negating the claimed benefits of this regimen. Hypertonic saline regimens induce some degree of cellular dehydration and depletion of intracellular water in excess of 15% is associated with impaired cellular function (Shimazaki et al., 1977). Comparisons between standard resuscitation protocols and hypertonic saline regimens have demonstrated no difference in the total amounts of sodium and volume administered. The tendency to develop hypernatraemia is promoted by evaporative water loss from the wound (Wilson and Moncrief, 1965) and the increased levels of renin–angiotensin and aldosterone which limit sodium excretion (Shirani et al., 1984). Hypernatraemic complications are seldom encountered in centres where 0.5% silver nitrate dressings are used in wound care, as significant transeschar leaching of sodium ions occurs. It would appear that only patients with significant limitations in cardiac reserve may benefit from resuscitation protocols using hypertonic saline.

The Modified Brooke Formula for burn resuscitation, which is recommended by the authors, uses no colloid or electrolyte free crystalloid solutions in the first 24 hours. Fluid needs are estimated at 2 or 3 ml of lactated Ringer's per kilogram body weight per percentage of the body surface area burned in adults and children respectively (Graves *et al.*, 1988). As previously mentioned, one-half of the fluid estimates are administered in the first 8 hours and the remainder over the subsequent 16-hour period. This formula serves only as a guide to fluid replacement and the actual volume administered depends upon the patient's clinical response.

In the second 24 hours, colloid-containing fluids are administered in an amount proportional to the extent of burn to help restore the plasma volume deficit:

30–50% BSA burns   0.3 ml/kg/% burn
50–70% BSA burns   0.4 ml/kg/% burn
>70% BSA burns   0.5 ml/kg/% burn

In addition, 5% dextrose in water is administered in quantities sufficient to maintain an adequate urine output. In paediatric patients less than 30 kg body weight, 5% dextrose in 0.45% saline rather than 5% dextrose in water is administered to avoid hyponatraemia and possible cerebral oedema.

The goal of fluid resuscitation is maintenance of organ perfusion and function and the adequacy of resuscitation is judged by the general status of the patient, the haemodynamic response, level of orientation, and, as a more objective indication of resuscitation, the urine output. A urinary output of 30–50 ml per hour is felt to reflect adequate resuscitation in most adult patients and 1 ml of urine output per kilogram of body weight per hour is the goal in patients weighing less than 30 kg. Special measures such as pulmonary artery catheterization and inotropes may be required, as mannitol may be required to clear haemochromagens in patients with high-voltage electrical injuries, patients with extensive burns in whom resuscitation is delayed, and patients with burns associated with soft tissue and muscle damage. The use of these agents invalidates the urine output as an indicator of the adequacy of resuscitation.

Insurance of adequate peripheral perfusion is another mandatory aspect of resuscitation therapy. Circumferentially burned extremities are at risk for restricted blood flow as subeschar oedema forms. If tissue pressure exceeds venous and capillary pressure, nutrient blood flow to distal tissue or deeper unburned areas on the extremity will be limited and, if reduced sufficiently, tissue death will occur. Prophylactic measures to avoid dangerous levels of oedema formation include extremity elevation and active exercise of the entire extremity for 5 minutes per hour (Salisbury *et al.*, 1973) and judicious fluid administration.

Clinical indicators such as distal cyanosis, impaired capillary refill, neurological deficits and constant deep tissue pain are unreliable. A Doppler flowmeter provides a more precise indication of peripheral perfusion. The distal palmar arch in the upper extremity and the posterior tibial artery in the lower extremity should be routinely monitored for alterations in flow (Moylan *et al.*, 1971). Absence of flow or a progressive diminution in Doppler signal intensity are indications for escharotomy, which can be performed at the patient's bedside without need for anaesthesia since the incisions are made through insensate full-thickness burns (Pruitt *et al.*, 1968a).

Escharotomy incisions are made in the midlateral and midmedial line of the involved extremity from the proximal to distal extent of burn (Figure 29.4). The depth of incision should be limited to the overlying eschar, allowing the wound edges to separate and thereby relieving the tension in the subjacent tissue. If performed correctly, minimal bleeding should be encountered. To delay eventual colonization and possible infection of the subcutaneous tissue exposed by the incisions, liberal quantities of topical antimicrobial agents should be applied to the wounds. Chest wall motion may be restricted by overlying circumferential eschar and

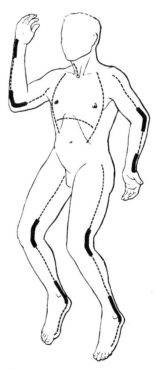

Figure 29.4 Illustration of the recommended locations of escharotomy incisions. Heavy lines emphasize the need to carry incisions across involved joints.

oedema formation, thereby impairing ventilation (Petroff and Pruitt, 1979). Should this occur, improvement in ventilatory status may be obtained by performing bilateral anterior axillary line escharotomies extending from the clavicles to the costal margins. Connecting these incisions with another incision at the costal margin may be necessary if the anterior abdominal wall is significantly burned.

Fasciotomies are rarely required to restore peripheral perfusion following thermal injury. The most common injuries requiring fasciotomy are those from high-voltage electrical discharges and concomitant blunt trauma.

POST RESUSCITATION FLUID AND ELECTROLYTE MANAGEMENT

As a consequence of resuscitation, the typical burn patient sustains a 10–20% weight gain. A diuresis spontaneously occurs on the second to seventh postburn day which parallels oedema fluid resorption. Optimally, a patient's resuscitative weight increase is reversed by 10% increments per day (Gump and Kinney, 1971). Excessive 'free' water loss (i.e a dilute urine) can contribute to the development of the most common electrolyte abnormality seen in these patients – hypernatraemia. Evaporative water loss via the burn wound and elevation of circulating levels of renin, angiotensin and aldosterone contribute to this. An estimation of total insensible water loss from the burn wound in millilitres per hour can be determined by the formula (Warden et al., 1973):

$$\text{Insensible water loss (ml/h)} = (25 + \%\text{BSA burn}) \times \text{total BSA in m}^2$$

Dehydration and hypernatraemia can also result from the osmotic diuretic effect of glycosuria caused by diabetes mellitus or excessive glucose administration. Excessive protein administration through nutritional support regimens can also promote an osmotic diuresis, as a consequence of the increased urea elimination.

Following fluid resuscitation, a mild hyponatraemia may be encountered as a consequence of the large volumes of lactated Ringer's infused. It is typically asymptomatic and corrects rapidly with an appropriate decrease in the rate of fluid administration. Patients treated with closed dressing techniques with 0.5% silver nitrate sustain significant transeschar sodium losses which may promote hyponatraemia (Batchelor et al., 1965).

Symptomatic hyponatraemia usually occurs when serum sodium values decrease to less than 120 mEq/l or when rapid changes in serum sodium concentrations occur. Cerebral oedema associated with hyponatraemia can cause seizures in children (McManus et al., 1975). Symptomatic hyponatraemia requires active correction of the free water

excess and sodium deficit by administering loop diuretics and hypertonic saline solutions.

Burn injury liberates potassium from damaged tissues and red blood cells; consequently, potassium supplementation is not indicated in the early postinjury phase. This tendency towards hyperkalaemia may be aggravated by a metabolic acidosis secondary to inadequate resuscitation. Elevation of the serum potassium above 5.5 mEq/l warrants active therapy.

Following resuscitation, during the postburn diuresis phase, hypokalaemia may become a problem and is complicated by hyperventilation-induced respiratory alkalosis. The use of mafenide acetate, a commonly employed topical antimicrobial agent, promotes kaliuresis, further aggravating this electrolyte abnormality (White and Asch, 1971). Silver nitrate dressings also cause significant transeschar losses of potassium (Moyer et al., 1965). Potassium repletion is indicated for patients with marked losses, with daily replacement based on serum and 24-hour urinary electrolyte measurements.

Total serum calcium levels are decreased following burn injury. This abnormal finding is attributed to a decrease in calcium binding proteins rather than an actual decrease in ionized calcium levels. Transeschar leaching of calcium cations can occur with the use of 0.5% silver nitrate dressings. The use of antacids as prophylaxis against Curling's ulcers may result in symptomatic hypophosphataemia. This commonly responds to a reduction in antacid doses or a discontinuation of phosphate-binding antacids and phosphate repletion. Adequate nutritional support should avoid the complications of both zinc deficiency, which adversely influences wound healing (Larson et al., 1970; Cohen et al., 1973), and magnesium depletion, which is associated with neuromuscular abnormalities (Broughton et al., 1968).

INHALATION INJURY

Inhalation injury is a frequent and often lethal concomitant injury in burns. The term includes carbon monoxide toxicity, direct thermal injury to the airway and chemical damage to the respiratory system. Carbon monoxide toxicity is quite common and occurs most often when there is a fire in an enclosed space. Direct thermal injury is infrequent and typically involves only the upper airways because of the effective heat-exchange capabilities of the nasopharynx and oropharynx. True thermal injury to the lower airway may occur from steam exposure which contains up to 4000 times the heat present in air. Products of incomplete combustion, such as hydrogen cyanide, ammonia, sulphur dioxide, aldehydes and esters, are typical causative agents of chemically induced inhalation injury (Wald and Balmes, 1987).

Inhalation injuries are most often diagnosed in patients injured within an enclosed space. The duration of exposure is often increased in patients who have sustained drug overdoses, ethanol intoxication or closed head trauma. Patients who present with burns about the head and neck, singed nasal vibrissae or swollen lips should be suspected of having sustained an inhalation injury. Hyperaemia of the hypopharynx, presence of carbonaceous sputum, hoarseness, stridor, dyspnoea and wheezing should prompt immediate evaluation of the airway (Figure 29.5).

Carbon monoxide is a byproduct of the combustion of organic material. It has 200 times greater affinity for haemoglobin than does oxygen which consequently decreases the blood's ability to deliver oxygen to the tissues (Stewart, 1975). Additionally, carbon monoxide produces a leftward shift in the oxygen–haemoglobin dissociation curve, further decreasing oxygen delivery to the tissues. Various laboratory investigations have confirmed that the mechanism of carbon monoxide toxicity is the consequence of impaired oxygen delivery and not a direct toxic effect on the tissues (Halebian *et al.*, 1986).

The predominant clinical manifestations of carbon monoxide toxicity are cardiac and neurological. The cardiac effects are those of myocardial ischaemia and, after prolonged exposure, efforts to improve cardiac performance with fluids or inotropic agents are usually unsuccessful. Central nervous system findings include confusion, agitation and loss of consciousness. About 10% of patients develop long-term sequelae of gait disturbance, mental deterioration and urinary incontinence (Richardson *et al.*, 1959). Similar problems are seen in patients who have sustained a significant anoxic brain injury (Plum *et al.*, 1962).

The most accurate method of diagnosing carbon monoxide toxicity is a direct carboxyhaemoglobin determination by oximetry. Levels exceeding 15% are consistent with some degree of carbon monoxide poisoning. The preferred treatment is administration of 100% oxygen via face-mask or endotracheal tube. The half-life of carboxyhaemoglobin decreases from 4 hours on room air to approximately 30 minutes with administration of 100% oxygen. Hyperbaric oxygen further speeds carbon monoxide removal, but has associated risks of oxygen toxicity and alterations in macrophage function (Hansborough *et al.*, 1980) and an improvement in survival or neurological sequelae has not been shown. Its overzealous use may delay the initiation of resuscitation. The administration of 100% oxygen during transport to a burn centre appears to be the most optimal treatment.

Chemical inhalation injury may include damage to the nasal cavity, pharynx, larynx, glottis, trachea and major bronchi. The most sensitive and expeditious diagnostic technique is direct evaluation of the airway using fibreoptic bronchoscopy (Moylan *et al.*, 1975). Bronchoscopic findings which support the diagnosis of inhalation injury include airway oedema, erythema, ulceration and carbonaceous debris distal to the level of the vocal cords.

Injury to the lower airways causes damage to the terminal bronchioles and alveoli. Mucosal sloughing which may obstruct the small airways increases the likelihood of developing bronchopneumonia. In a recent study at this Institute, inhalation injury alone was associated with a maximal increase in mortality of 20% and the presence of pneumonia alone was associated with up to a 40% increase in mortality. Combined inhalation injury and pneumonia were independent and additive in effect, resulting in up to a 60% increase in mortality (Shirani *et al.*, 1987).

Parenchymal injury is best demonstrated by abnormalities on [133]xenon ventilation perfusion scintigraphy performed within 24–48 hours following injury (Moylan *et al.*, 1972). Normally, complete washout of radioactivity from the lungs occurs within 90 seconds. A study, indicative of par-

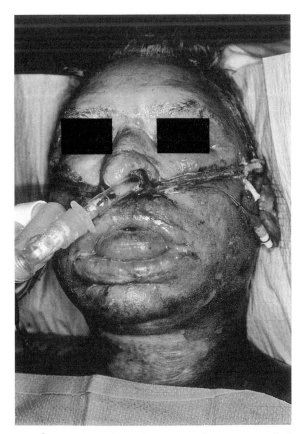

Figure 29.5 A patient demonstrating many of the features associated with inhalation injury, i.e. facial burns, circumoral swelling and carbonaceous oral secretions. A nasotracheal tube has been placed to maintain airway patency.

enchymal damage, has a regional or generalized delay in isotope elimination beyond 90 seconds. Beyond 48 hours, the hypermetabolic-induced hyperventilation causes a deceptively increased washout of [133]xenon from injured lung tissue. False-positive studies may be seen in patients with chronic obstructive pulmonary disease or those with significant atelectasis or pneumonia from other causes.

The current treatment of inhalation injury is supportive.

ELECTRICAL INJURY

Tissue damage from electrical injury results from the heat generated by electric current as well as direct thermal injury caused by the ignition of clothing (Hunt *et al.*, 1980). The severity of injury is dependent on voltage, whether the current is alternating or direct, the course of the current through the body and the duration of contact. Exposure to more than 1000 V is considered a high-voltage electrical injury. Alternating current, because of its propensity to stimulate cardiac arrest or arrhythmias and respiratory arrest, is more hazardous.

The body appears to behave as a volume conductor. The heat generated is proportional to the voltage drop and current flow per unit of cross-sectional area (Hunt *et al.*, 1976). Consequently, extremities tend to sustain severe injury, whereas truncal passage of current rarely produces severe complications. When contact with the electric current stops, the body functions as a volume radiator. Superficial tissues cool rapidly and sustain less injury than the deeper structures which retain heat (Zelt *et al.*, 1986).

Cardiac arrest often occurs following electrical contact and requires immediate cardiopulmonary resuscitation. Cardiac arrhythmias at 48–72 hours are also common (Solem *et al.*, 1977).

Patients sustaining high-voltage electrical injuries are at special risk for acute renal insufficiency (DiVincenti *et al.*, 1969a), either because of inadequate assessment and delivery of resuscitation fluids or from the liberation from damaged cells of myoglobin and haemoglobin which are potentially toxic to the renal tubules. Extensive tissue damage can produce hyperkalaemia requiring intervention to prevent adverse consequences.

The cutaneous manifestations of electrical injury are usually the consequence of direct contact and current arcing and may be deceptively slight by comparison with the extent of deeper injury. Subfascial oedema formation may lead to increasing tissue compartment pressures and features of inadequate distal tissue perfusion. High-voltage electrical injuries often produce such extensive tissue destruction that amputation is required (Figure 29.6). Arteriography, [133]xenon washout

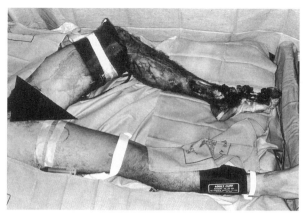

Figure 29.6 Profound tissue destruction of the left lower extremity due to high-voltage electrical injury. Note thrombosed vessels on the calf.

scans and technetium-99m pyrophosphate uptake have been recommended as techniques to determine tissue viability and to govern the extent of debridement (Hunt *et al.*, 1974, 1980; Clayton *et al.*, 1977).

Injuries to the nervous system due to high-voltage electrical contact can be immediate or delayed in presentation (Pruitt, 1979b). An accurate and well-documented neurological examination is essential on admission and at intervals during the period of recovery. Direct electrical injury to a nerve has a poor prognosis for recovery; however, functional deficits in nerves not directly damaged often recover (White *et al.*, 1983). Immediate cord deficits are usually transient and complete recovery typically ensues. Central deficits which appear later, such as quadriplegia, hemiplegia or transverse myelitis, are unfortunately usually permanent (Levine *et al.*, 1975). Radiographic examination of the vertebral column should be included in the initial evaluation, since tetanic contractions of paravertebral muscles can cause spinal fractures (Moncrief and Pruitt, 1970).

Cataract formation is common following high-voltage electrical injury, particularly in patients who have contact points on the head and neck region (Saffle *et al.*, 1985). This problem may be evident within hours of injury or appear as late as 3 years thereafter. Fundoscopic and slit-lamp examinations are indicated on admission and during follow-up.

A unique electrical injury sustained by young children is a burn of the oral commissure which occurs while chewing on an active electrical cord. These injuries can frequently lead to delayed haemorrhage from the labial arteries. Though these burns often appear full thickness, initial conservative management is usually rewarded by healing with minimal cosmetic distortion or a deformity which can be more successfully addressed later (Orgel *et al.*, 1975).

Patients struck by lightning are briefly subjected to currents of 12 000–200 000 A (Apfelberg *et al.*, 1974). The extent of injury is dependent upon entry and exit sites, the patient's position and the passage of the current to ground (earth). The major cause of death in these patients is cardiac arrhythmias or asystole. Surprisingly, permanent cardiac abnormalities are rare (Amy *et al.*, 1985). The neurological deficits that occur after the event usually resolve hours later. The cutaneous pattern of burn injury is often arborescent and frequently heals without the need for excision and grafting. With prompt institution of cardiopulmonary resuscitation and treatment of complications, approximately two-thirds of patients struck by lightning survive.

CHEMICAL INJURY

Chemical injuries are unique in that treatment priorities must be rearranged. The extent of tissue destruction is dependent upon the concentration and volume of the chemical and duration of exposure. Hence, the initial primary objective is to copiously lavage the wound, thereby effecting dilution and removal of the injurious agent. Use of neutralizing agents is contraindicated in managing these patients because the heat of the neutralization reaction may exceed the heat produced by the offending chemical itself.

Strong alkalis cause liquifactive necrosis of tissues. Powders or particles should be mechanically swept away before irrigation is begun. A common offending agent is pre-mixed Portland cement which accounts for 80% of the cement used in the USA. Calcium hydroxide is generated when the cement is reconstituted with water which yields a solution with a pH of 9.3 (Peters, 1984). Burns from phenol, which is poorly water soluble, are managed by lavage with glycerol or polyethylene glycol if available. Otherwise, copious amounts of water should be used to avoid delay (Pardoe *et al.*, 1976).

Acid burns typically result in coagulative necrosis of tissue. Copious water irrigation is also indicated for these patients. Burns from hydrofluoric acid, a chemical used in glassware etching, are of particular interest. Progressive tissue destruction occurs well after the removal of surface contamination and is characterized by constant deep pain. Local infiltration of 10% calcium gluconate neutralizes the acid by promoting the precipitation of calcium fluoride. The potential for delayed toxic effects of electrolyte imbalance and cardiac arrhythmia requires admission to hospital for hydrofluoric acid exposures which involve more than 50 cm^2.

Ocular exposure to strong acids or alkali are particularly catastrophic injuries. Continuous irrigation systems with conjunctival catheters or scleral lenses are used for prolonged irrigation.

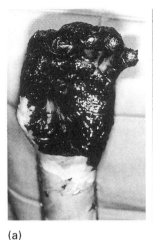 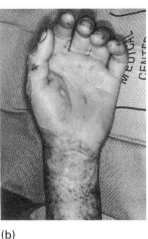

(a) (b)

Figure 29.7 (a) Patient with immersion of forearm and hand in hot tar. The tar was stripped from the forearm at the time of initial debridement prior to arrival at the burn centre. (b) Use of emulsifying agents facilitated removal of tar from the hand. Note deep burn wounds of the forearm and dorsum of thumb that required grafting. The integrity of the palmar skin reflects the protection afforded by early cooling of the tar and the thickness of that skin.

Immediate ophthalmological evaluation is indicated. Frequently ophthalmical antibiotic preparations and cycloplegic agents are used, in an attempt to minimize the devastating consequences of these exposures.

Contact with hot tar or asphalt is commonly seen in industrial settings. The initial objective is to cool the offending material and to stop the burning process. Most thermal injuries result from prolonged heat transfer because of the insulating effect of the material. Removal is best effected with the use of compounds that solubulize the tar such as Neosporin ointment, cold cream, Silvadene or petroleum jelly (Schiller, 1983; Stratta *et al.*, 1983). Most often the burn is of partial thickness and does not require skin grafting (Figure 29.7).

MANAGEMENT OF THE BURN WOUND

The scientific basis of the care of the burn wound is to avoid infection while allowing healing to take place by epithelial redevelopment in a partial-thickness injury, and early excision and skin replacement in a full-thickness injury. Infection is especially disadvantageous in a deep dermal burn in that it may destroy islets of surviving epithelium.

Loose non-viable tissue is removed as it forms a nidus for resident organisms and an antimicrobial barrier created which ideally prevents proliferation of bacteria at the surface of the wound and thus diminishes the incidence of invasive infection

TABLE 29.3

AGENTS IN COMMON USE FOR BURN-WOUND MANAGEMENT

Agent	Properties	Advantages	Problems
Mafenide acetate	Water soluble	Penetrates burn eschar. Wide antimicrobial spectrum	Transient pain on application. Metabolic acidosis
Silver sulphadiazine	Insoluble	Wide antimicrobial spectrum	Rapid development of resistance in gram-negative organisms. Poor eschar penetration
Silver nitrate 5%	Water soluble but Ag can precipitate	Wide antimicrobial spectrum	Staining of linen, etc. Electrolyte imbalance. Poor eschar penetration
Povidone iodine 5%	Water soluble	Active against both gram-negative and gram-positive organisms. Antimycotic	Raised serum iodine with depressed thyroid function. Metabolic acidosis; hypernatraemia. (Not to be used in burns > 30% BSA)

(Order and Moncrief, 1964). Because of the avascularity of the burn wound, parenteral antibiotics are ineffective (Pruitt et al., 1968b). The primary topical agents in clinical use today are mafenide acetate, silver sulfadiazine, 0.5% silver nitrate and 5% povidone iodine (Moyer et al., 1965; Wynn-Williams and Monballiu, 1965; Moncrief et al., 1966; Fox et al., 1969).

The agents in common use, and their drawbacks, are listed in Table 29.3.

Covering the wounds with a topical agent and leaving the patient otherwise exposed in a temperature- and humidity-controlled environment is our preferred technique. Exposure enables ready observation of the wound and promotes easy patient mobilization. By contrast, closed dressings may actually promote burn-wound infection by maintaining a moist, warm environment in which microorganisms can proliferate more rapidly.

DIAGNOSIS AND TREATMENT OF BURN WOUND INFECTION

Although the use of topical chemotherapeutic agents has decreased the incidence of invasive burn-wound infection, the problem has not been totally eradicated (Merrell et al., 1989). Impairment of host defences as well as rapid proliferation of bacteria within the eschar may permit the development of bacterial or fungal wound infection, a situation most commonly seen with burns of more than 30% of the body surface (Pruitt and Curreri, 1971).

Clinical signs of invasive burn wound infection include hyper- or hypothermia, tachycardia, tachypnoea, glucose intolerance and disorientation (Pruitt, 1984). Wound changes, such as focal dark-brown or black discoloration of the eschar, conversion of partial-thickness burn to full-thickness

injury and accelerated eschar separation are more reliable as signs of invasive burn-wound infection (Pruitt, 1984).

The most effective means of diagnosing invasive burn-wound infection is by histological and microbiological evaluation of a 500-mg lenticular burn-wound biopsy which includes subjacent or adjacent unburned tissue (Pruitt and Foley, 1973). A histological grading system developed at the US Army Institute of Surgical Research has been useful in quantifying the presence and extent of infection (Table 29.4). This system distinguishes between colonization and actual invasive burn-wound infection, as defined by the presence of organisms in healthy viable tissue.

The infecting organism determines the clinical presentation and progression of disease and thus determines the treatment regimen. Streptococcal infections do not deeply invade tissues and are usually manifested by surrounding erythema and lymphangitis. Staphylococcal infections can invade deeper tissues but often form a thick membrane

TABLE 29.4

HISTOLOGICAL GRADING SYSTEM DEVELOPED AT THE US ARMY INSTITUTE OF SURGICAL RESEARCH

Stage I: Wound colonization
 a. Superficial colonization
 b. Penetration of non-viable tissue
 c. Proliferation in viable tissue

Stage II: Invasive infection
 a. Microinvasion
 b. Generalized invasion
 c. Microvascular invasion

which prevents the further spread of infection and thereby limits the effectiveness of parenteral antibiotics. Consequently, local excision of the affected tissue is essential for adequate management. Pseudomonas species are the most common cause of invasive infection and have the propensity to spread widely via haematogenous and lymphatic routes (Teplitz, 1965). Diagnosis of this potentially lethal complication warrants immediate operative excision, preferably with immediate autografting, as soon as the patient's general condition permits.

Fungi and yeasts may also cause invasive burn-wound infections. Though Candida species commonly colonize wounds, they are rarely associated with invasion (Bruck et al., 1972). Aspergillus is the most common pathogenic fungus (Pruitt, 1979b). Typically, this process is localized and confined to tissue above the investing fascia (Pruitt, 1984). Wounds colonized by aspergillus can be treated with topical application of clotrimazole, whereas histological evidence of invasion should prompt surgical excision and systemic Amphotericin therapy.

BURN-WOUND EXCISION AND CLOSURE

Before 1970, burn-wound closure was accomplished by daily limited wound debridement and spontaneous eschar separation followed by the application of split-skin grafts to the underlying granulation tissue. Janzekovic introduced the technique of serial excision of tissue down to bleeding dermis or healthy subcutaneous fat, followed by application of split-thickness skin grafts (Janzekovic, 1970). This tangential excision method can be performed in the first week postburn once the patient is stable and resuscitation is complete. Although no statistical improvement in survival has been demonstrated with early excision, tangential excision has led to a significant decrease in the length of hospital stay (Burke et al., 1974). Unless extensive burn-wound infection indicates otherwise, the procedure should be limited to 20% of the body surface area, a blood loss which equals the patient's blood volume or 2 hours of operative time. Once an acceptable depth of excision is achieved the wound may be closed with autograft or temporarily closed with a biological dressing. If tangential excision results in a questionably viable wound bed, fascial excision may be indicated.

Fascial excision of burn wounds involves removal of all overlying tissue to the level of the investing muscle fascia. The advantages of this technique include the brevity of the procedure and significantly less blood loss than that encountered with tangential excision. Wound coverage is achieved either with autograft or biological dressings. The initial cosmetic defects seen with this technique diminish over the span of a year postinjury.

In the extensively burned patient, closure is optimally achieved with cutaneous autografts of 0.010–0.012 inch thickness following excision of the burn wound. Body areas with irregular contours can be harvested successfully by subcutaneous infiltration of a crystalloid solution to create a more uniform surface. The inner thighs and the inner aspect of the arms, areas that have thin skin and are difficult to keep dry, should if possible be avoided. Once obtained, these autografts can be meshed to provide expansion ratios of up to nine times the original surface area, though expansion ratios in excess of 4 : 1 are rarely utilized due to the length of time required for closure of the interstices (DiVincenti et al., 1969b).

Patients with large burn wounds often have insufficient donor sites available for autografting the entire burn wound at one operation. Multiple reharvesting over prolonged periods of time yields autografts of progressively inferior quality. Many burn centres are evaluating the efficacy of autologous derived cultured human epidermal cells (Gallico et al., 1984; Madden et al., 1986). Current culture techniques require 3 weeks or more of growth with a final product consisting of sheets six to eight cells thick. These epidermal sheets are quite fragile and susceptible to infection but success has been reported when they have been applied to freshly excised burn-wound beds. Unfortunately, patients with deep burn wounds devoid of dermal elements appear to develop considerable scarring when epidermal sheets are applied to the wound beds following excision of such burns.

Alternatively, large areas of excision can be covered with temporary biological dressings. Biological dressings prevent wound bed desiccation, minimize exudative protein loss and pain, and promote angiogenesis of granulation tissue. Fresh cadaver allograft is frequently used for this purpose and ultimately derives its blood supply from the underlying wound bed (Pruitt and Silverstein, 1971). Allograft typically remains adherent until surgically excised or rejected by the patient. Under normal conditions however, host rejection occurs within 1 week; however, in the burn patient, with varying degrees of immunosuppression, several weeks may pass before the applied allograft is rejected. The use of allograft is not without risk, as transmission of diseases such as hepatitis B, HIV or syphilis may occur.

Porcine cutaneous xenograft is another biological dressing. It is not vascularized by the host and adheres to the wound bed by fibrin bonding (Silverstein et al., 1971). For superficial partial-thickness wounds, application of porcine cutaneous xenografts can facilitate healing and provide the many benefits of biological dressings applied before significant wound colonization.

In an attempt to avoid the problems of disease transmission and storage requirements that are unique to biological dressings, several synthetic skin substitutes have been developed for temporary wound coverage. These materials are typically of a bilaminate configuration with an inner layer constructed to promote fibrovascular ingrowth from the wound bed and an outer layer which allows water-vapour transmission and prevents bacterial ingress (Pruitt and Levine, 1984). Additional requirements for synthetic skin substitutes include tissue compatibility and an elastic, conforming consistency.

NUTRITIONAL SUPPORT

The metabolic response to burn injury consists of several phases (Cuthbertson and Tilstone, 1969). Immediately following injury an 'ebb' phase develops. The ebb phase is characterized by cardiovascular instability, inadequate perfusion with impaired oxygen transport, a decrease in the metabolic rate, and an increase in autonomic activity. Following resuscitation, the patient enters the 'flow' phase of the metabolic response. This is marked by increased blood flow and improved oxygen transport. The anabolic phase is the final phase in the metabolic response to injury. Once wound closure is achieved and infectious foci are eradicated, the patient begins to replete fat and muscle stores.

The hypermetabolic response seen in the flow phase is characterized by a hyperdynamic cardiac response, muscle wasting and altered glucose metabolism creating relative glucose intolerance. This process is partially driven by neurohormonal influences of the hypothalamic-pituitary axis, as well as discharge from the autonomic nervous system. Antidiuretic hormone, β-endorphins and adrenocorticotropic hormone are released in increased amounts following thermal injury. Stimulation of the autonomic nervous system results in the release of catecholamines and glucagon which, along with cortisol, remain elevated during the hypermetabolic phase. The β-catecholamine response is associated with tachycardia, widened pulse pressure and increased cardiac output (Wilmore et al., 1974). The hyperdynamic circulation increases oxygen delivery to the peripheral tissues to meet the increased oxygen needs and support the elevated heat production. Associated with the hyperdynamic effects is an increase in glomerular filtration rate which accelerates the clearance of some drugs. Paralleling the increased consumption of oxygen is an increased production of carbon dioxide which results in an increase in minute ventilation. Administration of beta blocking agents can often blunt this phase of hypermetabolism but the resulting haemodynamic instability makes such treatment clinically impractical.

The burn-related hypermetabolic response is characterized by muscle protein breakdown which provides 3-carbon precursors for hepatic gluconeogenesis and the synthesis of acute-phase proteins. Significant nitrogen loss occurs, with 80–90% excreted in the form of urea (Wilmore, 1979). Administration of caloric supplements composed of at least 20% amino acids can diminish the extent of muscle wasting by improving protein synthesis.

Altered glucose metabolism is also a feature of the hypermetabolic response. Heptic gluconeogenesis is increased and uptake of glucose by insulin-dependent tissues is decreased in a milieu of relative insensitivity to insulin or insulin resistance (Allison et al., 1968; Wilmore et al., 1976b).

The overall metabolic response to injury represents the integration of the changes that occur in various organs and tissues. The wound anaerobically consumes glucose to fuel the cellular actions of removing necrotic tissue, containing and destroying microorganisms, and promoting cellular proliferation. In that glucose is primarily utilized by anaerobic pathways, an increase in lactate production occurs. Subsequently, lactate is converted to glucose by the liver via the Cori cycle, a process which requires energy expenditure. The liver is also capable of gluconeogenesis through the use of amino acids, principally alanine derived from skeletal muscle and the gut (Ruderman, 1975). The nitrogen from these amino acids is converted to urea which is excreted in the urine, thereby contributing to the negative nitrogen balance. Glutamine levels are also increased during the hypermetabolic phase and serve as a preferred substrate for the gut and a precursor for renal ammonia production. Glutamine is converted by the gut into alanine, which subsequently is transported to the liver by the portal circulation (Windmueller, 1982).

The concept that the gut plays a central role in the maintenance of a hypermetabolic response has recently gained substantial popularity. Failure to maintain mucosal integrity has been hypothesized to lead to the entry of endotoxin and bacteria into the portal system, which then modulates hepatic function. Glutamine supplementation in the diet, which decreases the catabolic demand for glutamine substrates by the gut, has been shown in experimental models to reverse the mucosal abnormalities and to prevent translocation of bacteria and endotoxin into the portal system (Ziegler et al., 1988).

The hypermetabolic response following injury is proportional to the extent of burn, plateauing at between two and two-and-a-half times normal in patients with burns of 50–60% of the body surface area (Wilmore et al., 1974) (Figure 29.8). The actual physiological response is influenced by the patient's age, pain and anxiety, environmental temperature, physical activity, the presence of infection, and health status prior to injury. Actual caloric needs can be determined by indirect calorimetry, involving the determination of oxygen

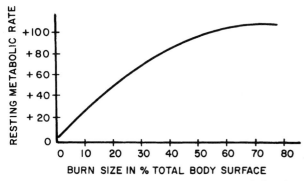

Figure 29.8 The hypermetabolic response following burn injury is proportional to the extent of burn, and plateaux at between about 2 and 2.5 times baseline in patients with burns of 50–60% of the body surface area.

consumption and carbon dioxide production, or estimated by utilizing various formulas. The Harris–Benedict equation (the most commonly used formula) takes into consideration body size, age and severity of injury to provide an estimate of the patient's metabolic rate and caloric needs. In extensive burns extra nutritional support is essential.

COMPLICATIONS

Sepsis is the most common complication. Dense bacterial colonization of the burn wound and the immunosuppression associated with significant injury increase the propensity of the burn patient to develop infectious complications. Pneumonia is the most frequent septic process encountered and since the advent of topical antimicrobials and control of burn-wound sepsis, bronchopneumonia has surpassed lobular haematogenous pneumonia as the predominant form (Pruitt *et al.*, 1970a). The emergence of pneumonia as the primary septic complication of burn patients also reflects improved management of critically ill patients in general and particularly those with inhalation injury who survive the initial insult.

Haematogenous pneumonias result from the systemic dissemination of the infecting organism from a primary septic focus. The radiographic hallmark is a solitary nodular pulmonary infiltrate which may progress to multiple nodular infiltrates throughout the lung fields. Common sources include foci of invasive wound infection, endocarditis, suppurative thrombophlebitis and prostatic abscess, all of which require immediate attention to prevent continued haematogenous dissemination (Pruitt *et al.*, 1970b).

Invasion of the blood stream by gram-negative organisms are associated with a poor prognosis and significantly increased mortality in relation to burn size (Mason *et al.*, 1986). A recent study has shown

that a significant positive correlation exists between the number of transfusions received by a patient and the infectious complications encountered during the hospital course (Graves *et al.*, 1989). This finding may indicate that the blood transfusions themselves contribute to the overall immunocompromised state of the burn patient or may simply reflect that a more seriously ill population of patients has greater impairment of host defences.

Pneumothorax is a frequently encountered iatrogenic complication. Central venous access and barotrauma from positive-pressure ventilation are the two most common causes. Rupture of a pneumatocele formed as a result of staphylococcal pneumonia can also cause pneumothorax.

Many gastrointestinal complications arise in relation to thermal injury. Punctate, shallow mucosal ulcerations throughout the stomach and duodenum may appear as early as 5 hours after a burn. In one series such lesions were documented in 86% of patients with burns of more than 35% of the body surface area (Czaja *et al.*, 1974). If unprotected by measures to reduce intraluminal acidity these lesions may progress to the frank ulcerations described by Curling. Progression of mucosal disease and significant bleeding from the resulting ulcerations have been largely eliminated through prophylactic measures utilizing antacids and H_2 blockers to keep the intragastric pH greater than 4.5 (McAlhany *et al.*, 1976), and the need to operate for bleeding and perforation is now extremely rare.

Acalculous cholecystitis can occur from direct haematogenous seeding of the gallbladder (Munster *et al.*, 1971) or as the consequence of dehydration, ileus or gallbladder atony, all of which may occur in critically ill patients.

Pseudo-obstruction of the colon occurs in about 1% of burn patients (Lescher *et al.*, 1978). If the caecal diameter exceeds 12–14 cm, the bowel is at significant risk for ischaemia and perforation.

Other potential gastrointestinal problems include the superior mesenteric artery syndrome which occurs in patients who sustain profound weight loss during their hospital course. The superior mesenteric artery obstructs the third part of the transverse duodenum when the patient is supine.

As previously mentioned, if resuscitation is effective, acute renal failure is seen infrequently in the early postburn period. Oliguria in the first 24 hours following injury typically reflects inadequate fluid replacement not intrinsic renal disease. Later sepsis and multiple organ system failure are the likely sources of renal insufficiency. Careful monitoring of plasma levels of nephrotoxic antibiotics can minimize the risk of acute tubular necrosis. Acute haemodialysis or haemofiltration should be utilized for the clinical criteria of volume overload, electrolyte imbalance or encephalopathy, rather than absolute elevated levels of blood urea or creatinine.

In the elderly or in patients with pre-existing cardiac disease, myocardial infarction is a potential complication. Most commonly, myocardial ischaemia occurs in the latter part of the first burn week when the hypermetabolic response peaks and tissue demand exceeds the capability of the heart to meet the hyperdynamic circulatory requirements and maintain myocardial perfusion.

SUMMARY

Burn trauma results in significant global physiological stress to all organ systems. Successful management of these critically ill patients is achieved most optimally with a multidisciplinary approach involving physicians, nurses and associated medical personnel. The great demands on clinical resources required for the successful care of these patients are best accommodated in the setting of a burn centre.

REFERENCES

Alexander F., Mathieson M., Teoh K.H. et al. (1984). Arachidonic acid metabolites mediate early burn edema. *J. Trauma*, **24**, 709–12.

Alexander J.W., Wixson D.P. (1970). Neutrophil dysfunction in sepsis in burn injury. *Surg. Gynecol. Obstet.*, **130**, 431–43.

Allen R.C., Pruitt B.A. Jr (1982). Humoral-phagocyte axis of-immune defense in burn patients. *Arch. Surg.*, **117**, 133–40.

Allison S.P., Hinton P., Chamberlain M.J. (1968). Intravenous glucose-tolerance, insulin, and free-fatty-acid levels in burned patients. *Lancet*, **ii**, 1113–16.

Amy B.W., McManus W.F., Goodwin C.W. Jr, Pruitt B.A. Jr (1985). Lightning injury with survival in five patients. *JAMA*, **253**, 243–5.

Apfelberg D.B., Masters F.W., Robinson D.W. (1974). Pathophysiology and treatment of lightning injuries. *J. Trauma*, **14**, 453–60.

Arturson G. (1961). Capillary permeability in burned and non-burned areas in dogs. *Acta Chir. Scand. (Suppl.)*, **274**, 55–103.

Asch M.J., Feldman R.J., Walker H.L. et al. (1973). Systemic and pulmonary hemodynamic changes accompanying thermal injury. *Ann. Surg.*, **178**, 218–21.

Aulick L.H., Goodwin C.W. Jr, Becker R.A., Wilmore D.W. (1981). Visceral blood flow following thermal injury. *Ann. Surg.*, **193**, 112–16.

Batchelor A.D.R., Sutherland A.B., Colver C. (1965). Sodium balance studies following thermal injury. *Br. J. Plast. Surg.*, **18**, 130–45.

Baxter C.R., Cook W.A., Shires G.T. (1966). Serum myocardial depressant factor of burn shock. *Surg. Forum*, **17**, 1–2.

Bjornson A.B., Bjornson H.S., Knippenberg, R.W. et al. (1986). Temporal relationships among immunologic alterations in a guinea pig model of thermal injury. *J. Infect. Dis.*, **153**, 1098–107.

Broughton A., Anderson I.R., Bowden C.H. (1968). Magnesium-deficiency syndrome in burns. *Lancet*, **ii**, 1156–8.

Bruck H.M., Nash G., Stein J.M., Lindberg R.B. (1972). Studies on the occurrence and significance of yeast and fungi in the burn wound. *Ann. Surg.*, **176**, 108–10.

Burke J.F., Bondoc C.C., Quinby W.C. (1974). Primary burn excision and immediate grafting: a method shortening illness. *J. Trauma*, **14**, 389–95.

Burleson D.G., Mason A.D. Jr, Pruitt B.A. Jr (1988). Lymphoid subpopulation changes after thermal injury and thermal injury with infection in an experimental model. *Ann. Surg.*, **207**, 208–12.

Cioffi W.G., Gamelli R.L., DeMueles J.E. (1986). The effects of burn injury and fluid resuscitation on cardiac function *in vitro*. *J. Trauma*, **26**, 638–42.

Cioffi W.G., Graves T.A., McManus W.F. et al. (1987). High frequency percussive ventilation in patients with inhalation injury. *J. Trauma*, **29**, 350–4.

Clayton J.M., Hayes A.C., Hammel J. et al. (1977). Xenon-133 determination of muscle blood flow in electrical injury. *J. Trauma*, **17**, 293–8.

Cohen I.K., Schechter P.J., Henkin R.I. (1973). Hypogeusia, anorexia, and altered zinc metabolism following thermal burn. *JAMA*, **223**, 914–16.

Curreri P.W., Katz A.J., Dotin L.N., Pruitt B.A. Jr (1970). Coagulation abnormalities in the thermally injured patient. *Curr. Top. Surg. Res.*, **2**, 401–11.

Curreri P.W., Wilterdink M.E., Baxter C.R. (1975). Characterization of elevated fibrin split products following thermal injury. *Ann. Surg.*, **181**, 157–60.

Cuthbertson D., Tilstone W.J. (1969). Metabolism during the postinjury period. *Adv. Clin. Chem.*, **12**, 1–55.

Czaja A.J., McAlhany J.C., Pruitt B.A. Jr (1974). Acute gastroduodenal disease after thermal injury: an endoscopic evaluation of incidence and natural history. *New. Engl. J. Med.*, **291**, 925–9.

Demling R.H., Kramer G.C., Gunther R., Nerlich M. (1984). Effect of non-protein colloid on postburn edema formation in soft tissues and lungs. *Surgery*, **95**, 593–602.

Demling R.H., Wong C., Jin L.J. et al. (1985). Early lung dysfunction after major burns: role of edema and vasoactive mediators. *J. Trauma*, **25**, 959–66.

DiVincenti F.C., Moncrief J.A., Pruitt B.A. Jr (1969a). Electrical injuries: a review of 65 cases. *J. Trauma*, **9**, 497–507.

DiVincenti F.C., Pruitt B.A. Jr, Curreri P.W. (1969b). Use of mesh skin autografts in the burn patient. *Plast. Reconstr. Surg.*, **44**, 464–7.

Dorethy J.W., Welch G.W., Treat R.C. et al. (1977). The hemodynamic response to thermal injury in burned soldiers. I. Sequential hemodynamic alterations in severe thermal injury in the military population – colloid-crystalloid vs. crystalloid fluid resuscitation. In *Annual Research Progress Report*. Fort Sam Houston, TX: US Army Institute of Surgical Research, pp. 120–38.

Evans E.I., Brooke J.W., Schmidt F.H. et al. (1955). Flash burn studies on human volunteers. *Surgery*, **37**, 280–97.

Fox C.L. Jr, Rappole B.W., Stanford W. (1969). Control of pseudomonas infection in burns by silver sulfadiazine. *Surg. Gynecol. Obstet.*, **128**, 1021–6.

Gallico G.G. III, O'Connor N.E., Compton C.C. et al. (1984). Permanent coverage of large burn wounds with autologous cultured epithelium. *N. Engl. J. Med.*, **311**, 448–51.

Graves T.A., Cioffi W.G., Mason A.D. Jr et al. (1988). Relationship of transfusion and infection in a burn population. *J. Trauma*, **29**, 948–53.

Gump F.E. and Vinney J.M. (1971). Energy balance and weight loss in burned patients. *Arch. Surg.*, **103**, 440–2.

Halebian P., Robinson N., Barie P. et al. (1986). Whole body oxygen utilization during carbon monoxide poisoning and isocapneic nitrogen hypoxia. *J. Trauma*, **26**, 110–17.

Hanback L.D., Rittenbury M.S. (1965). Response of the reticuloendothelial system in thermal injury. *Surg. Forum.*, **16**, 47–50.

Hansborough J.R., Piancentine J.G., Eiseman B. (1980). Immunosuppression by hyperbaric oxygen. *Surgery*, **87**, 662–7.

Herndon D.N., Abston S., Stein M.D. (1984). Increased thromboxane B$_2$ levels in the plasma of burned and septic burned patients. *Surg. Gynecol. Obstet.*, **159**, 210–13.

Hunt J.L., McManus W.F., Haney W.P. et al. (1974). Vascular lesions in acute electric injuries. *J. Trauma*, **14**, 461–73.

Hunt J.L., Mason A.D. Jr, Masterson T.S. et al. (1976). The pathophysiology of acute electric injuries. *J. Trauma*, **5**, 335–40.

Hunt J.L., Sato R.M., Baxter C.R. (1980). Acute electric burns. Current diagnostic and therapeutic approaches to management. *Arch. Surg.*, **115**, 434–8.

Jackson D.M. (1969). Second thought on the burn wound. *J. Trauma*, **9**, 839–62.

Janzekovic Z. (1970). A new concept in the early excision and immediate grafting of burns. *J. Trauma*, **10**, 1103–8.

Kupper T.S., Green D.R., Durum S.K., Baker C.C. (1985). Defective antigen presentation to a cloned T-helper cell by macrophages from burned mice can be restored with interleukin-I. *Surgery*, **98**, 199–206.

Kupper T.S., Deitch E.A., Baker C.C., Wong W.C. (1986). The human burn wound as a primary source of interleukin-1 activity. *Surgery*, **100**, 409–15.

Larson D.L., Maxwell R., Abston S., Dobrkovsky M. (1970). Zinc deficiency in burned children. *Plast. Reconstr. Surg.*, **46**, 13–21.

Lescher T.J., Teegarden D.K., Pruitt B.A. Jr (1978). Acute pseudo-obstruction of the colon in thermally injured patients. *Dis. Colon Rectum*, **21**, 618–22.

Levine B.A., Schwesinger W.H., Sirinek K.R. et al. (1978). Cimetidine prevents reduction in gastric muscosal blood flow during shock. *Surgery*, **84**, 113–19.

Levine N.S., Atkins A., McKeel D. Jr et al. (1975). Spinal cord injury following electrical accidents: case reports. *J. Trauma*, **15**, 459–63.

Madden M.R., Finkelstein J.L., Staiano-Crico L. et al. (1986). Grafting of cultured allogenic epidermis in second and third degree burn wounds on 26 patients. *J. Trauma*, **26**, 955–62.

Mason A.D. Jr (1980). The mathematics of resuscitation. *J. Trauma*, **20**, 1015–20.

Mason A.D. Jr, Pruitt B.A. Jr (1978). Epidemiology of burn injury. Paper presented at the Fifth International Congress on Burn Injuries, Stockholm, Sweden, 19 June.

Mason A.D. Jr, McManus A.T., Pruitt B.A. Jr (1986). Association of burn mortality and bacteremia: a 25 year review. *Arch. Surg.*, **121**, 1027–31.

McAhanny J.C., Crajn A.J., Pruitt B.A. Jr. (1976). Antacid control of complications from acute gastroduodenal after burns. *J. Trauma*, **16**, 645–9.

McElwee H.P., Sirinek K.R., Levine B.A. (1979). Cimetidine affords protection equal to antacids in prevention of stress ulceration following thermal injury. *Surgery*, **86**, 620–6.

MacIntyre N.R. (1986). Respiratory function during pressure support ventilation. *Chest*, **89**, 677–83.

McManus A.T. (1983). Examination of neutrophil function in a rat model of decreased host resistance following burn trauma. *Rev. Infect. Dis.*, **5**, S898–907.

McManus W.F., Hunt J.L., Pruitt B.A. Jr (1975). Postburn convulsive disorders in children. *J. Trauma*, **14**, 396–401.

Merrell S.W., Saffle J.R., Larson C.W., Sullivan J.J. (1989). The declining incidence of fatal sepsis following thermal injury. *J. Trauma*, **29**, 1362–6.

Moncrief J.A., Pruitt B.A. Jr (1970). Electric injury. *Postgrad. Med.*, **48**, 189–94.

Moncrief J.A., Lindberg R.B., Switzer W.E., Pruitt B.A. Jr (1966). The use of a topical sulfonamide in the control of burn wound sepsis. *J. Trauma*, **6**, 407–15.

Moyer C.A., Brentano L., Gravens D.L. et al. (1965). Treatment of large human burns with 0.5% silver nitrate solution. *Arch. Surg.*, **90**, 812–67.

Moylan J.A., Adib K., Burnbaum M. (1975). Fiberoptic bronchoscopy following thermal injury. *Surg. Gynecol. Obstet.*, **140**, 541–3.

Moylan J.A., Inge W.W. Jr, Pruitt B.A. Jr (1971). Circulatory changes following circumferential extremity burns evaluated by the ultrasonic flowmeter: an analysis of 60 thermally injured limbs. *J. Trauma*, **11**, 763–70.

Moylan J.A., Wilmore D.W., Mouton D.E. et al. (1972). Early diagnosis of inhalation injury using [133]Xenon lung scan. *Ann. Surg.*, **176**, 477–84.

Moylan J.A. Jr, Reckler J.M., Mason A.D. Jr (1973). Resuscitation with hypertonic lactate saline in thermal injury. *Am. J. Surg.*, **125**, 580–4.

Munster A.M., Goodwin M.N., Pruitt B.A. Jr. (1971) Acalculous cholecystitis in burned patients. *Am. J. Surgery*, **122**, 591–3.

O'Neill J.A. Jr, Pruitt B.A. Jr, Moncrief J.A. (1971). Studies of renal function during the early postburn period. In *Research in Burns* (Matter P., Barclay T.L., Konickova Z., eds). Bern: Hans Huber Publishers, pp. 95–9.

Order S.E., Moncrief J.A. (1964). Vascular destruction and revascularization in severe thermal injuries. *Surg. Forum*, **15**, 37–9.

Orgel M.G., Brown H.C., Woolhouse F.M. (1975). Electrical burns of the mouth in children: a method for assessing results. *J. Trauma*, **15**, 285.

Pardoe R., Minami R.T., Sato R.M., Schlesinger S.L. (1976). Phenol burns. *Burns*, **3**, 29–41.

Peters W.J. (1984). Alkali burns from wet cement. *Canad. Med. Assoc. J.*, **130**, 902–4.

Petroff P.A., Pruitt B.A. Jr (1979). Pulmonary disease in the burn patient. In *Burns: A Team Approach* (Artz C.P., Moncrief J.A., Pruitt B.A. Jr, eds). Philadelphia: W.B. Saunders, pp. 95–106.

Plum F., Posner J.B., Hain R.F. (1962). Delayed neurological deterioration after anoxia. *Arch. Intern. Med.*, **110**, 18–25.

Pruitt B.A. Jr (1979a). The burn patient. I. Initial care. *Curr. Prob. Surg.*, **16**, 1–55.

Pruitt B.A. Jr (1979b). The burn patient: II. Later care and complications of thermal injury. *Curr. Prob. Surg.*, **16**, 1–95.

Pruitt B.A. Jr (1984). The diagnosis and treatment of infection in the burn patient. *Burns*, **11**, 79–91.

Pruitt B.A. Jr, Levine N.S. (1984). Characteristics and uses of biologic dressings and skin substitutes. *Arch. Surg.*, **119**, 312–22.

Pruitt B.A. Jr, Mason A.D. Jr (1971). Hemodynamic studies of burned patients during resuscitation. In *Research in Burns* (Matter P., Barclay T.L., Konickova Z., eds). Bern: Hans Huber.

Pruitt B.A. Jr, Silverstein P. (1971). Methods of resurfacing denuded skin areas. *J. Transpl.*, **3**, 1537–45.

Pruitt B.A. and Curreri P.W. (1971). The burn wound and its care. *Arch. Surg.*, **103**, 461–8.

Pruitt B.A. amd Foley F.D. (1973). The use of biopsies burn patients care. *Surgery*, **73**, 887–97.

Pruitt B.A. Jr, Dowling J.A., Moncrief J.A. (1968a). Escharotomy in early burn care. *Arch. Surg.*, **96**, 502–7.

Pruitt B.A. Jr, O'Neill J.A. Jr, Moncrief J.A., Lindberg R.B. (1968b). Successful control of burn wound sepsis. *JAMA*, **203**, 1054–6.

Pruitt B.A. Jr, DiVincenti F.C., Mason A.D. Jr et al. (1970a). The occurrence and significance of pneumonia and other pulmonary complications in burn patients: comparison of conventional and topical treatment. *J. Trauma*, **10**, 519–31.

Pruitt B.A. Jr, Flemma R.J., DiVincenti F.C., Mason A.D. Jr (1970b). Pulmonary complications in burn patients: a comparative study of 697 patients. *J. Thorac. Cardiovasc. Surg.*, **59**, 7–20.

Pruitt B.A. Jr, Mason A.D. Jr, Moncrief J.A. (1971). Hemodynamic changes in the early postburn patient: the influence of fluid administration and of a vasodilator (Hydralazine). *J. Trauma*, **11**, 36–46.

Pruitt B.A. Jr, Erickson D.R., Morris A.H. (1975). Progressive pulmonary insufficiency and other pulmonary complications of thermal injury. *J. Trauma*, **15**, 369–79.

Pruitt B.A. Jr, Goodwin C.W. Jr (1983). Nutritional management of the seriously ill burned patient. In *Nutritional Support of the Seriously Ill Patient* (Winters R.W., ed.). New York: Academic, pp. 63–84.

Richardson J.C., Chambers R.A., Heywood P.M. (1959). Encephalopathies of anoxia and hypoglycemia. *Arch. Neurol.*, **1**, 178–90.

Ruderman N.B. (1975). Muscle amino acid metabolism and gluconeogenesis. *Annu. Rev. Med.*, **26**, 245–58.

Saffle J.R., Crandall A., Warden G.D. (1985). Cataracts: a long-term complication of electrical injury. *J. Trauma*, **25**, 17–21.

Salisbury R.E., Loveless S., Silverstein P. et al. (1973). Postburn edema of the upper extremity: evaluation of present treatment. *J. Trauma*, **13**, 857–62.

Schiller W.R. (1983). Tar burns in the southwest. *Surg. Gynecol. Obstet.*, **157**, 38–9.

Sevett S. (1957). *Burns, Pathology and Therapeutic Applications*. London: Butterworth.

Shea S.M., Caulfield J.B., Burke J.F. (1973). Microvascular ultrastructure in thermal injury: a reconsideration of the role of mediators. *Microvasc. Res.*, **5**, 87–96.

Shimazaki S., Yoshioka T., Tanaka N. et al. (1977). Body fluid changes during hypertonic lactated saline solution therapy for burn shock. *J. Trauma*, **17**, 38–43.

Shirani K.Z., Vaughan G.M., Mason A.D. Jr et al. (1984). Elevation of plasma renin activity, angiotensins I and II,

and aldosterone in burn patients: Na^+/volume-responsive but not volume-dependent. *Surg. Forum*, **35**, 62–3.

Shirani K.Z., Pruitt B.A., Mason A.D. (1987). The influence of inhalation injury and pneumonia on burn morality. *Ann. Surg.*, **205**, 82–7.

Silverstein P., Curreri P.W., Munster A.M. (1971). Evaluation of fresh, viable porcine cutaneous xenografts as a temporary burn wound cover. In *Ann. Res. Prog. Rep. U.S. Army Surg. Res. Unit Brooke Army Med. Ctr.*, 30 June. Washington, DC: US Printing Office.

Solem L., Fischer R.P., Strate R.G. (1977). The natural history of electrical injury. *J. Trauma*, **17**, 487–92.

Stewart R.D. (1975). The effect of carbon monoxide on humans. *Annu. Rev. Pharmacol.*, **15**, 409–23.

Stratta R.J., Saffle J.R., Kravitz M., Warden G.D. (1983). Management of tar and asphalt injuries. *Am. J. Surg.*, **146**, 766–9.

Teplitz C. (1965). Pathogenesis of *Pseudomonas* vasculitis and septic lesions. *Arch. Pathol.*, **80**, 297–307.

Wald P.H., Balmes J.R. (1987). Respiratory effects of short-term high-intensity toxic inhalations: smoke, gases, and fumes. *J. Intensiv. Care Med.*, **2**, 260–78.

Warden G.D., Wilmore D.W., Rogers P.W. et al. (1973). Hypernatremic state in hypermetabolic burn patients. *Arch. Surg.*, **106**, 420–7.

Warden G.D., Mason A.D. Jr, Pruitt B.A. Jr (1974). Evaluation of leukocyte chemotaxis *in vitro* in thermally injured patients. *J. Clin. Invest.*, **54**, 1001–4.

White J.W., Deitch E.A., Gillespie T.E. et al. (1983). Cerebellar ataxia after an electric injury: report of a case and review of the literature. *J. Burn Care Rehabil.*, **4**, 191–3.

White M.G., Asch M.J. (1971). Acid-base effects of topical mafenide acetate in the burned patient. *N. Engl. J. Med.*, **284**, 1281–6.

Wilmore D.W. (1979). Nutrition and metabolism following thermal injury. *Clin. Plast. Surg.*, **1**, 603–19.

Wilmore D.W., Long J.M., Mason A.D. Jr et al. (1974). Catecholamines: mediator of the hypermetabolic response to thermal injury. *Ann. Surg.*, **180**, 653–69.

Wilmore D.W., Mason A.D. Jr, Pruitt B.A. Jr (1976a). Impaired glucose flow in burn patients with gram-negative sepsis. *Surg. Gynecol. Obstet.*, **143**, 720–4.

Wilmore D.W., Mason A.D. Jr, Pruitt B.A. Jr (1976b). Insulin response to glucose in hypermetabolic burn patients. *Ann. Surg.*, **183**, 314–20.

Wilson J.S., Moncrief J.A. (1965). Vapor pressure of normal and burned skin. *Ann. Surg.*, **162**, 130–4.

Windmueller H.G. (1982). Glutamine utilization by the small intestine. *Adv. Enzymol.*, **53**, 201–5.

Wood J.J., O'Mahony J.B., Rodrick M.L. et al. (1986). Abnormalities of antibody production after thermal injury. *Arch. Surg.*, **121**, 108–15.

Wynn-Williams D., Monballiu G. (1965). The effects of povidone-iodine in the treatment of burns and traumatic losses of skin. *Br. J. Plast. Surg.*, **18**, 146–50.

Zelt R.G., Ballard P.A., Common A.A. et al. (1986). Experimental high-voltage electrical burns: role of progressive necrosis. *Surg. Forum*, **37**, 624–6.

Ziegler T.R., Smith R.J., O'Dwyer S.T. et al. (1988). Increased intestinal permeability associated with infection in burn patients. *Arch. Surg.*, **123**, 1313–19.

30. Mustard Gas Injuries: Skin

P. Rice

INTRODUCTION

Sulphur mustard is a powerful vesicant (blistering agent) in man and the descriptions of the casualties from the Gulf War of 1984–7, treated in various European medical centres, attest to the problems of the clinical management of both percutaneous and systemic sulphur mustard injuries (Mandl and Freilinger, 1984; Pauser et al., 1984; Colardyn et al., 1986; Willems, 1989). In addition to their association with large, pendulous fluid-filled blisters, the skin injuries differ in many other respects from thermal burns with which they are often compared. For example, the healing time is considerably longer than for comparable thermal injury and varies from species to species (Schrafl, 1938; Renshaw, 1940). Despite the obvious clinical importance, the biochemical basis of vesication in human skin remains largely undefined (Gales et al., 1989) (Figures 30.1 and 30.2).

Research to further elucidate the molecular mechanisms underlying vesication has been hampered by the lack of an appropriate animal model. In general, fur-bearing mammals do not produce blisters on challenge by either sulphur mustard liquid or vapour. This species variation in cutaneous response has long been known and several theories, none of which has yet been universally accepted, have been proposed to explain such differences (Flesch et al., 1952; McAdams, 1956). The reasons for differences in the healing time remain equally elusive (Papirmeister et al., 1984).

THE STRUCTURE AND FUNCTION OF NORMAL HUMAN SKIN

It is now more than 130 years since Rudulph Virchow portrayed the skin as essentially a protective covering for the delicate and functionally more sophisticated internal organs of the body (Virchow, 1860). At that time, the basic microscopic structure of the skin had been accurately described. It is now known that the skin is a far more complex organ in which many precisely regulated cellular and molecular interactions take place that govern many crucial responses to our immediate environment and the hazards within it. In addition to the protective role described by Virchow and others at the turn of the century, we now know that the skin is of vital importance for body temperature regulation, as an organ of excretion and as the most extensive sense organ of the body for the reception and detection of tactile, thermal and noxious stimuli.

Microscopic structure

The light and electron microscopic structure of the skin have been adequately reviewed elsewhere in the literature (Stenn, 1988; Urmacher, 1990) and will not be described here in more detail than that required to understand the pathogenesis of the sulphur mustard injury. Briefly, the structure of the skin can be divided into two interdependent layers: the epidermis, a specialized epithelium derived from the ectoderm supported by the dermis, a vascular, dense connective tissue layer which mer-

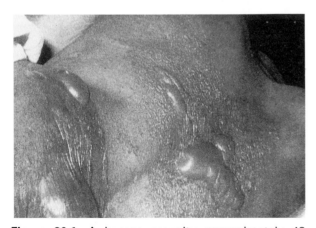

Figure 30.1 A human casualty approximately 48 hours after exposure to sulphur mustard vapour showing the formation of large, pendulous fluid blisters so characteristic of sulphur mustard exposure.

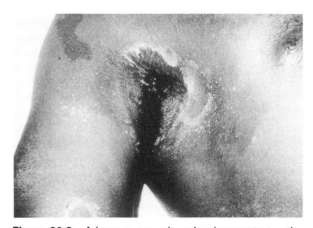

Figure 30.2 A human casualty who demonstrates the striking predilection of sulphur mustard burns to moist areas of the body, in this case the axillae. The lesion is at least 3 or 4 days old and shows rupture of the blister leaving a raw and ulcerated central zone.

ges with the deep subcutaneous adipose layer and is derived from mesoderm. Additionally, the skin also contains a variety of appendages, structures which represent specialized embryological down-growths of the surface epidermis and which in adult skin are recognized as hair shafts, sebaceous glands and sweat glands. Although the distribution, arrangement and detailed structure of these structures varies according to body region, they all conform to a basic tubular, three-dimensional structure.

The epidermis

The epidermis is composed of a stratified, squamous, keratinizing epithelium, the growth and differentiation of which ultimately results in the formation of a superficial layer of dead, keratinized cells or squames which are continually lost from the surface and balanced by replacement of cells that arise as a result of mitotic activity in the basal layer. This mitotic pressure displaces cells to higher and higher levels within the epidermis, a process which is accompanied by the production of increasing amounts of keratin. The structural organization of the epidermis into distinct layers which are visible at the microscopic level is, therefore, a reflection of a dynamic process (MacKenzie, 1972) involving both cell proliferation and differentiation (a change in phenotype) (Figure 30.3).

The overall thickness, in terms of the number of distinct cell layers, of the epidermis, varies according to body site, but in general the epidermis attains maximal thickness in those areas of the body where mechanical stress is greatest, that is, the soles of the feet and the palms of the hands. In these areas, it is clearly divisible into five distinct strata:

- *Stratum germinativum (basale)*. A single mitotically active layer of columnar cells in contact with the dermis through the basement membrane.
- *Stratum spinosum (prickle-cell layer)*. Several layers of irregular, polygonal cells characterized by surface membrane projections (prickles), which make contact with adjacent cells to form intercellular bridges.
- *Stratum granulosum*. Three to five layers of flattened, elongated cells whose cytoplasm contains irregular granules of keratohyalin, a precursor substance involved in the production of keratin. It is within this stratum that cells lose their cell contacts and undergo degenerative processes which ultimately result in their death.
- *Stratum lucidum*. A clear, translucent layer composed predominantly of cell envelopes containing the now semifluid substance, keratohyalin. The cell borders are indistinct and nuclei essentially absent.
- *Stratum corneum*. A layer of fused and flattened dead, scale-like cells, the nuclei of which are completely absent. The cytoplasm of the cells is completely replaced by keratin, a protein believed to be partly derived from tonafilament remnants.

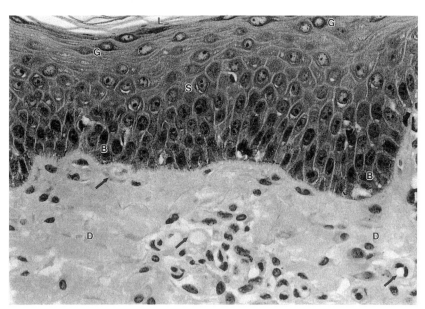

Figure 30.3 The histology of normal dorsal skin of the Yucatan mini-pig. Histologically, the skin is very similar in overall structure to that of human skin. The epidermis is composed of 8–12 cell layers and is clearly divisible into distinct layers: stratum germinativum (basale) (B), stratum spinosum (S), stratum granulosum (G) and stratum lucidum (L). The epidermis is supported by a well-vascularized papillary dermis (D). A complex network of capillaries (arrows) can be seen in the upper papillary dermis at several points. (Weigert's Haematoxylin & Eosin (WH&E), × 400.)

The epidermis covering other body areas is both thinner and simpler in structure than that of the soles and the palms, with less distinct and compressed strata; the stratum lucidum may be absent. The overall epidermal thickness in such areas is, in part, a reflection of the fact that keratinization at these sites is not marked and is probably incomplete.

The overall colour of the skin is dependent upon the interaction of three factors. First, the epidermis itself imparts a yellow colour due to the yellow/orange pigment carotene. The blood of the vascular dermis immediately below the epidermis confers a reddish/blue colour and the presence of varying quantities of melanin pigment (depending on race) gives rise to a brown colour. Melanin pigment is elaborated by specialized cells, the melanocytes, in the stratum germinativum and derived embryologically from the neural crest (neuroectoderm).

The dermis

The exact limits of the dermis are difficult to define since it merges, often imperceptibly, with the underlying subcutaneous soft tissues of the hypodermis. It is composed of connective tissue, predominantly collagen with occasional elastic fibres, and functions to support the overlying epidermis, the skin appendages (adnexae), blood vessels, lymphatics and nerves.

The dermis can be roughly divided into two zones; the advential or papillary dermis comprising the dermis immediately beneath the epidermis and that which invests the adnexal structures (the periadnexal dermis), and the reticular dermis which extends from below the origin of the skin adnexae to merge with the hypodermis below. The advential dermis is composed of a delicately woven matrix of type I and III collagen fibres which entrap a branching network of elastic fibres, ground substance (a semifluid gel composed of glycosaminoglycans), capillaries and fibroblasts. In contrast, the reticular dermis is a network of thick type I collagen and elastic fibres, the former arranged in arrays parallel to the surface.

In addition to fibroblasts, the cellularly sparse normal dermis also contains a small population of tissue histiocytes, cells which act as phagocytic scavengers, and mast cells which tend to aggregate around small blood vessels and capillaries. Although occasional small lymphocytes and neutrophil polymorphs may be identified within the advential dermis, their presence in greater numbers should always suggest the onset of a reactive or pathological process in the skin.

The biochemistry of normal skin

Mammalian skin is now known to be an active and dynamic tissue system with the various functional roles it serves being dependent upon the ability to synthesize and metabolize various macromolecules. The most important of these is the formation and deposition of keratin to form a significant superficial physical barrier in the skin; it is, however, not the only important synthetic pathway.

Lipogenesis and the role of epidermal lipid

Mammalian epidermis, including that of man, has been shown to synthesize short-chain fatty acids from glucose and acetate (Wheatley et al., 1970; Wilkinson, 1970) and the synthesis of these molecules is increased during hair growth (Brooks et al., 1968). By contrast, human epidermal cells synthesize little triacylglycerol fat directly (Jarrett, 1973); this type of fat is the main product of the sebaceous glands in mammals and the epidermis of birds (Wrench et al., 1980).

Complex lipids including phospholipids are important components of all cell membranes. Although many of the intermediate steps in phospholipid synthesis have not yet been identified in normal epidermis, there is evidence to suggest that fatty-acid-deficient rodents are able to incorporate topically applied linoleic acid into epidermal lecithin and, therefore, must possess some of the vital enzyme systems involved in the synthetic pathway (Prottey, 1977); evidence for the presence of similar synthetic pathways in human epidermis is still lacking. Complex, high-molecular-weight waxy esters present in the surface epidermal lipid layer are probably derived from the secretions of the sebaceous glands; there is little or no evidence of active synthesis by epidermal cells (Mier and Cotton, 1976). The epidermis has, however, been shown to actively synthesize the prostaglandins PGE_1, PGE_2 and PGF from arachidonic acid (Jouvenenaz et al., 1970; Greaves, 1972; Aso et al., 1975; Guilhou et al., 1978); their function is thought to be the regulation of the metabolism of cyclic nucleotides involved in transmembrane signalling.

Recent evidence suggests that lipogenesis is intimately involved with the process of normal epidermal keratinization. Human infants who are deficient in essential fatty acids produce thick, scaly layers of surface keratin; cutaneous applications of linoleic acid return the skin to normal (Skolnik et al., 1977). The main function of epidermal lipids, however, appears to be as a barrier to the diffusion of water across the epidermis. Whether this function is served solely by the horny surface layer of keratin remains uncertain (Kligman, 1964; Malkinson, 1964).

Epidermal protein metabolism

Both the epidermis and dermis have a role in producing the inherited characteristics of the skin. Spearman (1980) showed that the adult attributes of the epidermis are dependent on the continuous induction by the dermis; modulation of dermal characteristics has a profound effect on the regulation of normal epidermal biochemistry (Sengel, 1976; Goetinck, 1980). Dermal collagen not only provides support for the overlying basal epidermal cell layer but is essential for epidermal cell growth and differentiation; chick epidermal cells in culture fail to differentiate into keratinocytes in the absence of dermal fibroblasts (McLoughlin, 1963), and on the basis of some evidence, the antigen-presenting (Langerhans) cells of the epidermis may have a role in modulating normal keratinization (Jarrett and Spearman, 1964).

Keratinocytes manufacture proteins using polysomes, short chains of 2–20 coupled ribosomes associated with endoplasmic reticulum and small Golgi bodies. Protein synthesis is maximal in the mitotically active stratum germinativum and the anabolically active stratum spinosum (prickle-cell layer) where pre-keratins are produced. Frenkel *et al.* (1979) demonstrated that the epithelial cells of the hair follicle contain messenger ribonucleic acid (mRNA) for all the molecular sizes of keratin protein and were able to synthesize pre-keratins in cell-free systems from mRNA isolated from human scalp epidermis. Furthermore, there is now good evidence that the stratum spinosum can modulate pre-keratin structure prior to keratin stabilization (Fuchs and Green, 1980); the importance of trans-amidase enzymes in this process has been previously recognized (Mier and Cotton, 1976) and the presence of hydrolases within the stratum granulosum that modify keratin products are well documented (Magnus, 1956; Jarrett, 1973).

Epidermal keratinization

The keratinization of epidermal cells that begins in the stratum granulosum is a complex process, involving the stabilization of precursor pre-keratin proteins, thickening of cytoplasmic envelopes and the eventual disruption of cellular organelles by hydrolytic enzymes.

Keratin is an α-helical structure composed of three supercoiled filaments condensed together in microfibrillar structure (Fraser *et al.*, 1976); packed between the microfibrils are globular matrix proteins. The structure is stabilized by a combination of intramolecular disulphide bonds and attractive (ionic) and repulsive (Van der Waals) forces (Fraser and Macrae, 1980). The mechanical properties of the keratin complex are a direct result of its composite fibre-matrix structure. Keratins freely absorb water, and in doing so undergo a conformational structural change from a brittle and rigid to flexible state on hydration (Spearman, 1977).

Once keratin stabilization is complete, the cell membrane structure becomes altered, active transport across the membrane ceases and there is a loss of semipermeability. Membrane phospholipids are enzymatically degraded and the membrane becomes thickened by lateral extensions to the desmosomal plaque proteins (Brody, 1959). The establishment of a surface keratin structure is completed within the stratum granulosum with the formation of keratinized cell envelopes and the cytolysis of the nucleus, mitochondria, ribosomes and endoplasmic reticulum. A variety of hydrolytic (Jarrett and Spearman, 1964) and proteolytic (Yamura and Cormia, 1961; Lazarus *et al.*, 1975) enzymes responsible for this degradation have now been isolated from the epidermis.

THE HISTORY OF THE USE OF SULPHUR MUSTARD IN WAR

Sulphur mustard or 'mustard gas' is perhaps the most familiar member of the heterogeneous group of chemicals that are refered to as chemical warfare agents. The term 'king of the battle gases', thought to have been coined by Foulkes in his commentaries on the use of chemical warfare agents in the First World War (Foulkes, 1934), remains a relatively accurate and well-deserved description today.

The exact date of the first chemical synthesis of sulphur mustard is still disputed, but various dates between 1820 and 1854 have been quoted by a number of authors. In 1860, Guthrie (1860) reported the synthesis of sulphur mustard and noted some of its vesicant (blister-inducing) properties; this was followed by a report in 1886 detailing the synthesis of pure sulphur mustard (Meyer, 1886). There then followed a long period until the outbreak of the First World War, during which time little or no practical use for the compound was proposed. Although the British had successfully synthesized sulphur mustard by 1916, there were no plans to develop it as a chemical weapon. Germany, however, had recognized its potential military significance and, following initial development by Fritz Haber and industrial scale development by Lommel and Steinkopf (Papirmeister *et al.*, 1991), sulphur mustard was first deployed against the French troops at Ypres, Belgium on 12 July 1917 (Ireland, 1926).

During the first 3 weeks of its use, the British Army sustained more than 14 000 casualties, of whom approximately 500 subsequently died (*History of the Great War – Medical Services*, 1923). By the end of the war, sulphur mustard was being extensively used by both sides and the overall casualty figure had risen to 400 000 according to some authorities; the British alone reported in excess of 140 000 casualties (Foulkes, 1934). Despite these appallingly high figures, the mortality rate did not exceed 2–3% (Haldane, 1925); the much higher figure of 13–14% reported following the Bari Harbour incident in 1943 is now thought to be atypical of sulphur mustard exposure and may have been compounded by fatalities as a result of direct blast injury (Alexander, 1947).

Since the use of sulphur mustard in the 1914–18 war, there have been several allegations of its use around the world in numerous conflicts. Italian forces were reported to have used sulphur mustard against Abyssinian (Ethiopian) troops in 1936 and it was used, probably on several occasions, by the Japanese in China between 1937 and 1941 (Medema, 1986). Some evidence to support its use by Poland against Germany in 1939 and by Eygpt against the Yeman in 1963 to 1967 has also been reported (Medema, 1986). Much more recently, well-founded allegations of the use of mustard by Iraq against Iran (1984–7) were made and largely substantiated by independent specialists acting on behalf of the UN Secretary General (United Nations Security Council, 1984, 1986, 1987). During the period of the Iran–Iraq conflict, numerous Iranian casualties whose injuries were compatible with exposure to sulphur mustard arrived for hospital treatment in several Western European countries including the UK (Mandl and Freilinger, 1984; Pauser et al., 1984; Colardyn et al., 1986; Willems, 1989; Newman-Taylor, 1991).

CHEMICAL AND PHYSICAL PROPERTIES OF SULPHUR MUSTARD

The name 'mustard' was given to the compound by soldiers during the First World War, apparently because of the smell perceived during gas attacks; since this time, the odour has been variously described as similar to that of garlic, mustard, horseradish and leeks. Sulphur mustard itself should not be confused with mustard oil (Parry, 1921; Reynolds, 1977); the latter is allyl isothiocyanate and, interestingly, is also a powerful vesicant. Mustard is often refered to by the letter 'H'; it can also be denoted as 'HS' (representing **H**un**S**toff or 'German stuff'), 'HD' to imply distilled mustard, or 'LOST' believed to be a derivation of **LO**mmel and **ST**einkopf, the two German chemists responsible for its industrial-scale production. The compound remains referred to, particularly by the French, as Yperite in view of its initial use at Ypres.

Sulphur mustard is an oily, colourless to brown liquid at room temperature and has the chemical name bis(2-chloroethyl)sulphide; the chemical synonyms include 2,2'-dichlorodiethylsulphide, β, β'-dichloroethylsulphide, 1-chloro-2-(2-chloroethylthio)ethane and 1,1'-thiobis(2-chloroethane). Its physicochemical properties are summarized in the Table 30.1.

The vapour given off by a quantity of sulphur mustard has considerable penetrating ability; it rapidly passes through clothing to affect the underlying skin. Vapour will also penetrate substances such as wood and leather, albeit not as rapidly as cloth. Materials such as metal, glass and glazed ceramics are generally impervious; paint on metallic surfaces may, however, absorb mustard vapour and act as a potential source of a vapour hazard in the immediate vicinity.

TABLE 30.1

PHYSICOCHEMICAL PROPERTIES OF SULPHUR MUSTARD. SOURCE: US ARMY AND US AIR FORCE, (1975) WINDHOLZ AND BUDAVARI, (1983).

Parameter	Description/comments
1. Chemical structure	$S{<}^{CH_2 \cdot CH_2 \cdot Cl}_{CH_2 \cdot CH_2 \cdot Cl}$
	Molecular weight = 159
2. Boiling point	215–217°C
3. Melting point	14.4°C (for distilled mustard).
4. Specific gravity	1.27
5. Vapour pressure	*Temperature (°C)* *Pressure (mmHg)* 0 0.025 14 0.070 30 0.090 40 0.450
6. Solubility	Sparingly soluble in water, 0.68 g/l at 25°C. $t_{0.5} = 5$ min. In weak solutions, hydrolyses to the thiodiglycol, $S(CH_2 \cdot CH_2 \cdot OH)_2$. Freely soluble in animal oils, fats and organic solvents
7. Stability	Stable for many days under normal temperatures and pressures. Decomposes at high temperatures to give compounds with lachrymatory actions. Destroyed by strong oxidants such as hypochlorite to form the sulphoxide (O = $S[CH_2 \cdot CH_2 \cdot Cl]_2$) and the sulphone ($O_2 \cdot S[CH_2 \cdot CH_2 \cdot Cl]_2$)

THE INTERACTION OF SULPHUR MUSTARD WITH IMPORTANT BIOLOGICAL MACROMOLECULES

Sulphur mustard is a bifunctional alkylating agent capable of forming covalent linkages with nucleophilic groups in the cell (Mol *et al.*, 1989a). The ability of sulphur mustard to crosslink complementary strands of DNA has been extensively reviewed (Fox and Scott, 1980; Murname and Byfield, 1981), as well as its ability to bind to various important enzyme systems (Wheeler, 1962), collagen (Pirie, 1947) and keratin (Peters and Wakelin, 1947).

Reaction with DNA

The evidence that binding to DNA is a key mechanism underlying its potential to cause cell injury has slowly accumulated (Philips, 1950; Roberts *et al.*, 1968; Fox and Scott, 1980) since the elucidation of the structure and capacity for chemical reactions of DNA during the 1950s. The reaction with DNA is complex. As a bifunctional alkylating agent, sulphur mustard has two carbon chains that are capable of internal cyclization, a process which is necessary for alkylation to occur. Alkylation of complementary DNA bases by a single molecule of sulphur mustard is, therefore, possible and will lead to the formation of interstrand crosslinks. The important chemical steps are summarized below:

- First cyclization reaction

- Alkylation of DNA base (guanine)

- Second cyclization reaction

- Alkylation of complementary DNA base leading to interstrand crosslinking

Alkylated guanine residues have a tendency to form base pairs with thymine rather than cytosine (as normal), resulting in coding errors and inaccurate protein synthesis. This may ultimately lead to either non-production or excessive production of key metabolic enzymes and structural macromolecules. The effects on rapidly dividing tissues are particularly severe and have led to profound bone marrow suppression, gastrointestinal damage and spermatogenic arrest in human casualties (Rice and West, 1987; Willems, 1989).

Evidence is accumulating to suggest that damage to DNA is dependent on the mitotic state of the cell, so that DNA has a differential sensitivity to sulphur mustard depending on what part of the cell cycle it has entered. Savage and Brekon (1981) have shown that 12–16 hours after exposure to sulphur mustard, cultures of Syrian hamster fibroblasts produced a large number of chromatid aberrations due to substantial delay and disruption of the pre-S phase cells; most of these early S-phase cells failed to reach division within 36 hours. The greatest depression in the rate of DNA synthesis occurs in the late G1- and early S-phase, where the repair of DNA is severely reduced. Flow cytometric analysis of DNA has also shown blockage by sulphur mustard (and its monofunctional analogue, chloroethyl ethyl sulphide) in late G1- and early S-phase of the cell cycle of cultured human keratinocytes (Gales *et al.*, 1989) and human peripheral blood lymphocytes (Sanders *et al.*, 1989).

It is evident that for DNA replication to occur, the supercoiled material constituting the chromosomes must unwind; this potentially increases the accessibility of the genetic bases to alkylating agents such as sulphur mustard, and involves numerous enzymes which are critical to this process. According to Pardee (1989), in late G1-phase a number of enzymes involved in DNA synthesis appear; these include, DNA polymerase (DP), cyclin (proliferative cell nuclear antigen), thymidine kinase (TK), ribonucleotide reductase (RR) and dihydrofolate reductase (DR). The enzymes are translated at cytoplasmic ribosomes and subsequently undergo translocation to the nucleus at the end of the G1-phase. At the nucleus, the enzymes join together to form a multi-enzyme complex which contains RR and DR (required to catalyse precursor synthesis), TK (involved in thymidine salvage) and DP (required for the actual replication of the DNA strands). Finally, the DNA undergoes a conformational change at the replication origin. The G1- to S-phase transition is, therefore, very sensitive to all processes which inhibit protein synthesis.

Once the cell has reached the S-phase, the DNA is replicated very precisely in a matter of a few hours by the initiation of bidirectional replication at numerous points in every chromosome; if replication is not completed in the S-phase, breakage occurs at subsequent mitosis (Lasky *et al.*, 1989). The replication of chromosomes also requires that the conformation (three-dimensional structure) as well as the activity/non-activity of genes within the chromosome are conserved. The alkylation of any of the highly sensitive machinery associated with the processes surrounding DNA replication may, therefore, have a highly disruptive effect on the cell's metabolism.

Repair of DNA, whatever the initial cause, may also lead to further impairment of cellular function. An important aspect of the DNA repair mechanism involves the consumption of NAD^+ as a result of activation of poly (ADP-ribose)-polymerase (PRP), a DNA repair enzyme, in response to breaks occuring in the DNA backbone following alkylation of the DNA bases and the action of apurinic endonucleases. Other reports have also indicated that intracellular NAD^+ levels are decreased by DNA-damaging agents such as ionizing radiation, streptozotocin, neocarzinostatin and the mutagen, N-methyl-N'-nitro-N-nitrosoguanidine (Juarez-Salinas *et al.*, 1979).

PRP depletes cells of NAD^+ at vesicating doses of sulphur mustard, leading to the inhibition of glycolysis, stimulation of the NADP-dependent, hexose monophosphate shunt and cell death (Papirmeister *et al.*, 1984, 1985). Stimulation of this latter enzyme pathway has also been associated with enhancement of protease synthesis and release, resulting in localized subepidermal blister formation in the skin (Smulson, 1989).

The seemingly central role of depletion of cellular NAD^+ in sulphur mustard-induced cutaneous injury has, however, recently been questioned. Gross *et al.* (1985) found that by pretreating an athymic nude mouse grafted with human skin with 3-aminobenzamide (an inhibitor of PRP) they could protect the graft from sulphur mustard challenge by maintaining cellular NAD^+ levels. In a similar experiment, Mol *et al.* (1989b) found that maintenance of NAD^+ levels in cultures of human epidermal cells *did not* protect the cells' energy metabolism, as measured by impairment of glucose uptake, when exposed to sulphur mustard. The situation has only become more confused by the results of an experiment conducted by Meier *et al.* (1987), who showed that treatment with nicotinamide (an NAD^+ precursor) could protect cultured human leucocytes from sulphur mustard challenge. This apparent dichotomy of results has been interpreted as being attributable to the relatively high rate of turnover of cultured epidermal cells when compared to leucocytes (Mol *et al.*, 1989b), and once again emphasizes the importance of the cell cycle to sulphur mustard-induced DNA damage.

Reaction with tissue proteases

The link between the biochemical effects of sulphur mustard – such as its reaction with DNA and the subsequent inhibition of glycolysis – and its vesicant action still remains poorly defined, though the local release of tissue proteases may damage the dermo-epidermal junction (Einbinder, *et al.*, 1966; Kahl and Pearson, 1967; Briggamann *et al.*, 1984) and has been incorporated into the mechanistic schema proposed by Papirmeister (Papirmeister *et al.*, 1985).

The involvement of proteases in the vesication process is becoming less speculative, in the light of several papers that have established a crucial role for proteins such as plasminogen activator (PA) in pathological skin conditions such as psoriasis (Fraki *et al.*, 1983) and the blistering disorder of pemphigus (Hashimoto *et al.*, 1983; Singer *et al.*, 1985). Organ culture experiments have indicated that following exposure to sulphur mustard, tissue plasminogen levels increase and that the observed increases cannot be entirely explained in terms of either extravasation of serum or release from acute inflammatory cells (Woessner *et al.*, 1991). Furthermore, plasminogen has also been detected in the suprabasal, acantholytic cells of Darier's disease and in the degenerating basal cells of chronic cutaneous lupus erythematosis (Burge *et al.*, 1989); these observations suggest that the balance between protease activators and inhibitors, and between protease availability and location within the tissue, are important factors in the pathogenesis of these conditions.

Plasminogen activator (PA) is a serine protease which converts the proenzyme plasminogen into its active form plasmin by hydrolysing a single peptide bond in the precursor (Wun *et al.*, 1982). PA is found in a variety of cells and tissues, including keratinocytes. The hypothesis that keratinocyte PA may facilitate squame detachment (Myhre-Jensen and Astrup, 1971) is supported by the finding that cellular PA levels increase with increasing keratinocyte differentiation (Isserhof and Rifkin, 1983). According to Wilson and Reich (1978), PA secretion is a key mechanism underlying localized extracellular proteolysis.

PA is the main activator of latent collagenases in tissue (Werb and Gordon, 1975) and is able to induce the secretion of collagenase by fibroblasts as well as control the degradation of the extracellular matrix (ECM) and regulate the catabolism of tissue macromolecules (Liotta *et al.*, 1981). Human keratinocytes in culture synthesize and secrete two inhibitors of PA (PA inhibitor I and II); the latter is able to prevent intraepidermal blister formation induced by pemphigus IgG autoantibody in human skin grown in organ culture (Hashimoto *et al.*, 1989). Given, therefore, that PA is regulated by PA inhibitors (Leprince *et al.*, 1989), it follows that disruption of this negative control mechanism may lead to the loss of PA control *in vivo*. Any agent, such as sulphur mustard, which inhibits various components of cellular metabolism may also disrupt the proteolytic control mechanisms of the cell.

The role of inflammatory cells and the immune system in the release of tissue proteases

In addition to the direct effects which sulphur mustard may have in initiating proteolytic cascades, other sources of proteolytic enzymes have to be considered, the most important of these being the various inflammatory cell types that have been described as part of the sulphur mustard-induced cutaneous injury in various species (Papirmcister *et al.*, 1984; Vogt *et al.*, 1984; Mitcheltree *et al.*, 1989; Mershon *et al.*, 1990).

According to Sellers and Murphy (1981), in pathological situations involving significant infiltration of the tissues by neutrophils, elastase and cathepsin from these cells could contribute significantly to the lysis of collagen that is observed. Macrophages have the ability to degrade collagen intracellularly following phagocytosis of individual fibrils (Shoshan, 1981), and it is possible to speculate that these cells may play a role in the degradation of papillary dermal collagen that has been observed in rabbit skin following exposure to sulphur mustard (R. Knight and P. Rice, 1990, unpublished observations). Macrophages also secrete interleukin 1 (IL-1), which promotes the activation and multiplication of both B- and T-lymphocytes (Roitt *et al.*, 1988). On encountering the appropriate antigen, T-cells can secrete a preformed heparinase which degrades the heparin sulphate polysaccharide chains of the ECM proteoglycan scaffold; this allows T cells to traverse blood vessel walls and the endothelial ECM in order to reach their antigenic target sites. Macrophages also possess a pericellular heparinase which facilitates their penetration of the ECM, allowing access to all extravascular compartments (Savion *et al.*, 1987).

The exact roles for these cells and the immune system in the pathogenesis of sulphur mustard cutaneous injury remains largely unknown, although there is some evidence to suggest that the immunogenicity of various structural components of the skin, such as collagen, is altered following exposure to sulphur mustard (Berenblum and Wormall, 1939; Pirie, 1947; Jendryczko and Drozdz, 1985). Conversely, it is well known, that in high percutaneous and systemic doses, sulphur mustard is a powerful immunosuppressant (Vedder, 1925; Rice and West, 1987; Willems, 1989).

Reactions with the connective tissue matrices and components of the epidermal basement membrane.

Having considered the potential role of proteases in sulphur mustard-induced injury, it is necessary to consider the likely targets for protease activity in the skin. The two most important in this respect are the connective tissue matrices of the upper papillary dermis and the basement membrane, and its associated fibrils that lie at the interface of the former and the overlying epidermis (the dermoepidermal junction). The biochemical composition and ultrastructural organization of both these structures have been extensively reviewed previously (Martinez-Fernandez and Amenta, 1983; Katz, 1984; Lunstrum *et al.*, 1986; Keene *et al.*, 1987; Bosman *et al.*, 1989) but have, to the author's knowledge, received little or no attention in relation to being possible targets following exposure to sulphur mustard.

The connective tissue matrix
The connective tissue matrix of the papillary dermis is composed of collagens, elastin and other glycoproteins (Burgeson, 1988), as well as glycosaminoglycans (Lindahl and Hook, 1978). Normal adherent cells in culture, synthesize and deposit a connective tissue matrix which shows structural heterogeneity dependent on the cell phenotype and culture conditions (Leigh *et al.*, 1987). Type III collagen is essential for the normal tensile strength of the skin and accounts for 10–50% of the total collagen content in adult tissues such as the skin, large arteries, skeletal muscle and the lung. Type I collagen is the major collagen type of the adult skin, and together with type III fibres, entrap the n-terminal domains of the anchoring fibrils and their associated plaques (Keene *et al.*, 1987).

Basement membrane
Ultrastructurally, the basement membrane is composed of three distinct zones: the lamina lucida (or rara), the lamina densa and the lamina fibroreticularis.

The lamina lucida is an electronlucent layer adjacent to the plasma membrane of the adherent cell and is composed largely of laminin. Bullous pemphigoid antigen (a disease-specific glycoprotein recognized by an antibody that circulates in the serum of patients with the disease) and a number of poorly defined antigens that are recognized by circulating antibodies in patients with herpes gestationis and scarring pemphigoid (Katz, 1984) have also been demonstrated in the lamina lucida. Delicate anchoring filaments traverse this layer and insert themselves into the attachment plaques of the hemidesmosomes of the overlying basal epidermal cells (Bosman *et al.*, 1989).

The lamina densa is an electrondense layer situated at the stromal side of the lamina lucida and composed of type IV collagen and the KF-1 antigen, a non-collagenous antigen which appears to be restricted to the basement membranes of stratified squamous epithelia and is completely absent in patients with the autosomal recessive condition of dystrophic epidermolysis bullosa (Katz, 1984; Burgeson, 1988). Recent evidence suggests that the antigen is the 450-kDa, globular C-domain of type VII collagen (Lunstrum et al., 1986).

Finally, beneath the lamina densa is the lamina fibroreticularis or sub-basal lamina, a layer which appears to be restricted to basement membranes that support stratified, squamous epithelia (Bosman et al., 1989). The layer is composed of elastic fibres that interdigitate with the type I and III collagen fibres of the underlying connective tissue matrix, and anchoring fibrils. The latter are composed predominantly of type VII collagen (Lunstrum et al., 1986; Keene et al., 1987; Leigh et al., 1987) and stabilize the attachment of the basement membrane to the underlying stroma by forming a fibrous network; the C-terminal domains form globular structures which can be localized using immunoelectron microscopy of the inferior border of the lamina densa, cf. KF-1 antigen (Leigh et al., 1987).

The connective tissue matrix and basement membrane as targets for sulphur mustard attack

The cells of the epidermis are anchored to the underlying dermis by a complex network of intracytoplasmic filaments, hemidesmosomes, anchoring fibrils and basement membrane components. Protease release into any region of the basement membrane could disrupt the components of this meshwork structure and therefore, the structural integrity of the dermo-epidermal junction. This would, ultimately, lead to the separation of the epidermis from the dermis and vesicle (blister) formation. It is of interest to note that Mershon et al. (1990) have shown ultrastructural evidence of disruption of the anchoring fibrils, an observation that confirms the earlier reports of a similar lesion by Papirmeister et al. (1984). Careful inspection of the ultrastructural nature of these disruptions indicates that they are consistent with proteolytic cleavage of the type VII collagen molecule in the vicinity of the globular C-domain (P. Rice, 1989, unpublished observations). This observation clearly warrants further investigation.

In addition to providing support and a substratum for cell functions such as orientation and mitosis (Wessel, 1967; Rodriquez-Boulan and Nelson, 1989; Fleming, 1991), it has been suggested that the finite surface of the basement membrane may be an important factor in limiting the proliferation of cells (Vracko, 1974); in the event of injury that resulted in either the disruption or destruction of the basement membrane, healing would only occur by scar formation. This may have implication for

sulphur mustard-induced cutaneous injuries and their slow rate of healing (Schrafl, 1938; Renshaw, 1940).

Sulphur mustard and its effects on important cutaneous enzyme systems

Most of the work on skin biochemistry in relation to sulphur mustard burns was stimulated by the enzyme theory of vesication (Peters, 1936). It remains to be determined whether:

● Injury is primarily dependent upon a direct reaction of the agents with one or a few specific and highly important proteins or other molecular species, or
● There is more or less random reaction of the vesicant with reactive groups of numerous proteins producing the observed pathological effects.

Until fairly recently there was no convincing evidence that inactivation of any one enzyme or group of related enzymes has a causal relationship to the development of vesicant-induced burns. However, most of the earlier work concentrated on enzymes restricted to carbohydrate metabolism and many of the enzymes known today were undiscovered at the time of these early observations, e.g. adenosine triphosphatase (Jørgensen et al., 1971). Even if it is assumed that vesicants act by alkylating or disrupting a single enzyme or group of similar enzymes, since the reaction time, i.e. exposure to full alkylation, is so short, therapy would need to be directed towards prophylaxis rather than treatment.

Oxygen consumption and glycolysis

In 1935, Berenblum showed that cutaneous applications of dichloroethyl sulphide, dichlorodiethyl sulphone and other vesicants inhibited the development of cutaneous tumours evoked by the application of coal tar. Subsequently, he demonstrated that sulphur mustard in vitro caused a limited inhibition of $O_2(g)$ consumption by minced tumour tissue and a pronounced inhibition of its aerobic and anaerobic glycolysis (Berenblum et al., 1936).

Aerobic metabolism Normal skin is an actively respiring tissue; in young rats, oxygen consumption is as high as 4–5 mm³/h/mg of dry tissue (Needham and Dixon, 1941). Significant but limited inhibition of the basic respiratory rate does develop during the first 1–2 hours after poisoning with 20% sulphur mustard in alcohol (Thompson, 1940). Oxygen consumption of untreated skin is not influenced by the addition of glucose (Needham and Dixon, 1941) but is markedly increased by succinate (Thompson, 1940). Aerobic glycolysis of normal rat skin is low and unaffected by pyruvate. About 15 hours after 1.5 hours treatment with sulphur mustard, there is no significant change in the rate of acid production in the presence of glucose; but after 3 hours a marked decrease has occurred which is out of proportion to the fall in oxygen consumption (Needham and Dixon, 1941).

Anaerobic glycolysis Under anaerobic conditions, normal excised rat skin and skin extracts in the absence of added substrate produce lactic acid at a low rate. After treatment with sulphur mustard *in vivo*, residual glycolysis (i.e. no added substrate) of excised but otherwise intact skin remains unaltered. However, if glucose is added to the system, its conversion to lactic acid is almost completely inhibited (Dixon, 1943).

Tests of a large number of vesicant and non-vesicant substances has demonstrated a good correlation between the skin-damaging action of mustard and its inhibitory effect on the glycolysis of glucose by rat skin (Wheeler, 1962).

Observations and interpretations in terms of skin enzyme systems

The initial phosphorylation stages mediated by hexokinase are inhibited by sulphur mustard and other vesicant compounds (Dixon, 1943). Dixon demonstrated that treatment of skin with sulphur mustard *in vivo* results in the inhibition of the hexokinase system after a latency and according to a time-scale corresponding to that of glycolytic inhibition and the development of gross injury (12–24 hours). This parallel between hexokinase inhibition and the fall of anaerobic glycolysis on the one hand, and the development of serious injury on the other remains striking, but it is possible that these alterations are co-phenomena rather than cause and effect (Renshaw, 1940).

Inhibition of glycolysis in the rat by sulphur mustard is reversed by the chelating agent 2,3-dimercaptopropanol (British Anti-Lewisite or BAL) (Barron *et al.*, 1948), but it is known that long continued application of BAL, although preventing blister formation on H-treated human skin, does not prevent cellular injury or death. The possible relation of the pyruvate oxidase system to vesication was investigated by Peters (1936). He showed that the oxidation of pyruvate in chopped brain preparations is strikingly inhibited by sulphur mustard and other vesicant agents, including nitrogen mustard (HN_3), and that the effect did not depend upon inactivation of vitamin B_1 or glutathione. The significance of this enzyme system in the skin is as yet undetermined.

Cholinesterase is present in the skin and has been found to be inactivated by cutaneous applications of sulphur mustard and methyl N-(β-chloroethyl)-N-nitroso-carbamate (Thompson, 1942). The relevance of this to injury is not known.

FACTORS INFLUENCING THE INJURY-PRODUCING EFFECTIVENESS OF VESICANTS

There are numerous physical and biological variables which affect the efficiency of sulphur mustard as a chemical warfare agent; obviously the length of exposure and the total absorbed dose have profound effects on the resulting severity of injury, but biological variables such as age, size and body region exposed also influence the degree of injury in response to a given concentration of mustard.

Body region and degree of pigmentation

Reports on casualties from the First World War attested to the striking differences in susceptibility to sulphur mustard of various regions of the body (Warthin and Weller, 1919). Generally, the most sensitive regions are those that are naturally warm and moist and/or subject to friction (Marshall *et al.*, 1918; Renshaw, 1947). Thus, the genital regions, axillae, cubital and popliteal fossae are often the most severely affected.

Many previous investigations have highlighted the fact that black skin is more resistant than white to the blistering effects of similar doses of liquid and gaseous sulphur mustard. Thompson *et al.* (1945) found little difference in the severity of erythema between the two but blistering was four times more likely in the latter at liquid doses up to 65 µg. These observations held for exposure in temperate climates, but when white Americans were compared to Puerto Rican soldiers under tropical conditions, no statistical difference between them was noted (Renshaw, 1940). Similar conclusions were drawn from experiments in piebald pigs; no difference in severity of injury was found between pigmented and non-pigmented regions.

Age, size and nutritional status

Over the age range 17–35 years in man there are no correlations recorded between age and exposure to sulphur mustard. There is, however, some evidence in animals that age does modulate the response; Mirsky and Goldman (1943) were able to produce small blisters in the skin of ducklings up to 8 weeks of age. Thereafter, the response to mustard challenge was not characterized by the appearance of blisters; it is interesting to note that at 8 weeks of age the duckling develops the first of its mature feathers and some authors have suggested that the eruption of adnexal structures through the surface epidermis may be important in providing additional anchorage to the overlying epidermis.

There is little or no evidence that either fortified diets or certain nutritional deficiencies have any appreciable effect on the susceptibility of the skin to mustard-induced injury. It is well known, however, that the use of corticosteroids, deficiency of zinc and ascorbic acid, and infection due to generalized malnutrition all prolong wound healing, irrespective of cause (Crandon, 1940; Levenson 1950; Heldner and Hambridge, 1975).

Dose, exposure time and multiple exposures

There is evidence that the severity of cutaneous lesions produced by a given dose of sulphur mustard vapour is not significantly altered by an exposure time in the range 5–240 minutes (PCS (Project Co-ordination Staff), 1946). McNamara *et al.* (1975) quote the following guideline figures: the median incapacitating doses for percutaneous effects are $2000\,mg/min/m^{-3}$ at 70–80°F (21–27°C) and $1000\,mg/min/m^{-3}$ at 90°F (32°C). The Human Estimates Committee (1960) established an allowable Ct of $5\,mg/min/m^{-3}$ at 90°F (32°C) for unprotected skin.

Mustard is less effective on human skin when given in low concentrations over long exposure times (PCS (Project Co-ordination Staff), 1946). Exposure to a total Ct of $300\,mg/min/m^{-3}$ given as four exposures over 6–12 days causes similar lesions to those produced by $100\,mg/min/m^{-3}$ given as a single exposure (PCS (Project Co-ordination Staff), 1946). This type of data gives no indication of the time interval between exposures necessary to ensure that doses are not cumulative.

Physical state of the vesicating agent

Sulphur mustard may be applied to the skin as a liquid (consisting of large or small droplets or splashes), a vapour or as a particulate solid. The size and severity of the ensuing injuries produced by a given quantity of liquid mustard, for example, is affected by the degree to which the liquid is spread. This, of course, is dependent upon the mode of application and by any movement of the target site on application (McMaster *et al.*, 1945).

Environmental temperature and humidity, exercise and air flow

Most of the available evidence indicates that sulphur mustard (as either a liquid or a vapour) produces more severe cutaneous lesions at high rather than low temperatures, given that other environmental factors are kept constant. Increases in the relative (or absolute) humidity at constant temperatures increase the susceptibility of the skin to mustard, and these effects are even more pronounced when the skin surface is moist (Renshaw, 1947). Exercise acts to increase the susceptibility to challenge by causing sweating and hence moistening the skin (PCS (Project Co-ordination Staff), 1946). The direction and strength of air currents over the skin surface probably only assume importance in the development of a mustard lesion by causing drying of the skin surface.

MOLECULAR STRUCTURE IN RELATION TO VESICANCY

In order to produce blistering of the skin, a chemical agent must:

- Make contact with the skin surface.
- Penetrate the epidermis of the skin, and
- Possess the appropriate, inherent toxicity which results in cellular injury.

The readiness with which an agent can be brought into contact with the skin does not affect the mechanism by which it causes vesication but does have great practical importance in the choice of a vesicant agent for chemical warfare. Although there are numerous physical and chemical characteristics that have a bearing on vesicant potency, two are important:

- Solid vesicants, e.g. crystalline Q (Sesqui mustard), although possessing significant theoretical potency, are in practice relatively ineffective. They tend to be either rubbed or blown off the skin before penetration can occur (Geiling, 1944).
- There appears to be an inverse relationship between a vesicant's potency and its vapour pressure. Thus, vesicant compounds with high vapour pressures cannot be used effectively (Renshaw, 1940).

A compound may be an intrinsically potent cytotoxic agent when introduced into the body, but it may be entirely innocuous when applied to the skin if it lacks the ability to penetrate. An example here is the comparison between sulphur mustard and its selenium analogue, bis-(β-chloroethyl)-selenide. Both agents are equally toxic on the basis of LCt_{50} values in mice, but the selenide derivative is several times less toxic than mustard when applied to the skin (Young, 1944).

Nagy *et al.* (1946) studied the penetration of small quantities (up to 500 μg) of bis(β-chloroethyl)-sulphide (H), ethyl-bis(β-chloroethyl) amine (EBA), tris-(β-chloroethyl) amine (TBA) and β-chloroethyl-benzylsulphide (benzyl-H) into human skin at 21–23°C and 30–31°C. Their results can be summarized in Table 30.2.

Using these data, the authors calculated the amount of each vesicant that must penetrate the skin in order to produce vesication in 50% of the cutaneous sites challenged. This value was designated the V_{50} value for that particular compound. These values are shown in Table 30.3.

For sulphur mustards a number of empirical correlations between molecular structure and vesicancy have been derived (Geiling, 1944; Cull-

TABLE 30.2

PENETRATION OF VESICANT COMPOUNDS

Compound	Temperature °C	Relative humidity %	Penetration rate $\mu g.cm^{-2}.min^{-1}$
H	21–23	46	1.4
	30–31	47–49	2.7
EBA	22	50–52	2.8
	30–31	47–49	5.1
TBA	22–23	45–48	0.18
	30–31	47–49	0.29
Benzyl-H	22	55–60	0.35

After, J.M. Nagy et al. Journal of General Physiology. **29**: 441–69, 1946.

TABLE 30.3

CALCULATED V_{50} VALUES FOR VESICANT COMPOUNDS

Compound	Temperature °C	V_{50} $\mu g.cm^{-2}.min^{-1}$
H TBA	21–30	6.0
H TBA	30–31	4.0–5.0
EBA	22	26.0
	30–31	28.0

After, J.M. Nagy et al. Journal of General Physiology. **29**: 441–69, 1946.

umbine, 1947), and these can be summarized as follows;

- β-Chlorothioethers are the most effective vesicants. Rearrangement of the constituent chlorine atoms is associated with a fall in vesicant potency.
- Vesicancy is reduced by substituting iodine, cyano-, thiocyano-, acetoxy- or oximino- groups for the chloro- groups.
- Vesicancy of thioether is decreased by any change in structure which lessens the basicity of the central sulphur atom.
- Q (Sesqui mustard) and its analogues with the general formula:

$$Cl\cdot CH_2\cdot CH_2\cdot S\cdot(CH_2)_n\cdot S\cdot CH_2\cdot CH_2\cdot Cl$$

are more vesicant than sulphur mustard if n = 1–5. For values of n > 5, vesicancy falls markedly.
- All of the highly vesicant compounds exhibit considerable lipid solubility.

THE HISTOPATHOLOGY OF VESICANT-INJURED SKIN

The gross and microscopic descriptions of human skin injured by vesicant agents, and sulphur mustard in particular, have not altered in detail since the original descriptions by Warthin and Weller in 1919 and Cullumbine in 1947. Application of the relatively new techniques of enzyme histochemistry, molecular biology and immunohistochemistry to the study of the pathogenesis and resolution of mustard injury has only just begun. Compared to the research into the aetiology of similar human blistering diseases, such as epidermolysis bullosa (Eady, 1987; Lin and Carter, 1989) and lichen planus pemphigoides (Gawkrodger et al., 1989; Wilsteed et al., 1991); the elucidation of the molecular pathology of vesicant-induced blistering is in its early stages.

Since the early descriptions of human casualties, there have been numerous studies of vesication in experimental animals, the hope being the discovery of a model system in which the development and healing of mustard-induced cutaneous injury can be studied. Recently, three animal models have been proposed that have renewed optimism in finding appropriate methods to study the interaction between mustard and the skin. Papirmeister et al. (1984) have described well-formed blisters in human skin grafted to athymic nude mice, whilst Mershon et al. (1990) have produced microblisters in the skin of euthymic hairless guinea-pigs. The latter model responds in very similar ways to sulphur mustard challenge in domestic pigs, a model recently exploited by Mitcheltree et al. (1989). These three models clearly need further validation but are currently the only ones available.

Sulphur mustard cutaneous injury in animals

The most comprehensive description of the pathology of vesicant agents in animals was given by Vögt et al. (1984). This group studied the pathological effects of sulphur mustard on the skin of rabbits and guinea-pigs dosed with 25–250 $\mu g/cm^2$ liquid mustard. Their results can be summarized as follows:

- *Evolution of the visible lesion (macroscopy).* The treated cutaneous site showed erythema within 30–60 minutes of the application and spread beyond the treated site after 4 hours. The lesion became oedematous 5–8 hours postexposure, and by 8 hours, this feature had also spread well beyond the initially exposed site. The centre of the lesion showed blanching followed by petechial haemorrhage at 24–48 hours. Marked epidermal necrosis accompanied by a serofibrinous exudate was noted 48–72 hours postexposure (Figure 30.4).

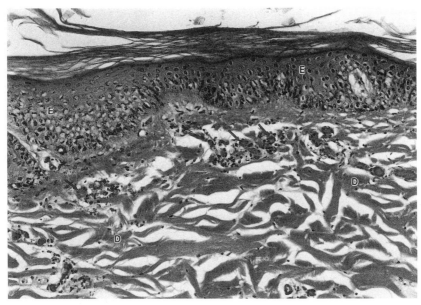

Figure 30.4 The early stages in the development of a sulphur mustard vapour injury in the Yucatan mini-pig at 24 hours post-exposure. The cells comprising the epidermis (E) already show advanced degeneration, nuclear pyknosis and focal cytoplasmic vacuolation. The individual collagen bundles of dermis (D) are forced apart by the accumulation of oedema fluid and the capillaries in the papillary dermis are congested and lined by degenerate endothelium (arrows). (Harris' Haematoxylin & Eosin (H&E), × 200.)

This surface exudate, along with the dead epidermis, had formed a well-circumscribed, adherent scab at 3–5 days; by this time erythema and oedema had subsided. Re-epithelialization began from the wound edges and undamaged hair follicles within the superficial reticular dermis and by 10–14 days had caused the surface scab to separate.

- *Microscopic observations.* The earliest changes were noted at 30–60 minutes postexposure and consisted of swelling of the basal epidermal cells and dilatation of the endoplasmic reticulum of fibroblasts within the papillary dermis. By 9 hours, cellular damage was profound with focal necrosis of the epidermis. A biphasic increase in vascular permeability was noted; the initial increase was short lived and appeared to involve only superficial postcapillary venules. A larger and more diffuse leakage ensued after a few hours and coincided with the oedematous phase noted macroscopically.

Early acute inflammatory changes were seen within 1 hour of exposure and consisted predominantly of the margination and emigration of neutrophil polymorphs; the magnitude of this reaction contrasts markedly to that described in humans by Renshaw (1940) and Rice and West (1987, unpublished observations). Migration of cells initially began from the postcapillary venules and in all other respects matched the classical descriptions of the acute inflammatory process (Ryan and Majno, 1977). Macrophages were not evident until 24–36 hours postexposure.

- *The effect of corticosteroids.* The experiments included the investigation of the effect of topically applied hydrocortisone. It was found that although it was possible to reduce the extent of the swelling around the injured sites, the application had no effect on the time-course of the development of the established lesion or its subsequent healing. It is well known that both topical and systemic steroids prolong the various stages of the healing process, and it is surprising that the healing time was not delayed in the treated animals.

Experiments conducted by the author using New Zealand white rabbits exposed to sulphur mustard vapour (at doses ranging from 32 to 320 µg/cm^2) have largely confirmed the results of Vögt *et al.* (1984). These studies have extended to encompass the healing phase of the lesion, and by the use of monoclonal, anti-human antibodies to basement membrane components (type-IV collagen and laminin) attempts have been made to study in detail the structural changes that underlie the development of the cutaneous lesion and its healing phase. The main conclusions of this work can be summarized as follows:

- In occasional animals examined at 9 hours postexposure small microblisters were produced that were similar in structure to those previously described in hairless guinea-pigs and domestic swine (Mitcheltree *et al.*, 1989; Mershon *et al.*, 1990). The blister roof was composed of intact but degenerating epidermal cells and, by the use of immunohistochemical techniques, it was demonstrated that the floor of the blister was formed by an intact basement membrane resting on immunologically altered papillary dermal collagen (Figures 30.5 and 30.6).

- Full-thickness epidermal and papillary dermal necrosis were evident by 48 hours postexposure. By 7 days, slender tongues of regenerative epidermis had begun to appear at the wound edges and were migrating towards the centre of the ulcer beneath the superficial surface scab.
- By 14 days postexposure, re-epithelialization of the lesion was complete. The regenerative

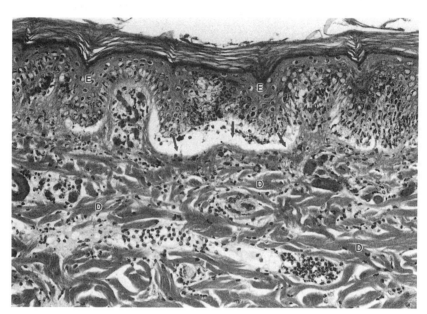

Figure 30.5 A more advanced sulphur mustard vapour injury at 48 hours postexposure. In addition to the features outlined in Figure 30.3, there is now a heavy acute inflammatory cell infiltrate throughout the dermis (D) and the epidermis (E) is focally separating from the underlying papillary dermis (arrows). (H&E, × 200.)

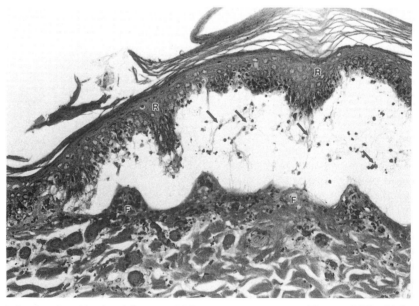

Figure 30.6 The fully developed microblister at 72 hours postexposure. The roof (R) of blister is composed of intact but degenerate epidermal cells and the floor (F) of degerate papillary dermal collagen and congested and necrotic papillary dermal capillaries. The blister cavity contains strands of cytoplasmic debris, red cells and occasional acute inflammatory cells (arrows). (H&E, × 200.)

epidermis at this time was hyperplastic showing acanthosis, hyperkeratosis, focal parakeratosis and dyskeratosis.

The lack of fully developed blistering in many experimental animal species has been appreciated for many years and many theories have been proposed to explain this difference in response between human and animal skin. McAdams (1956), like many other authors, stressed the general inability to duplicate the phenomenon of mustard vesication in laboratory and domestic animals. The experiments he conducted consisted of exposing suckling rats (hairless until the seventh day of life), rabbits and rats following chemical depilation and suckling pigs up to 10 days of age, to sulphur mustard using a vapour cup method: the subsequent lesions were examined histologically. McAdams concluded that the separation of the epidermis from the dermis was the result of basal cell destruction and that the differences between human and animal skin with respect to blistering was attributable to the action of the sweat glands. He commented upon the sparing of sweat glands, and the coiled ducts in particular, in human vesication. A similar observation had been made by Axelrod and Hamilton (1947) during their studies to localize mustard in the skin using autoradiography some 9 years earlier.

Flesch *et al.* (1952) believed that the relative thinness of the epidermis common to most laboratory animals, and the anchoring of the epidermis afforded by a high density of hair follicles, were important factors in explaining the differences in response to challenge between human and animal skin. However, although many laboratory animals do not blister when challenged, there are descriptions of blistering in perfused amphibian skin (Dixon and Needham, 1946) and in ducklings (Mirsky and Goldman, 1943).

The observation of focal blistering in the skin of a fur-bearing mammal such as a rabbit (R. Knight and P. Rice, 1990, unpublished observations), although not reproducible and of little use as an experimental model, is a unique and interesting observation.

Sulphur mustard injury in human skin

Gross pathology

Perhaps the best gross descriptions of human skin lesions are those of casualties from the First World War (Warthin and Weller, 1919; Winternitz and Finney, 1920; Schrafl, 1938; Cullumbine, 1947). More recently, the author has had the opportunity to observe the gross lesions and microscopy of several Iranian casualties injured during the recent conflict in the Middle East (P. Rice and T. West, 1987, unpublished observations). The appearances of such injuries may be summarized as follows:

- The lesion is a chemical burn and unlike that seen in thermal, electrical or corrosive (acid/alkali) burns. There is little or no thrombosis of vessels, but a great degree of moistness of the affected area. The coagulated appearance of thermal injuries is not a feature of vesicant injury (Pearson, 1964; Takigawa and Ofuji, 1977).
- The skin at first is pale but then becomes erythematous within a few hours of exposure. Vesication is not usually seen until the second day and progresses thereafter for several more days.
- Scab formation begins within 7 days once the early blisters begin to degenerate. The skin may be made to vesicate in areas of erythema by slight trauma, e.g. on rubbing, and this phenomenon is known as Nikolsky's sign. It does not imply the persistence of active vesicant (Sulzberger and Katz, 1943).
- Four to 6 days after exposure, necrosis is complete and separation of necrotic slough begins. The accompanying oedema and erythema may persist.
- By 16–20 days, separation of slough is complete and re-epithelialization has begun. Healing may take 3–8 weeks postexposure to be complete and the casualty is often left with depigmented areas surrounded by zones of hyperpigmentation.

Based on these descriptions it is possible to discern two striking differences between the lesions seen in animals and those observed in man. Firstly, the production of grossly visible blisters occurs regularly in man but not in animals. These blisters may enlarge by coalescence and may appear several days after the removal of the casualty from the affected environment. Secondly, the healing time in man is considerably longer than that seen in animals (Schrafl, 1938; Renshaw, 1940). Several attempts have been made to explain the differences between animal and human skin with respect to vesication, and these have been alluded to previously (Flesch *et al.*, 1952; McAdams, 1956). The reasons for the differences in healing time remain obscure (Papirmeister *et al.*, 1984).

Microscopy and ultrastructural observations of human vesicant injuries

Although microscopic descriptions of First World War vesicant-agent-induced lesions exist, more recently Papirmeister *et al.* (1985) have described a model (full-thickness human neonatal foreskin grafted to congenitally athymic nude mice) which appears to reproduce very accurately the findings previously described. The model has also allowed lesions to be studied at the ultrastructural level in an attempt to reveal additional information about the exact histogenesis of vesicant-induced cutaneous injuries. The observations made from this model can be summarized as follows;

General observations The severity of cutaneous injury appears to depend on the degree of alkylation occuring in the skin (Renshaw, 1940). Several dose regimens of liquid sulphur mustard were used, based on data derived from earlier studies by Renshaw (1947) as follows:

$20 \ \mu g/cm^2$ = mild injury
$60–120 \ \mu g/cm^2$ = moderate injury
$635 \ \mu g/cm^2$ = severe injury.

At these doses, no systemic effects were noted as the maximum dose only represented 25% of the percutaneous LD_{50} dose.

Microscopic observations

- There were minimal changes at 4 hours, consistent with the known latency for sulphur mustard cutaneous injuries. By 7 hours there was evidence of vacuolation of basal keratinocytes which had progressed to focal necrosis accompanied by congestion and oedema of the dermis by 12 hours.
- Widespread, multifocal necrosis of the epidermis accompanied by early acute inflammation was noted at 24 hours. By 48 hours, full-thickness necrosis had obliterated all normal cellular features, and there was a striking polymorph infiltrate at the base of the graft.
- Animals of the high-dose group showed dermo-epidermal separation at 24 hours with the formation of a subepidermal blister at 48 hours. The only deviation from true human injury was the impression of almost complete re-epithelialization of ulcerated lesions by 6 days postexposure.

Ultrastructural observations The use of the electron microscope confirmed and extended the observations outlined above and affirmed that the development of the injury was both dose and time dependant. A definite sequence of morphological changes was described:

- Condensation of heterochromatin and loss of euchromatin.
- Blebbing of the nuclear membrane with the formation of perinuclear vacuoles.
- Swelling of the endoplasmic reticulum and disintegration of polysomes.
- Loss of the integrity of the cell membrane.
- Leakage of organelles into the extracellular space.
- Disruption of the anchoring filaments of the hemidesmosomes.

The authors concluded that sulphur mustard injury to human skin commences at the level of the basal keratinocyte and thus confirmed the original theories of McAdams (1956). They also drew some parallels with thermal injury, which is also thought to act by disrupting the basal epidermal layer (Cullumbine, 1947).

RECENT DEVELOPMENTS

There is no specific therapy for sulphur mustard poisoning; the sole aim of clinical management in such cases is to maintain vital organ systems and alleviate symptoms. Skin burns may be severe and occupy extensive areas of the body surface. The naturally moist areas of the body such as the genitalia, perineal regions, groins, lower back and axillae often prove to be the most severely affected areas and crops of fresh blisters may appear at any time up to 2 weeks after exposure. The burns themselves tend to be superficial and will heal slowly without active treatment. However, experience in the clinical management of several Iranian casualties from the Iran–Iraq war (1984–7) demonstrated that those with severe burns will require weeks of hospital care followed by lengthy convalescence and that, despite the superficial nature of the burn, it is all too easy to underestimate the period of care for such patients.

The current clinical management strategy

The current clinical management of sulphur mustard cutaneous injury is essentially that for a similar degree of thermal burn (Mellor *et al.*, 1991) but it is always important to bear in mind that the signs and symptoms of injury will not be evident for several hours after exposure. The overall management can be summarized as follows:

- For areas of erythema and minor blistering, bland lotions such as calamine are useful.
- Topical bacteriostatic agents such as 1% silver sulphadiazine (Flamazine) cream were used on Iranian casualties to reduce the incidence of secondary infection once the blisters had ruptured.
- Moderately severe pain and itching are common problems once blisters have developed and may be managed by the use of mild analgesics, antihistamines and small doses of diazepam. Occasionally, some cases experience severe pain and these may require narcotic analgesics such as morphine. Newman-Taylor (1991) reported that carbamazapine proved valuable in alleviating pain in one patient and that its use allowed the withdrawal of narcotic analgesics.
- Dilute topical steroids have proved beneficial in relieving irritation and reducing the attendant oedema at exposed sites; their use in human casualties appeared to have little or no effect on the subsequent rate of healing of the lesions, so confirming the earlier observations made by Vögt *et al.* (1984).
- Fluid replacement is calculated in the same way as for a thermal burn although, unlike a thermal burn, large amounts of fluid loss will only occur once the blisters have formed, rather than in the first 24 hours.

- Although the time to healing may be long, the evidence suggests that the eventual scar is softer and more pliable than that seen in thermal injuries. Wound contracture does not appear to be a major problem in this context despite the predilection for the naturally moist areas such as the axillae and groin.
- Numerous other drugs and regimes, including bathing in fresh human breast milk, have been suggested (Hendrickx and Hendrickx, 1990), but there is no evidence that these have any therapeutic value in established cases.

Postexposure surgical intervention in the management of mustard burns

Based on our previous experiences with Iranian casualties and the previous literature (Shrafl, 1938; Renshaw, 1940; Willems, 1989), it was recognized that large, full-thickness burns heal very slowly and may ultimately require skin grafting to achieve epithelial coverage of the ulcerated site. The success of grafting, assessed either by an improvement in the healing time or by the survival of the graft, will be determined by the efficiency of the tangential excision in cutting back to healthy tissue not showing sulphur mustard-induced damage. To ensure that excision is complete both the depth and lateral extent of alkylation in the skin would need to be determined.

Histological examination of mustard-induced cutaneous injuries in rabbits (R. Knight and P. Rice, 1990, unpublished observations) has shown that the delayed rate of healing may be due, in part, to two distinct mechanisms:

- Alkylation of epidermal cells extends beyond the immediate region of exposure; although cells in this area may not ultimately die, the level of alkylation may be sufficient to delay or even prevent cell replication. Re-epithelialization of ulcerated lesions relies partly on the replication of cells from the undamaged epidermis at the edge of the lesion and partly from intact hair shafts in the base (Willems, 1989).
- In addition to achieving effective epidermal regeneration, re-epithelialization itself is dependent on the presence of an appropriate substrate on which regeneration can occur (Woodley *et al.*, 1985; Shakespeare and Shakespeare, 1987). The papillary dermis and basement membrane are vital in this respect and not only provide a structural scaffold for the epidermis but also act as signals for the subsequent differentiation of the overlying epidermis (Fleming, 1991). Immunohistochemical staining of the papillary dermis in rabbits has shown that the collagen at this site is altered by exposure to sulphur mustard, and in this altered state it may no longer function normally.

Recently, some preliminary wound healing studies, conducted in the author's laboratory using Yucatan miniature swine, have been directed towards establishing a more normal rate of wound healing by removing alkylated and sublethally injured epidermis and superficial papillary dermis. Rather than resorting to formal excision, the technique of dermal abrasion has been employed; the technique is currently used in cases of severe facial acne and is well recognized in the management of deep dermal burns (Holmes and Rayner, 1984). The Yucatan miniature swine was selected as the experimental model, on the basis that it has previously proved valid for a range of cutaneous toxicity tests (Khan, 1984), and preliminary experiments had shown that it was an appropriate model for vesication in human skin, responding to sulphur mustard challenge with full-thickness epidermal necrosis and microvesication. The preliminary results can be summarized as follows;

- Standardized sulphur mustard lesions are produced by exposure to 12 μmol/cm^2 mustard vapour under occluded conditions over a total exposure area of 10 cm^2. At 3 days postexposure, the established lesion is dermally abraded by gently scrubbing with wet emery cloth until breakthrough bleeding from viable capillary loops in the base of the lesion is achieved.
- During the dermabrasion procedure there is extension of erythema beyond the originally exposed site to given an ovoid mantle of acutely inflamed skin. Within this mantle, and during dermabrasion, we have witnessed the appearance of small, 0.2–0.3-cm-diameter blisters which on histological examination appear to be intra-epidermal. It is thought that these represent Nikolsky's sign and are a result of sublethal damage to the epidermis.
- Histological examination of the dermally abraded sites immediately after the procedure has confirmed that both the epidermis and papillary dermis are totally removed and that surface bleeding is occurring from intact healthy capillaries in the bed of the lesion.
- Comparison of abraded sites with those left untreated at 7 days postexposure has revealed that although the untreated site remains completely unhealed and covered by a surface layer of necrotic debris, the abraded site shows extensive re-epithelialization (up to 25% of the initial total exposed area).

Though these are preliminary results and further, longer-term studies are required, they are encouraging. The application of simple methods of treatment apparently enhances the rate of healing of mustard burns; if these results are confirmed in patients then an important step forward in the management of this form of chemical warfare injury will have been made.

Mustard gas was developed as a chemical warfare agent more than 75 years ago. Despite intensive study, little advance in the methods recommended for the management of skin lesions has been made. Recent studies which have involved a return to the study of the mechanics of wound healing have suggested that healing might be enhanced by the relatively simple measure of dermabrasion. The clinical value of such an approach will not be confirmed unless and until mustard gas is used again in war. Despite progress towards a Chemical Weapons Convention, such use cannot be ruled out.

REFERENCES

Alexander S.F. (1947). Medical report of the Bari harbour mustard casualties. *Milit. Surg.*, **101**, 1–17.

Aso K., Orenberg E.K., Farber E.M. (1975). Reduced epidermal cyclic AMP accumulation following prostaglandin stimulation: its possible role in the physiology of psoriasis. *J. Investi. Dermatol.*, **65**, 375–8.

Axelrod D.J., Hamilton J.G. (1947). Radio-autographic studies of the distribution of lewisite and mustard gas in skin and eye tissues. *Am. J. Pathol.*, **23**, 389–98.

Barron E.S.G., Meyer J., Miller Z.B. (1948). The metabolism of the skin. Effects of vesicants. *J. Invest. Dermatol.*, **11**, 97–118.

Berenblum I. (1935). Experimental inhibition of tumour induction by mustard gas and other compounds. *J. Pathol. Bacteriol.*, **40**, 549–58.

Berenblum I., Wormall A. (1939). The immunological properties of proteins treated with b,b'-dichlorodiethyl-sulphide and b,b'-dichlorodiethyl sulphone. *Biochem. J.*, **33**, 75–80.

Berenblum I., Kendal L.P., Orr J.W. (1936). Tumour metabolism in the presence of anti-carcinogenic substances. *J. Pathol. Bacteriol.*, **41**, 709–15.

Bosman F.T., Cleutgens J., Beek C., Havenith M. (1989). Basement membrane heterogeneity. *Histochem. J.*, **21**, 629–33.

Briggamann R.A., Schechter N.M., Fraki J., Lazarus G.S. (1984). Degradation of the epidermo-dermal junction by proteolytic enzymes from human skin and polymorphonuclear leucocytes. *J. Exp. Med.*, **160**, 1027–42.

Brody I. (1952). The ultrastructure of the tonofilaments in the keratinisation process of normal human epidermis. *J. Ultrastruct. Res.*, **2**, 482–511.

Brooks S.C., Lang L.K., Godefroi M.S. (1968). Metabolic studies on skin. III. Lipid metabolism in mouse skin during the hair growth cycle. *J. Invest. Dermatol.*, **50**, 161–70.

Burge S.M., Williams-Cederholm S., Ryan T.J. (1989). Plasminogen and plasminogen activators in human skin in health and disease. *Br. J. Dermatol.*, **120**, 307.

Burgeson R.E. (1988). Basement membranes. *Annu. Rev. Cell Biol.* **4**, 551–7.

Colardyn F., De Keyser H., Ringoir S., De Bersaques J. (1986). Clinical observation and therapy of injuries with vesicants. *J. Exp. Clin. Toxicol.*, **6**, 237–46.

Crandon J.H. (1940). Experimental human scurvy. *New Engl. J. Med.*, **223**, 353.

Cullumbine H. (1947). Medical aspects of mustard gas poisoning. *Nature (Lond.)*, **159**, 151.

Dixon M. (1943). *The Phosphokinase Theory of Vesication; Its Present Position. Report No. 19 (Y7483).* Cambridge: Cambridge Biochemistry Laboratory.

Dixon M., Needham D.M. (1946). Biomedical research on chemical warfare agents. *Nature (Lond.)*, **158**, 432–8.

Eady R.A. (1987). Babes, blisters and basement membranes: from sticky molecules to epidermolysis bullosa. *Clin. Exp. Dermatol.*, **12**, 161–70.

Einbinder J.M., Walzer R.A., Mandl I. (1966). Epidermo-dermal separation with proteolytic enzymes. *J. Investi. Dermatol.*, **46**, 492–504.

Fleming S. (1991). Cell adhesion and epithelial differentiation. *J. Pathol.*, **164**, 95–100.

Flesch P., Goldstone S.B., Weidman F.D. (1952). Blister formation and separation of the epidermis from the corium in laboratory animals. *J. Invest. Dermatol.*, **18**, 187–92.

Foulkes C.H. (1934). "Gas". *The Story of the Special Brigade*. London: William Blackwood and Son.

Fox M., Scott M. (1980). The genetic toxicology of nitrogen and sulphur mustard. *Mutat. Res.*, **75**, 131–68.

Fraki J.E., Lazarus G.S., Gilgor R.S. et al. (1983). Correlation of epidermal plasminogen activator activity with disease activity in psoriasis. *Br. J. Dermatol.*, **108**, 39–44.

Fraser R.D.B., MacRae T.P. (1980). In *The Skin of Vertebrates* (Spearman R.I., Riley P.A., eds). London: Academic, pp. 67–86.

Fraser R.D.B., MacRae T.P., Suzuki E. (1976). Structure of the alpha-keratin microfibril. *J. Molec. Biol.*, **108**, 432–5.

Frenkel M.J., Lock R.A., Rogers G.E. (1979). Studies on the ribonucleic acid coding for the keratin complex of hair. *Proc. Aust. Biochem. Soc.*, **12**, 89.

Fuchs E., Green H. (1980). Changes in keratin gene expression during terminal differentiation of the keratinocyte. *Cell*, **19**, 1033–42.

Gales K.A., Gross C.L., Krebs R.C., Smith W.J. (1989). In *Proceedings of the 1989 Medical Defence Bioscience Review (PMBR), USAMRDC, 15/17 August 1989. MD: USAMRICD*, pp. 437–40.

Gawkrodger D.J., Stavropoulos P.G., McLaren K.M., Buxton P.K. (1989). Bullous lichen planus and lichen planus pemphigoides – clinicopathological comparisons. *Clin. Exp. Dermatol.*, **14**, 150–3.

Geiling F.M. (1944). OSRD Informal Report. Division 9, National Defense Research Committee of the Office of Scientific Research and Development (OSRD).

Goetinck P.F. (1980). In *The Skin of Vertebrates* (Spearman R.I., Riley P.A., eds). London: Academic, pp. 169–84.

Greaves M.W. (1972). Prostaglandins and the epidermis. *Br. J. Dermatol.*, **87**, 161–2.

Gross C.L., Meier H.L., Papirmeister B. et al. (1985). Sulphur mustard lowers nicotinamide adenine dinucleotide levels in human skin grafted to athymic nude mice. *Toxicol. Appl. Pharmacol.*, **81**, 85–90.

Guilhou J.J., Meynadier J., Clot J. (1978). New concepts in the pathogenesis of psoriasis. *Br. J. Dermatol.*, **98**, 585–92.

Guthrie F. (1860). On some derivatives from the olefins. *J. Chem. Soc. (Lond.)*, **XII**, 109.

Haldane J.B.S. (1925). *Callinicus, A Defence of Chemical Warfare*. London: Kegan, Paul, Trench, Trubner.

Hashimoto K., Shafran K.M., Webber P.S. et al. (1983). Anti-cell surface autoantibody stimulates plasminogen activator activity of human epidermal cells. *J. Exp. Med.*, **157**, 259–72.

Hashimoto K., Wun T-C., Baird J. et al. (1989). Characterisation of keratinocyte plasminogen activator inhibitors and demonstration of prevention of pemphigus IgG-induced acantholysis by a purified plasminogen activator inhibitor. *J. Invest. Dermatol.*, **92**, 310–14.

Heldner K.M., Hambridge K.M. (1975). Zinc therapy. *New Engl. J. Med.*, **17**, 879.

Hendrickx A., Hendrickx B. (1990). Management of war gas casualties. *Lancet*, **336**, 1248.

Holmes J.D., Rayner C.R.W. (1984). The technique of late dermabrasion for deep dermal burns. Implications for planning treatment. *Burns*, **10**, 349–54.

History of the Great War – Medical Services (1923). *Diseases of the War*, Vol. II. London: HMSO, p. 291.

Human Estimates Committee (1960). Inclosure to Minutes of Meeting of CWL Committee on Human Estimates. 'The Use of the Detector Kit to Estimate Allowable Exposure Time Without Masks for Resting and Active Men'. March, 1960.

Ireland M.M. (1926). Medical aspects of gas warfare. In *The Medical Department of the United States Army in the World War*, Vd. XIV. Washington.

Isserhof R.R., Rifkin D.B. (1983). Plasminogen is present in the basal layer of the epidermis. *J. Invest. Dermatol.*, **80**, 217.

Jarrett A. (1973). *The Physiology and Pathophysiology of the Skin*. New York: Academic.

Jarrett A., Spearman R.I. (1964). *Histochemistry of the skin: Psoriasis*. London: Hodder.

Jendryczko A., Drozdz M. (1985). Action of phenylalanine mustard on collagen *in vivo*. *Biomed. Biochim. Acta*, **44**, 497–501.

Jørgensen P.L., Skou J.C., Solomonson L.P. (1971). Purification and characterisation of $(Na^+ + K^+)$-ATP_{ase}. *Biochim. Biophys. Acta*, **233**, 381–94.

Jouvenaz G.H., Nugteren D.H., Beerthuis A.M., van Dorp D.A. (1970). A sensitive method for the determination of prostaglandins by gas chromatography with electron capture detection. *Biochim. Biophys. Acta*, **202**, 231–4.

Juarez-Salinas H., Sims J.L., Jacobson M.K. (1979). Poly (ADP-ribose) levels in carcinogen-treated cells. *Nature (Lond.)*, **282**, 740–1.

Kahl F.R., Pearson R.D. (1967). Ultrastructural studies on experimental vesication. II. Collagenase. *J. Invest. Dermatol.*, **49**, 616–31.

Katz S.I. (1984). The epidermal basement membrane zone: structure, ontogeny and role in disease. *J. Am. Acad. Dermatol.*, **11**, 1025–37.

Keene D.R., Sakai L.Y., Lunstrum G.P. et al. (1987). Type-VII collagen forms an extended network of anchoring fibrils. *J. Cell Biol.*, **104**, 611–21.

Khan M.A. (1984). Mini-pig: advantages and disadvantages as a model in toxicity testing. *J. Am. Coll. Toxicol.*, **3**, 337–42.

Kligman A.M. (1964). In *The Epidermis* (Montagna W., Lobitz W.S., eds). New York: Academic, pp. 387–433.

Lasky R.A., Fairman P., Blow J.J. (1989). S-phase of the cell cycle. *Science*, **246**, 609–14.

Lazarus G.S., Hatcher V.B., Levine N. (1975). Lysosomes and the skin. *J. Invest. Dermatol.*, **65**, 259–71.

Leigh I.M., Purkis P.E., Bruckner-Tuderman L. (1987).

LH-7.2 monoclonal antibody detects type-VII collagen in the sublamina densa zone of ectodermally derived epithelia, including skin. *Epithelia*, **1**, 17–29.

Leprince P., Rogister B., Moonen G. (1989). A clorimetric assay for the stimultaneous measurement of plasminogen activators and plasminogen activator inhibitors in serum free conditioned media from cultured cells. *Ann. Biochem.*, **177**, 341–6.

Levenson S.M. (1950). The healing of soft tissue wounds: the effects of nutrition, anaemia and age. *Surgery*, **28**, 905.

Lin A.N., Carter D.M. (1989). Epidermolysis bullosa: when the skin falls apart. *J. Paediatr.*, **114**, 349–55.

Lindahl U., Hook M. (1978). Glycosaminoglycans and their binding to biological macromolecules. *Annu. Rev. Biochem.*, **47**, 385–417.

Liotta L.A., Goldfab R.H., Brundage R. (1981). Effect of plasminogen activator (urokinase), plasmin and thrombin on glycoprotein and collagenous components of basement membrane. *Cancer Res.*, **41**, 4629–36.

Lunstrum G.P., Sakai L.Y., Keene D.R. et al. (1986). Large complex globular domains of type-VII protocollagen contribute to the structure of anchoring fibrils. *J. Biochem. Chem.*, **261**, 9042–8.

MacKenzie I.C. (1969). Ordered structure of the stratum corneum of the mammalian skin. *Nature*, **222**, 881–3.

Magnus I.A. (1956). Observations on the thiol content of abnormal stratum corneum in psoriasis and other conditions. *Br. J. Dermatol.*, **68**, 243–51.

Malkinson F.D. (1964). In *The Epidermis* (Montagna W., Lobitz W.S., eds). New York: Academic, pp. 435–52.

Mandl H., Freilinger G. (1984). First report on victims of chemical warfare in the Gulf-war treated in Vienna. In *Proceedings of the First World Congress on Biological and Chemical Warfare, Ghent, Belgium*, pp. 330–40.

Marshall E.K., Lynch V., Smith H.W. (1918). On dichloroethylsulphide (mustard gas). II. Variations in susceptibility of the skin to dichloroethylsulphide. *J. Pharmacol. Exp. Ther.*, **12**, 291–301.

Martinez-Fernandez A., Amenta P. (1983). The basement membrane in pathology. *Lab. Invest.*, **48**, 656–77.

McAdams A.J. (1956). A study of mustard vesication. *J. Invest. Dermatol.*, **26**, 317–27.

McLoughlin C.B. (1963). In *Cell Differentiation* (Fogg G.E., ed.). Cambridge: Cambridge University Press, pp. 359–88.

McMaster P.C., Hogeboom G., Sulzberger M.B. et al. (1945). *Toxicological Basis for Controlling Levels of Sulphur Mustard in the environment*, Report No. OSRD 4853. Division 9, National Defense Research Committee of the Office of Scientific Research and Development (OSRD).

McNamara B.P., Owens E.J., Christensen M.K. et al. (1975). Special Publication No EB-SP-74030. DTIC No AD-A011 260. US Army Biomedical Laboratory, Aberdeen Proving Ground Maryland: 1975.

Medema J. (1982). Mustard gas: the science of H. *Nucl. Biol. Chem. Defence Technol. Int.*, **1**, (4), 66–71.

Meier H.L., Gross C.L., Papirmeister B. (1987). 2, 2'-Dichlorodiethyl sulfide (sulfur mustard) decreases NAD^+ levels in human keratinocytes. *Toxicol. Lett.*, **39**, 109–22.

Mellor S.G., Rice P., Cooper G.J. (1991). Vesicant burns. *Br. J. Plast. Surg.*, **44**, 434–7.

Mershon M.M., Mitcheltree L.W., Petrali J.P. et al. (1990). Hairless guinea-pig bioassay model for vesicant vapour exposure. *Fund. Appl. Toxicol.*, **15**, 622–30.

Meyer V. (1886). Versuche über die haltbarkeit von sublimatlosungen. *Berichte Deutsch. Chem. Gesellschaft.*, **1**, 1725–39.

Mier P.D., Cotton D.W.K. (1976). *The Molecular Biology of the Skin*. Oxford: Blackwell.

Mirsky I.A., Goldman L. (1943). The production of bullae in the skin of the duck. *Arch. Dermatol.*, **48**, 161–3.

Mitcheltree L.W., Mershon M.M., Wall H.G., Pulliman J.D. (1989). Microblister formation in vesicant-exposed pig skin. *J. Toxicol. (Cutan. Occ. Toxicol.)*, **8**, 309–19.

Mol M.A.E., Van de Ruit A-M., Kuivers A.W. (1989a). In *Proceedings of the 1989 Medical Defense Bioscience Review (PMBR), USAMRDC, 15/17 August 1989*, MD: USAMRICD, pp. 57–61.

Mol M.A.E., Van de Ruit A-M., Kluivers A.W. (1989b). NAD+ levels and glucose uptake of cured human epidermal cells exposed to sulphur mustard. *Toxicol. Appl. Pharmacol.*, **98**, 159–65.

Murnane J.C., Byfield J.E. (1981). Irreparable DNA cross-links and mammalian cell lethality with bifunctional alkylating agents. *Chem. Biol. Interac.*, **38**, 75–86.

Myhre-Jensen O., Astrup T. (1971). Fibrinolytic activity of squamous epithelium of the oral cavity and oesophagus of the rat, guinea-pig and rabbit. *Arch. Oral Biol.*, **16**, 1077.

Nagy S.M., Golumbic C., Stein W.H. et al. (1946). The penetration of vesicant vapours into human skin. *J. Gen. Physiol.*, **29**, 441–69.

Needham D.M., Dixon M. (1941). *The Metabolism of Normal and Vesicant Treated Skin*. Report No. 1 (U24815). Cambridge: Cambridge Biochemistry Laboratory.

Newman-Taylor A.J. (1991). Experience with mustard gas casualties. *Lancet*, **337**, 242.

Papirmeister B., Gross C.L., Petrali J.P., Hixson C.J. (1984). Pathology produced by sulphur mustard in human skin grafts on athymic nude mice. I. Gross and light microscopic changes. *J. Toxicol. (Cutan. Occul. Toxicol.)*, **3**, 371–91.

Papirmeister B., Gross C.L., Meier H.L. et al. (1985). Molecular basis for mustard-induced vesication. *Fund. Appl. Toxicol.*, **5**, (Suppl.), 134–49.

Papirmeister B., Feister A.J., Robinson S.I., Ford R.D. (eds.) (1991). Historical and Modern use of sulphur mustard in warfare. In *Medical Defense Against Mustard Gas*. Boston: CRC Press, pp. 1–9.

Pardee A.B. (1989). G_1 events and regulation of cell proliferation. *Science*, **246**, 603–8.

Parry E.J. (1921). In *The Chemistry of Essential Oils and Artificial Perfumes*, Vol. 1. London: Scott, Greenwood and Son.

Pauser G., Alloy A., Carvena M. et al. (1984). Lethal intoxication by wargases on Iranian soliders. Therapeutic interventions on survivors of mustard gas and mycotoxin immersion. In *Proceedings of the First World Congress on Biological and Chemical Warfare*, Ghent, Belgium, pp. 341–51.

PCS (Project Co-ordination Staff). (1946). *Technical Aspects of Chemical Warfare in the Field Parts 1 and 2*. Washington DC: Chemical Warfare Service.

Pearson R.W. (1964). Some observations on epidermolysis bullosa and experimental blisters. In *The Epidermis* (Montagna W., Lovitz W.C., eds.) New York: Academic, pp. 613–26.

Peters R.A. (1936). Effects of dichlorodiethyl-sulphone on brain respiration. *Nature (Lond.)*, **138**, 327–8.

Peters R.A., Wakelin R.W. (1947). Observations upon a compound of mustard gas and kerateine. *Biochem. J.*, **41**, 550–5.

Philips F.S. (1950). Recent contributions to the pharmacology of bis(2-haloethyl) amines and sulfides. *Pharmacol. Rev.*, **2**, 281–323.

Pirie A. (1947). The action of mustard gas on ox cornea collagen. *Biochem. J.*, **41**, 185–90.

Prottey C. (1977). Investigation of functions of essential fatty acids in the skin. *Br. J. Dermatol.*, **97**, 29–38.

Renshaw B. (1940). Mechanisms in the production of cutaneous injuries by sulphur and nitrogen mustards. In *Chemical Warfare Agents and Related Chemical Problems*, Vol. 1. Washington DC: US Office of Science Research and Development, National Defence Research Committee, pp. 479–518.

Renshaw B. (1947). Observations on the role of water in the susceptibility of human skin to injury by vesicant vapours. *J. Invest. Dermatol.*, **9**, 75–85.

Reynolds J.E. (ed.) (1977). Martindale. The Extra Pharmacopoeia, 27th edn. The Pharmaceutical Press.

Roberts J.J., Crathorn A.R., Brent T.P. (1968). Repair of alkylated DNA in mammalian cells. *Nature*, **218**, 970–2.

Rodriquez-Boulan E., Nelson W.J. (1989). Morphogenesis of the polarised epithelial cell phenotype. *Science*, **246**, 718–25.

Roitt I, Brostoff J, Male D. (eds.) (1988). Cell-mudiated immunology. In *Immunology*. Edinburgh: Churchill Livingstone, pp. 11.1–12.

Ryan G.B., Majno G. (1977). Acute Inflammation – a review. *Am. J. Pathol.*, **86**, 184–275.

Sanders K.M., Innace J.K., Gross C.L., Smith W.J. (1989). In *Proceedings of the 1989 Medical Defense Bioscience Review (PMBR), USAMRDC, 15/17 August 1989*. MD: USAMRICD, pp. 419–22.

Savage J.R., Brekon G. (1981). Differential effects of sulphur mustard on S-phase cells of primary fibroblast cultures from Syrian hamsters. *Mutat. Res.*, **34**, 375–87.

Savion N., Disatnik M-H., Nero Z. (1987). Murine macrophage heparanase: inhibition and comparison with metastatic tumour cells. *J. Cell. Physiol.*, **130**, 77–84.

Schrafl A. (1938). The symptoms, prophylaxis and the therapy of mustard injuries to the skin. *Protar*, **4**, 111–18.

Sellers A., Murphy G. (1981). In *International Review of Connective Tissue Research* (Hall D.A., Jackson D.S., eds.). New York: Academic, pp. 151–90.

Sengel P. (1976). Morphogenesis of Skin. Cambridge: Cambridge University Press.

Shakespeare V.A., Shakespeare P.G. (1987). Growth of cultured human keratinocytes on fibrous dermal collagen: a scanning electron microscopic study. *Burns*, **13**, 343.

Shoshan S. (1981). In *International Review of Connective Tissue Research*. (Hall D.A., Jackson D.S., eds.). New York: Academic, p. 426.

Singer K.H., Hashimoto K., Lensen P.K. et al. (1985). Pathogenesis of autoimmunity in pemphigus. *Annu. Rev. Immunol.*, **3**, 87.

Skolnik P., Eaglstein W.H., Ziboh V.A. (1977). Human essential fatty acid deficiency. *Arch. Dermatol.*, **113**, 939–41.

Smulson M.E. (1989). In *Proceedings of the 1989 Medical*

Defense Bioscience Review (PMBR), USAMRDC, 15/17 August 1989. MD: USAMRICD, pp. 361–71.

Spearman R.I. (1977). In *The Physiology and Pathophysiology of the Skin*, 4th (Jarrett, A., ed.). London: Academic, pp. 1495–513.

Spearman R.I. (1980). In *The Skin of Vertebrates* (Spearman R.I., Riley P.A., ed.). London: Academic, pp. 127–35.

Stenn K.S. (1988). In *Cell and Tissue Biology. A Textbook of Histology*. (Werss L., ed.), 6th edn. Baltimore: Urban and Schwarzenberg, pp. 540–72.

Sulzberger M.B., Katz J.H. (1943). The absence of skin irritants in the contents of vesicles. *US Navy Med. Bull.*, **43**, 1258–62.

Takigawa M., Ofuji S. (1977). Early changes in human epidermis following thermal burn: an electron microscopic study. *Acta Derm. (Stockh.)*, **57**, 187.

Thompson R.H.S. (1942). The significance of cholinesterase inhibition in poisoning by vesicants. Report No 62 (W8399). Oxford University.

Thompson J.F., Young H.D., Savit J. et al. (1945). In *Tests for Vesicancy on Human Skin*. Report No. OSRD 5194. Division 9, National Defense Research Committee of the Office of Scientific Research and Development (OSRD).

Thompson R.H.S. (1940). *The Respiration of Rat Skin after Damage with Sulphur Mustard*. Report U9434. Oxford: Department of Biochemistry, Oxford University.

Thompson R.H.S. (1947). The action of chemical vesicants on cholinesterase. *J. Physiol.*, **105**, 370–81.

United Nations Security Council (1984). *Report of the Specialists Appointed by the Secretary General to Investigate Allegations by the Islamic Republic of Iran Concerning the use of Chemical Weapons*, 26 March 1984. UN Report S\16433.

United Nations Security Council (1986). *Report of the Mission Dispatched by the Secretary General to Investigate Allegations of the Use of Chemical Weapons in the Conflict between Iran and Iraq*, 12 March 1986. UN Report S\17911.

United Nations Security Council (1987). *Report of the Mission Dispatched by the Secretary General to Investigate Allegations of the use of Chemical Weapons in the Conflict between the Islamic Republics of Iran and Iraq*, 08 May 1987. UN Report S\18852.

US Army and US Airforce (1945). Military chemistry and chemical compounds. Army Field Manual No 39, Airforce Regulations No. AFR 355–7. Washington, DC: Headquarters, Department of the Army.

Urmacher C. (1990). Histology of normal skin. *Am. J. Surg. Pathol.*, **14**, 671–86.

Vedder E.B. (1925). Medical aspects of chemical warfare. In *The Medical Aspects of Chemical Warfare*. Baltimore: Williams and Wilkins.

Virchow R. (1860). *Cellular Pathology*. London: John Churchill, p. 33.

Vögt R.F., Dannenberg A.M., Schofield B.H. et al. (1984). The pathogenesis of skin lesions caused by sulphur mustard. *Fund. Appl. Toxicol.*, **4** (Suppl.), 71–83.

Vrako R. (1974). Basal lamina scaffold: anatomy and significance for maintenance of orderly tissue structure. *Am. J. Pathol.*, **77**, 314–46.

Warthin A.S., Weller C.V. (1919). *The Medical Aspects of Mustard Gas Poisoning*. London: Henry Kimpton.

Werb Z., Gordon S. (1975). Secretion of a specific collagenase by stimulated macrophages. *J. Exp. Med.*, **142**, 346–60.

Wessel N.K. (1967). Differentiation of epidermis and epidermal derivatives. *New Engl. J. Medi.*, **277**, 21–33.

Wheatley V.R., Hodgins L.T., Coon W.M. (1970). Cutaneous lipogenesis. I. Evaluation of model systems and utilisation of acetate, citrate and glucose as compared with other tissues. *J. Invest. Dermatol.*, **54**, 288–97.

Wheeler G.P. (1962). Studies related to the mechanisms of action of cytotoxic alkylating agents. *Cancer Res.*, **22**, 651–88.

Wilkinson D.I. (1970). Incorporation of acetate-1-C^{14} into fatty acids of isolated epidermal cells. *J. Invest. Dermatol.*, **54**, 132–8.

Willems J.L. (1989). Clinical management of mustard gas casualties. *Ann. Med. Milit. (Belg.)*, **3** (suppl.), 1–61.

Wilson E.L., Reich E. (1978). Plasminogen activator in chick fibroblasts: induction of synthesis by retinoic acid; synergism with viral transformation and phorbol ester. *Cell*, **15**, 385–92.

Wilsteed E.M., Bhogal B.S., Das A.K. et al. (1991). Lichen planus pemphigoides: a clinicopathological study of nine cases. *Histopathology*, **19**, 147–54.

Windholz M., Budavari S. (1983). In *The Merck Index: An Encyclopaedia of Chemicals and Drugs, 9th edn.* (Windholz M., Budavari S., Stroumtsos L.Y., Fertig M.N., eds.). Rathway, Ng. Merck.

Winternitz M.C., Finney F.P. (1920). *The Pathology War Gas Poisoning*. New Haven: Yale University Press.

Woessner J.F., Dannenberg A.M., Pula P.J. et al. (1991). Extracellular collagenase, proteoglycanase and products of their activity, released in organ culture by intact dermal inflammatory lesions produced by sulphur mustard. *J. Invest. Dermatol.*, **95**, 717–26.

Woodley D.T., O'Keefe E.J., Prunieras M. (1985). Cutaneous wound healing: a model for cell-matrix interactions. *J. Am. Acad. Dermatol.*, **12**, 420.

Wrench R., Hardy J.A., Spearman R.I. (1980). Sebokeratocytes of avian skin with mammalian comparisons. In *The Skin of Vertebrates* (Spearman R.I., Riley P.A., eds.). London: Academic, pp. 47–56.

Wun T-C., Ossowski J. and Reich E. (1982). A pro-enzyme form of human urokinase. *J. Biological Chemistry*, **257(12)**, 7262–8.

Yamura T., Cormia F.E. (1961). Studies on human skin protease. *J. Invest. Dermatol.*, **37**, 121–4.

Young H.D. (1944). Report No. OSRD 4176. Division 9, National Defense Research Committee of the Office of Scientific Research and Development (OSRD).

31. Assessment of the Severity of Injury

D. W. Yates

INTRODUCTION

Measurement of the severity of an injury is an essential first step in its scientific evaluation. This chapter reviews the methods which have been proposed and those which are currently used to assess the size of the local response and, more particularly, the overall effect of the injury.

Scaling systems are used by a wide variety of professional groups (Table 31.1) to measure different aspects of the response to injury (Table 31.2). Whereas the practising clinician will use the measurement to guide further investigation and treatment and will therefore be more concerned with relative values and changes over time, the research worker will be chiefly concerned with comparing different groups of patients or their response to different forms of treatment. Common to all is the requirement for careful observation and accurate recording.

TABLE 31.1

WHO ASSESSES THE SEVERITY OF INJURY?

Prehospital care	Politician
Emergency medical service	Lawyer
Intensive care	Insurance agent
Operating theatre	Epidemiologist
Rehabilitation service	Bioengineer
Medical audit	Consumer safety officer
Medical scientist	Injury prevention researcher

TABLE 31.2

WHY ASSESS THE SEVERITY OF INJURY?

1. To improve prehospital triage
2. To assess the quality of hospital care
3. To measure response to treatment
4. To allow grouping of patients for comparative clinical research
5. To rank the severity of injury according to associated mortality and short- and long-term disability
6. To aid clinical audit

THE WOUND

Anatomical derangement

Early anatomical scoring systems were developed subjectively. They were, however, an improvement on previous clinical descriptors which had an infinite spectrum, were not standardized and defied computation. The Abbreviated Injury Scale, introduced in 1969 (Committee on Medical Aspects of Automotive Safety, 1971) evolved in this way but has been refined progressively by validation against survival or death so that it now provides a reasonably accurate way of ranking the severity of injury on a scale from 1 (minor) to 6 (maximum) (Table 31.3). Scores for over 1200 injuries are now available in a dictionary which has been revised on three occasions, the most recent edition being published in 1990. The scores are most appropriately used when applied retrospectively to large samples. They should not be employed for the prospective assessment of individual patients.

The Abbreviated Injury Scale (AIS) was first developed alongside the 'Comprehensive Research Injury Scale' (States, 1969). The latter scored each injury with respect of threat to life, energy dissipation, permanent impairment, treatment period and incidence. Experience with the use of both the Comprehensive and Abbreviated scales did not reveal any major value in retaining the former and the AIS is now widely accepted as the standard method of assessing the severity of anatomical damage. Although there is general consensus that AIS ranks severity of injury to individual organs and tissues, it does not claim to be an interval scale. For example the difference between AIS3 and AIS4 is not necessarily the same as the difference between AIS1 and AIS2.

Anatomical injury scaling is an inexact science. The extent of anatomical injury is most accurately described when autopsy reports are used in conjunction with clinical information, operation notes,

TABLE 31.3

EXAMPLE OF INJURIES SCORED BY THE ABBREVIATED INJURY SCALE

Injury	Score
Shoulder pain (no injury specified)	0
Wrist sprain	1 (minor)
Closed, undisplaced tibial fracture	2 (moderate)
Head injury – unconscious on admission but for less than 1 hour thereafter, no neurological deficit	3 (serious)
Major liver laceration, no loss of tissue	4 (severe)
Incomplete transection of the thoracic aorta	5 (critical)
Laceration of the brain stem	6 (maximum)

radiographs and CT scans. Clinical examination alone is insufficient. Streat and Civil (1989) reviewed 279 trauma deaths and found differences between clinical and post-mortem scores in 69% of cases. Most major differences – of two or more AIS grades – occurred in two body regions. In the head, injury scoring based on physiological features (e.g. coma) was often unsupported by evidence of anatomical injury. In the thorax, either treatment had abolished the evidence of the injury (e.g. pneumothorax) or injuries were discovered for the first time at autopsy.

Problems in the application of the AIS continue to arise. The initial orientation of the scale as a comprehensive measure of severity, including assessment of disability, has been replaced by the narrower concept of 'threat to life'. The current development of a separate 'disability scale' should help to clarify the situation. However the latter will probably have as long a gestation as the AIS and is unlikely to be used as a reliable indicator of disability before the end of the century. Both scales are monitored by a scaling committee of the Association for the Advancement of Automotive Medicine.

Functional impairment

Markers of organ dysfunction and of specific tissue disruption have also been proposed as methods of assessing the severity of injury of some organs. Pulmonary and renal function tests are used extensively in intensive care units but often reflect a more general response to trauma than primary damage to the lungs or kidneys. Markers of brain and muscle injury are not sufficiently specific to be used to measure severity of local injury. However, changes in cardiovascular and respiratory parameters and in level of consciousness can be used to reflect a more general functional impairment following injury.

THE GENERAL RESPONSE

The complex and interrelated responses to tissue damage and the activation of homeostatic mechanisms combine to frustrate attempts to characterize in simple terms the physiological response to and the severity of an injury. Initial clinical examination including measurements such as blood pressure and pulse do not reflect the extent of damage or the response to treatment. Nevertheless these and many other measurements are routinely collected and many analyses have been undertaken in order to identify those parameters which are most accurate in determining outcome. In 1980 Champion *et al.* published the results of an assessment of the association between 16 physiological variables and survival. These included systolic blood pressure, pulse rate and strength, capillary refill, lip colour,

respiratory rate and expansion, Glasgow Coma Scale and pupil size and reaction. By multivariate analysis of these recordings on 1084 patients, the authors refined the list to best reflect outcome whilst keeping data collection as simple as possible for out of hospital use. The resulting 'Triage Index' was based on respiratory expansion, capillary refill and the three elements of the Glasgow Coma Scale (eye opening, motor response and verbal response). Re-examination of the data set and the results of initial testing led to the inclusion of systolic blood pressure and respiratory rate in the list of measured variables and a change of name to the Trauma Score (Champion *et al.*, 1981). In 1989 a further revision was proposed (Champion *et al.*, 1989) because field use had shown that capillary refill and respiratory expansion were often difficult to measure. More importantly, independent audit by the 'Major Trauma Outcome Study' coordinated through the American College of Surgeons had shown that the Trauma Score tended to underestimate severity in some patients.

Boyd *et al.* (1987) also analysed the predictive value of the five elements of the original Trauma Score and determined that only three correlated independently with reasonable precision to mortality. These are the Glasgow Coma Scale, systolic blood pressure and the respiratory rate. They further argued that the total score should be derived from the relative value of these three elements as predictive indices. It was proposed that the observed measurements should be condensed into bands, each given a coded value and that these numbers should be weighted, according to their relative value in predicting outcome, before being added together to give a final score termed the Revised Trauma Score. The method is described in Table 31.4.

Cerebral function

The Glasgow Coma Scale, first introduced by Teasdale and Jennett in 1974, has become the accepted international standard for measuring neurological status. Previous descriptive systems were known to be inaccurate both between observers and also over time with the same observer. The Glasgow Coma Scale (GCS), in contrast, has been shown to be consistently applied by nurses and doctors working not only in different specialties but also in different countries.

Coma is defined as a GCS score of less than 8. A totally unresponsive patient would have a score of 3 and a fully conscious and alert patient a score of 15 (Table 31.5). However it can be difficult in some circumstances to ascribe a GCS score and, more importantly, to be sure that it reflects the degree of brain injury. Local eye injury or a subsequent swelling may preclude an assessment of eye opening. Therapeutic muscle paralysis and endotracheal

TABLE 31.4
REVISED TRAUMA SCORE

Physiological variable	Coded value	× Weight	= Score
Respiratory rate (breaths per minute)			
10–29	4		
> 29	3		
6–9	2	0.2908	____
1–5	1		
0	0		
Systolic blood pressure (mmHg)			
> 89	4		
76–89	3		
50–75	2	0.7326	____
1–49	1		
0	0		
Glasgow Coma Scale Score			
13–15	4		
9–12	3		
6–8	2	0.9368	____
4–5	1		
3	0		
Total = Revised Trauma Score			____

TABLE 31.5
GLASGOW COMA SCALE

Eyes open	Spontaneously	4
	To speech	3
	To pain	2
	Never	1
Motor response	Obeys commands	6
	Localizes pain	5
	Flexion withdrawal	4
	Decerebrate flexion	3
	Decerebrate extension	2
	No response	1
Best verbal response	Orientated	5
	Confused	4
	Inappropriate words	3
	Incomprehensible sounds	2
	Silent	1

TABLE 31.6
PROPOSED PAEDIATRIC GLASGOW COMA SCALE

Eyes open	As adult scale	(1–4)
Best motor response	As adult scale	(1–6)
Best verbal response	Appropriate words or social smiles, fixes on and follows objects	5
	Cries but is consolable	4
	Persistently irritable	3
	Restless, agitated	2
	Silent	1

intubation will clearly negate the entire exercise and, even if muscle paralysis has not been employed, the presence of an endotracheal tube will frustrate attempts to measure vocalization. The UK Intensive Care Society has recommended a convention for assessing Verbal Score in such circumstances: 5 if the patient appears orientated and able to converse; 3 if responsive but there is doubt about conversation potential; 1 if generally unresponsive.

Intoxication with alcohol or drugs will adversely affect the score. Hypoxia and hypovolaemia will depress cerebral function. Caution must be exercised therefore in analysing the results of surveys which involve the assessment of patients with associated problems. For example, in a group of patients with low GCS scores those who are initially inebriated with little brain damage will recover more quickly than their sober more seriously injured counterparts. This could be ascribed erroneously to the protective effects of alcohol.

There are also problems with its use in small children. They cannot normally achieve the highest score of the adult scale (Table 31.5). To accept a maximum achievable score commensurate with the child's biological age has the disadvantage of making more difficult the comparison of scores of patients with different ages. An alternative paediat-

ric modification retains the eye and motor scores of the adult scale but proposes new definitions for the scores for best verbal response (Table 31.6) (Swann and Yates, 1989).

Prehospital care

Measurement of severity of injury in the prehospital phase must rely on superficial clinical assessment with little or no equipment and no accurate knowledge of anatomical injury. Many scales have been proposed and the CRAMS Scale (Table 31.7) (Gormican, 1982), the Prehospital Index (Table 31.8) (Koehler et al., 1987) and the Trauma Score (Table 31.9) are the most widely used. Whilst some reports have been favourable (Moreau et al., 1985), others (Ornato et al., 1985; Koehler et al., 1987) have noted the inability of those scales to reliably predict serious injury in the majority of patients and hence their limited value as out-of-hospital triage tools.

TABLE 31.7
CRAMS SCALE

Circulation	
Respiration	Normal = 2
Abdomen	Abnormal = 1
Motor	Severely abnormal = 0
Speech	*Total Score = 0–10*

TABLE 31.8
PREHOSPITAL INDEX

Systolic blood pressure
More than 100	= 0
86–100	= 1
75–85	= 2
< 75	= 5

Pulse rate
Over 120	= 3
51–120	= 0
Less than 50	= 5

Respiratory status
Normal	= 0
Laboured/shallow	= 3
Less than 10, needs intubation	= 5

Level of consciousness
Normal	= 0
Confused/combative	= 3
No intelligible words	= 5

Add 4 for penetrating abdominal or chest wounds
0–3 = minor
4–24 = major

Scoring systems for intensive care

Physicians working in intensive care units have developed more comprehensive scales which can be applied to a wider spectrum of patients. They are of course applicable to the multiply-injured patient but the scores will inevitably represent the composite picture of primary tissue injury, the deleterious effects of secondary events and the benefits of homeostatic mechanisms and therapy. Although useful in the management of individual patients, such scoring systems cannot be used to indicate the true severity of the initial injury.

The Therapeutic Intervention Scoring System (Cullen *et al.*, 1974) ascribes a score of 1–4 on a daily basis for each of 80 possible interventions, from ECG monitoring to intra-aortic balloon counter pulsation. The computer-based scoring system (CARE) of Siegel *et al.* (1980) has been used as a teaching and auditing tool. These systems have largely been superseded by the Acute Physiology and Chronic Health Evaluation system (APACHE) introduced by Knaus in 1981. This uses measurements routinely obtained in intensive care units

TABLE 31.9
TRAUMA SCORE

Respiratory rate
10–24	= 4
25–35	= 3
> 35	= 2
< 10	= 1
0	= 0

Systolic blood pressure
> 90	= 4
70–90	= 3
50–69	= 2
< 50	= 1
0	= 0

Capillary refill
Less than 2 seconds	= 2
Greater than 2 seconds	= 1
None	= 0

Respiratory effort
Normal	= 1
Shallow/retractive	= 0

Glasgow Coma Scale
14–15	= 5
11–13	= 4
8–10	= 3
5–7	= 2
3–4	= 1

(Acute Physiology Score), together with the age and a measure of the previous health of the patient, to compute a score which can be used to monitor progress. Initially 34 variables were used, each scoring 0–4, to determine the Acute Physiology Score, but in APACHE II these were reduced to 12, using the worst value of each in the first 24 hours of admission to the intensive care unit (Knaus *et al.*, 1985). Chronic health status and age are incorporated into the final score (Table 31.10).

Much has been written about the ability of APACHE II to identify patients who can be expected to benefit from intensive care. Injured patients usually form a small subset in these reports. The subject has been reviewed recently by Waters and Nightingale (1990).

OUTSTANDING PROBLEMS

Most of the scales described above attempt to measure particular anatomical or physiological consequences of trauma. There are two outstanding deficiencies. None of the scales is able to encapsulate, in one score, the overall effect of the injury on the whole body and, secondly, when validation is attempted, it is always concerned with survival or death – disability is much more difficult to measure and has been largely overlooked.

TABLE 31.10
APACHE II

a. *Score 0–4 for each of the following:*
Core temperature
Mean arterial pressure
Heart rate
Respiratory rate
Arterial/alveolar oxygen gradient
pH
Plasma sodium
Plasma potassium
Plasma creatinine
Haematocrit
White blood count
Glasgow Coma Scale Score

b. *Score 0 for age less than 45, then increase incrementally to a score of 6 for age more than 75*

c. *Score 0–5 for chronic health status*

APACHE II Score = a + b + c

TABLE 31.11
INJURY SEVERITY SCORE

a. Use AIS90 dictionary to score every injury
b. Identify the highest AIS score in each of the following six areas:

head and neck	face
abdomen and pelvic contents	chest
bony pelvis and limbs	body surface

c. Summate the squares of the three highest area scores

Example:

Injury	AIS	Squares of 3 highest area scores
Colles fracture	2	4
Fracture of ribs 5–9 with flail segment	4	16
Elbow abrasions	1	
Head injury – unconscious for 15 min no neurological deficit	3	9
		29 = ISS

TABLE 31.12
TRISS METHODOLOGY

$$(Ps) = \frac{1}{1 + e^{-b}}$$

Where e = natural logarithm
$b = b_0 + b_1 (RTS) + b_2 (ISS) + b_3 (Age)$

b_{0-3} are weighted coefficients based on a large North American data set. These differ for blunt and penetrating injuries

Age score = 0 if the patient is less than 54 years
1 if equal to or more than 55 years

Overall scores

Two ways are currently used to ascribe an overall score to a multiply-injured patient. The Maximum AIS (MAIS) is often used by bioengineers. The highest AIS value is taken as a measure of applied force, irrespective of the number and distribution of all other injuries. In more widespread use is the method of Baker *et al.* (1974), which uses the AIS from the three most severely injured body areas. This Injury Severity Score (ISS) is obtained by adding together the squares of the three highest AIS scores in these areas (Table 31.11). By convention any individual injury which scores 6 on the AIS scale is given an ISS of 75. The score is non-linear and there is pronounced variation in the frequency of different scores. For example, 9 and 16 are common, 14 and 22 unusual, and 7 and 15 are unattainable. The overall ISS of a group of patients should therefore be identified by the median value and the range and not the mean. Non-parametric statistics should be used for analyses.

Although the ISS stands up reasonably well as a predictor of survival, it is not an ideal method for representing overall injury. In particular there are concerns that the threat to life posed by brain injuries are under-represented, those of the limbs over-represented. An alternative method, using the root sum squares of the AIS scores of the head and trunk, the 'Anatomic Profile', has been proposed (Copes *et al.*, 1989).

Combining a global measure of anatomical injury with a score which represents the associated physiological derangement will give a more comprehensive assessment of the severity of injury. Age must also be taken into account. The TRISS methodology combines these elements and provides a measure of the probability of survival. (The acronym is tortuously developed from TRauma score and Injury Severity Score.) The method is described in Table 31.12 and a complete case history with calculation of ISS, RTS and Probability of Survival is presented in Appendix 31.1. P_s is merely a mathematical calculation, it is not an absolute measure of mortality but only of the probability of survival (or death). For example, if a patient with a P_s value of 0.8 dies the outcome is unexpected in that four out of five patients with such a P_s value could be expected to survive. The fifth patient would be expected to die – and this could be the patient under study. The TRISS methodology is based on a large data set of North American patients collected

TABLE 31.13

WS SCORES AND 95% CONFIDENCE INTERVALS FOR A NUMBER OF UK HOSPITALS. VERTICAL LINE REPRESENTS UK MEAN. NUMBERS
REFER TO EXCESS SURVIVORS PER 100 PATIENTS ABOVE THE MEAN. DATA STANDARDIZED FOR CASE MIX

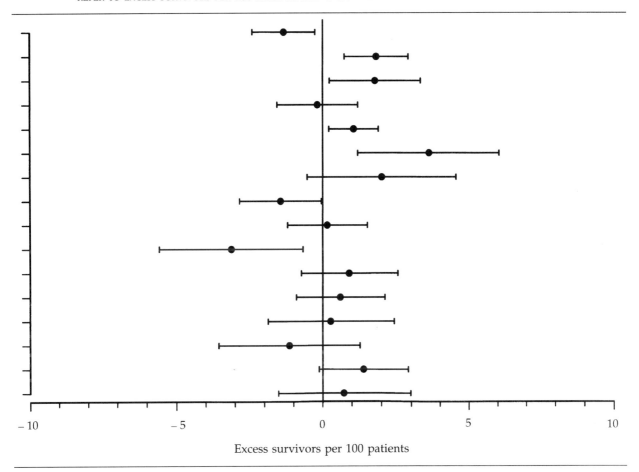

Excess survivors per 100 patients

at the Washington Hospital Centre (Boyd *et al.*, 1987) subsequently refined in the UK to take account of the improvements in anatomical scoring the 1990 edition of the AIS manual and to provide incremental correction for age over 55 (Woodford *et al.*, 1994).

The outcome of groups of patients treated by a particular hospital or a particular system of trauma care can be compared with the main data set if the input variables (ISS, RTS and age) and the type of wounding (blunt or penetrating) are compatible. The 'Z' statistic measures the significance of the difference between actual mortality in the study set and that predicted by reference to the main database. A significant difference is considered to be present if the Z statistic is outside the range -1.96 to $+1.96$. The W_S statistic provides a relative measure of performance (in terms of the number of deaths above or below the expected value, per 100 patients) standardized for case mix (Table 31.13) (Hollis, 1995).

This methodology is used increasingly in scientific publications. Computation is relatively

straightforward and many hospitals now carry out clinical audit using TRISS. However there are a number of problems. The data on which the calculations are based may not represent the direct effects of the injury (modification by homeostatic mechanisms and therapy are common), and the system used to combine descriptors of anatomical deficit and physiological status lacks absolute validation. But for the present the TRISS methodology has a reputation for consistency and reasonable prediction of outcome which has done much to improve our methods of recording the severity of injury.

Many institutions now use the system to audit patient care and compare performance between hospitals and over time. It is organized in the UK through the Major Trauma Outcome Study (North Western Injury Research Centre). An anonymous league table is compiled, comparing the Z and W statistics of all hospitals, so that participants can determine the relative position of their own institution. It should facilitate the scientific evaluation of different forms of trauma care and thereby promote the development of the best comprehensive system for the management of the multiply injured patient.

Impairment, disability and handicap

Measurement of outcome in terms of survival or death does not adequately represent the enormous effect of injury on society. There is an urgent need for scoring systems which measure impairment, disability and handicap. These specific terms are defined in Table 31.14.

The Glasgow Outcome Study measures the quality of long-term survival after brain injury (Jennett and Bond, 1975) and is chiefly concerned with major damage. However there are very many patients who sustain modest brain injury, with significant short-term disability and sometimes long-term psychomotor problems, who will be assessed as having fully recovered according to the Glasgow Outcome Scale. Musculoskeletal injuries also cause significant morbidity, yet there is no generally accepted method of measuring their effect. In contrast, thoracoabdominal injuries are frequently life threatening but rarely cause prolonged disability.

The idea of producing a single figure to represent the disability of a particular injury is very attractive but there are many problems to overcome. Assessment would be time consuming and difficult to standardize. Some activities would, presumably, be deemed more important than others and the need to weight results would have to be considered, with all the attendant problems. The distinction between impairment, disability and handicap is not well defined and the effects of environment, occupation

and motivation would have to be taken into account. Nevertheless, there is general agreement that some method of measuring morbidity is required and, as a first step an impairment scale based on professional consensus and peer review has been published by the authors of the AIS (Association for the Advancement of Automotive Medicine). Subsequent clinical measurement may enable it to be validated in a similar way to the AIS.

REFERENCES

American College of Surgeons Committee on Trauma (1989). Advanced Trauma Life Support Manual, p. 265.

Association for the Advancement of Automotive Medicine 2340 Des Plaines Avenue, Suite 106, Des Plaines, Illinois 60018, USA.

Baker S.P., O'Neill B., Haddon W., Long W.B. (1974). The injury severity score, a method for describing patients with multiple injuries and evaluating emergency care. *J. Trauma*, **14**, 187–96.

Boyd C.R., Tolson M.A., Copes W.S. (1987). Evaluating trauma care: the TRISS method. *J. Trauma*, **27**, 370–8.

Champion H.R., Sacco W.J., Hannan D.S. et al. (1980). Assessment of injury severity: the Triage Index. *Crit. Care Med.*, **8**, 201–8.

Champion H.R., Sacco W.J., Carnazzo A.J. et al. (1981). Trauma Score. *Crit. Care Med.*, **9**, 672–6.

Champion H.R., Sacco W.J., Copes W.S. et al. (1989). A revision of the trauma score. *J. Trauma*, **29**, 623–9.

Committee on Medical Aspects of Automotive Safety (1971). Rating the severity of tissue damage. I. The Abbreviated Scale. *JAMA*, **215**, 277–80.

Copes W.S., Sacco W.J., Champion H.R., Bain L.W. (1989). Progress in characterising anatomic injury. In *Proceedings of the 33rd Annual Meeting Association of the Advances in Automotive Medicine, Baltimore MA, USA*, pp. 205–18.

Cullen D.J., Civetta J.M., Briggs B.A. (1974). Therapeutic Intervention Scoring System: a method for quantitative comparison of patient care. *Crit. Care Med.*, **2**, 57–60.

Gormican S.P. (1982). CRAMS scale: field triage of trauma victims. *Ann. Emerg. Med.*, **11**, 132–5.

Hollis S., Woodford M., Yates D.W., Foster P. (1995). Standardised comparisons of performance indicators in trauma: a new approach to case mix variations. *J. Trauma*, **38**, 763.

Jennett B., Bond M. (1975). Assessment of outcome after severe brain damage. A practical scale. *Lancet*, **i**, 480–4.

Knaus W., Wagner D., Draper E. (1985). APACHE II: a severity of disease classification system. *Crit. Care Med.*, **13**, 818–29.

Koehler J.J., Malafa S.A., Millesland J. et al. (1987). A multicenter validation of the prehospital index. *Ann. Emerg. Med.*, **16**, 380–5.

Moreau M., Gainer P.S., Champion H.R., Sacco W.J. (1985). Application of the trauma score in the prehospital setting. *Ann. Emerg. Med.*, **14**, 1049–54.

Ornato J., Mlinek E.J., Craren E.J., Nelson N. (1985). Ineffectiveness of the Trauma Score and the CRAMS scale for accurately triaging patients to Trauma Centers. *Ann. Emerg. Med.*, **14**, 1061–4.

TABLE 31.14
DEFINITIONS OF IMPAIRMENT, DISABILITY AND HANDICAP

IMPAIRMENT	Has an anatomical or physiological basis and is usually a consequence of musculoskeletal or cerebral injury (e.g. an amputated finger, anosmia). It is easy to measure but variably related to the patient's activity
DISABILITY	Is a functional consequence of impairment so that the patient cannot perform activities of daily life. Its measurement is relevant to the patient's needs but it is influenced by the environment
HANDICAP	Refers to disability within the patient's social and professional environment. It reflects a change in lifestyle, but it is difficult to relate it to specific injury and is very difficult to measure

Siegel J.H., Cerra F.B., Moody E.A. et al. (1980). The effect on survival of critically ill and injured patients of an ICU teaching service organised about a computer based physiologic CARE system. *J. Trauma*, **20**, 558–79.

States J.D. (1969). The Abbreviated and the Comprehensive Research Injury Scales. In *Proceedings of the 13th STAPP Car Crash Conference, Society of Automotive Engineers, Warrendale PA*, pp. 282–4.

Streat S.J., Civil I.D. (1989). Injury scaling at autopsy: the comparison with premortem clinical data. In *Proceedings of the Proc 33rd Annual Meeting, Association for the Advancement of Automotive Medicine, Baltimore, MA, USA*, pp. 169–81.

Swann I., Yates D.W. (1989). *Mild Head Injury*. London: Chapman & Hall.

Teasdale G., Jennett B. (1974). Assessment of coma and impaired consciousness. A practical scale. *Lancet*, **ii**, 81–4.

Waters M., Nightingale P. (1990). Scoring and outcome audit systems relevant to emergency medicine. *Arch. Emerg. Med.*, **7**, 9–15.

Woodford M., Hollis S., Yates D.W. (1994). The translation of injuries from AIS85 to AIS90. *Acad. Energ. Med.*, **1**, 303.

APPENDIX 31.1

Case study

A 65-year-old pedestrian is knocked down, sustaining head, abdominal and leg injuries. On arrival in the accident and emergency department he has a Glasgow Coma Scale score of 9, respiratory rate of 35/min and systolic blood pressure of 80 mmHg. Computed tomography shows a small subdural haematoma with swelling of the right parietal lobe. There is a major laceration of the liver but no other intra-abdominal injury. Radiographs of the lower limbs show displaced fractures through both upper tibias.

Revised Trauma Score (Table 31.4)

Glasgow Coma Score = 9; coded value 3 × weighting 0.9368 = 2.8104
Respiratory rate = 35; coded value 3 × weighting 0.2908 = 0.8724
Blood pressure = 80; coded value 3 × weighting 0.7326 = 2.1978
$$RTS = 5.8806$$

Injury Severity Score (Table 31.11)

	Abbreviated injury score
Subdural haematoma (small)	4
[Parietal lobe swelling]	[3]
Liver laceration (major)	4
Upper tibial fracture (displaced)	3

$$ISS = 4^2 + 4^2 + 3^2 = 41$$

Coefficients from major trauma outcome study database for blunt injury:

$b_0 = -1.2470$
$b_1 = 0.9544$
$b_2 = -0.0768$
$b_3 = -1.9052$

$b = -1.2470 + (0.9544)(5.8806) = (-0.0768)(41) + (-1.9052)(1) = -0.6886$

$$P_s = \frac{1}{1 + e^{(0.6886)}} = 0.3343$$

PART 2
PATHOPHYSIOLOGY OF INJURY

SECTION 7
LOCAL RESPONSES

32. The Acute Inflammatory Response

G. Smedegård, J. Björk and C. Lundberg

INTRODUCTION

The Roman physician Celsus originally described the clinical signs of inflammation as rubor, tumour, calore and dolore, which translates into redness, swelling, heat, and pain. A fifth sign, loss of function, was later added by the German pathologist Virchow. The first-four signs can be seen in the wheal and flare reaction that follows a scratch to the skin. The scratch rapidly becomes red and swollen, pain is experienced, and there is a local rise in temperature. Loss of function is not very pronounced in this kind of mild trauma, but is evident, for example, when an ankle becomes inflamed following a sprain, and when normal joint function is lost in rheumatoid arthritis. An inflammatory response may be defined as a tissue reaction to a noxious stimulus, like a physical injury of various kinds or an infection. Every surgical procedure, for example, inevitably results in an inflammatory response. Inflammation of a particular tissue may occur without any obvious external noxious stimulus, for example when the immune recognition mechanism has failed to identify a tissue component as 'self' and a so-called autoimmune response has developed, resulting in a chronic disease state, such as rheumatoid arthritis or multiple sclerosis. Irrespective of the stimulus that initiates an acute inflammatory response, there is a common pattern of reaction leading to the cardinal signs of inflammation.

The acute inflammatory response following trauma can be looked upon as the initial preparative phase in the healing process. Microvascular events play a central role in the acute inflammatory reaction, as two of the key elements of acute inflammation, extravasation of plasma proteins and accumulation of inflammatory cells, involve microcirculatory alterations. After a general description of the acute inflammatory process, this chapter will focus on these two central events of inflammation – the vascular response and the interaction of leucocytes with the endothelium.

MECHANISMS OF THE ACUTE INFLAMMATORY RESPONSE

An acute inflammatory response is depicted schematically in Figure 32.1. When the skin is injured, blood vessels are damaged and haemorrhage occurs. This leads to a vascular reaction which is seen as vasoconstriction later followed by vasodilatation, mediated by various biologically active substances released from cells in the tissue. Inflammatory mediators cause increased vascular leakage of plasma from the blood into the extravascular space. Circulating neutrophils or polymorphonuclear leucocytes (PMNs) and the postcapillary endothelium in the inflamed area are activated to express specific adhesion molecules, resulting in adhesion of PMNs to the endothelium. The PMNs subsequently migrate from the vessel into the tissue, where they phagocytose dead tissue and foreign material. Lymphatic vessels are damaged by the injury, and this damage together with clotting of fibrin in the lymphatic vessels results in obstruction of lymph drainage from the injured area. This is later followed by activation of fibrinolysis and restoration of the drainage capacity (cf. Smedegård, 1985; Smedegård and Björk, 1985; Ward and Marks, 1989; Butcher, 1991).

An inflammatory reaction thus involves a variety of components, which can be referred to as either a humoral or a cellular response. These two types of responses act in concert and are necessary for the

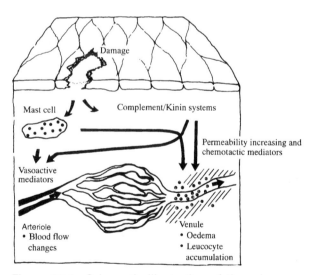

Figure 32.1 Schematic illustration of the microvascular effects of various vasoactive and chemotactic mediators following trauma. Arteriolar dilatation is induced by mediators such as prostaglandins and bradykinin. Permeability changes occur in the venules following exposure of mediators like histamine, bradykinin, C3a and leukotrienes. Chemotactic mediators such as leukotriene B_4 and C5a cause PMNs to adhere to the venular wall and extravasate. PMN adherence/extravasation is often followed by a PMN-dependent plasma leakage.

inflammatory process, the aim of which is to minimize damage to the body by rapid and efficient delimitation of the affected tissue, to eliminate damaged tissue and/or infectious agents, and to initiate the healing process.

The physiological events giving rise to the cardinal signs of inflammation can thus be summarized as follows. Dilatation of small arterioles increases the blood flow at the site of inflammation, causing redness and heat. An increase in the permeability of postcapillary venules leads to an enhanced transport of plasma proteins and water from the blood into the tissue, which together with an obstruction of lymphatic drainage results in oedema – swelling – and pain. Activated inflammatory cells migrate from the blood into the tissue, releasing products that cause vasodilatation and plasma leakage. Some of these products may also be deleterious to the tissue itself, which together with the oedema and pain impairs the functional capacity of the organ.

HUMORAL RESPONSE

Low-molecular-weight mediators

As shown in Table 32.1, there is an array of inflammatory mediators taking part in an inflam-matory reaction. Some are stored in cells and released in response to an inflammatory stimulus. For example, histamine is stored in mast cells, but when released it increases the permeability of small postcapillary venules to plasma proteins (Majno et al., 1961). Other mediators, synthesized and released from different types of cells during the inflammatory process, include arachidonic acid metabolites such as prostaglandins, thromboxanes and leukotrienes, as well as platelet-activating factor (PAF-acether) (Smedegård, 1985; Smedegård and Björk, 1985).

The cysteinyl-containing leukotrienes (LTC_4, LTD_4, LTE_4) are, like histamine, potent mediators of increased vascular permeability (Björk et al., 1983; Bray 1986). Another leukotriene, LTB_4, is a very strong chemotactic agent for PMNs (Björk et al., 1982; Bray 1986). Prostaglandins (PGE_2, PGI_2) cause vasodilatation of precapillary arterioles and by this means potentiate the plasma leakage induced, for example by histamine (Williams, 1983).

Plasma proteins

The complement, kinin, coagulation and fibrinolytic systems all participate in the inflammatory reaction (Cochrane et al., 1979). They consist of a series of plasma proteins which are sequentially

TABLE 32.1
PRIMARY EFFECTS OF SOME INFLAMMATORY MEDIATORS

	Source	Microvasculature	PMN leucocytes and monocytes
Histamine	Mast cells, basophils	Increases permeability	
PGE_2, PGI_2	Various cell types	Dilates arterioles	Inhibits migration and secretion
	(arachidonic acid–cyclooxygenase pathway)	Potentiate increased permeability	Inhibits adherence to endotheluim (PGI_2)
TXA_2	Various cell types (arachidonic acid – cyclooxygenase pathway)	Constricts arterioles	
LTC_4, LTD_4, LTE_4	Various cell types (arachidonic acid – lipoxygenase pathway)	Constricts/dilates arterioles Increases permeability	
LTB_4	Various cell types (Arachidonic acid – lipoxygenase pathway)	Increases permeability (PMN-dependent)	Activates PMNs Increases adherence to endothelium
PAF-acether	Various cell types	Constricts arterioles. Increases permeability (PMN–dependent and-independent)	Activates PMNs Increased adherence to endothelium
Bradykinin	Kinin system	Dilates arterioles Increases permeability	
C3b	Complement system		Facilitates phagocytosis
C3a	Complement system	Constricts arterioles Increases permeability	
C5a	Complement system	Constricts arterioles Increases permeability (PMN-dependent)	Activates PMNs Increases adherence to endothelium

activated, resulting in the generation of a variety of biologically active components. The complement system can be regarded as a non-specific defence mechanism against microorganisms, but may also play an important role in non-infectious inflammatory conditions. Immune complexes or cell surface polysaccharides on microorganisms may trigger the sequential activation of the complement plasma proteins that will ultimately lead to lysis of the microorganism. The cleavage fragments formed during the activation of the different complement factors exhibit a wide range of biological activities. These fragments include C3b, which opsonizes microorganisms and thereby facilitates phagocytosis. Other biologically active fragments are the anaphylatoxins C3a and C5a, both of which are vasoconstrictors and increase vascular permeability. C5a is, in addition, a chemotactic agent, participating in the accumulation of leucocytes at the inflammatory site (Hugli, 1981).

The kinin system, the coagulation system and the fibrinolytic system are all activated by the Hageman factor (factor XII), as is the complement system (Cochrane *et al.*, 1979). The Hageman factor is activated by contact with negatively charged surfaces, which are present in connective tissue. In the activated kinin system, kallikrein cleaves kininogen at two sites liberating bradykinin. This peptide is a vasodilator and in addition increases the permeability of small venules. The intrinsic coagulation pathway is triggered by activated factor XII and the extrinsic coagulation pathway by factor VII, which in turn has been activated by factor XII. The later stages of the coagulation system involve the conversion of fibrinogen to fibrin by thrombin. The fibrin is in turn degraded by plasmin in the fibrinolytic system. Peptides released during the degradation of fibrin may cause an increase in vascular permeability and activation of PMNs.

Cytokines

During the last decade a large number of cytokines have been described, each with a wide range of biological properties, most of which are related to immunoregulatory effects (not discussed here). These peptide mediators are released from various cell types involved in the inflammatory reaction, for example macrophages or lymphocytes, and can be considered as local mediators acting over small distances either in an autocrine or paracrine fashion (Arai *et al.*, 1990).

The cytokine interleukin-1 (IL-1) has a variety of effects in the inflammatory process. Although initially described as a product of activated macrophages, IL-1 is known to be produced by a variety of cells including fibroblasts, keratinocytes of the skin as well as lymphocytes. IL-1 appears to be a central molecule in inflammation by its ability to induce the release of other inflammatory factors such as PGE_2 and collagenase. Further, IL-1 increases the expression of adhesion molecules on endothelial cells, a property that IL-1 shares with tumour necrosis factor (TNFα) and interferon-gamma (IFN-gamma). TNFα also up-regulates the expression of adhesion molecules on PMNs. Interleukin 8, which belongs to the chemokine family, is important in the acute inflammatory process, activates and attracts PMNs to the inflammatory site (chemotaxis), activities similar to those of C5a and LTB_4.

In addition to their proinflammatory and immunoregulatory effects, some of the cytokines mediate systemic clinical symptoms such as fever and rises in acute-phase proteins.

CELLULAR RESPONSE

The influx and activation of various cell types are important features of acute inflammation. These cells include peripheral blood cells such as *PMNs*, *monocytes*, and, in chronic inflammatory conditions, also lymphocytes (the latter not discussed here) and stationary tissue cells such as *mast cells*.

PMNs represent 70% of the peripheral blood leucocytes in man and constitute the first line in our host defence system. The PMNs are among the first cell types to arrive at an inflammatory site. Accumulation of cells results from the local release of various chemotactic factors, such as LTB_4 or the anaphylatoxin C5a (Hugli, 1981; Bray, 1986). The primary function of the PMN is to phagocytose and destroy microorganisms and other foreign material as well as tissue debris. Phagocytosis is facilitated by opsonization of the foreign material, for example by immunoglobulins or complement factor C3b (Hugli, 1981). Thus, bacteria recognized by antibodies are readily phagocytosed and destroyed within the PMN in newly formed phagosomes. Destruction of microorganisms depends on the release of granule enzymes and on the generation and release of oxygen free radicals into the phagosome. The enzymes released include microbiocidal enzymes (lysozyme), proteases (collagenase, elastase, cathepsins), and proteins whose microbiocidal properties are non-enzymatic (cationic proteins). Oxygen free radicals are formed by the reduction of molecular oxygen by the action of NADPH-oxidase. These radicals include the superoxide ion (O_2^-), which, spontaneously or enzymatically (superoxide dismutase), is converted into hydrogen peroxide (H_2O_2). Under appropriate conditions, the extremely reactive oxidant, the hydroxyl radical (OH$^{\cdot}$), may be formed from O_2^- and H_2O_2. The PMN also generates the hypochlorite ion, OCl$^-$, by reaction of Cl$^-$ and H_2O_2. All these biologically active compounds, i.e. various enzymes and oxygen free radicals, are normally released intracellularly into the phagosome. Some of these products, however, are also released extracellularly and may thereby cause tissue destruction (Weissman, 1979).

An intact radical generating system is important for host defence. In patients with the genetic defect giving rise to chronic granulomatosis disease, the PMNs lack the ability to reduce O_2 to O_2^- leading to recurrent and sometimes fatal bacterial infections (Quie *et al.*, 1967).

Monocytes, like PMNs, are capable of both chemotaxis, phagocytosis, and release of enzymes and oxygen free radicals. Monocytes appear at the inflammatory site somewhat later than the PMNs. A cell type related to the monocytes is the macrophage. This is a tissue cell derived either from emigrated blood monocytes or from local precursors. Apart from their ability to phagocytose and destroy foreign material, macrophages can also present antigen to lymphocytes during an immune response, and by release of growth factors they can stimulates tissue repair.

The *mast cell*, unlike the PMN and the monocyte, is a stationary cell and is present in most tissues often in close association with the microvessels. These granulated cells release a number of mediators upon stimulation, such as histamine, serotonin and arachidonic acid metabolites.

VASCULAR RESPONSE

The microvasculature is the part of the circulation that interacts intimately with the tissue cells. The tissue microvasculature can be divided into three functionally distinct regions: the arteriolar part, which by an active change in vessel diameter regulates local blood flow and pressure; the capillary region, where nutrients and gases involved in the tissue metabolism are exchanged; and the venular part, where changes in vascular permeability and accumulation of PMNs in response to an inflammatory stimulus occur.

Vasoactive response

The initial response in an acute inflammatory situation is a constriction of the arterioles, which in the case of a traumatic insult minimizes loss of blood prior to activation of the coagulation system. This initial vasoconstriction is mediated both by neurological reflexes and by release of mediators with vasoconstrictor properties, e.g. the arachidonic acid metabolite thromboxane A_2 (TXA_2) (Samuelsson *et al.*, 1978). Following this transient constriction, dilatation occurs, increasing the blood flow and the intravascular pressure and thus delivery to the inflamed area of the various components involved in the inflammatory process. The dilatation and the local rise in blood pressure potentiate the plasma leakage induced by the released mediators which increase vascular permeability (Williams, 1983; Smedegård, 1985).

The local release of the nitric oxide (NO), previously known as 'endothelium-derived relaxing factor,' could account for the observed vasodilation, as several inflammatory mediators have been shown to activate nitric oxide synthetax (Billiar, 1995).

Vascular permeability

Under normal physiological conditions, the microvascular permeability to molecules larger than 10–20 kDa is restricted, whereas water and small solutes pass freely through the microvascular barrier, under homoeostatic control by the hydrostatic and colloid osmotic pressures in the intra- and extravascular compartments (Renkin, 1977). The microvasculature is not, however, a homogeneous entity in this respect, as permeability to both large and small molecules differs between the arteriolar and the venular regions (Ley and Arfors, 1986). This indicates that different segments of the microvascular bed exhibit important dissimilarities in physiological properties related to transmural exchange of fluid and solutes.

In an acute inflammatory situation, the permeability to macromolecules in postcapillary venules is dramatically enhanced. The increased extravascular protein content results in an increase in the colloid osmotic pressure, which is the main cause of the subsequent oedema. An increase in intravascular pressure and vascular surface area also contribute to tissue swelling. All these deviations from the normal physiological situation may be initiated by mediators (Table 32.1) that are formed or released in tissue subjected to a noxious stimulus.

The major barrier to macromolecular diffusion from blood to tissue appears to be the endothelial cell layer itself. The luminal surface of the endothelium and the basement membrane may, in addition, participate in the control of macromolecular permeability. The luminal surface of the endothelium, the glycocalyx, is a highly organized structure composed of a fibrous network of glycoproteins, sialoconjugates, proteoglycans and acidic glycoproteins (Simionescu *et al.*, 1982). This composition gives the glycocalyx a net negative charge and presumably contributes to the antiplatelet and anticoagulant properties of the endothelium.

The endothelial cells are attached to the basement membrane. This membrane is composed of collagen, glycosaminoglycans, elastin and laminin, and can act as a barrier to the passage of large colloidal particles (Siminonescu, 1983). Whether the passage of plasma proteins is restricted by the basement membrane is not known.

Mechanisms of increased macromolecular permeability

Electron microscopic studies have shown that the endothelial cell contains a large number of plasmalemmal vesicles, and it has been suggested that these vesicles may act as carriers of plasma proteins across the endothelium (Bruns and Palade, 1968). This may well be an important mechanism for macromolecular transport under physiological conditions. It is doubtful, however, whether this type of transmural transport plays any major role in an inflammatory situation as these vesicles are distributed regularly throughout the microvascular bed (Simionescu *et al.*, 1978), while macromolecular extravasation induced by inflammatory mediators is known to be restricted to the region of postcapillary venules (Majno *et al.*, 1961). This limited area of vascular leakage has probably evolved as the most functional site for inflammatory changes in permeability, as the intravascular pressure is lowest in the postcapillary venules, thus allowing optimal control of the vascular leakage via arteriolar constriction or dilatation. Furthermore, the postcapillary venule is the microvascular region where in an inflammatory situation PMNs specifically adhere and emigrate (see below). This region of the microvasculature is probably the optimal site of specific PMN adherence, as the blood flow and shear force are low in this area. The adhering PMNs may actively contribute to the vascular leakage. An increase in permeability induced by, for example, LTB_4 is fully dependent on the accumulation of PMNs, as no change in vascular leakage can be induced by this leukotriene in neutropenic animals (Björk *et al.*, 1982). This is in sharp contrast to the change in permeability induced by, e.g. histamine, which is not mediated via PMNs. Other mediators cause an increase in vascular leakage both via a PMN-independent and a PMN-dependent mechanism (cf. Figure 32.2 and Table 32.1).

Exposure of tissue to inflammatory mediators, e.g. histamine or bradykinin, results in the formation of interendothelial gaps (Majno *et al.*, 1961; Joris *et al.*, 1987). This phenomenon is restricted to the postcapillary venules. The intercellular junctions at the venular side of the microvasculature appear wider and looser than those at the arteriolar side, indicating a more fragile interendothelial attachment structure. The opening of these relatively loose junctions of the postcapillary venules dramatically increases the macromolecular permeability during an inflammatory response (cf. Figure 32.2. and Table 32.1, PMN-independent increased permeability).

The exact mechanism underlying the formation of interendothelial gaps is not known with certainty. It was originally proposed that inflammatory mediators induced contraction of endothelial cells, resulting in the formation of gaps. It has subsequently been shown that vascular endothelial cells contain actin and myosin as well as tropomyosin, organized into contractile elements, and closely associated with endothelial junctions. It is thus possible that the contractile elements of the endothelial cell may facilitate flattening and attachment of the endothelial cell to the substratum. The interendothelial gaps may, on the other hand, result from local cell membrane alterations such as membrane invaginations at the junctions. The pericytes, which are situated adjacent to the endothelial cells and also contain contractile elements, may participate in interendothelial gap formation. Contraction of the pericyte would thus result in a passive deformation of the endothelial cell by means of connecting interstitial matrix proteins (Miller and Sims, 1986). Although the exact mechanism of interendothelial gap formation is not completely resolved, it is clear that this process is dependent on active metabolism of the endothelial cells.

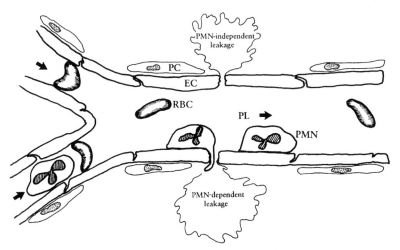

Figure 32.2 Schematic presentation of the two main mechanisms for induction of vascular leakage at postcapillary venules during inflammation. Top: PMN-independent leakage induced directly by an inflammatory mediator, as e.g. histamine or leukotriene C_4. Bottom: PMN-dependent leakage induced by PMNs stimulated to adhere/emigrate by a chemotactic mediator as, for example, leukotriene B_4. EC = endothelial cell; PC = pericyte; RBC = red blood cell; PMN = polymorphonuclear leukocyte.

PMN–ENDOTHELIUM INTERACTIONS

PMN accumulation at an inflammatory site is a process initiated by *rolling* of PMNs along the postcapillary wall, followed by their firm *adhesion* to the endothelium and *extravasation* through the blood vessel wall out into the tissue. These three events (Figure 32.3) are sequential and are all essential in PMN accumulation. The PMN is a suicidal cell which, after extravasation, phagocytosis and destruction of the offending agent, dies and disintegrates. A major component of pus is in fact dead PMNs. The process of PMN migration from the intravascular to the extravascular space requires an 'active' endothelial cell layer and may thus be regarded as an interaction between the two cell types. Distinct receptors on both the PMN and the endothelium are involved in the different events of the PMN–endothelium interaction (Figure 32.4). These receptor/ligands belong to three different families of cell-surface molecules: the immunoglobulin superfamily including ICAM-1, the integrin family with Mac-1 and the selectins with the three members E-, L- and P-selectin (Springer, 1990; Hogg, 1992). The latter family is different from the other two in that these members have a lectin domain and therefore bind carbohydrates.

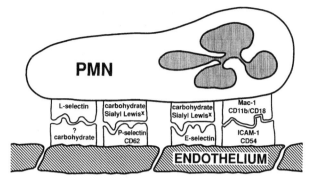

Figure 32.4 Illustration of adhesion-promoting cell-surface molecules on PMNs and endothelium.

Rolling

The PMN is normally transported in the blood stream with minimal contact with the vascular endothelium. In an inflamed region, however, the PMNs roll along the endothelium of postcapillary venules at a lower velocity than the other blood components, allowing time for the PMN to sense endothelial adhesion molecules and/or chemoattractants. The cell surface receptor(s) involved in the rolling phenomenon is distinct from that mediating adhesion. In the rolling process the highly glycosylated L-selectin on the PMN is of vital importance. Blockage of L-selectin has been shown to selectively inhibit rolling of PMNs along the walls of venules (Ley *et al.*, 1991; von Andrian *et al.*, 1991). L-selectin is present at high concentrations on circulating, resting PMNs and mediates their attachment to cytokinin-stimulated endothelial cells under flow conditions and in the absence of PMN activation. L-selectin is well suited for its function of mediating rolling as it is localized to microvillus sites on the PMN surface. Several ligands for L-section have been described including MadCAM-1, CD54 and GlyCAM (Carlos and Harlan, 1994). Another PMN surface molecule involved in rolling is the carbohydrate Sialyl Lewis[x], which serves as a ligand for endothelial E-selectin and P-selectin (CD62). The expression of both P-selectin and E-selectin on the endothelial cell is stimulated by various inflammatory factors. The expression of P-selectin, being immediate and short-lived, is induced by, for example, histamine and thrombin and that of E-selectin more delayed in time (1–2 h) and induced by cytokines such as IL-1 and TNF (Butcher, 1991; Hogg, 1992).

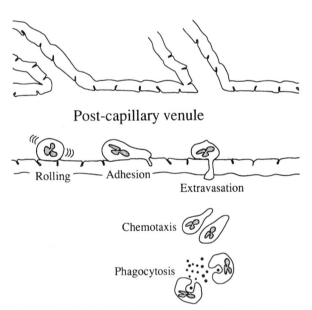

Post-capillary venule

Rolling — Adhesion

Extravasation

Chemotaxis

Phagocytosis

Figure 32.3 Schematic presentation of the different phases of PMN accumulation during an inflammatory response. In postcapillary venules, PMN roll along the vessel wall. Activation of the PMN results in its firm adhesion and in the presence of a chemotactic signal the PMNs migrate through the vessel wall. Outside the vessel they migrate towards the chemotactic signal and interaction with bacteria or tissue debris leads to stimulation and phagocytosis.

Adhesion

The next stage of the PMN–endothelium interaction process is the firm adherence of the PMN. This requires activation of the rolling PMN by a chemoattractant, e.g. C5a or LTB$_4$. Activation of the

PMN leads to shedding of the L-selectin and rapid upregulation and activation of the leucocyte integrin CD11b/CD18 (Mac-1), resulting in firm adhesion of the PMN to the endothelial cell (Patarnoyo *et al.*, 1990). The rolling/adhesion process is reversible and if no chemotactic gradient is present, the PMN detaches and re-enters the circulation.

Upregulation of Mac-1 is the result of a translocation of intracellular secondary and tertiary granules containing Mac-1 to the cell surface, leading to a 10-fold increase in expression. Mac-1 is activated by aggregation and/or re-conformation of this integrin on the cell surface (Carlos and Harlan, 1990). The ligand for Mac-1 on the endothelium has been identified as the intercellular adhesion molecule-1 (ICAM-1). This cell surface molecule is expressed on resting endothelium and increases following activation by cytokines such as IL-1, TNF and IFN-gamma.

Several of the normal functions of the PMN, such as chemotaxis, aggregation, phagocytosis, endothelial cell adherence, complement C3b binding and antibody-dependent cellular cytoxicity, are dependent on a functional expression of Mac-1 complex on the PMNs. The importance of the Mac-1 adhesion complex in PMN accumulation during the acute inflammatory response is evident in patients with leucocyte adhesion deficiency who are lacking the Mac-1 glycoprotein complex. This rare inherited condition is characterized by recurrent and often fatal bacterial infections. PMNs from these patients have marked defects in several PMN adhesion-related functions, which most probably account for the clinical manifestations of this disease (Arnout *et al.*, 1982; Anderson and Springer, 1987).

Extravasation

In the presence of a chemotactic gradient, the PMNs adhering to the endothelium penetrate the blood vessel wall and enter the extravascular compartment (Ward and Marks, 1989). PMNs most likely cross the endothelial barrier via the interendothelial junctions. The passage through the subendothelial basement membrane is achieved by the release of granular proteolytic enzymes. In the process of adhesion and migration, the PMN contributes to the plasma leakage observed at the inflammatory site (Figure 32.2). There are several mediators that promote this PMN-dependent plasma leakage (Table 32.1).

SUMMARY

The acute inflammatory response constitutes the first line in our host defence against a noxious stimulus and may be regarded as the initial stage in the healing process, and is therefore of vital importance. The beneficial aspects of an inflammatory reaction become apparent during the some-times fatal pathological, or drug-induced, states in which important inflammatory functions have become impaired, for example chronic granulomatosis, leucocyte adhesion deficiency and infections during steroid therapy. The inflammatory response is also, however, potentially deleterious to the host, and the balance may sometimes tilt from the beneficial to the destructive processes.

The pathophysiology underlying the five cardinal signs of inflammation – redness, heat, swelling, pain and loss of function – may be traced to the level of the microcirculation in any inflamed tissue. The changes at the venular part of the microvasculature, i.e. the increase in vascular permeability and the accumulation of PMNs, are of particular importance. The initiation of these changes at the microvascular level is a complex process involving several factors comprising both humoral and cellular responses. A multitude of factors is thus necessary for the development of a full inflammatory reaction and no individual mediator or receptor can be singled out. The different components act in synergy and the relative importance of any individual factor varies with the circumstances, such as the inciting agent, the tissue involved, and the stage of the inflammatory process.

REFERENCES

Anderson D.C., Springer T.A. (1987). Leukocyte adhesion deficiency: an inherited defect in the Mac-1, LFA-1 and p150, 95 glycoproteins. *Annu. Rev. Med.*, **38**, 175–94.

Arai K.I., Lee F., Miyajima A. et al. (1990). Cytokines: coordinators of immune and inflammatory process. *Annu. Rev. Biochem.*, **59**, 783–836.

Arnout M.A., Pitt J., Cohen H.J. et al. (1982). Deficiency of a granulocyte-membrane glycoprotein (gp 150) in a boy with recurrent bacterial infections. *N. Engl. J. Med.*, **306**, 693–9.

Billiar T.R. (1995). Nitric oxide, novel biology of clinical relevance. *Ann. of Surg.*, **221**, 339–49.

Björk J., Hedqvist P., Arfors K-E. (1982). Increase in vascular permeability induced by leukotriene B$_4$ and the role of polymorphonuclear leukocytes. *Inflammation*, **6**, 189–200.

Björk J., Dahlén S-E., Hedqvist P., Arfors K-E. (1983). Leukotriene B$_4$ and C$_4$ have distinct microcirculatory actions *in vivo*. In *Advances in Prostaglandin, Thromboxane and Leukotriene Research*, Vol. 12 (Samuelsson B., Paoletti R., and Ramwell P., eds). New York: Raven, pp. 1–6.

Bray M.A. (1986). Leukotrienes in inflammation. *Agents Actions*, **19**, 87–99.

Bruns R.R., Palade G.E. (1968). Studies on blood capillaries. II. Transport of ferritin molecules across the wall of muscle capillaries. *J. Cell Biol.*, **37**, 277–99.

Butcher E.C. (1991). Leukocyte–endothelial cell recognition: three (or more) steps to specificity and diversity. *Cell*, **67**, 1033–6.

Carlos T.M., Harlan J.M. (1990). Membrane proteins involved in phagocyte adherence to endothelium. *Immunol. Rev.*, **114**, 5–28.

Carlos T.M., Harlan J.M. (1994). Leukocyte-endothelial adhesion molecules. *Blood*, **84**, 2068–101.

Cochrane C.G., Revak S.D., Wiggins R.C., Griffin J.H. (1979). The Hageman factor system in inflammation. In *Advances in Inflammation Research*, Vol. 1 (Weissman G., Samuelsson B., Paoletti R., eds). New York: Raven, pp. 249–61.

Hogg N. (1992). Roll, roll roll your leukocyte gently down the vein.... *Immunol. Today*, **13**, 113–15.

Hugli T.E. (1981). The structural basis for anaphylatoxin and chemotactic functions of C3a, C4a and C5a. *Crit. Rev. Immunol.*, **1**, 321–66.

Joris I., Majno G., Corey E.J., Lewis R.A. (1987). The mechanism of vascular leakage induced by leukotriene E$_4$: endothelial contraction. *Am. J. Pathol.*, **126**, 19–24.

Ley K., Arfors K-E. (1986). Segmental differences of microvascular permeability for FITC-dextrans measured in the hamster cheek pouch. *Microvasc. Res.*, **31**, 84–99.

Ley K., Gathgens P., Fennie C. et al. (1991). Lectin-like cell adhesion molecule 1 mediates leukocyte rolling in mesenteric venules *in vivo*. *Blood*, **77**, 2553–5.

Majno G., Palade G.E., Schoefl G.I. (1961). Studies on inflammation. II. The site of action of histamine and serotonin along the vascular tree: a topographic study. *J. Biophys. Biochem. Cytol.*, **11**, 607–26.

Miller F.N., Sims D.E. (1986). Contractile elements in the regulation of macromolecular permeability. *Fed. Proc.*, **45**, 84–8.

Patarnoyo M., Prieto J., Rincon J. et al. (1990). Leukocyte-cell adhesion: a molecular process fundamental in leukocyte physiology. *Immunol. Rev.*, **114**, 67–108.

Quie P.G., White J.G., Holmes B., Good R.A. (1967) *In vitro* bactericidal capacity of human polymorphonuclear leukocytes: diminished activity in chronic granulomatous disease of childhood. *J. Clin. Invest.*, **46**, 668–79.

Renkin E.M. (1977). Multiple pathways of capillary permeability. *Circ. Res.*, **41**, 735–43.

Samuelsson B., Goldyne M., Granström E. et al. (1978). Prostaglandins and thromboxanes. *Annu. Rev. Biochem.*, **47**, 997–1029.

Simionescu M., Simionescu N., Palade G.E. (1982). Biochemically differentiated microdomains of the cell surface of capillary endothelium. *Ann. NY Acad. Sci.*, **401**, 9–24.

Simionescu N. (1983). Cellular aspects of transcapillary exchange. *Physiol. Rev.*, **63**, 1536–79.

Simionescu N., Simionescu M., Palade G.E. (1978). Structural basis of permeability in sequential segments of the microvasculature of the diaphragm. II. Pathways followed by microperoxidase across the endothelium. *Microvasc. Res.*, **15**, 17–36.

Smedegård G. (1985). Mediators of vascular permeability in inflammation. *Prog. Appl. Microcirc.*, **7**, 96–112.

Smedegård G., Björk J. (1985). Inflammation and the microvascular endothelium. In *Inflammation* (Veng P., Lindbom L., eds). Stockholm: Almqvist & Wiksell, pp. 25–46.

Springer T.A. (1990). Adhesion receptors of the immune system. *Nature*, **346**, 425–34.

von Andrian U.H., Chambers J.D., McEvoy L. et al. (1991). Two-step model of leukocyte–endothelial cell interaction in inflammation: distinct roles for LECAM-1 and the leukocyte beta$_2$ integrins *in vivo*. *Proc. Natl. Acad. Sci. USA*, **87**, 7538–42.

Ward P.A., Marks R.M. (1989). The acute inflammatory reaction. *Curr. Opin. Immunol.*, **2**, 5–9.

Weissman G., Korchak H.M., Perez H.D. et al. (1979). Leukocytes as secretory organs of inflammation. In *Advances in Inflammation*, Vol. 1 (Weissman G., Samuelsson B., Paoletti R., eds). New York: Raven, pp. 95–112.

Williams T.J. (1983). Interactions between prostaglandins, leukotrienes and other mediators of inflammation. *Br. Med. Bull.*, **39**, 239–42.

33. Macrophage–endothelial Cell Interactions

F. B. Cerra

INTRODUCTION

Tissue injury initiates a reaction characterized by redness, swelling, pain, temperature, and loss of function, an inflammatory response. This response can be manifest locally or systemically and can be initiated by direct injury (trauma), blood loss (trauma, ruptured abdominal aortic aneurysm), invading microorganisms (infection) or a non-specific inflammation (pancreatitis).

Generally, this response is associated with healing of the injury and has survival benefit for the host. In some settings, however, the response becomes severe and is associated with organ injury and dysfunction that becomes progressive and results in death.

This inflammatory response to injury or foreign antigens occurs as a result of the effects of individual cells, such as polymorphonuclear leucocytes (PMN), endothelial cells, macrophages; hormones such as cortisol and catecholamines; and modulating substances such as cytokines, eicosanoids, and nitric oxide.

This chapter will describe the systemic inflammatory response; its pathogenesis, with particular reference to the endothelial cell and macrophage, and then summarizes the current treatment approaches based on the current understanding of its pathogenesis.

THE SYSTEMIC INFLAMMATORY RESPONSE

The response to tissue injury follows a variety of patterns that are summarized in Figure 33.1. (Cerra, 1987). With a single, uncomplicated injury, the response tends to peak on days 3–5 postinjury and to abate by days 7–10. With a severe injury in a compromised host, the response can be a rapid death. In between, two other patterns emerge. In one, the response continues and organ dysfunction appears, and the process abates when the complication is corrected, as in the drainage of an abscess. In the second pattern, the response continues unabated, multiple organs fail and the patient expires.

These patterns were originally described following polytrauma (Baue, 1975), but have now been observed after severe infections and septic shock (Siegel et al., 1979; Pine et al., 1983; Cerra, 1987), severe hypovolaemia with or without shock (Tilney

et al., 1973), in the presence of inadequate resuscitation (Baker et al., 1980; Goris and Draisma, 1982) and in the presence of severe inflammation, as in pancreatitis (Cerra, 1987).

Once the patient responds to any one of these aetiologies, the clinical manifestations are indistinguishable (Siegel et al., 1979; Cerra, 1987). The local characteristics of an infection or an injury can clearly aid in diagnosis. However, when the response becomes systemic, the usual clinical signs, symptoms and laboratory tests are not helpful in distinguishing the presence or absence of infection, traumatic injury or perfusion-related injury. Hence, the concept of the systemic inflammatory response syndrome (SIRS) has evolved, with the term sepsis reserved for SIRS where there is evidence for a response to microorganisms or microorganisms in tissue where there should not be any (ACCP-SCCM Consensus Conference, 1992). Other synonyms for SIRS have included hypermetabolism, hyperdynamic state and sepsis syndrome.

When the systemic response occurs, two general clinical pathways are observed (Barton and Cerra, 1989; Cerra et al., 1990). (Figure 33.2) In the first, frequently seen after a primary pulmonary initiating event such as aspiration, the progressive multiple organ dysfunction is a terminal event, becoming manifest only within a few days of death. In the second form, commonly seen in septic shock with ARDS, the multiple organ dysfunction is present nearly from the time of injury and becomes progressive over 7–10 days. In both cases, there is a period of several days to weeks of relative stability (SIRS) and then progression of liver and renal failures.

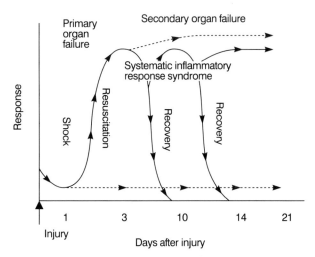

Figure 33.1 Trauma, shock, infection and tissue damage, when the injury is not severe enough to cause immediate death, induce a response best described as a systemic inflammatory response. Uncontrolled, this response appears able to induce multiple organ failure.

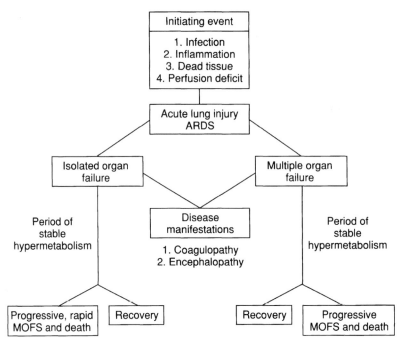

Figure 33.2 Two general types of clinical response have been observed. In one, the clinical picture is dominated by lung dysfunction; in the other, by multiple organ dysfunction.

Several clinical settings are associated with the transition from SIRS to the development of secondary organ dysfunction and progressive organ failure (Cerra *et al.*, 1980; Danek *et al.*, 1980; Moyer *et al.*, 1981a; Goris and Draisma, 1982; Gutierrez *et al.*, 1986; Bihari *et al.*, 1987). These include: a persistent perfusion deficit; an unrecognized perfusion deficit; persistent flow-dependent oxygen consumption; a persistent focus of infection; the combination of a perfusion deficit and a persistent or new septic focus; a persistent inflammatory focus in the absence of infection such as acute fulminant pancreatitis.

The transition to progressive MODS is a significant prognostic event. It heralds a change in mortality risk from the 40–60% range to the 90–100% range. The differentiation of early from late MODS is primarily a matter of the degree of liver and renal failure. The patients manifest abnormalities such as: progressive jaundice, biliary stasis, reduced hepatic amino acid extraction and reduced hepatic and total body protein synthesis in the presence of nutrition support, increased hepatic triglyceride production with reduced peripheral triglyceride clearance, increased ureagenesis even in the absence of protein loading, reduced hepatic redox potential as reflected in the betahydroxy-butyrate/acetoacetate ratio, and, terminally, a failure of glucose release and hypoglycaemia (Cerra *et al.*, 1979; Baker *et al.*, 1980; Moyer *et al.*, 1981a-c).

Patients who die are older, spend a longer time on a ventilator and a longer time in the intensive care unit (ICU), but do not spend a longer time in the hospital. On the other hand, survivors spend more time outside the ICU prior to hospital discharge while they restore sufficient body mass and function to allow effective discharge to occur. The admission APACHE score does not reliably discriminate subsequent survival or death (Cerra *et al.*, 1990c).

Thus, the clinical characterization of response is that it occurs in a setting of a defined injury that is associated with circulatory compromise followed by resuscitation. The postresuscitative response seen then depends on the severity of injury, the organ reserve of the patient at the time of injury, the time lapse in instituting effective treatment, the adequacy of the treatment instituted, and the number and severity of subsequent injuries and complications.

This postresuscitative inflammatory response is characterized by primary organ dysfunction, such as acute lung injury requiring mechanical ventilation. The severity of the organ dysfunctions and the development of secondary organ dysfunction can be ameliorated with treatment interventions such as source control, the restoration and maintenance of oxygen transport and nutrition/metabolic support.

Secondary injuries, perhaps from the inflammatory response itself, result in secondary organ dysfunction, principally in liver and kidney. New therapies are directed at ameliorating these responses, such as antibodies directed at lipopolysaccharide (LPS) or tumor necrosis factor (TNF) or

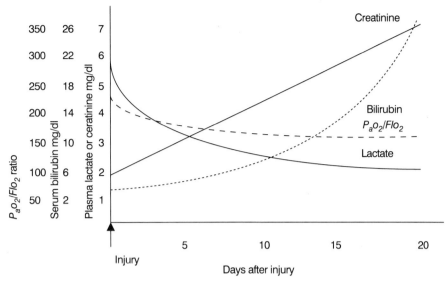

Figure 33.3 The most commonly observed blood chemistry pattern of failure syndrome is depicted. It manifests over time and is usually heralded by a progressive rise in serum bilirubin (secondary hepatic failure).

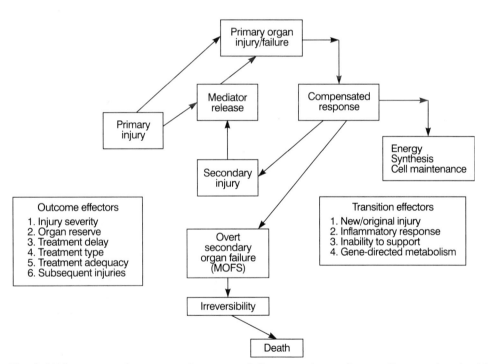

Figure 33.4 The initial response in progressive organ failure syndrome is usually associated with adequate energy availability, protein synthesis, and the maintenance of reasonable normal cellular functions. With secondary injury, secondary organ failure occurs.

interleukin 1 (IL-1) receptor antagonists (Figure 33.4).

Eventually, progressive organ failure and death ensue. The primary therapy for this form of the disease is prevention; the pathogenesis remains hypothesis.

The physiological and metabolic response have been studied and characterized over the years in a number of publications (Siegel *et al.*, 1979; Cerra, 1987; Barton and Cerra, 1989). These responses represent the clinical manifestations of the inflammatory process. As such, they serve several useful purposes:

1. Their manifestation indicates the presence of SIRS.

2. The characteristics of patients who survive the response process can be identified and serve as useful targets for therapeutic interventions.
3. These manifestations serve as outcomes to be explained by pathogenic mechanisms and as outcomes for evaluating the response to therapeutic intervention.

A detailed discussion of the responses is beyond the scope of this discussion. A summary of some of these manifestations is presented in Table 33.1.

Injury, then, manifests as alterations in structure and function of cells and organs. These alterations, if homeostatic and of short duration, are associated with survival. If they are prolonged or non-homeostatic however, progressive organ failure and death ensure (Figure 33.5).

PATHOGENESIS

Three general patterns of responses are observed (Cerra, 1987) (Figure 33.1). In one, the initial injury results in severe shock that produces sufficient direct tissue/cell injury so that resuscitation never compensates the anaerobic lactic acidosis and death occurs immediately or over the first few days postinjury. At the other end of the spectrum, the injury (even a severe one) induces just a local inflammatory response or a systemic one that abates in a few days with complete recovery. In between is the spectrum of persistent SIRS with MODS, whose pathogenesis will be discussed in this section.

The pathogenic mechanisms appear to change over time (Table 33.2). The initial event is an injury to tissue followed by reduced microcirculatory perfusion in the area of injury and systemically. The reduction in systemic perfusion is regional and dependent on the degree and type of injury and adequacy of the cardiovascular response. Vasoconstriction occurs first in the splanchnic viscera and skin; then in the extremities with preservation of the cardiocerebral axis when the low perfusion state becomes more severe; and finally, even to these latter organs in its most severe form. The injury produced in the tissue receiving direct impact and in these areas of underperfusion results from direct effects of oxygen deprivation, from activation of the coagulation and complement cascades, and from the release of eicosanoids, nitric oxide, endothelin and the inflammatory mediators (Figure 33.6).

Structural injury to endothelial cells occurs from the trauma and/or the microcirculatory underperfusion. Mast cells degranulate (Table 33.3), factor XII is activated by exposed collagen and basement membrane, resulting in activation of coagulation, complement and the kinin system. Platelets aggregate, releasing autocoids; PMNs adhere to endothelial cells and induce endothelial cell injury and activation with release of autocoids, cytokines and nitric oxide.

This process results in a local inflammatory response. The characteristics and mediators are summarized in Table 33.4. The observed response results from the net effects and varies by tissue bed. Some vascular beds, such as skeletal muscle, have a net dilatation response; some, such as the splanchnic viscera, have a net constriction response. In the microcirculation, the degree of loss of perfusion from a lack of volume and flow also influences the net response, as does the duration of perfusion shock and oxygen deprivation.

TABLE 33.1

CHARACTERISTICS OF THE SYSTEMIC INFLAMMATORY RESPONSE

Characteristic	Starvation	Systemic inflammation
Oxygen consumption	–	++
Cardiac output	–	++
Systemic vascular resistance	NC	–
Gluconeogenesis	–	+++
Ketonaemia	+++	–
Proteolysis	+	+++
Ureagenesis	+	++
Total nitrogen excretion	+	+++
Net catabolism	+	+++
Lipolysis	+	++
Acute-phase protein synthesis	+	++
Rate of malnutrition developing	+	+++
Neuroendocrine activation	–	++
Cytokine production	–	++

– = decreased;
+ = increased;
NC = no change.

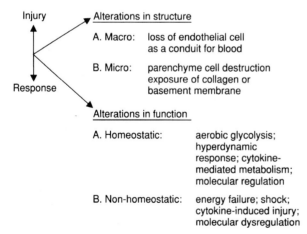

Figure 33.5 Traumatic injury produces alterations in structure and function. The functional injury may be related to the structural alterations, or to the response that occurs to the structural injury.

TABLE 33.2
SUMMARY OVERVIEW. (ADAPTED FROM CERRA, 1992)

Clinical presence	Reduced microcirculatory perfusion	Resuscitation	Systemic inflammatory response	Progressive organ failure

Pathogenesis/ mechanisms of regulation and injury	1. Oxygen deprivation
	2. Activation of complement, coagulation, PMNs, platelets endothelial cell; eicosinoids
	3. Macrohormone release
	4. Mechanical effects of the injury
		1. *Local injury –* oxygen radicals, cytokine, autocoid
		2. *Systemic injury –* endothelial cells, macrophage, LPS release from gut, nitric oxide, eicosanoids
			1. Macrohormone release
			2. *Cell – Cell communication –* endothelial cell; fixed macrophage; cytokines, eicosanoids
			3. Molecular regulation
				1. Dyshomeostatic cell–cell regulation
				2. Molecularly mediated death:
				    a. apoptosis
				    b. substrate competition

Therapy	1. Source control	1. Restore oxygen transport 2. Antibody against LPS and cytokine	1. Nutrition support 2. ω-3 PUFA, Arg, RNA 3. Monoclonal/ polyclonal antibody	1. Prevention

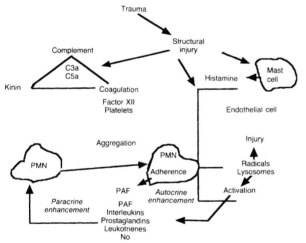

Figure 33.6 The local inflammatory response is mediated by the cellular elements of blood, endothelial cells, and the inherent reactive systems of blood. The process is regulated by autocrine and paracrine mechanisms; local injury usually results.

TABLE 33.3
PRODUCTS OF MAST CELL ACTIVATION

Compound released	Activity
Histamine	Vasodilatation, capillary leak
Heparin	Angiogenesis, complement inhibition, anticoagulation
Trypsin	Proteolysis, basement membrane collagen cleavage
Tumour necrosis factor	PMN activation, shock
Neutrophil chemotactic factor	PMN chemotaxis
Eicosanoids- prostaglandin, leukotriene, platelet activating factor	Vasodilatation, smooth muscle contraction, platelet activation

Thus, there is microcirculatory stagnation, coagulation, initiation of inflammation, and injury to endothelial cells and associated parenchyme cells (Holman, 1964; Barbul *et al.*, 1981; Van Buren *et al.*, 1983; Kremer *et al.*, 1985; Saito *et al.*, 1987; Billiar *et al.*, 1988).

There is also activation of the neurohumoral system with high autonomic tone, release of corti-sol, catecholamine, aldosterone, antidiuretic hormone, glucagon, insulin and other hormones (Vilcek, 1987; Clowes, 1988; Garrison and Cryer, 1988; Teupel *et al.*, 1988; Cook and Halushka, 1989; Ward *et al.*, 1989; Snyder and Cerra, in press). This neurohumoral response mediates the systemic physiological response and initiates the flow of metabolic substrate to support that response.

SUMMARY OF EICOSAINOID SYNTHESIS

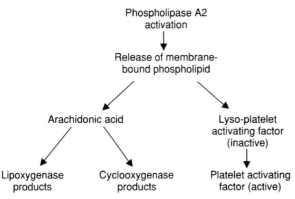

Figure 33.7 The autocoids are potent mediators of inflammation, physiology and metabolic function. They originate from membrane-bound phospholipids and are synthesized after precursor release by phospholipase A activation.

TABLE 33.4
CHARACTERISTICS OF THE INFLAMMATORY RESPONSE.
(ADAPTED FROM GALLIN, 1989)

Physiological response	Mediators
Vasodilatation	Hageman factor, bradykinin, lactate, acidosis, nitric oxide, prostacycline
Vasoconstriction	Thromboxane, leukotriene B4, C5a
Vascular permeability	PgE$_2$, C3a, C5a, leukotriene C and D, Hageman factor, bradykinin, prostacycline
PMN chemotaxis, adherence, phagocytosis	Interleukin 1, C3a, C5a, PAF, TNF, fibrinectin, heparin, collagen fragments, leukotriene, laminin
Fever	TNF, interleukin, PgE$_2$
Pain	PgE$_2$

TABLE 33.5
SYSTEMIC MANIFESTATION OF LOCAL INFLAMMATION

A. Local causes
  1. Continued injury
  2. New injury:
     a. infection
     b. decreased perfusion/oxygenation

B. Non-local causes
  1. Physiological response causes new injury, e.g. splanchnic vasoconstriction
  2. Reperfusion with systemic release of the local products and induction of injury distant from the local site

TABLE 33.6
EFFECTS OF SOME INFLAMMATORY MEDIATORS

Mediator	Effects
Hageman factor	1. Increased vascular permeability 2. Initiation of coagulation 3. Activation of the kinin system with plasminogen release and fibrinolysis and release of bradykinin
Complement	1. Bacterial opsonization 2. Cell lysis 3. Increased capillary permeability 4. Smooth muscle contraction 5. Anaphylatoxin activity (mast cell degranulation)
Platelet activating factor	1. Platelet aggregation and degranulation 2. Smooth muscle contraction 3. Leucocyte chemotaxis, aggregation and adherence 4. Increased vascular permeability 5. Hypotension 6. Myocardial contractile depression 7. Pulmonary hypertension

In the local area of injury, an inflammatory response occurs with capillary injury, interstitial oedema, the typical cellular response and the clinical manifestations of redness, swelling, pain and loss of function (Clowes, 1988; Cook *et al.*, 1989; Gallin, 1989; Ward *et al.*, 1989). The process can become systemically manifest under a number of situations, as summarized in Table 33.5.

There are a number of mediators of reperfusion injury: prostaglandins such as thromboxane; leukotrienes C, D, and B; nitric oxide and endothelin; PMN activation with oxygen radical release; release of platelet-activating factor and of endothelial-released cytokine such as IL-1 (Dinarello, 1984; Chang *et al.*, 1987; Clowes, 1988; Cook *et al.*, 1989;

Ward *et al.*, 1989) (Table 33.6). In some instances, additional toxic substances are released, such as endotoxin from the gut.

With reperfusion, the local response products become systemic, as do the products of tissue injury, such as peptides. A systemic response appears, generally manifest by changes in temperature, blood pressure, skin perfusion, WBC count and primary organ dysfunction such as acute lung injury. The injuries distant to site of direct trauma, infection or inflammation seem to originate from the products of the local injury response, in addition to the anatomical effects of the shock itself (Figure 33.8). Thus, the IL-1 released from the local site might induce systemic nitric oxide production

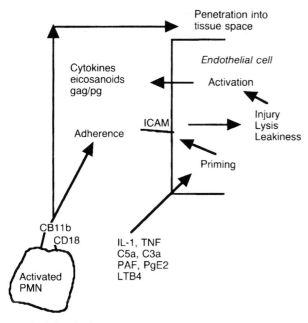

Figure 33.8 With resuscitation or reperfusion of areas of direct injury or areas of microcirculatory injury that result from the vascular response to injury, the local products are 'washed out' systemically. These products are capable of initiation of injury in vascular beds distal to the original injury.

from endothelial cells, causing a fall in systemic vascular resistance (Okusawa et al., 1988). The platelet activating factor (PAF) and IL-1, together with PMNs primed for adherence, i.e. manifestation of surface glycoproteins CD18 and CB11 a, b or c, can injure pulmonary endothelium and result in the manifestation of acute lung injury (Chang et al., 1987; Vercellotti, 1989). The leukotriene released with liver reperfusion could contribute to the pulmonary endothelial injury and the relative non-compliance of the ventricles of the heart. TNF released systemically may also contribute to vaso-dilatation and parenchyme cell injury (Dinarello, 1984).

Eventually, the macrophages become activated. A number of initiating mechanisms are present and include: LPS, bacteria, cytokines, hypoxia, PAF and interferon (Clowes et al., 1983; West et al., 1985; Mazuski et al., 1988; Meyer et al., 1988; Okusawa et al., 1988; Munro et al., 1989; Vercellotti, 1989). These phenomena set the stage for the persistence of the systemic inflammatory response.

One of the major controversies in the SIRS response is whether microcirculatory dysfunction persists after resuscitation has been completed. The data would suggest that some organs, particularly liver, do not have a return of normal perfusion for 2–3 days after resuscitation has been completed (Dahn et al., 1987), using systemic resuscitation

criteria. After that time, however, oxygen delivery and subsequent energy production and availability appear to be adequate, providing resuscitation is maintained (Del Maestro et al., 1981; McCord, 1983; Gutierrez et al., 1986; Bihari et al., 1987; Feuerstein et al., 1987; Tepliz et al., 1988; Vary et al., 1989; Vedder et al., 1989; Cain, 1991; Schlichtig et al., 1991; Thijs and Groenveld, 1991; Tracey, 1991). A fourth sub-group is now also being recognized that in whom oxygen consumption continues to rise with oxygen demand (Cain, 1989; Thijs and Gruenveld, 1989). Even in this subgroup, however, the biochemical and metabolic studies indicate aerobic glycolysis as the basis for energy production (Tilney et al., 1973; Baue, 1975; Siegel et al., 1979; Baker et al., 1980; Goris and Draisma, 1982; Pine et al., 1983; Cerra, 1987; Barton and Cerra, 1989; Cerra et al., 1990a; ACCP-SCCM Concesus Conferences, 1992) and appears to be a reflection of cytokine effects on the enzyme systems (post-translation regulation), par-ticularly the dehydrogenase enzymes that regulate the TCA cycle (Dinarello, 1984; Chang et al., 1987; Vary et al., 1989; Tracey, 1991).

The endothelial cells also become a major effector of cell–cell interaction through autocrine/paracrine mechanisms with the parenchyme cells in prox-imity (Del Maestro et al., 1981; McCord, 1983; Feuerstein and Hallenbeck, 1987; Tepliz, 1988; Vedder, 1989; Vercellotti, 1989). The endothelial cell essentially transforms into a macrophage. The

Macrophage-target cell interaction

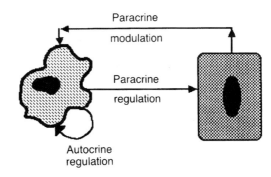

Advantages	Disadvantages
1. Specific immunity	1. Complexity
2. Host defense	2. Mechanism of injury
3. Protein synthesis	3. Organ dysfunction
4. Inflammation	

Figure 33.9 Cell–cell communication appears to be an important mechanism of regulating the inflamma-tory response and maintaining it in an activated state. Eventually, the process appears to be associated with cell metabolic failure that results in organ failure when enough cells become dysfunctional.

macrophages also become activated, release mediators and regulate the metabolic function of parenchyme cells. This is well studied in liver cells (Figure 33.9) with the regulation of hepatocellular protein synthesis. The activated macrophage releases cytokines (e.g. IL-1, IL-6, TNF) and prostaglandins (e.g. PgE$_2$) that simulate total hepatocellular protein synthesis and a relative increase in acute phase protein synthesis (e.g. C-reactive protein) (West *et al.*, 1985; Mazuski, 1988). When enough mediator is released, total hepatocellular protein synthesis decreases, mainly due to a decrease in non-acute-phase protein synthesis (e.g. albumin, transferrin). The liver cell is also actively involved and releases a number of mediators (e.g. nitric oxide, IL-6, GM-CSF) that maintain the Kupffer cell mediator release. Thus, a paracrine-regulated system is present that amplifies itself once it is initiated. The effects on liver cell protein synthesis persist for days, even if the mediators are removed from the system. In the clinical context, recurrent episodes of sepsis and circulatory insufficiency may act to maintain the activated macrophage cell–cell regulatory system.

Thus, a number of regulatory mechanisms are at play. As an example, liver cell protein synthesis is regulated by a number of mechanisms. The high amino acid delivery rate drives the synthesis by direct substrate induction of enzyme systems. Cortisol activates a soluble cell membrane receptor that then directly stimulates gene transcription. Interestingly, in this mechanism, the stimulation ceases soon after the cortisol is removed from the system. Cytokine activates the G-protein signal transduction system of the cell membrane and then modulates gene transcription through phosphorylation and protein kinase activity. This mechanism produces a sustained effect on protein synthesis that lasts for days after removal of the cytokine. In yet another way, protein kinase C, LPS can directly effect protein synthesis, presumably through transcriptional mechanisms (Mazuski, 1988).

The transition to progressive MODS remains the most problematical area of investigation. While the cell–cell interaction mechanisms are homeostatic, it has been difficult to prove that they are capable of causing irreversible cell injury and dysfunction in a manner that reproduces the clinical syndrome of progressive MODS. The mediator systems are also cytoprotective and promote survival and recovery. It is possible that toxic substances might be present, although their existence remains elusive in this late form of the disease. An area of great interest is that of molecular regulation and gene-mediated cell death. There are two lines of experimentation that are unfolding.

One hypothesis is that the accumulated injuries reach a threshold at which genetic self-destruction occurs, a phenomenon referred to as apoptosis (Buchman *et al.*, 1990; Barke *et al.*, 1991; De Maio *et*

al., 1991). Another hypothesis concerns itself with hierarchically regulated cell death. During the homeostatic response, the synthesis of constitutive proteins (e.g. enzymes, structural) and acute-phase proteins is expressed. When a threshold of injury occurs, the heat shock genes, which have metabolic salvage functions, become expressed. Their expression may then dominate at the expense of the constitutive function (Buchman *et al.*, 1990; Barke *et al.*, 1991; De Maio *et al.*, 1991). Cell injury and death could ensue.

It should also be emphasized that it is not necessary to hypothesize that individual cell death needs to occur in order to explain organism death from progressive MODS. Rather, only enough cell dysfunction needs to be present to interfere with organ function in a way that is incompatible with life in itself, or that upsets interorgan balance in a way that is not consistent with life.

THERAPEUTIC APPROACHES

The current therapy for SIRS–MODS focuses on prevention of organ injury and supportive care. Three types of therapy are emphasized: source control, restoration and maintenance of oxygen transport, and metabolic support (Figure 33.10). Whenever possible, complete removal of the cause of the inflammatory response is desirable, as in surgical control of bleeding, early drainage of an abscess, and full-thickness burn excision and skin grafting for third degree burns. When

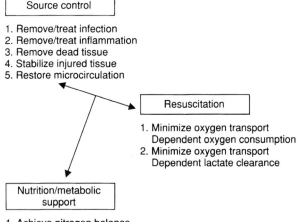

Figure 33.10 The general approach to therapy has prevention as its primary goal, and consists of control of the source, resuscitation, and the institution of appropriate nutritional support. This approach has resulted in major reductions in organ failure morbidity and mortality.

this is not possible, such as in primary pneumonias, pancreatitis, soft tissue injury and haemorrhagic suffusion, efforts to minimize the cause should be rapidly instituted, such as fracture fixation, appropriate antimicrobial agents, and altering dosing of immunosuppressive agents in patients with solid organ transplants during episodes of infection.

Rapid and effective resuscitation is a major therapeutic endpoint. With the recognition of subclinical flow-dependent oxygen consumption in such settings as hypovolaemic pancreatitis, ARDS, and septic and *volume* shock, and its relationship to SIRS–MODS, increased emphasis is placed on invasive techniques of resuscitation during the shock response, using oxygen consumption criteria. The usual clinical criteria of resuscitation (i.e. pulse, blood pressure, urine output, skin perfusion) do not appear sensitive enough to decide when oxygen delivery is equal to oxygen demand in these clinical settings. Rather, invasive monitoring during the shock-resuscitation phase with measurements of oxygen delivery and consumption appear to be necessary (Shoemaker, 1985; Cerra *et al.*, 1987; Shoemaker *et al.*, 1989).

Malnutrition is both a co-morbidity/co-mortality and a primary manifestation of SIRS–MODS. It seems increasingly clear that current nutrition support does not alter the course of the disease process itself, but is an effective way to manage single nutrient and generalized nutrient deficiency resulting in a reduction in morbidity and mortality. To effectively achieve these ends, several principles have evolved (Moore *et al.*, 1981; Cerra *et al.*, 1984; Bower *et al.*, 1986; Cerra *et al.*, 1988a; Berlauk *et al.*, 1991):

1. Providing 25–30 total calories/kg/day with 3–5 g/kg/day as glucose; maintain a respiratory quotient under 0.9.
2. Provide long-chain, polyunsaturated ω-6 fatty acids in doses less than 1.5 g/kg/day (Cerra *et al.*, 1988a).
3. Start amino acids, preferably the modified stress formulas at 1.5 g/kg/day. Promote nitrogen retention by adjusting the dose of amino acids every 5–7 days. Current clinical studies indicate that the modified amino acids are a more efficient protein source and can facilitate nitrogen retention with a higher rate of protein synthesis and less ureagenesis than the standard amino acid formulas (Moore *et al.*, 1981; Cerra *et al.*, 1984; Bower *et al.*, 1986; Cerra *et al.*, 1988b; Berlauk *et al.*, 1991).

The suppression of gut flora numbers by selective gut decontamination antibiotic regimens appears to be an effective means of reducing the incidence of nosocomial infections, and to be a cost-effective form of therapy (Tetteroo *et al.*, 1990). Use of regimen of prophylaxis for gastric stress ulceration and bleeding also appears to be both therapeutically effective and cost-efficient.

With the concept that the response to injury, i.e. the inflammatory response, may also contribute to the morbidity, mortality and resource costs, therapies are becoming directed at modulating the inflammatory response. These therapies are both specific and non-specific. Specific therapy is targeted against a defined mediator, such as endotoxin, IL-1 receptors or TNF. Non-specific therapy is directed at more generalized processes, such as second messenger generation.

One of the best studied specific therapies is the monoclonal antibody directed against endotoxin from gram-negative bacteria (Dunn and Ferguson, 1982; Ziegler *et al.*, 1991). When administered to new ICU admissions who have infection with sepsis and gram-negative bacteremia, a reduction in mortality was observed.

Currently, a number of monoclonal antibodies that are either in testing or going into testing, have been targeted to interfere with various points in the evolution of the inflammatory response. They include: antibodies designed to interfere with PMN adherence (anti CD 18 or CD 11) or IL-1 receptors, or to bind to TNF. Data are not yet available for analysis. However, a number of questions and concerns are present and are related to dosing, the timing of their use, adverse reactions, whether or not there will be reasonable efficacy because they are too well targeted, leaving many alternate mediator pathways available; and whether or not cost-effectiveness will be demonstrable.

For those latter reasons, less-targeted therapies are also being evaluated. In general, these non-specific therapies are targeted at general response mechanisms such as second messenger generation, eicosinoid release from cell membranes, and the molecular regulation of metabolism.

The best studied targeted nutrients are those whose use is designed to suppress the overactive macrophage and reduce the output of interleukin, TNF and eicosinoids such as PgE_2 and LTb_4, and designed to stimulate lymphocyte proliferation in response to specific antigen stimulation. The former would include ω-3 PUFA such as eicosapentanoic acid (EPA) and docasahexanoic acid (DHA); (Holman, 1964; Kremer *et al.*, 1985; Billiar *et al.*, 1988), and the latter would include arginine (Barbul *et al.*, 1981; Saito *et al.*, 1987), and uracil or ribonucleic acid (RNA) (Van Buren *et al.*, 1983; Kulkarni *et al.*, 1986).

Clinical trials with these agents as part of an enteral nutrition regimen have demonstrated restoration and enhancement of the *in vitro* tests of immune function; improved nutritional outcomes; and significant reductions in length of stay and nosocomial infection rates (Cerra *et al.*, 1990b; Lieberman *et al.*, 1990).

Unquestionably, combination therapies will be tested. These therapies will be designed to effect multiple points of the inflammatory response concurrently and sequentially, and specifically and non-specifically. Whether they will have efficacy and be reasonably cost-effective await clinical trials.

REFERENCES

ACCP–SCCM Consensus Conference (1992). Definitions for sepsis and organ failure and guidelines for the use of innovative therapies in sepsis. *Chest*, **101**, 1644–55.

Baker C.C., Oppenheimer L., Stephans B. et al. (1980). Epidemiology of trauma deaths. *Am. J. Surg.*, **140**, 144.

Bankey P., Fiegel B., Singh R. et al. (1989). Hypoxia and endotoxin induce macrophage-mediated suppression of fibroblast proliferation. *J. Trauma*, **29**, 972–80.

Barbul A., Sisto D.A., Wasserkrug H.L. et al. (1981). Arginine stimulates lymphocyte immune response in healthy humans. *Surgery*, **90**, 244–51.

Barke R.A., Brady P.S., Brady L.J. (1991). The effect of peritoneal sepsis on hepatic gene ession and hepatic mitochondrial long chain fatty acid oxidation in rats. *Forum*, **42**, 62–4.

Barton R., Cerra F.B. (1989). The hypermetabolism multiple system organ failure. *Chest*, **96**, 1153–60.

Baue A.E. (1975). Multiple, progressive or sequential systems failure: a syndrome of the 1970s. *Arch. Surg.*, **110**, 779–81.

Berlauk J.F., Abrams J.H., Gilmour I.J. et al. (1991). Preoperative optimization of cardiovascular hemodynamics improves outcome in peripheral vascular surgery. *Ann. Surg.*, **214**, 289–99.

Bihari D., Smithies M., Gimson A. et al. (1987). The effects of vasodilation with prostacyclin on oxygen delivery and uptake in critically ill patients. *New Engl. J. Med.*, **317**, 397.

Billiar T.J., Bankey P.E., Svingen B.A. et al. (1988). Fatty acid intake and kupfer cell function alters eicosanoid and monopkine production to endotoxin stimulation. *Surgery*, **104**, 343–9.

Bower R.H.R., Muggin-Sullam M., Fischer J. (1986). Branched chain amino acid-enriched solutions in the septic patient. *Ann. Surg.*, **203**, 13–21.

Buchman T.G., Cabin D.E., Vickers S. et al. (1990). Molecular biology of circulatory shock II: expression of four groups of hepatic genes is enhanced following resuscitation from cardiogenic shock. *Surgery*, **108**, 902–12.

Cain S.M. (1991). Physiologic and pathologic oxygen supply dependency. In *Update in Intensive Care and Emergency Medicine: tissue oxygen utilization* (Gutierrez G., Vincent J.L., eds). Berlin: Springer-Verlag, pp. 114–24.

Cerra F. (1987). Hypermetabolism, organ failure, and metabolic support. *Surgery*, **101**, 1–14.

Cerra F.B. (1992). Multiple Organ Failure Syndrome. *Disease of the Month*, **38**, 843–947.

Cerra F.B., Siegel J.H., Border J.R. et al. (1979). Correlations between metabolic and cardiopulmonary measurements in patients after trauma, general surgery and sepsis. *J. Trauma*, **19**, 621–9.

Cerra F.B., Siegel J.H., Coleman B. et al. (1980). Septic autocannibalism, a failure of exogenous nutritional support. *Ann. Surg.*, **192**, 570–80.

Cerra F.B., Mazuski J., Teasley K. (1984). Branched chain metabolic support. *Ann. Surg.*, **199**, 286–91.

Cerra F.B., Hirsch J., Mullen K. et al. (1987). The effect of stress level, amino acid formula, and nitrogen dose on nitrogen retention in traumatic and septic stress. *Ann. Surg.*, **205**, 282–7.

Cerra F.B., Alden P.A., Negro F. et al. (1988a). Sepsis and exogenous lipid modulation. *J. Parent. Entr. Nutr.*, **12**, 63S–9S.

Cerra F.B., McPherson J., Konstantinides F.N. et al. (1988b). Enteral nutrition does not prevent multiple organ failure syndrome after sepsis. *Surgery*, **104**, 727–33.

Cerra F.B., Negro F., Eyer S. (1990a). Multiple organ failure syndrome: patterns and effect of current therapy. In *Update in Intensive Care and Emergency Medicine* (Vincent J.L., ed.). Berlin: Springer-Verlag, pp. 22–31.

Cerra F.B., Lehman S., Konstantinides N. et al. (1990b). Effect of enteral nutrient on in vitro tests of immune function in ICU patients: a preliminary report. *Nutrition*, **6**, 84–7.

Cerra F.B., Abrams J., Negro F. (1990c). APACHE II score does not predict MOFS or mortality in postoperative patients. *Arch. Surg.*, **125**, 519–22.

Chang S., Feddersen C.O., Henson P.M. et al. (1987). Platelet-activating factor mediates hemodynamic changes and lung injury in endotoxin-treated rats. *J. Clin. Invest.*, **79**, 1498–509.

Clowes G.H.A. (1988). Stresses, mediators, and responses of survival. In *Trauma, Sepsis and Shock: the physiological basis of therapy* (Clowes, G.H.A. jr, ed.). New York: Marcel Dekker, pp. 1–53.

Clowes G.H.A., Georg B.C., Villu C.A. (1983). Muscle proteolysis induced by a circulating peptide in patients with trauma and sepsis. *New Engl. J. Med.*, **303**, 545.

Cook J.A., Halushka P.V. (1989). Arachidonic acid metabolism in septic shock. In *New Horizons: multiple organ failure* (Bihari D.J., Cerra F.B., eds). Fullerton, CA: Society of Critical Care Medicine, pp. 101–24.

Dahn M.S., Lange P., Lobdell K. et al. (1987). Splanchnic and total body oxygen consumption in septic and injury patients. *Surgery*, **101**, 69.

Danek S., Lynch J., Weg J. et al. (1980). The dependence of oxygen uptake on oxygen delivery in the adult respiratory distress syndrome. *Am. Rev. Resp. Dis.*, **122**, 387.

De Maio A., Buchman T. (1991). Molecular biology of circulatory shock IV: translation and secretion of HEP G2 cell proteins are independently attenuated during heat shock. *Surgery*, **34**, 329–35.

Del Maestro R.F., Björk J., Arfors K.E. (1981). Increase in microvascular permeability induced by enzymatically generated free radicals in *in vivo* studies. Microvasc. *Res.*, **22**, 255.

Dinarello (1984). Interleukin-1 and the pathogenesis of the acute-phase response. *New Engl. J. Med.*, **311**, 341–4.

Dunn D.L., Ferguson R.M. (1982). Immunotherapy of gram-negative sepsis: enhanced survival in a guinea pig model by use of rabbit antiserum to *Escherichia coli* J5. *Surgery*, **92**, 212.

Feuerstein G., Hallenbeck J.M. (1987). Prostaglandins, leukotrienes, and platelet activating factor in shock. *Annu. Rev. Pharmacol. Toxicol.*, **27**, 301.

Gallin J.I. (1989). Inflammation. In *Fundamentals of Immunology* (Paul W.E., ed.). New York: Raven Press, pp. 721–33.

Garrison R.N., Cryer H.M. (1988). Role of the microcirculation to skeletal muscle during shock. In *Perspectives in Shock Research: Progress in Clinical and Biological Research* (Bond R.F., Adams R., Chaudry I.H., eds). New York: Alan R. Liss, pp. 43–52.

Goris R.J.A., Draisma J. (1982). Causes of death after blunt trauma. *J. Trauma*, **22**, 141.

Gutierrez G., Pohil R. (1986). Oxygen consumption is linearly related to the oxygen supply in critically ill patients. *J. Crit. Care Med.*, **1**, 45.

Holman R.T. (1964). Nutritional and metabolic interrelationships between fatty acids. *Fed. Proc.*, **23**, 1062–7.

Kremer J.M., Michalek A.V., Kininger L. et al. (1985). Effect of manipulation of dietary fatty acids on clinical manifestations of rheumatoid arthritis. *Lancet*, **i**, 184–7.

Kulkarni A.D., Fanslow W.C., Rudolph F.B. et al. (1986). Effect of dietary nucleotides on response to bacterial infections. *J. Parent. Entr. Nutr.*, **10**, 169–71.

Lieberman M., Shou J., Torres B.S., Daly J. (1990). Effects of nutrient substrates on immune function. *Nutrition*, **6**, 88–92.

Mazuski J.E., Bankey P.E., Carlson A., Cerra F.B. (1988). Hepatocytes release factors that can modulate macrophage IL-1 secretion and proliferation. *Surg. Forum*.

Mazuski J.E., Platt J.L., West M.A. et al. (1988). Direct effects of endotoxin on hepatocytes. *Arch. Surg.*, **123**, 340–44.

Meyer J.D., Yurt R.W., Duhaney R. et al. (1988). Tumor necrosis factor-enhanced leukotriene B4 generation and chemotaxis in human neutrophils. *Arch. Surg.*, **123**, 1454.

Moore E.E., Dunn E.L., Jones T.N. (1981). Immediate jejunostomy feeding after major abdominal trauma. *Arch. Surg.*, **116**, 681.

Morris A., Henry W., Shearer J. et al. (1985). Macrophage interaction with skeletal muscle: a potential role of macrophages in determing the energy state of healing wounds. *J. Trauma*, **25**, 751.

Moyer E.D., Border J.R., Cerra F.B. et al. (1981a). Multiple systems organ failure VI: death predictors in the trauma-septic state – the most critical determinants. *J. Trauma*, **21**, 862–9.

Moyer E.D., Border J.R., Cerra F.B. (1981b). Multiple systems organ failure IV: Imbalances in plasma amino acids associated with exogenous albumin in the trauma-septic patient. *J. Trauma*, **21**, 543–7.

Moyer E.D., McMenamy R.H., Cerra F.B. et al. (1981c). Multiple systems organ failure III: contrasts in plasma amino acid profiles in septic trauma patients who subsequently survive and do not survive – effect of intravenous amino acids. *J. Trauma*, **21** 263–74.

Munro J.M., Pober J.S., Cotran R.S. (1989). Tumor necrosis factor and interferon-gamma induce distinct patterns of endothelial activation and associated leukocyte accumulation in skin of *Papio anubis*. *Am. J. Pathol.*, **135**, 121.

Okusawa S., Gelfand J.A., Ikejima T. et al. (1988). Interleukin-1 induces a shock-like state in rabbits. *J. Clin Invest.*, **81**, 1162–72.

Pine R.W., Wertz M.J., Lennard E.S. et al. (1983). Determinants of organ malfunction or death in patients with intraabdominal sepsis. *Arch. Surg.*, **118**, 242.

Saito H., Trocki O., Wang S. et al. (1987). Metabolic and immune effects of dietary arginine supplementation after burn. *Arch. Surg.*, **122**, 784–9.

Schlichtig R., Snyder J.V., Pinsky M.R. (1991). Multiple organ oxygen supply–demand relationships in redistributional flow. In *Update in Intensive Care and Emergency Medicine: tissue oxygen utilization* (Gutierrez G., Vincent J.L., eds). Berlin: Springer-Verlag, pp. 143–60.

Shoemaker W.C. (1985). Hemodynamic and oxygen transport patterns in septic shock: physiologic mechanisms and therapeutic implications. In *New Horizons: perspectives in sepsis and septic shock* (Sibbald W., Sprung C., eds). California: Society of Critical Care Medicine, pp. 203–34.

Shoemaker W., Appel P.L., Kram H.B. (1989). Tissue oxygen debt as a determinant of lethal and nonlethal postoperative organ failure. *J. Crit. Care Med.*, **16**, 1117–21.

Siegel J.H., Cerra F.B., Border J.R. et al. (1979). Physiological and metabolic correlation in human sepsis. *Surgery*, **806**, 409.

Snyder L., Cerra F. Shock. In *Surgery: scientific principles and practice* (Greenfield L.J., ed.). Philadelphia: JB Lippincott (in press).

Tepliz C. (1988). The pathology and ultrastructure of cellular injury and inflammation in the progression and outcome of trauma, sepsis, and shock. In *Trauma, Sepsis, and Shock, the Physiological Basis of Therapy* (Clowes G.H.A. Jr, ed.). New York: Marcel Dekker, p. 71.

Tetteroo G.W.M., Qagenvoort J.H.T., Castelein A. et al. (1990). SDD to reduce gram-negative colonization and infections after oesophageal resection. *Lancet*, **335**, 704–7.

Teupel G.E., Strong J.W., Wise W.C. et al. (1988). The role of eicosanoids in mediating blood flow in endotoxin shock. In *Perspectives in Shock Research: progress in clinical and biological research*, vol. 264 (Bond R.F., Adams R., Chaudry I.H., eds). New York: Alan R. Liss, pp. 27–42.

Thijs L.G., Groenveld A.B.J. (1991). Oxygen supply dependency in septic shock. In *Update in Intensive Care and Emergency Medicine: tissue oxygen utilization* (Gutierrez G., Vincent J.L., eds). Berlin: Springer-Verlag, pp. 217–27.

Tilney N., Bailey G., Morgan A. (1973). Sequential systems failure after rupture of abdominal aortic aneurysms. *Ann. Surg.*, **118**, 117.

Tracey K.J. (1991). Tumor necrosis factor (cachectin) in the biology of septic shock syndrome. *Circ. Shock*, **35**, 123–8.

Van Buren C.T., Kulkarni A.D., Rudolph F. (1983). Synergistic effect of a nucleotide-free diet and cyclosporine on allograft survival. *Transplant. Proc. Suppl.*, **1–2**, 2967–8.

Vary T.C., Siegel J.H., Placko R. et al. (1989). Effect of dichloroacetate on plasma and hepatic amino acids in sterile inflammation and sepsis. *Arch. Surg.*, **124**, 1071–7.

Vedder N.B., Winn R.K., Rico C.L., Harlan J.M. (1989). Neutrophil-mediated vascular injury in shock and multiple organ failure. In *Perspectives in Shock Research: metabolism, immunology, mediators, and models*. New York: Alan R. Liss, p. 181.

Vercellotti G.M. (1989). Role of netrophils in endotheleial injury. In *Multiple Organ Failure* (Bihari D., Cerra F.B., eds). Anaheim, CA: SCCM, pp. 77–91.

Vilcek L.E.J. (1987). Biology of disease TNF and IL-1: cytokines with multiple overlapping biological activities. *Lab. Invest.*, **56**, 234–48.

Ward P.A., Warren J.S., Remick D.G. et al. (1989). Cytokines and oxygen-radical-mediated tissue injury. In *New Horizons: multiple organ failure* (Bihari D.J., Cerra F.B., eds). Fullerton, CA: Society of Critical Care Medicine, pp. 93–100.

West M.A., Keller G., Hyland B. et al. (1985). Hepatocyte function in sepsis: Kupffer cells mediate a biphasic protein synthesis response in hepatocytes after endotoxin and killed *E. coli. Surgery*, **98**, 388–95.

Ziegler E.J. et al. (1991). Treatment of gram-negative bacteremia and septic shock with HA-1A human monoclonal antibody against endotoxin. *N. Engl. J. Med.*, **324**, 429–36.

34. Bacterial Toxins in Trauma and Sepsis

H. Redl, S. Bahrami, G. Leichtfried and G. Schlag

INTRODUCTION

Among intensive care patients, sepsis and the resulting multiorgan failure is the most common source of death. Despite the fact that sepsis is thought by many authors to be the result of bacteria, only a fraction of septic patients have positive blood cultures, e.g. in a recent study only 98 out of 226 (43%) had a positive culture (Martin *et al.*, 1991). In addition, sepsis is usually recognized clinically well before the bacteriological results are available (Bone *et al.*, 1989). Although gram-negative bacteria have been shown to be the most frequent source of infection in patients with sepsis syndrome, gram-positive bacteria have also been found to produce the same clinical signs. Beside the bacterial induction of sepsis, a generalized inflammatory reaction, e.g. after trauma, could also be responsible for sepsis induction (Goris, 1989). Whether such a reaction is with or without participation of bacteria is currently a matter of debate, since a lack of positive blood cultures does not necessarily mean non-participation of bacteria. Probably the most important aspect of bacterial action is the release of toxic products, *toxins*, the action of which might be the key to our understanding of the pathophysiology of the sepsis syndrome. Although there is the possibility of detecting such bacterial toxins in body fluids (e.g. endotoxin with the limulus assay), the absence of measurable amounts of circulating toxins (at specific time points) not full proof of the absence of bacterial participation in sepsis. Detection might be impossible because of the toxin release kinetics (short peaks), insensitive measurement techniques or very high potency of the toxins even at extremely low non-detectable concentrations.

On the other hand if there is a positive toxin measurement, it is a good indication that bacteria are involved, e.g. via bacterial translocation from the gut. The insensitivity of bacteria detection in blood might be due to the quick clearance by the body's reticulo-endothelial system (RES). In an experiment it has been demonstrated that a blood concentration of 10^5 CFU *E. coli* is reduced to 0 within 15 minutes after the infusion of *E. coli* is stopped (Schlag *et al.*, 1990).

TOXINS

Different types and amounts of bacterial toxins have to be dealt with depending on the type of bacteria and the composition of the bacterial cell membrane. The best known and studied toxins are the so-called *endotoxins* (lipopolysaccharides (LPS)), which in gram-negative bacteria account for about 80% of the cell wall mass. In contrast, gram-positive bacteria contain low LPS but possess a high percentage of *peptidoglycan*. Some bacteria, both gram negative and gram positive, are able to release *exotoxins* into the surrounding environment.

Endotoxin

The name endotoxin for the toxic principle of gram-negative bacteria originates from the historical view that toxicity is located within the bacterial cell. In subsequent studies it was shown that endotoxin is localized on the surface of bacterial cells as a part of the outer membrane and is chemically a lipopolysaccharide. These endotoxins represent immunoreactive surface antigens (O-antigens) and elicit antibody production in the host. The lipid component, lipid A, represents the second important part of LPS and is highly conserved among gram-negative bacteria. The structure is represented in Figure 34.1 and detailed structural principles are reviewed by Brade *et al.* (1988) and Rietschel *et al.* (1990). In contrast to this well-conserved lipid A region, the O-specific chain is species specific, and because of the diversity of the sugar and its linkages, enormous numbers of structures occur. This structural variability does not allow the production of therapeutically useful monoclonal antibodies against this region. In between the variable O-specific chain and the conserved lipid A structures is the core region which represents a hetero-oligosaccharide and is divided into inner and outer

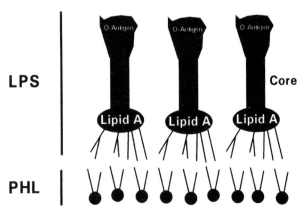

Figure 34.1 LPS in a section of the outer membrane of gram-negative bacteria, containing the lipid A, core and O-antigen portion. PHL-phospholipids of the outer membrane.

core parts. Therefore, several approaches have been made to produce cross-reacting antibodies for several bacterial species as a useful therapeutic approach.

The chemical structure of lipid A is known in great detail (e.g. Rietschel *et al.*, 1987, 1990) and principally contains a disaccharide, which carries two phosphoryl groups, and attached to this hydrophilic backbone acylated four to six fatty acids with a chain length between 12 and 16 carbon atoms with the distribution being specific and characteristic for the bacteria.

Lipid A is the endotoxic principle of LPS, and this has been postulated by Westphal and Lüderitz (1954) and confirmed experimentally by the work of Galanos and colleagues (Galanos *et al.*, 1977). The role of fatty acids for lipid A activity has been thoroughly studied by Rietschel and Brade (Brade *et al.*, 1988). According to present knowledge, endotoxin effects are maximal from molecules containing six acyl residues in a specific conformation, e.g. as in the *E. coli* lipid A. Slight modifications of the lipid A structure, e.g. changes in phosphoryl groups or the number of acyl groups, result in significant changes in lipid A bioactivity (Rietschel *et al.*, 1990). Thus the toxic principle seems to be based on a balance of hydrophilic and hydrophobic regions, which give lipid A a unique molecular conformation linked to endotoxic activity (Rietschel *et al.*, 1987).

Studies on lipid A also revealed lipid A analogues, which are less toxic but still express biological effects such as non-specific resistance to infections and are therefore of interest for prophylactic and therapeutic intervention (for review see Stütz and Liehl, 1991).

When injected into animals or volunteers, LPS can reproduce many of the pathological symptoms characteristic of septicaemia, including fever, leukopenia, haemodynamic changes, coagulopathies and complement activation. Therefore, it was suggested that endotoxins are important in the pathophysiology of gram-negative bacteraemia and septicaemia.

Lipopolysaccharide binding and clearance

When LPS is released from bacteria or injected into the body, it comes into contact with serum and reacts with serum in a complex interaction pattern which involves several serum components. Several serum proteins bind to LPS (for review see Tesh *et al.*, 1988). The important interaction is the binding of LPS to blood – and other organ-specific cells, which give rise to the body's host response. To initiate these reactions, LPS has to bind to cells. Some of the reaction partners have been characterized, such as lipopolysaccharide binding protein (LBP), which binds to LPS and the complex formed interacts with CD14 antigenic structures at the surface of monocyte/macrophages for example (Morrison and Ulevitch, 1978). While the overall LPS activity assessed by mouse lethality or limulus gelation is reduced after interaction with serum, some serum components like LBP have been shown to increase LPS activity and cytokine generation from cells.

The following factors are presently known to influence clearance: LPS antibodies, which inhibit binding of LPS to HDL and, thereby, augment the removal of LPS; the induction of LBP, which also decreases the rate of LPS/HDL complex formation and increases LPS clearance (Tobias and Ulevich, 1983; Freudenberg and Galanos, 1988; Tobias *et al.*, 1988). Probably the scavenger receptor of macrophages is also involved in plasma clearance of LPS (Hampton *et al.*, 1991).

It was found by Freudenberg and Galanos (1984) in the rat that liver is the main target organ which takes up LPS, and the sinusoidal cells, hepatocytes and granulocytes are involved. LPS may remain for a long time, but with chemical changes occurring e.g. through the processing by phagocytes (Munford, 1991). Munford demonstrated that phagocytes have enzymes that deacylate and dephosphorylate the toxic lipid A without destroying its immunogenicity. The net result might be that the detoxification prevents excessive inflammatory responses by promoting the development of bacterial immunity.

Currently clinical interest in endotoxin is increasing because of:

1. The improvement in the endotoxin assay.
2. The suggestion from experimental studies of translocation of bacteria and bacterial products, which might give an explanation of sepsis-like reactions in patients.
3. Drugs are now available which can be used as an effective anti-endotoxin measure.

Exotoxins

In contrast to the endotoxins, which are part of the bacterial outer membrane, some bacteria can also produce and release exotoxins. According to Bhakdi *et al.* (1989), these exotoxins can be divided in those which (a) damage the membrane of target cells, like endothelial cells, and (b) act intracellularly. Examples of (a) are cytolysins of *Staph. aureus* or streptococci while typical examples of (b) are toxins from diphtheria, cholera and neurotoxins. These membrane-damaging exotoxins are now described in more detail.

When the primarily water-soluble toxin molecules bind to the cell membrane, the toxins convert into integral membrane proteins via the lipophilic parts of the toxin molecule. By means of this integration of proteins within the membrane, transmembranous pores are formed, which allow a free

	Lipopoly-saccharide	Peptidoglycan
Pulmonary artery pressure	↑ ↑	↑ ↑
Thromboxane B$_2$	↑ ↑	↑ ↑
Lymph/plasma protein ratio × lymph flow	↑ ↑	=
P_aO_2	↓	=
Fever	↑ ↑	↑ ↑
Cardiac output	↑	more consistent ↑

transmembranous influx of small molecules (e.g. calcium) into the cell (Seydel *et al.*, 1989). This transmembranous pore formation is somewhat similar to that following terminal complement complex activation (C5b-9). The influx of Ca ions, initiates secondary reactions in the target cells such as the formation of cytokines (e.g. IL-1 – Bhakdi *et al.*, 1989), or the activation of arachidonic acid metabolism *in vitro* or in an *in vivo* model of alpha-toxin-induced permeability changes in chronically instrumented sheep. This alpha-toxin was the first identified bacterial pore forming toxin. The importance of this toxin might be, because it is able to react with endothelial cells at a very low concentration and leads, in a calcium-dependent fashion, to changes in the cytoskeleton and to sudden increases in permeability. Thus it was shown that alpha-toxin dramatically increased the filtration rate for water and decreased the reflection coefficient for albumin in porcine pulmonary artery endothelial cells grown on a membrane and sealed by pressure. These changes in permeability were accompanied by cell retraction and formation of large intercellular gaps. A similar effect was seen with *Pseudomonas aeruginosa* cytotoxin, but it was only one-third as effective as alpha-toxin (Suttorp *et al.*, 1988).

In accordance with the *in vitro* changes in endothelial cells, this process might also be relevant for the development of lung oedema in the isolated perfused rabbit lung. This development of lung oedema is parallelled by a release of prostaglandins, which initiates a steep increase in pulmonary arterial pressure. This is also seen *in vivo* in the chronically instrumented sheep.

Platelets also react on exposure to alpha-toxin with pore formation, an efflux of ATP and exocytosis of different vesicles which contain e.g., platelet factor 4 (PF4). These processes lead to the induction of blood coagulation, e.g. concentrations of 1 μg/ml

alpha-toxin lead to a significant reduction in coagulation time in recalcified plasma. Similarly monocytes are more sensitive to alpha-toxin and to LPS, with pore formation, loss of cellular ATP with synthesis of cytokines (IL-1), and the formation of procoagulatory activity. In contrast to the above mentioned cell types, human erythrocytes, granulocytes or lymphocytes have no high affinity binding sites for alpha-toxin and they react only at much higher toxin conconcentrations.

The importance of these exotoxins, which also influence myocardial cells (Reithmann *et al.*, 1989), resides in the following properties and facts: fast reaction kinetics, their influence on central cells of the sepsis response, the induction of cytokine and arachidonic acid metabolite synthesis as well as induction of coagulopathies.

These reactions might be especially relevant in severe staphylococcal infections. The *S. aureus* toxin (Berkowitz, 1989) might be the reason why, in a canine model of septic shock, *S. aureus* and *E. coli* challenges led to a very similar cardiovascular dysfunction. These findings indicate that bacteria both with or without endotoxin can activate a common pathway, resulting in cardiovascular injury and mortality (Natanson *et al.*, 1989).

Peptidoglycans

Peptidoglycans (PG) constitute the rigid succules of the cell wall of both gram-positive and gram-negative bacteria (Figure 34.2).

The PG content of gram-positive cell walls generally accounts for 50–80% of the weight of the wall (West and Apicella, 1985), as opposed to 1–10% of the total weight of the wall in gram-negative organisms.

In the cell walls of *S. aureus* strains, Hill (1968) found one of the many extracellular products that have been described as virulence factors. Such factors are thought to contain a mucopeptide (peptidoglycan) without teichoic acid and enhanced the lesions produced by a standard dose of *S. aureus* injected subcutaneously in mice.

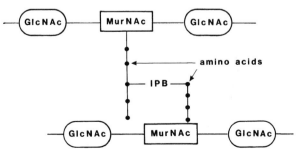

Figure 34.2 Schematic diagram of a peptidoglycan molecule. MurNAc = *N*-acetylglucosamine; Glc NAc = *N*-acetylmuramic acid; IPB = interpeptide bridge. (Adapted from Chetty and Schwab, 1984.)

The heteropolymer peptidoglycan was shown to possess different biological properties (Verhoef and Kalter, 1985) and to share a number of common properties with endotoxin, e.g. it activates the complement (Pryjma *et al.*, 1976) and the kallikrein systems (Kalter *et al.*, 1983; Chetty and Schwab, 1984), influences phagocyte function and platelets (Chetty and Schwab, 1984), and is haemodynamically reactive *in vivo*.

Since both gram-negative and gram-positive strains are involved in clinical septicaemia, haemodynamic and permeability properties of LPS and PG (from *B. subtilis*) were compared in the sheep. Small doses of endotoxin have been shown to increase pulmonary permeability in this species (Brigham *et al.*, 1979) and to increase cardiac output after 6 hours (Talke *et al.*, 1975; Traber *et al.*, 1987, 1988). We found haemodynamic and other effects of PG related to its 'endotoxin-like' properties which could not be attributed to LPS contamination. At the dose used (10 000 times the endotoxin dose on a weight basis), PG produced similar but less severe pulmonary microvascular changes than endotoxin.

Endotoxin-like properties of peptidoglycan can also be seen in the dose-dependent pyrogenic response (Rotta, 1975; Oken *et al.*, 1981; West and Apicella, 1985). A similar dose-dependent stimulation by PG of endogenous pyrogen production by human monocytes has also been shown (Oken et al., 1981). In the sheep experiments, mentioned above, the pyrogenic reaction was more severe and lasted longer in the PG group. These results are in accordance with previous studies, where the dose of PG required for a comparable pyrogenic response in rabbits was 100–10 000 times greater (Heymer and Rietschel, 1977) than LPS. A similar relationship was found in *in vitro* studies with macrophages (Pabst and Johnston, 1980).

PG produces a picture similar to that of endotoxin in the activation of major humoral and cellular systems during generalized inflammation, and is capable of inducing haemodynamic changes, e.g. increased MPAP and cardiac output, that are typical of the hyperdynamic phase of bacterial shock, but with LPS being 100–10 000-fold more potent. Therefore, the clinical role of PG remains to be established.

SOURCES OF TOXINS

Bacterial toxin translocation

The majority of ICU patients demonstrate the picture of clinical sepsis without a focus. In these patients, the gut may play an important part as a 'shock organ' involved in the subsequent development of sepsis. According to Fine *et al.* (1959), the intestine is the source of endotoxin (LPS). Ravin *et al.* (1960) demonstrated conclusively that endotoxin is absorbed from the gut during experimental haemorrhagic shock. This is in accordance with the report of Meakins and Marshall (1986), who state that the gastrointestinal tract is the motor of MOF. Usually, the intestinal mucosa is an effective barrier against micro-organisms and endotoxin. This natural barrier function can be lost in critical illness (Meakins and Marshall, 1986), with subsequent endotoxaemia and bacteraemia. Berg *et al.* (1988) and Deitch *et al.* (1987) have thoroughly addressed this concept, which could explain the hitherto unknown pathogenesis of septic events, where no focus could be identified.

The route of translocation to extraintestinal sites may vary (Wells, 1988); migration of bacteria through a disrupted intestinal epithelium is the most likely route. Translocation may reach the systemic circulation both via the bloodstream and the lymphatic system. Most studies reported so far rely on detection of viable bacteria in tissues or blood. However, Alexander (1991) noted that estimation of translocation by viable bacterial counts in tissues grossly underestimates the extent of translocation of bacteria and ignores the translocation of endotoxin.

The breakdown of the intestinal mucosa is due to hypoxia, reperfusion injury and granulocyte action. Endotoxin perpetuates this process by a positive feedback loop (Deitch *et al.*, 1987). In a series of experiments in awake sheep, Morris *et al.* (1990) found translocation after thermal and/or inhalation injury, and related translocation to the decreased cephalic mesenteric blood flow. Bacterial translocation was inhibited by sodium nitroprusside, suggesting a close relationship between relative mesenteric ischemia and translocation.

A baboon model of polytrauma has already been developed for the study of bacterial translocation, examining plasma endotoxin and blood as well as organ cultures in relationship to superior mesenteric artery flow, gut wall pH and histological changes (Schlag *et al.*, 1990). Positive blood cultures were obtained within 2–3 hours of the onset of shock. Plasma endotoxin levels demonstrated a continuous increase throughout the study (Figure 34.3). High endotoxin levels were not dependent on the reperfusion period. Bacterial translocation was noted in the mesenteric lymph nodes, liver and spleen in varying amounts. The colony forming unit (CFU) concentrations were highest in the mesenteric lymph nodes. All the traumatic shock animals revealed intestinal wall damage. Histological evaluation showed necrotic epithelium at the tip of the villi (Figure 34.4) and an accumulation of inflammatory cells with abundant macrophages and sometimes bacteria. Necrosis was always preceded by subepithelial oedema, which lifted the epithelium and may cause haemorrhage into the submucosa. Translocation of bacteria into the small vessels was also observed (Figure 34.5).

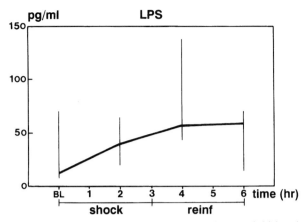

Figure 34.3 Endotoxin plasma levels in arterial blood samples of baboons with hypovolaemic traumatic shock measured by limulus assay. (Reproduced from G. Schlag *et al.*, 1990.)

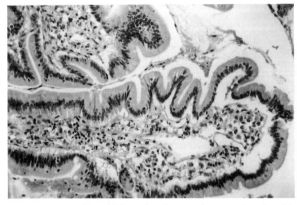

Figure 34.4 Semithin plastic section stained with toluidine blue of a baboon small intestine with mucosal oedema formation (arrow) after hypovolaemic-traumatic shock. (Reproduced from Schlag *et al.*, 1990.)

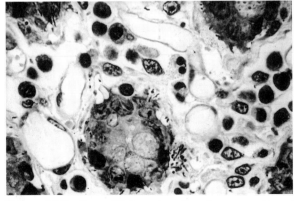

Figure 34.5 Bacterial translocation from cryptae of the colon in a baboon after hypovolaemic-traumatic shock. (Reproduced from Schlag *et al.*, 1990.)

During hypovolaemic-traumatic shock, the liver shows an overloading syndrome of the sinusoids with cell debris, which, to a certain extent, must be phagocytosed by Kupffer cells. The increased phagocytosis may lead to an inability of the Kupffer cells to detoxify endotoxin and/or bacteria. This could partly explain bacterial translocation via the portal vein and inferior vena cava into the systemic circulation during shock and reperfusion (Jiang *et al.*, 1985).

What is the exact cause of epithelial damage – hypoxia or reperfusion injury, or both? Haglund *et al.* (1984) have performed extensive experimental studies on hypoxia and gut damage during hypotension and shock. They observed that mucosal alterations developed during arterial hypotension secondary to increased oxygen 'shunting' in the countercurrent exchanger (Lundgren and Svanvik, 1973). The earliest time point we observed bacterial translocation was in the low-flow phase (shock) when positive blood cultures were obtained.

Some studies suggest that micro-organisms without LPS may also cause septicaemia by their impact on the mucosal barrier of the gut in the host, so that bacterial translocation or LPS leakage from the gut can occur (Bahrami *et al.*, 1995). It has been suggested by some authors that this could be the final common pathway of septic shock produced from different origin (Natanson *et al.*, 1989).

Septic foci

Other sources of endotoxin are septic foci, from which bacterial products are released into the circulation, sometimes related to the administration of antibiotics (Shenep and Morgan, 1984; Lingnau *et al.*, 1991). LPS may be released from intact bacteria in clinical infection, by natural death of the organism, by the action of the host defence system or by bacteriolysis induced by antibiotics. In a baboon model of bacteraemia, this antibiotic effect on endotoxin release and subsequent cytokine release was clearly evident (Figure 34.6).

DETECTION OF TOXINS

Detection and monitoring of toxins is currently restricted to LPS.

Monitoring of plasma endotoxin levels

The release of endotoxin can be monitored *in vivo* by measuring plasma endotoxin levels. For many years, the rabbit pyrogen test has been considered as a gold standard for detecting LPS. The discovery of limulus amoebocyte lysate (LAL) as a clotting system highly sensitive to endotoxin derived from various bacteria has led to the development of gel tests. Later, endpoint-chromogen test methods were developed using LAL combined with a chromo-

□ ng LPS/ml

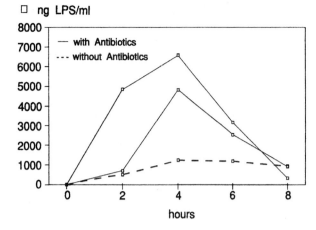

◇ pg IL1/ml

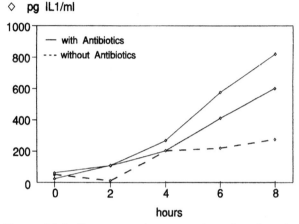

Figure 34.6 Representative examples of endotoxin and IL-1 plasma levels in baboon bacteraemia (live *E. coli* infusion 10^{10} CFU/kg) with (cefotaxime) (*n* = 2) or without (*n* = 1) antibiotic treatment.

genic substrate that allowed quantification of endotoxin. When endotoxin is added to LAL, the activation of clotting enzymes leads to gel formation or to release of p-nitroanilline (pNA) from the chromogen substrate. As the amount of pNA is exactly proportional to the endotoxin concentration, the endotoxin content of samples can be determined by reference to a standard curve (Bahrami *et al.*, 1991).

However, there are several objections to the limulus LPS measurement:

1. In plasma the test is not absolutely specific (even when a factor G free limulus preparation is used).
2. Contamination can easily occur during blood sampling and plasma preparation. To overcome this specific problem 'LPS' blood-sampling tubes have been developed to avoid LPS binding to vial walls and contamination due to the pyrogen content of the vials. This permits storage of samples after plasma and blood cell separation

in the freezer until the plasma samples are analysed (Redl *et al.*, 1992).
3. Endotoxin leaking into the circulation is quickly bound to plasma proteins and blood cells. Therefore the kinetics of infused endotoxin are characterized by a very short plasma half-life (Freudenberg *et al.*, 1984).
4. The activation of clotting enzymes is also possible by substances other than LPS and can lead to false-positive or -negative results. Therefore, various sample treatment methods are suggested to eliminate such interferences, e.g. extraction, precipitation, ultrafiltration, dilution and/or heat treatment. The latter combination of 1:10 dilution followed by heat treatment at 75°C has been suggested as the most convenient and useful method for plasma samples.
5. The presence of measurable amounts of endotoxin in the systemic circulation may reflect exhaustion of the RES, which no longer can fulfil its clearance capacity. This suggestion is supported by experimental studies. LPS is only detectable in the systemic circulation following gut ischaemia-reperfusion after partial resection of the liver (van Leeuwen *et al.*, 1991) or from studies in liver transplantation (Steininger *et al.*, 1990).

Clinical studies suggest that, except for systemic meningococcal disease with extremely high plasma LPS levels (Brandtzaeg *et al.*, 1989), endotoxaemia is often only a transient phenomenon even in severely septic patients. Thus a single measurement of endotoxin may be misleading. Hence in patients suffering from septic shock, endotoxin measurements were made at 4-hourly interval for 48 hours and daily thereafter for 4 weeks (Ledingham *et al.*, 1988). In a group of eight patients with septic shock, endotoxin levels tended to be highest during the first 24–48 hours, then declined, and subsequently showed marked variation in individual patients. In many instances endotoxaemia was seen transiently with LPS returning to undetectable levels for prolonged periods. Peaks of endotoxin often coincided with clinical events such as surgical interventions. In another study Ramsay *et al.* (1988) measured LPS concentrations in 15 consecutive admissions to the ICU with diagnosis of septic shock (10 deaths). All 15 patients had significant levels of LPS in the blood at least intermittently, but there was no significant difference in mean initial or peak levels between survivors and non-survivors. In all the studies it was shown, that there was no correlation between LPS measurements and blood cultures from these studies. It can be concluded that: (1) only sequential LPS measurements appear to relate to cardiopulmonary disturbance and (2) persistent endotoxaemia carries a bad prognosis.

It has recently been shown that anti-endotoxin antibodies are especially beneficial in those patients with a positive limulus test (Wortel *et al.*, 1991) but overall HA-1A antibody trials were not successful due to an inefficient drug. Measurement of plasma endotoxin levels might be useful for the critically ill and the relationship of such levels to the clinical manifestations of septic shock has been emphasized (Danner *et al.*, 1988). Limulus lysate (LAL) detectable (≥ 10 pg/ml) levels of endotoxin in plasma were found in 44% of critically ill patients (similar to a study of Aasen *et al.*, 1989). Organ failure (lung) occurred more often in patients with positive LAL and patients with documented septicaemia and positive LAL had a significantly higher mortality.

In a prospective trial in consecutive febrile patients with a low incidence of septicaemia, van Deventer *et al.* (1987) could demonstrate, with an optimized limulus assay, that analysis of LPS has clinically relevant positive and negative predictive values for the development of gram-negative septicaemia. They further demonstrated that endotoxaemia and gram-negative bacteraemia are separate clinical entities with different significance for the development of gram-negative septicaemia. A further study was performed (van Deventer *et al.*, 1988) in which patients with gram-negative infections of the urinary tract were studied regarding the predictive values of the limulus test for septicaemia. They found in 76 patients, of which 14 (18%) developed septicaemia, that 11 of these 14 patients were endotoxaemic overall. In 41% of the assays performed, a positive result (> 5 pg/ml) was found. The specificity and sensitivity of the limulus test for septicaemia were 79 and 95%, while in the febrile patients without septicaemia only 3% of the assays were > 5 pg/ml.

In contrast to these results Függer *et al.* (1990) found that endotoxin determination was not of prognostic significance in their patients, even though endotoxin levels were elevated in diffuse peritonitis and infected pancreatic necrosis.

Using a limulus test with a high sensitivity of 0.02 EU/ml, Berger and Beger (1991) studied several aspects of postoperative endotoxaemia. In 13 patients with peritonitis and operative treatment on continuous peritoneal lavage, they found maximum levels of LPS 1 day after the operation. Endotoxin plasma levels were decreasing over the next 4–5 days. They could also demonstrate in 33 patients an almost significant difference between those with septic shock (median 0.28 EU/ml) and those without (0.14 EU/ml). They further asked the question whether patients just with elective operations, which do not involve the gut region, would develop endotoxaemia as a result of bacterial translocation. Again they found at the first postoperative day a significantly increased LPS plasma level, even in patients with strumectomy.

Therefore probably, with sufficiently sensitive LPS assays more interesting data will appear and should further add to the question of the significance of LPS monitoring in patients.

MEDIATORS OF TOXIN-INDUCED DAMAGE AND ORGAN FAILURE

It has recently become clear that the deleterious effects of bacterial toxins are indirect and are caused by secondary mediators from *humoral* and *cellular* sources (Figure 34.7). For example, TNF antibodies have been shown to be protective both in gram-

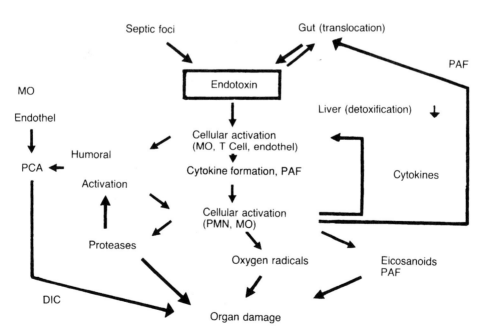

Figure 34.7 Schematic representation of LPS-induced reactions leading to organ damage. PCA = procoagulant activity; PAF = platelet activating factor; MO = macrophages. (Reproduced from Redl and Schlag, 1991.)

negative and gram-positive septicaemia (Hinshaw and Emerson, 1991). Probably the main differences between the different toxins lie in the primary event, e.g. the distinct action of pore-forming toxins. In the following, the relatively best studied toxin-LPS will be used as an example.

Humoral factors

LPS is known to be an activator of several cascade systems – coagulation, fibrinolysis and complement – via both the classical and alternative pathways (Vukajlovich et al., 1987) or only the alternative pathways (Keil et al., 1990).

These conclusions are usually derived from *in vitro* studies similar to others which require LPS in the μg/ml range to be effective. The reactions are probably also valid for *in vivo* studies with 'insensitive' laboratory animals like mice or rat, where mg/kg dosage is common. However, if one compares those 'industrial doses' with plasma levels currently found in clinical septic shock, it is evident that this direct humoral activation might be less likely *in vivo*. Therefore it is important to note that a single dose of endotoxin in humans produces, e.g., sustained PMN activation in the absence of complement activation (C3a and C5a measured) (Moore et al., 1987). Also in endotoxin-challenged volunteers with no complement activation, PMN activation (elastase release) was detected (van Deventer et al., 1990).

Cellular factors

Therefore the current research focus is on the products released by affected host cells (monocytes/macrophages, lymphocytes, granulocytes and endothelial cells).

Tumour necrosis factor

At present, the most prominent cellular mediator of the lethal effect of endotoxin is thought to be cachectin (Beutler and Cerami, 1986; Tracey et al., 1986), which is identical with the tumour necrotizing factor (TNF). TNF-cachectin is secreted by monocytes/macrophages (MO) in response to endotoxin (LPS).

Evidence for the mediator role of TNF is based on:

1. Studies in small animals, where application of TNF resulted in septic shock-like deaths (Tracey et al., 1986).
2. The use of antibodies to murine TNF, which protected animals subjected to otherwise lethal endotoxin shock (Beutler et al., 1985; Bahrami et al., 1991), haemorrhagic shock with endotoxin translocation (Bahrami et al., 1994a; Marzi et al.,

1995) or inhibition of TNF formation (Bahrami et al., 1992).
3. Clinical studies, where TNF plasma levels were found in certain types of sepsis (Waage et al., 1987).

Furthermore, it has been reported, that bolus endotoxin administration (4 ng/kg) to humans results in a rapid rise (up to 300 ± 150 ng/l) and fall in circulating TNF activity (Fromm et al., 1988; Michie et al., 1988; Zabel et al., 1989). Spriggs et al. (1988) further demonstrated that TNF administration in patients has effects similar to LPS infusion.

Studies in chronically instrumented sheep with lymph drainage revealed that human recombinant TNF (50 μg/kg) has similar biological activities to LPS (3 μg/kg) with regard to fever, leukopenia and microvascular permeability changes (Figure 34.8), but with different kinetics. This might be related to the fact that endogenous TNF has to be synthesized secondary to the LPS administration and/or that the applied TNF was a recombinant human material and/or that TNF is not solely responsible for all of the LPS effects.

Further evidence for the LPS mediator action of TNF can be seen in endotoxin-resistant strains of mice (CH3H/HeJ) (Beutler and Cerami, 1987) which are not resistant to TNF application (Lehmann et al., 1987). The protective effect of glucocorticoids in experimental endotoxin shock (Bahrami et al., 1987) is also related to the inhibition of TNF formation (Beutler and Cerami, 1987) and further parts of the cytokine cascade (Redl and Schlag, 1991).

While cytokines are not necessarily cytotoxic by themselves, organ damage with microvascular permeability changes may be mediated by indirect effects on endothelial cells. A distinct sequence of events occurs if the endothelial cells are activated by LPS or by cytokines. The endothelial induced changes induced by LPS and cytokines *in vitro* include cytokine expression, procoagulant activity, immunological functions and increased adhesiveness for leucocytes due to the expression of adherence molecules. These events are within the definition of 'endothelial activation' (Pober and Cotran, 1990). We demonstrated that a (*de novo*) expression of adhesion molecules occurs *in vivo* under septic conditions in non-human primate models by using antibodies to the ELAM-1 structure (Redl et al., 1991a), which seems to be TNF dependent (Redl et al. 1991b).

Interaction between endotoxin and haemostasis

Endotoxin stimulation of both monocytes and endothelial cells produces the procoagulant tissue factor, which may trigger disseminated intravascular coagulation (DIC) (Schorer et al., 1985; Bahrami et al., 1994). Tissue factor can initiate blood

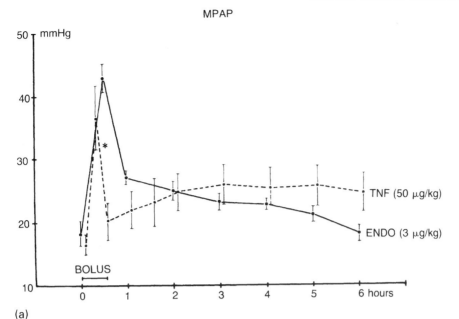

(a)

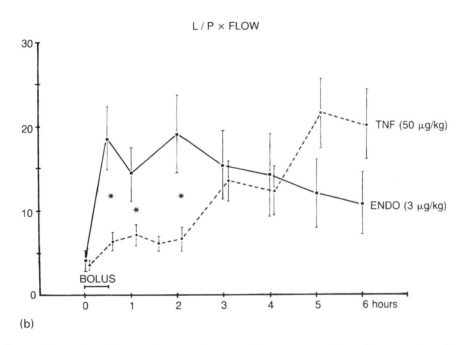

(b)

Figure 34.8 Comparison of cardiovascular reactions and lung permeability changes after either LPS or TNF infusion in a chronic ovine model. (a) MPAP = mean pulmonary arterial pressure. (b) L/P × Flow = protein clearance measured with chronic lymph drainage. (Reproduced from Redl *et al.*, 1989.)

coagulation (Colucci *et al.*, 1983; Lyberg *et al.*, 1983). In addition, endothelial cells may produce a plasminogen activator inhibitor (Colucci *et al.*, 1985), thus further disturbing the procoagulant–anticoagulant balance.

The thrombin formed acts directly on the endothelium, resulting in gap formation (Laposata *et al.*, 1983) and the release of IL-1, which induces procoagulant activity (Nawroth and Stern, 1986) and other IL-1 based endothelial reactions, such as

increased PMN adherence. Thus another feedback loop might exist.

The result of the induced coagulation (DIC) are fibrin deposits in direct contact with the endothelial cell. Fibrin can provoke separation and migration of endothelial cells, which requires contact between fibrin and the cells (Kadish *et al.*, 1979). Thus focal disruption of the microvascular endothelium and increased pulmonary vascular permeability might result.

THERAPY

Traditionally, the therapeutic approach in septicaemia has consisted of surgical removal of severely damaged tissues and bacterial foci, drainage of abscesses and antibiotic treatment. In addition, major efforts have been taken to support the circulation by fluid replacement and inotropic drugs, as well as ventilator support to improve the general condition of the ICU patient.

Despite these efforts, the mortality of septicaemia remains very high. Therefore, numerous efforts have been taken to improve the situation by interfering at the highest level in the mediator cascade of sepsis by binding and/or eliminating the bacterial toxins. These interventions can be divided into:

1. Physical elimination, e.g. plasmapheresis.
2. Binding by antibodies.
3. Binding by non-antigen–antibody interactions, e.g. bacterial permeability increasing protein (BPI).

The rationale for using plasmapheresis or other forms of extracorporeal treatment ((1) above) is the elimination of toxins and/or mediators of toxins by:

a. Total removal of 'sepsis' plasma = plasmapheresis (e.g. Werdan et al., 1991) and substitution.
b. Removal based on molecular size = haemofiltration (e.g. Zadrobilek et al., 1991).
c. Removal based on extracorporeal binding of toxins, e.g. endotoxin as shown with immobilized polymyxin B (e.g. Kodama et al., 1991; Staubach et al., 1991) or charcoal (Bertok, 1991).

Since no large prospective trials on physical elimination have been made concerning the efficacy of these treatment protocols, no final conclusions can be drawn.

When discussing anti-LPS antibody treatment modalities, one has to separate these antibodies according to *binding site* (O-antigen antibodies versus core antigen and lipid A antibodies), *type* of immunoglubulin (IgG, IgM) and *source* (polyclonal versus monoclonal).

Immunization with gram-negative bacteria elicits an antibody response, which is primarily directed against the immunodominant O-specific side chain. Animal studies have provided evidence that such antibodies are highly protective against infection by the bacterial strain LPS which was used for immunization, but do not provide cross-protection against other strains. Since there are several hundreds of serotypes, a species-specific antibody might not be a useful therapeutic approach. Therefore, as suggested by studies of Gaffin (1983), who found in about 10% of a normal population natural anti-LPS antibodies, the preparation of antisera which contain many different species-specific antibodies should be a valid approach. This 'natural' approach is easier in bacilli like *Pseudomonas aeroginosa*, where only a few serotypes occur as potential candidates. In patients with *P. aeruginosa* infections immunoglobulin therapy was shown to be promising (Pilz et al., 1991), and could be partially related to antitoxin effects. A specific anti-alpha-toxin antibody has been described by Bhakdi et al. (1989).

Since the core structure of LPS has parts which are common to most gram-negative bacteria, the administration of anti-core LPS antibodies was considered to be an attractive possibility for therapy. Such an approach is not only supported by experimental studies (Bahrami et al., 1993; Di Padova et al., 1993), but also by retrospective analysis of patients, which suggested that natural high titres of antibodies against LPS resulted in improved survival in patients with gram-negative bacteraemia (McCabe et al., 1972; Pollack et al., 1983), results which, however, could not be confirmed by Baumgartner et al. (1989). Nevertheless, therapeutic efforts in this direction have been taken first by application of *E. coli* polyclonal antiserum or an IgG preparation thereof. In patients with septic shock, the mortality rate was reduced from 77% to 44% with the J5 antiserum in a study of Ziegler et al. (1982), and reduced the development of gram-negative septic shock and its fatal outcome (Baumgartner et al., 1985). Mortality from gram-negative septic shock was not found to be influenced in another study with J5 IgG preparation (Calandra et al., 1988).

Since the production and collection of polyclonal anti-LPS antiserum is a difficult approach, much effort was placed in the development of monoclonal antibodies and many different groups have been involved in such a development. Two of these monoclonals, one murine and one human, both of IgM class, have been reported to bind to the lipid A part of LPS *in vitro* and some contradictory results have been reported on these monoclonals in animal models but are now considered as invalid approaches due to inefficient drugs and study design. For a more in-depth discussion of anti-LPS antibody treatment see Baumgartner and Glauser (1987).

Besides using the antibody approach, there are other ways to bind LPS, e.g. the use of antibiotic polymyxin B (Bannatyne, 1988), also in bound form, for extracorporeal elimination (Hanasawa et al., 1989). A further candidate for LPS binding is the bactericidal/permeability increasing protein (BPI) (Weiss and Olsson, 1987) derived from the group of antibiotic proteins of human neutrophils which has been cloned (Gray et al., 1989). This molecule (55 kDa) is remarkable for its strong affinity for the negatively charged LPS molecule (Marra et al., 1990), its sequence identity with the LPS binding protein (Schumann et al., 1990) and the likelihood that toxic lipid A is the reactive component.

The promise of therapeutic efficacy of BPI comes from the fact that it has been shown to be broadly effective both against rough and smooth LPS chemotypes *in vitro* and inhibited, among others, TNF release. The *in vivo* evidence for therapeutic value of BPI comes from rat studies with endotoxin shock, pseudomonas bacterial challenge in neutropenic animals as well as endotoxin shock experiments in mice. Within all three models, BPI reduced mortality substantially (Fisher *et al.*, 1991). These observations are corroborated by studies in shock-induced translocation, where BPI is an effective treatment modality (Yoo *et al.*, 1995). The observed release of BPI from stimulated PMN (Marra *et al.*, 1991) suggests that BPI might represent a promising natural approach for 'regulation' (therapy) of endotoxin action. In addition to BPI there are further molecules containing a lipid A binding site (Tobias *et al.*, 1988).

Because of the tremendous costs of drug treatment patient selection is critical. Therefore, the limulus assay or other parameter could probably be employed to select those patients at risk, who might benefit most from ante-LPS measures.

FINAL REMARKS

Despite clear evidence that toxins, especially endotoxin (LPS), are involved in septicaemia-related organ failure, there are reports which question such a role of endotoxin (e.g. Natanson *et al.*, 1989). Natanson found that *S. aureus* produced, over 7–10 days, a pattern of reversible cardiovascular dysfunction similar to that elicited by *E. coli*. However, whilst *E. coli* produced a significant endotoxaemia, this did not occur with *S. aureus*. Therefore, this study does not support the idea that it is necessary for endotoxin to leak from the intestine to cause the cardiovascular dysfunction induced by *S. aureus*. In these experiments, an *S. aureus* strain was used, which did not produce the exotoxin responsible for the toxic shock syndrome. These findings indicate that either local bacteria (septic focus) or another source of continuous inflammatory stimulation can activate the host response and elicit a similar pattern of response. Whether such reactions occur without the involvement of toxins or bacterial products cannot yet be elucidated. Current measurement techniques do not monitor the local release of toxins, which might be bound in the direct neighbourhood of a septic focus and thus elicit an inflammatory response without appearing in the systemic circulation. Toxic actions of toxins, e.g. LPS, are indirect, mediated primarily via blood–cell, macrophage and endothelial cell derived products. These mediators are responsible for the interaction of different cell types and for amplification effects through feedback cycles, finally leading to vascular permeability changes and organ damage.

REFERENCES

Aasen A.O., Rishovd A.L., Stadaas J.O. (1989). Role of endotoxin and proteases in multiple organ failure (MOF). In *Progress in Clinical and Biological Research*, Vol. 308, *Second Vienna Shock Forum* (Schlag G., Redl H., eds). New York: Alan R. Liss, pp. 315–22.

Alexander W.J. (1991), Translocation of endotoxin and bacteria from the gut following burn injury. *Circ. Shock*, **34**, 26.

Bahrami S., Leichtfried G., Redl H. et al. (1991). A kinetic-chromogenic method to determine endotoxin on microplates. *Eur. Clin. Lab.*, **October**, 8.

Bahrami S., Schlag G., Redl H. et al. (1987). Comparison of different corticosteroids in rat endotoxemia. In *Progress in Clinical and Biological Research*, Vol. 236. *First Vienna Shock Forum – Part B: Monitoring and treatment of shock* (Schlag G., Redl H., eds). New York: Alan R Liss, pp. 273–86.

Bahrami S., Redl H., Buurman W.A. et al. (1992). Influence of the xanthine derivate HWA138 on endotoxin-related coagulation disturbances: effect in non-sensitized vs D-galactosamine sensitized rats. *Thromb. Haemost.*, **68**, 418–23.

Bahrami S., Redl H., Leichtfried G. et al. (1994b). Similar cytokine but different coagulation responses to lipopolysaccharide injection in D-galactosamine sensitized versus nonsensitized rats. *Infect. Immun.*, **62**, 99–105.

Bahrami S., Schlag G., Yao A.M. et al. (1995). Significance of translocation/endotoxin in the development of systemic sepsis following trauma and/or haemorrhage. *Prog. Clin. Biol. Res.*, **392**, 197–208.

Bahrami S., Yao Y.M., Leichtfried G. *et al.* (1994a). Efficacy of monoclonal antibody (mab) to tumour necrosis factor (TNF) against haemorrhage-induced mortality in rats. *Intens. Care Med.*, **20**, Suppl. 1, S61.

Bannatyne R.M. (1988). Polymyxin B in gram-negative septicemia. *J. Infect. Dis.*, **157**, 1279.

Baumgartner J.D., Glauser M.P. (1987). Controversies in the passive immunotherapy of bacterial infections in the critically-ill patients. *Rev. Infect. Dis.*, **9**, 194–205.

Baumgartner J.D., Glauser M.P., McCutchan J.A. et al. (1985). Prevention of gram-negative shock and death in surgical patients by prophylactic antibody to endotoxin core glycolipid. *Lancet*, **ii**, 59–63.

Baumgartner J.D., Heumann D., Calandra T. et al. (1989). Antibodies to core LPS in patients with gram-negative septic shock: absence of correlation with outcome. In *Program and Abstracts of the 29th Interscience Conference on Antimicrobial Agents and Chemotherapy, Houston*. Washington: American Society for Microbiology, p. 175.

Berg R.D., Wommack E., Deitch E.A. (1988). Immunosuppression and intestinal bacterial overgrowth synergistically promote bacterial translocation. *Arch. Surg.*, **123**, 1359–64.

Berger D., Beger H.G. (1991). Neue Aspekte zur Pathogenese und Behandlung der Sepsis und des septischen Schocks. *Chirurg*, **62**, 4–8.

Berkowitz F.E. (1989). Bacterial exotoxins: how they work. *Pediatr. Infect. Dis.*, **8**, 42–7.

Bertok L. (1991). Prevention of septic/endotoxic shock by radiodetoxified endotoxin (tolerin-R) pretreatment. *Circ. Shock*, **34**, 122.

Beutler B., Cerami A. (1986). Cachectin and tumor necrosis factor as two sides of the same biological coin. *Nature*, **320**, 584–8.

Beutler B., Cerami A. (1987). Cachectin tumor necrosis factor: an endogenous mediator in shock and inflammation. *Immunol. Res.*, **5**, 281–93.

Beutler B., Milsark I.W., Cerami A.C. (1985). Passive immunization against cachectin/tumor necrosis factor protects mice from lethal effect of endotoxin. *Science*, **229**, 869–70.

Bhakdi S., Muhly M., Mannhardt U. et al. (1989). Bakterielle Exotoxine und ihre Relevanz für die Pathogenese des septischen Schocks. *Intensivmed. Notfallmed.*, **26**, (suppl.), 10–15.

Bone R.C., Fisher C.J., Clemmer T.P. et al. (1989). Sepsis syndrome: a valid clinical entity. *Crit. Care Med.*, **17**, 389–93.

Brade H., Brade L., Schade U. et al. (1988). Structure, endotoxicity, immunogenicity and antigenicity of bacterial lipopolysaccharides (endotoxins, O-antigens). In *Bacterial Endotoxins: pathophysiological effects, clinical significance, and pharmacological control* (Levin J., Büller H.R., ten Cate J.W. et al., eds). New York: Alan R. Liss, pp. 17–45.

Brandtzaeg P., Kierulf P., Saugstad P. et al. (1989). Plasma endotoxin as a predictor of multiple organ failure and death in systemic meningococcal disease. *J. Infect. Dis.*, **159**, 195–204.

Brigham K.L., Bowers R., Haynes J. (1979). Increased sheep lung vascular permeability caused by *Escherichia coli* endotoxin. *Circ. Res.*, **45**, 292–7.

Calandra T., Glauser M.P., Schellekens J. et al. (1988). Treatment of gram-negative septic shock with human IgG antibody to *Escherichia coli* J5: a prospective, double-blind, randomized study. *J. Infect. Dis.*, **158**, 312–19.

Chetty C., Schwab J.H. (1984). Endotoxin-like products of gram-positive bacteria. In *Handbook of Endotoxin. Chemistry of endotoxin* (Rietschel E.T. ed.). Elsevier, Amsterdam: Elsevier, p. 376.

Colucci M., Balconi R., Lorenzet R. et al. (1983). Cultured human endothelial cells generate tissue factor in response to endotoxin. *J. Clin. Invest.*, **71**, 1893–7.

Colucci M., Paramo J.A., Collen D. (1985). Generation in plasma of a fast-acting inhibitor of plasminogen activator in response to endotoxin stimulation. *J. Clin. Invest.*, **75**, 818–24.

Danner R.L., Elin R.J., Reilly J.M. et al. (1988). Endotoxemia in human septic shock. *Crit. Care Med.*, **16**, 397.

Deitch E.A., Berg R. (1987). Endotoxin but not malnutrition promotes bacterial translocation of the gut flora in burned mice. *J. Trauma*, **27**, 161–6.

Deitch E.A., Winterton J., Berg R. (1987). The gut as a portal of entry for bacteremia. *Ann. Surg.*, **205**, 681–92.

Di Padova F.E., Brade H., Barclay G.R. et al. (1993). A broadly cross-protective monoclonal antibody binding to *Escherichia coli* and Salmonella lipopolysaccharides. *Infect. Immun.*, **61**, 3863–72.

Fine J., Ruteburg S.H., Schweinburg F.B. (1959). The role of the RES in hemorrhagic shock. *J. Exp. Med.*, **110**, 547–51.

Fisher C.J., Opal S.M., Marra M.N. et al. (1991). Bactericidal/permeability-increasing protein (BPI) reduces mortality in experimental sepsis. *Circ. Shock*, **34**, 120A.

Freudenberg M.A., Galanos C. (1988). The metabolic fate of endotoxins. In *Bacterial Endotoxins: pathophysiological effects, clinical significance, and pharmacological control* (Levin J., Büller, H.R., ten Cate J.W. et al.). New York: Alan R. Liss, pp. 63–75.

Freudenberg M.A., Kleine B., Galanos C. (1984). The fate of lipopolysaccharide in rats: evidence for chemical alteration in the molecule. *Rev. Infect. Dis.*, **6**, 483–7.

Fromm R.E., Suffredini A.F., Kovacs J.A. et al. (1988). Circulating tumor necrosis factor in normal volunteers receiving endotoxin. *Crit. Care Med.*, **16**, 397.

Függer R., Hamilton G., Rogy M. et al. (1990). Prognostic significance of endotoxin determination in patients with severe intraabdominal infection. *J. Infect. Dis.*, **161**, 1314–15.

Gaffin S.L. (1983). Large scale production of anti gramnegative bacterial antibodies. *Lancet*, **ii**, 1420–1.

Galanos C., Lüderitz O., Rietschel E.T. et al. (1977). Newer aspects of the chemistry and biology of bacterial lipopolysaccharides, with special reference to their lipid A component. In *International Review of Biochemistry, Biochemistry of Lipids, II* Vol. 14 (Goodwin T.W., ed.). Baltimore: University Park Press, pp. 239–335.

Goris R.J.A. (1989). Multiple organ failure: whole body inflammation. *Schweiz. Med. Wochenschr.*, **119**, 347–53.

Gray P.W., Flaggs G., Leong S.R., Gumina R.J. (1989). Cloning of the cDNA of a human neutrophil bactericidal protein. Structural and functional correlations. *J. Biol. Chem.*, **264**, 9505–9.

Greenberg R.N., Wilson K.M., Kunz A.Y. et al. (1991). Randomized, double-blind phase II study of antiendotoxin antibody (E5) as adjuvant therapy in humans with serious gram-negative infectious. In *Bacterial Endotoxins: cytokines mediators and new therapies for sepsis* (Sturk A., van Deventer S.J.H., Wouter J. et al.). New York: Wiley-Liss, pp. 179–86.

Haglund U., Jodal M., Lundgren O. (1984). The small bowel in arterial hypotension and shock. In *Physiology of the Intestinal Circulation* (Shepard A.P., Granger D.N., eds.). New York: Raven, pp. 305–19.

Hampton R.Y., Golenbock D.T., Penman M. et al. (1991). Recognition and plasma clearance of endotoxin by scavenger receptors. *Nature*, **352**, 342–4.

Hanasawa K., Tani T., Kodama M. (1989). New approach to endotoxic and septic shock by means of polymyxin B immobilised fiber. *Surg. Gynecol. Obstet.*, **168**, 323–31.

Heymer B., Rietschel E.T. (1977). Biological properties of peptidoglycans. In *Microbiology, American Society for Microbiology* (Heymer B., ed.). Washington: American Society for Microbiology, p. 344.

Hill M.J. (1968). A staphylococcal aggressin. *J. Med. Microbiol.*, **1**, 33–43.

Hinshaw L.B., Emerson T.E. (1991). *Escherichia coli* and *Staphylococcus aureus* induced shock in the nonhuman primate: assessment of multiple organ failure. *Circ. Shock*, **34**, 61A.

Jiang J., Bahrami S., Leichtfried G. et al. (1995). Kinetics of endotoxin and tumor necrosais factor appearance in portal and systemic circulation after hemorrhagic shock in rats. *Ann. Surg.*, **221**, 100–6.

Kadish J.L., Butterfield C.E., Folkman J. (1979). The effect of fibrin on cultured vascular endothelial cells. *Tissue Cell*, **11**, 99–104.

Kalter E.S., Van Dijk W.C., Timmerman A. et al. (1983). Activation of purified human plasma prekallikrein triggered by cell wall fractions of *Escherichia coli* and *Staphylococcus aureus*. *J. Infect. Dis.*, **148**, 682–91.

Keil L.B., Gardiner J.S., DeBari V.A. (1990). Application of pathway-specific enzyme immunoassays to the study of complement activation by salmonella endotoxin. *J. Clin. Immunoassay*, **13**, 187–90.

Kodama M., Tani T., Aoki H. et al. (1991). Treatment of sepsis with extracorporeal elimination of endotoxin. *Circ. Shock*, **34**, 115.

Laposata M., Dovnarsky D.K., Shin H.S. (1983). Thrombin-induced gap formation in confluent endothelial cell monolayers *in vitro*. *Blood*, **62**, 549–56.

Ledingham I.McA., McCartney A.C., Ramsay G. et al. (1988). Endotoxins as mediators. In *Perspectives in Shock Research*, Vol. 264 (Bond R.F., Adams H.R., Chaudry I.H., eds). New York: Alan R. Liss, pp. 125–34.

Lehmann V., Freudenberg M.A., Galanos C. (1987). Lethal toxicity of lipopolysaccharide and tumor necrosis factor in normal and D-galactosamine treated mice. *J. Exp. Med.*, **165**, 657–63.

Lingnau W., Javorsky F., Duregger M. et al. (1991). Endotoxin levels and cytokine release in gram negative sepsis after starting antibiotic therapy. *Circ. Shock*, **34**, 123.

Lundgren O., Svanvik J. (1973). Mucosal hemodynamics in the small intestine of the cat during reduced perfusion pressure. *Acta Physiol. Scand.*, **88**, 551–63.

Lyberg T., Galdal K.S., Evensen S.A. et al. (1983). Cellular cooperation in endothelial cell thromboplastin synthesis. *Br. J. Haematol.*, **53**, 85–91.

Marra N.M., Wilde C.G., Griffith J.E. et al. (1990). Bactericidal/permeability-increasing protein has endotoxin-neutralizing activity. *J. Immunol.*, **144**, 662–6.

Marra M.N., Snable J.L., Scott R.W., Wilde C.G. (1991). Bactericidal/permeability-increasing protein: a naturally occurring lipopolysaccharide antagonist. *Circ. Shock*, **34**, 47A.

Martin A.M., Wenzel R.P., Gorelick K.J. (1991). Gram negative bacterial sepsis in natural history in the 1980s. In *Bacterial Endotoxins: cytokines mediators and new therapies for sepsis* (Sturk A., van Deventer S.J.H., Wouter ten Cate J. et al., eds). New York: Wiley-Liss, pp. 111–19.

Marzi I., Bauer M., Secchi A. et al. (1995). Effects of anti-tumour necrosis factor alpha on leukocyte adhesion in the liver after hemorrhagic shock: an intravital microscopic study in the rat. *Shock*, **3**, 27–33.

McCabe W.R., Kreger B.E., Johns M. (1972). Type-specific and cross-reactive antibodies in gram-negative bacteremia. *New Engl. J. Med.*, **287**, 261–7.

Meakins J.L., Marshall J.C. (1986). Multi-organ-failure syndrome. The gastrointestinal tract: the 'motor' of MOF. *Arch. Surg.*, **121**, 196–208.

Michie H.R., Manogue K.R., Spriggs D.R. et al. (1988). Detection of circulating tumor necrosis factor after endotoxin administration. *New Engl. J. Med.*, **3189**, 1481–6.

Moore F.D., Moss N.A., Revhaug A. et al. (1987). A single dose of endotoxin activates neutrophils without activating complement. *Surgery*, **102**, 200–5.

Morris S.E., Navaratnam N., Herndon D.N. (1990). Changes in mesenteric blood flow affect translocation in sheep. In *Shock Sepsis and Organ Failure (Austria, 1990)* (Schlag G., Redl H., Siegel J.H., Traber D.L., eds). Berlin: Springer-Verlag, pp. 548–67.

Morrison D.C., Ulevitch R.J. (1978). The interaction of bacterial endotoxins with cellular and humoral mediatior systems. *Am. J. Pathol.*, **93**, 527–618.

Munford R.S. (1991). How do animal phagocytes process bacterial lipopolysaccharides? *Acta Pathol. Microbiol. Scand.*, **99**, 487–91.

Natanson C., Danner R.L., Elin R.J. et al. (1989). Role of endotoxemia in cardiovascular dysfunction and mortality. *Escherichia coli* and *Staphylococcus aureus* challenges in a canine model of human septic shock. *J. Clin. Invest.*, **83**, 243–51.

Nawroth P.P., Stern D.M. (1986). Implication of thrombin formation on the endothelial cell surface. *Semin. Thromb. Hemostas.*, **12**, 197–9.

Oken M.M., Peterson P.K., Wilkinson B.J. (1981). Endogenous pyrogen production by human blood monocytes stimulated by staphylococcal cell wall components. *Infect. Immun.*, **31**, 208.

Pabst J., Johnston R.B. (1980). Increased production of superoxide anion by macrophages exposed *in vitro* to muramyl dipeptide or lipopolysaccharide. *J. Exp. Med.*, **152**, 1010.

Pilz G., Class I., Boekstegers P. et al. (1991). Pseudomonas immunoglobulin therapy in patients with pseudomonas sepsis and septic shock. *Antibiot. Chemother.*, **44**, 23–38.

Pober J.S., Cotran R.S. (1990). The role of endothelial cells in inflammation. *Transplantation*, **50**, 537–44.

Pohlman T.H., Stanness K.A., Beatty P.G. et al. (1986). An endothelial cell surface factor(s) induced *in vitro* by lipopolysaccharide, interleukin 1, and tumor necrosis factor-alpha increases neutrophil adherence by a CDw18-dependent mechanism. *J. Immunol.*, **136**, 4548–53.

Pollack M., Huang A.I., Prescott R.K. et al. (1983). Enhanced survival in *Pseudomonas aeruginosa* septicemia associated with high levels of circulating antibody to *Escherichia coli* endotoxin core. *J. Clin. Invest.*, **72**, 1874–81.

Pryjma K., Pryjma K., Grov A. et al. (1976). Immunological activity of staphylococcal cell wall antigens. In *Staphylococci and Staphylococcal Diseases* (Jeljaszewicz J., ed.). New York: Fischer, p. 873.

Ramsay G., Newman P.M., McCartney A.C. et al. (1988). Endotoxaemia in multiple organ failure due to sepsis. In *Bacterial Endotoxins: pathophysiological effects, clinical significance, and pharmacological control* (Levin J., Büller H.R., ten Cate J.W. et al., eds). New York: Alan R. Liss, pp. 237–46.

Ravin H.A., Jenkins C., Rowley D. et al. (1960). On the absorption of bacterial endotoxin from the gastrointestinal tract of the normal and shocked animal. *J. Exp. Med.*, **112**, 783–92.

Redl H., Leichtfried G., Bahrami S. et al. (1992). Special collection and storage tubes for blood endotoxin and cytokine measurements. *Clin. Chem.*, **38**, 764–5.

Redl H., Schlag G. (1991). Pathophysiological aspects of polytrauma, shock and organ failure. In *Molecular Aspects of Inflammation* (Sies H., Flohe L., Zimmer G., eds). Berlin: Springer-Verlag, 255–67.

Redl H., Schlag G., Lamche H. et al. (1989). TNF induced changes of lung vascular permeability: studies in unanesthetised sheep. *Circ. Shock*, **31**, 183–92.

Redl H., Schlag G., Dinges H.P. et al. (1991a). TNF dependent ELAM 1 expression and IL-8 release in baboon septicemia. *Circ. Shock*, **34**, 92A.

Redl H., Dinges H.P., Buurman W.A. et al. (1991b). Expression of endothelial leukocyte adhesion molecule 1 in septic but not traumatic hypovolemic shock in the baboon. *Am. J. Pathol.*, **139**, 461–6.

Reithmann C., Gierschik P., Werdan K. et al. (1989). Einfluß von Pseudomonas Exotoxin A auf die Regulation der Adenylatzyklase des Herzens – Blockade der Noradrenalin-induzierten heterologen Desensibilisierung in Rattenherzmuskelzellen. *Intensivmedizin*, **26**, 50–4.

Rietschel E.T., Brade H., Brade L. et al. (1987). Lipid A, the endotoxic center of bacterial lipopolysaccharide: relation of chemical structure to biological activity. In *Detection of Bacterial Endotoxins with the Limulus Amebocyte Lysate. Progress in Clinical and Biological Research*, Vol. 231 (Watson S.W., Levin J., Novitsky T., eds). New York: Alan R. Liss, pp. 25–53.

Rietschel E.T., Brade L., Holst O. et al. (1990). Molecular structure of bacterial endotoxin in relation to bioactivity. In *Cellular and Molecular Aspects of Endotoxin Reactions* (Nowoty A., Spitzer J.J., Ziegler E.J., eds). Amsterdam: Elsevier Science, pp. 15–32.

Rotta J.J. (1975). Endotoxin-like properties of the peptidoglycan. *Z. Immunitätsforsch. Exp. Klin. Immunol.*, **149**, 230.

Schlag G., Redl H., Dinges H.P. (1990). Bacterial translocation in a baboon model of hypovolemic-traumatic shock. In *Shock Sepsis and Organ Failure (Austria, 1990)* (Schlag G., Redl H., Siegel J.H., Traber D.L., eds). Berlin: Springer-Verlag, pp. 54–83.

Schorer A.E., Rick P.D., Swaim W.R. et al. (1985). Structural features of endotoxin required for stimulation of endothelial cell tissue factor production. Exposure of preformed tissue factor after oxidant-mediated endothelial cell injury. *J. Lab. Clin. Med.*, **106**, 38–42.

Schumann R.R., Leong S.R., Flaggs G.W. et al. (1990). Structure and function of lipopolysaccharide binding protein. *Science*, **249**, 1429–31.

Seydel U., Schröder G., Brandenburg K. (1989). Reconstitution of the lipid matrix of the outer membrane of gram-negative bacteria as asymmetric planar bilayer. *Membrane Biol.*, **109**, 95–103.

Shenep J.L., Morgan K.A. (1984). Kinetics of endotoxin release during antibiotic therapy for experimental gram-negative bacterial sepsis. *J. Infect. Dis.*, **150**, 380–8.

Spriggs D., Sherman M.L., Michie H. et al. (1988). Recombinant human tumor necrosis factor administered as a 24 hour intravenous infusion. A phase I and pharmacologic study. *J. Natl Cancer Inst.*, **80**, 1039–44.

Staubach K.H., Kooistra A., Otto V. et al. (1991). Extracorporal adsorption of endotoxin (ET) in blood – a feasible method in sepsis? *Circ. Shock*, **34**, 115.

Steininger R., Függer R., Hackl W. et al. (1990). Immediate graft function after orthotopic liver transplantation clears endotoxin. *Transplant. Proc.*, **22**, 180.

Stütz P., Liehl E. (1991). Lipid A analogs aimed at preventing the detrimental effects of endotoxin. *Infect. Dis. Clin. North Am.*, **5**, 847–73.

Suttorp N., Hessz T., Seeger W. et al. (1988). Bacterial exotoxins and endothelial permeability for water and albumin *in vitro. Am. J. Physiol.*, **255**, C368–76.

Talke P., Dunn A., Lawlis L. et al. (1975). A model of ovine endotoxemia characterized by an increased cardiac output. *Circ. Shock*, **17**, 103–8.

Tesh V.L., Vukajlovich S.W., Morrison D.C. (1988). Endotoxin interactions with serum proteins relationship to biological activity. In *Bacterial Endotoxins: pathophysiological effects, clinical significance, and pharmacological control* (Levin J., Büller H.R., ten Cate J.W., et al., eds). New York: Alan R. Liss, pp. 47–62.

Tobias P.S., Ulevitch R.J. (1983). Control of lipopolysaccharide-high density lipoprotein binding by acute phase proteins. *J. Immunol.*, **131**, 1913–16.

Tobias P.S., Mathison J.C., Ulevitch R.J. (1988). A family of lipopolysaccharide binding proteins involved in response to gram negative sepsis. *J. Biol. Chem.*, **263**, 13479–81.

Traber D.L., Schlag G., Redl H. et al. (1987). Pulmonary microvascular changes during hyperdynamic sepsis in an ovine model. *Circ. Shock*, **22**, 183–93.

Traber D.L., Redl H., Schlag G. et al. (1988). Cardiopulmonary responses to continuous administration of endotoxin. *Am. J. Physiol.*, **254**, H833–9.

Tracey K.J., Beutler B., Lowrey S.F. et al. (1986). Shock and tissue injury induced by recombinant human cachectin. *Science*, **234**, 470–4.

van Deventer S.J.H., Pauw W., ten Cate J.W. et al. (1987). Clinical evaluation in febrile patients of an optimized endotoxin assay in blood. In *Detection of Bacterial Endotoxins with the Limulus Lysate Test* (Watson S.W., Levin J., Novitsky T.J., eds). New York: Alan R. Liss, pp. 489–99.

van Deventer S.J.H., de Vries I., Statius L.W. et al. (1988). Endotoxemia, bacteremia and urosepsis. In *Bacterial Endotoxins: pathophysiological effects, clinical significance, and pharmacological control* (Levin J., Büller H.R., ten Cate J.W., et al.). New York: Alan R. Liss, pp. 213–24.

van Deventer S.J.H., Büller H.R., ten Cate J.W. et al. (1990). Experimental endotoxaemia in humans. Analysis of cytokine release and coagulation, fibrinolytic and complement pathways. *Blood*, **76**, 2520–6.

van Leeuwen P.A.M., Hong R.W., Rounds J.D. et al. (1991). Hepatic failure and coma following liver resection is reversed by manipulation of gut contents: the role of endotoxin. *Eur. Surg. Res.*, **23/S1**, 59–60.

Verhoef J., Kalter E. (1985). Endotoxic effect of peptidoglycan. In *Bacterial Endotoxins: structure, biomedical significance, and detection with the limulus amebocyte lysate test* (ten Cate J.W., Büller H.R., Sturk A., Levin J., eds). New York: Alan R. Liss, p. 101.

Vukajlovich S.W., Hoffman J., Morrison D.C. (1987). Activation of human serum complement by bacterial lipopolysaccharides structural requirements for antibody independent activation of the classical and alternative pathways. *Molec. Immunol.*, **24**, 319–31.

Waage A., Halstensen A., Expevik T. (1987). Association between tumor necrosis factor in serum and fatal outcome in patients with meningococcal disease. *Lancet*, **i**, 355–7.

Weiss J., Olsson I. (1987). Cellular and subcellular localization of the bactericidal/permeability-increasing protein of neutrophils. *Blood*, **69**, 652–9.

Wells C.L. (1988). Does the gut protect or injure? Expert commentary. In *Perspectives in Critical Care*, vol. 1 (Cerra F.B., ed.). St Louis: Quality Medical Publishing, pp. 25–31.

Werdan K., Pilz G., Kääb S. et al. (1991). Case reports on plasmapheresis (P) as supplemental treatment regimen in sepsis and septic shock. *Circ. Shock*, **34**, 114.

West T.E., Apicella M.A. (1985). Microbial factors in the pathogensis of sepsis. In *Septic Shock* (Root R.K., Sande M.A., eds). Edinburgh: Churchill Livingstone, pp. 27–35.

Westphal O., Lüderitz O. (1954). Chemische Erforschung von Lipopolysacchariden gram-negativer Bakterien. *Angew. Chem.*, **66**, 407–17.

Wortel C.H., Ziegler E.J., van Deventer S.J.H. (1991). Therapy of gram-negative sepsis in man with anti-endotoxin antibodies: a review. In *Bacterial Endotoxins: cytokines mediators and new therapies for sepsis* (Sturk A., van Deventer S.J.H., Wouter J. et al., eds). New York: Wiley-Liss, pp. 161–78.

Yao Y.M., Bahrami S., Leichtfried G. et al. (1995). Pathogenesis of hemorrhage-induced bacteria endotoxin translocation in rats. Effects of recombinant permeability increasing protein. *Ann. Surg.*, **221**, 398–405.

Zabel P., Schönharting M.M., Wolter D.T. et al. (1989). Oxpentifylline in endotoxaemia. *Lancet*, **ii**, 1474–7.

Zadrobilek E., Evstatieva V., Függer R. et al. (1991). Effects of hemofiltration on memodynamics, extravascular lung water, and gas exchange in patients with septic multiple organ failure. *Circ. Shock*, **34**, 115.

Ziegler E.J., McCutchan J.A., Fierer J. et al. (1982). Treatment of gram-negative bacteremia and shock with human antiserum to a mutant *Escherichia coli*. *New Engl. J. Med.*, **307**, 1225–30.

Ziegler E.J., Fisher C.J., Sprung C.L. et al. (1991). Treatment of gram negative bacteremia and septic shock with HA 1A human monoclonal antibody against endotoxin. A randomized double blind placebo controlled trial. *New Engl. J. Med.*, **324**, 429–36.

35. Eicosanoids, Platelet Activating Factor and Nitric Oxide as Mediators of Shock

B. L. Furman and
J. R. Parratt

INTRODUCTION

Numerous substances have been proposed as humoral mediators of shock. Over the past 10 years, abundant evidence has accumulated to implicate eicosanoids and platelet activating factor (PAF); more recent work has suggested an important role for nitric oxide. This chapter summarizes the evidence that these substances might have important functions as mediators of shock.

Much of the evidence has been derived from experimental models for shock. A detailed discussion of the models is beyond the scope of this chapter, but, to paraphrase Dr John Spitzer's words during his presentation at the Shock Society Meeting in Vienna in 1991: 'there are no bad models of shock, only bad interpretation of the data obtained using these models'. Thus extrapolation of the data to human shock must take into account the models from which the data were obtained. Information on the role of eicosanoids, PAF and nitric oxide has been obtained largely from two major types of shock models. First, experimental sepsis can be produced in various species by infusion of live organisms, by the intraperitoneal injection of faecal suspensions or, in rats, by caecal ligation and puncture. Second, there are models based on the assumption that the major pathological consequences of gram-negative septicaemia, which accounts for a large proportion of cases of septic shock, are mediated by bacterial endotoxin. In these models, shock is induced by the bolus injection, or slow infusion, of bacterial lipopolysaccharide derived from various organisms, most commonly *Escherichia coli*. The broad pattern of cardiovascular, metabolic and histopathological changes (e.g. hypotension and decreased cardiac output often preceded by a hyperdynamic phase, pulmonary, renal and mesenteric vasoconstriction; loss of plasma volume; thrombocytopenia; disseminated intravascular coagulation; hyperglycaemia followed by hypoglycaemia; increases in blood lactate; multiple organ failure), seen in septicaemia is observed in both types of models. However, some differences are seen depending on, for example, the animal species used and whether endotoxin is administered by bolus injection or by slow infusion over a period of hours or days. Some of the differences may explain conflicting data concerning the role of various mediators. Many of the changes seen in models of septic shock are also seen in models of shock produced by haemorrhage, burn injury and trauma and there may be common mediators and end mechanisms in all these forms of shock. There is also renewed interest in the concept that endotoxin may play an important role in many types of shock as a result of the breakdown of intestinal barrier function, allowing translocation of intestinal bacteria and access of endotoxin to the systemic circulation (e.g. see Deitch, 1991).

Another problem in extrapolating information from experimental studies to the human with shock arises from the measurement of survival to assess beneficial effects of drug intervention. In many studies survival has been measured over very short periods of time (< 24 hours to 1–2 days). Thus, 'improved survival' often means prolongation of the time to death, rather than an absolute decrease in mortality.

EICOSANOIDS

Eicosanoids are mainly formed from arachidonic acid (AA) which is derived from cell-wall phospholipids under the influence of phospholipase A_2. Metabolism of AA along both the cyclo-oxygenase and lipoxygenase pathways (Figure 35.1) yields a number of highly active molecules (see reviews by Lefer, 1983, 1985; Parratt, 1983, 1985; Ball et al., 1986; Feuerstein and Hallenbeck, 1987; Tracey and Lowry, 1990). Cyclo-oxygenase exists in two forms; a constitutive form (COX-1) and an inducible form (COX-2) (for references see Swierkosz et al., 1995).

Release of eicosanoids in shock

Increases in circulating concentrations of prostaglandin (PGE_2, $PGF_{2\alpha}$, 6-keto $PGF_{1\alpha}$ (the stable breakdown product of prostacyclin, PGI_2) and thromboxane TxB_2 (the stable breakdown product of thromboxane A_2), have been found following the administration of endotoxin to cats, rats, dogs, baboons, sheep and ponies. Moreover, similar increases in circulating concentrations of TxB_2 and 6-keto $PGF_{1\alpha}$ were found in sepsis/septic shock and following haemorrhage in a variety of species. Relatively few studies have been made in man, but raised blood concentrations and increased urinary excretion of $PGF_{2\alpha}$, TxB_2 and 6-keto $PGF_{1\alpha}$ were observed in patients with severe sepsis or septic shock (Parratt et al., 1982; Oettinger et al., 1987; Bernard et al., 1991).

Increases in lung lymph concentrations of 5-Hydroxyeicosatetraenoic acid (5-HETE) and LTB_4 were found after endotoxin administration to sheep. Endotoxin shock in the rat was associated with marked increases in plasma and bile concentrations of $LTEB_4$ and its *N*-acetyl metabolites

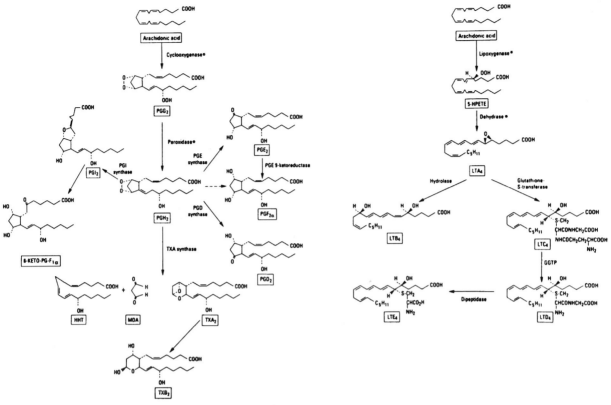

Figure 35.1   Metabolism of arachidonic acid along the cyclo-oxygenase (left panel) and lipoxygenase pathways. (Adapted from Foegh *et al.*, 1991 with permission.)

(Hagmann and Keppler 1982). Clinical studies in patients with ARDS (adult respiratory distress syndrome) showed increases in LTB_4 in blood and bronchoalveolar lavage fluid (Stephenson *et al.*, 1988; Antonelli *et al.*, 1989).

The cyclo-oxygenase products $PGF_{2\alpha}$ and $TxA_2(TxB_2)$ appear very rapidly in the circulation after administration of endotoxin, whereas the formation of prostacyclin is more gradual, with a delayed appearance of 6-keto $PGF_{1\alpha}$ in the circulation. The appearance of 5-HETE in sheep lung lymph was also markedly delayed after endotoxin administration. The time-course of the appearance of $PGF_{2\alpha}$ and TxA_2 is such that they could mediate the initial rapid effects of endotoxin (e.g. the increase in pulmonary artery pressure) and there is evidence in patients with sepsis both for TxA_2 release from the lungs and for a reduced release following improvements of pulmonary function (Parratt *et al.*, 1982). It is possible that later effects of endotoxin (e.g. increase in pulmonary vascular permeability; pulmonary neutrophil accumulation) involve 5-lipoxygenase products.

The source of AA metabolites in shock is uncertain, although they can probably be generated by all tissues. Endotoxin may have direct effects on pulmonary vascular smooth muscle cells, neu-

trophils and endothelial cells to increase production of prostacyclin, thromboxanes and leukotriene C_4. On the other hand, its effects on platelets, and possibly on other tissues, appear to require the presence of white blood cells, suggesting an indirect action mediated via a white cell product, such as interleukin I (IL-1). Very marked direct effects of endotoxin were found on prostanoid production by peritoneal macrophages (Cook *et al.*, 1982). The macrophage may be the most important source of AA metabolites following endotoxin administration, either directly or via the generation of cytokines (tumour necrosis factor (TNF), IL-1), which then influence other cells. Both endotoxin and cytokines induce COX-2. This enzyme may be responsible for the more delayed appearance of prostanoids in endotoxaemia/septic shock.

Ability of arachidonic acid metabolites to mimic various aspects of shock

Although effects may vary among different species, $PGF_{2\alpha}$, TxA_2 and the peptidoleukotrienes, LTC_4 and LTD_4, are potent vasoconstrictor agents, contract a variety of non-vascular smooth muscles and aggregate platelets and white cells (Lefer, 1985; Parratt, 1985). Thus they could variously mediate the

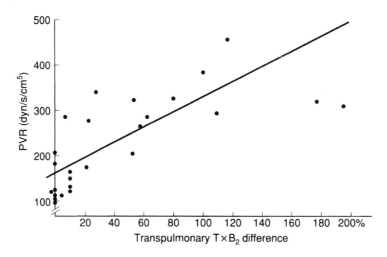

Figure 35.2 Linear correlation of transpulmonary TXB_2 difference and pulmonary vascular resistance (PVR) derived from data of 27 patients in phase I (preshock patients) and phase II (patients with fully pronounced shock syndrome). The thromboxane release is calculated from arterial mixed-venous concentration differences and is given as a percentage of mixed-venous concentrations ($r = 0.70$; $P < 0.001$). (Reproduced from Oettinger *et al.*, 1987, with permission.)

pulmonary, mesenteric and renal vasoconstriction seen after endotoxin administration or in sepsis. Clinical studies have shown a significant correlation between pulmonary vascular resistance and the plasma concentrations of TxB_2 (Oettinger *et al.*, 1987) (Figure 35.2) and between TxB_2 and $PGF_{2\alpha}$ and alveolar–arterial oxygen tension difference (Parratt *et al.*, 1982). Prostacyclin, on the other hand, is a potent vasodilator and could contribute to endotoxin-induced hypotension. The vasodilator, platelet antiaggregatory and cytoprotective properties of prostacyclin (Lefer, 1983) may also ameliorate the harmful effects of other eicosanoids or of other humoral mediators released concurrently in shock. For example, the synthetic prostacyclin analogue, iloprost, can reduce endotoxin-induced pulmonary vasoconstriction. Various eicosanoids (PGE_2, TxA_2 and especially the leukotrienes) increase vascular permeability, leading to pronounced plasma extravasation and reduction in blood volume which are prominent features of endotoxic/septic shock. The leukotrienes, especially LTB_4, have marked effects in promoting leucocyte migration into the tissues, which is also seen, for example, in the lung, after endotoxin administration and in other types of shock. Finally, TxA_2 is an extremely potent aggregator of platelets thus promoting microthrombi formation in the kidney, lung and mesenteric circulations. Such an effect could contribute to the thrombocytopenia and disseminated intravascular coagulation of shock.

It should be noted that some actions of leukotrienes may be indirectly mediated by increased formation of cyclo-oxygenase products.

Modification of shock by inhibition of the synthesis of arachidonic acid metabolites

Effects of inhibitors of cyclo-oxygenase

Northover and Subramanian (1962) were the first to show a beneficial action of acetylsalicyclic acid in canine endotoxin shock. Since then several studies have shown prolongation of survival in endotoxicosis, or in experimental septic shock, after administration of aspirin or other cyclo-oxygenase inhibitors, such as ibuprofen or indomethacin. However, not all studies have reported a beneficial effect and there is some evidence that cyclo-oxygenase inhibitors may actually be detrimental.

The characteristic endotoxin-induced increase in pulmonary artery pressure, as well as the initial and delayed reductions in systemic arterial pressure, in the cat, dog, sheep and pony, are markedly reduced by pretreatment with the cyclo-oxygenase inhibitors indomethacin, flurbiprofen or sodium meclofenamate (Figure 35.3). Endotoxin-induced thrombocytopenia, pulmonary platelet trapping, diarrhoea and increases in haematocrit are also prevented or reduced. Most data have been derived from studies in which animals were *pretreated* with cyclo-oxygenase inhibitors and there is little information on the effect of administering these drugs *after* the induction of shock.

Although ibuprofen, naproxen and indomethacin each showed anti-inflammatory activity in a rat model of ARDS they did not reduce mortality (Turner *et al.*, 1991b) and there is some indication that these drugs might actually enhance inflammatory white cell infiltration in the lung.

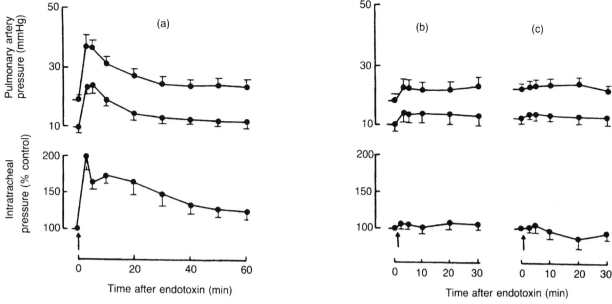

Figure 35.3 Changes in pulmonary artery pressure (upper panels) and intratracheal pressure (lower panels) after endotoxin in control animals (a) and in animals treated with flurbiprofen 100 μg/kg (b) and 250 μg/kg (c). Endotoxin was injected at the arrows. This cyclo-oxygenase inhibitor almost completely abolished the increase in pulmonary artery pressure and intratracheal pressure produced by endotoxin. Values are means ± s.e.m. (Adapted from Parratt and Sturgess, 1976, with permission.)

Endotoxin administration and experimental sepsis depress vascular reactivity to endogenous vasoconstrictors such as noradrenaline and angiotensin II, and this may contribute importantly to peripheral circulatory failure of shock. This disturbance could be rectified by treatment with cyclo-oxygenase inhibitors and could be mimicked by PGE_2 (Gray *et al.*, 1990), thus suggesting an important role for cyclo-oxygenase products. However, other factors are probably of greater importance (see later).

There are predictably few clinical studies using these drugs in shocked patients. In a double-blind, placebo-controlled study, a single dose of indomethacin significantly, but transiently, improved lung function in patients with ARDS (Steinberg *et al.*, 1990). A similarly controlled investigation showed ibuprofen (three doses at 4-hour intervals) to reduce temperature, heart rate and to improve airways function coincident with the reduction in urinary concentrations of AA metabolites (Bernard *et al.*, 1991).

Although the above generally supports a beneficial role for cyclo-oxygenase inhibitors in endotoxaemia/sepsis, it must be pointed out that these drugs are not entirely specific for cyclo-oxygenase inhibition. Large doses may inhibit lipoxygenase (Parratt, 1985). Moreover, such drugs may block calcium entry into white blood cells and inhibit lysosomal enzyme release, actions that may be independent of cyclo-oxygenase inhibition. As 'classical' calcium entry blockers may be beneficial

in endotoxin shock, the beneficial effects of drugs such as indomethacin must be interpreted cautiously.

Another problem may arise from shunting of AA along the lipoxygenase pathway by inhibitors of cyclo-oxygenase. This may explain, for example, the paradoxical enhancement of white cell infiltration in the lung and the failure of cyclo-oxygenase inhibitors to show beneficial effects in some studies. Finally, loss of certain beneficial prostaglandins (e.g. prostacyclin) or loss of prostaglandins in certain tissues may be detrimental to survival. It is well established that renal prostaglandins play an important part in maintaining renal blood flow, particularly when the kidney is exposed to vasoconstrictor stimuli. Thus, the loss of vasodilator prostaglandins may seriously compromise renal function in shock, in which renal blood flow may be already markedly reduced.

Thromboxane synthesis inhibition

Some, but not all, studies have shown that specific inhibition of thromboxane synthesis using imidazole, dazoxiben or dazmegrel improved survival in rats treated with bolus doses of endotoxin and reduced endotoxin-induced thrombocytopenia and hypoglycaemia. No beneficial effect was obtained in experimental sepsis or in studies where endotoxin was given by slow infusion, a situation which may mimic more closely the pattern of endotoxaemia seen in experimental, or indeed clinical, sepsis. Although there is uncertainty about the role

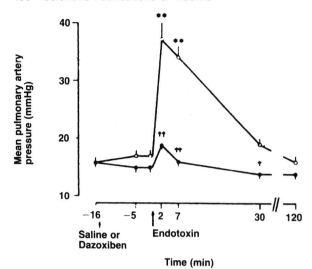

Figure 35.4 Effect of pretreatment with saline (○) and dazoxiben 5 mg/kg (−15 min) (●) on increase in mean pulmonary artery pressure elicited by endotoxin 2 mg/kg given at time zero. Values are means ± s.e.m.; n = 12 (saline group) and 10 (dazoxiben group). ** $P < 0.01$, compared to −1 min value. ++ $P < 0.01$, + $P < 0.05$, compared to corresponding value in saline group. (From Ball et al., 1983, with permission.)

Interpretation of data from experiments using thromboxane synthesis inhibitors may be complicated by two factors. First, 'shunting' may occur from the cyclic endoperoxides towards other prostaglandins or prostacyclin. As prostacyclin is a vasodilator, cytoprotective and inhibits platelet aggregation, beneficial effects of thromboxane synthetase inhibition may be due to increased formation of prostacyclin. Second, cyclic endoperoxides have thromboxane-mimetic properties. Thus specific inhibition of thromboxane synthesis may not eliminate thromboxane-like substances, which may explain the absence of a beneficial effect of thromboxane synthetase inhibitors in some studies.

Lipoxygenase inhibition

Studies using dual cyclo-oxygenase/lipoxygenase inhibitors such as BW 755C and SK&F 86002 have yielded conflicting results and are, of course, difficult to interpret because their use leads to global inhibition of AA metabolism. Selective lipoxygenase inhibitors such as U-66855 (1-naphthalenol, 2, 3, diethyl-4-methoxy-acetate) and SK&F 103842 significantly reduced certain endotoxin-induced changes such as renal microthrombosis, fibrin deposition in glomerular capillaries (Schaub et al., 1987) and lung protein permeability in rat ARDS (Turner et al., 1991a). Mortality and other aspects of lung inflammation were not altered. Again, the interpretation may be difficult as a result of shunting along other pathways of AA metabolism, although this has not been considered experimentally.

Glucocorticoids

Glucocorticoids may have beneficial effects in experimental endotoxicosis and sepsis and in human septic shock (Sprung et al., 1984), although this is still controversial. Glucocorticoids inhibit the formation of AA by induction of an endogenous inhibitor (lipocortin) of phospholipase A_2 (Flower and Blackwell, 1979) and also inhibit the induction of COX-2 by cytokines and by endotoxin (see Swierkosz et al., 1995). Thus, their beneficial effects

of thromboxanes in the lethal outcome of endotoxicosis or sepsis, there is strong evidence for their role in the specific pathophysiological changes occuring in shock. Thus, the specific thromboxane synthesis inhibitors dazoxiben and dazmegrel markedly reduced the increase in pulmonary arterial pressure seen in porcine and feline models of sepsis and endotoxaemia (Figure 35.4). There is also strong evidence for a role of thromboxane in the reduced hepatic perfusion and renal fibrin deposition seen in experimental septic/endotoxic shock, and also in endotoxin-induced gastrointestinal damage. Gastrointestinal damage was markedly diminished by pretreatment with two different thromboxane synthesis inhibitors (OKY 1581 and 1-benzyl imidazole) (Boughton-Smith et al., 1989).

TABLE 35.1

THE EFFECTS OF 4-HOUR INFUSION OF E. COLI ENDOTOXIN (41.7 MG/KG/MIN IV) ON PLASMA CONCENTRATIONS OF THROMBOXANE B_2 AND PROSTAGLANDIN 6-KETO PGF_{1A} IN NORMAL RATS, RATS TREATED WITH METHYLPREDNISOLONE (30 MG/KG^{-1} IV 20 MIN BEFORE COMMENCING THE ENDOTOXIN INFUSION) OR WITH BW755C (50 MG/KG PO 1 HOUR BEFORE COMMENCING THE ENDOTOXIN INFUSION)*. (REPRODUCED FROM MCKECHNIE ET AL. 1985, WITH PERMISSION)

Treatment	Plasma thromboxane B_2	Plasma prostaglandin 6-keto $F_{1\alpha}$
Control (saline infusion)	169 ± 43 (6)	Undetectable (6)
Endotoxin alone	903 ± 127 (6)	4775 ± 622 (6)
Endotoxin + methylprednisolone	783 ± 109(5)	1946 ± 285** (5)
Endotoxin + BW755C	185 ± 38** (6)	78 ± 48** (6)

*Each value is the mean ± s.e.m. of the number of observations shown in parentheses.
**Statistically significant differences from the endotoxin alone value ($P < 0.05$).

in septic shock could be explained by prevention of the formation of both cyclo-oxygenase and lipoxygenase products of AA metabolism. However, this is not supported by experimental data. Despite producing a significant improvement in 96-hour survival rate in rats receiving endotoxin infusion, methylprednisolone produced only a 13% and non-significant decrease in plasma TxB_2 concentrations, which was markedly elevated after endotoxin in this model (Table 35.1). 6-Keto PGF_{1a} concentrations were, moreover, also reduced by methylprednisolone (by 50%; Table 35.1). The TxB_2 concentrations after methylprednisolone were still indicative of the formation of harmful amounts of thromboxane. Dissociation of the beneficial effects of methylprednisolone from effects on eicosanoid formation was also seen in a porcine sepsis model, in which methylprednisolone improved cardiac index whilst producing no significant reduction in TxA_2 formation (Harvey et al., 1987). 6-Keto $PGF_{1\alpha}$ concentrations were reduced, although not significantly. It is interesting that methylprednisolone reduced 6-keto $PGF_{1\alpha}$ concentrations by 50% in either endotoxicosis or in sepsis in the rat. However, it is unclear if this reflects an action on phospholipase A_2 or is secondary to a protective effect of the steroid on the vascular endothelium. Steroids have other actions that might be relevant to their beneficial effects in shock, for example by preventing nitric oxide synthase enzyme induction by endotoxin (see below).

Effects of pharmacological antagonism of arachidonic acid metabolites in shock

Theoretically, the use of specific pharmacological antagonists of AA metabolites should overcome problems of interpretation caused by 'shunting' and should enable the more clear definition of the role of particular AA metabolites in shock.

The specific thromboxane receptor antagonist AH23848 prevented completely the increases in pulmonary artery pressure and intratracheal pressure produced by endotoxin in the cat. Another selective thromboxane receptor antagonist completely prevented mortality in a rat model of ARDS, although, paradoxically, it increased pulmonary inflammation (Turner et al., 1991b). These data thus support findings using thromboxane synthetase inhibitors.

Several leukotriene antagonists have been developed and studied in shock. It is difficult to make any firm conclusions, since the agents differ in their selectivities for the various leukotriene receptors. Moreover, the various studies have used *different* agents in *different* species to examine *different* parameters of shock in *different* shock models! However, the peptidoleukotriene (LTC_4, LTD_4, LTE_4) antagonists FPL55712, FPL57231, LY171883 and SK&F 106203 protected against the lethal

effects of endotoxin, improved renal blood flow during endotoxin shock, blunted endotoxin-induced decreases in cardiac output and in myocardial and gastrointestinal blood flow, improved endotoxin-induced acute hypotension, leukopenia and haemoconcentration, reduced small bowel infarction, diminished the effect of endotoxin on pulmonary artery pressure and reduced pulmonary inflammatory changes in a rat ARDS model (Hagmann and Keppler, 1982; Etemadi et al., 1987; Pacitti et al., 1987; Krausz et al., 1988; Turner et al., 1991a) (Figure 35.5). Prevention of endotoxin-induced hypotension in the rat and reductions in the lymphocytopenia, leucopenia and thrombocytopenia were also reported with the selective LTB_4 receptor blocking drug, LY255283 (Li et al., 1991). In general, the evidence using specific antagonists appears to strongly support a role for leukotrienes in endotoxaemia. However, this information requires cautious interpretation since there are few corroborative studies and the drugs used may not be specific in their antagonism of leukotrienes. For example, in cats FPL 57231 also antagonized the pulmonary effects of $PGF_{2\alpha}$ and of the thromboxanemimetic U46619 and prevented endotoxin-induced increases in TxB_2 and 6-keto $PGF_{1\alpha}$ concentrations (Pacitti et al., 1987). However, in other species this drug appears to show greater specificity. The specificity of other leukotriene antagonists in the doses used and under particular experimental circumstances has only rarely been examined.

Summary and conclusions

To date, the evidence supports a role for AA metabolites as contributory mediators in septic shock. There is clear evidence for increased circulating levels of prostaglandins, thromboxanes, prostacyclin and leukotrienes in various models of septic and endotoxic shock. Inhibition of cyclo-oxygenase generally confers beneficial effects. However, the beneficial effects of eliminating some cyclo-oxygenase products may be offset by shunting to deleterious lipoxygenase products or by the loss of the protective effect of, for example, prostacyclin and prostaglandins of the E series. As beneficial effects of prostacyclin have been found in endotoxin shock, one useful strategy might be concurrent cyclo-oxygenase inhibition and prostacyclin administration. The use of specific thromboxane synthesis inhibitors and, more recently, specific thromboxane antagonists, has provided strong evidence for a role for thromboxanes in the acute pulmonary effects of sepsis and endotoxin. However, it remains to be determined if they have a role in the more long-term lung damage of septic shock. Similarly, it seems likely that there is an important role for lipoxygenase products of AA metabolism.

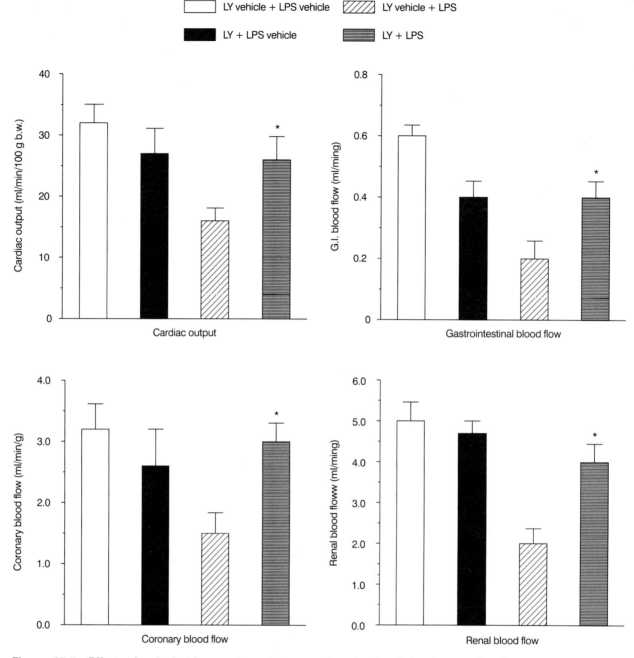

Figure 35.5 Effect of a leukotriene antagonist on endotoxin shock in the rat. Cardiac output, coronary, gastrointestinal and renal blood flow 30 min after endotoxin (15 mg/kg IV). The leukotriene (LTD$_4$, LTE$_4$, LTC$_4$) antagonist LYH1883 (LY) (30 mg/kg i.p.) was administered 10 min prior to LPS or vehicle. Bars represent mean ± s.e.m. of 4–6 rats per group. *$P < 0.05$ compared to vehicle + endotoxin (LPS) group. (Adapted from Etemadi *et al.*, 1987, with permission.)

Apart from the production of eicosanoids, the metabolism of AA yields oxygen-centred free radicals which are implicated in producing tissue damage in several pathological conditions. The lipid-soluble antioxidant α-tocopherol and the hydrophobic spin trapping agent phenyl-*tert*-butyl-nitrone improved survival in endotoxicosis in conscious rats (McKechnie *et al.*, 1986), although the natural free radical scavenger, superoxide dismutase, infused alone, or with catalase, did not modify survival in this model (McKechnie *et al.*, 1986), it did reduce gastric mucosal damage in cats with sepsis (Arvidsson *et al.*, 1985). Thus, there is some evidence for a role for oxygen free radicals in the pathophysiology of endotoxicosis and sepsis and other forms of shock (Siegel, 1991). Further work is required in this area. Prevention of AA metabolism, or formation, may confer benefit by reducing the formation of oxygen free radicals and thus the consequent lipid-peroxidation-induced tissue damage.

PLATELET ACTIVATING FACTOR

Platelet activating factor (PAF, PAF-acether) is formed, via lyso-PAF, from cell membrane phospholipids under the influence of phospholipase A_2 (Figure 35.6; Braquet et al., 1987). It is released from many cell types, including platelets, monocytes, macrophages, mast cells and endothelial cells. PAF is rapidly degraded in plasma to lyso-PAF.

Release of platelet activating factor in shock

The high lability of PAF in the circulation and problems in obtaining sufficiently sensitive and specific assays have made it difficult to determine the release of PAF in shock. However, patients with sepsis show elevated plasma concentrations of PAF

(Leaver et al., 1990). Administration of endotoxin to rats leads to increased concentrations of PAF in plasma (Tracey and Lowry, 1990) and markedly elevated PAF concentrations were detected in the peritoneal fluid of rats subjected to traumatic shock (Noble-Collip drum). Human monocytes incubated in vitro responded to low concentrations of endotoxin with an increase in PAF release (Leaver et al., 1990). Endotoxin administration to anaesthetized rats produced a dose-dependent increase in jejunal PAF content (Boughton-Smith et al., 1989) (Figure 35.7).

Ability of platelet activating factor to mimic pathophysiological changes seen in shock

The consequences of PAF administration to various species resemble closely the changes seen in septic/endotoxic shock. Thus PAF produces hypotension, acute circulatory collapse, impaired cardiac function, increased vascular permeability, platelet activation and aggregation, bronchoconstriction, long-lasting lung inflammation, gastrointestinal damage and endothelial cell swelling (Braquet et al., 1987).

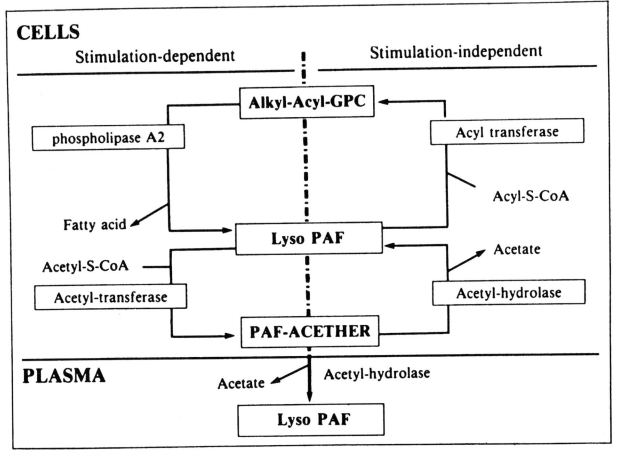

Figure 35.6 Biosynthesis and degradation of PAF-acether. (Adapted from Braquet et al., 1987, with permission.)

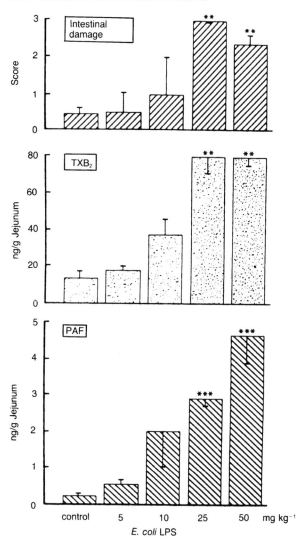

Figure 35.7 Induction of jejunal damage and the stimulation of formation of PAF and TXB_2, 10 min following challenge by *E. coli* lipopolysaccharide (LPS; 5–50 mg/kg IV) in the rat. Jejunal damage was scored macroscopically in a blinded manner using a 0–3 scale. Jejunal formation of PAF and TXB_2 is expressed as ng/g of tissue. Results are the mean ± s.e.m. of (5) rats where statistical significance from the control group is shown as ** $P < 0.01$ and *** $P < 0.001$. (Reproduced from Boughton-Smith *et al.*, 1989, with permission.)

Modification of shock by platelet activating factor antagonists

Several specific antagonists of PAF at its receptors have been identified and studied in various models of shock. The PAF antagonists CV-3988, SRI 63441, BN 50739, BN 52021, ONO-6240, kadsurenone and WEB 2086 reduced endotoxin-induced hypotension and prolonged survival (Braquet *et al.*, 1987; Tracey and Lowry, 1990). PAF antagonists were very effective in suppressing endotoxin-induced gastrointestinal damage in the rat (Boughton-Smith *et al.*,

1989). In a double-blind, placebo-controlled study, the PAF antagonist Ro 24–4736 reduced symptoms (rigors and myalgia) as well as peak concentrations of cortisol and adrenaline during experimental endotoxaemia in man (Thompson *et al.*, 1994).

Although the above evidence clearly supports a role for PAF in endotoxin-induced shock, it remains unclear if the actions of PAF are direct or are mediated by other substances. PAF increases the release of thromboxane and there is indirect evidence that thromboxane may mediate the effects of PAF in inducing gastrointestinal damage (Boughton-Smith *et al.*, 1989). PAF-receptor antagonists (BN 52021, BN 50739) prevented endotoxin-induced increases in plasma thromboxane and PGE_2 concentrations (Rabinovici *et al.*, 1990). Moreover, BN 50739 markedly reduced TNF-induced mortality in rats (Rabinovici *et al.*, 1990). TNF, along with other cytokines, may be pivotal in mediating shock in response to bacterial endotoxin (Tracey and Lowry, 1990; Tracey, 1991). PAF antagonists were also found to reduce plasma TNF concentrations in endotoxin-treated rats and mice (Rabinovici *et al.* 1990) (Figure 35.8). However, in human experimental endotoxaemia Ro 24–4736 produced its effects without modifying cytokine concentrations (Thompson *et al.*, 1994).

Summary and conclusions

There is strong evidence implicating PAF as a mediator of endotoxic shock. PAF formation is stimulated by phospholipase A_2 and both PAF and AA may be derived from the same cell wall phospholipids. Moreover, PAF appears to release further AA metabolites. It remains to be established if PAF plays a central role in eicosanoid formation in endotoxaemia. There do not appear to be any clinical studies of PAF antagonists in patients with the sepsis syndrome.

NITRIC OXIDE

The discovery of endothelium-derived relaxant factor by Furchgott (for references see Fleming *et al.*, 1991a) was followed by a period of intensive research which resulted in the characterization of this factor as nitric oxide or a nitric oxide-like material (for references see Fleming *et al.*, 1991a). Nitric oxide can be produced by a variety of cell types from L-arginine under the influence of the enzyme nitric oxide synthase. It activates soluble guanylate cyclase in various tissues, thereby elevating the cytosolic concentration of cyclic 3′5′ guanosine monophosphate (cGMP). There are at least two different types of nitric oxide synthase, characterized by their dependency upon Ca^{2+}, ability to use different substrates and sensitivity to inhibition by various substances. The constitutive, calcium-dependent nitric oxide synthase is present in

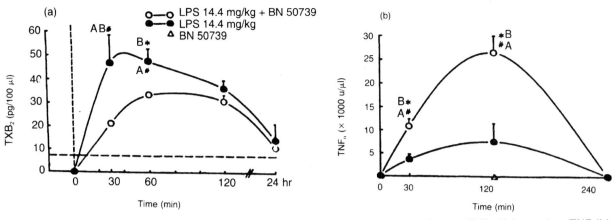

Figure 35.8   Effect of pretreatment with the PAF antagonist BN50739 (10 mg/kg) on TXB_2 ((a), $n = 6$ or TNF (b), $n = 5$) response to LPS. The horizontal dashed line represents the minimum detecting level of TXB_2 assay (7.8 pg/ 100 μl), *$P < 0.05$, # $P < 0.01$, A vs baseline; B, vs other group. (Reproduced from Rabinovici et al., 1990, with permission.)

endothelial cells and brain (Knowles et al., 1990) and is rapidly activated in response to endothelium-dependent vasodilators, such as acetylcholine and bradykinin. The second type is present in lung, liver, macrophages and smooth muscle (Knowles et al., 1990) and is an inducible enzyme, activity being dependent upon protein synthesis. There is strong evidence that endotoxin induces the second type of enzyme, resulting in a long-lasting production of nitric oxide (Knowles et al., 1990; Rees et al., 1990; Fleming et al., 1991a,b), probably via release of the cytokines TNF and IL-1 (McKenna, 1991). The consequent elevation of cGMP in vascular smooth muscle leads to a marked loss of vascular responsiveness to endogenous vasoconstrictors (Fleming et al., 1991a). Nitrovasodilators, such as sodium nitroprusside, exert their effects by liberating nitric oxide within the vascular smooth muscle cells. These agents mimic endotoxin in producing a loss of reactivity to vasoconstrictor agents (Fleming et al., 1991a).

Effects of inhibition of nitric oxide synthesis or antagonism of nitric oxide in shock

Nitric oxide synthesis from L-arginine can be stereospecifically inhibited by a variety of analogues of L-arginine, including N^G-monomethyl-L-arginine (LNMMA) and N^G-nitro-L-arginine. These agents were found to reverse endotoxin-induced hypotension and to restore vascular responsiveness to vasoconstrictors and to sympathetic nerve stimulation, both in vivo and in vitro (Kilbourn et al., 1990; Fleming et al., 1991a) (Figure 35.9). These effects of inhibitors are stereospecific and can be overcome by addition of an excess of L-arginine (but not of D-arginine). Glucocorticoids, which can restore blood pressure, at least in experimental shock (McKechnie et al., 1985), were

found to prevent endotoxin-mediated induction of nitric oxide synthase in vascular smooth muscle and to prevent endotoxin-induced impairment of vascular responsiveness (Rees et al., 1990).

Prevention of the action of nitric oxide using inhibitors of soluble guanylate cyclase (methylene blue, LY 83583 (6-anilino-5, 8-quinolinedione)) was also effective in restoring vascular responsiveness in tissues removed from endotoxin-treated animals (Fleming et al., 1991b).

Pathophysiological significance of nitric oxide in shock

Although cardiac function is clearly impaired in shock, many patients die with a normal or elevated cardiac output. Thus, the unrelenting hypotension of shock may be largely due to peripheral vascular failure. A marked and prolonged elevation in nitric oxide production would render the peripheral vasculature unresponsive to both endogenous and exogenous vasoconstrictors. Additionally, nitric oxide derived from hepatic Kupffer cells probably plays an essential role in inducing the synthesis of acute-phase proteins in hepatocytes. These proteins may play an important part in activating the complement system and contributing to the cell damage of shock (Siegel, 1991). Inhibition of this elevated nitric oxide production would appear to be a potentially useful strategy for reversing shock. Simple inhibition of the L-arginine pathway using L-arginine analogues certainly elevates blood pressure in shocked patients (Petros et al., 1994). However, this may well be detrimental to tissue perfusion and could therefore exacerbate shock. Such an outcome is supported by findings in rats, in which L-NMMA markedly enhanced endotoxin-induced jejunal damage, an effect which was prevented by concurrent administration of the

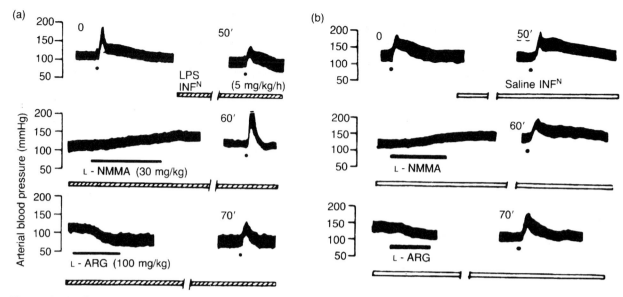

Figure 35.9 Representative traces showing the effect of L-NMMA and L-arginine on continuously recorded arterial blood pressure and the pressor response to noradrenaline in anaesthetized rats during infusion of LPS (5 mg kg/h, (a)) or solvent (saline (b)). The pressor response to noradrenaline (1 mg/kg, injected at.) was measured before and after 50 min of infusion of LPS or saline (upper panels). In the continued presence of LPS or solvent, further pressor responses to noradrenaline were obtained in the presence of L-NMMA (30 mg/kg, lower panels). The time relative to beginning the infusion is indicated in minutes beside each response. (Reproduced from Julou-Schaeffer *et al.*, 1990, with permission.)

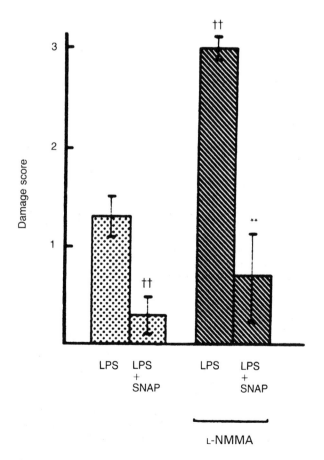

Figure 35.10 Effect of SNAP (*S*-nitroso-*N*-acetyl penicillamine, a nitric oxide donor), 10 μg kg/min IV, on the jejunal damage induced by *E. coli* LPS (50 mg/kg IV) and on enhanced damage produced by pretreatment with L-NMMA (50 mg/kg IV), an inhibitor of nitric oxide synthesis. Macroscopic damage of the jejunum induced 15 min after LPS was scored (0–3 scale) in a randomized manner. SNAP infusion was started 10 min before LPS. Results are means ± s.e.m. of six rats per experimental group. Statistical difference from LPS is shown as $^{++}P < 0.01$ and from L-NMMA and LPS as $^{**}P < 0.01$.

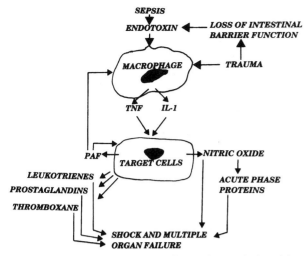

Figure 35.11 Some possible interrelationships between eicosanoids, PAF and nitric oxide in the production of shock.

nitric oxide donor, *S*-nitroso-*N*-acetyl penicillamine (Boughton-Smith *et al.*, 1990) (Figure 35.10). An important approach will be to selectively prevent the induction of nitric oxide synthase without interfering with the protective effect of the constitutive enzyme. Glucocorticoids probably do this but their clinical effectiveness in shock remains controversial. More selective approaches are required. Recently, a novel class of potent isothiourea nitric oxide synthase inhibitors has been developed (Southan *et al.*, 1995). Some of these, for example, 5-methyl-isothiourea, show selectivity for the inducible enzyme and produce beneficial effects and improved survival in experimental endotoxaemia.

OVERALL SUMMARY AND CONCLUSIONS

There is strong evidence that eicosanoids, PAF and nitric oxide fulfil the criteria as putative mediators of shock. Thus, they are released in various forms of shock and antagonism of their effects at receptor level, or inhibition of their synthesis, ameliorate some features of the shock state. There are certainly important interrelationships between these substances; some of these are well documented, some have yet to be unravelled. For example, PAF produces some of its actions through the increased formation of eicosanoids, whereas leukotrienes work partly through the liberation of cyclo-oxygenase products and partly on endothelial cells to increase the formation of PAF. PAF can also induce nitric oxide synthase, possibly via cytokines. On the other hand, nitric oxide can reduce the expression of COX-2, as well as its activity (Swierkosz *et al.*, 1995). It is highly likely that the formation of all three groups of mediators in shock is initiated to an important extent by the activity of cytokines (TNF,

IL-1) released from monocyte/macrophages. In the case of septic shock the initial trigger is endotoxin, which may also be an important mediator of non-infective trauma, as a result of bacterial (or bacterial product) translocation. TNF may also be released in response to PAF, acting on the monocyte/macrophage in a positive feedback manner. We have attempted to summarize some of these relationships in a simple fashion in Figure 35.11.

The question remains as to whether one should attempt to inhibit or antagonize any one or groups of these mediators in the therapy of shock. Some at least have important roles in host-defence mechanisms and their antagonism is unlikely to be without cost in terms of compromising these mechanisms or other physiological functions. As the cytokines are probably central to the release of all the mediators discussed in this chapter, perhaps the rational therapeutic approach should be focused on that area. This is discussed elsewhere in this volume.

REFERENCES

Antonelli A., Bufi M., De Blasi R.A. et al. (1989). Detection of leukotriene B_4, C_4 and of their isomers in arterial, mixed venous blood and bronchoalveolar lavage fluid from ARDS patients. *Intensive Care Med.*, **15**, 296–301.

Arvidsson S., Falt K., Marklund S., Haglund U. (1985). Role of oxygen free radicals in the development of gastrointestinal mucosal damage in *Eschericia coli* sepsis. *Circ. Shock*, **16**, 383–94.

Ball H.A., Cook J.A., Wise W.C., Halushka P.V. (1986). Role of thromboxane, prostaglandins and leukotrienes in endotoxic and septic shock. *Intensive Care Med.*, **12**, 116–26.

Ball H.A., Parratt J.R., Zeitlin I.J. (1983). The effect of dazoxiben, a specific inhibitor of thromboxane, on acute pulmonary responses to *E Coli* endotoxin in anaesthetised cats. *Br. J. Clin. Pharmacol.*, **15**, 1275–1315.

Bernard G.R., Swindell B.B., Higgins S. et al. (1991). Role and modification of eicosanoids in human sepsis syndrome. *Circ. Shock*, **34**, 159.

Boughton-Smith N.K., Hutcheson I., Whittle B.J.R. (1989). Relationship between PAF-acether and thromboxane A_2 biosynthesis in endotoxin-induced intestinal damage in the rat. *Prostaglandins*, **38**, 319–33.

Boughton-Smith N.K., Hutcheson I.R., Deakin A.M. et al. (1990). Protective effect of *S* nitroso-*N*-acetyl-penicillamine in endotoxin-induced acute intestinal damage in the rat. *Eur. J. Pharmacol.*, **191**, 485–8.

Braquet P., Mencia-Huerta J.M., Chabrier P.E. et al. (1987). The promise of platelet activating factor. *ISI Atlas Sci. Pharmacol.*, **1**, 187–98.

Cook J.A., Halushka P.V., Wise W.C. (1982). Modulation of macrophage arachidonic acid metabolism: potential role in the susceptibility of rats to endotoxin shock. *Circ. Shock*, **9**, 605–12.

Deitch E.A. (1991). Experimental evidence of bacterial translocation in trauma. In *Shock, Sepsis and Trauma. Second Bernard Wiggers Conference* (Schlag G., Redl H.,

Siegel J.H., Traber D.L., eds). Berlin: Springer-Verlag, pp. 23–47.

Etemadi A.R., Tempel G.E., Farah B.A. et al. (1987). Beneficial effects of leukotriene antagonist on endotoxin-induced haemodynamic alterations. *Circ. Shock*, **22**, 55–64.

Feuerstein G., Hallenbeck J.M. (1987). Prostaglandins, leukotrienes and platelet-activating factor in shock. *Ann. Rev. Pharmacol. Toxicol.*, **27**, 301–13.

Fleming I., Furman B.L., Gray G.A. et al. (1991a). Mechanisms of vascular impairment during endotoxaemia with special reference to the role of the L-arginine pathway. In *Shock, Sepsis and Organ Failure. Second Bernard Wiggers Conference* (Schlag G., Redl H., Siegel J.H., Traber D.L., eds). Berlin: Springer-Verlag, pp. 399–424.

Fleming I., Julou-Schaeffer G., Gray G.A. et al. (1991b). Evidence that an L-arginine/nitric oxide dependent elevation in tissue cyclic GMP content is involved in depression of vascular reactivity by endotoxin. *Br. J. Pharmacol.*, **103**, 1047–52.

Flower R.J., Blackwell G.J. (1979). Anti-inflammatory steroids induce biosynthesis of a phospholipase A_2 inhibitor which prevents prostaglandin generation. *Nature*, **278**, 456–9.

Foegh M.L., Fletcher M., Rasswell P.W. et al. (1991). The eicosanoids: Proslaglandins, thromboxones, leukolrienes and related compounds. In *Basic and Clinical Endocrinology* (Greenspan F.S., ed.). New York: Prentice-Hall, pp. 55–6.

Gray G.A., Furman B.L., Parratt J.R. (1990). Endotoxin-induced impairment of vascular reactivity in the pithed rat: role of arachidonic acid metabolites. *Circ. Shock.*, **31**, 395–406.

Hagmann W., Keppler D. (1982). Leukotriene antagonists prevent endotoxin lethality. *Naturwissenschaften*, **69**, 594–5.

Harvey C.F., Sugerman H.J., Tatum J.L. et al. (1987). Ibuprofen and methylprednisolone in a pig pseudomonas ARDS model. *Circ. Shock*, **21**, 175–84.

Julou-Schaeffer G., Gray G.A., Fleming I., Schott C., Parratt J.R., Stodet J-C. (1990). Loss of vascular responsiveness induced by endotoxin involves the L-arginine pathway. *Am. J. Physiol.*, **259**, H1038–43.

Kilbourn R.G., Jubran A., Gross S.S. et al. (1990). Reversal of endotoxin-mediated shock by N^G-methyl-L-arginine an inhibitor of nitric oxide synthesis. *Biochem. Biophys. Res. Commun.*, **172**, 1132–8.

Knowles R.G., Merrett M., Salter M., Moncada S. (1990). Differential induction of brain, lung and liver nitric oxide synthase by endotoxin in the rat. *Biochem. J.*, **270**, 833–6.

Krausz M.M., Dahan J.B., Gross D. (1988). Effect of the leukotriene receptor antagonist LY-171883 on endotoxaemia in awake sheep. *Circ. Shock*, **26**, 431–42.

Leaver H.A., Qu J.M., Smith G. et al. (1990). Endotoxin releases platelet-activating factor from human monocytes *in vitro. Immunopharmacology*, **20**, 105–13.

Lefer A.M. (1983). Role of prostaglandins and thromboxanes in shock states. In *Handbook of Shock and Trauma*, Vol. 1: *basic science* (Altura B.M., Lefer A.M., Schumer W., eds). New York: Raven, pp. 355–76.

Lefer A.M. (1985). Eicosanoids as mediators of ischaemia and shock. *Fed. Proc.*, **44**, 275–80.

Li E.J., Cook J.A., Wise W.C. et al. (1991). Effect of LTB_4 receptor antagonists in endotoxin shock in the rat. *Circ.*

Shock, **34**, 385–92.

McKechnie K., Furman B.L., Parratt J.R. (1985). Metabolic and cardiovascular effects of endotoxin infusion in conscious unrestrained rats: effects of methylprednisolone and BW755c. *Circ. Shock*, **15**, 205–15.

McKechnie K., Furman B.L., Parratt J.R. (1986). Modification by oxygen free radical scavengers of the metabolic and cardiovascular effects of endotoxin infusion in conscious rats. *Circ. Shock*, **19**, 429–39.

McKenna P.M. (1990). Prolonged exposure of rat aorta to low levels of endotoxin *in vitro* results in impaired contractility. *J. Clin. Invest.*, **86**, 160–8.

Northover B.J., Subramanian G. (1962). Analgesic antipyretic drugs as antagonists of endotoxic shock in dogs. *J. Pathol. Backeriol.*, **83**, 463–8.

Oettinger W., Berger D., Beger H.G. (1987). The clinical significance of prostaglandins and thromboxane as mediators of septic shock. *Klin. Wochenschr.*, **65**, 61–8.

Pacitti N., Bryson S.E., McKechnie K. et al. (1987). Leukotriene antagonist FPL 57231 prevents the acute pulmonary effects of *Eschericia coli* endotoxin in cats. *Circ. Shock*, **21**, 155–68.

Parratt J.R. (1983). Pulmonary function in experimental endotoxin shock – an examination of the role of chemical mediators. In *Shock Research* (Lewis D.H., Hagland U., eds). Amsterdam: Elsevier Science, pp. 129–45.

Parratt J.R. (1985). The role of arachidonic acid metabolites in endotoxin shock I: lipoxygenase products. In *Handbook of Endotoxin*, vol. 2; *Pathophysiology of Endotoxin* (Hinshaw L.B., ed.). Amsterdam: Elsevier Science, pp. 203–36.

Parratt J.R., Coker S.J., Hughes B. et al. (1982). The possible roles of prostaglandins and thromboxane in the pulmonary consequences of experimental endotoxin shock and clinical sepsis. In *Role of Chemical Mediators in the Pathophysiology of Acute Illness and Injury* (McConn R., ed.). New York: Raven, pp. 195–218.

Parratt J.R., Sturgess R.M. (1976). The effect of a new anti-inflamatory drug flurbiprofen, on the respiratory, haemodynamic and metabolic responses to *E. Coli* endotoxin shock in the cat. *Br. J. Pharmacol.*, **58**, 547–52.

Petros A., Lamb G., Leone A. et al. (1994). Effect of a nitric oxide synthase inhibitor in human with septic shock. *Cardiovasc. Res.*, **28**, 34–9.

Rabinovici R., Yue T-L., Farhat M. et al. (1990). Platelet activating factor (PAF) and tumour necrosis factor-α (TNF_α) interactions in endotoxemic shock: studies with BN50739, a novel PAF antagonist. *J. Pharmacol. Exp. Ther.*, **255**, 256–63.

Rees D.D., Cellek S., Palmer R.M.J., Moncada S. (1990). Dexamethasone prevents the induction by endotoxin of a nitric oxide synthase and the associated effects on vascular tone: an insight into endotoxin shock. *Biochem. Biophys. Res. Commun.*, **173**, 541–7.

Schaub R.G., Ochoa R., Simmons C.A., Lincoln K.L. (1987). Renal microthrombosis following endotoxin infusion may be mediated by lipoxygenase products. *Circ. Shock*, **21**, 261–70.

Siegel J.M. (1991). The liver as a modulator of the host defense response: most defense failure disease as a manifestation of hepatic decompensation. In *Shock, Sepsis and Organ Failure. Second Bernard Wiggers Conference* (Schlag G., Redl H., Siegel J.H., Traber D.L., eds).

Amsterdam: Springer-Verlag, pp. 149–202.

Southan G.J., Szabo C., Thierermann C. (1995). Isothioureas: potent inhibitors of nitric oxide synthases with variable isoform selectivity. *Br. J. Pharmacol.*, **114**, 510–16.

Sprung C.L., Caralis P.V., Marcial E.H. et al. (1984). The effects of high-dose corticosteroids in patients with septic shock. A prospective study. *N. Engl. J. Med.*, **311**, 1137–43.

Steinberg S.M., Rodriguez J.G., Bitzer L.G. et al. (1990). Indomethacin treatment of human adult respiratory syndrome. *Circ. Shock*, **30**, 375–84.

Stephenson A.M., Lonifro A.J., Hyers T.M. et al. (1988). Increased concentrations of leukotrienes in bronchoalveolar lavage fluid of patients with ARDS or at risk of ARDS. *Am. Rev. Resp. Dis.*, **138**, 714–19.

Swierkosz A., Mitchell J.A., Warner T.D. et al. (1995). Co-induction of nitric oxide synthase and cyclo-oxygenase: interactions between nitric oxide and prostanoids. *Br. J. Pharmacol.*, **114**, 1335–42.

Thompson W.A., Coyle S., Van Zee K. et al. (1994). The metabolic effects of platelet activating factor antagonism in endotoxaemic man. *Arch. Surg.*, **129**, 72–9.

Tracey K.J. (1991). Tumour necrosis factor (cachectin) in the biology of septic shock syndrome. *Circ. Shock.*, **35**, 123–8.

Tracey K.J., Lowry S.F. (1990). The role of cytokine mediators in septic shock. *Adv. Surg.*, **23**, 21–56.

Turner C.R., Lackey M.N., Quinlan M.F. et al. (1991a). Therapeutic interactions in a rat model of adult respiratory distress syndrome: II Lipoxygenase pathway inhibition. *Circ. Shock*, **34**, 263–9.

Turner C.R., Lackey M.N., Quinlan M.F. et al. (1991b). Therapeutic interventions in a rat model of adult respiratory distress syndrome: III cyclooxygenase pathway inhibition. *Circ. Shock*, **34**, 270–7.

36. Opioids: Physiology, Pharmacology and Therapeutics

R. G. Evans and
J. Ludbrook

INTRODUCTION

Knowledge of the psychoactive properties of opium dates back to the ancient Babylonians at least 4000 years BC. However, it is only since the mid 1970s that the diverse actions of opioids have come to be appreciated. This explosion of our understanding of their pharmacology, physiology and pathophysiology was stimulated by two major discoveries. The first was the demonstration that opioids attach themselves to membrane-bound receptors to produce their effects (Pert and Snyder, 1973). The second was the discovery in 1975 of the existence of endogenous opioid peptides (Bloom, 1983). These events led to the realization that endogenous opioids are important mediators of a range of physiological responses, particularly in stress and trauma. This chapter concentrates on the importance of endogenous opioid mechanisms in the response to trauma, and the use of exogenous opioids in the treatment of the injured patient, with particular reference to new possibilities in opioid therapy. In addition, some of the effects of exogenous opioids which should be taken into account when they are used after injury are discussed.

First, an overview of the current understanding of the pharmacology and biochemistry of opioids is presented. The complexity of opioid systems results from multiple endogenous ligands, receptor subtypes, signal transduction mechanisms and sites of action involved.

BASIC PHARMACOLOGY AND BIOCHEMISTRY OF OPIOID SYSTEMS

Opioid receptors and signal transduction

It is generally accepted that there are three main types of opioid receptor, designated μ, κ and δ after the prototype agonists morphine, ketocyclazocine and D-Ala-D-Leu-enkephalin (Table 36.1). Selective agonists and antagonists for these receptors have been developed (Table 36.1; Zimmerman and Leander, 1990). Recent studies have provided excellent evidence for further subdivision of these receptors (Table 36.1). The first to be subclassified was the μ-receptor. Pasternak and Wood (1986) demonstrated that the μ_1-site had a high affinity both for enkephalins and morphine, while the μ_2-site had a high affinity only for morphine. They postulated that many of the side-effects of morphine, such as

TABLE 36.1
CHARACTERISTICS OF OPIOID RECEPTORS

Receptor type	Endogenous agonists	Selective agonists	Selective antagonists	Signal transduction*	Proposed subtypes[†]
μ (mu)	β-endorphin met-enkephalin	DAMGO sufentanil morphine	β-FNA CTP naloxonazine	Reduced K^+ conductance at low concentrations Increased K^+ and reduced Ca^{++} conductance at higher concentrations	μ_1, μ_2
δ (delta)	leu-enkephalin met-enkephalin	DPDPE [D-Ala^2]-deltorphin II	ICI 174864 naltrindole BNTX DALCE	Reduced K^+ conductance at low concentrations Increased K^+ and reduced Ca^{++} conductance at higher concentrations	δ_1, δ_2
κ (kappa)	dynorphin (1–19)	U50, 488H	nor-binaltorphimine	Increased Ca^{++} conductance at low concentrations Reduced Ca^+ conductance at higher concentrations	k_1, k_2

Abbreviations: CTP = D-Phe-Cys-Tyr-D-Trp-Lys-The-Phen-The-NH$_2$; DAMGO = [D-Ala^2, Me-Phe^4, Gly-ol^5]-enkephalin; DPDPE = [D-Pen^2, D-Pen^5]-enkephalin; ICI 174,864 = N, N-diallyl-Tyr-Aib-Leu-OH; BNTX = 7-benzylidene-naltrexone; DALCE = [D-Ala^2, Leu^5, Cys^6] enkephalin.

* Activation of all three types of opioid receptor causes inhibition of adenyl cyclase activity and inhibition of cyclic AMP formation. This probably contributes to the longer-term effects of opioids (Di Chiara and North, 1992).

[†] Functional studies provide definitive evidence for two subtypes of each of the opioid receptor types. Radioligand binding studies suggest that further subtypes exist (see 'Opioid receptors and signal transduction').

respiratory depression and physical dependence, were mediated through activation of the μ_2-receptor, whereas μ_1-receptors mediated supraspinal analgesia. Radioligand-binding studies have provided evidence for up to four κ-receptor subtypes, designated as κ_{1A}, κ_{1B}, κ_{2A} and κ_{2B} (Rothman et al., 1990). However, only two κ subtypes have been identified so far in functional studies (Wollemann et al., 1993). There is also evidence for at least two subtypes of the δ-receptor, based on the differential antagonism of δ-agonist antinociception by [D-Ala^2, Leu^5, Cys^6]enkephalin and naltrindole 5'-isothiocyanate (Jiang et al., 1991). A complete understanding of the range of membrane-bound receptors at which exogenous and endogenous opioids act must, however, await their full molecular characterization (see below).

The cellular effects of activating opioid receptors include modulation of the release of a wide range of neurotransmitters and hormones (Illes, 1989), through interactions with guanine nucleotide binding regulatory proteins of the G_1/G_0 type (Uhl et al., 1994). In general, receptor activation, particularly by higher (μM) concentrations of opioid, inhibits neuronal activity. Activation of μ- or δ-receptors causes an increase in the potassium conductance of the neuronal membrane, while activation of all three types can lead to a reduction in voltage-dependent calcium conductance (Di Chiara and North, 1992). These effects, depending on the circumstances, could either lead to an inhibition of firing or a reduction in transmitter release for any particular rate of firing (North, 1986). There have also been reports of excitatory effects of opioids on neuronal activity (Crain and Shen, 1990). Thus, activation of μ-, κ- and δ-receptors by low (nM) concentrations of opioids can elicit excitatory modulation of the action potentials of sensory neurones isolated in culture. These excitatory effects, as is the case with the inhibitory effects, can be prevented by the opioid antagonist naloxone. The excitatory effects of opioids appear to be mediated by actions opposite to those that mediate their inhibitory effects: that is, a decrease in potassium conductance in the case of μ- and δ-receptors and an increase in calcium conductance in the case of κ-receptors. This putative duality of opioid effects may explain the paradoxical hyperalgesic and aversive effects of opioids under some experimental conditions, and some aspects of opioid tolerance and addiction. Receptors of the three major opioid receptor types can also inhibit adenyl cyclase in various tissues, though how this is related to the cellular and integrated responses evoked by opioid agonists is not clear (Di Chiara and North, 1992).

Opioid receptors of the δ-, κ- and μ-types have recently been cloned (Reisine and Bell, 1993; Knapp et al., 1995). They are closely interrelated members of a super-family of seven-transmembrane spanning receptors (about 50% of the amino acids are identical in all three cloned receptors). In the near future, the molecular biological approach should provide precise information about the diversity of opioid receptor subtypes, and on the cellular expression of opioid receptors in different tissues and in various physiological and pathological states (Mansour et al., 1995).

Endogenous opioid peptides

The known mammalian endogenous opioid peptides are derived from three different precursor molecules: pro-opiomelanocortin, pro-enkephalin (also known as pro-enkephalin A) and pro-neo-endorphin (also known as either pro-dynorphin or pro-enkephalin B). These precursor peptides are in turn derived from 'pre-pro-peptides' translated from three separate genes.

A wide range of opioid peptides, with differing affinities for the various opioid receptors, are formed from the cleavage of these precursor molecules. These post-translational processes are tissue dependent. Thus, in the anterior lobe of the pituitary, pro-opiomelanocortin is processed to yield adrenocorticotrophic hormone (ACTH) and β-endorphin, and in the intermediate lobe α-melanocyte stimulating hormone and β-endorphin (Khachaturian et al., 1985). Apart from the pituitary, which is the major site of synthesis of pro-opiomelanocortin, there are two other major cell groups in the brain (of rats) which produce β-endorphin/ACTH. One is in the arcuate nucleus in the medial basal hypothalamus, which projects to many areas of the limbic system and brain stem. The other is found in the brain stem, in the nucleus tractus solitarus and nucleus commissuralis.

In contrast to pro-opiomelanocortin, all of the known biologically active peptides derived from pro-enkephalin are opioids. Pro-enkephalin is processed to yield four copies of methionine-enkephalin, two different carboxyl extended methionine-enkephalin analogues and one copy of leucine-enkephalin (Gubler et al., 1982; Noda et al., 1982). The pro-enkephalin pathways in the brain are widespread (Akil et al., 1984). Peripherally, pro-enkephalin-derived peptides are found in the adrenal medulla, gastrointestinal tract, and several other structures (Akil et al., 1984; Weisenger, 1995).

A number of leucine-enkephalin-containing peptides are derived from pro-neoendorphin-dynorphin. These include α- and β-neoendorphin, dynorphin A and dynorphin B. Pro-neoendorphin-dynorphin is found in the gut, posterior pituitary and brain (Khachaturian et al., 1985).

All the peptides that contain pro-enkephalin show some selective affinity for δ-receptors and differing degrees of activity at μ-receptors (Lord et al., 1977; Akil et al., 1984). Pro-neoendorphin-dynorphin fragments, particularly the longer chain peptides, have selective affinity for κ-receptors (Oka *et al.*, 1982), but dynorphin A (1–8) has some activity at δ-receptors and dynorphin A (1–13) is a potent μ-agonist. Beta-endorphin has a slight preference for δ as opposed to μ-receptors (Akil *et al.*, 1984).

These data do not, however, necessarily indicate at which receptors these peptides act *in vivo*, since this depends on the types of receptor available in the biophase. Thus, endogenous opioid function is dependent on the nature of the opioid gene being expressed in a particular neurone, post-translational processes, the function and site of the neurone, and the opioid receptor types present in the biophase.

OPIOID MECHANISMS IN TRAUMA

Pain pathways

The neural pathways involved in the perception of pain have been reviewed in great detail by others (Wall and Melzack, 1984; Yaksh, 1988). Therefore, only the briefest outline will be provided to introduce the reader to the anatomical sites at which opioids may mediate analgesia (see 'Sites and mechanisms in opioid analgesia' below).

Information about the presence of injury is transmitted to the central nervous system by afferent nerves. Some small diameter fibres (A δ and C) fire only in response to noxious (electrical, mechanical, thermal or chemical) stimuli, whereas others fire tonically but increase their firing rate when stimuli reach noxious levels. The Aδ-fibres, which have conduction velocities of 12–30 m/s, are probably responsible for the initial perception of pain when tissues first come into contact with an injurious stimulus. The slower (0.5–2 m/s) conducting C-fibres are probably responsible for the aching or diffuse pain that follows.

These pain fibres enter the central nervous system via the dorsal horn of the spinal cord. Nociceptive-specific cells have been found not only in lamina I, but also laminae II, IV–VIII and X (Willis, 1988). Nociceptive information is then transmitted in a number of well-defined tracts. In man, the most important are the spinothalamic tract, from lamina I and laminae IV–VI directly to the contralateral thalamus and medial thalamus; and the spinoreticular system, from spinal cord to regions of the brain stem and reticular formation. Other pathways include the dorsal columns, from cord to ipsilateral dorsal column nuclei, and the spinocervical tract to the lateral cervical nucleus. Other polysynaptic pathways also exist.

The Melzack and Wall gate theory of pain (Wall and Melzack, 1984) proposes that the perception of pain depends not only on peripheral stimulation of nociceptors, but also on modulation occurring in the spinal cord and supraspinal regions of the central nervous system. Thus, cells in the spinal cord or fifth nerve nucleus which are excited by noxious stimuli are facilitated or inhibited by activity in other, non-nociceptive, sensory nerve fibres. There are also descending inhibitory pathways from the brain stem reticular formation, the thalamus (periaqueductal grey and lateral reticular formation) and the hypothalamus (Willis, 1988). Other descending inhibitory pathways have been proposed on the basis of neuroanatomical studies, though functional evidence is lacking at present (Holstege, 1988). Most evidence suggests that the thalamus is the main region responsible for the integration of pain input. However, cortical areas appear to be concerned with the subjective interpretation of pain.

Sites and mechanisms in opioid analgesia

There have been reports that activation of any of the three types of opioid receptor can, at least in some circumstances, result in analgesia. Conceptually, there are four sites/mechanisms by which opioids might produce analgesia: a direct effect in the brain to reduce the perception of pain; a direct effect in the spinal cord to reduce the activity in ascending pain pathway; an action in the brain to increase the activity in descending inhibitory pathways, and a peripheral effect to reduce the excitability of nociceptors. In this section the evidence is reviewed for effects of opioids on these four possible mechanisms, and the roles that they may play in the analgesia resulting from systemic opioid administration.

Antinociception can be achieved in laboratory animals by the administration of morphine into the lateral ventricle. The sites at which morphine acts to produce this effect are primarily the periaqueductal and periventricular grey matter, the lateral mesencephalic reticular formation and the nucleus gigantocellularis of the bulbar reticular formation (Advokat, 1988). Spinal administration of morphine also causes antinociception, and an inhibition of the response of sensory neurones to nociceptive stimuli (Advokat, 1988). There is also considerable evidence that morphine and other μ-agonists directly inhibit the activity of nociceptive nerve endings (Junien and Wettstein, 1992). Thus, μ-opioid analgesia probably results from the combined activation of receptors in the periphery, spinal cord and at supraspinal sites. There is considerable controversy, however, as to the nature of supraspinal μ-opioid analgesia. There is evidence that morphine administration actually decreases descending inhibition of spinal cord nociceptive neurones, so that supraspinal μ-opioid analgesia is probably due only to a direct effect within the brain to reduce the perception of pain (Advokat, 1988). There is also evidence that spinal and supraspinal μ-opioid analgesia may be mediated by different receptor subtypes, spinal analgesia resulting from activation of μ_2-receptors and supraspinal analgesia from activation of μ_1-receptors (Paul *et al.*, 1989).

Opioid δ- and κ-agonists also appear to exert their antinociceptive actions at peripheral, spinal and probably also supraspinal sites, though the relative contributions of these sites to the analgesic action of systemically administered δ- and κ-opioids remains a matter of controversy (Heyman *et al.*, 1988; Stein *et al.*, 1989; Millan, 1990).

There is great interest in the possibility that δ- or (especially) κ-opioid agonists might provide alternative opioid analgesic agents that lack some of the undesirable side-effects of morphine-like analgesics. Kappa-agonists do not cause respiratory depression (see 'Opioids and respiration' below), constipation, nausea and vomiting, or pruritus, though they do have diuretic (see 'Opioids and the kidney' below) and sedative effects. They also lack the potential for abuse of morphine-like compounds, since withdrawal symptoms in experimental animals are very mild and κ-agonists do not have the euphorigenic effects of morphine-like drugs. However, they have dysphoric and psychotomimetic effects that may limit their therapeutic utility. Several κ-opioid analgesics have just progressed to clinical trial, so that an informed decision about their clinical usefulness may not be too far away. There has also been recent interest in the possible synergistic actions of δ-agonists on μ- and κ-opioid analgesia (Miaskowski *et al.*, 1990; Porreca *et al.*, 1990; Traynor and Elliot, 1993). Thus, the development of opioid agonists with selectivity for the various opioid receptors has rekindled interest in the development of novel analgesic therapies that lack the drawbacks of conventional morphine-like treatments.

Quite apart from the development and trial of various types and subtypes of opioid agonists for pain relief, major advances have already been made by using novel routes and delivery systems for existing drugs such as morphine (Junien and Wettstein, 1992; Dray *et al.*, 1994; Siddall and Cousins, 1995), some of which are relevant to the effects and after-effects of surgical or accidental trauma. Continuous intravenous or subcutaneous infusion of morphine (or patient-controlled bolus injection by either route) provides better analgesia at lower doses than when morphine is given by regular intermittent injection of fixed doses. Intrathecal opioids (or α_2-adrenoceptor agonists) can provide very effective spinal analgesia in the short term, and can even be used as long-term treatment for the neuropathic pain that can follow amputation or spinal cord injury. Local administration of morphine can provide satisfactory analgesia after knee-joint surgery (Stein *et al.*, 1991). A great advantage of these therapeutic strategies is that unwanted side-effects, especially physical dependence, can be minimized (Di Chiara and North, 1992).

Opioids and the immune system

There is convincing evidence, from studies in experimental animals and humans, that both exogenous and endogenous opioids are capable of profoundly altering immune function. Endogenous opioid release, into both the plasma and cerebrospinal fluid, is increased during various forms of experimental stress (Ader *et al.*, 1990). Lymphocytes have been shown both to contain opioid peptides (Ader *et al.*, 1990; Stein *et al.*, 1990), and to have opioid receptors on their plasma membranes (Ader *et al.*, 1990). Moreover, activation of lymphocyte opioid receptors modifies their function *in vitro* (Ader *et al.*, 1990). Opioids are also known to affect the hypothalamic–pituitary–adrenal (HPA) axis so as to modulate the release of adrenocorticotrophin and thereby immunosuppressive glucocorticoids (Pechnick, 1993). However, the clinical relevance of opioid effects on the HPA axis is not clear. For instance, in humans they are inhibitory, in rodents excitatory.

Thus, mechanisms exist by which endogenous and exogenous opioids might modulate immune function following injury. On the basis of recent studies in laboratory animals demonstrating effects of exogenous and endogenous opioids on immune function *in vivo* (Adora *et al.*, 1990; Stein *et al.*, 1990), it seems appropriate that similar, prospective, studies should be carried out in humans. At present, the main information about opioid-induced immune dysfunction in humans comes from observations on opioid addicts (Kreek, 1989; McLachlan *et al.*, 1993). These suggest that the immunosuppression observed in heroin users is more likely the result of a drug-using lifestyle than of opioid receptor activation.

Opioids and the haemodynamic consequences of acute blood loss

Exogenous and endogenous opioids are known to have profound effects on circulatory control. In the injured patient, the most commonly observed cardiovascular disturbance is that of circulatory shock resulting from acute blood loss. Recent studies have provided convincing evidence that endogenous opioids play a pivotal role in circulatory control under hypovolaemic conditions. Discussion here will be limited to the role of endogenous opioids in the haemodynamic response to acute central hypovolaemia, and the possibility of new forms of exogenous opioid treatment for circulatory shock. For further information on the haemodynamic and neurohumoral responses to acute hypovolaemia in conscious animals and man, refer to recent reviews (Schadt and Ludbrook, 1991; Ludbrook, 1993).

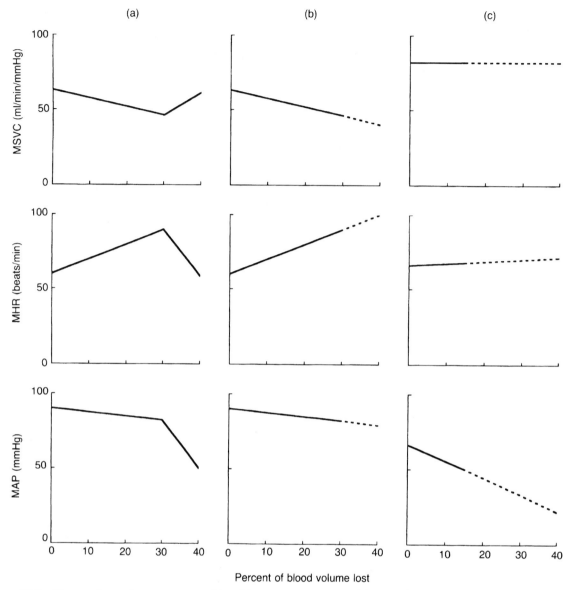

Figure 36.1 Haemodynamic response to blood loss or acute central hypovolaemia and effects of treatments. Solid lines, human studies; dashed lines, extrapolated from studies in rabbits. MAP = mean arterial pressure; MHR = mean heart rate; MSVC = mean systemic vascular conductance. (a) The normal response (see Schadt and Ludbrook, 1991; Ludbrook, 1993). The first, compensatory, phase is followed by an abrupt decompensatory phase in which MSVC rises steeply and MAP and MHR plummet. (b) After administration of δ-opioid receptor antagonists or μ-receptor agonists, including μ-opioid anaesthetic agents such as alfentanil and fentanyl. Compensation is normal but prolonged. No decompensatory phase occurs. (c) During halothane anaesthesia at 1.25 times the minimal alveolar concentration (Ebert *et al.*, 1985). Other anaesthetic agents such as ketamine and propofol have a similar effect (van Leeuwen *et al.*, 1990). Baseline systemic vascular conductance is high and arterial pressure low. There is no compensatory phase.

In all conscious animals in which it has been tested, including man, the haemodynamic response to acute central hypovolaemia consists of two quite distinct phases (Figure 36.1). During the first phase, arterial pressure is well maintained by an increase in vascular resistance (fall in vascular conductance) and heart rate. This vasoconstriction is selective, in that vascular resistance in the coronary and cerebral circulation changes little so that the overall effect is to conserve blood flow to the heart and brain. When central blood volume has been critically reduced, arterial pressure drops precipitately due to a decrease in vascular resistance. It is only during this second, decompensatory phase that the blood flow to the heart and brain is compromised. Studies in conscious dogs and rabbits have shown that during the initial, compensatory phase there is a progressive increase in sympathetic vasoconstrictor drive, which in most species is chiefly attributable to the actions of unloading arterial baroreceptors. In humans, there is evidence for a contribution by cardiopulmonary receptors as well. During the second, decompensatory phase, sympathetic drive (except to the adrenal medulla) falls abruptly. Thus, the two phases of the response to acute central hypovolaemia can be described as sympathoexcitatory and sympathoinhibitory respectively (Schadt and Ludbrook, 1991).

The first evidence that endogenous opioids might play a role in hypovolaemic shock came from the work of Faden and Holaday (1979), who showed that intravenous naloxone had a pressor effect in conscious rats that had been made hypotensive by haemorrhage. Only in the last few years has the nature of this effect been elucidated.

When conscious rabbits are subjected to haemorrhage, or when haemorrhage is simulated by gradual inflation of a cuff around the thoracic inferior vena cava, a biphasic haemodynamic response is observed. Thus, progressive vasoconstriction maintains arterial pressure at near normal levels until cardiac output falls to about 50% of its baseline level, at which stage vascular resistance and arterial pressure fall abruptly. Intravenous administration of the universal opioid receptor antagonist naloxone (4–8 mg/kg) prevents the decompensatory phase without affecting the compensatory phase. Administration of naloxone into the 4th cerebral ventricle at doses 100- to 1000-fold less than required by the intravenous route has the same effect (Evans *et al.*, 1989a). Furthermore, only opioid antagonists with high affinity for the δ_1-opioid receptor have this effect (Evans *et al.*, 1989b; Ludbrook and Ventura, 1994). Thus, there is strong evidence that an endogenous δ_1-opioid receptor mechanism in the brain stem is an essential element in the decompensatory phase of the response to acute hypovolaemia in rabbits. The most likely site for this mechanism is the nucleus tractus solitarus, situated near the dorsal surface of the medulla oblongata very close to the tip of a 4th ventricular catheter and which, at least in rabbits, contains a large population of δ-opioid receptor binding sites (May *et al.*, 1989). No attempt appears to have been made to repeat these experiments in other mammalian species.

Much interest has focused on the possibility of using opioid antagonists in the treatment of hypovolaemic shock in humans, at least as a first-aid measure. A non-specific antagonist such as naloxone would not be clinically efficacious, since doses that would block the δ-opioid receptors would also prevent the analgesic effect of exogenous μ-agonists such as morphine. Until recently, the highly selective δ-antagonists that have been developed are peptides, which do not cross the blood–brain

barrier after systemic administration. Non-peptide δ-receptor antagonists have now been developed, including BNTX which acts on the δ_1 receptor (Table 36.1; Portoghese *et al.*, 1992). However, it is not yet established that BNTX would be effective if given systemically rather than into the fourth ventricle (Ludbrook and Ventura, 1994).

A number of other treatments prevent the decompensatory phase of the response to acute hypovolaemia in unanaesthetized rabbits. These include high mesencephalic decerebration, indicating that suprapontine brain centres might also play a role in this failure of reflex vasoconstriction (Evans *et al.*, 1991). It is tempting to suggest that the same higher brain centres might be involved in the vasovagal syncope associated with emotional fainting in humans.

Agonists with high affinity at the 5-hydroxy-tryptamine$_{1A}$ receptor also prevent the decompensatory phase in conscious rabbits (Evans *et al.*, 1993). The recent development of selective agonists for this receptor might also provide a therapeutic avenue for improving reflex vasoconstriction during hypovolaemic shock. Adrenocorticotrophin (ACTH), which is normally released during hypotensive haemorrhage, also prevents the decompensatory phase of acute hypovolaemia in rabbits by a central action (Ludbrook and Ventura, 1995). ACTH has the additional property of acting peripherally as a vasodilator, a property that might be useful if it were to be used therapeutically in haemorrhagic shock.

Of special interest in trauma with acute blood loss are the effects of anaesthetic agents. All anaesthetics distort the haemodynamic response to acute hypovolaemia. Anaesthetic doses of agents such as pentobarbitone sodium, ketamine, propofol and, in particular, halothane attenuate, or even completely extinguish, the vasoconstriction which is characteristic of the compensatory phase of the response (Figure 36.1). Though it is presumed that these effects are mediated in the central nervous system, some contribution may arise peripherally, particularly in the case of halothane which depresses myocardial contractility and is a direct vasodilator. Exceptions to this rule are the μ-opioid anaesthetics fentanyl and alfentanil, which do not affect the compensatory phase. Moreover μ-agonists also prevent the decompensatory phase in rabbits (van Leeuwen *et al.*, 1990). This action is probably mediated in the brain stem, since low doses of alfentanil and DAMGO (Table 36.1) injected into the 4th ventricle also prevent the decompensatory phase in conscious rabbits, without causing respiratory depression (Evans and Ludbrook, 1990; Van Leeuwen *et al.*, 1990). Thus, μ-opioid anaesthetics may have a special place in surgical patients in whom acute blood loss is expected or has occurred, since they might be expected to preserve blood flow to the brain and heart even when blood loss has exceeded that which triggers the failure of reflex vasoconstriction (Figure 36.1).

Opioids and the kidney

Opioids have profound effects on urine production and composition. Though the exact nature of these is still a matter of controversy, recent advances have shed some light on the mechanisms involved. Since urine production is often used as an index of adequacy of intravascular volume, the effects of opioids on urine production and the mechanisms thought to be involved are briefly summarized.

Administration of μ-agonists such as morphine causes a fall in urine production in both humans and laboratory animals. This overall effect results from actions at multiple sites. At least in rats, morphine and other μ-opioid receptor agonists reduce plasma levels of arginine vasopressin (AVP) (Evans *et al.*, 1989c), which would tend to promote the production of larger volumes of more dilute urine, though they also increase plasma levels of atrial natriuretic peptide (Vollmar *et al.*, 1987). Morphine enhances the tubular reabsorption of sodium, probably by enhancing sympathetic neurotransmission within the kidney (El-Awady and Walker, 1990; Kapusta 1991). Morphine also inhibits bladder motility through a central action (Dray and Metsch, 1984), so that the frequency of micturition decreases (Abrahams *et al.*, 1986). The relative contributions of these effects to the overall antidiuretic and antinatriuretic effects of morphine and other μ-agonists remains a matter of controversy (Kapusta, 1995).

Opioid κ-agonists have a diuretic effect which has recently been the subject of interest. Rats and humans to whom κ-agonists have been administered excrete large volumes of dilute urine. In rats, this effect appears to depend on inhibition of neurohypophyseal AVP release, since plasma levels of AVP are reduced after κ-agonist administration (Evans *et al.*, 1989c), and κ-agonists do not affect urine volume in Brattleboro rats which are congenitally deficient in neurohypophyseal AVP (Abrahams *et al.*, 1986). The effects of opioids on AVP release, however, do not appear to be directly mediated at the level of the neurohypophysis. Recent experiments have provided convincing evidence that a blood-borne factor released from the adrenal medulla is an essential link between activation of κ-receptors and polyuria (Borkowski, 1989). Kappa-opioid agonists also have an antinatriuretic action which appears to depend on enhanced sympathetic drive to the kidney (Kapusta and Obih, 1993). The treatment of a patient suffering from chronic inappropriate antidiuresis resulting from head injury with the partial κ-agonist oxilorphan was described by Miller and Moses (1976). During the period of treatment there was a progressive increase in urinary volume and improvement in the ability to excrete a water load.

There is limited information regarding the effects of δ-agonists on urine production, though unlike μ- and δ-agonists, they do not appear to affect neurohypophyseal hormone release (Van de Heijning, 1991; Kapusta, 1995).

Opioids and respiration

Of all of the side-effects of μ-opioid agonists such as morphine, pethidine and fentanil, respiratory depression is the most life threatening. This appears to be mediated exclusively by activation of μ₂-receptors (Pasternak and Wood, 1986) on pontomedullary respiratory neurones, chiefly in the nuclei tractus solitarus, nucleus ambiguus and nucleus parabrachialis medialis, and on neurones in the anterior hypothalamus (Denavit-Saubié *et al.*, 1978; Dewey *et al.*, 1987). Activation of these μ₂-receptors leads to an inhibition of the neuronal activity responsible for respiratory drive (Denavit-Saubié *et al.*, 1978). Activation of μ₁-, δ- or κ-receptors on the other hand does not lead to respiratory depression (Pasternak and Wood, 1986; May *et al.*, 1989). This is of particular interest in terms of the recent interest in κ- and δ-agonists as alternative agents for the relief of pain (*see* Sites and mechanisms in opioid analgesia above).

Opioids and temperature regulation

Thermoregulation is a complex integrative function involving multiple peripheral sensors, central nervous system integrators (primarily the preoptic anterior hypothalamus (POAH)) and peripheral effector mechanisms. The effects of opioids on thermoregulation are dependent on species as well as on experimental conditions such as the ambient temperature, whether the animals are restrained, route of administration and other factors (Adler *et al.*, 1988).

In unrestrained conscious rats and mice, μ-agonists cause hyperthermia when given in low doses, probably through upward resetting of the hypothalamic set point and subsequent vasoconstriction in skin which decreases heat loss. At higher doses, hypothermia is sometimes observed, related to a fall in oxygen consumption without change in skin blood flow. These effects are probably mediated by direct actions in the POAH, though spinal actions may also be involved (Adler *et al.*, 1988). Activation of κ-receptors in conscious unrestrained rats usually results in hypothermia. Most evidence indicates that this is mediated either in the spinal cord or outside the brain. At present, there is no evidence for the involvement of δ-receptors in thermoregulation (Adler *et al.*, 1988).

Opioids and neurotrauma

Recently, there has been intense interest in the effects of opioid agonists and antagonists in experi-

TABLE 36.2
EFFECTS OF EXOGENOUS AND ENDOGENOUS OPIOIDS

Receptor type	Analgesia	Immune system	Blood loss	Kidney function	Respiration	Thermoregulation	Neurotrauma	Other side-effects
μ (mu)	Spinal, supraspinal and peripheral sites. Used clinically	Exogenous and endogenous μ-agonists reduce plasma levels of cortisol in man. Other effects have been proposed	Exogenous agonists prevent decompensation. No endogenous role	Exogenous agonists cause antidiuresis and antinatriuresis. No known endogenous role	Exogenous μ$_2$ agonists cause respiratory depression	Exogenous agonists mainly cause hyperthermia	Endogenous μ-agonists may be neuroprotective	Euphoria, severe physical dependence, sedation, nausea and vomiting, pruritus, constipation
δ (delta)	Spinal, peripheral and perhaps also supraspinal sites. No studies in humans	Unknown, though some actions have been proposed	Endogenous brain stem mechanism necessary for decompensation	No known effect of exogenous agonists. No proposed endogenous role	No effect	No effect	No known effect	Unknown
κ (kappa)	Spinal, supraspinal and peripheral sites. Progressed to clinical trial	Unknown, though some actions have been proposed	Exogenous agonists prevent decompensation. No endogenous role	Exogenous agonists cause diuresis and antinatriuresis. No known endogenous role	No effect	Exogenous agonists cause hypothermia	Endogenous agonists may exacerbate neuronal damage	Sedation, dysphoria hallucination

mental brain injury, and the possibility that endogenous opioids play some role in the pathogenesis of traumatic and ischaemic brain injury. Unfortunately, there is little agreement as to the effects of opioids, which seem to depend on the model of brain injury being studied (Faden, 1983; Hayes *et al.*, 1990; Faden and Salzman, 1992).

There is considerable experimental evidence for a role of dynorphin in the pathophysiology of brain and spinal cord injury, though a good deal of controversy about the receptors (opioid and non-opioid) involved (Faden and Salzman, 1992; Shukla and Lemaire, 1994). Moreover, there are still no clinical data demonstrating benefit from opioid antagonist treatment of central nervous system injury (Faden and Salzman, 1992).

NEW APPROACHES AND CONSIDERATIONS FOR OPIOID THERAPY IN INJURED PATIENTS

From the above discussion, it can be seen that exogenous and endogenous opioids have profound effects on a whole range of integrative physiological functions which bear on the management of the injured patient (Table 36.2). However, none of these areas of scientific endeavour has yet resulted in new therapies for use in clinical practice. There have been, in recent years, some developments in the range of treatments available for the treatment of pain. Spinal opioid analgesia has proved to be, in many circumstances, a useful alternative to systemic opioid administration (Morgan, 1989; Siddall and Cousins, 1995), with the advantage of less respiratory depression and other side-effects (Table 36.2). Partial-agonist opioids such as buprenorphine, which lack much of the physical dependence and respiratory depression associated with more conventional μ-agonists, have also been useful (Lasagna, 1987; Rosow, 1987). In years to come, κ-or δ-agonists (or peripherally acting μ-agonists) might provide other forms of analgesic treatment. The possible use of opioid agonists or antagonists for the treatment of haemorrhagic shock, traumatic or ischaemic brain injury, or in the modulation of fluid balance, immune function or body temperature, still remains highly speculative.

REFERENCES

Abrahams J.M., Boura A.L.A., Evans R.G. et al. (1986). The effects of N-(cyclopropylmethyl)-19-isopentylnororvinol (M320), a potent agonist at κ- and μ-opiate receptors, on urine excretion of rats. *Br. J. Pharmacol.*, **89**, 759–67.

Ader R., Felten D., Cohen N. (1990). Interactions between the brain and the immune system. *Annu. Rev. Pharmacol. Toxicol.*, **30**, 561–602.

Adler M.W., Geller E.B., Rosow C.E., Cochin J. (1988). The opioid system and temperature regulation. *Annu. Rev. Pharmacol. Toxicol.*, **28**, 429–49.

Adora P.K., Fride E., Petitto J. et al. (1990). Morphine-induced immune alterations *in vivo*. *Cell. Immunol.*, **126**, 343–53.

Advokat C. (1988). The role of descending inhibition in morphine-induced analgesia. *Trends Pharmacol. Sci.*, **9**, 330–4.

Akil H., Watson S.J., Young E. et al. (1984). Endogenous opioids: biology and function. *Annu. Rev. Neurosci.*, **7**, 223–55.

Bloom F.E. (1983). The endorphins. A growing family of biologically pertinent peptides. *Annu. Rev. Pharmacol. Toxicol.*, **23**, 151–70.

Borkowski K.R. (1989). Studies on the adrenomedullary dependence of κ-opioid agonist-induced diuresis in conscious rats. *Br. J. Pharmacol.*, **98**, 1151–6.

Crain S.M., Shen K.-F. (1990). Opioids can evoke direct receptor-mediated excitatory effects on sensory neurons. *Trends Pharmacol. Sci.*, **11**, 77–81.

Denavit-Saubié M., Champagnat J., Zieglgänsberger W. (1978). Effects of opiates and methionine-enkephalin on pontine and bulbar respiratory neurones of the cat. *Brain Res.*, **155**, 55–67.

Dewey W., Morris D., Brase D., Meyer E. (1987). The role of β-endorphin in respiratory disorders in man. In *Problems of Drug Dependence 1987 National Institute of Drug Abuse (U.S.A) Research Monograph Series* Vol. 81 (Harris L.S., ed.). Maryland: US Department of Health and Human Services, pp. 181–7.

Di Chiara G., North R.A. (1992). Neurobiology of opiate abuse. *Trends Pharmacol. Sci.*, **13**, 185–93.

Dray A., Metsch R. (1984). Opioid receptor subtypes involved in the central inhibition of urinary bladder motility. *Eur. J. Pharmacol.*, **104**, 47–53.

Dray A., Urban L., Dickenson A. (1994). Pharmacology of chronic pain. *Trends Pharmacol. Sci.*, **15**, 190–7.

Ebert T.J., Kotrly K.J., Vucins E.J. et al. (1985). Halothane anesthesia attenuates cardiopulmonary baroreflex control of peripheral resistance in humans. *Anesthesiology*, **63**, 668–74.

El-Awady E-L., Walker L.A. (1990). Effects of morphine on the renal handling of sodium and lithium in conscious rabbits. *J. Pharmacol. Exp. Ther.*, **254**, 957–61.

Evans R.G., Ludbrook J. (1990). Effects of μ-opioid receptor agonists on circulatory responses to simulated haemorrhage in conscious rabbits. *Br. J. Pharmacol.*, **100**, 421–6.

Evans R.G., Ludbrook J., Potocnik S.J. (1989a). Intracisternal naloxone and cardiac nerve blockade prevent vasodilatation during simulated haemorrhage in awake rabbits. *J. Physiol.*, **409**, 1–14.

Evans R.G., Ludbrook J., Van Leeuwen A.F. (1989b). Role of central opiate receptor subtypes in the circulatory responses of awake rabbits to graded caval occlusions. *J. Physiol.*, **419**, 15–31.

Evans R.G., Olley J.E., Rice G.E., Abrahams J.M. (1989c). μ-and κ-opiate receptor agonists reduce plasma neurohypophysial hormone concentrations in water-deprived and normally-hydrated rats. *Clin. Exp. Pharmacol. Physiol.*, **16**, 191–7.

Evans R.G., Ludbrook J., Woods R.L., Casley D. (1991). Influence of higher brain centres and vasopressin on the haemodynamic response to acute central hypovolaemia in rabbits. *J. Auton. Nerv. Syst.*, **35**, 1–14.

Evans R.G., Haynes J.M., Ludbrook J. (1993). Effects of 5-HT-receptor and α₂-adrenoceptor ligands on the haemodynamic response to acute hypovolaemia in conscious rabbits. *Br. J. Pharmacol.*, **109**, 37–47.

Faden A.I. (1983). Neuropeptides and stroke: current status and potential application. *Stroke*, **14**, 169–72.

Faden A.I., Holaday J.W. (1979). Opiate antagonists: a role in the treatment of hypovolemic shock. *Science*, **205**, 317–18.

Faden A.I., Salzman S. (1992). Pharmacological strategies in CNS trauma. *Trends Pharmacol. Sci.*, **13**, 29–35.

Gubler U., Seeburg P., Hoffman B.J. et al. (1982). Molecular cloning establishes proenkephalin as precursor of enkephalin-containing peptides. *Nature*, **295**, 205–8.

Hayes R.L., Lyeth B.G., Jenkins L.W. et al. (1990). Possible protective effect of endogenous opioids in traumatic brain injury. *J. Neurosurg.*, **72**, 252–61.

Heyman J.S., Vaught J.L., Raffa R.B., Porreca F. (1988). Can supraspinal δ-opioid receptors mediate antinociception? *Trends Pharmacol. Sci.*, **9**, 134–8.

Holstege G. (1988). Direct and indirect pathways to lamina I in the medulla oblongata and spinal cord of the cat. In *Pain Modulation, Progress in Brain Research*, vol. **77** (Fields H.L., Besson J-M., eds). Amsterdam: Elsevier, pp. 47–94.

Illes P. (1989). Modulation of transmitter and hormone release by multiple neuronal opioid receptors. *Rev. Physiol. Biochem. Pharmacol.*, **112**, 139–233.

Jiang Q., Takemori A.E., Sultana M. et al. (1991). Differential antagonism of opioid *delta* antinociception by [D-Ala^2, Leu^5, Cys^6] enkephalin and naltrindole 5'-isothiocyanate: evidence for *delta* receptor subtypes. *J. Pharmacol. Exp. Ther.*, **257**, 1069–75.

Junien J.L., Wettstein J.G. (1992). Role of opioids in peripheral analgesia. *Life Sci.*, **51**, 2009–18.

Kapusta D.R., Obih J.C. (1993). Central *kappa* opioid receptor-evoked changes in renal function in conscious rats: participation of renal nerves. *J. Pharmacol. Exp. Ther.*, **267**, 197–204.

Kapusta D.R. (1995). Opioid mechanisms controlling renal function. *Clin. Exp. Pharmacol. Physiol.*, **22**, 891–902.

Kapusta D.R., Jones S.Y., DiBona G.F. (1991). Renal *mu* opioid receptor mechanisms in regulation of renal function in rats. *J. Pharmacol. Exp. Ther.*, **258**, 111–17.

Khachaturian H., Lewis M.E., Schafer M.K-H., Watson S.J. (1985). Anatomy of the CNS opioid systems. *Trends Neurosci.*, **8**, 111–19.

Knapp R.J., Malatynska E., Collins N., Fang L., Wang J.Y., Hruby V.J., Roeske W.R., Yamamura H.I. (1995). Molecular biology and pharmacology of cloned opioid receptors. *FASE B. J. L.*, **9**, 516–25.

Kreek M.J. (1989). Immunological approaches to clinical issues in drug abuse. In *Problems of Drug Dependence, 1988, National Institute of Drug Abuse (USA) Research Monograph Series*, vol. 90 (Harris L.S., ed.). Maryland: US Department of Health and Human Services, pp. 77–86.

Lasagna L. (1987). Benefit-risk ratio of agonist–antagonist analgesics. *Drug Alcohol Depend.*, **20**, 385–93.

Lord J.A.H., Waterfield A.A., Hughes J., Kosterlitz H.W. (1977). Endogenous opioid peptides: multiple agonists and receptors. *Nature*, **267**, 495–9.

Ludbrook J. (1993). Haemorrhage and shock. In *Cardiovascular Reflex Control in Health and Disease* (Hainsworth R., Mark A.L., eds). London W.B. Saunders, pp. 463–90.

Ludbrook J., Ventura S. (1994). The decompensatory phase of acute hypovolaemia in rabbits involves a central δ$_1$-opioid receptor. *Eur. J. Pharmacol.*, **252**, 113–16.

Ludbrook J., Ventura S. (1995). ACTH-(1–24) blocks the decompensatory phase of the haemodynamic response to acute hypovolaemia. *Eur. J. Pharmacol.*, **275**, 267–75.

McLachlan C., Crofts, N., Wodak A., Crowe S. (1993). The effects of methadone on immune function among injecting drug users: a review. *Addiction*, **88**, 257–63.

Mansour A., Fox C.A., Akil H., Watson S.J. (1995). Opioid-receptor mRNA expression in the rat CNS: anatomical and functional implications. *Trends Neurosci.*, **18**, 22–9.

May C.N., Dashwood M.R., Whitehead C.J., Mathias C.J. (1989). Differential cardiovascular and respiratory responses to central administration of selective opioid agonists in conscious rabbits: correlation with receptor distribution. *Br. J. Pharmacol.*, **98**, 903–13.

Miaskowski C., Taiwo Y.O., Levine J.D. (1990). κ- and δ-opioid agonists synergize to produce potent analgesia. *Brain Res.*, **509**, 165–8.

Millan M.J. (1990). κ-Opioid receptors and analgesia. *Trends Pharmacol. Sci.*, **11**, 70–6.

Miller M., Moses A.M. (1976). Drug induced states of impaired water excretion. *Kidney Int.*, **10**, 96–103.

Morgan M. (1989). The rational use of intrathecal and extradural opioids. *Br. J. Anaesthesia*, **63**, 165–88.

Noda M., Teranishi Y., Takahashi H. et al. (1982). Isolation and structural organization of the human preproenkephalin gene. *Nature*, **297**, 431–4.

North R.A. (1986). Opioid receptor types and membrane ion channels. *Trends Neurosci.*, **9**, 114–17.

Oka T., Negishi K., Kajiwara M. et al. (1982). The choice of opiate receptor subtype by neo-endorphins. *Eur. J. Pharmacol.*, **79**, 301–5.

Pasternak G.W., Wood P.J. (1986). Minireview: multiple my opiate receptors. *Life Sci.*, **38**, 1889–98.

Paul D., Bodnar R.J., Gistrak M.A., Pasternak G.W. (1989). Different μ receptor subtypes mediate spinal and supraspinal analgesia in mice. *Eur. J. Pharmacol.*, **168**, 307–14.

Pechnick R.N. (1993). Effects of opioids on the hypothalamo-pituitary-adrenal axis. *Annu. Rev. Pharmacol. Toxicol.*, **32**, 353–82.

Pert C.B., Snyder S.H. (1973). Opiate receptor: demonstration in nervous tissue. *Science*, **179**, 1011–14.

Porreca F., Jiang Q., Tallarida R.J. (1990). Modulation of morphine antinociception by peripheral [Leu^5] enkephalin: a synergistic interaction. *Eur. J. Pharmacol.*, **179**, 463–8.

Portoghese P.S., Sultana M., Nagase H., Takemori A.E. (1992). A highly selective δ$_1$-opioid receptor antagonist: 7-benzylidene-naltrexone. *Eur. J. Pharmacol.*, **218**, 195–96.

Reisine T., Bell G.I. (1993). Molecular biology of opioid receptors. *Trends Neurosci.*, **16**, 506–10.

Rosow C.E. (1987). The clinical usefulness of agonist–antagonist analgesics in acute pain. *Drug Alcohol Depend.*, **20**, 329–37.

Rothman R.B., Bykov V., De Costa B.R. et al. (1990). Interaction of endogenous opioid peptides and other drugs with four kappa opioid binding sites in guinea pig brain. *Peptides*, **11**, 311–31.

Schadt J.C., Ludbrook J. (1991). Hemodynamic and neurohumoral responses to acute hypovolemia in conscious mammals. *Am. J. Physiol.*, **260**, H305–18.

Shukla V.K., Lemaire S. (1994). Non-opioid effects of

dynorphins: possible role of the NMDA receptor. *Trends Pharmacol. Sci.*, **15**, 420–4.

Siddall P.J., Cousins M.J. (1995). Pain mechanisms and management: an update. *Clin. Exp. Pharmacol. Physiol.*, **22**, 679–88.

Stein C., Millan M.J., Shippenberg T.S. et al. (1989). Peripheral opioid receptors mediating antinociception in inflammation. Evidence for involvement of mu, delta and kappa receptors. *J. Pharmacol. Exp. Ther.*, **248**, 1269–75.

Stein C., Hassan A.H.S., Przewioki R. et al. (1990). Opioids from immunocytes interact with receptors on sensory nerves to inhibit nociception in inflammation. *Proc. Nat. Acad. Sci. (USA)*, **87**, 5935–9.

Stein C., Comisel K., Haimerl E. et al. (1991). Analgesic effect of intraarticular morphine after arthroscopic knee surgery. *New Engl. J. Med.*, **325**, 1123–6.

Traynor J.R., Elliot J. (1993). δ-opioid receptor subtypes and cross-talk with μ-receptors. *Trends Pharmacol. Sci.*, **14**, 84–6.

Uhl G.R., Childers S., Pasternak G. (1994). An opiate-receptor gene family reunion. *Trends Neurosci.*, **17**, 89–93.

Van de Heijning H.J.M. (1991). Opioid Control of the Vasopressin and Oxytocin Release in the Rat. PhD Thesis. Rudolf Magnus Institute, University of Utrecht, The Netherlands.

Van Leeuwen A.F., Evans R.G., Ludbrook J. (1990). Effects of halothane, ketamine, propofol and alfentanil anaesthesia on circulatory control in rabbits. *Clin. Exp. Pharmacol. Physiol.*, **17**, 781–98.

Vollmar A.M., Arendt R.M., Schulz R. (1987). The effect of opioids on rat plasma natriuretic peptide. *Eur. J. Pharmacol.*, **143**, 315–21.

Wall P.D., Melzack R. (1984). *Textbook of Pain*. Edinburgh: Churchill Livingstone.

Weisenger G. (1995). The transcriptional regulation of the preproenkephalingene. *Biochem. J.*, **307**, 617–29.

Willis W.D. (1988). Anatomy and physiology of descending control of nociceptive responses of dorsal horn neurons: comprehensive review. In *Pain Modulation Progress in Brain Research*, vol. 77 (Fields H.L., Besson J-M., eds). Amsterdam: Elsevier, pp. 1–32.

Wollemann M., Benyhe S., Simon J. (1993). The kappa-opioid receptor: evidence for the different subtypes. *Life Sci.*, **52**, 599–611.

Yaksh T.L. (1988). Neurologic mechanisms in pain. In *Neural Blockade in Clinical Anesthesia and Management of Pain 2nd edn* (Cousins M.J., Bridenbaugh P.O., eds). Philadelphia, PA. Lippincott.

Zimmerman D.M., Leander J.D. (1990). Selective opioid receptor agonists and antagonists: research tools and potential therapeutic agents. *J. Med. Chem.*, **33**, 895–902.

37. Mechanisms of Cellular Damage

M. S. Mulligan and
P. A. Ward

INTRODUCTION

The vascular endothelium plays a critical role in the regulation of acute inflammation. In response to cytokines and other stimuli released during inflammatory reactions, the endothelial cell surface expresses proteins that promote adhesive interactions with circulating leucocytes. It is now assumed that initiation of an inflammatory response involving migration of leucocytes is intimately linked to the endothelium, involving changes which appear to be a prerequisite for emigration of leucocytes. One of the first signals of a developing inflammatory reaction occurs when the movement of leucocytes shifts from a rapid laminar type of flow to a process of slow rolling as leucocytes 'marginate' and begin to come into contact with the endothelial surface. These events predate leucocytic emigration from the confines of the vascular lumen. The ability to interrupt or modulate this process would have broad clinical utility. On the basis of current knowledge, molecules that mediate adhesive interactions between leucocytes and endothelial cells are essential for the sequence of events leading to the acute inflammatory response.

The resistance of the vascular barrier to permeation by water, electrolytes and protein may be diminished either by functional or structural changes in the endothelium. In the former case, vasopermeability factors (such as histamine, bradykinin or 'platelet activating factor') can cause reversible opening of junctions between endothelial cells, resulting in permeability changes. Structural changes reflective of damage to endothelial cells result in a more persistent increase in vascular permeability and are also frequently associated with intravascular thrombosis and haemorrhage into the extravascular space. These changes often occur as an early phase of the acute inflammatory response when neutrophils come into physical contact with endothelial cells whose adhesion molecules have been upregulated. If neutrophils have been stimulated as a result of contact with a variety of mediators, their generation and release of toxic products may injure the endothelial cells. Toxic factors released from neutrophils include oxygen products and proteases, which can interact in a synergistic manner to damage or kill endothelial cells. The generation of chemotactic factors in tissues as well as amplification of the inflammatory response by cytokines and other mediators often leads to accumulation of leucocytes in the extravascular compartment. The ability to interrupt the early phases of the inflammatory response by blocking adhesive interactions between leucocytes and endothelial cells represents a new and promising approach to anti-inflammatory therapy. The mechanisms of leucocyte–endothelial adhesive and cytotoxic interactions will be briefly discussed.

DETERMINANTS OF LEUCOCYTES–ENDOTHELIAL CELL ADHESIVE INTERACTIONS

As indicated above, adhesive molecules can be expressed on endothelial cells in a manner that can enhance adhesive interactions with leucocytes. In a like manner, leucocytes express and can upregulate certain adhesion molecules that promote adhesive interactions with endothelial cells. One series of glycoproteins expressed on surfaces of leucocytes are the β2 integrins, which represent the major adhesion molecules on these cells. β2 integrins are composed of a common β subunit (CD18) and one of three paired α subunits (CD11a, b, or c). CD11a/CD18 is commonly referred to as LFA-1, CD11b/CD18 is also known as Mo-1 or Mac-1, and CD11c/CD18 is designated p150/95. Mo-1 and p150/95 are present on neutrophils, monocytes and NK cells while LFA-1 is also present on monocytes and T and B lymphocytes. Endothelial cell ICAM-1 is a ligand for LFA-1 and Mo-1 while the ligand for p150/95 has not been characterized. ICAM-2 is also a ligand for LFA-1. Adhesive interactions between activated neutrophils and endothelial cell monolayers can be nearly completely blocked by antibodies to CD18, significantly blocked with antibodies to CD11b and inhibited to lesser degrees with antibodies to CD11c or CD11a. As is the case with endothelial cell adhesion molecules that are constitutively expressed (ICAM-1) or can be upregulated (ICAM-1,2, ELAM-1 and VCAM-1), β2 integrins are constitutively expressed but can also be upregulated on neutrophils which have been activated by a variety of stimuli. The same stimuli that upregulate β2 integrins on neutrophils can also induce neutrophil degranulation and initiate the respiratory burst, leading to the generation of toxic oxygen species (Varani et al., 1985; Arnout et al., 1988). In addition to their roles in the promotion of adhesion of neutrophils to endothelial cells, the β2 integrins also mediate monocyte attachment to the endothelium. Among the β2 integrins, CD11a appears to be the more common mediator of monocyte–endothelial adhesive interactions (Arnout et al., 1988; Cavender et al., 1991).

In addition to the β2 integrins, the *selectin* family of adhesion molecules plays important roles in adhesive interactions between leucocytes and endothelial cells. *Selectins* are adhesion-promoting molecules that interact with complementary molecules that are carbohydrates. E-selectin is also known as ELAM-1 and is a major upregulatable adhesion-promoting molecule on endothelial cells, demonstrating reactivity with neutrophils, monocytes and T cells. The carbohydrate moiety on the neutrophil interactive with ELAM-1 has been identified as the carbohydrate, sialyl-Le^x. Recently L-selectin, which is a molecule on leucocytes and is also known as LECAM-1, has been shown to contain the sialyl-Le^x molecule which is interactive with ELAM-1 (Picken *et al.*, 1991). It is currently thought that interaction of neutrophil L-selection with ELAM-1 on upregulated endothelial cells is the initial adhesion-promoting event under conditions of shear stress, resulting in neutrophil adhesion to endothelial cells, following which CD18-dependent pathways are brought into play to facilitate leucocyte transmigration (Hallmann *et al.*, 1991). Therefore, the CD18 and the selectin family of adhesion molecules are likely to work in concert. As indicated above, L-selectin is an adhesion molecule present on neutrophils and T cells and is also known as LECAM-1, MEL-14 or LAM-1. It is constitutively expressed on neutrophils and is rapidly shed when neutrophil activation occurs. P-selectin, also known as GMP-140, is transiently expressed on platelets and endothelial cells and is stored within granules of the cytoplasm. The molecule on the neutrophil or monocyte reactive with P-selection is LECAM-1 (Picken *et al.*, 1991).

Like the β2 integrins, the E-selectin molecules of endothelial cells are upregulated in response to cytokines. In the case of platelets, P-selectin is rapidly expressed on the platelet surface following contact with platelet activating factor and other stimuli. P-selectin is also expressed transiently on endothelial cells after their stimulation with various agonists. Most endothelial leucocyte adhesion-promoting molecules are not normally expressed and are upregulated when endothelial cells come in contact with TNFα, IL-1 or endotoxin. The family of adhesion molecules on endothelial cells includes ICAM-1,2, ELAM-1 and VCAM-1 (INCAM-1) (Bevilacqua *et al.*, 1985, 1987; Dustin *et al.*, 1986; Pober *et al.*, 1986). The patterns of upregulation are distinct for each of these molecules. P-selectin is transiently expressed and then rapidly lost from the endothelial cell surface in response to cytokine stimulation. ELAM-1 (E-selectin) is not constitutively expressed on human endothelial cells and is maximally upregulated 4 hours after stimulation with TNFα. By 24 hours, expression of ELAM-1 is completely lost, even in the continued presence of cytokine stimulation. ICAM-1 is constitutively expressed on endothelial cells but greatly increased expression is induced by cell contact with TNFα and IL-1, peaking at 4 hours, but with the upregulation being maintained for 12–24 hours. VCAM-1 expression

does not occur on non-stimulated endothelial cells but the pattern of expression for VCAM-1 is similar to that for ICAM-1 after interaction of endothelial cells with cytokines or endotoxin. However, the level of constitutive expression of VCAM-1 may be slightly lower.

As mentioned, LFA-1 and Mac (Mo-1) interact with ICAM-1 on endothelial cells (Marlin and Springer, 1987). The leucocyte ligand for VCAM-1 is VLA-4, which is found on lymphocytes and monocytes but not on neutrophils. As already indicated, ELAM-1 binds to the carbohydrate moiety sialyl-Le^x on neutrophils (Phillips *et al.*, 1990). Other carbohydrate ligands for ELAM-1 may be present in monocytes and lymphocytes. Because P-selectin is present in alpha platelet granules of platelets, in alpha granules of endothelial cells, it is mobilized to the cell surface within seconds of stimulation and is rapidly shed with continued stimulation of platelets or endothelial cells. Thus, P-selectin may mediate rapidly evolving leucocyte–endothelial cell adhesion interactions in a manner that is complementary to ELAM-1. As mentioned, the neutrophil ligand for P-selectin is L-selectin (LECAM-1) (Picken *et al.*, 1991).

NEUTROPHIL MEDIATED INJURY OF ENDOTHELIAL CELLS

Non-toxic injury

Neutrophils kill invading microorganisms by a variety of mechanisms, including generation of toxic oxygen radicals, or release of proteases and cationic proteins. These same mechanisms, when improperly controlled, can cause inflammatory tissue injury. The vascular endothelium appears to be a common target for the cytotoxic effects of neutrophils. Endothelial cell damage leads to a compromise of vascular integrity resulting in a loss of the soluble constituents of plasma (water, ions, proteins). If the endothelial damage is of sufficient severity, the passage of RBC beyond the vascular barrier will also occur. Neutrophil-mediated endothelial cell injury is not necessarily lethal but is almost always disruptive of normal endothelial cell function. Monolayers of human umbilical vein endothelial cells can be perturbed, leading to a lifting off from the monolayer in a non-cytolytic manner, resulting in a loss of fluid-retaining features of the monolayer (Hartan *et al.*, 1981, 1985). *In vivo*, the release of proteolytic enzymes by activated neutrophils may cause the release from basement membrane of endothelial cells, leading to an accumulation in the interstitium of fluids (Simon *et al.*, 1986). These changes are inhibited by proteinase inhibitors. Antibodies to CD18, but not superoxide dismutase (a 'scavenger' of O_2^-) or catalase (a scavenger of H_2O_2), will block the ability of the activated neutrophil to cause the proteolytic release of endothelial cells from basement membrane. It therefore appears that adherent neutrophils release proteases that mediate this type of vascular injury. The lifting off of endothelial cells from their basement membrane anchor on the vascular wall will lead to a sustained increase in vascular permeability. It is also likely that in such circumstances contact of the denuded basement membrane with platelets and a variety of plasma proteins can lead to the activation of these cells or proteins. For instance, when platelets are exposed to basement membrane, they aggregate and release factors such as P-selectin and adenine nucleotides. Basement membrane that has been denuded of its endothelial cell lining can also react with plasma proteins to initiate the cascade of events leading to coagulation and complement activation. Thus, vascular denudation due to leucocytic protease, toxic oxygen products or the combination, is potentially highly damaging to the vessel wall.

Cytotoxic injury

Activated neutrophils produce substantial amounts of toxic oxygen products following contact with a variety of stimuli (chemotactic factors, immune complexes, etc.). These neutrophil products injure and kill endothelial cells. The first evidence of neutrophil-mediated endothelial cell cytotoxicity was found when activated neutrophils were shown to damage endothelial cells *in vitro* (Sacks *et al.*, 1978). Myeloperoxidase inhibitors were subsequently found to augment this injury, indicating that halide producers of H_2O_2, such as hypochlorous acid (HOCl), are not linked to the killing process (Weiss *et al.*, 1981). Neutrophil-generated H_2O_2 will kill bovine aortic and rat pulmonary endothelial cells (Martin, 1984; Varani *et al.*, 1985). Hydroxic radical scavengers (DMSO, DMTU) and the iron chelator deferoxamine were protective, suggesting the conversion of H_2O_2 to the hydroxyl radical ($\cdot$OH) by the iron-dependent Fenton reaction was an important factor associated with endothelial cell cytotoxicity. Given the highly reactive nature of $\cdot$OH and its short half-life, it is likely that it is formed in close proximity to intracellular targets. The source of the iron required for the conversion of leucocytic H_2O_2 to $\cdot$OH by the Fenton reaction appears to be the endothelial cell itself. Pretreatment of endothelial cells with deferoxamine, followed by washing before addition of the activated neutrophils, nearly completely eliminated killing (Gannon *et al.*, 1987). Conversely, pretreatment of neutrophils with deferoxamine is not protective. It appears that the protective effects of deferoxamine can be linked to its chelation of endothelial cell-derived iron. Most intracellular iron is stored as Fe^{3+} in ferritin and it must be reduced to Fe^{2+} so that it can participate in the reduction of H_2O_2. Recent evidence suggests that O_2^- may be responsible for the reduction of Fe^{3+} (see below).

Neutrophil-mediated killing of endothelial cells is enhanced if the latter are first exposed to TNFα or IL-1. The most likely explanation for this increased killing is the upregulation on endothelial cells of adhesion-promoting molecules (ELAM-1, ICAM-1,2). As is the case with the iron requirement, which is provided by endothelial cells for their killing by activated neutrophils, generation of O_2^- by endothelial cells is another important contribution in their ultimate killing by activated neutrophils. This has most clearly been shown by the ability of superoxide dismutase (SOD) to protect endothelial cells from neutrophil-mediated killing (Markey *et al.*, 1990). It is important to stress that the protective effects of SOD are related to the requirement that SOD is endothelial cell-associated, most likely intracellular. Thus, endothelial cells preloaded with SOD are protected, whereas the addition of the enzyme to the culture fluid bathing the endothelial cells at the time of addition of neutrophils is not protective. Thus, SOD apparently must gain entry to the endothelial cell to have protective effects. It now seems likely that the source in the endothelial cell of O_2^- is xanthine oxidase (XO), which is a cytosolic enzyme. XO is activated by reversible oxidation of xanthine dehydrogenase (XD) or by limited proteolytic cleavage of XD. In the case of rat pulmonary endothelial cells, in which the enzyme content of XD and XO is present in a ratio of approximately 2 : 1, this ratio is reversed by endothelial cell contact with activated neutrophils (in which case neutrophil elastase appears to be the responsible factor) or by endothelial cell contact with nM concentrations of TNFα, C5a or formyl chemotactic peptides (Varani *et al.*, 1985; Friedl *et al.*, 1989; Phan *et al.*, 1989). Although data suggest that $\cdot$OH is responsible for lethal injury of endothelial cells that have come in contact with endothelial cells, proof for this conclusion is not forthcoming. Furthermore, the precise mechanism by which $\cdot$OH and other radicals cause damage to critical intracellular targets is not known.

Protease-mediated endothelial cell injury

Under certain conditions, neutrophil proteases can bring about cytotoxic injury of endothelial cells. Human neutrophils from normal human subjects and from patients with chronic granulomatous disease of childhood each demonstrate a degree of endothelial cell killing that is not inhibited by the presence of antioxidants (Smedley *et al.*, 1986). Killing of endothelial cells can also be induced with purified neutrophil elastase and reversed by the presence of an elastase inhibitor. On balance, it appears that proteases are acting in concert with oxidants, since pretreatment of endothelial cells with XO inhibitors is protective against protease-mediated injury (Rodell *et al.*, 1987). Exposure sequentially or simultaneously of endothelial cells to H_2O_2 and proteases results in cell killing at concentrations of reactants which, alone, are not cytotoxic (Varani *et al.*, 1989). Little is known about the mechanism of synergy involved in the killing of endothelial cells by the combination of H_2O_2 and protease (trypsin, cathapsin G, elastase). Inasmuch as the order of exposure (i.e. protease followed by H_2O_2, or vice versa) of endothelial cells does not alter the outcome of enhanced injury, it has been difficult to determine the sequence of events involved in the cytotoxic process. Although the mechanisms are currently poorly understood, exposure of endothelial cells to other combinations by substances also enhances the cytotoxic outcome. For instance, cationic substances and lysophosphatides also enhance the killing of endothelial cells by activated neutrophils. However, these factors also augment O_2^- production by neutrophils (Ginsburg *et al.*, 1989a,b). TNFα also sensitizes endothelial cells to neutrophil-mediated cytotoxicity. This may be explained by the ability of this cytokine to induce adhesion molecule expression in the endothelial cell (Bevilacqua *et al.*, 1985, 1987; Dustin *et al.*, 1986; Pober *et al.*, 1986) and to enhance the catalytic activity of XO (Varani *et al.*, 1989a), as described above.

Mechanisms of *in vivo* vascular injury

Tissue injury developing after deposition of IgG immune complexes is known to be complement and neutrophil dependent (Johnson and Ward, 1974) and mediated by toxic oxygen metabolites, and perhaps nitrogen (Johnson and Ward, 1981). Included among these toxic products is the nitrogen-centred radical, nitric oxide (·NO). Studies employing the L-arginine analogue, N^G-monomethyl-L-arginine acetate, have shown that inhibition of ·NO synthase and diminished ·NO production attenuates immune complex-induced injury in lung and skin without affecting neutrophil influx (Mulligan *et al.*, 1991a). Histological features of IgG immune complex-induced alveolitis include endothelial cell blebbing and destruction, interstitial oedema, fibrin deposition, neutrophil accumulation and haemorrhage. TNFα, IL-1 and platelet activating factor (PAF) have all been shown to be important mediators for the full development of this type of lung injury. Recently, it has been shown that TNFα is capable of upregulating ELAM-1 expression in the rat pulmonary vasculature (Mulligan *et al.*, 1991b). The lung vasculature does not normally express ELAM-1, whereas at 1 hour and 3 hours after TNFα exposure (via intratracheal instillation), the intensity of ELAM-1 expression steadily increases. Deposition of IgG immune complexes in lung and the associated induction of ELAM-1 appears to be followed by adhesion of neutrophils to the vascular endothelium

and the ultimate transmigration of neutrophil and accumulation in lung (Mulligan *et al.*, 1991c). Upregulation of endothelial ICAM-1 and neutrophilic CD18/CD11b also promote neutrophil adhesion and transmigration into inflammatory foci (Warren *et al.*, 1989). While elaboration of TNFα, IL-1 and PAF are important in lung following deposition of IgG immune complexes (Strieter *et al.*, 1989; Warren *et al.*, 1990; Warren, 1991), in skin IL-1 but not TNFα appears to be required, its source apparently the resident tissue macrophage.

In the lung there is extensive cytokine 'networking'. TNFα and IL-1 are capable of mediating the upregulation of endothelial adhesion molecules. These cytokines are also capable of stimulating production of a number of proinflammatory mediators such as neutrophil chemotactic factor (NCF, IL-8) and PAF, which is chemotactic for neutrophils (Bussolino *et al.*, 1988; Strieter *et al.*, 1988; Warren *et al.*, 1990). In skin, however, for the reasons stated above, the cytokine networking appears to be more restricted. Perhaps the skin has the capacity to produce fewer cytokines. Also, inflammatory reactions in skin may be more compartmentalized secondary to anatomical and structural constraints.

In summary, a likely sequence of the pathological events leading to IgG immune complex-induced lung injury is as follows: IgG immune complex deposition and complement activation stimulate alveolar macrophages to produce cytokines (TNFα and IL-8); complement activation products (C5a) also activate neutrophils and act as chemoattractants; TNFα and IL-1 induce adhesion molecule expression on the vascular endothelium (i.e. ELAM-1) and, in response, neutrophils emigrate from the vasculature in a CD18-dependent manner, ultimately releasing tissue damaging oxygen radicals and proteins.

REFERENCES

Arnout M.A., Lanier L.L., Faller D.V. (1988). Relative contribution of the leukocyte molecules Mo-l, LFA-1 and p150,95 (LeuM5) in adhesion of granulocytes and monocytes to vascular endothelium is tissue- and stimulus-specific. *J. Cell Physiol.*, **137**, 305–9.

Bevilacqua M.P., Pober J.S., Wheeler M.E. et al. (1985). Interleukin 1 acts on cultured human vascular endothelium to increase the adhesion of polymorphonuclear leukocytes, monocytes, and related leukocyte cell lines. *J. Clin. Invest.*, **76**, 2003–11.

Bevilacqua M.P., Pober J.S., Mendrick D.L., et al. (1987). Identification of an inducible endothelial-leukocyte adhesion molecule. *Proc. Natl. Acad. Sci. USA*, **84**, 9238–42.

Bussolino F., Camussi G., Baglioni C. (1988). Synthesis and release of platelet-activating factor by human vascular endothelial cells treated with tumor necrosis factor or interleukin 1 α. *J. Biol. Chem.*, **263**, 11856–61.

Cavender D.E., Edelbaum D., Welkovich L. (1991). Effects of inflammatory cytokines and phorbol esters on the adhesion of U937 cells, a human monocyte-like cell line, to endothelial cell monolayers and extracellular matrix proteins. *J. Leukoc. Biol.*, **49**, 566–78.

Dustin M.L., Rothlein R., Bhan A.K. et al. (1986). A human intercellular adhesion molecule (ICAM-1) distance from LFA-1. *J. Immunol.*, **137**, 1270–4.

Friedl H.P., Till G.O., Ryan U.S., Ward P.A. (1989). Mediators-induced activation of xanthine oxidase in endothelial cells. *FASEB J.*, **3**, 2512–18.

Gannon D.E., Varani J., Phan S.H. et al. (1987). Source of iron in neutrophil-mediated killing of endothelial cells. *Lab. Invest.*, **57**, 37–44.

Ginsburg I., Gibbs D.F., Schuger L. et al. (1989a). Vascular endothelial cell killing by combinations of membrane active agents and hydrogen peroxide. *Free Rad. Biol. Med.*, **7**, 369–76.

Ginsburg I., Ward P.A., Varani J. (1989b). Lysophosphatides enhance superoxide responses of stimulated human neutrophils. *Inflammation*, **13**, 163–79.

Hallmann R., Jutila M.A., Smith C.W. et al. (1991). The peripheral lymph node homing receptor, LECAM-1 is involved in CD18-independent adhesion of human neutrophils to endothelium. *Biochemn. Biophys. Res. Commun.*, **174**(1), 236–43.

Harlan J.M., Killen P.D., Harker L.A. et al. (1981). Neutrophil-mediated endothelial injury *in vitro* mechanisms of cell detachment. *J. Clin. Invest.*, **68**, 1394–403.

Harlan J.M., Schwartz B.R., Reidy M.A. et al. (1985). Activated neutrophils disrupt endothelial monolayer integrity by an oxygen radical-independent mechanism. *Lab. Invest.*, **52**, 141–50.

Johnson K.J., Ward P.A. (1974). Acute immunologic pulmonary alveolitis. *J. Clin. Invest.*, **54**, 349–57.

Johnson K.J., Ward P.A. (1981). Role of oxygen metabolites in immune complex injury of lung. *J. Immunol.*, **126**, 2365–9.

Marlin S.D., Springer T.A. (1987). Purified intercellular adhesion molecule-1 (ICAM-1) is a ligand for lymphocyte function-associated antigen 1 (LFA-1). *Cell*, **51**, 813–19.

Markey B.A., Phan S.H., Varani J. et al. (1990). Inhibition of cytotoxicity by intracellular superoxide dismutase supplementation. *Free Rad. Biol. Med.*, **9**, 307–14.

Martin W.J. (1984). Neutrophils kill pulmonary endothelial cells by a hydrogen-peroxide-dependent pathway. An *in vitro* model of neutrophil-mediated lung injury. Am. Rev. *Resp. Dis.*, **130**, 209–13.

Mulligan M.S., Hevel J.M., Marletta M.A., Ward P.A. (1991a). Tissue injury following deposition of immune complexes is L-arginine dependent. *Proc. Natl. Acad. Sci. USA*, **88**, 6338–42.

Mulligan M.S., Smith C.W., Anderson D.C., Ward P.A. (1991b). Induction of ELAM-1 in the rat pulomonary microvasculature. *FASEB J.*, **5**, A526.

Mulligan M.S., Varani J., Dame M.K. et al. (1991c). Role of ELAM-1 in neutrophil mediated lung injury in rats. *J. Clin. Invest.*, **88**, 1396–406.

Phan S.H., Gannon D.E., Varani J. et al. (1989). Xanthine oxidase activity in rat pulmonary artery endothelial cells and its modulation by activated neutrophils. *Am.J. Pathol.*, **134**, 1201–11.

Phillips M.L., Nudelman E., Gaeta F.C. et al. (1990). ELAM-1 mediates cell adhesion by recognition of a carbohydrate ligand, sialyl-Lex. *Science*, **250**, 1130–2.

Picken L.J., Warnock R.A., Burns A.R. et al. (1991). The neutrophil selectin ELCAM-1 prevents carbohydrate

ligands to the vascular selectins ELAM-1 and GMP-140. *Cell*, **66**, 921–33.

Pober J.S., Bevilacqua M.P., Mendrick D.L. et al. (1986). Two distinct monokines, interleukin 1 and tumor necrosis factor, each independently induce biosynthesis and transient expression of the same antigen on the surface of cultured human vascular endothelial cells. *J. Immunol.*, **136**, 1680–7.

Rodell T.C., Cheronis J.C., Ohnemus C.L. et al. (1987). Xanthine oxidase mediates elastase induced injury to isolated lungs and endothelium. *J. Appl. Physiol.*, **63**, 2159–63.

Sacks T., Moldow C.F., Craddock P.R. et al. (1978). Oxygen radicals mediate endothelial cell damage by complement-stimulated granulocytes. An *in vitro* model of immune vascular damage. *J. Clin. Invest.*, **61**, 1161–7.

Simon R.H., DeHart P.D., Todd R.F. III. (1986). Neutrophil-induced injury of rat pulmonary alveolar epithelial cells. *J. Clin. Invest.*, **78**, 1375–86.

Smedly L.A., Tonnesen M.G., Sandhaus R.A. et al. (1986). Neutrophil-mediated injury to endothelial cells. Enhancement by endotoxin and essential role of neutrophil elastase. *J. Clin. Invest.*, **77**, 1233–43.

Strieter R.M., Kunkel S.L., Showell H.J., Marks R.M. (1988). Monokine-induced gene expression of a human endothelial cell-derived neutrophil chemotactic factor. *Biochem. Biophys. Res. Commun.*, **156**, 1340–5.

Strieter R.M., Kunkel S.L., Showell H. et al. (1989). Human endothelial cell gene expression of a neutrophil chemotactic factor by TNFα, LPS, IL-1β. *Science, (Wash DC)* **243**, 1467–9.

Varani J., Fligiel S.E.G., Till G.O. et al. (1985). Pulmonary endothelial cell killing by human neutrophils: possible involvement of the hydroxyl radical. *Lab. Invest.*, **53**, 656–63.

Varani J., Bendelow M.J., Sealey D.E. et al. (1989a). Tumor necrosis factor enhances suspectibility of vascular endothelial cells to neutrophil-mediated killing. *Lab. Invest.*, **59**, 292–4.

Varani J., Ginsburg I., Schuger L. et al. (1989b). Endothelial cell killing by neutrophils: synergistic interaction of oxygen products and proteases. *Am. J. Pathol.*, **135**, 435–8.

Varani J., Phan S.H., Gibbs D.F. et al. (1990). H_2O_2-mediated cytotoxicity of rat pulmonary endothelial cells: changes in adenosine triphosphate and purine products and effects of protective interventions. *Lab. Invest.*, **63**, 683–9.

Varani J., Stoolman L., Wang T.L., Ward, P.A. (1991). Thrombospondin production and thrombospondin-mediated adhesion in U937 cells. *Exp. Cell Res.*, **195**(1), 177–82.

Warren J.S. (1991). Intrapulmonary interleukin-1 mediates acute immune complex alveolitis in rats. *Biochem. Biophys. Res. Commun.*, **175**, 604–10.

Warren J.S., Yabroff K.R., Remick D.G. et al. (1989). Tumor necrosis factor participated in the pathogenesis of acute immune complex alveolitis in the rat. *J. Clin. Invest.*, **84**, 1873–82.

Warren J.S., Barton P.A., Mandel D.M., Matosic K. (1990). Intrapulmonary tumor necrosis factor triggers local platelet-activating factor production in rat immune complex alveolitis. *Lab. Invest.*, **63**, 746–54.

Weiss S.J., Young J., LoBuglio A.F. et al. (1981). Role of hydrogen peroxide in neutrophil-mediated destruction of cultured endothelial cells. *J. Clin. Invest.*, **68**, 714–21.

38. The Wound-organ

D. W. Wilmore and H. B. Stoner

The idea that a wound has a significant effect on the body is not new. It was suggested long ago (Moore, 1959) that a wound could produce 'hormones' which were necessary for wound healing. Recently, a wider concept has been proposed (Wilmore, 1986), namely that the wound acts as a separate organ added to the body; this 'new organ' interacts with the body by sending signals to alter host responses. In addition, the wound parasitizes oxygen and other essential nutrients to facilitate repair. This idea was developed from the study of burn patients but it has a much more general application. However, before this two-way relationship between the 'wound-organ' and the rest of the body is considered, the composition of the wound itself should be examined.

THE WOUND

In the creation of the wound, cells are destroyed and blood is extravasated into both necrotic and partially injured tissue. Tissue destruction may continue after the initial insult through the inadequate oxygenation of potentially viable cells in the damaged area and by the liberation of toxic metabolites. Blood vessels may be transected or become occluded in various ways; by thrombi, by oedema, by haematomas, by abscess formation or by badly applied splints and bandages. The concept of primary and secondary tissue damage is usually applied to the brain (Mendelow and Teasdale, 1983; Stoner and Cremer, 1985), but this concept may be applicable to all tissues. However, the primary effect of the local changes associated with the injury is tissue hypoxia which will lead to a series of biochemical changes ending in the death of the cell if the hypoxia is sufficiently severe and prolonged.

The biochemical effects of cellular hypoxia have been frequently reviewed (e.g. Heath, 1985). They may be summarized as an increased uptake of glucose, anaerobic glycolysis leading to an accumulation of lactate, a fall in tissue pH, loss of any energy stores such as glycogen, phosphocreatine and ATP, failure of ATP generation, failure of ion pumps with loss of intracellular K^+ and entry of Na^+ and Ca^{2+}, mitochondrial disintegration, increased membrane permeability and loss of cell constituents (myoglobin, creatine, enzymes, etc.). It has been shown in brain that partial ischaemia can be more deleterious than total ischaemia (Hossmann and Kliehues, 1973; Siesjö, 1984), since by preserving a supply of glucose it allows the continuing production of lactate and depression of pH. Others have suggested that the generation of free oxygen radicals during hypoperfusion or reperfusion accounts for many of the deleterious effects on cell and structure and function (Iles and Poole-Wilson, 1990; Lunec and Blake, 1990). These principles probably apply generally and may be particularly relevant when hyperglycaemia, hypoperfusion or reperfusion is present.

In ischaemic tissue, the pH falls to between 6.5 and 6.8 (Stoner and Green, 1948; Siesjö, 1984), and this can be important for two reasons. It will lead to the activation of proteolytic enzymes in damaged tissue (Stoner and Green, 1948) and it will also create a suitable environment for the growth of anaerobic bacteria such as *Clostridium perfringens* (Oakley, 1954).

Tissue damage initiates an inflammatory response (Jose, 1990). Local mediators such as prostaglandins, histamine and bradykinin are produced as a consequence of cell injury and result in vasodilatation, increased microvascular permeability and oedema formation. The capillary endothelium generates a variety of proinflammatory mediators and this facilitates the attachment of circulating neutrophils and monocytes to the vessel and allows their subsequent migration from the vascular compartment into the area of tissue injury. Foreign protein and microorganisms are highly effective chemoattractants and soon a large number of inflammatory cells will migrate into those parts of the wound which retain a blood supply. While fixed tissue macrophages, mast cells and vascular endothelium serve as the initial sources of wound mediators, infiltrating macrophages and neutrophils are potent factors for the production of prostaglandins, interleukins, tumour necrosis factor and macrophage colony stimulating factor, and all of these substances have been recovered from experimental healing wounds (Ford *et al.*, 1989).

These responses will occur even if the wound remains sterile, but the cellular infiltrate will be much greater if the wound is contaminated or becomes infected. The cellular pattern in the wound will depend on its age and the nature of any infecting organisms. Because infection heightens the inflammatory response, the presence of microorganisms prolongs the life of the wound.

Wound infection has been widely studied (e.g. Williams and Miles, 1949). Mostly the infection comes from without but self-contamination is frequent. Human and rat tissues are normally sterile, but this is not the case in all species; for example dog and goat, and that must be taken into account when interpreting experimental results. The presence of bacteria in a wound can lead to the elaboration of a variety of microbial products. Gram-positive organisms can elaborate exotoxins, some with enzymatic properties. An example of this effect is the collagenase of the α-toxin of *Clostridium perfringens* which will have destructive effects on the surrounding tissues. Gram-negative organisms, on the other hand, produce endotoxins which will be liberated on the death of the organism. While these substances initiate extremely potent local responses (such as microthrombosis), if these gain access to the body, they will produce a variety of toxic effects such as fever, a pituitary adrenal stress response and, in some cases, shock (see Chapter 34).

Endotoxins are normally present in large amount in the lumen of the gut but these substances are retained there by the intact gut wall and its associated lymphoid elements. Any small amount which reaches the portal circulation will be inactivated by the Küppfer cells of the liver. However, any process which reduces the effectiveness of these two barriers will allow increased entrance of endotoxin into the bloodstream; this may exert a deleterious impact on liver function and may also allow endotoxin to appear in the peripheral circulation and exert systemic effects.

Wound requirements

Attempts at tissue repair will commence soon after the creation of the wound. As the early inflammatory changes subside, granulation tissue will form. This mixture of leucocytes, macrophages, fibroblasts and newly formed blood vessels forms the base on which repair will occur. Skin epithelium can be replaced fairly rapidly but the repair of muscle and bone takes much longer. Repair requires an adequate supply of oxygen, nutrients and co-factors such as vitamins and trace metals (Hunt, 1987). Unless the body can supply these substances, wound healing will be delayed. However, the vasculature may not only serve to transport substances to the wound, but its endothelium may secrete growth factors to promote tissue remodelling and wound healing.

These requirements give some idea of the demands which the wound is going to make on the body. The main ones are probably related to the supply of blood. The newly formed capillary bed may greatly increase the size of the vascular compartment. Because this vascular network is not innervated, it behaves physiologically like an arteriovenous fistula; the wound decreases peripheral resistance which requires an increase in cardiac output to maintain blood pressure. Flow is also varied by local metabolic factors and is not generally subservient to systemic demands.

These changes will develop at different rates over a variable time-span depending on the size of the wound and its rate of healing. They will probably reach a maximum in the second week.

In one sense the size of the wound is determined by the initial insult – the extent and depth of a burn, the number and type of fractures, the presence of associated soft tissue injuries, etc. For this reason the late ('flow phase' (Cuthbertson, 1942)) changes observed in the body are closely and positively related to the Injury Severity Score (Threlfall *et al.*, 1984). However, the size of the wound requires some further consideration, particularly if we are going to generalize about wounds produced in different ways. For this purpose, the size of the wound should be equated to the amount of the granulation tissue (e.g. capillary surface area), as that is the common factor for comparison. Thus, size is obvious in the case of the healing burn injury where a thick layer of granulation tissue covers the base of the burn. It may not be so obvious in patients with intra-abdominal sepsis or multiple fractures (Stoner, 1987). However, there is a large amount of granulation tissue at these sites, in the walls of abscesses and as the callus of healing fractures. Its presence is seen when the distribution of intravenously injected radioactive markers (labelled leucocytes, etc.) are studied with a gamma camera. It is this newly formed granulation tissue which forms the bulk of the new 'wound-organ'.

SYSTEMIC EFFECTS OF THE WOUND

The changes in the body produced by this mass of granulation tissue can be divided into those which reflect the 'pull' of the new organ (e.g. tissue demand) and those which can be attributed to the 'push' of the metabolites, autacoids and cytokines elaborated in it – the 'wound hormones' of old (Figure 38.1). The effect of these factors will now be considered, particularly in relation to the changes in energy metabolism which have long been used to assess the effect of an injury.

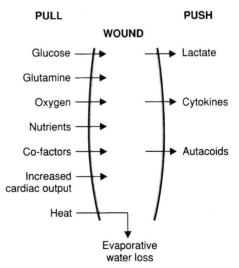

Figure 38.1 Diagram to show the 'pull' and 'push' of the wound on the body.

TABLE 38.1

CALORIC COST AND EQUIVALENT OXYGEN CONSUMPTION OF PROCESSES INVOLVED IN THE BODY'S RESPONSE TO THE WOUND.

Response	Caloric cost	Oxygen equivalent
Increased cardiac output $\times$ 2	–	46 ml/min (normal* 23 ml/min)
Hepatic gluconeogensis[†] (2 lactate $\rightarrow$ glucose)	0.38 Kcal/kg/min	–
Q_{10} effect of pyrexia	–	+10–13% per °C rise in body temp.
Evaporation of water from wound[‡]	0.58 Kcal per g H_2O	circa. 116 ml per g H_2O

* From Wilmore (1977).
[†] From Wolfe et al. (1987).
[‡] from Clark and Edholm (1985).

'Pull'

Cardiovascular factors

The presence of a large amount of highly vascularized granulation tissue where the vessels are not under nervous control increases the intravascular space of the body and calls for an increase in blood volume and cardiac output. The restoration of the blood volume to an adequate level should be achieved by resuscitation. Then, cardiac output can more than double after serious injury (Sibbald, 1986; Wilmore, 1986). The ensuing increase in cardiac work (Table 38.1) will further raise the demand for oxygen and this will be one of a number of factors leading to the increase in the patient's total oxygen consumption.

Fluid loss

The main loss of fluid from the body usually occurs at the time of the accident but fluid loss may continue throughout convalescence. Apart from delayed or secondary haemorrhage, there may be continuing drainage from the wound. This loss may become important when there is wound infection or if an enterocutaneous fistula develops. Another route for fluid loss is by evaporation, in which case there will also be loss of heat.

The evaporative loss of water from normal, non-sweating skin is small, <10 g/m^2/h, and will be increased some three-fold by the onset of sweating. However, the evaporative loss from the exposed, wet surface of a burn or granulation tissue is very much greater, and 10-fold increases have been reported (Childs et al., 1992). Since the evaporation of a gram of water from the surface extracts 0.58 Kcal of heat from the body (Clark and Edholm, 1985), this can represent an important route of heat loss. This is not just confined to the raw, exposed surface of a burn, for evaporation is not reduced by the formation of a burn eschar which is freely permeable to water. Increased evaporative loss will occur from the exposed surface of any wound and could become important when this is large, as in some patients after laparostomy. The loss of heat,

although not necessarily that of fluid, by this route may be considerably reduced by wound dressings (Childs et al., 1992).

Substrate utilization

From the point of view of energy substrate the wound utilizes glucose as the main energy source which supplies at least 70% of its requirement (Wilmore, 1986). Fortunately, the cells of the wound are not insulin dependent, so that they are not affected by the insulin resistance which impacts on other tissues of the body following injury, such as skeletal muscle, adipose tissue and liver (Black et al., 1982; Henderson et al., 1991). In the wound, ATP is generated by glycolysis rather than by oxidative phosphorylation, even in the presence of oxygen (the process of aerobic glycolysis). Because so much less ATP is produced by the partial breakdown of glucose than in its complete combustion in mitochondrial oxidative phosphorylation, a large amount of glucose has to be taken up by the wound and converted to lactate to meet the demand. This lactate is then returned to the host via the circulation (see below).

Although the wound produces a large portion of its ATP in this manner, it also consumes oxygen. In view of the large number of leucocytes in its cellular composition, an additionally important substrate for oxidation is probably glutamine (Newsholme et al., 1985). The use of both glucose and glutamine could be related to the bursts of oxygen consumption associated with phagocytosis, which must be a major activity in the wound. Oxygen is also required for the oxidation of fat and amino acids and for the conversion of proline to hydroxyproline in collagen synthesis.

'Push'

The wound manufactures signals to alter host response and thus optimize an environment for tissue repair. Since the wound in large part is without innervation, these signals must be circulating factors. To insure a warm environment, blood flow to the wound is enhanced, and this effect is augmented by pyrexia – an elevation in total body temperature.

Metabolic products

The main metabolic product of the wound is lactate. As shown above, this is produced in large amounts from glucose. Some of the lactate entering the body from the wound will be oxidized by organs such as the heart and skeletal muscle but the majority will be extracted by the liver and converted back to glucose. This is an oxygen-consuming process (Table 38.1). The symbiosis of the wound with its host will therefore depend on the host being adequately oxygenated, with appropriate blood flow to essential organs.

Autacoids and cytokines

The cells which form the wound elaborate a range of substances which act both locally and at a distance. These substances include the various inflammatory mediators, various derivatives of arachidonic acid, prostaglandins, etc. and, most importantly, cytokines. These substances are small peptide products produced by a variety of activated inflammatory cells. The activated macrophages which may be the main producers of wound cytokines will only migrate into the wound some hours after its creation and reach a maximum after about 48 hours. These inflammatory cells will continue to be present and active as long as the wound remains. The pharmacological actions of these compounds are described in Chapters 32, 33 and 34. IL-1, IL-6 and TNF (tumour necross factor) are particularly important, since they are pyrogens, and mediate other acute-phase responses. These substances also activate the pituitary–adrenal response which participates in skeletal muscle protein breakdown and augments the hepatic acute-phase response. When the appropriate organisms are present in the wound, microbial products will also be produced. An important member of this group is endotoxin, which enhances the production of cytokines.

WOUND–HOST INTERACTIONS

The changes after trauma usually reach a maximum during the second week after the injury and then gradually decline as the wound heals and the patient recovers. These changes may be much more prolonged in the burns patient where there is a large skin deficit to replace or when a wound becomes infected. Much the same changes are seen in surgical patients with postoperative sepsis. The changes in the host during the 'flow phase' as it was named by Cuthbertson (1942) are well known, essentially an increase in metabolic rate with increased nitrogen loss and negative nitrogen balance. The question, therefore, is how far these changes can be explained by the 'push and pull' of the wound.

In a detailed study of a group of severely burned patients being treated by exposure and showing an increase of up to three-fold in resting energy expenditure, Henane et al. (1981) showed that up to 70% of the excess oxygen consumption was being used to meet the heat losses from the exposed burn. When the burn is covered with dressings preparatory to early tangential excision and skin grafting, heat loss by this route is reduced but not eliminated (Childs et al., 1992). In units practising this technique the enormous increases in oxygen consumption after burns are no longer seen, although the metabolic rate is still significantly elevated in these patients.

Can we explain the 30% of the oxygen consumption unaccounted for by Henane et al. (1981) and, of course, the increases observed in patients with other forms of injury where there has been no abnormal increase in heat loss? There are, indeed, a number of factors in the wound which could be involved. Greater oxygen uptake will be needed to meet the demands of the heart because of the increase in cardiac output, of the liver because of the increase in gluconeogenesis, an energy-demanding process (Krebs, 1954), and of the wound itself. Respiratory work will be increased which will require a further increase in oxygen uptake. Many of the patients at this stage have a raised body temperature and this in turn will increase oxygen consumption through a Q_{10} effect on the biochemical reactions of the body. The rise in body temperature may be due to alterations in thermoregulatory mechanisms produced by pyrogens (e.g. cytokines) originating in the wound. There are, therefore, plenty of reasons for thinking that the increase in metabolic rate in the injured patient could be due to the 'push and pull' of the wound itself. The question then is whether or not the changes produced by these factors are large enough to account for the effects observed.

The increases in resting energy expenditure currently being observed in injured patients are not large. After an elective abdominal operation uncomplicated by sepsis, an increase of 10% might be expected, whereas in patients with multiple musculoskeletal injuries increases of around 30% are usually found (Frayn et al., 1984). The large changes reported in some patients with head injuries (e.g. Fruin et al., 1986) probably reflect increased muscle tone and spasm, i.e. the patients are not strictly resting. The effects of the various factors are summarized in Table 38.1. From this it can be seen that the hypermetabolism of the 'flow phase' may well be accounted for by the 'push and pull' of the new organ added to the body by the injury, namely the wound.

This conclusion has therapeutic implications. If this response is needed to meet the requirements of the wound, treatment must not be aimed at reducing the response but at reducing the size of the wound so as to reduce the need for the response. A reduction in the response not secondary to a reduction in the size of the wound might well impede the rate of recovery. This is, in fact, seen when the patient is unable to mount an adequate response because of pre-existing or concurrent disease (Sibbald, 1986).

Although the changes in energy metabolism during the 'flow phase' can probably be explained, full understanding of the other feature of the phase, the negative nitrogen balance, still eludes us. It may be that this too is mediated by the wound through the action of substances such as TNF (see Chapter 46). However, the work of Clague (1981) and Rennie (1985) suggests that there may be more than one mechanism involved in the imbalance between protein synthesis and breakdown. Increased breakdown certainly occurs after severe injuries, partly to remove damaged tissue at the site of the injury but mainly as a later response in the rest of the body. Attempts to correct this negative balance are never very successful. Our attempts to correct it are hindered by two factors: (1) lack of knowledge of the biochemical mechanism involved and (2) lack of understanding of the aim of the effect, if, indeed, it has one. Various teleological suggestions have been made, for example that body protein is broken down in a search for rare amino acids required by the wound for its repair, but until we have a much clearer understanding of the matter it will be difficult to take effective measures to curtail the loss of muscle mass that can be so debilitating for the injured patient.

VARIATIONS ON THE RESPONSE

Some of the features of the host which could alter the response to the wound-organ have already been mentioned. Existing cardiovascular or respiratory disease will obviously reduce the ability of the body to respond to the challenge of the wound, which may precipitate a fatal outcome after an injury which could have been overcome by a fit person. Changes of this type are most likely to be present in elderly patients and may be a reason for the greater morbidity and mortality after trauma in this group (Horan *et al.*, 1988). However, on the whole, the acute metabolic response to trauma in the elderly is not very different from that in younger patients (Horan *et al.*, 1992). Nevertheless there are differences in the 'flow phase' where the endocrine and metabolic disturbance persist much longer than expected (Frayn *et al.*, 1983; Roberts *et al.*, 1990). The explanation for this is unclear and it does not seem to be attributable to the immobility of many of the elderly as at first thought.

The necessity for adequate oxygen transport to the tissues of the body if they are to meet the demands of the wound satisfactorily has already been pointed out. If this is to be achieved there must be very full resuscitation in the early stages and the blood volume must continue to be fully maintained to allow for the increase in cardiac output. Appreciation of these needs is the basis for Shoemaker's advocacy of vigorous resuscitation to supranormal levels of oxygen delivery (Shoemaker *et al.*, 1985).

The response to trauma in children is only now being studied in detail. Some differences from the adult response have been reported. For instance, Childs (1988) has shown that pyrexia is common in the burned child during the first 48 hours after the injury, i.e. at a stage when it is not seen in the adult. The reasons for this are not fully understood. The pyrexia is accompanied by an increase in heat production and a decrease in heat loss from the acral skin (Childs and Little, 1994) and there is evidence that it is related to the concentration of IL-6 in the plasma (Childs *et al.*, 1990a). It may reflect the greater effect of this pyrogen on an immature thermoregulatory system (Childs *et al.*, 1989). Whatever the mechanism, the ensuing weight loss in these burned children is important as a fall in their weight centile position is not quickly restored (Childs *et al.*, 1990b).

Further work is needed on the variations in the responses to the wound if we are to fulfil our obligations to the patient.

CONCLUSION

John Hunter (1794) proposed that the body's reaction to injury was aimed at aiding recovery. This proposal has been the subject of much argument but now we begin to understand that some, at least, of the changes which occur are a response by the body to the presence of what may be looked on as a new organ, namely the wound. Hunter's views are, at least partially, vindicated.

REFERENCES

Black P.R., Brooks D.C., Bessey P.Q. et al. (1982). Mechanisms of insulin resistance following injury. *Ann. Surg.*, **196**, 420–35.

Childs C. (1988). Fever in burned children. *Burns*, **14**, 1–6.

Childs C., Little R.A. (1994). Acute changes in oxygen consumption and body temperature after burn injury. *Arch. Dis. Child.*, **71**, 31–4.

Childs C., Stoner H.B., Little R.A., Davenport P.J. (1989). A comparison of some thermoregulatory responses in healthy children and in children with burn injury. *Clin. Sci.*, **77**, 425–9.

Childs C., Ratcliffe R.J., Holt I. et al. (1990b). The relationship between Interleukin-1, Interleukin-6 and pyrexia in burned children. In *The Physiological and Pathological Effects of Cytokines. Progress in Leucocyte Biology*, 10 B. (Dinarello C.A., Kluger M.J., Powanda

M.C., Oppenheim J.J., eds). New York: Wiley-Liss, pp. 295–300.

Childs C., Hall T., Davenport P.J., Little R.A. (1990b). Dietary intake and changes in body weight in burned children. *Burns*, **16**, 418–22.

Childs C., Stoner H.B., Little R.A. (1992). Cutaneous heat loss shortly after burn injury in children. *Clin. Sci.*, **83**, 117–26.

Clague M.B. (1981). Turnover in pathological states. In *Nitrogen Metabolism in Man* (Waterlow J.C., Stephen J.M.L., eds). London: Applied Science, pp. 525–39.

Clark R.P., Edholm O.G. (1985). *Man and his Thermal Environment*. London: Arnold, p. 109.

Cuthbertson D.P. (1942). Post-shock metabolic response. *Lancet*, **i**, 433–7.

Ford H.R., Hoffman R.A., Wing E.J. et al. (1989). Characterization of wound cytokines in the sponge matric model. *Arch. Surg.*, **124**, 1422–8.

Frayn K.N., Stoner H.B., Barton R.N. et al. (1983). Persistence of high plasma glucose, insulin and cortisol concentrations in elderly patients with proximal femoral fractures. *Age Aging*, **12**, 70–6.

Frayn K.N., Little R.A., Stoner H.B., Galasko C.S.B. (1984). Metabolic control in non-septic patients with musculoskeletal injuries. *Injury*, **16**, 73–9.

Fruin A.N., Taylor C., Pettis M.S. (1986). Caloric requirements in patients with severe head injuries. *Surg. Neurol.*, **25**, 25.

Heath D.F. (1985). Subcellular aspects of the response to trauma. *Br. Med. Bull.*, **41**, 240–5.

Henane R., Bittel J., Banssillon V. (1981). Partitional calorimetry measurements of energy exchanges in severely burned patients. *Burns*, **7**, 180–9.

Henderson A.A., Frayn K.N., Galasko C.S.B., Little R.A. (1991). Dose–response relationships for the effects of insulin on glucose and fat metabolism in injured patients and control subjects. *Clin. Sci.*, **80**, 25–32.

Horan M.A., Barton R.N., Little R.A. (1988). Ageing and the response to injury. In *Advanced Geriatric Medicine*, vol. 7 (Evans J.G., Caird J.I., eds). Bristol: Wright, pp. 101–35.

Horan M.A., Roberts N.A., Barton R.N., Little R.A. (1992). Injury responses in old age. In *Oxford Textbook of Geriatric Medicine* (Evans J.G., Williams T.F., eds). Oxford University Press, pp. 88–93.

Hossman K.A., Kleihues P. (1973). Reversibility of ischemic brain damage. *Arch. Neurol.*, **29**, 375–84.

Hunt T.K. (1987). A retrospective prospective on the nature of wounds. In *Growth Factors and other Aspects of Wound Healing* (Barbul A., Pines E., Caldwell M., Hunt T.K., eds). New York: Alan R. Liss, pp. 1–18.

Hunter J. (1794). *A Treatise on the Blood, Inflammation and Gunshot Wounds*. London.

Iles R.A., Poole-Wilson P.A. (1990). Ischaemia, hypoxia and reperfusion. In *The Metabolic and Molecular Basis of Acquired Disease*, vol. 1 (Cohen R.D., Lewis B., Alberti K.G.M.M., Denman A.M., eds). London: Baillière Tindall, pp. 322–41.

Jose P.J. (1990). Inflammation. In *The Metabolic and Molecular Basis of Acquired Disease*, vol. 1 (Cohen R.D., Lewis B., Alberti K.G.M.M., Denman A.M., eds).

London: Baillière Tindall, pp. 342–62.

Krebs H.A. (1954). Considerations concerning the pathways of synthesis in living matter. *Bull Johns Hopkins Hosp.*, **95**, 19.

Lunec J., Blake D. (1990). Oxygen free radicals: their relevance to disease processes. In *The Metabolic and Molecular Basis of Acquired Disease*, vol. 1 (Cohen R.D., Lewis B., Alberti K.G.M.M., Denman A.M., eds). London: Baillière Tindall, pp. 189–212.

Mendelow A.D., Teasdale G.M. (1983). Pathophysiology of head injuries. *Br. J. Surg.*, **70**, 641–50.

Moore F.D. (1959). *Metabolic Care of the Surgical Patient*. Philadelphia: W.B. Saunders.

Newsholme E.A., Crabtree B., Ardawi M.S.M. (1985). Glutamine metabolism in lymphocytes, its biochemical, physiological and clinical importance. *Q.J. Exp. Physiol.*, **70**, 473–89.

Oakely C.L. (1954). Gas gangrene. *Br. Med. Bull.*, **10**, 52–8.

Rennie M.J. (1985). Muscle protein turnover and the wasting due to injury and disease. *Br. Med. Bull.*, **41**, 257–64.

Roberts N.A., Barton R.N., Horan M.A., White A. (1990). Adrenal function after upper femoral fracture in elderly people: persistence of stimulation and the roles of adrenocorticotrophic hormone and immobility. *Age Aging*, **19**, 304–10.

Shoemaker W.C., Bland R.D., Appel P.L. (1985). Therapy of critically ill post-operative patients based on outcome prediction and prospective clinical trials. *Surg. Clin North Am.*, **65**, 811–33.

Sibbald W.J. (1986). The influence of cardiopulmonary complications of severe trauma on the systemic response to trauma. In *The Scientific Basis for the Care of the Critically Ill* (Little R.A., Frayn K.N., eds). Manchester: Manchester University Press, pp. 275–92.

Siesjö, B.K. (1984). Cerebral circulation and metabolism. *J. Neurosurg.*, **60**, 883–908.

Stoner H.B. (1987). Interpretation of the metabolic effect of trauma and sepsis. *J. Clin. Pathol.*, **40**, 1108–17.

Stoner H.B., Cremer, J.E. (1985). Maintenance of metabolic integrity in the brain after trauma. *Br. Med. Bull.*, **41**, 246–50.

Stoner H.B., Green H.N. (1948). Bodily reactions to trauma. The effect of ischaemia on muscle protein. *Br. J. Exp. Pathol.*, **29**, 121–32.

Threlfall C.J., Maxwell A.R., Stoner H.B. (1984). Post-traumatic creatinuria. *J. Trauma*, **24**, 516–32.

Williams R.E.O., Miles A.A. (1949). *Infection and Sepsis in Industrial Wounds of the Hand*. Medical Research Council Special Report Series No. 266. London: HMSO.

Wilmore D.W. (1977). *The Metabolic Management of the Critically Ill*. New York: Plenum.

Wilmore D.W. (1986). The wound as an organ. In *The Scientific Basis for the Care of the Critically Ill* (Little R.A., Frayn K.N., eds). Manchester: Manchester University Press, pp. 45–60.

Wolfe R.R., Herndon D.N., Jahoor F. et al. (1987). Effect of severe burn injury on substrate cycling by glucose and fatty acids. *New Engl. J. Med.*, **317**, 403–8.

39. Wound Healing

T. K. Hunt, H. W. Hopf and R. V. Mueller

INTRODUCTION

An era of physiological measurement of seriously ill patients has forced improved explanations for old observations about wounds. A number of new methods of clinical management, many of which are based on circulatory and endocrinological support, have been the result. At the same time the chemical contributions made by wounds to the metabolic response are being defined.

INJURY AND RESPONSE

Injury profoundly disrupts the normal architecture and chemical environment of tissue. The postinjury environment is marked by impaired perfusion coincident with inflammation. The subsequent struggle to restore normality, that is 'wound healing', or, 'repair', is a sequence of overlapping processes which starts when vessels are cut, endothelial cells are injured, inflammation is activated and coagulation begins. These events lead to the assembly of a chemoattractive and growth-promoting environment. Cell movement and replication follow with the onset of angiogenesis and fibroplasia. Healing tissue then acquires a characteristic architecture which assures that the new cells will deposit a fibrous matrix to support the new vessels and epithelium to cover the injury until the metabolic consequences of injury are alleviated. Later, the provisional matrix will be turned over, rearranged and strengthened.

The major components of repair are shown in Figure 39.1. The lines in this figure indicate signalling processes which include cytokines, growth factors, complement, and other classical inflammatory mediators, and in some cases metabolic signals such as hypoxia and accumulated lactate. Often several signals capable of exciting any given step are present. The conclusion to be drawn from this is that pathways of wound healing are replicated. Many details, especially of growth factor actions, cannot yet be put into the perspective of actual wound healing.

COAGULATION AND INFLAMMATION

Immediately after injury, coagulation is the prominent component. Fibrin, fibrinopeptides and fibrin-split-products instantaneously begin to attract inflammatory cells, particularly macrophages. Platelets and thrombin are activated. Platelets release growth factors such as platelet-derived growth factor (PDGF), insulin-like growth factor (IGF-I) and transforming growth factor alpha and beta (TGF-α, TGF-β) which attract a variety of cells into the injured area and prepare them to multiply (Ross et al., 1974; Deuel et al., 1981; Assoian et al., 1983; Senior et al., 1983; Zwaal et al., 1986; Gallin et al., 1988; Karey et al., 1989; Tuddenham et al., 1989). Thrombin and fibrinopeptides also contribute growth stimuli (Chen et al., 1975, 1976; Bar-shavit et al., 1983).

Damaged endothelium expresses receptors for so-called 'integrin' molecules on the cell membranes of leucocytes (Mentzer et al., 1986; Kishimoto et al., 1989), and complement factors generated in response to the injury cause leucocytes to adhere and migrate into tissue. Inflammatory components such as histamine, serotonin and bradykinin, cause vessels first to constrict to control haemostasis, and then to dilate and become so porous that blood plasma and inflammatory cells move freely into the injured area (Knighton et al., 1982; Hunt et al., 1988; Knighton et al., 1988; Rabkin and Hunt, 1988).

Microvascular injury severely distorts the local environment because it not only impairs perfusion and oxygenation but also leads to increased cell density and oedema. Consequently, the oxygen concentration falls. Carbon dioxide and lactate accumulate (Hunt et al., 1967, 1978; Knighton et al., 1984).

Enzymes released by leucocyte granules and activated by the local acid pH, many of them proteolytic, begin to distort the local macromolecular structure. These include collagenase, amylase, elastase and ß-glucuronidase. Fibrinolysin appears to release a growth factor peptide sequence from fibrin. Fibrinopeptide C attracts macrophages, and fibrin activates them to produce angiogenic factors (Paty et al., 1987).

The appearance of macrophages both starts the synthetic phase of healing and ensures its continuation, because at this stage, as the flood of coagulation-mediated growth-promoting substances begins to ebb, macrophages assume control of the local environment. Macrophages release large amounts of lactate, even in the presence of oxygen (Paty, 1988). As will be detailed later, accumulated lactate and hypoxia stimulate macrophages to release growth and chemoattractant substances such as TGF-α and -β (D. Ladine, E. Amento, T. Hunt, 1991, unpublished data), TNF-α and IL-1 (Ghezzi et al., 1991). Many of these prepare fibroblasts both to grow and synthesize collagen, and some stimulate angiogenesis. Here, relationships become even more complex since IL-1, for instance, becomes mitogenic to fibroblasts only by inducing PDGF.

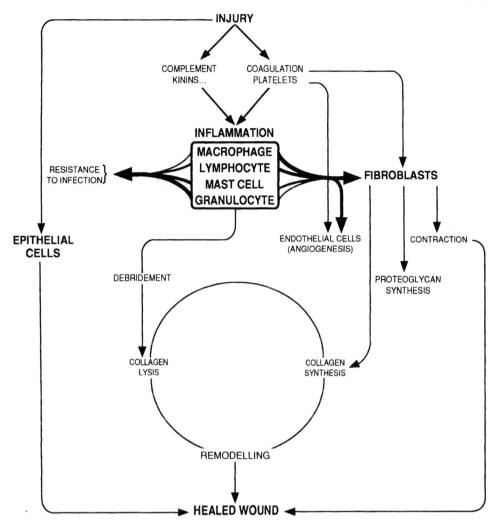

Figure 39.1 A schema of wound healing. (Reproduced from Levenson *et al.*, 1979, with permission.)

The large concentrations of lactate in the extracellular fluid of wounds, often reaching 15 mmol (as opposed to 1 mmol in blood), seem to be a cardinal property. The hypothesis has been proposed that they act as a metabolic signal, assuring that healing will continue until the local microvasculature is sufficiently repaired to carry away the excess and provide enough oxygen to prevent re-accumulation (Jensen *et al.*, 1986b).

THE WOUND ENVIRONMENT AND THE 'WOUND MODULE'

Growth and chemoattractant factors released during coagulation and inflammation rearrange the local cell population, so that by the third or fourth day after injury the cells involved in repair are loosely arranged in a characteristic spatial relationship which is shown in Figure 39.2 (Hunt *et al.*, 1985). Unless the wound is infected, the granulocyte population which dominated on the first day has diminished. Macrophages cover the cut surface.

Immature fibroblasts lie just beneath. More mature fibroblasts are scattered behind with small vessels beginning to appear among them. These relationships, not clear in ordinary microscopic sections of wounds, become clear when healing tissue is forced to grow across a narrow space bounded by optically clear membranes. In this constricting apparatus, wound cells must proceed in a coherent single-file order, leaders first, followers next. In the rabbit ear chamber illustrated in Figure 39.2, healing wounds may be observed in the living state and later fixed, stained and examined (Hunt *et al.*, 1985). The arrangement of cells seen in electron microscopic sections is characteristic. The leading macrophages lie in an area of hypoxia and accumulated lactate. Just behind are youthful fibroblasts and budding microvessels. Farther back in the healing tissue are mature fibroblasts synthesizing and depositing new collagen in an environment which is still rich in lactate but rather better oxygenated than is the zone in which macrophages collect. These are the conditions in which the new matrix molecules, collagen,

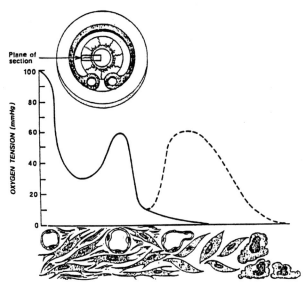

Figure 39.2 Oxygen tension profile of a rabbit ear chamber wound measured by microelectrodes. The solid line represents the profile in hypovolaemia, as opposed to normovolaemia represented by the dashed line. The distal-most capillary shuts down as a result of volume loss, and the fragile leading edge of the wound literally becomes anoxic. (Reproduced from Hunt, 1979a, with permission.)

proteoglycans and fibronectin, are best synthesized, deposited and remodelled. Most of the dividing fibroblasts are seen on the wound side of the last functioning vessels where oxygen tension is 'normally' about 40 mmHg. This Po_2 is optimal for fibroblast replication in cell culture (Bradley *et al.*, 1978).

This 'module' moves across the ear chamber using the area of mitotic fibroblasts and budding vessels as a growth point and leaving behind a relatively acellular, sparsely vascular, fibro-fatty tissue. The fine new blood vessels which remain behind coalesce to form larger vessels separated by longer distances (Schoefl, 1963). In this manner, so-called granulation tissue forms and wound spaces fill with new tissue. Primary repair is similar except that the 'module' is quickly formed, little tissue replacement is necessary, and resolution occurs more quickly.

CELL GROWTH AND REPLICATION: I. FIBROPLASIA

Fibroplasia, i.e. the replication and accumulation of fibroblasts, is stimulated by multiple mechanisms starting when platelet-derived growth factors are released, continuing with fibrin-related growth factor sequences, and remaining until macrophages and lymphocytes stop releasing growth-promoting cytokines and growth factors. PDGF (Scher *et al.*,

1979), interleukins 1, 2, 6 and 8, tumour necrosis factor, fibroblast growth factor (FGF) (Baird, 1989; Klagsbrun, 1989; Gospodarowicz, 1990), TGF-α and β (Roberts *et al.*, 1985; Burgess *et al.*, 1989), IGF-I (Gilmour *et al.*, 1988), and other leucocyte-derived growth factors (Magee *et al.*, 1977; Matsuoka and Grotendorst, 1989) all seem to be potential contributors. All appear to be released locally from platelets, lymphocytes and macrophages, as well as from binding sites on local connective tissue and even from fibroblasts themselves (Rappolee *et al.*, 1988; Baird and Walicke, 1989). Locally released growth substances are joined by counterparts derived from blood, such as epidermal growth factor (EGF) (very much like TGF-α) and IGF-I (Sbarra, 1988; Spencer, 1988).

The precise nature of the progenitor cells of fibroblasts is not clear. If there is such a thing as a 'fibrocyte', it is not well recognized. Smooth muscle cells seem to be a likely source. Fibroblasts seem to stream from the adventitia and media of vessels. Lipocytes (which produce collagen in injured liver), pericytes, and others are also candidates. Fibroblasts seem to multiply best at a Po_2 of about 40 mmHg (Bradley *et al.*, 1978), which is above the attainable levels in some ischaemic wounds.

CELL GROWTH AND REPLICATION: II. ANGIOGENESIS

Angiogenesis becomes visible by about 4 days after injury but begins 2 or 3 days earlier when new capillaries 'bud' out of pre-existing venules and grow toward the injury in response to chemoattractants. The migrating epithelial cells send out cytoplasmic processes from time to time and establish contact with other cells. On making contact, the cells seem to flow together and establish continuity of lumens. The process by which lumens are established is not clear.

In primarily closed wounds, budding vessels soon encounter similar cells migrating from the other side of the wound and circulation forms across the wound cleft. In unclosed wounds, or those not closed well, the new capillaries fuse only with neighbours migrating in the same direction and 'granulation tissue' is formed instead.

Chemoattractants to endothelial cells include the BB homodimer of platelet-derived growth factor (Fiegel *et al.*, 1991) and a macrophage-derived growth factor whose identity is not yet fully established (J. Feng, Z. Hussain, T. Hunt, 1991, unpublished data). Although many of the so-called growth factors are capable of stimulating angiogenesis, animal experiments indicate that the dominant factor in wounds is derived from macrophages in response to hypoxia or lactate accumulation (Knighton *et al.*, 1981, 1983; Jensen *et al.*, 1986a). Its precise identity has not been established.

Angiogenesis arising from metabolic need is well known in biology and medicine. Physical conditioning, for instance, leads to new vessel formation. Reducing conditions, such as elevated lactate, are one expression of metabolic need. Macrophages cultured in 10 mM lactate or in simple hypoxia (0–30 mmHg or so) release angiogenic factor(s) which are chemoattractive to endothelial cells (Jensen *et al.*, 1986a). In such reducing conditions, NAD^+ is converted to NADH and the concentration of NAD^+ falls. This changes a normal flux in which some NAD^+ (specifically) is metabolized (by removal of the nicotinamide moiety) to ADP ribose (ADPR), which governs a variety of cell functions. When the NAD^+ pool shrinks, the ADP ribose pool shrinks as well (Hussain *et al.*, 1989).

Apparently, ADPR normally controls synthesis or release of factors which elicit angiogenesis, because when the enzymes which convert NAD^+ to ADPR are inhibited or when lactate removes the NAD^+, which is their only substrate, angiogenic factor(s) result (J. Feng, Z. Hussain, T. Hunt, 1991, unpublished data). The concentration of lactate in wound fluid, the environment of wound macrophages, rises to about 10 mM early, before angiogenesis becomes established, and remains high until repair ceases. It is not certain how the diminished ADPR leads to angiogenesis. However, this mechanism is remarkably similar and complementary to that which governs collagen synthesis and is known in greater detail (below).

CELL GROWTH AND REPLICATION: III. EPITHELIZATION

Epithelial cells respond to many of the same stimuli as do fibroblasts and endothelial cells. A number of growth factors enhance replication of epithelial cells and others are probably chemoattractants (Aaronson *et al.*, 1990, Anderson *et al.*, 1990; Mckay and Leigh, 1991). Transforming growth factor β for instance, tends to prevent epithelial cells from differentiating and thus appears to potentiate and perpetuate mitogenesis though it is not, itself, mitogenic (Moses *et al.*, 1991). Hypoxia causes keratinocytes to secrete TGF-β (Falanga *et al.*, 1991). Epidermal growth factor (EGF or TGF alpha) is a mitogen for epithelial cells as well as for fibroblasts (Burgess, 1989).

Epithelialization proceeds in a somewhat curious manner. The first mitoses appear a few cells away from the edge of epithelial wounds. The new cells migrate into the unepithelialized area and anchor, forming a new edge. The next new cells migrate over the last and anchor at the new edge. Though it has not been measured, Po_2 under the leading epithelial cells is likely to be low and therefore stimulatory to TGF-ß production.

New epithelial cells must differentiate in order to regain normal epithelial functions. Very little is known of this process in wound healing, but deposition of basement membrane is an early component. This requires collagen and laminin synthesis, and this, as well as cell replication, is dependent upon oxygen tension.

Squamous epithelialization and probably differentiation proceed at maximal rate when local Po_2 approaches about 700 mmHg (Medawar, 1948). Local oxygen can accelerate epithelialization but only if the underlying surface is suitable for anchoring and movement and an appropriate growth environment has been assembled.

Epithelialization is also more rapid when surface wounds are kept moist. Contrary to classical thought, even short periods of drying can impair it. The exudate from acute, uninfected superficial wounds is essentially the same as fluid taken from a closed wound. It contains growth factors and lactate and therefore recapitulates the growth environment found internally. Lactate levels in acute burn wound exudate are low, however, possibly due to the large concentration of LDH derived from disintegrating cells. Fluid from chronic, non-healing surface wounds is notably poor in growth factors (G. Schultz, 1991, personal communication).

MATRIX DEPOSITION

Collagen (together with proteoglycans) is the only protein which can provide the strength and flexibility needed for human connective tissue function. Its synthesis is not a constitutive property of fibroblasts. It must be stimulated.

The mechanisms of stimulation and synthesis are not clear. Some growth factors, TGF-β and IGF-I for example, seem to simulate it through gene transcription (Ignotz *et al.*, 1987; Goldstein *et al.*, 1989; Thiebaud *et al.*, 1990). More basic, however, is the finding that mere accumulation of lactate in the environment stimulates transcription of collagen genes and mRNA synthesis and posttranslational modification of the collagen molecule itself in a manner similar to stimulation of angiogenesis. This mechanism is not pH dependent, but rests instead on the cellular pool of adenosine diphosphoribose (ADPR), the molecule that remains when the nicotinamide is removed from NAD^+ (Figure 39.3). Accumulation of lactate converts NAD^+ to NADH. As a consequence, less NAD^+ is available to have its nicotinamide moiety removed and thus be converted to ADPR (which logically should be called AD^+). This reaction, which can occur only to NAD^+ and not to NADH, yields monomeric ADPR in the cytoplasm and polymeric ADPR (pADPR) in the nucleus. In the nucleus, this molecule normally, and by means

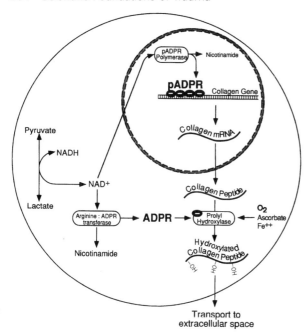

Figure 39.3 The regulation of collagen synthesis by ADP ribose (ADPR). Increased ADPR concentration decreases collagen gene expression and inhibits prolyl hydroxylase enzyme activity, thereby decreasing collagen peptide production.

unknown, represses collagen gene transcription. When, for any reason, the pADPR pool is diminished, as it is when the NAD^+ pool is diminished, collagen mRNA production is increased. The cause of decreased NAD^+ can be hypoxia, inhibition of enzymes of the respiratory chain, or accumulation of lactate by rapid or aerobic glycolysis to the extent that it cannot be removed by the still regenerating microcirculation. The same effect is achieved by interfering with the conversion of NAD^+ to pADPR by adding nicotinamide for instance. Conversely, the artefactual increase of the NAD^+ pool by simple addition of NAD^+ inhibits transcription of the collagen gene (Hussain *et al.*, 1988, 1989).

Indications are that the increase in collagen mRNAs is passed on to an increase in the quantity of procollagen peptide. However, these events by themselves are still not sufficient to accelerate extracellular collagen deposition because procollagen peptide cannot be transported from the cell until a certain number of its prolines are hydroxylated. This reaction is performed by a dioxygenase called prolyl hydroxylase which inserts an oxygen atom (to form a hydroxyl group) onto the required number of collagen prolines in the presence of molecular oxygen, ascorbic acid, iron and alphaketoglutarate. The activity of this enzyme normally is suppressed by monomeric, cytoplasmic ADPR. Thus, accumulation of lactate, or any other process which leads to reduction of the NAD^+ pool,

causes: (1) the production of collagen mRNAs; (2) increased collagen peptide formation; and (3) increased post-translational modification with release of collagen into the extracellular space, provided that enough ascorbate and oxygen are present (Hussain *et al.*, 1989).

Another dioxygenase, lysyl hydroxylase (with the same requirements as prolyl hydroxylase), hydroxylates a number of the procollagen lysines, and sets the stage for later intramolecular cross-binding of extracellular collagen molecules which is necessary for development of their characteristic strength. Details of its regulation are not known.

This mechanism appears complex at first appearance. However, the parallelism between lactate stimulation of macrophages with release of angiogenic factors and collagen synthesis is striking and simple. As elegant as this process is, however, it is vulnerable. For instance, ascorbate, as noted, is a necessary cofactor for prolyl- and lysyl-hydroxylase. Ascorbic acid deficiency (scurvy) inhibits collagen deposition because it impairs prolyl and lysyl hydroxylation, and the underhydroxylated collagen can neither be transported from the cell nor hydroxylated. Hypoxia can be considered a subset of scurvy in this sense.

The kinetics of prolyl hydroxylase are such that prolyl hydroxylation reaches its most rapid rate only when P_{O_2} reaches about 200 mmHg (Figure 39.4). As oxygen tension falls from that level, collagen processing falls, reaching half-maximal velocity (K_m) at slightly above 20 mmHg, and zero velocity at zero P_{O_2} (Hutton *et al.*, 1967; Myllyla *et al.*, 1977). Thus, this critical element of extracellular collagen deposition is highly influenced by circulatory factors (Figure 39.5).

The oxygen tension in fluid trapped in human wound dead spaces, especially those on the lower extremity, is often as low as zero to 20 mmHg, even when arterial P_{O_2} is elevated by administration of

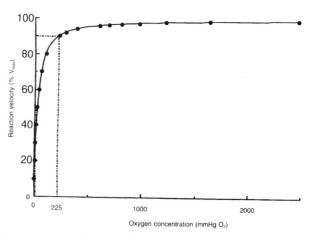

Figure 39.4 The kinetics of the prolyl hydroxylase. $K_m = 25$ mmHg O_2.

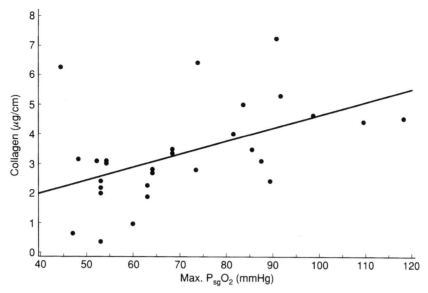

Figure 39.5 Collagen deposition, measured in human subjects on postoperative day 5 using expanded polytetrafluoroethylene tubes implanted subcutaneously in the lateral upper arm during surgery, is proportional to the subcutaneous tissue Po_2 (subject breathing 50% oxygen) on the first 3 days after surgery. Note that the relationship holds even at a Po_2 above 100% saturation of haemoglobin with oxygen. (Reproduced from Jonsson *et al.*, 1991, with permission.)

supplemental oxygen (Hunt *et al.*, 1967, 1978; Douglas *et al.*, 1973; Niinikoski *et al.*, 1973; Knighton *et al.*, 1984). Where there is less tissue damage, in needle wounds for instance, Po_2 is often in the region of 30 or 40 mmHg, and even higher in central and head wounds (Niinikoski *et al.*, 1972; Heppenstall *et al.*, 1974; Chang *et al.*, 1983). All indications are that in normal cases at sea level or above, collagen may never be deposited at the maximum possible rate. More importantly, each successive decrement of Po_2 has a greater effect than the last on collagen deposition. Since collagen is the only source of significant strength in tissue, the entire process of restructuring wounded tissue becomes exceptionally vulnerable to circulatory and respiratory parameters.

On superficial examination, the above seems contradictory. It would seem that lactate concentration, the signal to collagen synthesis, would be greatest in the absence of oxygen and the least in its presence. In fact, although wound extracellular lactate concentration can be increased by hypoxia, systemic hyperoxia does not significantly lower it (Hussain *et al.*, 1988). This is explained by the fact that macrophages and fibroblasts make considerable lactate even in aerobic conditions. Most rapidly replicating cell systems release excess amounts of lactate under the influence of growth factors.

The above considerations have two important consequences. First, they imply that the lactate-mediated stimulus to angiogenesis and collagen synthesis will remain until the inflammation which produces much of the lactate subsides and until the

new microcirculation is sufficiently competent to remove it. Meanwhile, collagen synthesis can be enhanced by raising oxygen tension in the zone of rapid collagen synthesis (Figure 39.2).

The proclivity of wound cells for lactate production is important in patients with burns or other large injuries. Wounds produce so much lactate that some inevitably reaches the general circulation. The quantity of lactate returned to the liver can be quite large. The liver must then convert lactate back to glucose which it exports back to the wound. This cycle is energetically inefficient, and is part of the cause of the hypermetabolism which accompanies serious injuries (Wilmore *et al.*, 1977; Wilmore, 1990, 1991; Wolfe *et al.*, 1991).

COLLAGEN MATURATION, REMODELLING AND CONTRACTION

Fibroblasts in healing wounds lie in a series of provisional extracellular matrices. At first, the matrix is largely fibrin and fibronectin which is deposited during coagulation. Fibroblasts and inflammatory cells degrade this and replace it with a hastily secreted mixture of collagen and proteoglycans. Later this will be replaced by collagen deposited in a more mature and stronger pattern.

Fibre formation, together with the more slowly developing intramolecular cross-linking that gives mature collagen its strength, occurs as a result of the actions of several extracellular enzymes, at least one of which is Po_2 dependent. Collagen leaves fibroblasts in a monomeric form with terminal extension peptides in place that must be cleaved away before the nuclear monomer can be polymerized into mature fibrils. In the absence of the enzymes which do this, collagen gains no strength. When the monomers are put in place, cross-linking and strengthening occurs by a variety of means, one of the most important being condensation of adjacent lysines by lysyl oxidase. This is also an oxygen-consuming step.

At first, collagen fibres are rapidly formed in a disorderly, brittle and weak pattern of small fibres. Collagenases secreted by fibroblasts and leucocytes slowly degrade this provisional matrix and fibroblasts replace it with a mature matrix which more closely resembles normal collagenous structure. During this time, wounds lose mass and gain strength. This process is called 'remodelling'. Proteoglycans appear to create an environment for orderly polymerization.

Even after minor wounds, collagen turnover can be detected chemically as long as 18 months. During this time, due to the provisional nature of the new extracellular matrix, wounds are vulnerable to contraction, stretching and weakening. 'Contraction' is a component of closure of open wounds in which normal tissue is drawn into the space previously occupied by the wound. Fibroblasts provide the motive force. Fibroblasts are mobile cells, and on vital microscopy can be seen to ruffle their membranes as they move, shortening them by segments. Receptors in their membranes attach to collagen fibres and gradually pull the collagen fibres together. The fibres then cross-link in the shortened dimensions. Both open and closed wounds tend to contract if not subjected to a superior distorting force. This phenomenon is best seen in surface wounds which in areas of loose skin, often close by 90% or more by contraction alone (Figure 39.6). The result of a large wound on the back of the neck may be a very small area of re-epithelialization surrounded by normal skin which has 'contracted' centripetally as if by an invisible purse-string. The major force of contraction is exerted in the periphery of the wound. Excision of the wound contents exclusive of the periphery does not impair it.

Contraction is usually a beneficial process to be relied upon for healing of open wounds on the back, the buttock or the neck, whereas around the eye and about the mobile joints, its results are often disabling and disfiguring and are called contractures. Skin grafts, especially thick ones, impede but do not totally stop contraction. Dynamic splints, passive or active stretching, or insertion of flaps containing dermis and subdermis are often necessary to correct contractures. The force can be extremely strong, though severely contractured joints can usually be straightened out with traction, even after months of healing. It seems self-evident that the force of contraction in fibroblasts has limits

and cannot overcome a determined effort to lengthen the scar. If, however, wounds are traumatized when they are stretched, contraction may continue for long periods and may become troublesome.

The plasticity of scar also has its drawbacks. Wounds also stretch when tension is great enough to overcome contraction. This may account for the laxity of scars in some ligaments and the tendency for hernia formation in abdominal wounds of obese patients – all examples of continuous, mild and repeated stretching.

The result of adult healing is a scar, but it contains some features of regeneration. Wounds in fetal skin during the first two trimesters of fetal life are significantly different. They repair in the collagenous pattern of normal growth (Longaker and Adzick, 1991). The mechanism of this 'scarless' healing, still obscure, is becoming a kind of holy grail for those who study wound mechanisms.

SYSTEMIC CONSEQUENCES OF INJURY AND HYPOXIA

The systemic consequences of injury are well known although the mechanisms are not clear. Normally, cytokines released by wounded and inflamed tissues probably serve a useful purpose by assembling reparative cells and preparing local cells to resist infection. As the extent of injury increases, cytokines reach the systemic circulation and divert the liver, for instance, to synthesize and release acute-phase proteins. As injury increases still further, however, more leucocytes and macrophages are recruited and more denatured, hypoxic tissue and fibrin activate them to release cytokines to the extent that they may become harmful. IL-1 is found in large quantities early in even clean wounds, and it undoubtedly leaks into the circulation, probably accompanied by TNF (Ford et al., 1989; Kaplan et al., 1989; Fahey et al., 1990; Marano et al., 1990). This probably explains why fever, for instance, is often an early feature of pancreatitis, some burns, and large operations. In many cases of severe trauma, fever, acute-phase protein responses, and even multiorgan failure occur in the absence of any objective proof of infection. Certainly, when infection becomes established in wounds, fever and other signs of cytokine release develop in proportion to the number of reticuloendothelial cells which are recruited and to the degree to which they are stimulated. For instance, burns recruit them in proportion to the area of burn and thereafter the denatured burned tissue continues to stimulate them. This concept underscores the importance of debridement of damaged tissue and rapid immobilization of fractures (Border and Bone, 1988). The consequence of failure to debride major amounts of

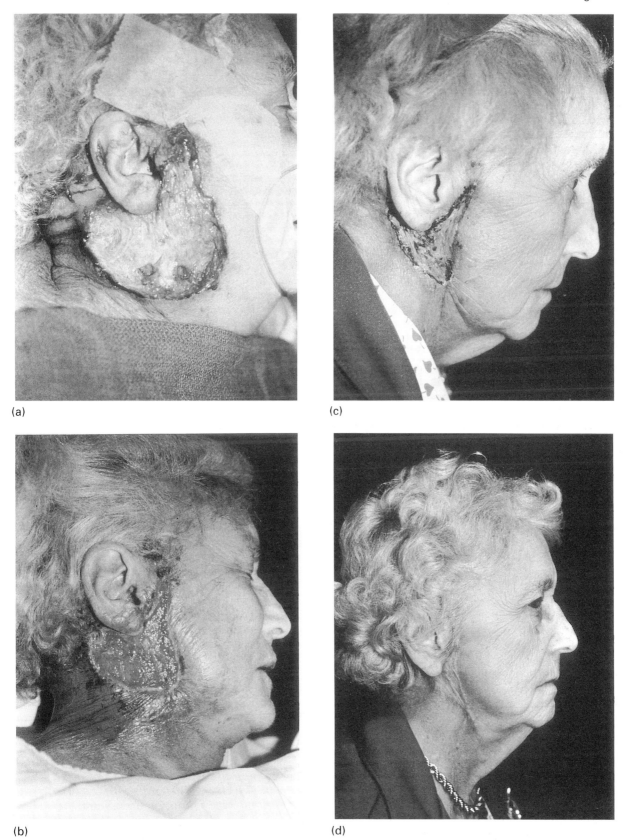

(a)

(c)

(b)

(d)

Figure 39.6   (a) Large cheek wound due to tissue slough caused by extravasated calcium solution. (b) Wound contraction. (c) Wound covered with split-thickness skin graft and still shrinking. (d) Fully contracted wound. (Reproduced from Rudolph *et al.*, 1992, with permission.)

injured tissue can be days of excess fever, susceptibility to infection, and even the full syndrome of the so-called SIRS (or systemic inflammatory response syndrome) including multiple organ failure even in the absence of complicating infection. Catabolic metabolic responses then follow and malnutrition becomes a problem (Brown *et al.*, 1989a). Necrotic tissue is easily infected, and superimposition of infection on injury potentiates the inflammatory response.

HEALING IS VULNERABLE TO DISORDERS OF INFLAMMATION

Growth signals and lytic enzymes released by inflammatory cells are necessary for repair, yet excessive release is detrimental. If inflammation is prevented, repair suffers. Failure to heal is a common problem in patients taking anti-inflammatory steroids, other immune suppressants or cancer chemotherapy. Open wounds suffer more than primarily healing ones. Introduction of these agents after inflammation is established is less detrimental, though second-intention healing will decelerate. Vitamin A potentiates the normal inflammatory response (Ehrlich and Hunt, 1968, 1969). Healing impaired by steroids can be accelerated by vitamin A given systemically or locally. Many growth factors also can mitigate steroid-related healing, but at this moment none are cleared for therapeutic use (Amento and Beck, 1991; Mueller *et al.*, 1991).

The destructive aspects of inflammation are not always appropriate to the needs of repair. Excessive inflammatory responses are troublesome locally as well as systemically, because growth factors and cytokines have a diphasic action. High concentrations induce excessive release of proteolytic enzymes from macrophages and fibroblasts which lyse both new and old collagen to the detriment of wound strength. This kind of process may even impair 'normal' healing in some tissues. For instance, administration of inhibitors of inflammatory proteolytic enzymes enhances the development of strength of intestinal anastomoses in normal animals, presumably by inhibiting 'normal' lysis (Jonsson and Jiborn, 1987).

More vigorous proteolytic responses literally digest normal tissues. This accounts for the digestion of skin in pyoderma gangrenosum, a disastrous ulcerative (but not infectious) condition which sometimes accompanies ulcerative colitis and other immunological disorders. Every experienced surgeon has seen peri-wound tissue literally melt away in response to local infections. Past logic has placed the onus on the bacteria. These newer concepts challenge that interpretation and assign more blame to cytokine release. Interestingly, anti-inflammatory steroids accelerate healing of pyoderma gangrenosum (Prystowsky *et al.*, 1991)!

Prolonged, mild stimulation of inflammatory cells might also prolong repair by continuing growth factor and lactate release past the point of usefulness. Though no proof of this hypothesis currently exists, the recently appreciated power of the inflammatory response clearly indicates its plausibility. Such a mechanism could account totally for hypertrophic scarring. It might also contribute to keloid formation, but one would expect that other, particularly genetic, factors would also contribute. To establish such a hypothesis would require identification of a stimulant. Unfortunately, there are probably many.

CAN WOUNDS BE 'MANAGED'?

Healing, in contrast to the traditional view, is a malleable process. It can be modified in a number of ways and is vulnerable to a large number of often subtle influences. Surgeons have learned to accept a standard of adequate healing less than that which may realistically be reached. Many possibilities for improvement already exist. Proteolytic enzymes may enhance development of tensile strength in intestinal wounds. Vitamin A can overcome steroid suppression. Steroids, colchicine, alpha interferon and others can theoretically retard excessive collagen deposition. Diphenylhydantoin can impair excessive collagenase activity. Few of these have been exploited.

Everyone agrees that healing can be supported and protected. Deliberate manipulation is now the goal. This is a new area which undoubtedly will grow. The question of manipulation currently revolves around growth factors which, in animals, can accelerate even normal collagen deposition and epithelization. Epidermal growth factor (EGF) (Buckley *et al.*, 1987; Brown *et al.*, 1988, 1989b, 1991), PDGF (Grotendorst *et al.*, 1985; Pierce *et al.*, 1988, 1989), TGF-β (Sporn *et al.*, 1983; Mustoe *et al.*, 1987; Quaglino *et al.*, 1990; Amento *et al.*, 1991) and IGF-I (Mueller *et al.*, 1986; Spencer, 1988; Steenfos *et al.*, 1989) have been tested. The effects are greater in retarded wounds. The impression is that wounds in highly vascular areas appear to approach the maximum possible biological rate, although even this is not proved.

One interesting contemporary question is whether systemically given growth factors may enhance wound healing in seriously injured patients. The first few indications are that growth hormone (GH) and, therefore, IGF-I will be beneficial in seriously injured and burned patients whose levels of IGF-I and GH are characteristically depressed (Eichler *et al.*, 1988; Belcher *et al.*, 1989; Christensen *et al.*, 1990; Herndon *et al.*, 1990; Strock *et al.*, 1990; Zaizen *et al.*, 1990; Gottardis *et al.*, 1991; Nielsen *et al.*, 1991).

NUTRITION

Surgery and trauma induce a catabolic state, with elevated glucagon, glucocorticoid and catecholamine levels, and decreased insulin levels. This hypermetabolism increases oxygen consumption (Wolfe *et al.*, 1991). The increase in basal energy expenditure is proportional to the severity of injury, ranging from 20–30% with isolated long bone fractures, to 50–80% with multiple trauma and sepsis, and 100–150% with extensive thermal injury (Jensen *et al.*, 1982). Maximal nutritional support cannot restore an anabolic state until the levels of stress hormones return toward normal (Muller *et al.*, 1986). Clearly, nutritional maintenance and repletion is critical; however, specific nutritional therapy remains controversial.

Vitamin and mineral requirements

Vitamin C (ascorbic acid) is required for the hydroxylation of proline and lysine during post-translational modification of collagen (Barnes and Kodicek, 1972). Requirements increase after injury, from 20–30 mg/day to 100–2000 mg/day, depending on the severity of injury (Goodson and Hunt, 1988; Orgill and Demling, 1988). Deficiency (scurvy) profoundly impairs healing.

Deficiencies of the B vitamins have been shown to impair wound strength, antibody production and bacterial killing (Levenson *et al.*, 1977). Vitamin A deficiency impairs epithelialization (Weber, 1983), collagen synthesis (Ehrlich, 1971) and cross-linking (Mohanram *et al.*, 1976), and wound contraction (Levenson *et al.*, 1977). Routine supplementation is recommended for surgical and trauma patients.

Magnesium is a cofactor for many enzymes involved in protein synthesis (Wacker and Parisi, 1968), and thus is essential for healing. Zinc is a cofactor for RNA (Scrutton *et al.*, 1971) and DNA (Slater *et al.*, 1971) polymerase and many other enzymes (Riordan and Vallee, 1976). Steroid therapy and trauma deplete serum zinc levels. Zinc levels below 100 μg/dl impair wound healing and immune function (Goodson and Hunt, 1988). Deficiency is uncommon in the absence of alcoholism, malabsorption or recent starvation (Levenson *et al.*, 1977).

Copper is a cofactor for many enzymes, including lysyl oxidase (Goodson and Hunt, 1988). Manganese is a cofactor for superoxide dismutase (McCord, 1976). Deficiency of these trace minerals is uncommon, except with long-term, unsupplemented parenteral nutrition. Molybdenum, cobalt, chromium, selenium, vanadium and tin are all essential at very low levels. Little is known about their roles in healing (Levenson *et al.*, 1977). Iron (Fe^{2+}) is required for hydroxylation of proline and lysine. Deficiency is common in trauma and surgery patients, and should be corrected, although it has been shown to impair healing only in children (Levenson *et al.*, 1977).

Nutrition as a practical matter

Up to 50% of elective surgery patients suffer from chronic protein-calorie malnutrition (Bistrian *et al.*, 1974; Jenson *et al.*, 1982; Warnold and Lundholm, 1984; Streat and Hill, 1987). Protein-calorie malnutrition frequently develops in trauma patients as a result of increased metabolism combined with decreased caloric intake. Poor diet immediately prior to injury seems to affect repair more than chronic defects. There is disagreement on the best way to evaluate nutritional status. At present, the most accurate, yet easily measured markers include serum albumin (< 3 mg/dl) and total lymphocyte count (< 1500) (Freed *et al.*, 1982; Jensen *et al.*, 1982; Dickhaut *et al.*, 1984; Pettigrew *et al.*, 1986). Weight loss (> 10%) is predictive only when associated with clear physical impairment (Dionigi *et al.*, 1977; Windsor and Hill, 1988).

Nutritional support improves measures of wound healing in animals and man (Haydock and Hill, 1987). Both parenteral and enteral supplementation may cause complications, however, so the decision to implement perioperative nutritional support requires weighing the benefits (improved wound healing and resistance to infection) against the risks. This requires outcome studies on the effect of different nutritional regimens. There is growing evidence that in certain well-defined populations, particularly recently starved patients, preoperative nutritional repletion may reduce surgical complications.

In patients with *severe* protein-calorie malnutrition there is good evidence that preoperative nutritional repletion for 1–2 weeks is beneficial (Williams *et al.*, 1976; Muller *et al.*, 1980; Muller *et al.*, 1986; Buzby, 1990). These patients suffered a slightly higher rate of infectious complications (catheter sepsis, UTI, pneumonia), which was more than offset by the decrease in wound complications. In patients with only mild to moderate malnutrition, delay of surgery is not indicated, as a small decrease in wound complications is overwhelmed by a large increase in infectious complications of the technique itself (Buzby, 1990).

Postoperative nutritional support may be indicated. Enteral nutrition, if feasible, is clearly superior to parenteral, as the enteral route helps maintain gut integrity and may decrease bacterial translocation (Moore *et al.*, 1989). Immediate postoperative use of enteral feeding is often feasible, and routine use is advocated by some (Moore and James, 1986; Schroeder *et al.*, 1991).

Nutritional support with vitamins and minerals is clearly indicated in trauma patients who are not expected to be able to take adequate oral nutrition for 3–4 days.

Other low-risk, specific nutritional interventions are currently receiving attention and may prove valuable. Arginine, for example, shows promise as a routine supplement. Arginine-deficient rats show impaired wound strength and collagen deposition (Seifter *et al.*, 1978), while arginine supplementation improves these variables even in the absence of arginine deficiency (Barbul *et al.*, 1985). Oral arginine improved collagen deposition in PTFE tubes implanted subcutaneously in non-operated volunteers. Lymphocyte function was also improved in these subjects (Barbul *et al.*, 1981, 1990). The beneficial effects of arginine are likely to be multifactorial (Barbul *et al.*, 1983).

Some controversy about the value of total patenteral nutrition (TPN) has arisen in studies of preoperative nutrition for cancer patients in which little clinical value for preoperative TPN has been found. This may result from specific effects of cancer itself. At the moment, these studies should be interpreted as being specific to cancer patients.

RESISTANCE TO INFECTION

Well-made, well-tended wounds in vascularized tissues are amazingly resistant to infection. Wounds made in ischaemic tissue are notoriously susceptible. Wounds made in the feet and hands of even normal individuals often become infected. Those made in the face, tongue, heart and anus rarely are. Superficial anal wounds rarely host invasive infections despite massive contamination. The heart, face and anus do not have a superior immune system, but they do have greater blood perfusion. The assumption once grew that circulation becomes adequate or inadequate at some critical point, but we now know that any interference with circulation or oxygen delivery to any degree will increase susceptibility to infection. The converse is also true, and this surprises many surgeons. Increasing the circulation and oxygenation of injured tissue even to supranormal levels enhances resistance to infection.

Immunity is generally conceived to consist of two major but not quite distinct systems, a non-specific component which depends upon phagocytosis and intracellular killing and is not influenced by prior exposure to the infecting agent, and a specific system, often called 'cellular immunity', which depends on prior exposure and antibody formation.

Tissue trauma and shock impair cellular immunity (Howard and Simmons, 1974). However, it is difficult to determine the clinical significance of this observation, since there are few studies which examine clinical infection as an outcome. One must interpret the evidence with a broad perspective. Defects of cellular immunity lead to infections with opportunistic fungi, bacteria and viruses, but not those due to staphylococcus, bacteriodes or clostridia, for instance (Meakins, 1988). Moreover, opportunistic infections arise more often as a result of immune suppression by major burns and prior infection. They more often involve major organs, and are widespread rather than focused in injured tissue. They occur late after injury.

Natural or non-specific immunity is the critical portion of host defences at the time and place of acute injury (Knighton and Hunt, 1988). It is the principal means by which wounds defend against *Staphylococcus aureus*, for example, and it is modulated by changes in leucocyte number, mobility, ability to adhere to organisms, and ingest and kill them (Hohn *et al.*, 1977). Migration and adherence are facilitated by activation of complement. Margination, migration, opsonization and phagocytosis can be accomplished in astonishingly deprived environments on energy derived solely from glycolysis (Knighton and Hunt, 1988). The major hazards to this part of non-specific defence are the use of anti-inflammatory steroids (Claman, 1972), poor leucocyte number or mobility (Klebanoff and Clark, 1978; Boxer *et al.*, 1983) and regional blood supply poor enough to impair phagocytic functions (Moelleken *et al.*, 1991) or to limit leucocyte access (Baker *et al.*, 1982). The hazards of corticosteroid therapy can be lessened by diminishing dose, substituting the less anti-inflammatory cortisone for drugs such as prednisolone, and using vitamin A to restimulate inflammation (Ehrlich and Hunt, 1968, 1969).

Disorders of leucotaxis are a common though ill-defined consequence of major trauma, significant malnutrition and pre-existing infection. Attempts to enhance leucocyte mobility directly have resisted intensive research, but draining or otherwise effectively treating pre-existing infection and repairing nutritional deficits are usually rewarded by improvement. Leucocyte mobility can be measured in the patient by response to skin test antigens. This is ordinarily regarded as a test of cellular immunity, but in the end it depends on leucocytes migrating to the area of immune reaction. These tests are not specific enough for screening, but they have value in the individual patient who is not healing or resisting infection appropriately. Leucotaxis can also be measured in Boyden chambers or agarose-well cultures (Boyden, 1962; Nelson *et al.*, 1975). Immobility measured in the laboratory correlates to failure to respond to skin test antigens; that is 'anergy'. This in turn has been related on a statistical basis to increased susceptibility to infection (Hohn, 1988; Anderson *et al.*, 1989) on the one hand and decrement of body cell mass due to malnutrition (Law *et al.*, 1974; Christou, 1990) on the other.

Natural and specific immune mechanisms overlap at the level of opsonization. Leucocytes recognize and ingest organisms opsonized by specific antibodies or by non-specific means such as fibronectin. Evidence conflicts as to whether opsonic activity is normally deficient in the wound environment. Opsonization (and thus phagocytosis and killing) of some bacteria may be impaired, particularly in wounds with a large dead-space, or a seroma (Peterson *et al.*, 1977). Opsonophagocytosis of *Staphylococcus aureus, Pseudomonas aeruginosa* and *Escherichia coli* is impaired in neutrophils and monocytes incubated in wound fluid (mastectomy wounds) compared with normal serum (Bridges *et al.*, 1987). Fibronectin and complement (C3b) are decreased in this seroma fluid. Blister fluid from burn patients did not support opsonophagocytosis of *P. aeruginosa*, although in these experiments, killing of *S. aureus* was not impaired (Deitch, 1983; Deitch *et al.*, 1987). Fibronectin is concentrated in non-dead-space incisional wounds to levels higher than that of plasma (Clark, 1988; Martin *et al.*, 1988). It is not clear that these data apply to all wounds.

Disorders of phagocytosis are rarely a problem. Requisite energy can be derived from anaerobic metabolism, but even anaerobic energy sources are limited in some patients, for example, poorly controlled insulinopenic diabetics (Knighton and Hunt, 1988).

Regional blood supply problems can be attacked through debridement of devascularized and infectable tissue; or, when feasible, vascular surgery by repairing injured vessels, transplanting a vascular system with myocutaneous flaps or omentum, and by assuring maximum possible perfusion of the vulnerable tissue.

Intracellular killing appears to be the most vulnerable link in non-specific immunity, and this is because an important component of it is Po_2 dependent. Once leucocytes have internalized bacteria, they must kill them. Killing mechanisms are generally divided into two categories, oxygen dependent and oxygen independent. The oxygen-independent system operates through antibacterial enzymes poured onto ingested bacteria as cytoplasmic granules fuse with phagosomes. Lysosyme, cationic protein, myeloperoxidase and other enzymes participate. These enzymes are prepackaged in the cell, and if the cell ingests an organism, the mechanism proceeds as programmed (McRipley *et al.*, 1967; Hohn, 1988). Specific genetic disorders are known but rare (Wolff *et al.*, 1972; Babior, 1988; Ganz *et al.*, 1988). This enzymatic mechanism kills many types of organisms which arrive in wounds. However, it is insufficient by itself to kill most wound pathogens efficiently.

The second mechanism, oxygen-dependent killing (Figure 39.7), requires consumption and reduction of atmospheric oxygen. It is set in motion by phagocytosis which stimulates a 10- to 25-fold increase in oxygen consumption by leucocytes. Some of the oxygen is used for energy and the rest is converted first into superoxide (O_2^-) and peroxide (H_2O_2), and thence to a variety of high-energy free radicals, including active aldehydes, hydroxyl radical, singlet oxygen, hypohalites and others, which exert their lethal effects on bacterial membranes. A mixture of hydrogen peroxide, myeloperoxidase (an enzyme found in large quantities in the azurophilic granules of white cells) and a small amount of chloride or iodide is lethal to many organisms (Selvaraj *et al.*, 1966; McRipley and Sbarra, 1967; Hohn *et al.*, 1976; Babior, 1978; Klebanoff, 1980).

This oxidative mechanism fails in anoxic conditions. Figure 39.8 shows the effect of varying oxygen atmospheres on the killing of staphylo-

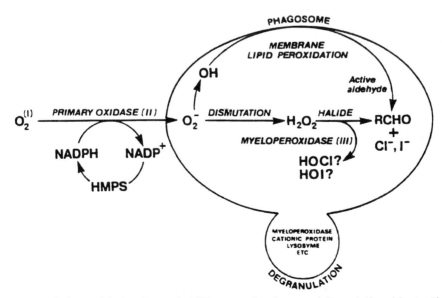

Figure 39.7 Schema of the oxidative bacteria-killing mechanism and its relationship to the non-oxidative mechanism. (Reproduced from Hunt, 1975, with permission.)

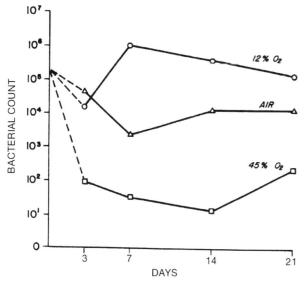

Figure 39.8 Mean bacteria counts in wound fluid obtained from stainless steel mesh cylinders implanted subcutaneously in rabbits and inoculated with 10^6 bacteria. (Reproduced from Hunt, 1979a, with permission.)

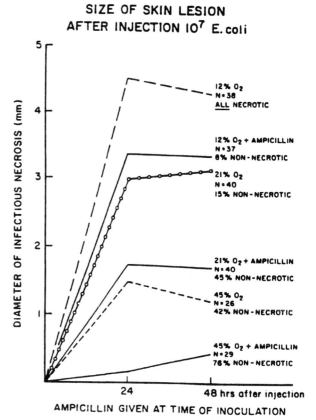

Figure 39.9 Effect of ambient FiO^2 and/or antibiotic on lesion diameter after intradermal injection of bacteria into guinea-pigs. (Reproduced from Hunt *et al.*, 1988, with permission.)

coccus in dead-space wounds in animals. The effect is also shown by injecting live bacteria into the skin of animals and measuring the subsequent indurated or necrotic area (Figure 39.9). The average lesion size is far smaller in animals breathing 50% oxygen than those kept at 12% oxygen, and many injection sites show no evidence of infection at all (75%), as opposed to hypoxic animals (15%). The change from 12% oxygen to air produces an effect comparable to specific antibiotics, except that the period of time in which oxygen can be used efficaciously (the 'critical period') is greater than the few hours to which antibiotics are limited. The antibacterial effects of hyperoxia and antibiotics are independent and additive (Knighton *et al.*, 1984).

The oxygen effect is best understood in the framework of the rare, inherited defect called chronic granulomatous disease (CGD). Without antibiotics, children with this disorder die of infection in their first few years. The defect is the absence of the primary oxygenase which reduces dissolved oxygen to superoxide (Woeff *et al.*, 1972; Babior, 1988; Ganz *et al.*, 1988). By definition, the absence of the substrate, oxygen, is equivalent to the absence of the oxygen-reducing enzyme. Therefore, when white cells fall into hypoxic wounds they 'acquire' a degree of CGD.

The rate of superoxide production depends on oxygen tension, and bacterial killing seems to decrease sharply as oxygen tension falls below about 30 mmHg. Normal granulocytes become equivalent to CGD granulocytes at zero Po_2 (Wolff

et al., 1972; Babior, 1988; Ganz *et al.*, 1988). Oxygen tensions in the 20–50 mmHg range are often found in human wounds. Significant trauma at a distance from the wound lowers the wound Po_2 and increases susceptibility to infection (Zederfeldt and Hunt, 1969; Heppenstall *et al.*, 1974), as does local injection of catecholamines (Magee *et al.*, 1977; Jensen *et al.*, 1985), increasing viscosity of blood with high-molecular-weight dextran (Heughan *et al.*, 1972), arterial hypoxia (Jonsson *et al.*, 1986, 1988; Gottrup *et al.*, 1987) and hypovolaemia (Kwan and Hunt, 1973; Maxwell *et al.*, 1973; Gottrup *et al.*, 1987; Gosain *et al.*, 1991).

The significance of blood and oxygen supply to infectability is illustrated by a series of experiments on skin flaps in dogs. Two skin flaps were elevated simultaneously. One was myocutaneous (with excellent blood flow and tissue oxygenation throughout its length) and the other random pattern (with progressively poorer perfusion and oxygenation from base to tip). Bacteria introduced into the flaps survive, multiply and cause visible lesions, whose size and depth are in inverse relation to both blood flow and tissue oxygen tension as measured locally in the flaps and in normal skin. The myocutaneous flap is perfused as well as normal skin and resists infection just as well. On the other hand, infection literally destroys the distal portion of random pattern flaps where tissue P_{O_2} falls to about 15 mmHg. Infectious necrosis in all sites is significantly lessened by breathing 50% oxygen, and is increased by breathing 12% oxygen. In these experiments, an average of about 60% of the random pattern flaps became necrotic during arterial hypoxia, while less than 30% died in animals breathing hyperoxic mixtures. The only explanation is that immune function increased in proportion to P_{O_2} (Niinikoski *et al.*, 1972; Gottrup *et al.*, 1984).

WOUND PHYSIOLOGY AND OXYGEN: THE POWER OF PERFUSION

In energy metabolism, oxygen is used mainly at the terminal end of the respiratory chain on the mitochondrial membrane, specifically by cytochrome oxidase for the reaction $4H^+ + O_2 \rightarrow 2H_2O$. The affinity of cytochrome oxidase for oxygen is so great that its rate is slowed only when oxygen tension in the environment of the cell falls below about 10 mmHg and mitochondrial P_{O_2} falls to below 1 mmHg (Denison, 1989). Many oxygenases (enzymes which use molecular oxygen as a substrate) have considerably lesser affinity, among them, prolyl and lysyl hydroxylases as noted above (Prockup *et al.*, 1962; Hutton *et al.*, 1967; Chvapil *et al.*, 1968; Hunt and Pai, 1972; Uitto and Prockup, 1974; Myllyla *et al.*, 1977; Pietila *et al.*, 1984), and the NADPH-linked oxygenase of leucocytes which produces superoxide (Babior, 1978). There are many more examples. This inability of important reparative processes to capture vital oxygen would disastrously limit life were it not for the fact that perfusion of vital tissues can be increased enough to maintain P_{O_2} at a high level despite increased consumption. Fortunately, healing wounds consume relatively little oxygen (Evans and Naylor, 1966). Since they require it to be delivered, however, at a high P_{O_2}, the rate at which blood perfuses the healing tissue becomes extremely important to healing and resistance to infection.

Under ambient conditions at sea level, only increased perfusion can raise wound-tissue P_{O_2} to the levels necessary for hydroxylating proline in collagen and producing superoxide. If perfusion can be maintained at a high level, the oxygen needs of healing can be met at haematocrits as low as 15% (Zederfeldt, 1957; Nasution and Taylor, 1981; Jensen *et al.*, 1986a; Jonsson *et al.*, 1991). Compensation to this degree requires a patient to raise cardiac output by several fold. The regional vasculature must, of course, be able to support increased flow. *Flow must be increased.* Adding oxygen to the breathing mix-

ture further enhances repair and resistance to infection.

In practice, maintaining flow is not simply replacing blood and fluid losses. Injury frequently occurs also in the setting of hypothermia, pain and fear, all of which stimulate microvascular constriction via the sympathetic nervous system. It is important to correct these, particularly hypothermia which contracts vascular capacity. When the patient rewarms, vascular capacitance expands and more fluid is required to fill it. New pain-control techniques seem also to provide an advantage in perfusion, although this has not yet been proved.

PERFUSION OF WOUNDS AS A PRACTICAL MATTER

Tissue perfusion and *tissue* oxygenation are poorly established concepts in patient care. Few surgeons have ever measured them. The idea of blood moving rapidly and in good volume through tissue is intuitively easy and attractive, but assessing it quantitatively is not a skill taught in medical school or surgical residency.

Practising surgeons, anaesthesiologists, internists and intensivists alike equate perfusion with pulse, blood pressure, urine output, skin color and skin temperature. Of these, urine output is normally thought to be the best index of perfusion. Numerous experiments have shown that when resuscitation fluids are given to the point at which blood pressure and urine output are normalized, perfusion of the 'peripheral' connective tissues remains well below normal, thus leaving repair and resistance to infection unprotected (Jensen *et al.*, 1987; Jonsson *et al.*, 1987a, 1988; Gosain *et al.*, 1991). Though this conflicts with surgical dogma, it is predictable in a physiological sense for the following reason: one action of the sympathetic nervous system is to direct perfusion away from connective tissues, which are normally 'dispensable' during 'stress' in order to direct it toward the kidneys, liver, brain and heart, which are temporarily far more important (Mellander *et al.*, 1960). In other words, perfusion of connective tissue and bone where wounds must heal is sacrificed to maintain perfusion of other organs. The kidneys, therefore, maintain urine output even after wounded skin and fascia have lost perfusion. How common is this? The only answer available now is that about one-third to one-half of the patients undergoing elective abdominal surgery in the authors' institution reach the ward with measurably poor tissue perfusion until more fluid was given than originally planned by the surgical team, and until the patient was warm and relatively free of pain.

One can estimate perfusion by a systematic clinical examination (Jonsson *et al.*, 1987a). Clearly, this examination gives a better assessment than urine output alone. The steps in it are:

1. Capillary return in the skin between and just above the eyes should be less than 1.5 seconds (count 'one thousand one...').
2. Eye turgor should equal the examiner's.
3. Mucous membranes should be moist and the patient should not be thirsty. Many patients can distinguish between true thirst, which is a sign of hypovolaemia, and dry mouth, which is not.
4. The skin should be normally moist. Patients in shock often perspire excessively. Dehydrated patients feel dry.
5. Skin temperature over the patellae should be equal to or barely less then the thighs and calves. Capillary return there should be less than 5 seconds. Measurements in blood banks have shown that lowered skin temperature in the legs is the first noticeable sign of mild volume deficit.
6. Pulse or blood pressure should change only momentarily on standing from a lying position. Compensation due to postural change should be complete within seconds unless the patient is heavily narcotized.

If all these tests are satisfied and urine output is over about 1 ml/kg/h, wound perfusion will be fairly close to satisfactory, and extra oxygen breathed may reach and have its effect on the wound. This last point has been determined by actual measurement (Jonsson et al., 1987a).

Unfortunately, clinical assessment is inferior to actual measurement. Several methods to measure peripheral perfusion have been used in patients: mucosal pH in the stomach (Fiddian-Green and Baker, 1987), laser Doppler (Holloway and Watkins, 1977), transcutaneous P_{O_2} (Podolsky et al., 1982), subcutaneous oxygen tension (Jonsson et al., 1991), conjunctival oxygen tension (Smith and Abraham, 1986), and postcapillary venous pressure and oxygenation (Sheldon et al., 1983). There is little doubt that one or more of these techniques will eventually contribute to intensive care of trauma victims. At the moment, subcutaneous oximetry by an optode technique is the most available.

In the subcutaneous technique, an oxygen-sensitive optode system is placed under the skin of the upper arm – a small wound. Normal values in air-breathing volunteers are about 60–80 mmHg, and approximately double with the administration of about 50% oxygen. In postoperative patients, the baseline value is less (35–60 mmHg), and the response to supplemental oxygen is also diminished. A rise of 20% on breathing oxygen indicates adequate perfusion (Hopf et al., 1988; Jonsson et al., 1987a, 1991; Jensen et al., 1991). The best definition of wound hypoperfusion available today is failure of subcutaneous oxygen tension to rise in response to a significant increment in arterial oxygen tension.

In practice, one rarely needs to measure these values simultaneously more than once or twice in order to solve patient problems. If there is doubt, a rapid infusion of 250–500 ml of saline can be given. It will raise P_{O_2}, at least temporarily, in hypovolaemic patients (Jonsson et al., 1987a).

Clinical assessment of perfusion is usually over-optimistic. The tissue P_{O_2} of many of our patients who have been assessed clinically as being normally perfused immediately after major operations has been improved with the infusion of small amounts of electrolyte solutions and correction of mild hypothermia. Commonly, even patients given huge amounts of necessary fluid may malperfuse because therapy still lags behind losses by only a few hundred millilitres. Patients with compromised cardiac function may respond to infusion of saline with a decrement of tissue oxygenation. This indicates overload, and the infusion should be stopped. The ideal is not to give the right total volume of fluid over a long period, but instead to give it at the right rate early after injury. It is entirely possible to give a great deal of fluid so late that wounds and fractures remain underperfused for days during the critically vulnerable period, and the patient becomes overloaded when third space losses are mobilized.

PRACTICAL DECISIONS IN WOUND CARE OF TRAUMA PATIENTS

One of the elements of judgement is to be able to assess risk. The surgeon who can assess the risk of poor healing and/or infection is one step ahead because there are effective precautions to be taken. Antibiotics can be given, ideally within 2 hours of incision (Polk and Malangoni, 1988). Cultures and smears can be taken. Debridement can be aggressive. Body cavities can be closed with mass suture techniques to prevent dehisence. Colostomies and other diverting procedures can be undertaken. Delayed primary closures can be used. In the latter technique, the vulnerable subcutaneous tissue wound is left open and closed no earlier than the fifth postinjury day if inspection of the wound reveals no sign of necrotic tissue or infection.

A useful guide for risk assessment in elective surgery has been constructed by the Center for Disease Control (Haley et al., 1985). Using logistic regression, it was found that four major factors contributed about equally to the risk of wound infection after elective surgery, and from them a risk score can be calculated. A patient receives one point for each of the following: abdominal site of operation, surgery lasting 2 or more hours, contaminated or dirty wound (III or IV by the standard wound classification system), and three or more discharge diagnoses (excluding wound infection). For a total score of zero, the infection risk is no greater than 1%. The risks for scores of 1, 2, 3 and 4 are 4%, 9%, 17% and 27%, respectively. This system is less adequate for clinical decision making in trauma surgery. However, the score correlates with subcutaneous P_{O_2} and together the two illustrate the basic principles of wound management in trauma: prompt and complete debridement, protection from contamination, circulatory support and management of underlying health problems.

ACKNOWLEDGEMENTS

Supported by NIH Grant no. GM27345.

REFERENCES

Aaronson S.A., Rubin J.S., Finch P.W. et al. (1990). Growth factor-regulated pathways in epithelial cell proliferation. *Am. Rev. Resp. Dis.*, **142**(6 pt 2), S7–10.

Amento E.P., Beck L.S. (1991). TGF-beta and wound healing. *Ciba Found. Symp.*, **157**, 115–23, discussion 123–9.

Anderson D., Smith C., Springer T. (1989). Leukocyte adhesion deficiency and other disorders of leukocyte motility. In *The Metabolic Basis of Inherited Disease II*, 6 ed. (Scriver C., Beaudet A., Sly W., Valle D., eds). New York: McGraw-Hill, pp. 2751–77.

Anderson T.L., Gorstein F., Osteen K.G. (1990). Stromal-epithelial cell communication, growth factors, and tissue regulation. *Lab. Invest.*, **62**, 519–21.

Assoian R., Komoriya A., Myers C. (1983). Transforming growth factor-beta in human platelets. *J. Biol. Chem.*, **258**, 7155–60.

Babior B. (1978). Oxygen-dependent microbial killing by phagocytes. *New Engl. J. Med.*, **298**, 659–68.

Babior B. (1988). Disorders of neutrophil function. In *Cecil Textbook of Medicine*; 18 ed. (Wyngaarden J., Smith L., ed.). Philadelphia: W.B. Saunders, pp. 957–61.

Baird A., Walicke P.A. (1989). Fibroblast growth factors. *Br. Med. Bull.*, **45**, 438–52.

Barbul A., Sisto D., Wasserkrug H., Efron G. (1981). Arginine stimulates lymphocyte immune response in healthy human beings. *Surgery*, **90**, 244–51.

Barbul A., Rettura G., Levenson S., Seifter E. (1983). Wound healing and thymotropic effects of arginine: a pituitary mechanism of action. *Am. J. Clin. Nutr.*, **37**, 786–94.

Barbul A., Fishel R., Shimazu S. et al. (1985). Intravenous hyperalimentation with high arginine levels improves wound healing and immune function. *J. Surg. Res.*, **38**, 328–34.

Barbul A., Lazarou S., Efron D. et al. (1990). Arginine enhances wound healing and lymphocyte immune responses in humans. *Surgery*, **108**, 331–7.

Barker W., Rodeheaver G., Edgerton M., Edlich R. (1982). Damage to tissue defenses by a topical anesthetic agent. *Ann. Emerg. Med.*, **11**, 307–10.

Barnes M., Kodicek E. (1972). Biological hydroxylations and ascorbic acid with special regard to collagen metabolism. *Vitamins and Hormones*, **30**, 1–43.

Bar-shavit R., Kahn A., Wilner G. (1983). Monocyte chemotaxis: stimulation by specific exosite region in thrombin. *Science*, **220**, 728–31.

Belcher H.J., Mercer D., Judkins K.C. et al. (1989). Biosynthetic human growth hormone in burned patients: a pilot study. *Burns* **15**, 99–107. (Published erratum appears in Burns 1989; **15**, 273.)

Bistrian B., Blackburn G., Hallowell E., Heddle R. (1974). Protein status of general surgical patients. *JAMA*, **230**, 858–60.

Border J.R., Bone L.B. (1988). Multiple trauma: major extremity wounds; their immediate management and its consequences. *Adv. Surg.*, **21**, 263–91.

Boxer L., Stossel T. (1983). Qualitative abnormalities of neutrophils. In *Hematology*, 3rd edn (Williams W., Beutler E., Erslev A., Lichtman M., eds). New York: McGraw-Hill, p. 802.

Boyden S. (1962). The chemotactic effect of mixtures of antibody and antigen on polymorphonuclear leukocytes. *J. Exp. Med.*, **115**, 453–66.

Bradley T., Hodgson G., Rosendaal M. (1978). The effect of oxygen tension on haemopoietic and fibroblast cell proliferation *in vitro*. *J. Cell Physiol.*, **97**(3 pt 2 Suppl 1), 517–22.

Bridges M., Morris D., Hall J., Deitch E. (1987). Effects of wound exudates on *in vitro* immune parameters. *J. Surg. Res.*, **43**, 133–8.

Brown G., Curtsinger L., White M. (1988). Accleration of tensile strength of incisions treated with EGF and TGF-b. *Ann. Surg.*, **208**, 788–94.

Brown J., Grosso M., Harken A. (1989a). Cytokines, sepsis and the surgeon. *Surg. Gynecol. Obstet.*, **169**, 568–75.

Brown G.L., Nanney L.B., Griffen J. et al. (1989b). Enhancement of wound healing by topical treatment with epidermal growth factor [see comments]. *N. Engl. J. Med.*, **321**, 76–9.

Brown G.L., Curtsinger L., Jurkiewicz M.J. et al. (1991). Stimulation of healing of chronic wounds by epidermal growth factor. *Plast. Reconstr. Surg.*, **88**, 189–94; discussion 195–6.

Buckley A., Davidson J., Kamerath C. (1987). Epidermal growth factor increases granulation tissue formation dose dependently. *J. Surg. Res.*, **43**, 322–8.

Burgess A.W. (1989). Epidermal growth factor and transforming growth factor alpha. *Br. Med. Bull.*, **45**, 401–24.

Buzby G. (1990). Perioperative nutritional support. *J. Parenter. Enter. Nutr.*, **14**, 197–9S.

Chang N., Goodson W., Gottrup F., Hunt T. (1983). Direct measurement of wound and tissue oxygen tension in postoperative patients. *Ann. Surg.*, **197**, 470–8.

Chen L., Buchanan J. (1975). Mitogenic activity of blood components. I. Thrombin and prothrombin. *Proc. Natt. Acad. Sci. USA*, **72**, 131–5.

Chen L., Teng N., Buchanan J. (1976). Mitogenicity of thrombin and surface alterations on mouse splenocytes. *Exp. Cell Res.*, **101**, 41–6.

Christensen H., Oxlund H., Laurberg S. (1990). Growth hormone increases the bursting strength of colonic anastomoses. An experimental study in the rat. *Int. J. Colorectal Dis.*, **5**, 130–4.

Christou N. (1990). Perioperative nutritional support: immunologic defects. *J. Parenter. Enter. Nutr.*, **14**, (suppl.), 186–92S.

Chvapil M., Hurych J., Ehrlichova E. (1968). The influence of various oxygen tensions upon proline hydroxylation and the metabolism of collagenous and noncollagenous proteins in skin slices. *Z. Physiol. Chem.*, **349**, 211–17.

Claman H. (1972). Corticosteroids and lymphoid cells. *New End. J. Med.*, **287**, 388–97.

Clark R. (1988). Potential roles of fibronectin in cutaneous wound repair. *Arch. Dermatol*, **124**, 201–6.

Deitch E. (1983). Opsonic activity of blister fluid from burn patients. *Infect. Immunol.*, **41**, 1184–9.

Deitch E., Bridges R., Dobke M., McDonald J. (1987). Burn wound sepsis may be promoted by a failure of local antibacterial host defenses. *Ann.Surg.*, **206**, 340–8.

Denison D. (1989). Oxygen supply and uses in tissues. In *Clinical Aspects of O_2 Transport and Tissue Oxygenation* (Reinhart K., Eyrich K., eds). Berlin: Springer-Verlag, pp. 37–43.

Deuel T., Senior R., Chang D. et al. (1981). Platelet factor 4 is chemotactic for neutrophils and monocytes. *Proc. Natl. Acad. Sci. USA*, **78**, 4584–7.

Dickhaut S., DeLee J., Page C. (1984). Nutritional status: importance in predicting wound healing after amputation. *J. Bone Joint Surg.*, **66A**, 71–5.

Dionigi R., Zonta A., Dominioni L. et al. (1977). The effects of total parenteral nutrition on immunodepression due to malnutrition. *Ann. Surg.*, **185**, 467–74.

Douglas N., Twomey P., Hunt T., Dunphy J. (1973). Effect of exposure to 94% oxygen on the metabolism of wounds. *Bull. Soc. Int. Chir.*, **32**, 178–85.

Ehrlich H. (1971). Effects of beta-carotene, vitamin A and glucocorticoids on collagen synthesis in wounds. *Proc. Soc. Exp. Biol. Med.*, **137**, 936–8.

Ehrlich H., Hunt T. (1968). Effects of cortisone and vitamin A on wound healing. *Ann. Surg.*, **167**, 324–8.

Ehrlich H., Hunt T. (1969). The effects of cortisone and anabolic steroids on the tensile strength of healing wounds. *Ann. Surg.*, **170**, 203–6.

Eichler I., Frisch H., Eichler H.G., Soukop W. (1988). Isolated growth hormone deficiency after severe head trauma. *J. Endocrinol. Invest.*, **11**, 409–11.

Evans N., Naylor P. (1966). Steady states of oxygen tension in human dermis. *Resp. Physiol.*, **2**, 46–60.

Fahey T., Sherry B., Tracey K.J. et al. (1990). Cytokine production in a model of wound healing: the appearance of MIP-1, MIP-2, cachectin/TNF and IL-1. *Cytokine*, **2**, 92–9.

Falanga V., Qian S.W., Danielpour D. et al. (1991). Hypoxia upregulates the synthesis of TGF-beta 1 by human dermal fibroblasts. *J. Invest-Dermatol.*, **97**, 634–7.

Fiddian-Green R., Baker S. (1987). The predictive value of measurements of pH in the wall of the stomach for complications after cardiac sturgery: a comparison with other forms of monitoring. *Crit. Care Med.*, **15**, 153–6.

Fiegel V., Penner B., Wohl R., Knighton D. (1991). PDGF-BB induces wound capillary endothelial cell chemotaxis. In *The Wound Healing Society 1st Annual Scientific Meeting. Galveston Island, Texas*, p. 23.

Ford H.R., Hoffman R.A., Wing E.J. et al. (1989). Characterization of wound cytokines in the sponge matrix model. *Arch. Surg.*, **124**, 1422–8.

Freed B., Corliss R., Bergman R. et al. (1982). Albumin level and total lymphocyte count as predictors of morbidity and mortality in patients undergoing abdominal surgery. *J. Parenter. Enter. Nutr.*, **6**, 584.

Gallin J., Goldstein I., Snyderman R. (eds) (1988). *Inflammation: basic principles and clinical correlates*. New York: Raven, p. 995.

Ganz T., Metcalf J., Gallin J. et al. (1988). Microbicidal/cytotoxic proteins of neutrophils are deficient in two disorders: Chediak–Higashi syndrome and 'Specific' granule deficiency. *J. Clin. Invest.*, **82**, 552–6.

Ghezzi P., Dinarello C.A., Bianchi M. et al. (1991). Hypoxia increases production of interleukin-1 and tumor necrosis factor by human mononuclear cells. *Cytokine*, **3**, 189–94.

Gilmour R.S., Prosser C.G., Fleet I.R. et al. (1988). From animal to molecule: aspects of the biology of insulin-like growth factors. *Br. J. Cancer Suppl.*, **9**, 23–30.

Goldstein R.H., Poliks C.F., Pilch P.F. et al. (1989). Stimulation of collagen formation by insulin and insulin-like growth factor I in cultures of human lung fibroblasts. *Endocrinology*, **124**, 964–70.

Goodson W., Hunt T. (1988). Wound healing and nutrition. In *Nutrition and Metabolism in Patient Care* (Kinney J., Jeejeebhoy K., Kill G. et al. eds). Philadelphia: W.B. Saunders, pp. 635–42.

Gosain A., Rabkin J., Reymond J-P. et al. (1991). Tissue oxygen tension and other indicators of blood loss or organ perfusion during graded hemorrhage. *Surgery*, **109**, 523–32.

Gospodarowicz D. (1990). Fibroblast growth factor. Chemical structure and biologic function. *Clin. Orthop.*, **257**, 231–48.

Gottardis M., Benzer A., Koller W. et al. (1991). Improvement of septic syndrome after administration of recombinant human growth hormone (rhGH)? *J. Trauma*, **31**, 81–6.

Gottrup F., Firmin R., Hunt T.K., Mathes S.J. (1984). The dynamic properties of tissue oxygen in healing flaps. *Surgery*, **95**, 527–36.

Gottrup F., Firmin R., Rabkin J. et al. (1987). Directly measured tissue oxygen tension and arterial oxygen tension assess tissue perfusion. *Crit. Care Med.*, **15**, 1030–6.

Grotendorst G., Martin G., Pencev D. (1985). Stimulation of granulation tissue formation by platelet derived growth factor in normal and diabetic rats. *J. Clin. Invest.*, **76**, 2323–9.

Haley R., Culver D., Morgan W. et al. (1985). Identifying patients at high risk of surgical wound infection: a simple multivariate index of patient susceptibility and wound contamination. *Am. J. Epidemiol.*, **121**, 206–15.

Haydock D., Hill G. (1987). Improved wound healing response in surgical patients receiving intravenous nutrition. *Br. J. Surg.*, **74**, 320–3.

Heppenstall R.B., Littooy F.N., Fuchs R. et al. (1974). Gas tensions in healing tissues of traumatized patients. *Surgery*, **75**, 874–80.

Herndon D.N., Barrow R.E., Kunkel K.R. et al. (1990). Effects of recombinant human growth hormone on donor-site healing in severely burned children. *Ann. Surg.*, **212**, 424–9; discussion 430–1.

Heughan C., Zederfeldt B., Grislis G., Hunt T.K. (1972). Effect of dextran solutions on oxygen transport in wound tissue. An experimental study in rabbits. *Acta Chir. Scand.*, **138**, 639–43.

Hohn D. (1988). The phagocytes. In *Surgical Infectious Disease*, 2 eds. Norwalk, Connecticut: Appleton & Lange, p. 158.

Hohn D.C., MacKay R.D., Halliday B., Hunt T.K. (1976). Effect of O_2 tension on microbicidal function of leukocytes in wounds and *in vitro*. *Surg. Forum*, **27**, 18–20.

Hohn D., Ponce B., Burton R., Hunt T. (1977). Antimicrobial systems of the surgical wound. I. A comparison of oxidative metabolism and microbicidal capacity of phagocytes from wounds and from peripheral blood. *Am. J. Surg*, **133**, 597–600.

Holloway G., Watkins D. (1977). Laser Doppler measurement of cutanous blood flow. *J. Invest. Dermatol.*, **69**, 306–9.

Hopf H., Hunt T., Jensen J. (1988). Calculation of subcutaneous tissue blood flow. *Surg. Forum*, **34**, 33–6.

Howard R., Simmons R. (1974). Acquired immunologic deficiencies after trauma and surgical procedures. *Surg. Gynecol. Obstet.*, **139**, 771–82.

Hunt T. (1975). The effect of differing ambient oxygen tensions on wound infection. *Ann. Surg.*, **181**, 35–9.

Hunt T. (1979a). Disorders of wound repair and their management. In *Fundamentals of Wound Management* (Hunt T., Dunphy J., eds). New York: Appleton-Century-Crofts, p. 85.

Hunt T. (1979b). Disorders of repair and their management. In *Fundamentals of Wound Management* (Hunt T., Dunphy J., eds). New York: Appleton-Century-Crofts, p. 99.

Hunt T. (1988). Physiology of wound healing. In *Trauma, Sepsis and Shock. The physiological basis of therapy* (Clowes G, ed.). New York: Marcel Dekker, pp. 443–71.

Hunt T., Pai M. (1972). Effect of varying ambient oxygen tensions on wound metabolism and collagen synthesis. *Surg. Gynecol. Obstet.*, **135**, 257–60.

Hunt T.K., Twomey P., Zederfeldt B., Dunphy J.E. (1967). Respiratory gas tensions and pH in healing wounds. *Am. J. Surg.*, **114**, 302–7.

Hunt T.K., Conolly W.B., Aronson S.B., Goldstein P. (1978). Anaerobic metabolism and wound healing: an hypothesis for the initiation and cessation of collagen synthesis in wounds. *Am. J. Surg.*, **135**, 328–32.

Hunt T., Banda M., Silver I. (1985). Cell interations in post-traumatic fibrosis. In *Fibrosis. Ciba Foundation Symposium 114* (Evered D., Whelan J., eds). London: Pitman, pp. 127–9.

Hunt T., Halliday B., Knighton D. et al. (1988). Oxygen in the prevention and treatment of infection. In *Contemporary Issues in Infectious Diseases*. vol. 6. *Focus on infection: new surgical and medical approaches* (Root R., Trunkey D., Sande M., eds). New York: Churchill Livingstone, p. 8.

Hussain M.Z., Hunt T.K., Bhatnagar R.S. (1988). Metabolic regulation of prolyl hydroxylase activation. *Prog. Clin. Biol. Res.*, **266**, 229–36.

Hussain M.Z., Ghani Q.P., Hunt T.K. (1989). Inhibition of prolyl hydroxylase by poly(ADP-ribose) and phosphoribosyl-AMP. Possible role of ADP-ribosylation in intracellular prolyl hydroxylase regulation. *J. Biol. Chem.*, **264**, 7850–5.

Hutton J., Tapel A., Udenfriend S. (1967). Cofactor and substrate requirements of collagen proline hydroxylase. *Arch. Biochem.*, **118**, 231.

Ignotz R., Endo T., Massague J. (1987). Regulation of fibronectin and type I collagen mRNA levels by transforming growth factor-β. *J.Biol. Chem.*, **262**, 6443–6.

Jensen J., Jensen T., Smith T. et al. (1982). Nutrition in orthopaedic surgery. *J. Bone Joint Surg.*, **64A**, 1263–72.

Jensen J.A., Jonsson K., Goodson W. et al. (1985). Epinephrine lowers subcutaneous wound oxygen tension. *Curr. Surg.*, **42**, 472–4.

Jensen J.A., Goodson W., Vasconez L.O., Hunt T.K. (1986a). Wound healing in anemia. *West. J. Med.*, **144**, 465–7.

Jensen J.A., Hunt T.K., Scheuenstuhl H., Banda M.J. (1986b). Effect of lactate, pyruvate, and pH on secretion of angiogenesis and mitogenesis factors by macrophages. *Lab. Invest.*, **54**, 574–8.

Jensen J., Riggs K., Vasconez L. et al. (1987). Clinical assessment of postoperative peripheral perfusion. *Surg. Forum*, **38**, (66–7).

Jensen J.A., Goodson W.H., Hopf H.W., Hunt T.K. (1991). Cigarette smoking decreases tissue oxygen. *Arch Surg.*, **126**, 1131–4.

Jonsson K., Jensen J.A., Goodson W.H.I. et al. (1986). Wound healing in subcutaneous tissue in surgical patients in relation to oxygen availability. *Surg. Forum*, **37**, 86–8.

Jonsson K., Jensen J.A., Goodson W. et al. (1987a). Assessment of perfusion in postoperative patients using tissue oxygen measurements. *Br. J. Surg.*, **74**, 263–7.

Jonsson K., Jiborn H., Zederfeldt B. (1987b). Collagen metabolism in small intestinal anastomosis. *Am. J. Surg.*,288–91.

Jonsson K., Hunt T., Mathes S. (1988). Oxygen as an isolated variable influences resistance to infection. *Ann. Surg.*, **208**, 783.

Jonsson K., Jensen J., Goodson W. et al. (1991). Tissue oxygenation, anemia and perfusion in relation to wound healing in surgical patients. *Ann. Surg.*, **214**, 605–13.

Kaplan E., Dinarello C.A., Gelfand J.A. (1989). Interleukin-1 and the response to injury. *Immunol. Res.*, **8**, 118–29.

Karey K.P., Sirbasku D.A. (1989). Human platelet-derived mitogens. II. Subcellular localization of insulinolike growth factor I to the alpha-granule and release in response to thrombin. *Blood*, **74**, 1093–100.

Kishimoto T.K., Larson R.S., Corbi A.L. et al. (1989). The leukocyte integrins. *Adv. Immunol.*, **46**, 149–82.

Klagsbrun M. (1989). The fibroblast growth factor family: structural and biological properties. *Prog. Growth Factor Res.*, **1**, 207–35.

Klebanoff S. (1980). Oxygen metabolism and the toxic properties of phagocytes. *Ann. Intern. Med.*, **93**, 480–9.

Klebanoff S., Clark R. (1978). Cellular defects. In *The Neutrophil: function and clinical disorders* (Klebanoff S., Clark R., eds). New York: North-Holland Publishing Company, p. 553.

Knighton D., Hunt T. (1988). The defenses of the wound. In *Surgical Infectious Diseases* (Howard R., Simmons R., eds) 2 edn. Norwalk, CT: Appleton and Lange, pp. 188–93.

Knighton D.R., Silver I.A., Hunt T.K. (1981). Regulation of wound-healing angiogenesis – effect of oxygen gradients and inspired oxygen concentration. *Surgery*, **90**, 262–70.

Knighton D., Hunt T., Thrakral K., Goodson W. (1982). Role of platelets and fibrin in the healing sequence. *Ann. Surg.*, **196**, 379–88.

Knighton D.R., Hunt T.K., Scheuenstuhl H. et al. (1983). Oxygen tension regulates the expression of angiogenesis factor by macrophages. *Science*, **221**, 1283–5.

Knighton D.R., Halliday B., Hunt T.K. (1984). Oxygen as an antibiotic: the effect of inspired oxygen on infection. *Arch. Surg.*, **119**, 199–204.

Kwan M.R., Hunt T.K. (1973). Continous tissue oxygen tension measurements during acute blood loss. *J. Surg. Res.*, **14**, 420–5.

Law D., Dudrick S., Abdon N. (1974). The effects of protein calorie malnutrition on immune competence of the surgical patient. *Surg. Gynecol. Obstet.*, **139**, 257–66.

Levenson S., Seifter E., Winkle W.V. (1977). Nutrition. In *Fundamentals of Wound Management in Surgery*. New Jersey: Chirurgecom.

Levenson S., Seifter E., Winkle E.V. (1979). Nutrition. In *Fundamentals of Wound Management* (Hunt T., Dunphy J., (eds). New York: Appleton-Century-Crofts, p. 286.

Longaker M.T., Adzick N.S. (1991). The biology of fetal wound healing: a review. *Plast. Reconstr. Surg.*, **87**, 788–98.

Magee C., Rodeheaver G., Edgerton M. et al. (1977). Studies of the mechanisms by which epinephrine damages tissue defenses. *J. Surg. Res.*, **23**, 126–31.

Marano M.A., Fong Y., Moldawer L.L. et al. (1990). Serum cachectin/tumor necrosis factor in critically ill patients with burns correlates with infection and mortality. *Surg. Gynecol. Obstet.*, **170**, 32–8.

Martin D., Reece M., Maher J., Reese A. (1988). Tissue debris at the injury site is coated by plasma fibronectin and subsequently removed by tissue macrophages. *Arch. Dermatol.*, **124**, 226–9.

Matsuoka J., Grotendorst G.R. (1989). Two peptides related to platelet-derived growth factor are present in human wound fluid. *Proc. Natl. Acad. Sci. USA*, **86**, 4416–20.

Maxwell T.M., Lim R.C., Fuchs R., Hunt T.K. (1973). Continuous monitoring of tissue gas tensions and pH in hemorrhagic shock. *Am. J. Surg.*, **141**, 235–9.

McCord J. (1976). Iron and manganese containing super-oxide dismutase: structure, distribution, and evolutionary relationships. *Adv. Exp. Med. Biol.*, **74**, 540.

Mckay I., Leigh I. (1991). Epidermal cytokines and their roles in cutaneous wound healing. *Br. J. Dermatol.*, **124**, 513–18.

McRipley R., Sbarra A. (1967). Role of the phagocyte in host–parasite interactions: XII. Hydrogen peroxide-myeloperoxidase bactericidal system in the phagocyte. *J. Bacteriol.*, **94**, 1425–30.

Meakins J. (1988). Alterations of host defenses in the surgical patient. In *Surgical Infectious Diseases*, 2 ed (Howard R., Simmons R., eds). Norwalk, CT: Appleton and Lange, pp. 193–9.

Medawar P. (1948). The cultivation of adult mammalian skin epithelium. *Q. J. Micr. Sci.*, **89**, 187.

Mellander S. (1960). Comparative studies on the adrenergic neurohormonal control of resistance and capacitance of blood vessels in the cat. *Acta Physiol. Scand.*, **50**, (suppl), 1–86.

Mentzer S.J., Burakoff S.J., Faller D.V. (1986). Adhesion of T lymphocytes to human endothelial cells is regulated by the LFA-1 membrane molecule. *J. Cell. Physiol.*, **126**, 285.

Moelleken B., Mathes S., Amerhauser A. et al. (1991). An adverse wound environment activates leukocytes prematurely. *Arch. Surg.*, **126**, 225–30.

Mohanram M., Rucker R., Hodges R., Ney D. (1976). Vitamin A deficiency and the metabolism of glycosaminoglycans and ascobic acid in the rat. *J. Nutr.*, **106**, 471–7.

Moore E., Jones T. (1986). Benefits of immediate jejunostomy feeding after major abdominal trauma – a prospective, randomized study. *J. Trauma*, **26**, 874–81.

Moore F., Moore E., Jones T. et al. (1989). TEN versus TPN following major abdominal trauma–reduced septic morbidity. *J. Trauma*, **29**, 916–23.

Moses H.L., Yang E.Y., Pietenpol J.A. (1991). Regulation of epithelial proliferation by TGF-beta. *Ciba Found. Symp.*, **157**, 66–74; discussion 75–80.

Mueller R., Spencer E., Sommer A. et al. (1991). The role of IGF-I and IGFBP-3 in wound healing. In *Modern Concepts of Insulin-Like Growth Factors* (Spencer EM, ed.). New York: Elsevier Science, pp. 185–92.

Mullen J., Buzby G., Matthews D. et al. (1980). Reduction of operative morbidity and mortality by combined preoperative and postoperative nutritional support. *Ann. Surg.*, 192.

Muller J., Keller H., Brenner U. et al. (1986). Indications and effects of preoperative parenteral nutrition. *World J. Surg.*, **10**, 53–63.

Mustoe T.A., Pierce G.F., Thomason A. et al. (1987). Accelerated healing of incisional wounds in rats induced by transforming growth factor-beta. *Science*, **237**, 1333–6.

Myllyla R., Tuderman L., Kivirikko K. (1977). Mechanism of the prolyl hydroxylase reaction. 2. Kinetic analysis of the reaction sequence. *Eur. J. Biochem.*, **80**, 349–57.

Nasution A., Taylor D. (1981). The effect of acute haemorrhage and of delayed blood replacement on wound healing. *Br. J. Surg.*, **68**, 306–9.

Nelson R., Quie P., Simmons R. (1975). Chemotaxis under agarose: a new and simple method for measuring chemotaxis and spontaneous migration of human polymorphonuclear leukocytes and monocytes. *J. Immunol.*, **115**, 1650–6.

Nielsen H.M., Bak B., Jorgensen P.H., Andreassen T.T. (1991). Growth hormone promotes healing of tibial fractures in the rat. *Acta Orthop. Scand.*, **62**, 244–7.

Niinikoski J., Heughan C., Hunt T.K. (1972). Oxygen tensions in human wounds. *J. Surg. Res.*, **12**, 77–82.

Niinikoski J., Jussila P., Vihersaari T. (1973). Radical mastectomy wound as a model for studies of human wound metabolism. *Am. J. Surg.*, **126**, 53–8.

Orgill D., Demling R. (1988). Current concepts and approaches to wound healing. *Crit. Care Med.*, **16**, 899–908.

Paty P. (1988). Activation of macrophages by L-lactic acid. *Surg. Forum*, **39**, 27–8.

Paty P., Banda M., Hunt T. (1987). Fibrin activation of macrophages: one mechanism of angiogenesis in wound healing. *Highlights of Second Internation Forum*. In *Fibrinolysis and Angiogenesis* (Steward A., Cederholm-Williams S., Terrence J., Lydon M., eds). San Antonio, TX: Amsterdam, Excerpta Medica, pp. 36–9.

Peterson P., Verhoef J., Schmeling D., Quie P. (1977). Kinetics of phagocytosis and bacterial killing by human polymorphonuclear leukocytes and monocytes. *J. Infect. Dis.*, **136**, 502–8.

Pettigrew R., Hill G. (1986). Indicators of surgical risk and clinical judgement. *Br. J. Surg.*, **73**, 47–51.

Pierce G., Mustoe T. (1988). *In vivo* incisional wound healing augmentaed by platelet-dervied growth factor and recombinant c-*sis* gene homodimeric proteins. *J. Exp. Med.*, **167**, 974–87.

Pierce G., Mustoe T., Lingelbach J. (1989). Platelet-derived growth factor and transforming growth factor-b enhance tissue repair by unique mechanisms. *J. Cell Biol.*, **109**, 429–40.

Pietila K., Jaakkola O. (1984). Effect of hypoxia on the synthesis of glycosaminoglycans and collagen by rabbit aortic smooth muscle cells in culture. *Atheros*, **50**, 183–90.

Podolsky S., Baraff L., Geehr E. (1982). Transcutaneous oximetry measurements during acute blood loss. *Ann. Emerg. Med.*, **11**, 523–5.

Polk H., Malangoni M. (1988). Chemoprophylaxis of wound infections. In *Surgical Infectious Diseases*, 2 ed (Howard R., Simmons R., eds). Norwalk, CT: Appleton and Lange, pp. 351–61.

Prockop D., Kaplan A., Udenfriend S. (1962). Oxygen-18 studies on the conversion of proline to hydroxyproline. *Biochem. Biophys. Res. Commun.*, **9**, 162–6.

Prystowsky J.H., Kahn S.N., Lazarus G.S. (1989). Present status of pyoderma gangrenosum. Review of 21 cases. *Arch. Dermatol.*, **125**, 57–64.

Quaglino D.J., Nanney L.B., Kennedy R., Davidson J.M. (1990). Transforming growth factor-beta stimulates wound healing and modulates extracellular matrix gene expression in pig skin. I. Excisional wound model. *Lab. Invest.*, **63**, 307–19.

Rabkin J., Hunt T.K. (1988). Infection and oxygen. In *Problem Wounds: the role of oxygen* (Davis J., Hunt T.K., ed.). New York: Elsevier, pp. 1–16.

Rappolee D.A., Mark D., Banda M.J., Werb Z. (1988). Wound macrophages express TGF-alpha and other growth factors *in vivo*: analysis by mRNA phenotyping. *Science*, **241**, 708–12.

Riordan J., Vallee B. (1976). Structure and function of zinc metalloenzymes. In *Trace Elements in Human Health and Disease*, Vol. I (Prasad A., Oberleas D., ed.). New York: Academic Press, pp. 27–56.

Roberts A., Anzano M., Wakefield L. et al. (1985). Type β transforming growth factor: a bifunctional regulator of cellular growth. *Proc. Natl. Acad. Sci. USA*, **82**, 119–23.

Ross R., Glomset J., Kariy B. (1974). A platelet dependant serum factor that stimulates the proliferation of arterial smooth muscle cells *in vitro*. *Proc. Natl. Acad. Sci. USA*, **71**, 1207–10.

Rudolph R., VandeBerg J., Ehrlich H. (1992). Wound contraction and scar contracture. In *Wound Healing: Biochemical and Clinical Aspects* (Cohen I., Diegelmann R., Lindblad W., eds). Philadelphia: W.B. Saunders, p. 97.

Sbarra A., Strauss R. (1988). *The respiratory burst and its physiologic significance*. New York: Plenum Press.

Scher C., Shephard R., Antoniades H., Stiles C. (1979). Platelet-derived growth factor and the regulation of the mammalian fibroblast cell cycle. *Biochem. Biophys. Acta*, **560**, 212–41.

Schoefl G. (1963). Studies in inflammation. III. Growing capillaries: their structure and permeability. *Virchows Arch. Pathol. Anat.*, **33**, 97.

Schroeder D., Gillanders L., Mahr K., Hill G. (1991). Effects of immediate postoperative enteral nutrition on body composition, muscle function, and wound healing. *J. Parenter. Enter. Nutr.*, **15**, 376–83.

Scrutton M., Wu C., Goldwait P. (1971). The presence and possible role of zinc in RNA polymerase obtained from *Eschericia coli*. *Proc. Natl. Acad. Sci. USA*, **68**, 2497–501.

Seifter E., Rettura G., Barbul A., Levenson S. (1978). Arginine: an essential amino acid for injured rats. *Surgery*, **84**, 224–30.

Selvaraj R., Sbarra A. (1966). Relationship of glycolytic and oxidative metabolism to particle entry and destruction in phagocytosing cells. *Nature*, **211**, 1272–6.

Senior R., Griffin G., Huang J. et al. (1983). Chemotactic activity of platelet alpha granule proteins for fibroblasts. *J. Cell Biol.*, **96**, 382–5.

Sheldon C., Cerra F., Bohnhoff N. et al. (1983). Peripheral postcapillary venous pressure: a new, more senstive monitor of effective blood volume during hemorrhagic shock and resuscitation. *Surgery*, **94**, 399.

Slater J., Mildvan A., Loeb L. (1971). Zinc in DNA polymerase. *Biochim. Biophys. Res. Commun.*, **44**, 37.

Smith M., Abraham E. (1986). Conjunctival oxygen tension monitoring during hemorrhage. *J. Trauma*, **26**, 217–24.

Spencer E.M. (1988). Somatomedins: do they play a pivotal role in wound healing? In *Symposium on Tissue Repair* (Hunt TK, ed.). New York: Alan R. Liss, pp. 103–16.

Sporn M., Roberts A., Shull J. (1983). Polypeptide transforming growth factors isolated from bovine sources and used for wound healing *in vivo*. *Science*, **219**, 1329–31.

Steenfos H., Spencer E., Hunt T. (1989). Insulin-like growth factor has a major role in wound healing. *Surg. Forum*, **40**, 68–70.

Streat S., Hill G. (1987). Nutritional support in the management of critically ill patients in surgical intensive care. *World J. Surg.*, **11**, 194–201.

Strock L.L., Singh H., Abdullah A. et al. (1990). The effect of insulin-like growth factor I on postburn hypermetabolism. *Surgery*, **108**, 161–4.

Thiebaud D., Ng K.W., Findlay D.M. et al. (1990). Insulinlike growth factor 1 regulates mRNA levels of osteonectin and pro-alpha 1(I)-collagen in clonal pre-osteoblastic calvarial cells. *J. Bone Miner. Res.*, **5**, 761–7.

Tuddenham E. (ed.) (1989). *The Molecular Biology of Coagulation. Bailliere's Clinical Haematology: international practice and research*. London: Ballière Tindall, pp. 787–1046.

Uitto J, Prockop D. (1974). Synthesis and secretion of underhydroxylated procollagen at various temperatures by cells subject to temporary anoxia. *Biochem. Biophy. Res. Commun.*, **60**, 414–23.

Wacker W., Parisi A. (1968). Medical progress: magnesium metabolism. *N. Engl. J. Med.*, **278**, 658–63.

Warnold I., Lundholm K. (1984). Clinical significance of preoperative nutritional status in 215 non-cancer patients. *Ann. Surg.*, **199**, 299–305.

Weber F. (1983). Biochemical mechanisms of vitamin action. *Proc. Nutr. Soc.*, **42**, 31–41.

Williams R., Heatley R., Lewis M. (1976). A randomized controlled trial of preoperative intravenous nutrition in patients with stomach cancer. *Br. J. Surg.*, **63**, 667.

Wilmore D.W. (1990). Pathophysiology of the hypermetabolic response to burn injury. *J. Trauma*, **30**(12 suppl 1), S4–6.

Wilmore D.W. (1991). Catabolic illness. Strategies for enhancing recovery. *N. Engl. J. Med.*, **325**, 695–702.

Wilmore D., Aulick L. Jr. (1977). Influences of the burn wound on local and systemic responses to injury. *Ann. Surg.*, **186**, 444.

Windsor J., Hill G. (1988). Weight loss with physiologic impairment. *Ann. Surg.*, **207**, 290–6.

.Wolfe R.R., Jahoor F., Herndon D.N., Miyoshi H. (1991). Isotopic evaluation of the metabolism of pyruvate and related substrates in normal adult volunteers and severely burned children: effect of dichloroacetate and glucose infusion. *Surgery*, **110**, 54–67.

Wolff S., Dale D., Clark R. et al. (1972). The Chediak–Higashi syndrome: studies of host defenses. *Ann. Intern. Med.*, **76**, 293–306.

Zaizen Y., Ford E.G., Costin G., Atkinson J.B. (1990). The effect of perioperative exogenous growth hormone on wound bursting strength in normal and malnourished rats. *J. Pediatr. Surg.*, **25**, 70–4.

Zederfeldt B. (1957). Studies on wound healing and trauma. *Acta Chir. Scand. Suppl.*, **224**, 1–85.

Zederfeldt B., Hunt T. (1970). Effect of Dextran solution on respiratory gas tension in wound fluid and on granulation tissue formation after trauma. *Eur. Surg. Research*, **2**, 251–62.

Zwaal R., Hemker H. (eds). *Blood Coagulation. New Comprehensive Biochemistry*, vol. 13. New York: Elsevier Science, p. 321.

40. Cardiovascular Control After Injury
R. A. Little and E. Kirkman

The ability to compensate for fluid loss (haemorrhage) from the circulation is arguably the most important factor in determining resistance to the acute effects of injury. The cardiovascular reflexes are vital to such homoeostasis and this chapter is a discussion of the organization of those reflexes involved in the maintenance of blood pressure and tissue oxygen delivery. Special attention will be given to their central organization and how that might interact with the pathways concerned with nociception and antinociception. This is very relevant to the clinical situation where haemorrhage is most commonly accompanied by tissue damage which generates somatic afferent (nociceptive) impulses. The patterns of cardiovascular response elicited by haemorrhage and nociceptive stimulation alone and in combination will be compared. The consequences of such interactions and their implications for therapy will also be discussed.

CARDIOVASCULAR REFLEXES INVOLVED IN THE RESPONSE TO HAEMORRHAGE

A number of reflexes are involved in the cardiovascular response to haemorrhage. In this section three of these reflexes will be discussed: the arterial baroreceptor and chemoreceptor reflexes, and that elicited by stimulation of cardiac vagal C-fibre afferents. There will then follow a description of how these reflexes are organized to produce a cardiovascular response to a progressive haemorrhage.

The arterial baroreceptor reflex

This reflex serves to minimize moment to moment variations in blood pressure around a given 'set-point' which itself can be altered (Cowley et al., 1973). The baroreceptor endings are found in parts of the arterial system with an elastic structure, mainly the aortic arch and carotid sinus, although others have been found at the origin of the subclavian arteries and along the common carotid arteries (Kirchheim, 1976). These endings, situated in the medio-adventitial border of the arterial wall, are slowly adapting mechanoreceptors which respond to the degree of stretch of the arterial wall (e.g. Angell-James, 1971). The baroreceptors respond to the rate of change of arterial blood pressure as well as to its absolute level, and so can transduce information about pulse pressure and heart rate as well as mean arterial blood pressure (Angell-James and Daly, 1970). Afferent information from the baroreceptors in the aortic arch is mainly carried in the vagi, while that from those in the carotid sinus travels in the sinus nerve, a branch of the glossopharyngeal nerve (Heymans and Neil, 1958; Kirchheim, 1976).

The baroreceptor afferent fibres terminate within the nucleus of the tractus solitarius in the brain stem (Spyer, 1984). The efferent limb of the baroreceptor reflex is carried in both the parasympathetic nerves (vagi) to the heart and the sympathetic supply to the heart and peripheral vasculature. The cell bodies of the vagal cardiac preganglionic motor neurones are located in the nucleus ambiguus and dorsal vagal motor nucleus (McAllen and Spyer, 1976; Jordan et al., 1982). The sympathetic preganglionic cell bodies are found in the intermediolateral columns of the thoracic and upper lumbar segments of the spinal cord (Henry and Calaresu, 1972).

Activation of the baroreceptor reflex by a fall in arterial blood pressure elicits a reflex withdrawal of vagal tone to the heart and reflex increase in sympathetic drive to the heart and peripheral vasculature. The result is an increase in cardiac output and total peripheral resistance, both of which tend to restore arterial blood pressure. The balance of pressures across the microvascular endothelium is also changed in such a way that fluid moves from the extravascular to the intravascular compartment. It should be emphasized that the activation of the sympathetic supply to the various vascular beds is not uniform, with some experiencing a more intense vasoconstriction than others (Kirchheim, 1976). Thus the baroreceptor reflex serves to maintain blood flow to tissues critically dependent on oxygen delivery (e.g. brain) at the expense of flow to other organs (e.g. skeletal muscle) where oxygen delivery is less critical, at least in the short term.

The activity of the baroreceptor reflex can be reset by sustained rises or falls in arterial blood pressure (e.g. Kunze, 1981); this ensures that the range of pressures over which the reflex is most effective follows the 'chronic' level of blood pressure. The efficiency of the baroreflex can also be manipulated by changes in its sensitivity, defined as the response (e.g. change in heart rate) elicited by a given change in stimulus (e.g. blood pressure) (Scott, 1983).

The arterial chemoreceptor reflex

The arterial chemoreceptors are found in the carotid and aortic bodies close to the carotid sinus and aortic arch respectively. They respond to changes in oxygen tension, a fall in oxygen tension increasing chemoreceptor afferent activity, and as they have a large oxygen consumption relative to their size they are well placed to monitor the oxygenation of arterial blood. In addition, increases in carbon dioxide tension and falls in arterial blood pH increase the sensitivity of the arterial chemo-receptors to hypoxia (Biscoe *et al.*, 1970). The afferent neural pathways, primary central termina-tion, and some of the central projections for the chemoreceptors are similar to those for the arterial baroreceptors (Donoghue *et al.*, 1984; Izzo *et al.*, 1988).

Stimulation of arterial chemoreceptors produces an increase in respiration (Heymans and Neil, 1958), while the primary cardiovascular effects are a vagally mediated bradycardia and a vasoconstric-tion in, for example, skeletal muscle which is due to increased sympathetic vasoconstrictor-activity (Daly, 1983). This pattern of response is subse-quently modified by the increased respiratory activity which tends to inhibit both the increased vagal activity to the heart and sympathetic vaso-constrictor activity (Spyer, 1984). Thus, in species which show a marked increase in respiration, the primary bradycardia and vasoconstriction can be reversed to a tachycardia and a vasodilatation. This interaction between the respiratory and cardiovas-cular responses to chemoreceptor stimulation may have implications for the treatment of injured patients. For example, procedures such as intuba-tion which inhibit respiratory activity could unmask a dangerous bradycardia (e.g. Angell-James and Daly, 1975).

There is good evidence that arterial chemo-receptors are stimulated during haemorrhage and contribute to the maintenance of blood pressure (Kenney and Neil, 1951). The activation of the chemoreceptors is due to the reduction in blood flow through the carotid and aortic bodies second-ary to the fall in arterial blood pressure, and to sympathetic vasoconstriction in the bodies them-selves (Daly *et al.*, 1954; Acker and O'Regan, 1981).

The cardiac 'C-fibre afferent' reflex

The cardiac vagal C-fibre afferents are unlikely to be involved in the regulation of blood pressure under normal circumstances, but they may be involved in pathophysiological situations. Until recently these afferents were thought to be involved in the response to severe haemorrhage, although there is now increasing evidence against this possibility.

The afferent pathway of this reflex is carried in vagal C-fibres arising from receptors located mainly in the wall of the left ventricle. Although the receptors can be activated by chemical and/or mechanical stimuli the reflex response elicited is the same, namely a profound bradycardia, hypotension

and reduction in skeletal muscle and renal vascular resistance (Öberg and Thorén, 1973; Daly *et al.*, 1988). The bradycardia is due to increased vagal cardiac efferent activity, while the reduction in vascular resistance is due to a withdrawal of sympathetic vasoconstrictor tone (Öberg and Tho-rén, 1973; Daly *et al.*, 1988). It has been suggested that this 'depressor' reflex may serve to protect the heart by reducing cardiac work at a time when coronary blood flow is compromised.

THE CARDIOVASCULAR RESPONSE TO A PROGRESSIVE HAEMORRHAGE

It is almost axiomatic that haemorrhage induces a progressive increase in heart rate and vascular resistance as a result of activation of the baro-receptor reflex (e.g. Secher and Bie, 1985). In the presence of blood losses of up to 10–15% of blood volume this mechanism will maintain a mean arterial blood pressure close to prehaemorrhage levels (Figure 40.1(a)). The activity of the baro-receptor reflex at this time is augmented by a concomitant increase in its sensitivity (Little *et al.*, 1984). The mechanism of this increase in sensitivity is unknown, although it may be due to the increases

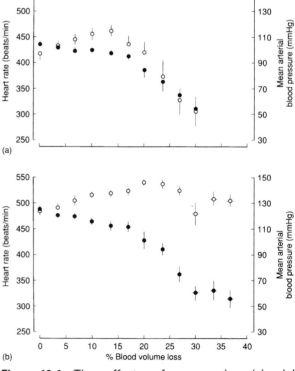

Figure 40.1 The effects of progressive 'simple' haemorrhage (a) and haemorrhage in the presence of bilateral hind-limb ischaemia (b) on heart rate (○) and mean arterial blood pressure (●) in the rat. Values shown are mean ± standard error.

in the plasma levels of vasopressin and renin activity which occur after haemorrhage (Kirkman and Scott, 1983; Cowley *et al.*, 1984).

As the severity of haemorrhage increases and exceeds 20% of the blood volume a very different pattern of response is elicited; a marked brady-cardia and peripheral vasodilatation accompanied by a precipitous fall in blood pressure which may lead to syncope (Barcroft *et al.*, 1944). This depressor response is not due to a sudden failure of the baroreflex or the imminent demise of the heart, it has been suggested that it is due to activation of a second reflex as a result of stimulating the cardiac C-fibre afferents by deformation of the ventricular wall as the heart contracts vigorously around an incompletely filled chamber (Öberg and Thorén, 1972; Little *et al.*, 1989). However recent studies have questioned the afferent pathway mediating the 'depressor' response to severe haemorrhage since such a response has been reported in con-scious dogs subjected to cardiac denervation or acute cardiac nerve blockade (Shen *et al.*, 1990). Furthermore there is a case of sympathoinhibition following the infusion of a vasodilator agent in a cardiac transplant patient with no ventricular innervation (Scherrer *et al.*, 1990). Also, although the depressor response elicited by chemical stim-ulation of cardiopulmonary receptors (including the cardiac afferent C-fibres) can be prevented by the central injection of the 5HT-antagonist methio-thepin (Bogle *et al.*, 1990), that associated with severe haemorrhage is unaffected (Kirkman *et al.*, 1994).

The third reflex important in the cardiovascular response to haemorrhage is the arterial chemo-receptor reflex. The arterial chemoreceptors will be activated following large falls in blood pressure which produce stagnant hypoxia due to a reduced blood flow through the chemoreceptors. Under these circumstances they may prevent arterial blood pressure falling even further and may also be responsible for the increase in respiration noted following severe haemorrhage (D'Silva *et al.*, 1966). Since an increase in respiratory activity has been shown to reduce the reflex bradycardia produced by stimulation of cardiac C-fibre afferents (Daly *et al.*, 1988), it is possible that the enhanced respiratory activity seen following a severe haemorrhage may attenuate the bradycardia seen under these circum-stances. The role of the chemoreceptors in helping to maintain blood pressure will, of course, be increased in the injured patient with thoracic injuries which may impair pulmonary function.

THE ROLE OF ENDOGENOUS OPIOIDS IN THE RESPONSE TO HAEMORRHAGE

There is strong evidence suggesting that the endog-enous opioid system may be involved in both the sympathoinhibitory and bradycardic responses to severe hypovolaemia. Thus the opioid antagonist naloxone, when given intravenously, attenuated the reduction in sympathetic efferent activity and the hypotension associated with severe haemorrhage (Burke and Dorward, 1988; Ludbrook and Rutter, 1988). In these studies it has been assumed that naloxone is exerting its effects via an antagonistic action at δ-opioid receptors within the medulla, possibly the nucleus tractus solitarius which con-tains a dense population of δ-opioid receptors.

In addition to the δ-opioid receptors, the μ and κ receptors are also capable of modifing the response to severe hypovolaemia. Thus, activation of μ and κ receptors can prevent the reflex sympathoinhibition (Evans *et al.*, 1989; Evans and Ludbrook, 1990) and morphine, presumably acting at μ opioid receptors within the medulla, can block the bradycardia as well as the depressor response associated with severe blood loss (Ohnishi *et al.*, 1996).

THE CARDIOVASCULAR RESPONSE TO TISSUE INJURY

In direct contrast to haemorrhage, tissue injury/ ischaemia produces an increase in arterial blood pressure accompanied by a tachycardia (Alam and Smirk, 1937, 1938). The increase in arterial blood pressure which accompanies injury is largely medi-ated by an increase in sympathetic outflow to the vasculature and a consequent increase in total peripheral resistance. Thus the injury-induced pressor response is unaffected by complete cardiac autonomic blockade, but is abolished by the α-adre-noceptor antagonist phentolamine (Redfern, 1981). This intense sympathetically mediated vasocon-striction induced by injury could lead to a reduction in blood flow to vital organs such as the gut and kidney and possibly lead to ischaemic damage of those organs (Overman and Wang, 1947), hence contributing to the pathophysiology of the response to injury and its sequelae such as multiple organ failure.

The injury-induced pressor response is accom-panied by a tachycardia, rather than a bradycardia which would be expected were the baroreflex (see above) functioning normally. This pattern of response is possible because there is a concomitant reduction in the sensitivity and a rightward reset-ting (i.e. towards a higher arterial blood pressure) of the baroreflex following injury (Redfern *et al.*, 1984). The reduction in baroreflex sensitivity in man is evident within 3 hours of injury of moderate severity (e.g. fracture of a long bone) and is persistent such that only partial recovery has occurred at 14 days after injury (Anderson *et al.*, 1990) (Figure 40.2). This impairment of the baro-reflex is accompanied by a persistent tachycardia which is not related to hypovolaemia, and a reduction in the variation in heart rate induced by respiration. Many of the victims of accidental injury

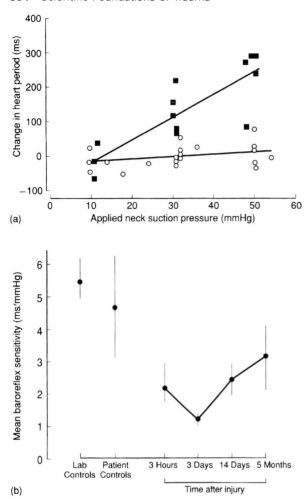

(a)

(b)

Figure 40.2 (a) The relationship between changes in heart period and negative pressure applied to the carotid sinus region of the neck in an injured patient. ○, 2 hours after fracture of the right tibia and fibula; ■, 10 days later. The relationships shown are the lines of best fit calculated by the technique of least mean squares. (b) Baroreflex sensitivity (the gradient of the line relating change in heart period to applied neck suction pressure) in control groups and in patients tested at different times after injury (ISS range 9–17; median 9). Values are shown as mean ± standard error.

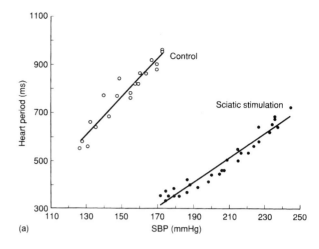

(a)

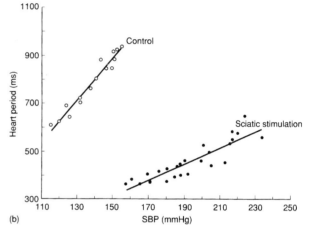

(b)

Figure 40.3 The effects of stimulating electrically the central cut end of the sciatic nerve to mimic injury on the relationship between systolic blood pressure (SBP) and heart period (HP) in a dog anaesthetized with propofol. The slope of this relationship is an index of baroreflex sensitivity, while a lateral displacement indicates a resetting of the reflex. (a) Assessment during 'control' conditions. (b) Assessment during the intravenous infusion of ethanol sufficient to produce a blood ethanol level of 152.1 mg% in the same animal.

have significantly raised plasma ethanol levels (e.g. 100–200 mg%), and although there is no convincing evidence that ethanol consistently modifies baroreflex function (Anderson *et al.*, 1988), it does seem to potentiate the baroreflex impairment elicited by injury (Figure 40.3). Raised plasma ethanol levels also markedly increase the bradycardia elicited by stimulation of the cardiac C-fibre afferents (Kirkman *et al.*, 1990), an interaction which might explain the association between acute alcoholism and hypotension without a tachycardia following relatively minor trauma (Swan *et al.*, 1977).

The afferent pathway of the response to injury appears to run in somatic (including nociceptive) fibres arising in the damaged tissues. Afferent information then ascends in the spinal cord (probably via the spinothalamic tract) to the brain (Redfern *et al.*, 1984). The precise mechanism of the reduction in the sensitivity of the baroreflex is unknown but the response is reminiscent of the visceral alerting response of the defence reaction (Quest and Gebber, 1972). Indeed, lesions of the periaqueductal grey (PAG; an area known to integrate the defence reaction; Hilton and Redfern, 1986) in the rat prevent the reduction in baroreflex sensitivity normally elicited by tissue injury (Jones *et al.*, 1990). Furthermore, the PAG contains cell bodies and nerve terminals which synthesize the opioid met-enkephalin (Uhl *et al.*, 1979), and it has been demonstrated in experimental studies that some of the effects of injury on the baroreflex can be mimicked by the central administration of a long-lasting analogue of met-enkephalin (d-ala^2-met^5-enkephalinamide; Little *et al.*, 1988). Conversely, the administration of naloxone, either centrally or peripherally, can prevent or reverse the reduction in baroreflex sensitivity produced by injury (Eltrafi *et al.*, 1989; Wyatt *et al.*, 1995b). Further studies have indicated that it is μ-opioid receptors and not the δ-receptor subtype which are responsible for the 'injury'-induced reduction in baroreflex sensitivity (Wyatt *et al.*, 1995a).

Many of the responses to injury can be reproduced by the central injection of the neuropeptide corticotrophin releasing factor (CRF). For example, CRF injected intracerebroventricularly reduces baroreflex sensitivity, an effect which can be blocked by pretreatment with the synthetic analogue α-helical CRF$_{9-41}$, which antagonizes the actions of CRF. The same antagonist also prevents the acute (10 min) reduction in baroreflex sensitivity produced by tissue injury, in the propofol anaesthetized rat (Turnbull *et al.*, 1993). Thus it seems possible that there are at least two mechanisms mediating the effects of injury on the baroreflex: an early (10 min) mechanism mediated by CRF followed by a later (30 min) mechanism involving the endogenous opioids acting at μ receptors.

The above discussion has been limited to the effects of injury to peripheral tissues on cardiovascular control. Less detail is known of the effects of head injury on cardiovascular control. However, there is evidence that head injury produces a detrimental effect on the autoregulation of cerebral blood flow (Cold *et al.*, 1977). Additionally, the raised intracranial pressure induced by a head injury produces a resetting of the baroreceptor reflex to a higher working blood pressure in an attempt to maintain cerebral perfusion (Little and Öberg, 1981).

Central nervous pathways organizing the cardiovascular response to injury

The most striking aspects of the response to peripheral injury include the cardiovascular changes and antinociception. Some of the cardiovascular changes have been described in a previous section (see above), while there are numerous anecdotal accounts of the antinociceptive effects of injury. Unfortunately, there is very little in the literature regarding the central nervous organization of these responses to injury. There is, however, a wealth of information concerning pathways which can modulate both cardiovascular function and nociception. One group of central nervous pathways which produce such changes are those involved in the

visceral alerting response of the defence reaction (Lovick, 1985a).

It has been suggested that the response to injury is reminiscent of the visceral alerting response (see above). Activation of the visceral alerting response produces a simultaneous increase in heart rate and blood pressure, and an attenuation of the baroreflex, similar to the changes induced by injury (see above). Furthermore, stimulation within central nervous loci known to be involved in the visceral alerting response also produce antinociception (Duggan and Morton, 1983), again reminiscent of the response to injury. There are also a number of other pathways which may play a role in the response to injury. These pathways, and those involved in the visceral alerting response, will be reviewed briefly in the following section, together with ways in which they may be modulated either pharmacologically or by interaction with other reflex pathways.

Pathways involved in integrating the visceral alerting response of the defence reaction

The visceral alerting response of the defence reaction can be induced by electrical stimulation at a number of sites, including an area in the hypothalamus ventral to the fornix and in the dorsomedial periaqueductal grey (PAG; Yardley and Hilton, 1986). Of these areas, only the dorsomedial PAG appears capable of fully integrating the defence reaction (Hilton and Redfern, 1986), whereas the region in the hypothalamus identified by electrical stimulation (Yardley and Hilton, 1986) may contain fibres of passage from a number of more rostral sites in the hypothalamus which together can integrate the defence reaction (Lovick, 1985b). There is evidence to suggest that the PAG may be involved in the response to injury (see above). This area is known to process afferent nociceptive information (Basbaum and Fields, 1978), and was shown to display increased neuronal activity following injury (Jones, 1989).

The cardiovascular response to injury involves a modulation of two efferent autonomic pathways – the vagal control of heart rate (involved in the baroreflex, see above), and the sympathetic control of the heart and vasculature. For reasons of clarity the effects of the 'defence pathways' on these two efferent pathways will be discussed separately in the following sections, although it must be stressed that the control of the two efferent limbs of the autonomic nervous system are intimately linked.

(a) Modulation of vagal cardiac efferent activity.
The cell bodies of the vagal preganglionic motor-neurones which supply the heart are found in two brain stem nuclei – the nucleus ambiguus and the dorsal vagal motor nucleus (see above). When the baroreceptors are stimulated, activity in the vagal cardiac motorneurones is increased via two main

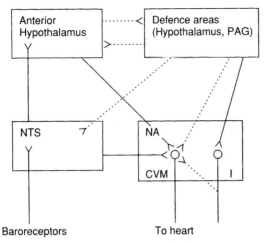

Baroreceptors   To heart

Figure 40.4 Schematic diagram indicating some of the pathways whereby activity in the defence areas (stimulated following injury?) can modify the baroreflex control of vagal efferent activity to the heart. Excitatory pathways are shown as solid lines, inhibitory pathways as broken lines. PAG = periaqueductal grey; NTS = nucleus tractus solitarius; NA = nucleus ambiguus; CVM = cardiac vagal motorneurone; I = inspiratory neurone. See text for details. (Modified from Spyer, 1984.)

excitatory pathways: from the nucleus of the tractus solitarius (NTS, which is the primary relay of the baroreceptor afferents, see above) there is both a 'segmental' pathway within the medulla and a pathway ascending to relay in the anterior hypothalamus before descending again to the vagal nuclei (Spyer, 1984; Figure 40.4). Activity in the 'defence pathways' can inhibit vagal efferent activity by a number of mechanisms. Firstly, there are inhibitory GABA-ergic projections from the defence areas onto the vagal cardiac motorneurones (Jordan et al., 1980). Secondly, activation of the defence reaction can cause an inhibition within the NTS (McAllen, 1976; Mifflin et al., 1988), where GABA has been shown to act as an inhibitory transmitter (Bennett et al., 1987). Also activation of somatic afferent Aδ fibres can lead to inhibition of baroreflex-sensitive neurones within the nucleus of the tractus solitarius and nucleus ambiguus via GABA-ergic mechanisms (e.g. McMahon et al., 1992). The GABA-receptor antagonist bicuculline injected into the fourth cerebral ventricle prevents the injury-induced reduction in baroreflex sensitivity (Wyatt et al., 1994). Thirdly, activation of the defence reaction can lead to an excitation of inspiratory neurones within the nucleus ambiguus (Spyer, 1984), which in turn send an inhibitory cholinergic collateral onto the vagal cardiac preganglionic motorneurones (Garcia et al., 1978). These pathways are summarized in Figure 40.4. The inhibition by the defence reaction may not be restricted to an attenuation of baroreflex-elicited vagal efferent

activity, but may also affect vagal activity generated by other reflexes, for example, by activation of cardiac C-fibre afferents.

(b) Modulation of sympathetic efferent activity. The increase in arterial blood pressure during the visceral alerting response is partly mediated by a sympathetically induced increase in total peripheral resistance. However, the increase in total peripheral resistance is not the result of an indiscriminate vasoconstriction, but rather is due to a highly organized pattern involving increased resistance in vascular beds such as the renal and mesenteric, and a reduction in skeletal muscle vascular resistance. There is sufficient differentiation within the PAG to organize these changes, since it contains groups of cells which are viscerotopically organized with respect to their control over various vascular beds (Carrive et al., 1989).

In addition to the cardiovascular effects, stimulation within the dorsomedial PAG produces an antinociceptive effect (Duggan and Morton, 1983). The efferent pathways mediating the cardiovascular and antinociceptive effects relay in the nucleus paragigantocellularis lateralis (PGL) in the ventrolateral medulla (Hilton et al., 1983; Lovick, 1985a, 1986a).

The PGL appears to integrate the efferent activity of a number of cardiovascular reflexes and response patterns (Lovick, 1987a, 1988a), since it receives inputs from a number of sites which are known to be involved in cardiovascular and somatosensory control. These sites include the hypothalamic and PAG defence areas, the lateral hypothalamus, the nucleus of the solitary tract (NTS), the caudal ventrolateral medulla (CVLM), nucleus raphe magnus (NRM) and obscurus (NRO) and the nucleus parabrachialis (NPB) (Andrezik et al., 1981; Lovick, 1986b, 1988a), many of which converge onto the same neurone in the PGL (Lovick, 1988a). The PGL, in turn, sends an efferent output to the intermediolateral column (Ross et al., 1984; modulation of sympathetic efferent activity) and the dorsal horn (Martin et al., 1979; modulation of nociception) of the spinal cord. Stimulation within the PGL therefore produces sympathoexcitation (McAllen and Dampney, 1990) and antinociception (Lovick, 1987b). However, the sympathoexcitatory and antinociceptive effects are not mediated by the same pool of neurones within the PGL (Lovick, 1987b; Siddall and Dampney, 1989). Indeed, in animals such as the cat the cardiovascular sympathoexcitatory drive originates from a specialized subnucleus, the subretrofacial nucleus (Siddall and Dampney, 1989), where the neurones are arranged topographically according to the type of vascular bed that they control (McAllen and Dampney, 1990), and receive an equally well organized projection from equivalent areas within the PAG (Carrive et al., 1989). Both the cardiovascular and antinociceptive neurones (at least in the rat) are subject to a tonic GABA-ergic inhibition (Lovick, 1987b). However, since different neurones mediate the cardiovascular and anti-nociceptive effects there is a possibility of differentially modulating the two effects. Thus the sympathoexcitatory, but not the antinociceptive drive from the PGL is subject to a tonic cholinergic inhibition (Lovick, 1987b) and can be inhibited by 5-hydroxytryptamine (5HT) injected into the PGL during both 'resting' conditions (Lovick, 1989a), and when enhanced by stimulation of the dorsal PAG (Lovick, 1989b). However, it is possible that 5HT is acting on different cells in the two situations since the latency of the depressor response to 5HT injected into the PGL was much longer when the PAG was stimulated. Additionally, the pressor response elicited by stimulation of the dorsal PAG can be attenuated at the level of the synaptic relay in the PGL by electrical stimulation of the nucleus raphe obscurus (Gong and Li, 1989), which may lead to a release of 5HT within the PGL. Whether 5HT, either injected or released within the PGL, inhibits the sympathoexcitatory cells directly, or via a GABA-ergic interneurone (Lovick, 1988b; McCall, 1988), is unknown (Figure 40.5).

Finally, it has been shown that the activity of the tonically active sympathoexcitatory cells within the PGL is modulated by activity in somatic afferent fibres from skin and muscle (Terui *et al.*, 1987). Interestingly, the sympathoexcitatory cells are inhibited by group III and IV muscle afferent fibres (Terui *et al.*, 1987), which is somewhat surprising since these muscle afferents have been implicated in the response to injury (Redfern *et al.*, 1984). One possible explanation is that whereas these effects of cutaneous and muscle afferents were studied on barosensitive units in the PGL, other non-baro-sensitive units may not behave in the same way.

Involvement of the raphe pathways in the response to injury

There is evidence that peripheral injury also induces an increased neuronal activity within the nucleus raphe magnus (Jones, 1989). In addition, this nucleus has been implicated in modulating sympathetic output to the cardiovascular system and in antinociception. Thus, the nucleus raphe

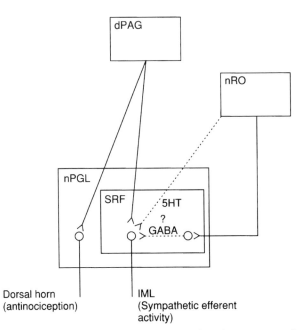

Figure 40.5 Schematic diagram showing some of the possible pathways whereby activity in the dorsal periaqueductal grey may produce sympathoexcitation and antinociception, and how these pathways may be modulated by activation of the raphe. Excitatory pathways are shown as solid lines, inhibitory pathways as broken lines. dPAG = dorsal periaqueductal grey; nRO = nucleus raphe obscurus; nPGL = nucleus paragigantocellularis lateralis; SRF = sub-retrofacial nucleus; IML = intermediolateral cell column of spinal cord. See text for details.

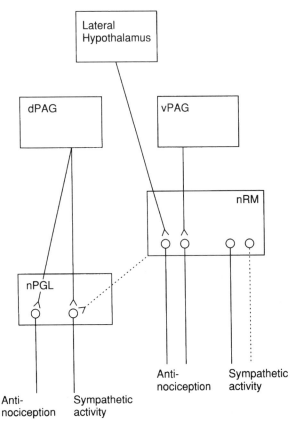

Figure 40.6 Schematic diagram showing possible pathways involving the raphe magnus in modulating sympathetic efferent activity and nociception. Excitatory pathways are shown as solid lines, inhibitory pathways as broken lines. dPAG = dorsal periaqueductal grey; vPAG = ventral periaqueductal grey; nRM = nucleus raphe magnus; nPGL = nucleus paragigantocellularis lateralis. See text for details.

magnus is thought to act as a relay in anti-nociceptive pathways originating in both the lateral hypothalamus (Aimone and Gebhart, 1988) and ventral (but not dorsal) PAG (Praag and Frenk, 1990). Electrical stimulation within the raphe can produce both increases and decreases in blood pressure, the pressor and depressor areas being topographically organized within the nucleus raphe magnus (Adair *et al.*, 1977). The nucleus raphe magnus has been shown to send projections to both the PGL (which are inhibitory, Lovick, 1988a) and to the spinal cord (inhibitory and excitatory, McCall, 1984), and can modulate cardio-vascular activity and nociception. It has therefore been suggested that there are two parallel systems in the medulla each of which controls cardiovascular and somatosensory activity (Lovick, 1988a). When cells in the nucleus raphe magnus are activated they may attenuate activity in the PGL pathway possibly via a GABA-ergic mechanism (Lovick, 1988b; McCall, 1988) to allow the action of the raphe system to predominate (Lovick, 1988a), as shown in Figure 40.6.

There are therefore a number of central nervous pathways which *may* be involved in the cardiovascular response to injury. Further studies, both of these central pathways and of the precise haemodynamic response to injury, are required to determine which, if any, *are* involved in the response to injury.

THE CARDIOVASCULAR RESPONSE TO COMBINED HAEMORRHAGE AND TISSUE INJURY

The cardiovascular changes elicited by a progressive haemorrhage are markedly attenuated by the presence of concomitant tissue injury (Little *et al.*, 1989). The initial tachycardia following a loss of 10–15% blood volume is reduced, and the vagal bradycardia following greater losses prevented (Figure 40.1(b)). This may result from a central inhibition of vagal cardiac preganglionic motor-neurones, since a long-lasting inhibition of such neurones in the nucleus ambiguus has been demonstrated following electrical stimulation of nociceptive afferent fibres (Wang *et al.*, 1988). Somatic afferent stimulation (e.g. of the sciatic nerve) is also able to block the vagal bradycardia evoked by stimulation of either the NTS (Wang *et al.*, 1988) or cardiac C-fibre afferents (E. Kirkman and R.A. Little, unpublished). This attenuation of the heart rate changes normally associated with blood loss seems to offer some degree of protection against the hypotensive effects of a severe haemorrhage (Little *et al.*, 1989). However this protection may be more apparent than real, as a lower survival rate has been demonstrated in animals subjected to haemorrhage and concomitant electrical stimulation of the sciatic nerve (to simulate injury) compared to animals subjected to haemorrhage alone (Overman and Wang, 1947). It is possible that the better maintenance of blood pressure is achieved at the expense of intense peripheral vasoconstriction leading to ischaemic organ damage which will exacerbate the severity of injury. It is tempting to speculate that the splanchnic circulation may be selectively vulnerable to such ischaemic damage leading to the release of blood-borne factors which may impair cardiovascular function (c.f. Chapter 42). There is evidence that when haemorrhage is superimposed on a background of somatic afferent stimulation (to mimic injury) there is a relative redistribution of blood flow from the gut towards skeletal muscle (in contrast to the pattern seen with simple haemorrhage) (Mackway-Jones *et al.*, 1994). This diversion of blood flow (oxygen delivery) away from metabolically active organs (such as the gut) towards relatively inactive resting skeletal muscle may explain the increase in critical oxygen delivery elicited by somatic afferent nerve stimulation (Kirkman *et al.*, 1995). Intestinal permeability may also be increased, leading to enhanced translocation of bacteria and endotoxin (e.g. Wilmore *et al.*, 1988; Deitch, 1990), a suggestion that is reminiscent of Fine's endotoxin theory of shock (Fine, 1961).

The complexity of the interaction between the responses to haemorrhage and to injury is further illustrated by studies which show that the blood loss required to achieve a given reduction in cardiac function and tissue oxygen delivery is less if haemorrhage is superimposed on somatic afferent nerve stimulation compared to haemorrhage alone (Rady *et al.*, 1991). If the haemorrhage is super-

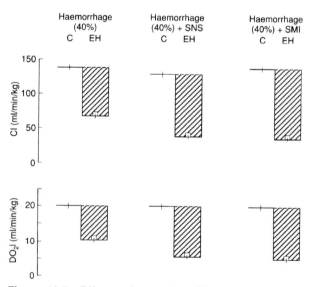

Figure 40.7 Effects of somatic afferent nerve stimulation (SNS) and skeletal muscle injury (SMI) on the changes in cardiac output (expressed as cardiac index, CI) and oxygen delivery index (DO₂I) produced by a haemorrhage of 40% of estimated blood volume in pigs anaesthetized with isoflurane.

imposed on real rather than simulated tissue injury the tolerance to blood loss is reduced even further (Figure 40.7).

CLINICAL IMPLICATIONS

It is, perhaps, premature to consider pharmacological modification of the response to haemorrhage. Although it is apparant that μ-receptor agonists (e.g. morphine and also, perhaps, fentanyl and alfentanyl) or even atropine can prevent the depressor response to severe haemorrhage (see above), it is unclear whether such a manoeuvre would be beneficial or detrimental. It has been suggested that the depressor response may serve to protect the heart by reducing cardiac work at a time when coronary blood flow is compromised. Indeed there have been reports that the administration of atropine in such situations can jeopardize survival (Barriot *et al.*, 1987). The logical treatment is to restore blood volume and hence reduce the activation of the reflex whereupon the bradycardia should correct itself.

The apparently detrimental effect that tissue injury has on the cardiovascular response to fluid loss from the circulation is clinically relevant because haemorrhage is seen most commonly as a consequence of tissue damage. Thus the classical descriptions of the heart rate response to 'simple' haemorrhage may not be applicable to clinical practice except, perhaps, in cases such as bleeding from ruptured varices or aneurysms where direct tissue damage is minimal. The interactions discussed above may explain the limited value of heart rate and blood pressure as signs of hypovolaemia, and why a failure to recognize the presence and/or extent of fluid loss is an important factor in many of the avoidable deaths associated with trauma (West *et al.*, 1979; Anderson *et al.*, 1988b).

The limited usefulness of clinical signs such as heart rate and blood pressure are further illustrated by data collected as early as the First World War. Cowell (1919) observed that traumatic shock was not always accompanied by a tachycardia, and it was concluded that 'blood pressure is of assistance in judging blood volume only when it is below a certain point, for there may be a considerable reduction in blood volume without any appreciable drop in pressure' (Robertson and Bock, 1919). A study of air-raid casualties during the Second World War was also instructive (Grant and Reeve, 1941). All cases studied were classified as shocked, and were described on initial observation as hypertensive (9%), normotensive (28%) or hypotensive (63%). It was emphasized that the normotensive group had sustained severe injuries and blood loss, and had a mortality rate of 25%. The hypotensive group (systolic blood pressure less than 100 mmHg) were further divided into those with a bradycardia (<70 beats/min – 14%), normal pulse rate (43%) or

tachycardia (>100 beats/min – 43%). Overall only 27% of patients observed within the first few hours after severe injury showed the classical signs of hypotension and tachycardia. In a summary of a large amount of data from the Second World War it was concluded that pulse rate was of no value in determining blood volume or the degree of oligaemia (Grant and Reeve, 1951). Systolic blood pressure was considered to be of some use but not as good as the 'measurement' of wound site assessed as imprecisely as 'hands full' of tissue damage.

Analysis of data from the Vietnam conflict confirmed the limited value of pulse rate as an indicator of blood loss. For example, no difference in pulse rate could be found between shocked and non-shocked battlefield casualties with penetrating intraperitoneal wounds as their only significant injuries (Vayer *et al.*, 1988). Indeed of the three casualties studied who died, two had 'normal' pulse rates (68–74 beats/min; Vayer *et al.*, 1988). A similar finding of a relative bradycardia following major injury has been made in a number of studies of civilian trauma (e.g. Sander-Jensen *et al.*, 1986; Barriot and Riou, 1987; Thompson *et al.*, 1990).

The obvious short-comings of blood pressure and pulse rate for assessing hypovolaemia led to the development of the Shock Index (SI), calculated by dividing pulse rate by the systolic blood pressure (Allgöwer and Burri, 1967). It was hoped that combining the changes in pulse rate and blood pressure would give a more sensitive indication of blood loss and a low flow state than either variable used alone. Initial studies showed a direct relationship between SI and the magnitude of blood loss in a

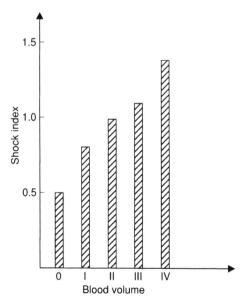

Figure 40.8 The relationship between Shock Index and the magnitude of blood volume loss (O = no loss; I = 10–20% loss; II = 20–30% loss; III = 30–40% loss; IV = 40–50% loss) in man. (Reproduced from Allgöwer and Burri, 1967.)

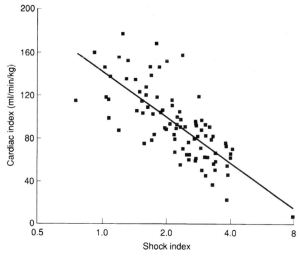

Figure 40.9 The relationship between cardiac output (expressed as cardiac index) and shock index in the isoflurane anaesthetized pig during haemorrhage at a rate of 0.7 ml/min/kg body weight up to a total of 30 ml/kg (approximately 40% of estimated blood volume).

group of patients with either gastrointestinal bleeding, open wounds or intra-abdominal/thoracic bleeding following blunt trauma (Figure 40.8). The SI on admission to hospital was also directly related to subsequent mortality (Allgöwer and Burri, 1967). More recent studies have confirmed the usefulness of SI and suggested that it may be a more sensitive indicator of physiological status after injury than more commonly used indices such as the Revised Trauma Score. Thus in a group of 160 trauma victims with a normal Revised Trauma Score, 69 (43%) had an abnormal SI (Little *et al.*, 1990).

The SI has been further validated in a number of experimental studies. For example, despite the markedly biphasic heart response elicited by 'simple' haemorrhage in the rat, a progressive increase in SI was found as the magnitude of blood loss increased (Little *et al.*, 1990); a relationship that did not appear to be modified by the presence of concomitant tissue injury. It is important to decide what aspect of cardiovascular activity SI is reflecting; further consideration of its calculation suggests that it may be an inverse function of cardiac work and this is confirmed by the finding, during haemorrhage in anaesthetized pigs, of a negative relationship between SI and both left ventricular stroke volume and cardiac output (Figure 40.9). Thus SI seems to be a simple, non-invasive, means of evaluating cardiac function during acute hypovolaemia.

CONCLUSIONS

There is clearly a very complex interaction between the cardiovascular responses to haemorrhage and

to tissue injury which is integrated centrally. Recognition of these changes will improve our ability to appreciate the magnitude of post-traumatic fluid loss, aid the development of more sensitive indicators of such losses and enable the efficacy of resuscitation to be monitored more accurately.

Experimental studies indicate that these interactions may not be beneficial, when considered in terms of survival, and seem to confirm the clinical impression that patients are better able to tolerate blood loss from a 'simple' intestinal haemorrhage than that associated with tissue injury (Tibbs, 1956). The interactions may, however, be beneficial in the short term and help maintain arterial blood pressure and, for example, cerebral blood flow, thereby buying extra time until appropriate therapy can be introduced. The reduction in baroreflex sensitivity induced by injury means that the pressor activity of hormones (e.g. vasopressin) released at this time will not be buffered and will therefore contribute to the immediate homoeostatic response to fluid loss.

If at some time in the future it is deemed desirable to modify these interactions then the pharmacological mediators involved will have to be identified. There is evidence that the endogenous opioids have an important role but it is important that the receptor subtypes involved are identified if the cardiovascular changes are to be modified whilst maintaining analgesia. It may be possible to manipulate the cardiovascular and antinociceptive responses to injury using 5HT agonists and antagonists, but such a possibility lies someway ahead.

REFERENCES

Acker H., O'Regan R.G. (1981). The effects of stimulation of autonomic nerves on carotid body blood flow in the cat. *J. Physiol.*, **315**, 99–110.

Adair J.R., Hamilton B.L., Scappaticci K.A. et al. (1977). Cardiovascular responses to electrical stimulation of the medullary raphe area of the cat. *Brain Res.*, **128**, 141–5.

Aimone L.D., Gebhart G.F. (1988). Serotonin and/or an excitatory amino acid mediates stimulation produced antinociception from the lateral hypothalamus in the rat. *Brain Res.*, **450**, 170–80.

Alam M., Smirk F.H. (1937). Observations in man upon a blood pressure raising reflex arising from the voluntary muscles. *J. Physiol.*, **89**, 372–83.

Alam M., Smirk F.H. (1938). Observations in man upon a pulse accelerating reflex from the voluntary muscles of the legs. *J. Physiol.*, **92**, 167–77.

Allgöwer M., Burri C. (1967). Schockindex. *Deutsche Med. Wochensch.*, **43**, 1–10.

Anderson I.D., Fairhurst J., Heath D.F., Little R.A. (1988a). Effects of acute ethanol ingestion on the arterial baroreflex in man. *J. Physiol.*, **403**, 85P.

Anderson I.D., Woodford M., DeDombal F.T., Irving M.H. (1988b). Retrospective study of 1000 deaths from injury in England and Wales. *Br. Med. J.*, **296**, 1305–8.

Anderson I.D., Little R.A., Irving M.H. (1990). An effect of trauma on human cardiovascular control: baroreflex suppression. *J. Trauma*, **30**, 974–82.

Andrezik J.A., Chan-Palay V., Palay S.L. (1981). The nucleus paragigantocellularis lateralis in the rat. Demonstration of afferents by retrograde transport of horseradish peroxidase. *Anat. Embryol.*, **161**, 373–90.

Angell-James J.E. (1971). The effects of changes in extramural, 'intrathoracic', pressure on aortic-arch baroreceptors. *J. Physiol.*, **214**, 84–103.

Angell-James J.E., Daly M. de B. (1970). Comparison of the reflex vasomotor responses to separate and combined stimulation of the carotid sinus and aortic arch baroreceptors by pulsatile and non-pulsatile pressures in the dog. *J. Physiol.*, **209**, 257–93.

Angell-James J.E., Daly M. de B. (1975). Some aspects of upper respiratory tract reflexes. *Acta Otolaryngol.*, **79**, 242–52.

Barcroft H., Edholm O.G., McMichael J., Sharpey-Schafer E.P. (1944). Posthaemorrhagic fainting. Study by cardiac output and forearm flow. *Lancet*, **i**, 489–91.

Barriot P., Riou B. (1987). Hemorrhagic shock with paradoxical bradycardia. *Int. Care Med.*, **13**, 203–7.

Barriot P., Riou B., Buffat J-J. (1987). Pre-hospital management of severe haemorrhagic shock. In *Update in Intensive Care and Emergency Medicine*, vol. 3 (Vincent J-L., ed.). Berlin: Springer-Verlag, pp. 377–84.

Basbaum A.I., Fields H.L. (1978). Endogenous pain control mechanisms: review and hypothesis. *Ann. Neurol.*, **4**, 451–62.

Bennett J.A., McWilliam P.N., Shepheard S.L. (1987). A gamma-aminobutyric-acid-mediated inhibition of neurones in the nucleus tractus solitarius of the cat. *J. Physiol.*, **392**, 417–30.

Biscoe T.J., Purves M.J., Sampson S.R. (1970). The frequency of nerve impulses in single carotid body chemoreceptor afferent fibres recorded *in vivo* with intact circulation. *J. Physiol.*, **208**, 121–31.

Bogle R.G., Pires J.G., Ramage A.G. (1990). Evidence that central 5-HT1A-receptors play a role in the von Bezold–Jarisch reflex in the rat. *Br. J. Pharmacol.*, **100**, 757–60.

Burke S.L., Dorward P.K. (1988). Influence of endogenous opiates and cardiac baroreceptors on renal nerve activity during haemorrhage in conscious rabbits. *J. Physiol.*, **402**, 9–27.

Carrive P., Bandler R., Dampney R.A.L. (1989). Vis100cerotopic control of regional vascular beds by discrete groups of neurons within the midbrain periaqueductal gray. *Brain Res.*, **493**, 385–90.

Cold G.E., Jensen F.T., Malmros R. (1977). The cerebrovascular CO_2 reactivity during the acute phase of brain injury. *Acta Anaesthesiol. Scand.*, **21**, 222–31.

Cowell E.M. (1919). The initiation of wound shock. Special report series. *Med. Res. Committee*, **25**, 99.

Cowley A.W., Liard J.F., Guyton A.C. (1973). Role of baroreceptor reflex in daily control of arterial blood pressure and other variables in dogs. *Circ. Res.*, **32**, 564–76.

Cowley A.W., Merrill D., Osborn J., Barber B.J. (1984). Influence of vasopressin and angiotensin baroreflexes in the dog. *Circ. Res.*, **54**, 163–72.

Daly M. de B. (1983). Peripheral arterial chemoreceptors and the cardiovascular system. In *Physiology of the Peripheral Arterial Chemoreceptors* (Acker H., O'Regan R.G., eds). Amsterdam: Elsevier Science, pp. 325–93.

Daly M. de B., Lambertsen C.J., Schweitzer A. (1954). Observations on the volume of blood flow and oxygen utilization of the carotid body in the cat. *J. Physiol.*, **125**, 67–89.

Daly M. de B., Kirkman E., Wood L.M. (1988). Cardiovascular responses to stimulation of cardiac receptors in the cat and their modification by changes in respiration. *J. Physiol.*, **407**, 349–62.

Deitch E.A. (1990). Intestinal permeability is increased in burn patients shortly after injury. *Surgery*, **107**, 411–16.

Donoghue S., Felder R.B., Jordan D., Spyer K.M. (1984). The central projections of the carotid baroreceptors and chemoreceptors in the cat: a neurophysiological study. *J. Physiol.*, **347**, 397–409.

D'Silva J.L., Gill D., Mendel D. (1966). The effects of acute haemorrhage on respiration in the cat. *J. Physiol.*, **187**, 369–77.

Duggan A.W., Morton C.R. (1983). Periaqueductal grey stimulation: an association between selective inhibition of dorsal horn neurones and changes in peripheral circulation. *Pain*, **15**, 237–48.

Eltrafi A., Kirkman E., Little R.A. (1989). Reversal of the injury induced reduction in baroreflex sensitivity by naloxone in the conscious rat. *Br. J. Pharmacol.*, **96**, 145P.

Evans R.G., Ludbrook J. (1990). Effects of mu-opioid receptor agonists on circulatory responses to simulated haemorrhage in conscious rabbits. *Br. J. Pharmacol.*, **100**, 421–6.

Evans R.G., Ludbrook J., van Leeuwen A.F. (1989). Role of central opiate receptor subtypes in the circulatory responses of awake rabbits to graded caval occlusions. *J. Physiol.*, **419**, 15–31.

Fine J. (1961). Endotoxins in traumatic shock. *Fed. Proc.*, **20**, (suppl. 9), 166–72.

Garcia M., Jordan D., Spyer K.M. (1978). Studies on the properties of cardiac vagal neurones. *Neurosci. Lett. (Suppl.)*, **1**, S16.

Gong Q.L., Li P. (1989). Inhibitory effect of nucleus raphe obscurus on the pressor response to stimulation of the hypothalamic and midbrain defence areas in the anaesthetized rabbit. *J. Physiol.*, **418**, 85P.

Grant R.T., Reeve E.B. (1941). Clinical observations on air-raid casualties. *Br. Med. J.*, **2**, 293.

Grant R.T., Reeve E.B. (1951). Observations on the general effects of injury in man with special reference to wound shock. Special report series. *Med. Res. Committee*, **277**.

Henry J.L., Calaresu F.R. (1972). Topography and numerical distribution of neurons of the thoraco-lumbar intermediolateral nucleus in the cat. *J. Comp. Neurol.*, **144**, 205–14.

Heymans C., Neil E. (1958). *Reflexogenic Areas of the Cardiovascular System*. London: Churchill.

Hilton S.M., Redfern W.S. (1986). A search for brain stem cell groups integrating the defence reaction in the rat. *J. Physiol.*, **378**, 213–28.

Hilton S.M., Marshall J.M., Timms R.J. (1983). Ventral medullary relay neurones in the pathway from the defence areas of the cat and their effect on blood pressure. *J. Physiol.*, **345**, 149–66.

Izzo P.N., Lin R.J., Richter D.W., Spyer K.M. (1988). Physiological and morphological identification of neurones receiving arterial chemoreceptor afferent input in the nucleus tractus solitarius of the cat. *J. Physiol.*, **399**, 31P.

Jones R.O. (1989). The Identification of the Brain Areas Involved in the Interaction Between Peripheral Injuries and Baroreceptor Reflex Activity in the Rat. PhD Thesis, University of Manchester.

Jones R.O., Kirkman E., Little R.A. (1990). The involvement of the midbrain periaqueductal grey in the cardiovascular response to injury in the conscious and anaesthetized rat. *Exp. Physiol.*, **75**, 483–95.

Jordan D., Khalid M.E.M., Schneiderman N., Spyer K.M. (1980). The inhibitory control of vagal cardiomotor neurones. *J. Physiol.*, **301**, 54P.

Jordan D., Khalid M.E.M., Schneiderman N., Spyer K.M. (1982). The location and properties of preganglionic vagal cardiomotor neurones in rabbit. *Pflügers Arch.*, **395**, 244–50.

Kenney R.A., Neil E. (1951). The contribution of aortic chemoreceptor mechanisms to the maintenance of arterial blood pressure of cats and dogs after haemorrhage. *J. Physiol.*, **112**, 223–81.

Kirchheim H. (1976). Systemic arterial baroreceptor reflexes. *Physiol. Rev.*, **56**, 100–77.

Kirkman E., Scott E.M. (1983). The effect of changes in plasma renin activity on the baroreceptor reflex arc in the cat. *J. Physiol.*, **342**, 73P.

Kirkman E., Marshall H.W., Heyworth J., Little R.A. (1990). Ethanol potentiates the reflex bradycardia elicited by stimulating cardiac C-fibre afferents in the anaesthetised dog. *Br. J. Pharmacol.*, **99**, 22P.

Kirkman E., Shiozaki T., Little R.A. (1994). Methiothepin does not attenuate the bradycardia associated with severe haemorrhage in the anaesthetised rat. *Br. J. Pharmacol.*, **112**, 111P.

Kirkman E., Zhang H., Spapen H. et al. (1995). Effects of afferent neural stimulation on critical oxygen delivery: a hemodynamic explanation. *Am. J. Physiol.*, **38**, R1448–54.

Kunze D.L. (1981). Rapid resetting of the carotid baroreceptor reflex in the cat. *Am. J. Physiol.*, **241**, H802–6.

Little R.A., Öberg B. (1981). Arterial baroreceptor reflex function during elevation of intracranial pressure. *Acta Physiol. Scand.*, **112**, 27–32.

Little R.A., Randall P.E., Redfern W.S. et al. (1984). Components of injury (haemorrhage and tissue ischaemia) affecting cardiovascular reflexes in man and rat. *Q.J. Exp. Physiol.*, **69**, 753–62.

Little R.A., Jones, R.O., Eltraifi A.E. (1988). Cardiovascular reflex function after injury. In *Perspectives in Shock Research. Progress in Clinical and Biological Research*, vol. 264 (Bond R.F., Adams H.R., Chaudry I.H., eds). New York: Liss, pp. 191–200.

Little R.A., Marshall H.W., Kirkman E. (1989). Attenuation of the acute cardiovascular responses to haemorrhage by tissue injury in the conscious rat. *Q.J. Exp. Physiol.*, **74**, 825–33.

Little R.A., Gorman D., Allgöwer M. (1990) The shock index revisited. In *Update in Intensive Care and Emergency Medicine*, vol. 10 (Vincent J.L., ed.). Berlin: Springer-Verlag, pp. 505–12.

Lovick T.A. (1985a). Ventrolateral medullary lesions block the antinociceptive and cardiovascular responses elicited by stimulating the dorsal periaqueductal grey matter in rats. *Pain*, **21**, 241–52.

Lovick T.A. (1985b). Projections from the diencephalon and mesencephalon to nucleus paragigantocellularis lateralis in the cat. *Neuroscience*, **14**, 853–61.

Lovick T.A. (1986a). Analgesia and the cardiovascular changes evoked by stimulating neurones in the ventrolateral medulla in rats. *Pain*, **25**, 259–68.

Lovick T.A. (1986b). Projections from brainstem nuclei to the nucleus paragigantocellularis lateralis in the cat. *J. Auton. Nerv. Syst.*, **16**, 1–11.

Lovick T.A. (1987a). Differential control of cardiac and vasomotor activity by neurones in nucleus paragigantocellularis lateralis in the cat. *J. Physiol.*, **389**, 23–35.

Lovick T.A. (1987b). Tonic GABAergic and cholinergic influences on pain control and cardiovascular control neurones in nucleus paragigantocellularis lateralis in the rat. *Pain*, **31**, 401–9.

Lovick T.A. (1988a). Convergent afferent imports to neurones in nucleus paragigantocellularis lateralis in the cat. *Brain Res.*, **456**, 183–7.

Lovick T.A. (1988b). GABA-mediated inhibition in nucleus paragigantocellularis lateralis in the cat. *Neurosci. Lett.*, **92**, 182.

Lovick T.A. (1989a) Cardiovascular response to 5HT in the ventrolateral medulla of the rat. *J. Auton. Nerv. Syst.*, **28**, 35–41.

Lovick T.A. (1989b). Effect of 5HT in the ventrolateral medulla on the pressor response and analgesia evoked by stimulation of the dorsal periqueductal grey matter in anaesthetized rats. *J. Physiol.*, **418**, 84P.

Ludbrook J., Rutter P.C. (1988). Effect of naloxone on haemodynamic responses to acute blood loss in unanaesthetized rabbits. *J. Physiol.*, **400**, 1–14.

Martin G.F., Humbertson A.O., Laxson C., Panneton W.M. (1979). Evidence for direct bulbospinal projections to laminae IX, X and the intermediolateral cell column. Studies using axonal transport techniques in the North American opossum. *Brain Res.*, **170**, 165–71.

McAllen R.M. (1976). Inhibition of the baroreceptor input to the medulla by stimulation of the hypothalamic defence area. *J. Physiol.*, **257**, 45P.

McAllen R.M., Dampney R.A. (1990). Vasomotor neurons in the rostral ventrolateral medulla are organized topographically with respect to type of vascular bed but not body region. *Neurosci. Lett.*, **110**, 91–6.

McAllen R.M., Spyer K.M. (1976). The location of cardiac vagal preganglionic motorneurones projecting to the heart and lungs. *J. Physiol.*, **282**, 353–64.

McCall R.B. (1984). Evidence for a serotonergically mediated sympathoexcitatory response to stimulation of medullary raphe nuclei. *Brain Res.*, **311**, 131–9.

McCall R.B. (1988). GABA-mediated inhibition of sympathoexcitatory neurons by midline medullary stimulation. *Am. J. Physiol.*, **255**, R605–15.

McMahon S.E., McWilliam P.N., Robertson J., Kaye J.C. (1992). Inhibition of carotid sinus baroreceptor neurones in the nucleus tractus solitarius of the anaesthetized cat by electrical stimulation of hind-limb afferent fibres. *J. Physiol.*, **452**, 224P.

Mackway-Jones K., Foëx B., Kirkman E., Little R.A. (1994). Modification of the haemodynamic response to blood loss by somatic afferent stimulation. *Shock*, **2**, 17.

Mifflin S.W., Spyer K.M., Withington-Wray D.J. (1988). Baroreceptor inputs to the nucleus tractus solitarius in the cat: modulation by the hypothalamus. *J. Physiol.*, **399**, 369–87.

Öberg B., Thorén P. (1972). Increased activity in left ventricular receptors during haemorrhage or occlusion of the caval veins in the cat. A possible cause of the vasovagal reaction. *Acta Physiol. Scand.*, **85**, 164–73.

Öberg B., Thorén P. (1973). Circulatory response to stimulation of left ventricular receptors in the cat. *Acta Physiol. Scand.*, **88**, 8–22.

Ohnishi M., Kirkman E., Marshall H.W., Little R.A. (1996). Morphine blocks the reflex bradycardia associated with severe haemorrhage. *Shock*.

Overman R.R., Wang S.C. (1947). The contributory role of the afferent nervous factor in experimental shock: sublethal haemorrhage and sciatic nerve stimulation. *Am. J. Physiol.*, **148**, 289–95.

Praag H., Frenk H. (1990). The role of glutamate in opiate descending inhibition of nociceptive spinal reflexes. *Brain Res.*, **524**, 101–5.

Quest J.A., Gebber G.L. (1972). Modulation of baroreceptor reflexes by somatic afferent nerve stimulation. *Am. J. Physiol.*, **222**, 1251–9.

Rady M., Little R.A., Edwards J.D. et al. (1991). The effect of nociceptive stimulation on the changes in hemodynamics and oxygen transport induced by hemorrhage in anesthetized pigs. *J. Trauma*, **31**, 617–21.

Redfern W.S. (1981). Effects of Limb Ischaemia on the Cardiac Component of the Baroreceptor Reflex in the Unanaesthetized Rat – afferent, central and efferent mechanisms. PhD Thesis, University of Manchester.

Redfern W.S., Little R.A., Stoner H.B., Marshall H.W. (1984). Effect of limb ischaemia on blood pressure and the blood pressure–heart rate reflex in the rat. *Q.J. Exp. Physiol.*, **69**, 763–79.

Robertson O.H., Bock A.V. (1919). Memorandum on blood volume after haemorrhage. Special report series. *Med. Res. Committee*, **25**, 213–44.

Ross C.A., Ruggiero D.A., Joh T.H. et al. (1984). Rostral ventrolateral medulla: selective projections to the thoracic autonomic cell column from the region containing C_1 adrenaline neurons. *J. Comp. Neurol.*, **228**, 168–85.

Sander-Jensen K., Secher N.H., Bie P. et al. (1986). Vagal slowing of the heart during haemorrhage: observations from 20 consecutive hypotensive patients. *Br. Med. J.*, **292**, 364–6.

Scherrer U., Vissing, S., Morgan B. et al. (1990). Vasovagal syncope after infusion of a vasodilator in a heart-transplant recipient. *New Engl. J. Med.*, **322**, 602–4.

Scott, E.M. (1983). Reflex control of the cardiovascular system and its modification – some implications for pharmacologists. *J. Auton. Pharmacol.*, **3**, 113–26.

Secher N.H., Bie P. (1985). Bradycardia during reversible haemorrhagic shock – a forgotten observation? *Clin. Physiol.*, **5**, 315–23.

Shen Y.T., Knight D.R., Thomas J.X., Vatner S.F. (1990). Relative roles of cardiac receptors and arterial baroreceptors during haemorrhage in conscious dogs. *Circ. Res.*, **66**, 397.

Siddall P.J., Dampney R.A. (1989). Relationship between cardiovascular neurones and descending antinociceptive pathways in the rostral ventrolateral medulla of the cat. *Pain*, **37**, 347–55.

Spyer K.M. (1984). Central control of the cardiovascular system. *Recent Adv. Physiol.*, **10**, 163.

Swan K.G., Vidaver R.M., Lavigne J.E., Brown C.S. (1977). Acute alcoholism, minor trauma and 'shock'. *J. Trauma*, **17**, 215–18.

Terui N., Saeki Y., Kumada M. (1987). Confluence of barosensory and nonbarosensory inputs at neurons in the ventrolateral medulla in rabbits. *Can. J. Physiol. Pharmacol.*, **65**, 1584–90.

Thompson D., Adams S.L., Barrett J. (1990). Relative bradycardia in patients with isolated penetrating abdominal trauma and isolated extremity trauma. *Ann. Emerg. Med.*, **19**, 268.

Tibbs D.J. (1956). Blood volumes in gastroduodenal haemorrhage. *Lancet*, **ii**, 266–74.

Turnbull A.V., Kirkman E., Rothwell N.J., Little R.A. (1993). Corticotrophin-releasing factor (CRF) is involved in the modulation of the baroreflex following bilateral hindlimb ischaemia in the propofol anaesthetized rat. *J. Physiol.*, **468**, 529–41.

Uhl G.R., Goodman R.R., Kuhar M.J. et al. (1979). Immunohistochemical mapping of enkephalin containing cell bodies, fibres and nerve terminals in the brain stem of the rat. *Brain Res.*, **166**, 75–94.

Vayer J.S., Henderson J.V., Bellamy R.F., Galper A.R. (1988). Absence of a tachycardic response to shock in penetrating intraperitoneal injury. *Ann. Emerg. Med.*, **17**, 227–31.

Wang Q., Guo X-Q., Li P. (1988). The inhibitory effects of somatic input on the excitatory responses of vagal cardiomotor neurones to stimulation of the nucleus tractus solitarius in rabbits. *Brain Res.*, **439**, 350–3.

West J., Trunkey D.D., Lim R.C. (1979). Systems of trauma care. *Arch. Surg.*, **114**, 455–60.

Wilmore D.W., Smith R.J., O'Dwyer S.T. et al. (1988). The gut: a central organ after surgical stress. *Surgery*, **104**, 917–23.

Wyatt J., Kirkman E., Little R.A. (1994). 'Injury'-induced decreases in baroreflex sensitivity are mediated via endogenous GABA. *Shock*, **2**, 50.

Wyatt J., Kirkman E., Little R.A. (1995a). Reversal of injury induced reductions in baroreflex sensitivity by β-funaltrexamine in the anaesthetised rat. *Physiol. Zool.*, **68**, 67.

Wyatt J., Kirkman E., Little R.A. (1995b). Reversal of the 'injury'-induced reductions in baroreflex sensitivity by naloxone. *Fund. Clin. Pharmacol.*

Yardley C.P., Hilton S.M. (1986). The hypothalamic and brainstem areas from which the cardiovascular and behavioural components of the defence reaction are elicited in the rat. *J. Auton. Nerv. Syst.*, **15**, 227–44.

41. Cardiac Responses to Injury

R. D. Goldfarb, J. Flor and R. R. Gandhi

INTRODUCTION

Shock, trauma, burns and sepsis lead to the dysfunction of many organ systems, a process which, if not treated, leads to the development of multiorgan system failure and death. As the technology to immediately resuscitate trauma and burn victims becomes widely available, incidence of multiple organ failure secondary to trauma has become a leading cause of death in intensive care facilities. There is overwhelming evidence that ventricular performance is depressed during shock or systemic sepsis in patients and experimental models of sepsis (Cunnion et al., 1986; Natanson et al., 1986, Abel, 1989; Parker et al., 1989). This chapter will review the physiology of cardiac contraction, in vivo evaluation of cardiac contraction, cardiac performance during human shock, trauma, burns or sepsis and review the appropriate experimental models. Furthermore, potential mechanisms for loss of cardiac inotropism during these states will be discussed.

The heart's role in the biological response to shock, burns or sepsis has been of intensive interest, and only now has a consensus been reached that ventricular function is compromised during these conditions. As late as 1983 when Downing (1983) reviewed the then current literature evaluating cardiac function in shock, he stated that although most studies indicated that shock was associated with myocardial structural and functional damage, many investigators held that pump failure contributed little to multiorgan failure of shock. Six years later, Abel (1989) was able to state that overwhelming evidence existed for the concept that sepsis and endotoxin challenge induce significant myocardial damage and this damage was coincident with development of multiorgan systems failure. This conclusion was supported by newly developed assessments of cardiac inotropism which were independent of loading conditions, especially the slope of the end-systolic pressure–volume relationship (ESPVR; Sagawa, 1978). Indeed, Cunnion and Parrillo suggested that cardiac failure was the major cause of death in 10–15% of trauma patients and a major contributor in another 20–30% (Cunnion and Parrillo, 1989). The disparate results from initial studies were caused by differing experimental species, differing models of experimental trauma or sepsis, etc. However, many insupportable conclusions were reached by use of indices of cardiac dynamics that were not load independent (reviewed in Goldfarb, 1982b). In the early 1980s use of load independent assessments of cardiac inotropism became widespread and these results supported Abel's statement 'overwhelming evidence that the performance of the myocardium is depressed...' (Abel, 1989).

In order to understand mechanisms by which cardiac inotropism is affected by sepsis, trauma or burns, it will be necessary to review fundamental principles of cardiac contraction. A brief discussion of cardiac ultrastructure, molecular interactions which generate force, determinants of cardiac performance and technical means to assess cardiac function are presented below. A fuller description of these topics can be found in Katz (1992).

REVIEW OF CARDIAC PHYSIOLOGY

Cardiac ultrastructure

The functional unit of a myocardial cell is the sarcomere, consisting of parallel arrays of overlapping thick and thin filaments. Each thin filament of sarcomere consists of filamentous actin, tropomyosin and troponin. A thin filament's backbone is F-actin, two strands of polymerized G-actin molecules in a double helix. Tropomyosin, an elongated protein, lies in the grooves of the F-actin helix and troponin, a complex of three proteins, is bound to tropomyosin. The thick filament consists of myosin, a high-molecular-weight protein consisting of three pairs of chains: two heavy and one light chain. Two heavy chains form a supercoil that produces two globular heads and a long rigid tail. During contraction, the heads of the myosin molecules, the cross-bridges, interact with active sites on actin.

Cardiac contraction

Contraction of cardiac fibres is initiated by electrical excitation of cardiac membranes. In cardiac muscle cells, depolarization is initiated by opening of fast Na^+ channels which allows entry of Na^+ ions depolarizing the cardiac membrane. Increased membrane potential opens a second cationic channel, slow Ca^{++} channel, which allows entry of Ca^{++} into the myocyte initiating contraction through several different Ca^{++} pools. Contraction is mediated by variation in $[Ca^{++}]_i$: at low $[Ca^{++}]_i$, troponin and tropomyosin block interactions of actin and myosin; at high $[Ca^{++}]_i$, Ca^{++} binds troponin causing a conformational change in the troponin–tropomyosin complex exposing myosin binding sites of actin. Attachment of myosin to actin, cross-bridging, produces a conformational change that pulls thin filaments towards each other shortening the sarcomere. Energy for cross-bridge cycling appears to be consumed during formation of the actin–myosin interaction. Upon complete cycling, ADP and P_i are released, with a net result that one complete cross-bridge cycle results in one ATP hydrolysed, energy liberated, force generated and sarcomere shortening. Myosin light chains regulate the rate of ATP hydrolysis and, thus, all expressions of energy liberation. Relaxation occurs as Ca^{++} is pumped out of the cells and less becomes available for cross-bridging. Cross-bridges are broken and not re-formed, ending contraction and beginning relaxation.

The flux of Ca^{++} across the plasma membrane during excitation is not sufficient to activate contraction. Activator Ca^{++}, the Ca^{++} which binds to troponin, comes from the sarcoplasmic reticulum (SR) which also initiates and completes removal of intracellular Ca^{++} so that relaxation can occur. The SR is a calcium sequestering organelle with a large surface area for rapid release and reuptake of Ca^{++}. It consists of two sections, terminal cisternae coupled to long, thin longitudinal sections. Terminal cisternae are in close proximity to sarcolemma and this is where Ca^{++} is initially released during an action potential. Calsequestrin, a Ca^{++} binding protein, is present in the SR and it enhances the rate of reuptake by lowering the $[Ca^{++}]_i$ of SR, thus maintaining the Ca^{++} gradient between the cytosol and SR.

The SR flux of Ca^{++} across the SR during the cardiac cycle is vastly important to the dynamics of cardiac contraction. In contrast to skeletal muscles, the amount of Ca^{++} released for binding with cardiac troponin C can be modulated during excitation. Thus, force generation can be modulated by external influences. It is this property of the cardiac muscle, modulation of SR released Ca^{++} for binding to troponin C, which is the molecular basis of inotropism.

Physiological basis of inotropism

Cardiac muscle, in contrast to skeletal muscle, has an intrinsic ability to modify its strength of contraction without a change in its initial fibre length. 'Inotropic state' refers to quantification of this ability. Thus, cardiac muscle can change its force-generating capacity by two mechanisms; by changing its initial length so that an altered number of actin–myosin binding sites become available for cross-bridging and by altering the amount of sarcoplasmic reticulum released Ca^{++} during excitation so that more cross-bridges per unit length of sarcomere can be formed.

Cardiac inotropism is subject to physiological regulation by sympathetic and parasympathetic systems due to their ability to alter sarcolemmal conductance to Ca^{++}. The sympathetic system releases norepinephrine locally or humorally which stimulate β-adrenergic receptors on cardiac cells, stimulating adenyl cyclase to increase intracellular cAMP which augments conductance of cardiac cells to Ca^{++}. This increased intracellular Ca^{++} permits increased cross-bridge formation and increased force generation at fixed sarcomere length. The parasympathetic system releases acetylcholine which stimulates guanyl cyclase forming cGMP which inhibits Ca^{++} conductance of cardiac cells. Acetylcholine also can presynaptically inhibit sympathetic neuron release of catecholamines. Thus, the parasympathetic system has several mechanisms by which it can decrease contractile force, with the final pathway a decrease in the availability of intracellular Ca^{++} upon excitation.

Determinants of cardiac performance

Inotropism, discussed above, is only one of four determinants of cardiac performance. Other determinants are heart rate, preload (initial fibre length) and afterload. Interrelationships between these determinants are complex, but must be understood in order to properly evaluate cardiac performance *in vivo*. Understanding these complexities is necessary because cardiac contraction *in vivo* is isotonic; it develops force (pressure) until ventricular pressure overcomes its afterload (aortic diastolic pressure), its aortic valve opens and then ventricular shortening proceeds at a relatively constant pressure. Each of these determinants are under

TABLE 41.1
DEFINITIONS OF TERMS EMPLOYED IN CARDIAC MECHANICS

Determinants of cardiac performance:
  Cardiac performance:
    quantification of cardiac pumping action
  Preload:
    force acting on ventricle at end-diastole – often assessed by ventricular fibre length at end-diastole
  Afterload:
    force preventing the ventricle from emptying – pressure in the aorta at end-diastole
  Rate:
    number of heart beats per minute
  Inotropic state:
    ability of cardiac muscle to change developed force or work *without* a change in diastolic fibre length

Inotropic agent – an agent that can alter inotropic state
  A *positive* inotrope *increases* inotropic state
  A *negative* inotrope *decreases* inotropic state

Venous return – rate of blood flow to heart per unit time (ml/s; l/min)

  E_{max} or E_{es} = maximal value of ratio of ventricular pressure to volume during a cardiac cycle which occurs at end-systole

ESPVR (end-systolic pressure–volume relationship) – relationship of pressure and volume at sequential E_{es} points obtained under different loading conditions

Starling relationship – regression of stroke work to end-diastolic volume over several beats

independant control but alteration of one determinant will affect others (Table 41.1).

Cardiac performance *in vivo* is quantification of the cardiac cycle's contractile phase which must be made in physical terms; for example, stroke volume, pressure generation, stroke work, etc. However, the ventricle is in a closed cardiac-vascular system where each part of the system effects the other parts. Other parts of this system include: heart, large arteries, arterioles, capillaries, venules and large veins. All of these components are modulated by sympathetic and parasympathetic neurohormonal systems, blood volume, as well as other regulatory systems.

The magnitude of *in vivo* cardiac performance, a physical measurement, is determined by afterload, preload, heart rate and inotropic state (Figure 41.1). Preload is a force which distends the ventricle prior to contraction – end-diastolic pressure. It determines myocardial fibre length, and thus thin-thick filament overlap, before contraction and is a function of diastolic filling rate and heart rate. Therefore, venous compliance, which is dependent on sympathetic tone, contributes to ventricular performance by regulating venous return per unit time. Blood volume also affects preload; decreases in blood volume will decrease venous return. Afterload is a force which the ventricle must generate in order to shorten, quantified by the pressure at aortic valve opening. It is dependent upon arterial vasculature impedance, large artery elastance and arteriolar resistance. Increases in α-sympathetic tone will increase afterload by increasing arterial elastance and arteriolar resistance restricting cardiac performance. Heart rate

changes can also affect cardiac performance. As heart rate increases, time for removal of Ca^{++} from the myoplasm is reduced so that upon subsequent contractions $[Ca^{++}]_i$ is increased, increasing the rate of cross-bridge formation. Thus, each precondition of cardiac contraction can affect cardiac performance independently.

The fourth determinant of cardiac performance is inotropic state, the quantification of ability of cardiac muscle to alter force generation without a change in resting fibre length. An increase in inotropic state increases force generation at every point of the length–tension relationship. Cardiac muscle, unlike skeletal muscle, does not generate maximal force upon stimulation. Combining this ability to alter force generation at a constant initial length with length-dependant changes in force, allows a ventricle to adjust to widely varying alterations of loading conditions and rate that occur constantly.

In vivo, the heart acts as a demand pump; that is, its performance, quantified by stroke work, is matched to peripheral demand so each contraction is unique. Beat-to-beat variations in stroke work are due to an interaction of subtle alterations of preload, end-diastolic volume, and afterload, end-diastolic aortic pressure. Heart rate is modulated by autonomic influences on SA nodal pacemaker cells. For example, subtle alterations in autonomic outflow occur on sequential beats due to respiration. Centrally induced sympathetic stimulation, caused by neurogenic influences (fright, flight of fight responses), exercise tachycardia or shock will cause heart rate to accelerate to over 200 bpm in man. As heart rate rises, unless venous return rate increases in equal magnitude, stroke volume will fall. An increased inotropic state induced by sympathetic drive in isolation should increase cardiac performance, stroke work. However, *in vivo*, increased inotropism will increase cardiac emptying so unless venous return also increases, preload will decrease on subsequent beats so that stroke volume will remain constant, albeit at lower end-diastolic and end-systolic volumes. Even this simple example demonstrates that an accurate understanding of the interrelationship between the four determinants of cardiac performance can be difficult to achieve. Analysis of cardiac pressure–volume diagrams has proved to be helpful in achieving this understanding, both in theory and in practice (Figure 41.2).

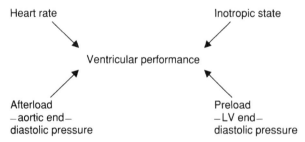

Determinants of cardiac performance

Figure 41.1 Ventricular performance, defined as work done on the vascular system by the ventricle, is determined by four factors: heart rate, inotropic state, preload (ventricular distending force immediately prior to contraction) and afterload (force the ventricle must generate in order to empty). A change in any one of these determinants will alter ventricular performance or work as well as other determinants of performance. For instance, an increase in afterload will reduce ventricular emptying, increasing ventricular residual volume so that, if diastolic filling rate remains constant, preload will increase.

In Vivo assessments of cardiac performance and inotropic state

Evaluation of cardiac performance can be made relatively easily since it is a physical quantity, stroke work. This evaluation allows one to determine whether the heart is meeting peripheral demands. Three preconditions of contraction, preload, afterload and rate, are quite easily meas-

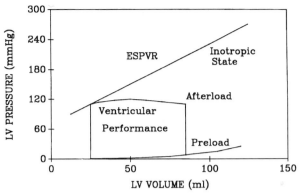

Figure 41.2 Ventricular performance and its determinants are presented within the ventricular pressure–volume loop diagram. Ventricular function is the area within the P–V loop, quantified by stroke work. Preload for each cardiac cycle is the point on the diastolic filling curve (bottom curve) when contraction begins. Afterload is the pressure at which ventricular emptying begins and isotonic contraction commences. Ejection ends when ventricular pressure and volume intercept the top curve, end-systolic pressure–volume relationship (ESPVR). The degree of emptying is determined by the slope of ESPVR, indicative of inotropic state. An increased inotropic state rotates ESPVR counter-clockwise so that ejection is more complete.

ured. However, the fourth, inotropism, is not so easily measured, and indeed much investigation has been conducted to find an easy and appropriate method for its evaluation. The paradox is that all assessments of inotropism are physical measures of cardiac performance and are, thus, more or less dependent upon the other three preconditions of cardiac contraction. Evaluation of inotropism needs to be made by measuring a physical performance relationship that is independent of the other preconditions of cardiac contraction. For example, the Starling relationship relates cardiac work to preload at fixed afterload and rate so that an increased slope indicates an increased inotropic state. This relationship is an extension of the isometric length–tension relationship which assumes a fixed, infinite afterload. *In vivo*, alterations in afterload will change the slope of the Starling curve so that it may be an unreliable index of inotropism.

Several multi-beat relationships describing cardiac performance have been suggested to assess inotropic state accurately. The relationship between stroke work and end-diastolic volume, the classic Starling relationship first observed in frog ventricle, has been used extensively in clinical and experimental studies (Parker *et al.*, 1984; Sibbald and Drieger, 1985; Natanson *et al.*, 1986). A similar relationship between maximal dP/dt and end-diastolic volume has also been proposed

as an accurate assessor of inotropic state. However, these assessments of ventricular inotropic state *in vivo* are complicated by an inability to experimentally fix preload, afterload and heart rate *in vivo*. Therefore, an accurate assessment of inotropic state will vary with altered inotropism but be independent of altered preload, afterload and rate. The Starling relationship (Starling 1918), a mathematical regression between ventricular performance and preload, is based upon the fundamental relationship of isovolumetric length–tension. However, the heart contracts isotonically *in vivo* so that this approach is limited.

The slope of the end-systolic pressure–diameter relationship (ESPDR) has been proposed as an accurate assessor of inotropism despite changes in preload and afterload. The concept that the relationship between left ventricular pressure and volume at end-systole accurately reflects inotropism is founded on the analysis of isotonic contraction. It was found that the magnitude of the slope of the end-systolic pressure–volume relationship (ESPVR) was determined almost entirely by the inotropic state of the ventricle and that preload and afterload had minimal effects within physiological ranges (Sagawa, 1978). Initial studies reported ESPVR to be a linear, sensitive measure of inotropism that is insensitive to heart rate, preload and afterload (Sagawa, 1978; Goldfarb *et al.*, 1989). These studies were performed using excised, intact ventricles, with artificial loading systems for filling and with ejection into a computer-simulated servomechanism, simulating a Windkessel model. The slope of ESPVR was constant despite changes in 'aortic' resistance, capacitance, or characteristic impedance (Sagawa, 1978).

Andrejuk *et al.* (1991) demonstrated that ESPDR was a most robust measurement of inotropism *in vivo* during large changes of preload and afterload. Their study also demonstrated that simplified one-dimension measurement of the slopes of both ESPDR and SWEDD (stroke work to end-diastolic diameter) were valid for assessment of cardiac performance in altered loading conditions. Of the three relations (ESPDR, DPEDD and SWEDD), ESPDR had the best linearity with both caval occlusion and aortic occlusion producing slopes that were consistently positive, but not necessarily equal. SWEDD had good linearity with preload reduction but not with increased afterload. The most unexpected observation was that DPEDD (the relationship between dP/dt_{max} and end-diastolic diameter) was parabolic, with the peak at steady state, and positive slopes during caval occlusion and negative slopes during aortic occlusion. In addition, ESPDR and SWEDD were more repeatable with less variation in steady state than DPEDD in a relatively stable open-chest animal preparation.

CARDIAC DYNAMICS DURING SHOCK AND TRAUMA

Definitions of trauma, burn, sepsis and shock

Shock can be defined as circulatory collapse leading to decreased tissue oxygenation (Waxman, 1986) and is initiated by an insult to the organism. Some frequent insults are: trauma – wounding of soft tissue (Stoner, 1987), burn – thermal injury extending to a full-thickness lesion of the dermis, sepsis – systemic infection, discrete mechanical cardiac failure such as dilated cardiomyopathy of cardiac tamponade, or neurogenic failure. Despite the variety of initial insults, shock develops via a common path. These initiating insults lead to loss of circulating vascular volume and release of toxic mediators such as cytokines, prostaglandins, catecholamines, vasopressin, ACTH, glucagon, cortisol and reactive oxidants. If the degree and duration of an initial insult is severe and prolonged, compensatory mechanisms are not sufficient to restore homoeostasis, so that shock, prolonged cardiovascular system failure to meet peripheral needs, develops. Multiple organ dysfunction results from prolonged circulatory collapse as evidenced by decreased circulating volume and decrements in tissue oxygenation.

Burn is an injury to the skin caused by high thermal loads accompanied by fluid loss due to evaporation and/or extrusion of fluid through the burn wound. In addition, many tissue-generated substances which mediate cardiovascular dysfunction are released into the circulation. Circulatory collapse following burn injury is due to systemic vascular volume depletion exacerbated by the deficit of tissue oxygenation, due to the failure to meet the increased tissue oxygen demand of the regenerative process.

Sepsis remains a subject of intensive investigation because it has become a common cause of death in the modern hospital setting (Goodwin and Schaer, 1989; Cunnion and Parrillo, 1989). The biological response to systemic infection is multiphasic. The severity of the response to vascular invasion by bacteria is dependant upon numbers of bacteria entering the vascular system and the temporal dynamics of this invasion. The initial cardiovascular response is termed 'hyperdynamic' and is characterized by decreased peripheral resistance, increased heart rate, body temperature, cardiac output and cardiac work. This period of hyperdynamism can persist for extended periods and is resolved by recovery or development of a second phase; 'hypodynamic' sepsis. Hypodynamic sepsis is characterized by decreased cardiac output and cardiac work, increased peripheral resistance and very high heart rates. Often, hypodynamic sepsis leads to death. Clinical features of sepsis include signs and symptoms of an infection such as chills, fever (Luce, 1987), tachycardia, tachypnoea, leukocytosis, thrombocytopenia, nausea, vomiting, decreased urine output, decreased mentation and other signs of decreased organ perfusion (Robie, 1984; Goodwin and Schaer, 1989). In addition, there may be respiratory alkalosis and metabolic acidosis in the early stages.

The discussion that follows is largely based on studies in sepsis or endotoxaemia but it is still relevant to a consideration of the responses to trauma/burns. In the early response to accidental injuries of the skin and perhaps even of the gut barrier, function is compromised and microorganisms and their associated toxins gain access to the circulation. Following the acute phase, a hypermetabolic flow phase sepsis is a common complication and can be a prominent feature of multiple organ failure.

Sepsis and cardiovascular function

Many experimental models of sepsis have been used in attempts to mimic human sepsis. In many such models a component of the bacterial cell wall, endotoxin, is used. Endotoxin, or lipopolysaccharide, is composed of three parts: an O antigen side chain which is unique to each phenotype, R cone antigen and lipid antigen. The biological response to endotoxin mimics sepsis only when it is administered over an extended time duration rather than as a bolus. An experimental model of human systemic sepsis was developed by Fish and Spitzer (1984) for rats and modified by Lee et al. for larger animals (1988a,b). This model which uses a continuous intravenous infusion of endotoxin from an implanted osmotic infusion pump induces hypermetabolism, elevated cardiac outputs, reduced peripheral resistance, increased heart rate and decreased inotropism (Fish and Spitzer, 1984; Lee et al., 1988a,b), thereby replicating many of the responses of human systemic sepsis (Parker et al., 1984; Cunnion et al., 1986; Natanson et al., 1986). Previously sepsis had been mimicked by the bolus administration of endotoxin which leads to acute decreases in cardiac output and blood pressure, which elicit increased adrenergic tone and elevated peripheral resistance (Goldfarb et al., 1986). The results of these studies demonstrate that the responses to 'bolus' endotoxaemia are unlike those to systemic sepsis primarily because of the rapid onset of insult.

The model of Fish and Spitzer (1984) was adapted for evaluation of myocardial inotropism and coronary flow regulation in pigs (Lee et al., 1988a,b). High cardiac output, heart rate and dP/dt_{max} were associated with reduced myocardial inotropism (reduced end-systolic pressure–diameter relationship (ESPDR) and % diameter shortening). Percentage shortening, a measure of inotropic state independent of ESPDR, confirmed these data. Despite intensive research, causes of prolonged cardiac impairment in sepsis have not been established definitively. One proposed mechanism for reduced inotropism was inadequate coronary flow (Goldfarb *et al.*, 1986; Abel, 1989). Lee *et al.* measured coronary flow and flow to work ratios in endotoxaemic pigs with elevated cardiac outputs, and found that the myocardium was hyperperfused rather than underperfused (Lee *et al.*, 1988b). Studies in septic patients (Goldfarb *et al.*, 1986) support these observations.

Sepsis generates cardiovascular responses which impose maximal cardiac stresses. To understand the results of these stresses on cardiac function, one needs to discern effects of altered loading conditions and rate on cardiac function as distinguished from altered inotropism. Bacteraemia leads to an initial development of hyperdynamic cardiovascular function characterized by increased cardiac output and heart rate. Bacteraemia causes peripheral vasodilatation, possibly caused by direct vascular effects of bacteria and/or indirectly by inducing hypermetabolic vasodilatation in systemic tissues. In these circumstances, preconditions of cardiac performance (Figure 41.1) change radically and simultaneously. For example, peripheral vasodilatation produces decreased cardiac afterload and increased venous return, possibly increasing preload (only if heart rate increase is proportionally less than increased venous return). These circumstances, plotted on a pressure–volume (P–V) diagram (Figure 41.2), will show increased width of the P–V loop and a slightly lowered top (as afterload is reduced). Stroke volume will increase (area of P–V loop) but whether inotropism is altered cannot be defined. Indeed, endotoxin infusion in healthy humans decreases stroke–volume index, stroke–volume index normalized to end-diastolic volume, and ratio of peak systolic pressure to end-systolic volume index (Suffredini *et al.*, 1989). Thus, use of indices of cardiac performance that are independent of preload, afterload and rate but sensitive to inotropic state must be used in sepsis otherwise deceptive results can be obtained.

Clinical evaluation of cardiac function

Cardiac inotropism during sepsis is not easily assessed in a patient, although some parameters of cardiac performance can be measured at the bedside. Non-invasive techniques (Sharpe *et al.*, 1985) can be used but may be inaccurate, while invasive techniques can be accurate but many have deleterious effects on the patient including infection and serious blood loss. Vital signs are among the most common noninvasive techniques including pulse rate and blood pressure (Waxman, 1986). While the results from these simple studies may suggest sepsis, they are non-specific. Blood pressure may increase but this increase does not necessarily mean an increase in cardiac output; for example, increased vascular resistance (increased afterload) actually decreasing the cardiac output. The 12-lead electrocardiogram is a non-invasive tool for monitoring cardiac performance. The ECG can diagnose ischaemic heart disease due to acute myocardial infarction, congestive heart failure and hypoxia.

Radiological tests are also used to obtain data for cardiovascular evaluation. Chest X-rays may help diagnose displacement of the heart, congestive heart failure, cardiac chamber hypertrophy, dilatation and restrictive filling of the heart. Heart disease may be diagnosed if the cardiothoracic ratio (maximum transverse cardiac diameter/maximum transverse thoracic diameter) is greater than 55%. However the quality of the X-ray may be compromised by, for example, less than optimal degrees of exposure of the film, degree of rotation, exposure at maximal lung inflation, and the amount of PEEP a patient is receiving.

Echocardiography is a novel non-invasive technique which can evaluate cardiac dynamics with great sophistication. This technique may be able to detect pericardial effusion, pressure/volume overload, mitral stenosis, mitral insufficiency, mitral regurgitation, prolapsing mitral valve, aortic stenosis, bicuspid insufficiency, intracardiac tumours, cardiomyopathy, congenital heart disease, left ventricular volume (Weiss *et al.*, 1983), right ventricular volume (Linker *et al.*, 1986), vegetation in endocarditis and traumatic myocardial contusion. Unfortunately, the mathematical models to date are not always accurate and cannot reliably provide data concerning right ventricular performance.

Invasive techniques are powerful tools for obtaining accurate, minute to minute information but have risks to the patient not associated with non-invasive techniques. Catheterization of an artery allows monitoring of blood pressure as well as easy access to arterial blood for blood gas measurements. Pulmonary artery catheterization has become routine for measurement of central venous pressure, pulmonary artery systolic and diastolic pressures, pulmonary artery wedge pressure (which is related to left ventricular stroke work but is dependent on ventricular contractility, Waxman, 1986), mixed venous oxygen tension, serial monitoring of right ventricular function (Dhainaut *et al.*, 1987) and cardiac output. Measurement of cardiac output is fairly accurate (Kay *et al.*, 1983; Vincent *et al.*, 1986) and can help to evaluate shock. Hypovolaemic shock is characterized by a low pulmonary artery wedge pressure while cardiogenic shock has a high pulmonary artery wedge pressure. While these invasive techniques are useful for obtaining accurate, reliable information, they have many risks to the patient. These include arrhythmias, bundle branch block, thrombosis, pulmonary infarction, artery rupture, pneumothorax, haemothorax, cardiac complications, knotting of the cannula, haemorrhage, embolism, and infection.

Management by mechanism-oriented therapy

Since shock entails decreased tissue oxygenation, it has been hypothesized that an appropriate treatment would be to increase blood oxygenation. This increased oxygenation may be achieved by increasing blood oxygen carrying capacity by 'artificial blood', increasing haematocrit by transfusion of synthetic blood products. Since blood volume is decreased in shock, crystalloid solutions have been employed to increase vascular volume (Rackow et al., 1988). Since the host response to sepsis and shock is responsible for the mediator release and subsequent decline in cardiovascular function, control of bacteraemia and infection is essential, possibly combined with immunosuppression. Immunosuppressive therapy with steroids has been tried, but with little success, possibly because the doses were too high and continued for a longer period of time than necessary – indeed a relatively small, one-time dose may be more effective (Sheagren et al., 1989; Putterman, 1990). Non-steroidal anti-inflammatory therapy may also help and be associated with less side-effects than steroid therapy. Finally, since toxic oxygen radicals have been suspected as causes of tissue damage, toxic oxygen radical scavengers may be used as part of shock therapy. Cardiovascular inotropism can be increased with various agents such as dobutamine (Schremmer and Dhainaut, 1990), but vasopressor should be used with caution since they are two-edged swords that increase blood pressure by increasing total peripheral resistance and therefore also increase afterload (Luce, 1987). Fibronectin, a protein that participates in host defence, has been used therapeutically to decrease vascular permeability and increase host defence during sepsis (Putterman, 1990). Immunotherapy in the forms of anti-LPS or other antibodies may be important in the future but at present there is little evidence of its usefulness (Putterman, 1990). Another possibility is administration of acute-phase reactants that increase degradation and removal of LPS or other endotoxin remnants (Siegel et al., 1979; Warren and Chedid, 1987).

MECHANISMS OF REDUCED INOTROPICITY DURING TRAUMA AND SHOCK

Role of reduced coronary flow

In the normal heart, perfusion and function are closely related. Perfusion is determined by the combined effects of extravascular compression, vascular tone of the coronary vessels, perfusion pressure and metabolic demand. In the normal heart, perfusion pressure is sufficient to provide flow. Extravascular compression prevents perfusion during systole, but the time duration of diastole allows for complete transmural perfusion. Vascular tone is modified by adrenergic innervation, but in the normal heart, blocking α-adrenergic constrictor tone allows perfusion to increase by only 10–15%. In the normal heart, the major determinant of coronary perfusion is metabolic demand. This is expressed by the high oxygen extraction, approaching 75%, and the strong relationship between perfusion and cardiac energy expenditure, measured as cardiac work. Thus, the most appropriate question to resolve is not whether absolute cardiac flow is reduced, but whether myocardial perfusion is adequate to support the underlying cardiac workload demanded by the peripheral circulation.

In shock, burns, trauma or sepsis, the interrelationships between these determinants of coronary perfusion are significantly altered. In studies which sought to model sepsis with endotoxin bolus infusion, it was found that coronary perfusion decreased significantly, and decreased significantly below metabolic demand. This led to the hypothesis that endotoxin and, by extension, sepsis, caused myocardial depression by direct coronary vascular constriction. However, direct infusion of endotoxin into coronary arteries, if pH adjusted, did not demonstrate any vascular or contractile effects. Indirect evidence to indicate that endotoxin may indirectly cause coronary vasoconstriction included altered transmural perfusion and reduced coronary flow to cardiac work ratio following endotoxin injection. Interpretation of these results, however, is complicated by the peripheral vascular effects of acute endotoxin injection, especially the massive vasodilatation and venous pooling induced, thereby lowering arterial perfusion pressure. In models of sepsis that do not include the acute vasodilatation, it has been repeatedly demonstrated that coronary perfusion is elevated absolutely and in proportion to coincident cardiac work (reviewed by Adams et al., 1990).

In conclusion, numerous clinical and experimental studies support the concept that coronary perfusion is adequate in human trauma, burns and sepsis. In fact, coronary perfusion may be elevated and the extraction of nutrients may be reduced, inducing a situation of physiological shunting. If, however, the clinical state progresses to where the perfusion pressure decreases below the autoregulatory capacity of the myocardial vascular bed, then maldistribution and/or actual ischaemia may induce loss of contractile function in the heart. But, at this time, the organism is in the terminal stages of shock so that all organs are failing simultaneously.

Role of reactive oxygen metabolites

Significant data exist to indicate that the toxic effects of endotoxin may be mediated by reactive oxygen metabolites (Manson and Hess, 1983; Bernard *et al.*, 1984; McKechnie *et al.*, 1986; Kunimoto *et al.*, 1987, Chang *et al.*, 1988; Chen *et al.*, 1988). Endotoxin interacts with a large number of cell types *in vivo* and *in vitro* to stimulate the inflammatory process (Wilson, 1985; Weiss, 1986; Movat *et al.*, 1987). These cell types include neutrophils, macrophages and endothelial cells, and the products of this stimulation include cytokines, arachidonic acid metabolites, tumour necrosis factor, tissue procoagulant activity, chemotaxis factors, etc. (reviewed in Movat *et al.*, 1987). One major by-product of macrophage and neutrophil stimulation is the uncontrolled production of reactive oxygen intermediates and is a major extracellular source of reactive oxidants. Additionally, the large increase in cardiac work in sepsis and the possibility of decoupling of oxidative phosphorylation in sepsis suggests that the intracellular generation of reactive oxidants are also increased, further stressing the intracellular antioxidant mechanisms.

Considerable evidence suggests that reactive oxidant generation occurs during endotoxaemia and is important in the cellular and systemic alterations during the syndrome. The origin of these reactive oxygen species remains incompletely understood but appears to arise from sources intrinsic and extrinsic to the myocardium. The major intrinsic source consists of the xanthine oxidase pathway (McCord, 1985), whereas activated neutrophils have been implicated as the important extrinsic source (Wilson, 1985; Movat *et al.*, 1987). In addition, based on *in vitro* results with phorbol myristate-activated leucocytes, Kukreja *et al.* (1991) recently reported that oxygen free radicals inhibit Ca^{++} sequestration and adenosine triphosphatase activity of cardiac sarcoplasmic reticulum. Hess and Krause (1981) hypothesized that this or an analogous reactive oxidant generating pathway might account for the myocardial contractile failure and circulatory collapse occurring during endotoxaemia. Further support of the idea of reactive oxidant involvement in endotoxaemia was provided by Kunimoto *et al.* (1987). They reported that endotoxin toxicity was diminished in rats by exogenous superoxide dismutase, a free radical scavenging enzyme that catalyses dismutation of superoxide anion to H_2O_2.

The most important antioxidant system in the heart is glutathione (GSH)–glutathione peroxidase (Simmons and Jamall, 1989), having a larger antioxidant capacity than superoxide dismutase or catalase systems. GSH-peroxidase reduces H_2O_2 and GSH to water and glutathione disulfide (GSSH). GSH is resynthesized from GSSH and NADPH by GSH-reductase. If sufficient NADPH is unavailable, GSSH is exported from the cell (Meister and Anderson, 1983; Meister, 1984). In models of septic shock, reduced tissue levels of GSH (Chen *et al.*, 1988) and increased levels of plasma GSSH (Chang *et al.*, 1988) have been reported, suggesting that sepsis induces significant oxidant stress. Reduced myocardial GSH levels have been reported following ischaemia and reperfusion of the postischaemic myocardium via the local generation of reactive oxygen intermediates (Ferrari *et al.*, 1985; Singh *et al.*, 1989).

The hypothesis that reactive oxidants mediate sepsis-induced loss of cardiac inotropism is supported by several lines of evidence. Recent evidence has drawn attention to important pathophysiological similarities between endotoxin-induced cytotoxic responses and cytotoxic changes evoked by reactive oxidants induced experimentally or *in vivo*. Shared effects include microvascular permeability defects (Traber *et al.*, 1985), ischaemic-related tissue damage in different vital organs (Manson and Hess, 1983; McKechnie *et al.*, 1986) and lipid peroxidation of cell membrane constituents (Julicher *et al.*, 1984). Such similarities have supported the hypothesis that endotoxin evokes increased generation of oxygen radicals, with the latter causing adverse cellular and systemic reactions to endotoxaemia (Manson and Hess, 1983; McKechnie *et al.*, 1986; Kunimoto *et al.*, 1987).

Endotoxin challenge reduced myocardial glutathione significantly, suggesting that endotoxin challenge induced a significant oxidant stress on the myocardium (Chang *et al.*, 1988; Chen *et al.*, 1988). It has been reported that circulating levels of GSSH are elevated (Chang *et al.*, 1988) and tissue GSH levels reduced (Chen *et al.*, 1988) in endotoxin challenged models. The decrease in myocardial GSH levels noted may be due to the combination of increased metabolic use and leakage of GSS from the myocardium. Regardless of the cause, this depletion should make the myocardium more vulnerable to oxidant-induced injury. Such observations have been made in reperfused postischaemic myocardium (Singh *et al.*, 1989). Thus, the endotoxin-induced reduction in GSH levels suggests that an oxidant stress is being placed upon the myocardium by endotoxin challenge.

Several recent studies were based on the premise that drugs shown to inhibit xanthine oxidase- and/or neutrophil-derived oxidant events in other circulatory disorders should ameliorate responses to endotoxin, if the latter depend on reactive oxygen metabolites for pathogenesis then of cardiovascular changes (Bernard *et al.*, 1984; McKechnie *et al.*, 1986; Kunimoto *et al.*, 1987; Chang *et al.*, 1988). Despite speculation in favour of this relationship, data to support this hypothesis have not been decisive. Kukreja *et al.* (1991) described basic similarities between endotoxin-induced and leucocyte-induced disorder of Ca^{++} uptake in cardiac sarcoplasmic reticulum. However, that study was based on phorbol myristate-activated leucocytes *in vitro*. It is not known whether leucocytes activated during endotoxaemia exert similar effects in the *in vivo* heart. Traber *et al.* (1985) studied intact sheep and found that superoxide dismutase enhanced pulmonary vascular damage resulting from endotoxin. This finding was interpreted as evidence that H_2O_2 and HO, rather than superoxide anion itself, were responsible for the tissue damage associated with endotoxaemia. Kunimoto and colleagues (1987) indicated that superoxide dismutase with and without catalase were effective during endotoxaemia. In contrast, McKechnie *et al.* (1986) found that similar treatment of endotoxin rats was not efficacious.

The hypothesis that continuous endotoxaemia induced loss of cardiac inotropism via reactive oxygen metabolites has been tested by altering cardiac levels of glutathione, prior to and during endotoxin challenge (Lee *et al.*, 1995). A heart depleted of glutathione should be more vulnerable to oxidant injury and, conversely, a heart with augmented glutathione levels should be resistant to the injurious effects of endotoxaemia. Cardiac GSH was reduced by prior treatment with buthionine sulfoximine (BSO), a potent-inhibitor of cellular GSH synthesis (Calvin *et al.*, 1986). Cellular GSH was increased by constant infusion of N-acetylcysteine which crosses the cell membrane and provides cysteine for GSH synthesis (Meister and Anderson, 1983; Mulligan *et al.*, 1991).

The experimental treatment regimens were successful in their modulation of myocardial GSH levels. Buthionine sulfoximine (BSO) treatment reduced cardiac GSH by 50%. N-Acetylcysteine (NAC) treatment maintained cardiac GSH at basal levels during continuous endotoxaemia. Despite the success of experimentally manipulating cardiac GSH levels before and during endotoxin challenge, no relationship between altered myocardial GSH and cardiac dynamic or cardiovascular profiles during endotoxin challenge was detected. The finding that cardiac injury was unrelated to GSH levels in endotoxin challenge was opposite to the finding that, following perfusion of the post-ischaemic myocardium, the infarcted area of myocardium was inversely correlated to experimentally modulated myocardial GSH levels (Bernard *et al.*, 1984). It is well known that reactive oxidants are produced during ischaemia and upon reperfusion (Julicher *et al.*, 1984; McCord, 1985; Weiss, 1986; Simpson *et al.*, 1987; Cochrane *et al.*, 1988).

The finding that reactive oxidants may not play major roles in the early development of porcine endotoxaemia was unusual. However, these findings do not eliminate the possibility that reactive oxidants may participate in middle and late development of cardiac injury of endotoxaemia or sepsis. These results do suggest that because of the diversity of mediator systems induced by sepsis, successful therapeutic interventions cannot be designed to inhibit a single mediator system. Protective effects of NAC have been used as evidence that reactive oxygen metabolites are important factors in endotoxaemia (Bernard *et al.*, 1984). Ferrari *et al.* (1985) have suggested that depleting myocardial GSH, along with other antioxidants, may contribute to myocardial injury.

Role of cardiac cellular bioenergetics

All of the potential molecular mechanisms for sepsis-induced loss of inotropism are dependent upon appropriate myocardial high-energy phosphate metabolism. These processes include abnormalities of actin–myosin interaction, membrane integrity, ion channel and/or adrenergic receptor architecture, excitation–contraction coupling and Ca^{++} homoeostasis. Therefore, in order to determine the molecular mechanism that is responsible for sepsis-induced loss of inotropism, the central role of high-energy phosphate metabolism must be elucidated. Assessment of cardiac high-energy phosphate metabolism during human systemic sepsis and experimental models of sepsis has commenced.

Whether or not the decrement of cardiac bioenergetics is the molecular mechanism responsible for loss of cardiac inotropy in sepsis, time-dependent collection of all appropriate data is essential, because sepsis is time-dependent. The combination of two technologies, P-31 NMR spectroscopy for the repetitive evaluation of cardiac high-energy phosphate levels along with repetitive measurement of mechanical function and perfusion via sonomicrometry and computerized data reduction (Dziuban and Goldfarb, 1987), provides a powerful approach for evaluating the *time course* of metabolic, perfusional and mechanical events during periods of increased cardiac work induced in basal states or by continuous endotoxin challenge.

Cardiac performance during the initial stages of human systemic sepsis is driven by the demands of the periphery so that cardiac output rises to provide sufficient oxygen delivery to support the elevated systemic oxygen consumption. Until recently, it was uncertain whether or not this elevated cardiac output reflected an elevated inotropic state. This uncertainty arose because many of the techniques used to assess inotropic state were either load or rate sensitive. With the development of improved inotropic assessments, it has become apparent that the initial response to human systemic sepsis includes a significant reduction in inotropic state, despite elevated cardiac outputs (Parker *et al.*, 1984; Sibbald, 1985; Goldfarb *et al.*, 1986; Lee *et al.*, 1988a).

The relationship between cardiac bioenergetics, regulation of perfusion and mechanical function has been explored in various models of normal and abnormal states (reviewed in Balban and Heineman, 1989). In the normal heart, although increased cardiac external work causes an increase in ATP synthesis and utilization rates, cellular concentrations of ATP, ADP,P_i and PCr remain relatively unchanged (Balban and Heineman, 1989; Martin *et al.*, 1989). *In vivo* ATP, inorganic phosphate (P_i) and phosphocreatine (PCr) levels as measured by NMR spectroscopy did not change markedly during three-fold increases in work and coronary blood flow induced by pacing, epinephrine or phenylephrine infusion (Balban and Heineman, 1989). These data imply that a feedback mechanism exists between myofibril ATPase activity and mitochondrial function *in the normal heart*. These results are similar to findings in the isolated heart and other *in vivo* studies (reviewed in Sako *et al.*, 1988; Balban and Heineman, 1989). Thus, the simple kinetic model in which increases in ADP and/or P_i regulate ATP synthesis cannot adequately explain respiratory control in the normal heart. There are several other mechanisms which may regulate respiration *in vivo*: oxygen delivery via altered coronary vasomotion, mitochondrial redox state or mitochondrial membrane potential. These mechanisms are currently under investigation.

The relationship between myocardial bioenergetics and inotropic state has not been well explored. A reduction in myocardial respiration (reduced ATP synthesis rate) can reduce the inotropic state by at least two mechanisms: (1) a decrease in the amount of ATP available for myosin ATPases which develop tension, or (2) reduction in the amount of ATP available for Ca^{++} ATPases which control Ca^{++} homoeostasis. It has recently been suggested that cytosolic Ca^{++} may be a cytosolic transduction mechanism for control of mitochondrial phosphorylation (Balban and Heineman, 1989).

The linkage between metabolic and mechanical performance, strongly coupled in the normal heart, can be uncoupled by injury. There is substantial evidence that a reduction in ATP or total adenine nucleotide content can lead to loss of ventricular function. Abnormal states, such as ischaemia followed by reperfusion, cause degradation of cardiac bioenergetics coincident with reduced mechanical function (Koretsky *et al.*, 1983; Guth *et al.*, 1987; Camacho *et al.*, 1988; Robitaille *et al.*, 1989; Wolfe *et al.*, 1989).

The loss of ATP and PCr has generally been assumed to be the link between metabolic and functional abnormalities. Camacho *et al.* (1988) reported that the temporal relationship of metabolic and mechanical alterations following brief periods of ischaemia may be mediated by acute increases in inorganic phosphate, pH or both, rather than a loss of ATP. Thus, the finding that cardiac ATP is unaltered may not indicate an absence of metabolic injury.

There is a strong correlation between loss of high-energy phosphate content and ventricular performance by global ischaemia followed by reperfusion. The ischaemic and postischaemic myocardium, studied with NMR spectroscopy (Robitaille *et al.*, 1989), contained less ATP and PCr than normal. These decreases were dependent on ischaemic time period. Recovery of ATP + PCr after ischaemia was also time dependent (Wolfe *et al.*, 1989). Further studies suggest that mitochondrial uncoupling may not be a cause of postischaemic dysfunction, rather ischaemia-induced inefficiency of ATP utilization may exist (Sako *et al.*, 1988); Guth *et al.* (1987) examined the relationship between regional metabolism, perfusion and function during ischaemia and reperfusion. This study found that ischaemia rapidly depleted all high-energy phosphates. Upon reperfusion all but ATP were repleted. The recovery of ATP correlated (in time) with the recovery of mechanical function. However, these authors concluded that loss of ATP did not *cause* mechanical dysfunction. Rather, these data were consistent with the hypothesis that reduced energy utilization by the myofibril occurs during reperfusion of the postischaemic myocardium. Zimmer *et al.* (1989) studied isolated perfused rat hearts and suggested that altered myocardial respiration could limit maximal postischaemic myocardial mechanical performance. They reported that reperfused postischaemic myocardium resulted in alteration of the site of respiratory regulation from a non-ADP mode to an 'ADP:P_i limited' domain along with reduced maximal oxygen consumption. These data strongly suggest that one form of injury to the heart, ischaemia/reperfusion, significantly impacts upon the relationship between cardiac bioenergetics and performance.

Assessment of cardiac high-energy phosphate metabolism during human systemic sepsis or in experimental models of sepsis has just commenced. Several studies have examined the interrelationship between perfusion, work and inotropic state in sepsis. The normal heart is highly capable of regulating coronary perfusion and high-energy phosphate levels to match metabolic demand (Balban and Heineman, 1989), but in sepsis the matching of perfusion to work is lost (Lee *et al.*, 1988b; Tresadern *et al.*, 1988; Cunnion *et al.*, 1990). Natanson *et al.* (1986) demonstrated in septic patients, as we have with continuous endotoxin challenged pigs (Lee *et al.*, 1988b), that coronary perfusion is two to three times higher than external work, a sign of metabolic injury. High-energy phosphate in the hearts of animals exposed to bolus doses of endotoxin demonstrate little or no change in ATP or PCr levels but significant reductions in other adenine nucleotides as well as NAD/NADH (Astiz *et al.*, 1988; Rumsey *et al.*, 1988) have been observed. Since, as reviewed above, in a normal heart, ATP, PCr, etc. levels are generally well regulated

(Julicher *et al.*, 1984), observed alterations in the levels of these compounds should be interpreted as signs of metabolic injury. But the temporal relationship between metabolic and mechanical injury in sepsis remains unresolved.

That altered cardiac bioenergetics may participate in the biological response to sepsis can be inferred from data obtained from skeletal muscle in septic patients and animals which demonstrate alterations in high-energy phosphate metabolism. Jacobs *et al.* (1988) reported that rats subjected to caecal ligation and puncture had significantly reduced PCr/P_i and ATP/P_i ratios despite unchanged ATP, indicating that skeletal muscle metabolism was rapidly altered upon infection (results via ^{31}P NMR spectroscopy) (Jacobs *et al.*, 1988). Astiz *et al.* (1988) found reduced muscle high-energy phosphate levels despite maintained tissue oxygenation following caecal ligation and perforation. Tresadern *et al.* (1988) reported similar findings of reduced high-energy phosphates (via muscle biopsy) in septic patients. These changes were not indexed to nutritional state, however. In studies of acutely challenged endotoxaemic animals no consistent findings of reduced high-energy phosphate compounds were reported. This suggested that bolus infusion of endotoxin may not model sepsis accurately.

Cardiac inotropic state is decreased in sepsis (Parker *et al.*, 1984; Lee *et al.*, 1988a) and continuous endotoxin challenge (Lee *et al.*, 1988a). The underlying mechanism for this loss of inotropism has not been elucidated. It is well known that sepsis induces a state of high cardiac output and cardiac work, termed 'hyperdynamic' sepsis. The normal heart is highly capable of regulating coronary perfusion and high-energy phosphate levels to match metabolic demand (Katz *et al.*, 1989), but in sepsis, the matching of perfusion to work is lost (Cunnion *et al.*, 1986; Lee *et al.*, 1988a). Several studies have suggested that sepsis leads to an early metabolic injury in heart (Rumsey *et al.*, 1988) and skeletal muscle (Jacobs *et al.*, 1988; Tresadern *et al.*, 1988). Most studies on myocardial bioenergetics have been performed via biopsy sampling, an approach that has many disadvantages for cardiac stability and repetitive assessments which make time-dependent correlations difficult if not impossible. Future studies need to employ repetitive ^{31}P NMR spectroscopy to determine the effect of continuous endotoxin challenge upon cardiac high-energy phosphate metabolism and to correlate time-varying bioenergetic state to time-varying levels of external cardiac work, perfusion and oxygen delivery and inotropic state. Determination of the interrelationships among energetics, perfusion and mechanics is essential because bioenergetics are central to many of the molecular mechanisms potentially responsible for cardiac mechanical dysfunction, e.g. Ca^{++} homoeostasis, membrane electrical potential, excitation-contraction coupling, etc.

Role of circulating cardiodepressant compounds

The existence of shock-induced circulating compounds which exert negative inotropic effects are widespread. The majority of these reports indicate that these negative inotropic compounds are relatively low molecular weight, are released into the circulation upon shock, and are assayed by isolated cardiac muscle strips. However, only a few investigators have attempted to isolate and identify these compounds, a task that is necessarily very difficult.

It has been proposed by Lefer *et al.* (1970) that endotoxaemia results in a decreased perfusion of the pancreas, resulting in the production of a cardiotoxic peptide. Despite much evidence that would support the concept of a shock-induced circulating cardiodepressant substance, especially the data reviewed by Lefer *et al.* (1970), this concept has not been generally accepted. Many reasons have been advanced for rejecting this concept, including the failure to detect significant cardiac depression in shock states and the failure to detect cardiodepressant activity in shock plasma. However, it has been the inability to isolate, purify, identify and characterize a specific shock-induced cardiodepressant substance that has most often provided the rationale for rejecting the shock-induced circulating toxic substance concept.

Reports of the existence of a cardiodepressant substances are widespread, several groups reporting complete or partial isolation of several species of cardiodepressant substances (reviewed in Goldfarb, 1982a). The range of chemical characteristics varies widely but the means of detecting the presence of these compounds in a bioassay of some sort, usually the isometrically beating right ventricular papillary muscle of cat or rabbit. Low- and high-molecular-weight cardiodepressant substances were reported by several groups. The typical technique for the isolation of biologically active components is to first filter through a 1000 MW cut-off membrane. If cardiodepressant activity was present in shock plasma ultrafiltrate but absent in normal plasma ultrafiltrates, the plasma ultrafiltrate was further fractionated by gel filtration to resolve one biologically active fraction, which might be then subjected to amino acid analysis. The biological activity of isolated samples was assayed by the cat papillary muscle bioassay system.

In 1977, Greene *et al.* reported the isolation of myocardial depressant factor (MDF) from dogs in haemorrhagic shock. They used 3 litres of plasma recovered from dogs in the terminal stage of cardiovascular collapse induced by haemorrhagic shock. They proceeded to fractionate the recovered plasma by trichloracetic acid (TCA) precipitation of proteins followed by ether extraction, gel filtration with Sephadex G25, equilibrium and gradient elution chromatography on Dowex 50 × 2, equilibrium chromatography on QAE-Sephadex at pH 5.0, step elution chromatography on QAE-Sephadex, analytical gel filtration on Sephadex G25, or high-voltage paper electrophoresis to achieve purification of biologically active materials. These separation steps yielded two compounds with biological activity (assayed by the use of isolated feline papillary muscles). Amino acid analysis revealed that MDF A_1 consisted of glutamate, glycine, serine, and one unidentified amino acid in ratios of 1.13 : 1.00 : 0.67 : 0.74. MDF A_2 consisted of glycine and the same unidentified amino acid in the ratio of 1.00 : 1.25. These investigators reported that they isolated a peptide with biological activity indicated by the absence of free amino acids in the purified samples not subjected to 6 N HCl hydrolysis. Unfortunately, owing to the small amounts of purified material obtained, amino acid sequencing was not performed. However, these data raise one serious caveat, as expressed by Greene *et al.* (1977); that is, the amino acids identified in the active fractions include significant amounts of serine and glycine, both of which were contaminants in their laboratory solvents and in the paper used in the last purification step of high-voltage paper electrophoresis.

Some investigators have reported that cardiodepressant activity resides in the higher-molecular-weight fractions of plasma or serum obtained from shocked animals or man. The presence of cardiodepressant activity in plasma obtained from cats subjected to a simulated shock condition has been reported. The cardiodepressant activity was separable into high- and low-molecular-weight components. Additionally, cardiotoxic substances in the sera of severely burned patients have been reported. This cardiotoxic factor appeared to have a molecular weight of about 8000 daltons. The direct cardiotoxic effects of this substance were illustrated *in vivo* and in cultured myocardial cells.

Goldfarb has reported results concerning our attempts to identify shock-induced cardiodepressant factors. Initial studies have concentrated on the low-molecular-weight fraction of serum collected from shocked animals. The isolation procedures were sequential deproteinization, ultrafiltration, gel filtration, repeated ion exchange chromatography and amino acid analysis. These procedures resulted in one fraction containing most of the cardiodepressant activity of the initial starting material. Using amino acid analysis with hydrolysed and non-hydrolysed samples, we discovered that the active fraction contained a mixture of leucine and isoleucine. With testing of both amino acids in the papillary muscle system, it was apparent that only leucine could exhibit a cardiodepressant effect.

Since the presence of a high-molecular-weight cardiodepressant compound has been reported, we examined the high-molecular-weight fraction (> 10 000 daltons) of plasma obtained from dogs in irreversible shock. We found that whole serum from unshocked dogs caused no cardiodepression, but whole serum from splanchnic artery occlusion-shocked (SAO-shocked) dogs exerted high cardiodepression (49 ± 10 cardiodepressant activity units (CDAU)). After ultrafiltration the ultrafiltrand (> 10 000 MW) of 'shock' serum had cardiodepressant activity (33 ± 4 CDAU), whereas normal serum ultrafiltrand (> 10 000 MW) had little activity (5.3 ± 1.5 CDAU). The ultrafiltrate (> 10 000 MW) of shocked serum also had significant activity. To fractionate the UM-10 ultrafiltrand further, it was subjected to $(NH_4)_2SO_4$ fractionation.

Cardiodepressant activity was associated with several ammonium sulphate fractions (80–100% saturation precipitates). Further studies are being conducted to determine the identity of the substance that exerts this MDF-like activity. The finding that depressant activity was found in the 80–100% $(NH_4)_2SO_4$ supernatant indicates that the proteins that exert this activity are of relatively low molecular weight.

Recently, Hallstrom *et al.* (1990) reported the possible occurrence of net negative inotropic activity in plasma and that the generation of negative inotropism may play a role in the development of irreversible circulatory shock. In summary, they were able to detect cardiodepressant activity in the low-molecular-weight fraction of plasma obtained from dogs subjected to severe hypovolaemic traumatic shock. These authors were very careful to remove shock plasma fractions from all sources of contamination. These contaminants included the byproducts of anaesthesia and ionic concentrations. They reported no difference between ionic calcium concentrations and pH as compared to the bioassay solution, nor a lack of energy substrates. Part of the negative inotropic activity was ascribed to high shock-induced potassium concentrations accounting for 10–30% of the depression, depending on its individual concentration in shock blood. Lactate showed no inotropic effect in shock relevant concentrations, because the authors excluded the depressive effect of lactate H^+. The fact that the depressive effect of the plasma obtained from shocked dogs was maintained after addition of glucose to shock ultrafiltrates indicates no lack of energy substrate.

Furthermore, Hallstrom *et al.* (1990) were able to isolate two inotropic factors (salt-free) with opposite inotropic action from shock plasma. Thus, the resulting negative inotropic (MDF) activity in prolonged hypovolaemic traumatic shock seems to represent the net physiological effect of inotropically active plasma components in shock. These authors are currently attempting to isolate and characterize all the inotropic factors generated by the shock syndrome. This would be the first step towards determining the distribution and individual concentration of these compounds in various states of circulatory shock, which may improve our understanding of their possible influence on cardiac deterioration. Endogenous positive inotropic factors may even be beneficial as they could correct a negative 'inotropic status' of plasma in shock.

Other humoral compounds

Cytokines

Cytokines are a family of polypeptide hormones that are reported to mediate the body's response to microbial invasion, inflammation, immunological reactions and tissue injury (Dinarello, 1988). The primary sources of cytokines include macrophages and endothelial, lymphoid, epidermal and vascular tissues. This family of polypeptides includes interleukins, of which many forms have been recently identified, and tumour necrosis factor (TNF). In the first hours of infection or tissue injury, several types of interleukins are generated and released, especially interleukin-1 (IL-1). IL-1 has extensive systemic actions including fever and sleep induction, increased ACTH production, neutrophilia, lymphopenia, and increased tumour killing. Cells that produce IL-1 *in vitro*, when exposed to IL-1 will increase IL-1, IL-2, interferon, IL-3, and IL-6 production. At the vascular wall, IL-1 causes leucocyte adherence, increased PGI_2 and PGE_2 production, increased procoagulant and plasminogen activator inhibitor activities. IL-1 is a key mediator of host response to infection and injury. This molecule functions at several levels; to signal onset of disease and to trigger defensive mechanisms necessary for the host to fight bacterial invasion. However, the defensive measures taken to ensure host defence can contribute to the pathological processes of infection or inflammation and, if not regulated, become detrimental to the host.

Tumour necrosis factor (cachectin) is a cytokine of 17 000 molecular weight produced by stimulated reticuloendothelial cells, macrophages and monocytes. There are now increasing data supporting the concept that endotoxaemia or sepsis induces a marked increase in circulating levels of TNF and that TNF can mediate many of the symptoms of endotoxaemia (reviewed in Michie *et al.*, 1988). TNF has been reported in the circulation of laboratory animals following injection of lethal doses of endotoxin, infusion of TNF into laboratory animals caused many of the physiological changes associated with systemic sepsis, and passive immunization of endotoxin-sensitive mice with antisera to TNF substantially reduced the lethality of injected endotoxin. TNF has also been detected in the plasma of septic patients, albeit inconsistently. The injection of endotoxin into normal, human volunteers (Michie *et al.*, 1988) revealed that TNF is

generated in large quantities early in the response to endotoxin, having a peak at 1 hour and duration of appearance in the plasma of 4 hours. This rapid plasma appearance and disappearance is confirmed by *in vitro* studies of macrophages. When stimulated by endotoxin, macrophages rapidly synthesize and release TNF. After an initial stimulus, macrophages become insensitive to further stimulation. TNF appearance coincided with clinical manifestations of sepsis – fever, chills, headache, myalgia and nausea (Michie *et al.*, 1988).

Significant data have been presented to establish that TNF mediates many toxic effects of endotoxaemia or systemic sepsis. In addition to appearing in septic patients and upon experimental infusion of endotoxin, TNF when infused into experimental animals and humans induces many of the clinical signs and symptoms of sepsis. TNF infusion, in large doses, can induce circulatory collapse in mice. In smaller doses, it induces signs of hyperdynamic sepsis including fever, hypermetabolism, hypotension, acidosis and increased stress hormone elaboration (Michie *et al.*, 1989). When infused in humans, TNF induces fever, anorexia and fluid retention. Because TNF elaboration is rapid and pulsatile upon the onset of sepsis, therapies must be initiated as soon as a clear diagnosis is made. However, further clinical and experimental studies are needed to take clinical advantage of experimental data linking TNF production with lethality of sepsis.

Neutophil activation via up-regulation of adhesion protein expression

The appearance of LPS in the circulation has profound effects upon numerous cell types. The biological response to LPS is multi-faceted and redundant. Many systems are activated, all of which participate in host-defence responses. For instance, in plasma, LPS activates the complement system with generation of C3a and C5a producing a systemic inflammatory response. However, it is LPS's interaction with numerous cell types that mediates its biological effects. LPS activation of PMNs, monocytic cells, platelet, lymphocytes and endothelial cells have been demonstrated through specific receptors, lipid–lipid and lipid–plasma protein interactions.

LPS's interaction with monocytes/macrophages produce large amounts of immunoregulatory molecules such as TNF, IL-1 and IL-6, as well as eicosanoids (prostaglandins and leukotrienes). It has been demonstrated to induce macrophage up-regulation of cytokines, including TNF and IL-1 within 1 hour of exposure (Ulich *et al.*, 1991). Interaction of LPS and PMN are equally profound inducing activation, margination and adherence to endothelial cells. This interaction of activated neutrophils with endothelial cells has been linked to development of sepsis-induced vascular injury.

Interactions between macrophage, neutrophil and endothelial cells induced by LPS seem to be crucial to the development of sepsis-induced vascular and organ injury. The process by which neutrophils and endothelial cells are activated, neutrophils marginate onto endothelium, attach and finally diapedesis into the interstitium are beginning to be defined, mostly *in vitro*. LPS stimulates macrophage release of TNF which triggers endothelial cell hyperadhesivity for neutrophils. The adhesion of blood-borne cells to endothelium depends upon the increased expression of complementary proteins on circulating cells and endothelium. For example, TNF causes PMNs to express ICAM-1 and endothelial cells to express ELAM-1 (E-selectin). Additionally, LPS stimulates macrophage to release IL-1 and IL-6 which are strong up-regulators of endothelial cell expression of P- and E-selectins (Furie and McHugh, 1989). In addition, these cytokines can induce up-regulation of neutrophil b2 integrins, including Mac-1 and LFA-1 (Smith *et al.*, 1989). Von Asmuth *et al.* (1991) demonstrated that a specific CD11B/CD18-mediated signal triggers TNF-activated neutrophil cytotoxicity. It is the process of neutrophil adhesion, diapedesis and activation which can cause tissue injury; in the heart, this injury is expressed as cardiac mechanical dysfunction (Smith *et al.*, 1991). The same cytokine mediators (TNF, IL-1 and IL-6) that cause PMNs to adhere to endothelium, cause myocytes to up-regulate and release adhesion molecules and chemotaxis factors, such as PAF or LTB4, which stimulate PMN diapedesis and activation on myocytes so that they release their granular contents and reactive oxidants inducing massive tissue injury.

However, these data were largely obtained *in vitro*, whence cell biology can be influenced by artificial media, extraneous growth factors, as well as by a limited source of cells. In the case of endothelial cells, *in vivo* there appears to be significant differences from site to site such that cells isolated from one site can respond differently than those from another site. Therefore, data must be generated *in vivo* to support the concept that cell adhesion, mediated by selectins, mediates tissue injury and bacteraemia-induced cardiac injury.

Acute lung injury is a model in which endothelial cell injury and consequent expression of adhesion molecules has been studied (Mulligan *et al.*, 1991; Fukushima *et al.*, 1992). Lung injury induced by intravenous infusion of BSA and anti-BSA (Mulligan *et al.*, 1991), or via inhalation of *A. suum* extract (Gundel *et al.*, 1991), induced *in vivo* upregulation of ELAM-1 in primates. Airway inflammation was associated with neutrophil infiltration and onset of late-phase airway obstruction. ICAM-1 was not upregulated in this preparation nor was anti-ICAM-1 effective in reducing airway inflammation. These data suggest that ELAM-1 expression *in vivo*

may modulate the late-phase response of airway inflammation in a neutrophil-dependent fashion. In lungs undergoing IgG immune complex-induced vascular injury, ELAM-1 upregulation was marked in venules and interstitial capillaries, with peak intensity occurring at 3–4 hours after challenge with immune complexes. Expression of ELAM-1 is coincident with neutrophil infiltration in rat lungs after immune complex challenge. Furthermore, Mulligan *et al.* (1991) presented data that suggests that TNF release serves as the trigger for ELAM-1 expression. Data to support this conclusion includes: TNF appears simultaneously in lavage fluid with lung injury, antibodies to TNF when infused into the lung attenuate lung injury, and TNF *in vitro* can upregulate pulmonary endothelial cells to express ELAM-1.

Currently there is little *in vivo* evidence (pro or con) that endothelium undergoes marked alterations in its adhesiveness in sepsis or that this mechanism accounts for organ function deterioration observed in sepsis. Redl *et al.* (1991) evaluated *de novo* expression of ELAM-1 in septic baboons. In animals made septic by infusion of *E. coli* endotoxin, there was widespread expression of ELAM-1 in most tissues, including liver, lung and kidneys. These authors also reported ELAM-1 expression in capillaries, arterioles and arteries as well as venules, suggesting that all endothelial cells responded to extremely high levels of cytokines that are released by endotoxin challenge. Although these results are consistent with the possibility that ELAM-1 and other adhesive proteins contribute to leucocyte adhesion and eventual organ damage in sepsis, only when the availability of specific blocking agents are available can such studies be performed.

The concept that cardiovascular dysfunction induced by sepsis is initiated by macrophage recognition of bacteria and/or endotoxin producing cytokine release, which upregulates endothelial cell expression of adhesive proteins mediating neutrophil margination and ultimate diapedesis and activation, has received extensive support from *in vitro* experimentation. However, proof of this concept can only be obtained *in vivo*.

SUMMARY

There is now abundant evidence, from both clinical and experimental studies, that myocardial performance is depressed in most forms of shock, trauma and sepsis. These conclusions are based upon re-examination of cardiac dynamics with estimates of cardiac inotropism that are relatively independent of loading conditions. Use of newly developed estimators, such as ESPVR and ejection fraction, in these syndromes are necessary because shock, trauma and sepsis alter markedly the preconditions of cardiac contraction, i.e. preload, afterload and rate as well as inotropic state. Mechanisms which cause loss of cardiac inotropism in these syndromes are not firmly established. In models where severe hypotension is a feature, cardiac perfusion may be compromised, thereby leading to relative myocardial ischaemia. However, cardiac hypoperfusion is not noted in syndromes in which hypotension is not apparent, such as burns and sepsis.

An early theory to explain loss of organ function in disease was generation of 'toxic humors'. Although the practice of bleeding has been abandoned, endogenous generation of toxic factors still has experimental support. Recently, Hallstrom *et al.* (1990) defined plasma-borne factors which exerted significant negative inotropic effects. Several other components of the cytokine family, such as tumour necrosis factor, IL-1 and IL-6, have been implicated in the deterioration of cardiac and organ function in shock, trauma and sepsis.

Sepsis has recently been defined as Systemic Inflammatory Response Syndrome (SIRS), implying that sepsis-induced organ injury is mediated by uncontrolled systemic inflammation. *In vitro* work indicates that bacterial or endotoxin activation of circulating macrophages may be a key trigger step towards induction of organ injury. Uncontrolled and system-wide stimulation of macrophages and other circulating host-defence cells promotes general upregulation of endothelial cell expression of adhesion proteins, leading to attachment and subsequent activation of neutrophils which can then lead to localized tissue injury. The mechanism by which neutrophils injure tissues appears to be endogenous generation of reactive oxygen metabolites which participate in loss of inotropism. However, recent studies suggest that this mechanism may not be responsible for loss of inotropism in sepsis.

Attempts to discern mechanisms for sepsis-induced cardiac injury need to discriminate between initiating reactions from consequences of these reactions. Studies conducted *in vitro* cannot make this discrimination, but are extremely valuable in defining potential interactions *in vivo*. However, *in vivo* studies of sepsis are complex because a wide variety of interactions occur almost simultaneously so that discrimination of initiating versus responding reactions are difficult. In general, it is safe to assert that the biological response to bacteraemia is redundant

REFERENCES

Abel F.L. (1989). Myocardial function in sepsis and endotoxin shock. *Am. J. Physiol.*, **257**, R1265–81.

Adams H.R., Parker J.L., Laughlin M.H. (1990). Intrinsic myocardial dysfunction during endotoxemia: dependent or independent of myocardial ischemia? *Circ. Shock*, **30**, 63–76.

Andrejuk T., Goldfarb R.D., Lee K.J., Dziuban S.W. Jr (1991). Characterization of three left ventricular performance curves derived by manipulation of preload and afterload. (Unpublished observations.)

Astiz M., Rackowe, E.C., Weil M.H., Schumer, W. (1988). Early impairment of oxidative metabolism and energy production in severe sepsis. *Circ. Shock*, **26**, 311–20.

Balban R.S., Heineman F.W. (1980). Interaction of oxidative phosphorylation and work in the heart, *in vivo*. *News Physiol. Sci.*, **4**, 215–18.

Bernard G.R., Lucht W.D., Niedermeyer M.E. et al. (1984). Effect of N-acetylcysteine on the pulmonary response to endotoxin in the awake sheep and upon *in vitro* granulocyte function. *J. Clin. Invest.*, **73**, 1772–84.

Calvin H.I., Medvedovsky C., Worgul B.V. (1986). Near total glutathione depletion and age specific cataracts induced by buthionine sulfoximine in mice. *Science*, **273**, 553–6.

Camacho S.A., Lanzer P., Toy B.J. et al. (1988). *In vivo* alterations of high energy phosphates and intracellular pH during reversible ischemia in pigs: A P-31 magnetic resonance spectroscopy study. *Am. Heart J.*, **116**, 701–8.

Chang S.W., Lanterburg B.H., Voehel, N.F. (1988). Endotoxin causes a neutrophil independent oxidant stress in rats. *J. Appl. Physiol.*, **65**, 358–67.

Chen M.F., Chen L.T., Boyce H.W. (1988). Effect of endotoxin on the rat colon glutathione level. *Biochem. Biophys. Res. Common.*, **151**, 844–50.

Cochrane C.G., Schraufstatter I.U., Hyslop P., Jackson J. (1988). Cellular and biochemical events in oxidant injury. In *Oxygen Radicals and Tissue Injury* (Halliwell B., ed.). Bethesda: FASEB, pp. 49–6.

Cunnion R.E., Parrillo J.E. (1989). Myocardial dysfunction in sepsis: Recent insights. *Chest.*, **95**, 941–5.

Cunnion R.E., Shaer G.L., Parker M.M. et al. (1986). The coronary circulation in human septic shock. *Circulation*, **73**, 637–44.

Dhainaut J-F., Brunet F., Monsallier J.F. et al. (1987). Bedside evaluation of right ventricular performance using a rapid computerized thermodilution method. *Crit. Care Med.*, **15**, 148–52.

Dinarello C.A. (1988). Biology of interleukin 1. *FASEB J.*, 2108–15.

Downing S.E. (1983). The heart in shock. In *Handbook of Shock and Trauma: Basic Science* Vol. 1 (Altura B.M., Lefer A.M., Schumer W. eds). New York: Raven Press, pp. 5–28.

Dziuban S.W. Jr, Goldfarb R.D. (1987). Beat profile approach to computerized cardiac wave-form analysis. *Fed. Proc.*, **46**, 497.

Ferrari R., Ceconi C., Currello C. et al. (1985). Oxygen-mediated myocardial damage during ischemia and reperfusion: role of the cellular defenses against oxygen toxicity. *J. Mol. Cell Cardiol.*, **41**, 42–3.

Fish R.E., Spitzer J.A. (1984). Continuous infusion of endotoxin from an osmotic pump in the conscious, unrestrained rat: a unique model of chronic endotoxemia. *Circ. Shock*, **12**, 135–49.

Fukushima R., Saito H., Taniwaka K. et al. (1992). Different roles of IL-1 and TNF on hemodynamics and interorgan amino acid metabolism in awake dogs. *Am. J. Physiol.*, **262**, E275–81.

Furie M.B., McHugh D.D. (1989). Migration of neutrophils across endothelial monolayer is stimulated by treatment of the monolayer with IL-1 or TNFa. *J. Immunol.*, **143**, 3309.

Goldfarb R.D. (1982a). Cardiac dynamics following shock. *Circ Shock*, **9**, 317–34.

Goldfarb R.D. (1982b). Cardiac mechanical performance in circulatory shock. *Circ. Shock*, **9**, 633–53.

Goldfarb R.D., Nightingale L.M., Kish P. et al. (1986). Left ventricular function during lethal and sublethal endotoxemia in swine. *Am. J. Physiol.*, **251**, H364–73.

Goldfarb R.D., Lee K.J., Dziuban S.W. Jr (1989). Variation in end-systolic pressure-diameter relationship using dP/dt min or P/Dmax as a definition of end-systole in chronic endotoxemic pigs. *Circ. Shock*, **28**, 109–19.

Goodwin J-K., Schaer M. (1989). Septic shock. *Vet. Clin. Natl. Am.*, **19**, 1239–58.

Greene L.J., Shapanka R., Glenn T.M., Lefer A.M. (1977). Isolation of a myocardial depressant factor from plasma of dogs in hemorrhagic shock. *Biochem. Biophys. Acta.*, **491**, 275–85.

Gundel R.H., Wegner C.D., Torcellini C.A. et al. (1991). ELAM-1 mediates antigen induced acute airway inflammation and late phase airway obstruction in monkeys. *J. Clin. Invest.*, **88**, 1407–11.

Guth B.D., Martin J.F., Heusch G., Ross J. Jr (1987). Regional myocardial blood flow, function and metabolism using P-31 NMR spectroscopy during ischemia and reperfusion in the dog. *J. Am. Coll. Cardiol.*, **10**, 673–81.

Hallstrom S., Vogl C., Redl H., Schlag G. (1990). Net inotropic plasma activity in canine hypovolemic shock traumatic shock. *Circ. Shock*, **30**, 129–44.

Hess M.L., Krause S.M. (1981). Contractile protein dysfunction as a determinant of depressed cardiac contractility during endotoxin shock. *J. Mol. Cell Cardiol.*, **13**(8), 715–23.

Jacobs D.O., Maris J., Fried R. et al. (1988). In vivo phosphorous 31 magnetic resonance spectroscopy of rat hind limb skeletal muscle during sepsis. *Arch. Surg.*, **123**, 1425–8.

Julicher R.H.M., Tijburg L.B.M., Sterrenberg L. et al. (1984). Decreased defense against free radicals in rat heart during normal reperfusion after hypoxic, ischemic and calcium-free perfusion. *Life Sci.*, **35**, 1281–8.

Katz L.A., Swain J.A., Portman M.A., Balaban R.S. (1989). Relation between phosphate metabolites and oxygen consumption of heart in vivo. *Am. J. Physiol.*, **256**, H265–74.

Katz L.A. (1992). *Physiology of the Heart*, 2nd edn. New York: Raven Press.

Kay H.R., Afshari M., Barash P. et al. (1983). Measurement of ejection fraction by thermal dilution techniques. *J. Surg. Res.*, **34**, 337–46.

Koretsky A.P., Wang S., Murphy-Boesch J. et al. (1983). P-31 NMR spectroscopy of rat organs, in situ, using chronically implanted radiofrequency coils. *Proc. Natl. Acad. Sci. USA*, **80**, 7491–5.

Kukreja R.C., Weaver A.B., Hess M.L. (1989). Stimulated human neutrophils damage cardiac sarcoplasmic reticulum function by generation of oxidants. *Biochem. Biophys. Acta.*, **990**, 198–205.

Kunimoto F., Morita T., Ogawa R., Fujita T. (1987). Inhibition of lipid peroxidation improves survival rate of endotoxemic rats. *Circ. Shock*, **21**, 15–22.

Lee K., van der Zee H., Dziuban S.W. et al. (1988a). Left ventricular function during chronic endotoxemia in swine. *Am. J. Physiol.*, **254**, H324–30.

Lee K.J., Dziuban S.W., van der Zee H., Goldfarb RD. (1988b). Cardiac function and coronary flow in chronic endotoxemia pigs. *Proc. Soc. Exp. Biol.*, **189**, 245–52.

Lee K.J., Dziuban S.W. Jr, Andrejuk T., Goldfarb R.D. (1995). Deleterious effects of buthionine sulfoxide on cardiac function during continuous endotoxin infusion. *Proc. Soc. Exptl. Biol. Med.*, **209**, 178–84.

Lefer A.M. (1970). The role of a MDF in the pathogenisis of circulatory shock. *Fed. Proc.*, **29**, 1836–7.

Linker D.T., Moritz W.E., Pearlman A.S. (1986). A new three-dimensional echocardiographic method of right ventricular volume measurement: in vitro validation. *J. Am. Coll. Cardiol.*, **8**, 101–6.

Luce J.M. (1987). Pathogenesis and management of septic shock. *Chest*, **91**, 883–8.

Manson N.H., Hess M.L. (1983). Interaction of oxygen free radicals and cardiac sarcoplasmic reticulum: proposed role in the pathogenesis of endotoxin shock. *Circ. Shock*, **10**, 205–13.

Martin J.F., Guth B.D., Griffey R.H., Hoekenga D.E. (1989). Myocardial creatine kinase exchange rates and 31-P NMR relaxation rates in intact pigs. *Magn. Reson. Med.*, **11**, 64–72.

McCord J.M. (1985). Oxygen-derived free radicals in post-ischemic tissue injury. *N. Engl. J. Med.*, **312**, 159–63.

McKechnie K., Furman B.L., Parratt J.R. (1986). Modification by free radical scavengers of the metabolic and cardiovascular effects of endotoxin infusion in conscious rats. *Circ. Shock*, **19**, 429–39.

Meister A. (1984). New aspects of glutathione biochemistry and transport: selective alteration of glutathione metabolism. *Fed. Proc.*, **43**, 3031–42.

Meister A., Anderson M.E. (1983). Glutathione. *Anna. Rev. Biochem.*, **52**, 711–60.

Michie H.R., Manoque K.R., Spriggs D.R. et al. (1988). Detection of cirulating tumor necrosis factor after endotoxin administration. *New Engl. J. Med.*, **318**, 1481–6.

Michie H.R., Guillou P.J., Gillmore D.W. (1989). Tumor necrosis factor and bacterial sepsis. *Br. J. Surg.*, **76**, 670–1.

Movat H.Z., Cybulsky M.I., Colditz I.G et al. (1987). Acute inflammation in gram-negative infection: endotoxin, interleukin-1, tumor necrosis factor, and neutrophils. *Fed. Proc.*, **46**, 97–104.

Mulligan M.S., Varani J., Dame M.K. et al. (1991). Role of endothelial-leukocyte adhesion molecule (ELAM-1) in neutrophil mediated lung injury in rats. *J. Clin. Invest.*, **88**, 1396–406.

Natanson C., Fink M.P., Ballantyne H.K. et al. (1986). Gram negative bacteremia produces both severe systolic and diastolic cardiac dysfunction in a canine model that simulates human septic shock. *J. Clin. Invest.*, **78**, 259–70.

Parker M.M., Shelhamer J.H. et al. (1984). Profound but reversible myocardial depression in patients with septic shock. *Ann. Intern. Med.*, **100**, 483–90.

Putterman C. (1990). Modern approaches to the therapy of septic shock. *Am. J. Emerg. Med.*, **8**, 152–61.

Rackow E.C., Astiz M.E., Weil M.H. (1988). Cellular oxygen metabolism during sepsis and shock. *JAMA*, **259**, 1989–93.

Redl H., Dinges H.P., Buurman W.A. et al. (1991). Expression of ELAM-1 in septic but not traumatic/ hemorrhagic shock in the baboon. *Am. J. Pathol.*, **139**, 461–6.

Robie N.W. (1984). Controversial evidence regarding the functional importance of presynaptic alpha receptors. *Fed. Proc.*, **43**, 1371–4.

Robitaille P-M., Lew B., Merkle H. et al. (1989). Transmural metabolite distribution in regional myocardial ischemia as studied with P-31 NMR. *Mag. Res. Med.*, **10**, 108–18.

Rumsey W.L., Kilpatrick L., Wilson D.F., Erecinska M. (1988). Myocardial metabolism and coronary flow: effects of endotoxemia. *Am. J. Physiol.*, **255**, H1295–304.

Sako E.Y., Kingsley-Hickman P.B., From A.H.L. et al. (1988). ATP synthesis kinetics and mitochondrial function in the post-ischemic myocardium as studied by P-31 NMR. *J. Biol. Chem.*, **263**, 10600–7.

Sagawa K. (1978). The ventricular pressure–volume diagram revisited. *Circ. Res.*, **43**, 677–87.

Schremmer B., Dhainant J.F. (1990). Heart failure in septic shock: effect of inotropic support. *Crit. Care Med.*, **18**, 549–55.

Sharpe M., Driedger A.A., Sibbald W.J. (1985). Noninvasive clinical investigation of the cardiovascular system in the critically ill. *Crit. Care Clin.*, **1**, 507–32.

Sheagren J.N. (1989). Mechanism-oriented therapy for multiple systems organ failure. *Crit. Care Clin.*, **5**, 393–409.

Sibbald W.J., Drieger A.A. (1985). Myocardial function in the critically ill: factors influencing left and right ventricular performance in patients with sepsis and trauma. *Surg. Clinics North America*, **65**, 867–93.

Siegel J.H., Cerra F.B., Coleman B. et al. (1979). Physiological and metabolic correlations in human sepsis. *Surgery*, **86**, 163–93.

Simmons T.W., Jamall I.S. (1989). Relative importance of intracellular glutathione peroxidase and catalase *in vivo* for prevention of peroxidation to the heart. *Cardiovasc. Res.*, **23**, 774–9.

Simpson P.J., Mickelson J., Lucchesi B.R. (1987). Free radical scavengers in myocardial ischemia. *Fed. Proc.*, **46**, 2413–21.

Singh A., Lee K.J., Lee C.Y. et al. (1989). Relation between myocardial glutathione content and extent of ischemia-reperfusion injury. *Circulation*, **80**, 1795–804.

Smith C.W., Marlin S.D., Rothlein R. et al. (1989). Cooperative interactions of LFA-1 and Mac-1 with intercellular adhesion molecule-1 in facilitating adherence and trans-endothelial migration of human neutrophils *in vitro. J. Clin. Invest.*, **83**, 2008–17.

Smith C.W., Entman M.L., Lane C.L. et al. (1991). Adherence of neutrophils to canine cardiac myocytes in vitro is dependant on ICAM-1. *J. Clinical Invest.*, **88**, 1216–23.

Starling E.H. (1918). *Linacre Lecture on the Law of the Heart.* London: Longman.

Stoner H.B. (1987). Interpretation of the metabolic effects of trauma and sepsis. *J. Clin. Pathol.*, **40**, 1108–17.

Suffredini A.F., Fromm R.E., Parker M.M. et al. (1989). The cardiovascular response of normal humans to the administration of endotoxin. *New Engl. J. Med.*, **321**, 280–7.

Traber D.L., Adams T., Sziebert L. et al. (1985). Potentiation of lung vascular response to endotoxin by superoxide dismutase. *J. Appl. Physiol.*, **58**, 1005–9.

Tresadern J.C., Threlfall C.J., Wilford K., Irving M.H. (1988). Muscle adenosine 5-triphosphate and creatine phosphate concentrations in relation to nutritional status and sepsis in man. *Clin. Sci.*, **75**, 233–42.

Ulich T.R., Watson L.R., Yin S.M. et al. (1991). The intratracheal administration of endotoxin and cytokines. *Am. J. Pathol.*, **138**, 1485–96.

Vincent J-L., Thirion M., Brimioulle S. et al. (1986). Thermodilution measurement of right ventricular ejection fraction with a modified pulmonary artery catheter. *Intens. Care Med.*, **12**, 33–8.

von Asmuth E.J., van der Linden C.J., Leeuwenberg J.F., Buurman W.A. (1991). Tumour necrosis factor-alpha induces neutrophil-mediated inury of cultured endothelial cells. *Scand. J. Immunol.*, **34**, 197–206.

Warren H.S., Chedid L.A. (1987). Strategies for the treatment of endotoxemia: significance of the acute-phase response. *Rev. Infect. Dis.*, **9**, (suppl. 3) S630–8.

Waxman K. (1986). Invasive cardiorespiratory monitoring. *Emerg. Med. Clin. North. Am.*, **4**, 775–89.

Weiss S.J. (1986). Oxygen, ischemia and inflammation. *Acta Physiol. Scand. Suppl.*, 548: 9–37, 1986.

Weiss J.L., Eaton L.W., Kallman C.H., Maughan W.L. (1983). Accuracy of volume determination by two-dimensional echocardiography: defining requirements under controlled conditions in the ejecting canine left ventricle. *Circulation*, **67**, 889–95.

Wilson M.E. (1985). Effects of bacterial endotoxins on neutrophil function. *Rev. Infect. Dis.*, **7**, 404–18.

Wolfe C.L., Moseley M.E., Wikstrom M.G. et al. (1989). Assessment of myocardial salvage after ischemia and reperfusion using NMR imaging and spectroscopy. *Circulation*, **80**, 969–82.

Zimmer S.D., Ugugbil, K., Michurski S.P. *et al.* (1989). Alterations in oxidative function and respiratory regulation in the post-ischemic myocardium. *J. Biol. Chem.*, **264**, 12402–11.

42. The Response of the Splanchnic Circulation to Injury

P. M. Reilly, H. J. Schiller, T. G. Buchman, U. Haglund and G. B. Bulkley

Circulatory shock affects all organs in general, but the mesenteric organs in particular. The prioritization of systemic over mesenteric organ function results in disproportionate mesenteric ischaemia during shock, thereby rendering the gastrointestinal tract a particular target for injury. This mesenteric ischaemia may lead to splanchnic organ injury which may, in turn, be transduced to systemic organs.

The conventional view of the function of the gastrointestinal tract focuses on digestion, of which secretion, decomposition, absorption and excretion are the major components. However, since 1856 when Claude Bernard proposed the concept of a mucosal defensive barrier which prevented the autodigestion of the stomach by acid, a second, and no less fundamental function of the gastrointestinal tract has been appreciated: the gastrointestinal wall in general, and the mucosa in particular, provide a remarkably efficient protective barrier between the outside environment (i.e. the toxic contents of the lumen) and the organism's internal *milieu*. The mesenteric haemodynamic response to circulatory shock adversely affects all of these functions of the gastrointestinal tract, while initially sustaining systemic haemodynamics. Therefore it is important to consider not only the positive haemodynamic effects of that response, but also the adverse consequences, both for the gut itself, and ultimately for the organism as a whole. Such consideration is based upon the unique anatomy and physiology of the mesenteric vascular bed.

NORMAL MESENTERIC HAEMODYNAMICS

Anatomy

It is helpful to consider the mesenteric vasculature as composed of several vascular circuits coupled both in series and in parallel (Figure 42.1) (Folkow, 1967). The three primary parallel circuits serve the muscularis propria, the submucosa and the mucosa respectively. Each of these circuits is itself composed of five series-coupled components:

1. The *resistance arterioles* are the primary determinants of vascular resistance and thereby regulate blood flow both to the splanchnic bed as a whole and through each parallel circuit. The flow is inversely proportional to the resistance, and proportional to the arterial (inflow) pressure.
2. The *precapillary sphincters*, located distal in the cascade to the resistance arterioles, contribute little to vascular resistance; however, they do play an important role in the regulation of transcapillary exchange, determining capillary bed patency, and thereby perfused capillary density.
3. The *capillary exchange* vessels allow fluid, solute and metabolic exchange at the tissue level.
4. The *postcapillary sphincters*, while having little effect on total vascular resistance, do greatly influence the postcapillary to precapillary resistance ratio. This ratio, which determines mean hydrostatic capillary pressure, strongly influences net fluid filtration across the proximal exchange vessels.
5. The tone of the distal *venous capacitance vessels* (venules and small collecting veins) determines the overall volume of blood sequestered within the splanchnic bed. In the adult, this may comprise as much as 30% of the total circulating blood volume (Guyton, 1981). This highly elastic compartment plays an important role in the mesenteric haemodynamic response to shock.

The vascular architecture of the intestinal villus is unique. The villus is supplied by a single, unbranched arterial vessel which arborizes at the tip into a network of surface capillaries which coalesce to form a central venule which runs back down the centre of the villus (Figure 42.2). This parallel arrangement of arterioles and venules provides a site for the villous countercurrent exchange (Lundgren and Haglund, 1978). The anatomical arrangement of this system allows the passage of rapidly diffusible small molecules, such as oxygen, directly from arteriole to venule, short-circuiting the capillary bed at the villus tip. While in the non-hypoxic state, the countercurrent exchanger may or may not play an important role in the absorption of water and solutes from the intestinal lumen; in ischaemic states, it makes the villus tips much more susceptible to hypoxic injury (Haglund *et al.*, 1975).

Physiology

The splanchnic circulation receives from 20 to 30% of the cardiac output under normal conditions (Guyton, 1981). Most of this is distributed to the small intestine, where resting flows of 20–50 ml/min^{-1}/100g^{-1} are seen. These flows are 1.5–2.0 times greater than those seen in the colon. Within the intestine, the mucosal-submucosal region receives approximately 70% of splanchnic blood flow, with the superficial villus region, the primary

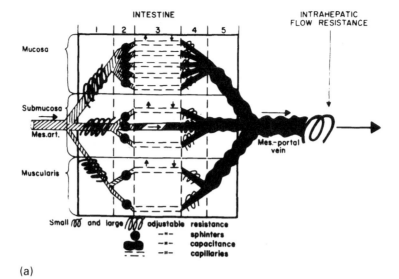

(a)

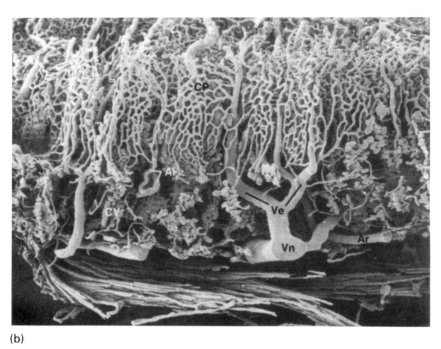

(b)

Figure 42.1 Microvascular anatomy of the mesenteric circulation. (a) The fundamental anatomical arrangement of the intestinal microvasculature is in three parallel circuits serving the muscularis propria, the submucosa and the mucosa respectively. Each circuit is composed of five series-coupled components: 1 = precapillary arterioles; 2 = precapillary sphincters; 3 = capillary exchange vessels; 4 = postcapillary venules; 5 = collecting veins. (Reproduced from Folkow, 1967, with permission.) (b) Scanning electron micrograph of a methacrylate-injected, digested specimen of the rat jejunum. Although oriented at 90 degrees from (a), the anatomical basis for the parallel-coupled vascular bed is evident. (Reproduced from Kessek *et al.*, 1979, with permission.)

site of absorption, receiving nearly half of this (Redfors *et al.*, 1984). In addition, the splanchnic organs demonstrate a striking functional hyperaemia in response to feeding. This response consists of an increase in blood flow as well as an increase in oxygen uptake, reflecting the region's increased level of metabolic activity. This functional hyperaemia is limited to regions where functional activity is increased, and at any single point in time, is not a uniform phenomenon along the length of the gut.

Pressure-flow autoregulation

A decrease in vascular resistance in response to reductions in arterial perfusion pressure (Figure 42.3(a)) has been observed in nearly all splanchnic

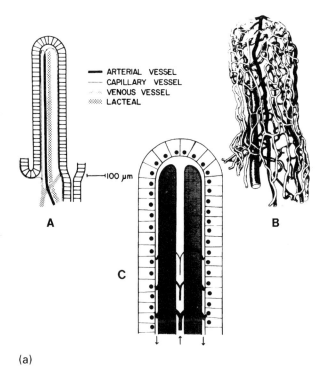

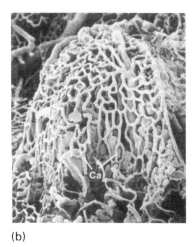

(a)

(b)

Figure 42.2 Villous microvascular anatomy. (a) The villus is fundamentally a longitudinal structure, containing a central arteriole which arborizes near the villus tip to form a network of surface capillaries. Blood draining from these capillaries is collected into a central venule. In the schematic diagram of the countercurrent exchange, the arteriole and venule are antiparallel, allowing the diffusion of small molecules, such as oxygen, directly from arteriole to venule, thereby shunting oxygen away from the villus tip. (Reproduced from Lundgren, 1967, with permission.) (b) Injected specimen of the rat villus prepared as in Figure 42.1(b). The central arteriole, collecting venule and surface capillaries (Ca) can be seen. (Reproduced from Kessek and Kardon, 1979, with permission.)

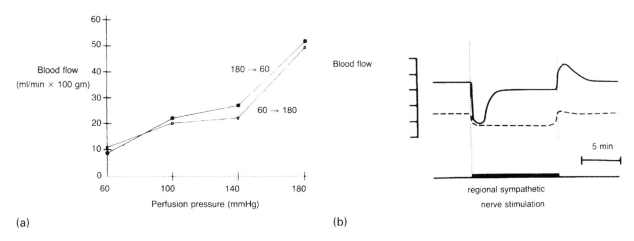

(a)

(b)

Figure 42.3 Autoregulation of blood flow. (a) Pressure–flow autoregulation. As perfusion pressure is varied independently in an isolated loop of dog small intestine, the commensurate changes in blood flow are disproportionately smaller than would be seen in a passive system of rigid conduits. (Reproduced from Shepherd and Granger, 1984, with permission.) (b) Autoregulatory escape. When perfusion pressure is reduced suddenly, the initial ischaemia is rapidly ameliorated by compensatory vasodilatation in response to the sudden decrease in perfusion pressure (myogenic response) and the accumulation of local ischaemic metabolites (metabolic response). Note also the reactive hyperaemia on reperfusion. (Reproduced from Bulkley *et al.*, 1987, with permission.)

organs, including the stomach, small intestine, colon, pancreas and liver (Kvietys, 1984; Lautt, 1985). This phenomenon, termed autoregulation of blood flow, means that the fall in perfusion is disproportionately smaller than the fall in perfusion pressure, and thereby serves as a local protective mechanism. In the fasted state, this autoregulation is not as pronounced as that seen in the brain or kidney; blood flow still falls to a substantial degree, despite the decrease in vascular resistance. However, in areas of enhanced functional activity, this autoregulation may be more marked. Moreover, as perfusion pressure falls, flow is also redistributed among the various layers of the intestine, with an increase in flow to the more metabolically active superficial mucosa. The capacity to autoregulate blood flow is also reflected in the phenomenon of autoregulatory escape (Figure 42.3(b)), where the degree of blood flow reduction seen initially, in response to a fixed reduction in perfusion pressure, becomes substantially ameliorated over the next few minutes (Folkow, 1967). This compensatory vasodilatation may also be manifest as a transient reactive hyperaemia which is seen when the occlusion is released. This intestinal autoregulatory response is mediated primarily by the precapillary arterioles. The mechanism underlying this autoregulation of flow is partially understood: Metabolites, including adenosine, and oxygen tension, cause arteriolar vasodilatation when their levels increase (adenosine) or decrease (oxygen tension) in response to decreased blood flow. This 'metabolic' response accounts for part of the compensatory vasodilatation seen during partial ischaemia (Shepherd, 1978). Relaxation of vascular smooth muscle as a direct, reflex response to the decreased perfusion pressure, characterized as the 'myogenic' response, is also a factor in this vasoregulation (Johnson, 1980).

Autoregulation of oxygen consumption

Further local protection from mesenteric ischaemia is provided by the autoregulation of oxygen consumption. As blood flow is reduced, tissue oxygen extraction is increased reciprocally, such that oxygen consumption is maintained constant over a wide range of blood flows (Figure 42.4). This has been observed in most mesenteric organs to compensate for blood flows as low as 25ml/min 1100 g (Granger and Norris, 1980). This increase in the extraction of oxygen is presumably the result of the opening of precapillary sphincters, thereby increasing the surface area for capillary exchange and decreasing the distance for diffusion. However, if flow falls below a critical level, the ability to increase oxygen extraction is surpassed and oxygen consumption falls precipitously (Figure 42.5). This autoregulation of oxygen consumption is protective for the bowel during periods of hypoperfusion

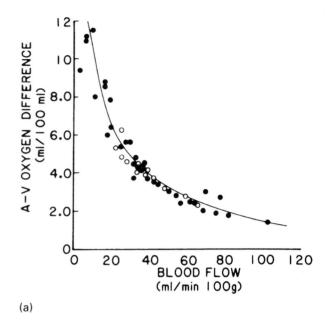

(a)

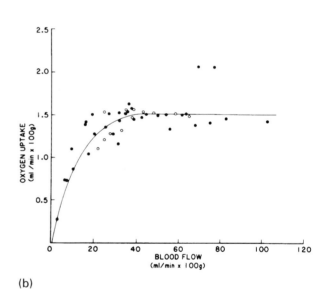

(b)

Figure 42.4 Maintenance of oxygen consumption. (a) As blood flow is reduced, oxygen extraction (A-V oxygen difference) increases reciprocally. (b) As a result, oxygen consumption (uptake) is maintained constant over a wide range of blood flows. Only when flow falls below a critical level does oxygen consumption fall, and hypoxia develop. (Reproduced from Bulkley *et al.*, 1983, with permission.)

(Bulkley *et al.*, 1985). This important mechanism of protection is provided without haemodynamic 'cost' to the systemic circulation, for, unlike pressure-flow autoregulation, it does not compete with the rest of the organism for a greater proportion of the cardiac output. It does, however, reduce the oxygen available to the liver via the portal venous inflow.

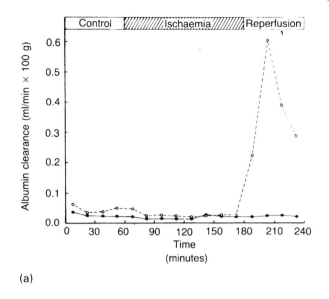

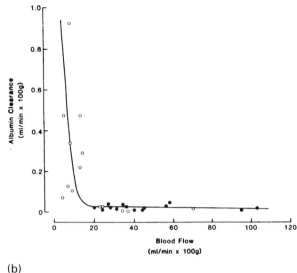

(a)   (b)

Figure 42.5 Protection from ischaemic injury by the maintenance of oxygen consumption. In these experiments in the canine jejunum, the clearance of ^{125}I-albumin from the interstitium into the lumen was used to measure mucosal permeability as an index of mucosal injury. (a) Transmucosal albumin clearance before, during and after 2 hours of partial arterial occlusion. In one loop (broken line) blood flow was reduced beyond the capability of the intestine to compensate by maintaining oxygen consumption. This loop shows evidence of injury at reperfusion. The other loop (solid line) sustained a lesser degree of ischaemia, and oxygen consumption was maintained. No injury was seen. (b) When a series of these experiments are plotted on a single figure, it is evident that there is no injury whatsoever unless blood flow has been reduced below 20 ml·min^{-1}·100g^{-1}. When compared to (b), it is evident that this threshold is below that at which oxygen consumption starts to decline. (Reproduced from Bulkley *et al.*, 1985, with permission.)

THE SPLANCHNIC HAEMODYNAMIC RESPONSE TO SHOCK

Cardiogenic shock

Resistance vessels

A number of neural and humoral agents play important roles in the systemic and mesenteric vasoconstriction associated with cardiogenic shock (Table 42.1). The mesenteric response to cardiogenic shock reflects the systemic neurohumoral response superimposed upon, and largely overriding, the above local haemodynamic control mechanisms, especially with respect to the precapillary resistance vessels. As a result, marked mesenteric vasoconstriction occurs in an effort to maintain vital organ perfusion – in essence the 'fight or flight' response described by Walter B. Cannon (1920). In shock states, the major vascular resistance response of the body as a whole is mediated in the gut. This response is one of the primary means by which systemic blood pressure is maintained. In fact, nearly 40% of the increase in total peripheral resistance seen during cardiogenic shock is mediated through the mesenteric vascular bed (Reilly *et al.*, 1992).

Sympathetic nervous system Stimulation of the alpha adrenergic receptors, either by splanchnic nerve stimulation, or by the release of circulating catecholamines, produces marked constriction of the precapillary splanchnic resistance vessels, with consequent reductions in arterial inflow that quantitatively parallel changes in the somatic vasculature. As a consequence, the mesenteric vasoconstrictor response to activation of the neural and humoral components of the sympathetic nervous system in response to shock is a vasoconstriction of the splanchnic resistance vessels that is approximately *proportional* to that of the systemic (non-mesenteric) circulation (McNeill *et al.*, 1977; Gershon and Erde, 1981; Bulkley *et al.*, 1985).

The parasympathetic nervous system also innervates splanchnic organs extensively, but no direct innervation of the splanchnic vasculature has been demonstrated in mammals. Cholinergic sympathetic nerves and purinergic nerves have also not yet been identified as mediators of the physiological or pathophysiological response of the mesenteric circulation to shock.

Vasoactive mediators Angiotensin II causes a selective, disproportionate splanchnic vasoconstriction at physiological and pathophysiological blood levels (Figure 42.6) (McNeill *et al.*, 1977; Said, 1983; Bulkley *et al.*, 1985; Bailey *et al.*, 1986b, 1987a,b; Reilly *et al.*, 1992). In fact, most of the systemic response to angiotensin II at such levels is mediated

TABLE 42.1

VASOCONSTRICTOR ACTIONS IN THE SPLANCHNIC VASCULAR BED. (REPORTED FROM PORTER *ET AL.*, 1989, WITH PERMISSION)

Agent	Dose	Action	Significance
Autonomic nervous system			
Sympathomimetics			Mediates non-selective arteriolar vasoconstriction
Norepinephrine	$0.01–1.0\,\mu g/kg/min^{-1}$	1°	Mediates ambient arteriolar tone
Epinephrine	$0.1–1.0\,\mu g$	1°	(Does not mediate selective vasoconstriction)
Dopamine	$5–20\,\mu g/kg/min$	1°	Mediates post-capillary venous vasoconstriction
Sympatholytics (Propanolol)	$0.1\,\mu g/kg$ bolus	2°	Blocks ambient β-vasodilator tone
Parasympatholytics (atropine)	$50\,\mu g/kg$ bolus	2°	Blocks ambient cholinergic vasodilator tone
Parasympathomimetics			
Physostigimine	$0.15–0.9\,\mu g/kg/min$	2°	Blood flow reduction 2° to muscular contraction
Vasoconstrictor peptides			
Vasopressin	$0.7–50\,mU/kg$	1°	Potent, selective, important to shock
Angiotensin II	$0.01–0.05\,\mu g/kg/min$	1°	Very potent, highly selective, primary mediator of selective splanchnic vasoconstriction in shock
Gastrointestinal polypeptides			
Vasoactive Intestinal Peptide	$1.75–175\,ng/min$	?2°	Many act via renin release
Glucagon	$50\,\mu g/kg/h$	?	Usually a dilator, may act as a constrictor
Miscellaneous peptides			
Prolactin	$0.6\,\mu g/h$	?	Unknown
Thyrotropin releasing hormone	$2\,mg/kg$	?	Unknown
Arachnidonic acid metabolites			
Prostaglandin $F_{2}\alpha$	$12.5–50\,\mu g/min$	1°	Potent, selective
Prostaglandin B_2	$12.5–50\,\mu g/min$	1°	Selective
Prostaglandin D_2	$0.1–0.3\,\mu g$ bolus	1°	Selective
Thromboxane (U46619)	$0.01–0.1\,\mu g$ bolus, i.a.	?	Selective
Leukotrienes C_4 and D_4	$0.3–3.0\,\mu g$ bolus, i.a.	?	Selective
Indomethacin	$8\,kmg$ bolus	2°	Blocks ambient vasodilator tone
Aspirin	$100\,mg/kg$ bolus	2°	Due to prostaglandins
Meclofenamate		2°	
Digitalis glycosides			
Ouabain	$5\,\mu g/min$	1°	Potent, selective
Digoxin	$50\,\mu/kg$ bolus	1°	Role in non-occlusive mesenteric ischemia
Serotonin	$30–100\,\mu g/kg/min$	?1°	Unknown

by the mesenteric vascular bed; the response of the non-mesenteric circulation, as a whole, is minimal (except at pharmacological levels). This is clinically quite important, as the splanchnic hypersensitivity to angiotensin II, generated via renin release by the kidney in response to hypotension, appears to be the fundamental mechanism underlying non-occlusive mesenteric ischaemia and other syndromes of mesenteric organ injury frequently seen following profound shock (see below) (Bailey *et al.*, 1986b, 1987a,b). In pigs and dogs subjected to cardiogenic shock via pericardial tamponade, we have observed profound, disproportionate mesenteric ischaemia due to severe, selective splanchnic vasospasm (Figure 42.7(a)) (Bulkley *et al.*, 1985; Bailey *et al.*, 1986b, 1987a,b). While this response is unaffected by blockade of the sympathetic nervous system, it is virtually abolished by ablation of the renin–

angiotensin axis (Figure 42.7(b)). Furthermore, these haemodynamic changes correlate closely with plasma renin activity, and can be reproduced, in the absence of shock, by the intravenous infusion of angiotensin II.

Vasopressin, a vasoconstrictor peptide, also affects primarily the mesenteric resistance vasculature (McNeill *et al.*, 1977; Said, 1983). The response of the mesenteric vascular bed is disproportionately greater than that of the systemic resistance vessels. (This differential in splanchnic vasoconstriction is used to advantage therapeutically to control gastrointestinal haemorrhage.) In one shock model of cardiogenic shock, vasopressin and angiotensin II played significant, reciprocal (see below) roles in the disproportionate mesenteric vasoconstriction observed 24 hours after the induction of myocardial injury (Arnolda *et al.*, 1991). However, in another

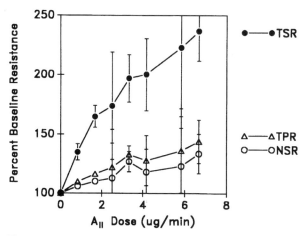

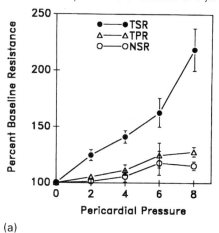

(a)

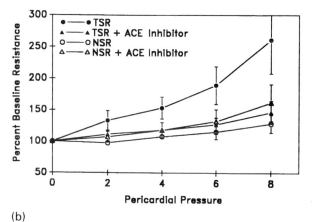

(b)

Figure 42.6 Angiotensin II infusion. In the absence of shock, the mesenteric vascular bed responds disproportionately to a central intravenous infusion of angiotensin II. TSR = total splanchnic resistance; TPR = total peripheral resistance; NSR = non-splanchnic resistance. Reproduced from Reilly *et al.*, 1991a, with permission.)

model of cardiogenic shock employing cardiac tamponade, the roles of vasopressin and angiotensin II do not seem to be reciprocal. In this latter model, blockade of both the renin–angiotensin axis and the vasopressin axis added little to renin–angiotensin axis blockade alone (Reilly *et al.*, 1992).

Other humoral agents, such as glucagon, vasoactive intestinal peptide (VIP) and cholecystokinin (CCK), may reduce mesenteric blood flow at pharmacological doses, but they are primarily vasodilators at physiological concentrations. Thyrotropin releasing hormone (TRH) also produces vasoconstriction in the splanchnic bed. The action of TRH may be related to the fact that its amino acid sequence is somewhat similar to those of angiotensin II and vasopressin (Said, 1983). Many arachidonic acid metabolites (eicosanoids) are mesenteric vasodilators or vasoconstrictors (Table 42.1). Their role, as well as those of VIP, CCK and TRH in the mesenteric vasoconstriction associated with circulatory shock, is currently under investigation.

Digitalis glycosides produce significant and selective mesenteric vasoconstriction at clinically relevant pharmacological doses (Bynum and Hanley, 1982). While once thought to be the cause of non-occlusive mesenteric ischaemia, they most likely contribute, but are not primary mediators in this disorder.

Capacitance vessels

Sympathetic nervous system The capacitance vessels of the body as a whole, and the gut in particular, contain a large percentage of the circulating blood volume. Constriction of the postcapillary

Figure 42.7 Vascular resistance in cardiogenic shock. (a) In a porcine model of cardiogenic shock produced by cardiac tamponade, as pericardial pressure is increased (and cardiac output thereby decreased), total splanchnic vascular resistance (TSR) increases to a much greater extent than total peripheral vascular resistance (TPR). Non-splanchnic resistance (NSR), the vascular resistance of the rest of the body, increases to a lesser degree, reflecting the quantitative importance of the splanchnic component of the systemic response to cardiogenic shock. (b) In this same model, ablation of the renin–angiotensin axis largely blocks the rise in splanchnic vascular resistance, and thereby blocks the selective splanchnic haemodynamic response to shock. (Reproduced from Reilly *et al.*, 1991a, with permission.)

(venous) capacitance vessels in response to the sympathetic nervous system effectively decreases the volume of blood pooled in the mesenteric vascular bed (Granger *et al.*, 1980; Rothe, 1983). This redistribution of blood into the systemic circulation will act to increase 'preload' and thereby improve cardiac output by the Starling mechanism. While this may inotropically support the failing heart in cardiogenic shock, it probably has its greatest effect in supporting cardiac output during hypovolaemic shock.

Haemorrhagic shock

Resistance vessels

The response of the mesenteric resistance vasculature to hypovolaemic shock is very similar to the response of the mesenteric vascular bed to cardiogenic shock. Graded haemorrhage causes a disproportionate increase in mesenteric vascular resistance, and consequent selective decrease in mesenteric perfusion as described above (Figure 42.8) (McNeill *et al.*, 1970, 1977). As a result, profound ischaemia occurs in the stomach, small intestine, pancreas, liver and gall bladder in order to maintain adequate perfusion of vital organs such as the brain and heart.

Sympathetic nervous system As with cardiogenic shock, blockade of the sympathetic nervous system does *not* block this disproportionate mesenteric response (McNeill *et al.*, 1970, 1977). α-Adrenergic stimulation only leads to proportionate increases in nonmesenteric and mesenteric vascular resistance. While the sympathetic nervous system does largely regulate ambient vascular tone (in conjunction with nitric oxide), and does play an important role in the overall increase in total peripheral resistance seen in response to hypovolaemic shock, it does not mediate this disproportionate mesenteric vasoconstriction.

Vasoactive mediators As with cardiogenic shock, the selective mesenteric vasospasm seen in response to haemorrhage is largely mediated by the vasoactive mediators, angiotensin II and vasopressin. However, in contrast to the mesenteric vascular response to cardiac tamponade, the mesenteric response to haemorrhage is not blocked by ablation of the renin–angiotensin axis (or vasopressin system) alone (McNeill *et al.*, 1970, 1977). Only ablation of both the angiotensin and vasopressin systems in combination effectively ameliorates the disproportionate mesenteric vasospasm seen in response to hypovolaemia. This has led McNeil and colleagues to term the renin–angiotensin axis and the vasopressin system 'reciprocal mechanisms' of mesenteric vasoconstriction (McNeill *et al.*, 1977). While these two vasoactive hormones appear to be the principal mediators of this disproportionate response, a number of other mediators, including the eicosanoids, nitric oxide and endothelin, all may play some role in the local response of the mesenteric vascular bed to hypovolaemic shock.

Capacitance vessels

Sympathetic nervous system At any given time the adult mesenteric circulation contains approximately 1400 ml, or about 30% of the circulating blood volume. Thus alterations in mesenteric blood volume distribution will clearly have a systemic effect. Constriction of the postcapillary (venous) capacitance vessels effectively decreases the volume of blood pooled in the mesenteric vascular bed (Granger *et al.*, 1980; Rotle, 1983). The result is an 'autotransfusion' which increases cardiac 'preload' and maintains cardiac output. This haemodynamic mechanism, mediated largely by the sympathetic nervous system, serves as a first line of defence against acute hypovolaemia, helping to maintain perfusion of such vital organs as the brain, heart and kidneys at no expense to nutrient blood flow in the gut. In fact, this redistribution of blood back into the systemic circulation may be the single most important contribution of the sympathetic nervous system to systemic haemodynamics during haemorrhagic shock.

Septic shock

The situation in sepsis differs considerably from that in other forms of shock. In sepsis, not only is blood flow (oxygen delivery) affected, but there is a striking increase in metabolic demand which is reflected in increased tissue oxygen consumption and extraction (Dahn *et al.*, 1987; Arvidsson *et al.*, 1991b).

Resistance vessels

In many forms of experimental septic shock the mesenteric vascular resistance is not elevated (Fink, 1989). This has also been clearly documented in

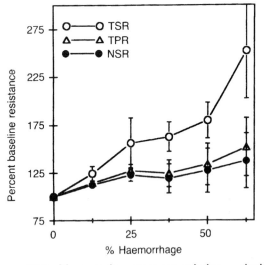

Figure 42.8 Mesenteric vasoconstriction during haemorrhage. Graded haemorrhage results in marked increases in both systemic and mesenteric vascular resistances. However, the increase in total splanchnic vascular resistance (TSR) is disproportionate when compared to the increase in total peripheral resistance (TPR).

some cases of clinical sepsis. In some experimental models, particularly when septicaemia coincides with significant hypovolaemia, splanchnic vasoconstriction has also been reported. Recently Arvidsson *et al.* (1991a), using an experimental protocol based on faecal peritonitis without aggressive volume resuscitation, documented that splanchnic vascular resistance did increase with time. However, if volume (Ringer's lactate) was supplied to the animals in order to maintain a constant and normal haematocrit, splanchnic vascular resistance remained in the preseptic range. In other series, where aggressive fluid therapy has followed the induction of sepsis, an increased cardiac output and a decreased splanchnic vascular resistance have been reported (Fink, 1989). There are indications that the sympathetic nervous system plays a fairly insignificant role in the development of increased resistance in the splanchnic vasculature during sepsis (Swan *et al.*, 1971; Jacobsen, 1972).

Mediators

The mediators responsible for splanchnic vasodilatation during septicaemia have not been identified. Macrophage-produced mediators such as tumour necrosis factor (TNF) and interleukins may be involved, as may platelet activating factor (PAF) and other eicosanoids (Dal Nogare, 1991). The relative hypoxia encountered by the splanchnic organs during septicaemia (Dahn *et al.*, 1987; Fink *et al.*, 1989; Arvidsson *et al.*, 1991b), itself probably an effect of mediators released by macrophages, may in itself account for the vasodilatation.

Capacitance vessels

The reaction of the capacitance vessels in sepsis has been less thoroughly studied. In a septic shock model induced by intravenous infusion of live *E. coli* bacteria, Falk *et al.* (1980) found a small, transient increase in intestinal vascular resistance, an initial increase in the intestinal capillary filtration coefficient, reflecting the net effect of changes in capillary permeability and the number of capillaries open to flow. Infusion of bacteria did not induce any change in mean capillary hydrostatic pressure nor any change in the tone of the capacitance vessels. Except for a very transient and small initial increase, portal venous pressure remained in the normal range in these experiments (Falk *et al.*, 1980). In the previously described faecal peritonitis-induced septic shock protocol (Arvidsson *et al.*, 1991a), increments of portal venous pressure of the magnitude of 2–3 mmHg were found with and without aggressive fluid resuscitation. A very significant increase in portal venous pressure has been reported following bolus injection of endotoxin but not in more clinically relevant models of septic shock.

CONSEQUENCES OF THE MESENTERIC HAEMODYNAMIC RESPONSE TO SHOCK

Mesenteric organ injury

As a consequence of the pathophysiological prioritization of systemic over local mesenteric haemodynamic needs, the response of the mesenteric vasculature to circulatory shock often leads to mesenteric organ ischaemic injury, as the gut seems to be sacrificed to preserve perfusion of the organism as a whole. The histological consequences of short periods of vascular occlusion or non-occlusive ischaemia in the small intestine are characterized by patchy necrosis of the superficial epithelium, seen initially at the tips of the villi (Bulkley *et al.*, 1987). More severe degrees of injury can result in more extensive epithelial loss. As ischaemia progresses, the remainder of the mucosa, and still deeper layers of the intestinal wall, are affected (Figure 42.9). Only when severe, prolonged ischaemia results in transmural infarction does the bowel become non-viable.

Other mesenteric organs may also be affected by the selective vasospasm induced by circulatory shock. Ischaemic colitis (Bailey *et al.*, 1986b) and stress ulceration of the stomach (Bailey *et al.*, 1987b) have both been produced experimentally in response to circulatory shock and found to be a direct consequence of the hypersensitivity of the mesenteric vasculature to the renin–angiotensin axis. Additionally, ischaemic hepatitis ('shock liver'), characterized histologically by centrilobular necrosis, and functionally by evidence of hepatocellular necrosis and a loss of synthetic and detoxification capabilities, can be reproduced (Bailey *et al.*, 1986a). (Ischaemic pancreatitis and some cases of acalculous cholecystitis may also be manifestations of this selective mesenteric vasoconstriction, although the extension of this concept to these latter two organs is primarily by analogy, and not yet based upon experimental data.) All of these experimentally produced mesenteric lesions, while unresponsive to adrenergic ablation, can be prevented by the prior ablation of the renin–angiotensin axis, either by nephrectomy or pharmacological blockade (Bailey *et al.*, 1986a,b; 1987a,b).

Non-occlusive mesenteric ischaemia

The fundamental mechanism which leads to non-occlusive mesenteric ischaemia (NOMI) is a selective mesenteric vasospasm which overwhelms the normal autoregulation of blood flow in the intestinal microvasculature (Bailey *et al.*, 1987a). Severe mesenteric vasoconstriction occurs in the setting of haemorrhagic or cardiogenic shock and other forms of severe physiological stress. A neonatal form of NOMI, neonatal necrotizing enterocolitis, also may be largely a manifestation of profound mesenteric vasoconstriction (Bailey and Bulkley, 1987). As discussed above, humoral mediators, particularly

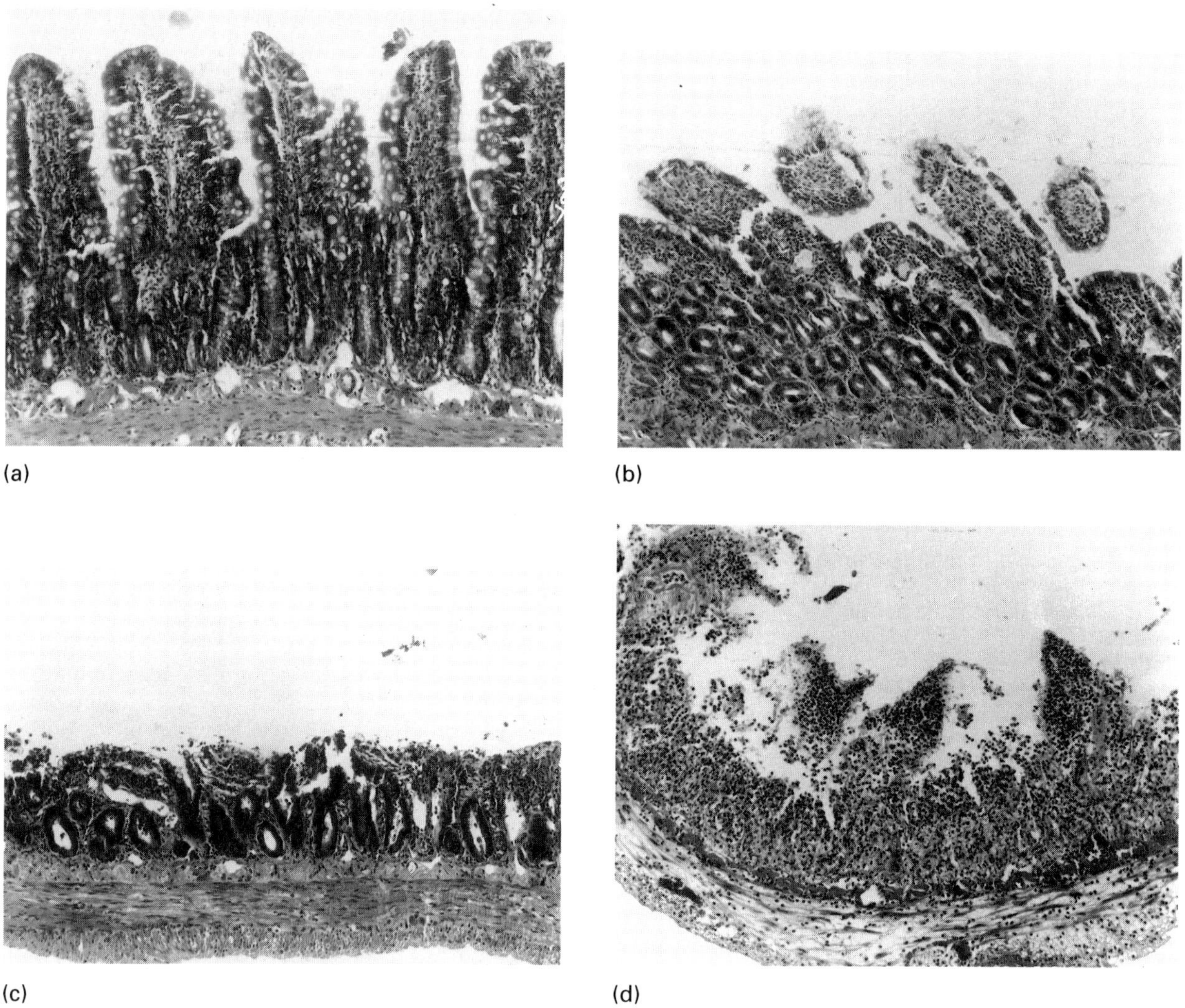

(a)

(b)

(c)

(d)

Figure 42.9 The spectrum of intestinal ischaemic injury. Haematoxylin and eosin sections of the rat small intestine. (a) Normal villi. (b) Villus tip injury. (c) Complete villus loss with extension into the crypt layer. (d) Transmucosal necrosis with extension into the muscularis propria. (Reproduced from Bulkley *et al.*, 1987, with permission.)

angiotensin II and vasopressin, directly mediate this response (McNeill *et al.*, 1977; Bailey *et al.*, 1987a).

Presenting signs and symptoms of NOMI are a gradual onset of an initially crampy, periumbilical abdominal pain, which changes to a constant, dull ache as the ischaemic insult progresses. However, the progression to a frank ischaemic insult is not necessary for a significant injury to occur. Lesser degrees of ischaemia may result in mucosal, but not full-thickness, necrosis. This loss of the mucosal barrier, which normally prevents the translocation of bacteria, endotoxin and other noxious luminal contents, may result in the systemic transduction of an (initially) isolated mesenteric injury. The consequences of such a subclinical injury are discussed below.

Experimentally, just such a lesion in the pig small intestine can be produced by 4 hours of cardiogenic shock and 2 hours of resuscitation (Bailey *et al.*, 1987a). Blockade of the sympathetic nervous system in this model does not prevent small intestinal hypoperfusion nor injury. On the other hand, ablation of the renin–angiotensin axis results in a marked improvement in small intestinal perfusion during shock, and a consequent prevention of this small intestinal injury after resuscitation (Figure 42.10) (Bailey *et al.*, 1987a).

Ischaemic colitis

Ischaemic colitis has become increasingly recognized during the 1960s with the advent of aortic aneurysm surgery. A clinical spectrum of colonic ischaemic pathology may develop, secondary to a

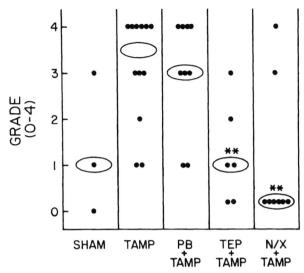

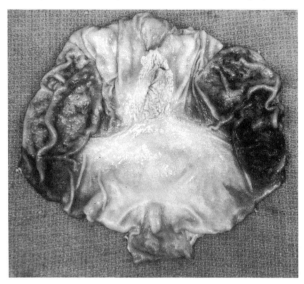

(a)

Figure 42.10 Small intestinal mucosal injury. The severity of histological injury in pigs exposed to 4 hours of cardiogenic shock (tamponade) and 2 hours of resuscitation is illustrated by blinded grading of the intestinal mucosa. The grading scale ranges from 0 (no injury) to 4 (full-thickness mucosal necrosis), and is based on the severity of necrosis and inflammation within the mucosal layer. The median grades for each group are circled. Renin–angiotensin axis blockade significantly lessened the injury seen consequent to shock, but prior alpha-adrenergic blockade had no protective effect. TAMP = tamponade; PB = phenoxybenzamine; TEP = teprotide; N/X = nephrectomy. (*******P*< 0.05 vs tamponade alone by Wilcoxan.) (Reproduced from Bailey *et al.*, 1987a, with permission.)

variety of causes, including iatrogenic arterial injury, low flow states, increased intraluminal pressure or spontaneous vascular thrombosis. The ischaemic colitis which occurs following a low flow state is largely mediated by mesenteric vasospasm (Bailey *et al.*, 1986). These spontaneous cases of colonic ischaemia tend to occur in severely ill and compromised patients, often suffering from systemic illnesses which contribute to low flow states. Pathologically, the colon demonstrates thickening, mucosal ulceration and stenosis. There may be a gradient of injury from the mucosa to the muscularis propria. Fortunately, supportive care is most often adequate for these patients.

As in the small intestine, the vasoconstriction which may lead to ischaemic colitis is mediated largely by the renin–angiotensin axis (Bailey *et al.*, 1986). Experimentally, lesions similar to those seen in patients with ischaemic colitis have been produced in the porcine model of cardiogenic shock described above. As with the small intestinal lesions, ablation of the renin–angiotensin axis results in a marked amelioration of these lesions, largely due to an improvement in perfusion during the shock period.

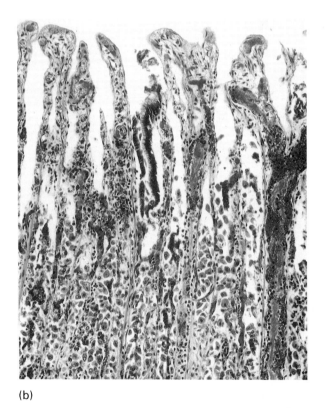

(b)

Figure 42.11 Ischaemic gastritis. (a) Specimen of pig stomach demonstrating the gross findings of ischaemic gastritis. The lesion is characteristically confined to the corpus, with antral sparing. (b) The histological specimen reveals mucosal injury and local haemorrhage. Although often described as an 'ulcer', the lesion in 'stress' gastritis is actually confined to the superficial mucosa, as seen here. (Reproduced from Bailey *et al.*, 1987b, with permission.)

Acute erosive 'stress' gastritis

Many patients who have suffered severe physiological stress (hypotension, multiple trauma, major burns) develop acute erosions in the gastric mucosa, often within hours, but usually several days after the acute event (Figure 42.11). In fact, endoscopic surveillance of critically ill intensive care unit patients demonstrates that virtually 100% will have some evidence of mucosal ulceration. Most of these lesions disappear within 7–14 days, but massive bleeding may occur if the erosions persist (Czaja *et al.*, 1974; Zinner *et al.*, 1981).

Although the aetiology of stress ulceration is multifactorial (Silen *et al.*, 1981), an angiotensin-mediated decrease in gastric mucosal blood flow seems to be the primary underlying factor (Bailey *et al.*, 1987b). Lesions similar to those seen in patients with stress ulceration can be experimentally produced in a porcine model of cardiogenic shock, and blocked by ablation of the renin–angiotensin axis. Toxic oxygen metabolites generated at reperfusion also seem to play a role in the development of these lesions. The consequence of this ischaemia and reperfusion is a loss of mucosal resistance to acid

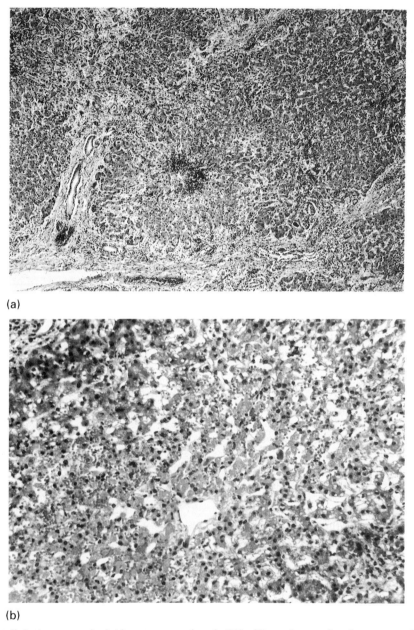

(a)

(b)

Figure 42.12 Centrilobular necrosis. (a) Low-power view (×80) of liver shows classic pattern of necrosis localized to the centrilobular region. Here there is substantial haemorrhage within these necrotic areas. (b) High power (×175) view from the same liver, taken at biopsy 5 days prior to death. The centrilobular necrosis is present, but the haemorrhage has not yet occurred. (Reproduced from Vickers *et al.*, 1989, with permission.)

back diffusion. When acid production returns to the stomach, the injury is promoted and massive bleeding may occur. As a result, the maintenance of the intragastric pH above 4.0 has been shown to markedly reduce the incidence of bleeding.

Ischaemic hepatitis
Ischaemic hepatitis is defined as hepatic insufficiency associated with centrilobular necrosis which appears after a period of circulatory shock (Figure 42.12). Also known as shock liver or post-traumatic hepatic insufficiency, this entity has quite specific histopathological features (Champion *et al.*, 1976). Two major groups of patients are at risk for ischaemic hepatitis: (1) those with underlying cardiovascular disease, manifest as either cardiac failure or arrhythmias, and (2) those with hypotension secondary to haemorrhage, dehydration or sepsis. The reported incidence varies widely, but a significant elevation of bilirubin has been seen in nearly 33% of those patients who have experienced major hypotensive episodes (Birgens *et al.*, 1978).

The liver is unique among mesenteric organs in that it derives its blood supply from two sources which differ markedly in their relative oxygen content, but not in their response to ischaemia. Approximately two-thirds of the blood supply is provided by the portal circulation which, under resting conditions, has a mixed venous oxygen saturation of 35–50%. During shock, this drops to as low as 6–10%, owing largely to increased oxygen extraction upstream in the mesenteric vascular bed (McMichael, 1937). In addition, both hepatic artery and portal vein blood flows decrease (disproportionately) in response to shock (Bailey *et al.*, 1986a). While, under normovolaemic conditions, the isolated occlusion of either the hepatic artery or portal vein is associated experimentally with compensatory vasodilatation in the bed of the other vessel (termed the hepatic arterial buffer response), both beds are compromised in parallel during shock as this homeostatic mechanism is overwhelmed by the selective response of both vascular beds to angiotensin II. As a result, the liver, a metabolically active organ with a high oxygen demand, is ill suited to tolerate prolonged periods of shock. Experimentally, ischaemic hepatitis can be produced in a porcine model of cardiogenic shock. As with the other mesenteric organ injury syndromes described above, blockade of the renin–angiotensin axis largely ameliorates this injury (Bailey *et al.*, 1986a).

Although the initiating factor is ischaemic anoxia, it appears that the generation of toxic oxygen metabolites at reperfusion may play an important role as well. The liver is rich in xanthine oxidase (XO), both in the hepatocyte and the vascular endothelium (Della Corte *et al.*, 1969). Therefore the enzyme (XO), as well as its substrates (O_2, hypoxanthine), are in excess during reperfusion.

Ischaemic pancreatitis
The mesenteric ischaemia which occurs in association with shock or hypotension has been implicated in the initiation of some cases of clinical pancreatic disease. This ischaemic pancreatitis may be defined as acute pancreatitis developing after a period of circulatory compromise, when no other predisposing factors are found.

Many factors have been suggested in the aetiology of ischaemic pancreatitis, including hypovolaemia, thromboembolism, splanchnic vasoconstriction, diuretics, atheroembolism, hypercalcaemia and operative trauma (Warshaw and O'Hara, 1978). Cardiopulmonary bypass (CPB) may predispose to pancreatitis because of low-flow, non-pulsatile perfusion, hypothermia, and venous sludging. While there are no studies evaluating directly the role of vasopressors in the aetiology of ischaemic pancreatitis, it is interesting to note that the renin–angiotensin axis is strongly activated by the non-pulsatile perfusion of CPB, the clinical situation most commonly associated with ischaemic pancreatitis (Taylor *et al.*, 1979). Recently, disproportionate vasoconstriction in the pancreatic vascular bed in response to cardiogenic shock has been demonstrated (Reilly *et al.*, 1991b). This pancreatic vasospasm is ameliorated by renin–angiotrensin axis blockade, but not by blockade of the sympathetic nervous system nor the vasopressin system.

Acalculous cholecystitis
Acalculous cholecystitis is necrotic cholecystitis occurring in the absence of demonstrable gallstones. It often, although not always, occurs in the setting of critically ill, shocked, traumatized or postoperative patients. The aetiology of acalculous cholecystitis is clearly multifactorial, but it appears that non-occlusive ischaemia may play a fundamental role in a number of cases (Haglund and Arvidsson, 1989). The disproportionate increase in vascular resistance in the bed of the gall bladder, and consequent selective decrease in gall bladder blood flow seen experimentally in response to cardiogenic shock, is mediated by angiotensin II. Obstruction of the cystic duct, narcotics and numerous other factors (thromboxane A_2, leukotrienes, platelet activating factor, tumour necrosis factor) have also been implicated. Biliary stasis, as occurs with prolonged fasting and parenteral nutrition, most likely accounts for some cases as well.

Mechanisms of ischaemic mesenteric organ injury

Ischaemia (hypoxia) has long been considered the primary mechanism of mesenteric organ injury resulting from hypoperfusion. A number of other mechanisms have been found to also play important roles: toxic oxygen metabolites, neutrophils, toxic luminal proteases, bacteria and toxins.

Hypoxic injury

Hypoxia itself may contribute significantly to the injury that is seen after ischaemia. In perfused segments of canine jejunum, reductions in blood flow do not result in intestinal mucosal injury unless they are severe enough to compromise oxygen uptake (Bulkley *et al.*, 1985). In addition, the perfusion of a segment of intestine with oxygenated saline can substantially ameliorate the injury seen in ischaemic segments (Haglund *et al.*, 1976). These studies provide evidence that the critical event is the impairment of oxygen consumption (i.e. hypoxia) in the underperfused vascular bed, not the reduction of flow *per se*. Although several biochemical mechanisms underlying hypoxic injury have been postulated, including increased calcium influx and cellular acidosis, the precise mechanisms whereby hypoxia leads to tissue injury remain unknown.

Gradient of injury A gradient of injury develops from the most superficial layers of the bowel wall (the villus tip) to the deeper layers (muscularis propria) as an ischaemic insult progresses (Figure 42.13) (Bulkley *et al.*, 1987). The earliest manifestation of this injury is an increase in capillary permeability to large molecules. Subsequently the mucosal epithelial layer allows leakage of large molecules through a normally selective barrier. More severe or prolonged ischaemia produces a subepithelial oedema, followed by an actual shedding of epithelial cells, initially from the villus tip. Even more prolonged ischaemia eventually leads to full mucosal necrosis, followed by disruption of the submucosa, and eventually of the muscularis propria, producing transmural necrosis. The preferential sensitivity of the mucosa in general, and of the villus tip in particular, to ischaemic injury is probably related to its distal location in the arborization of the vascular tree. The countercurrent diffusion of oxygen from arteriole to venule, with its consequent shunting away from the villus tip, may explain this (see above) (Haglund *et al.*, 1975; Lundgren and Haglund, 1978). The explanation for increased mucosal susceptibility may also be explained by the presence of higher concentrations of xanthine oxidase within the villus tip enterocyte, and the presence of digestive enzymes, toxins and microorganisms within the lumen.

Reperfusion injury

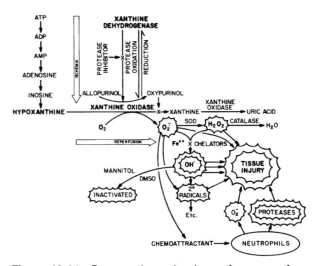

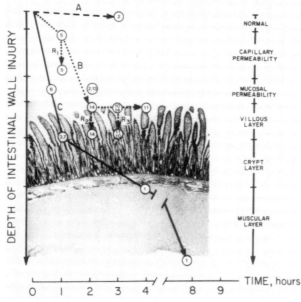

Figure 42.13 Gradient of Injury. A, B, and C represent mild, moderate and total vascular occlusions, respectively. Numbers in circles indicate specific studies, referenced in Haglund *et al.* (1987). Data are compiled from various species in a number of laboratories. Note that increasing degrees of ischaemia produce progressive injury, from the villus tips inward, ultimately to the muscularis propria. (Reproduced from Haglund *et al.*, 1987, with permission.)

Figure 42.14 Proposed mechanism of oxygen free radical production. (a) During ischaemia, the breakdown of high-energy phosphate compounds results in the accumulation of purine bases, including hypoxanthine and xanthine. At the same time, xanthine oxidoreductase is converted from a non-radical generating form, xanthine dehydrogenase, to the superoxide radical generating form, xanthine oxidase. At reperfusion, oxygen is reintroduced suddenly and in excess, allowing the oxidation of hypoxanthine and xanthine to uric acid, with the secondary generation of the superoxide free radical. This can then secondarily generate the highly toxic hydroxyl radical (OH·). In addition, free radical generation may lead to neutrophil accumulation and activation. Consequent tissue injury may be mediated by xanthine oxidase-generated radicals, neutrophil-generated radicals or neutrophil proteases. Selected free radical inhibitors are also listed where they would interrupt this cascade. (Modified from Granger D.N. *et al.*, 1981.) (Reproduced from Susman *et al.*, 1991, with permission.)

While hypoxia may play a role in organ injury during hypoperfusion, much of the injury is often sustained not during the period of ischaemia itself, but during reperfusion (Figure 42.14) (Granger et al., 1981). The net catabolism of ATP during ischaemia results in increased concentrations of hypoxanthine and xanthine. Simultaneously, ischaemia mediates the conversion of xanthine dehydrogenase to xanthine oxidase, the latter enzyme using O_2 as an electron acceptor and thereby generating the superoxide free radical O_2^- as a byproduct of the oxidation of these purines to uric acid. At the time of reperfusion, oxygen is added suddenly and in excess. The burst of superoxide generated by xanthine oxidase then triggers a free radical chain reaction. These radicals and other toxic oxygen metabolites may directly cause injury, and/or act as a chemo-attractant for neutrophils which accumulate and mediate further injury, in part through free radical mechanisms (Hernandez et al., 1987). Endothelial cells, which contain xanthine oxidase, may serve as a ubiquitous initiator of free radical-mediated reperfusion injury in many organs (endothelial cell trigger mechanism) (Ratych et al., 1987).

Gastric acid

In 1855 Claude Bernard first demonstrated that the ability of the stomach to resist digestion by gastric acid was not an inherent property of living tissue, but a highly specialized function of the stomach lining. The relationship between splanchnic ischaemia and mucosal integrity was first proposed by Virchow in 1853, and is now firmly based on numerous studies. It now seems clear that the gastric mucosa sustains a severe ischaemic (and reperfusion) injury during a period of severe physiological stress as a consequence of a profound and disproportionate vasoconstriction of the mesenteric vascular bed (see above). Gastric haemorrhage, the clinical manifestation of mucosal ulceration, usually does not appear until several days after the insult, probably reflecting the effects of the resumed secretion of gastric acid upon a mucosa which has lost its barrier (protective) capability (Mersereau and Hinchey, 1973). The fact that neutralization of gastric acid can largely prevent the haemorrhage seen in this clinical syndrome is not inconsistent with this hypothesis.

Proteases

Included among the digestive enzymes are proteases that catalyse the hydrolysis of the peptide bonds. The pancreas secretes approximately 5–10 g of proteases each day, mostly of the serine variety. Experimentally, ligation of the pancreatic duct or intraluminal administration of aprotinin or soybean trypsin inhibitor markedly attenuates the injury seen during periods of ischaemia (Bou-nous et al., 1977). Moreover, intraluminal administration of the proteases trypsin or elastase aggravate the lesions (Bounous, 1986). Isolation of the ischaemic segment from the intestinal stream also protects against ischaemic injury.

Bacteria and toxins

The normal human intestinal tract is colonized with large quantities of aerobic and anaerobic bacteria. The concentrations of these bacteria increase from the duodenum to the colon. The concept that these bacteria (or their products) may play a role in mucosal injury during ischaemia is not novel; unfortunately, it is difficult to demonstrate experimentally. Patients with subclinical mesenteric ischaemia (and subsequent loss of the gut epithelial barrier) are at an increased risk for 'bacterial translocation' from the gut lumen to the gut wall, mesenteric lymph nodes, portal circulation, liver, and even the systemic circulation. Evidence is emerging that enteral feeding, especially of glutamine, may play an important role in the prevention of pneumonia, hypermetabolism, organ failure and perhaps even death by maintaining the gut mucosal barrier (Cerra et al., 1985; McAnena et al., 1991).

Stasis and ischaemia promote overgrowth of bacteria which serve as a rich source of toxins which subsequently have easy access to ischaemic mucosal segments. High concentrations of endotoxin have been documented on the mucosal surface of ischaemic segments of bowel (Deitch and Berg, 1987). Here endotoxin can act on mucosal cellular function, activate complement and coagulation pathways, and stimulate neutrophils and monocytes which further elaborate cytokine production. The net result may be a marked inflammatory response, and/or systemic dissemination.

Recovery following ischaemic injury

The determinate factor in tissue recovery is not tissue viability, but the patency of the intestinal microvasculature. If ischaemia proceeds long enough for microvascular injury and consequent thrombosis to occur, irreversible progressive necrosis results. However, if thrombosis is prevented by pretreatment with an anticoagulant, the small intestine can tolerate much longer periods of complete ischaemia with complete recovery (Amano et al., 1980). (Clinically, this microvascular patency is used in the intraoperative determination of bowel viability.)

After flow is restored, the mucosal injury caused by mild to moderate degrees of ischaemia resembles a second degree burn of the skin, and epithelial integrity can be restored over the course of 1–3 weeks from regeneration of deeply situated epithelial elements (crypts).

Distant organ injury

Multiple organ failure syndrome

The syndrome of multisystem organ failure (MSOF) affects a wide variety of critically ill or injured patients. The complex includes initial tissue injury, adult respiratory distress syndrome (ARDS) and hypermetabolism, followed by sequential organ failure (Table 42.2). It accounts for most prolonged intensive care unit stays and for over 90% of the deaths in many SICUs. The care of these patients consumes major human and financial resources.

The inciting events which subsequently lead to MSOF are local injury from trauma, infection or hypoperfusion (Cerra, 1987). A local inflammatory response subsequently occurs, probably as a result of endothelial injury, platelet and clotting cascade activation, and the release of inflammatory mediators. As a result, a hypermetabolic state develops, characterized by a marked increase in O_2 consumption and, therefore, demand (Figure 42.15). Often the lung is the first organ to fail, producing a picture of ARDS, and resulting in prolonged ventilator dependence. Failure of the kidneys, immune system, gastrointestinal tract and liver follows, resulting ultimately in sepsis, cardiovascular collapse, and death.

Controversy exists as to whether this syndrome is necessarily associated with a septic state. Although the haemodynamic and metabolic characteristics of MSOF mimic those seen with sepsis, many of the patients have no identifiable septic source and are repeatedly culture negative. Even with optimal management of bacterial contamination and septic sources, a syndrome of sequential organ failure may develop and progress. Clearly some of these patients do have an ongoing, endogenous source of sepsis, perhaps secondary to persistent bacteraemia and endotoxaemia from their own gastrointestinal tract.

There is increasing evidence that the gastrointestinal tract may play a central role in the development and maintenance of the full-blown MSOF syndrome (Meakins and Marshall, 1989). The breakdown of the gastrointestinal mucosal barrier allows a portal of entry for not only bacteria, but endotoxin, and other luminal factors that may contribute to a systemic inflammatory response and distant organ injury (see below). Indeed it has been recently suggested that maintaining the intestinal mucosal barrier via enteral feedings may provide a mechanism for decreased mortality in the critical care setting, whereas parenteral nutritional support may actually increase the incidence of bacterial translocation by promoting gut atrophy (Cerra *et al.*, 1985).

Of all the proposed aetiologies for MSOF, ischaemia reperfusion injury to the superficial gut mucosal barrier seems the most likely. Patients subjected to circulatory shock, hypoxia, sepsis and other initial forms of severe physiological stress

TABLE 42.2

MULTIPLE SYSTEM ORGAN FAILURE ORGAN INVOLVEMENT.
(REPRODUCED FROM PETERS *ET AL.*, 1981, WITH PERMISSION)

Gastrointestinal organs
    Small intestine – non-occlusive mucosal ischaemia
    Large intestine – ischaemic colitis
    Stomach – stress gastritis
    Liver – ischaemic hepatitis
    Gall Bladder – acalculous cholecystitis
    Pancreas – ischaemic pancreatitis

Non-gastrointestinal Organs
    Lung – ARDS
    Heart – decreased myocardial contractility
    Kidney – renal failure
    CNS – obtundation
    Clotting system – DIC
    Immune system – activation of inflammatory
                mediators
                – immunosuppression

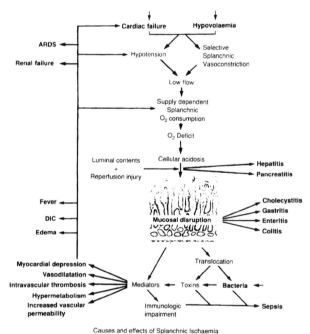

Causes and effects of Splanchnic Ischaemia

Figure 42.15 Causes and effects of mesenteric ischaemia. The interrelationship between mesenteric ischaemia and organ failure (both mesenteric and distant) is represented in this diagram. While initially mesenteric ischaemia may be caused by an isolated physiological stress, the consequences of this ischaemia may actually lead to a further ischaemic insult. As a result, a vicious cycle of mesenteric hypoxia is set up which often cannot be disrupted until the patient is no longer salvageable. (Reproduced from Marston *et al.*, 1989, with permission.)

may sustain a mild, non-occlusive ischaemia of the gut that does not progress to frank bowel necrosis. Although this is not recognized clinically, it may result in mucosal damage, with the subsequent loss of the barrier function of the epithelium. Indeed, critically ill patients coming to autopsy have long been recognized to have these lesions, but they are often signed out as 'autolysis' and not recognized as a premortem change.

Once the barrier function has been lost, the translocation of bacteria, and perhaps other luminal toxins, is facilitated. In rats subjected to haemorrhagic shock, the full sequence of events is seen, and is prevented by pretreatment with allopurinol, suggesting that free radicals, generated from xanthine oxidase at reperfusion, play an important role (Deitch et al., 1988). It is not known whether it is the bacteria, toxins, digestive enzymes or another mediator which mediates this systemic injury, or whether these agents merely trigger the release of inflammatory mediators from the gut itself, the liver or from elsewhere. In any case, the loss of this barrier function is probably the basis for the fact that the 'gut is the motor of multiple organ failure'.

Circulating mediators of mesenteric origin

Considerable attention has been focused recently on the role of the gastrointestinal tract in promoting and maintaining this hypermetabolic state seen in severe stress and surgical illness. Once thought a 'passive' organ, the gut may play a central role in the pathophysiology of such illness. As the gut mucosal barrier fails, multiple gut-derived factors gain entry into the portal and perhaps the systemic circulation. The consequences may be not only systemic haemodynamic alterations, but also distant, non-mesenteric organ injury.

Bacteria and bacterial toxins

As discussed above, intestinal bacteria may 'translocate' from the gut lumen to the bowel wall, the mesenteric lymph nodes, the liver, the portal (and even systemic) circulation. The initial pathophysiological event may be the 'leak' of endotoxin, rather than bacterial translocation itself. In experimental studies, ileal ischaemia resulted in death only in those rats with normal ileal flora, while the germ-free rats uniformly survived (Wells et al., 1987). Human studies have also documented portal bacteraemia in as many as 30% of patients subjected to surgical stress (Ambrose et al., 1984). In addition, portal, as well as systemic levels of endotoxin are markedly increased in critically ill animals and humans. All of these findings give credence to the hypothesis that normal intestinal bacteria are responsible, in part, for the lethal effects of intestinal ischaemia.

Myocardial depressant factor

It has been recognized for some time that fluid shifts alone cannot account for the cardiovascular changes observed in patients with intestinal ischaemia. The most likely explanation is that humoral substances exist which may actually be 'cardiotoxic'. The exact nature of this humoral substance(s) remains unclear, but a great deal of work has focused on a proported 'Myocardial Depressant Factor' (MDF) (see Chapter 41).

Other gut-derived inflammatory mediators

Ischaemic injury may result in the systemic release of a number of inflammatory mediators that may contribute to distant organ injury. The most extensively studied model is that of adult respiratory distress syndrome in which oxygen-derived free radicals and complement fragments (especially C5a) have been implicated as mediators of this injury. Arachidonic acid metabolites, the generation of which may also be triggered by oxidants, have also been implicated as mediators of systemic effects of ischaemic gut injury. Thus it is becoming increasingly likely that local injury caused by toxic oxygen metabolites can produce other inflammatory mediators that then act systemically to cause distant organ injury. Some of the most important candidate mediators are tumour necrosis factor, and the interleukins 1 and 2.

Tumour necrosis factor

Tumour necrosis factor (TNF) is a proinflammatory cytokine produced by macrophages in response to stimulation by bacterial endotoxin, gram-positive bacterial cell wall components and by interleukin 2 (IL-2) produced by activated lymphocytes (Dal Nogare, 1991). TNF is capable of producing haemodynamic alterations consistent with those of septic shock, including hypotension, low systemic vascular resistance and elevated cardiac index (Dinarello, 1991). In addition, TNF has been shown to directly damage endothelial cell monolayers and induce endothelial production of other mediators, including interleukin 1 (IL-1), platelet activating factor (PAF) and prostacyclin (Dal Nogare, 1991; Dinarello, 1991). One of its most interesting properties in this context is its ability to activate xanthine oxidase from xanthine dehydrogenase in endothelial cells. Pretreatment of animals with antibodies against TNF have been shown to prevent the metabolic and haemodynamic derangements observed after intravenous infusion of live bacteria, endotoxin or TNF itself (Dal Nogare, 1991), and antibodies against endotoxin have recently been introduced for the treatment of septic shock (Ziegler et al., 1991).

Interleukin 1

Interleukin 1 (IL-1), formerly known as endogenous pyrogen, is another proinflammatory cytokine which shares many of the actions of TNF (Dal Nogare, 1991; Dinarello, 1991). It is released from macrophages and endothelial cells in response to TNF or endotoxin and, like TNF, also produces the haemodynamic alterations associated with septic shock. Indeed, IL-1 potentiates the effects of TNF (Dal Nogare, 1991; Dinarello, 1991).

Interleukin 2

Interleukin 2 (IL-2) is a cytokine released from lymphocytes in response to gram-positive toxins (Dal Nogare, 1991). Its primary effect is the activation of lymphocytes. IL-2 activated cells are also known to release TNF. IL-2 also induces a haemodynamic picture consistent with septic shock, as well as an increase in vascular permeability (Dal Nogare, 1991).

SUMMARY

The mesenteric haemodynamic response to circulatory shock has evolved as a protective, homeostatic mechanism that serves to favour the survival of the organism from mild to moderate levels of circulatory shock. The redistribution of blood flow to the heart, kidneys and brain, and away from the digestive organs, in response to mild to moderate blood loss would be a natural selective advantage, leaving an animal awake and alive, able to engage or escape – the 'fight or flight' response described by Walter B. Cannon in 1920. When this is exaggerated in response to more severe injury, it can itself lead to the demise of a patient, often several days after successful resuscitation from the initial shock episode. One can easily imagine, that in an era before emergency rooms, blood banks and intensive care units, such patients would not have survived long enough to sustain this later injury, and therefore no negative natural selective pressure would have been brought to bear on the genome, thus allowing the exaggerated form of this homeostatic mechanism to develop into a pathological extreme.

The number of patients who suffer from mesenteric ischaemia may well be underestimated. We tend to readily identify only the uncommon, classical patient with severe ischaemia and consequent transmural necrosis and peritonitis, and not those patients suffering from initially subclinical levels of (non-occlusive) intestinal ischaemia. While the use of pulmonary artery catheters and vasodilators to maximize cardiac output in the management of cardiogenic shock, and the development of a trauma system and rapid infusion devices to promptly correct hypovolaemia, appear to have reduced the overall incidence of this non-occlusive mesenteric ischaemia, this entity still plays an important role in the pathophysiology of mesenteric ischaemia.

Otherwise subclinical levels of intestinal ischaemia, again usually of the non-occlusive type, may well lead to the destruction of the protective barrier of the intestinal mucosa, leading to the systemic absorption of bacteria and luminal toxins and progression to the multiple organ failure syndrome. As our ability to resuscitate the severely ill patient improves, the scope of this problem may well increase. The use of tonometry to identify subclinical levels of mucosal ischaemia, of angiotensin converting enzyme inhibitors to block the selective vasospasm of the mesenteric vasculature, or of free radical ablation to diminish mucosal injury during reperfusion, may prove to be an important approach to the care of patients with circulatory shock. When we can come to better understand the pathophysiological mechanisms by which this ischaemic gut lesion is transduced to distant organ injury, new, and perhaps more effective means of prevention and treatment of multiple organ failure will undoubtedly be developed for the care of patients following circulatory shock.

REFERENCES

Amano H., Bulkley G.B., Gorey T. et al. (1980). The role of microvascular patency in the recovery of small intestine from ischemic injury. *Surg. Forum*, **XXXI**, 157–9.

Arnolda L., McGrath B.P., Johnston C.I. (1991). Systemic and regional effects of vasopressin and angiotensin in acute left ventricular failure. *Am. J. Physiol.*, **260**, H499–506.

Arvidsson D., Almqvist P., Haglund U. (1991a). Effects of positive end expiratory pressure on splanchnic circulation and function in experimental peritonitis. *Arch. Surg.*, **126** 631–6.

Arvidsson D., Rasmussen I., Almqvist P. et al. (1991b). Splanchnic oxygen consumption in septic and hemorrhagic shock. *Surgery*, **109**, 190–7.

Bailey R.W., Bulkley G.B., Hamilton S.R. (1986a). Protection of the liver from ischemic injury due to cardiogenic shock. *Gastroenterology*, **90**, 1708.

Bailey R.W., Bulkley G.B., Hamilton S.R. et al. (1986b). Pathogenesis of nonocclusive ischemic colitis. *Ann. Surg.*, **203**, 590–9.

Bailey R.W., Bulkley G.B. (1987). Role of the circulation in NEC. In *Pathophysiology of the Splanchnic Circulation* (Kvietys P.R., Barrowman J.A., Granger D.N., eds). Boca Raton: CRC Press, pp. 141–64.

Bailey R.W., Bulkley G.B., Hamilton S.R. et al. (1987a). Protection of the small intestine from nonocclusive mesenteric ischemia injury due to cardiogenic shock. *Am. J. Surg.*, **153**, 108–16.

Bailey R.W., Bulkley G.B., Hamilton S.R. et al. (1987b). The fundamental hemodynamic mechanism underlying gastric 'stress ulceration' in cardiogenic shock. *Ann. Surg.*, **205**, 597–612.

Birgens H.S., Henriksen J., Matzen P., Paulsen H. (1978). The shock liver: clinical and biochemical findings in patients with centrilobular liver necrosis following cardiogenic shock. *Acta Med. Scand.*, **204**, 417–21.

Bounous G. (1986). Pancreatic proteases and oxygen-derived free radicals in acute ischemic enteropathy. *Surgery*, **99**, 99–4.

Bounous G., Menard D., De Medicis E. (1977). Role of pancreatic proteases in the pathogenesis of ischemic enteropathy. *Gastroenterology*, **73**, 102–8.

Bulkley G.B., Kvietys P.R., Perry M.A. (1983). Effects of cardiac tamponade on colonic hemodynamics and oxygen uptake. *Am. J. Physiol.*, **244**, G605–12.

Bulkley G.B., Kvietys P.R., Parks D.A. et al. (1985). Relationship of blood flow and oxygen consumption to ischemic injury in the canine small intestine. *Gastroenterology*, **89**, 852–7.

Bulkley G.B., Haglund U.H., Morris J.B. (1987). Mesenteric blood flow and the pathophysiology of mesenteric ischemia. In *Vascular Surgical Emergencies* (Bergan J.J., Yao S.T., eds). Orlando, FL: Grune and Stratton, pp. 25–41.

Bynum T.E., Hanley H.G. (1982). Effect of digitalis on estimated splanchnic blood flow. *J. Lab Clin Med.*, **99**, 84–91.

Cannon W.B. (1920). *Bodily changes in pain, hunger, fear and rage: an account of recent researches into the function of emotional excitement*. New York: D. Appleton.

Cerra F.B. (1987). The hypermetabolism organ failure complex. *World J. Surg.*, **11**, 173–83.

Cerra F.B., Shronts E.P., Konstantinides N.N. et al. (1985). Enteral feeding in sepsis; a prospective randomized double blind trial. *Surgery*, **98**, 632–9.

Champion H.R., Jones R.T., Trump B.F. et al. (1976). A clinicopathologic study of hepatic dysfunction following shock. *Surg. Gyneal. Obste.*, **142**, 657–63.

Czaja A.J., McAlhany J.C., Pruit B.A. (1974). Acute gastroduodenal disease after thermal injury: an endoscopic evaluation of incidence and natural history. *N. Engl. J. Med.*, **291**, 925–9.

Dahn M.S., Lange P., Lobdell H.B. et al. (1987). Splanchnic and total body oxygen consumption differences in septic and injured patients. *Surgery*, **101**, 69–80.

Dal Nogare A.R. (1991). Septic Shock. *Am. J. Med. Sci.*, **302**, 50–65.

Della Corte F., Gozzetti G., Novello F., Stirpe F. (1969). Properties of the xanthine oxidase from human liver. *Biochim. Biophys. Acta*, **191**, 164–6.

Deitch E., Berg R.D. (1987). Endotoxin but not malnutrition promotes bacterial translocation of the gut flora in burned mice. *J. Trauma*, **27**, 161–66.

Deitch E.A., Bridges W., Baker J. et al. (1988). Hemorrhagic shock-induced bacterial translocation is reduced by xanthine oxidase inhibition or inactivation. *Surgery*, **104**, 191–8.

Dinarello C.A. (1991). The proinflammatory cytokines interleukin-1 and tumor necrosis factor and treatment of the septic shock syndrome. *J. Infect Dis.*, **163**, 1177–84.

Falk A., Kaijser B., Myrvold H.E., Haglund U. (1980). Intestinal vascular and central hemodynamic responses in the cat following i.v. infusion of live *E. coli* bacteria. *Circ. Shock*, **17**, 239–50.

Fink M.P. (1989). Systemic and splanchnic hemodynamic derangements in the sepsis syndrome. In *Splanchnic Ischemia and Multiple Organ Failure* (Marston A., Bulkley G.B., Fiddian-Green R.G., Haglund U.H., eds). London: Edward Arnold, pp. 101–6.

Fink M.P., Cohn S.M., Lee P.C. et al. (1989). Effect of lipopolysaccharide on intestinal intramucosal hydrogen ion concentration in pigs: evidence of gut ischemia in a normodynamic model of septic shock. *Crit. Care Med.*, **17**, 641–6.

Folkow B. (1967). Regional adjustments of intestinal blood flow. *Gastroenterology*, **52**, 423–32.

Gershon M.D., Erde S.M. (1981). The nervous system of the gut. *Gastroenterology*, **80**, 1571–94.

Granger H.J., Norris C.P. (1980). Intrinsic regulation of intestinal oxygenation in the anesthetized dog. *Am. J. Physiol.*, **238**, H836–43.

Granger D.N., Richardson P.D.I., Kvietys P.R., Mortillaro N.A. (1980). Intestinal blood flow. *Gastroenterology*, **78**, 837–63.

Granger D.N., Rutili G., McCord J.M. (1981). Superoxide radicals in feline intestinal ischemia. *Gastroenterology*, **81**, 22–9.

Guyton A.C. (1981). *Textbook of Medical Physiology 6th edn.* Philadelphia: W.B. Saunders, pp. 349–52.

Haglund U., Arvidsson D. (1989). Acute acalculous cholecystitis. In *Splanchnic Ischemia and Multiple Organ Failure* (Marston A., Bulkley G.B., Fiddian-Green R.G., Haglund U.H., eds). London: Edward Arnold, pp. 269–77.

Haglund U., Hulten L., Lundgren O., Ahern C. (1975). Mucosal lesions in the human small intestine in shock. *Gut.*, **16**, 979–84.

Haglund U., Abe T., Ahren C. et al. (1976). The intestinal mucosal lesions in shock I: Studies on the pathogenisis. *Eur. Surg. Res.*, **8**, 435–47.

Haglund U., Bulkley G.B., Granger D.N. (1987). On the pathophysiology of intestinal ischemic injury. *Acta Chir. Scand.*, **153**, 321–4.

Hernandez L.A., Grisham M.B., Twohig B. et al. (1987). Role of neutrophils in ischemia-reperfusion induced microvascular injury. *Am. J. Physiol.*, **253**, H699–703.

Jacobsen E.D. (1972). Are adrenergic overactivity and splanchnic vasoconstriction the prime pathophysiological events in shock? In *The Fundamental Mechanisms of Shock* (Hinshaw L.B., Cox B.G., eds). New York: Plenum, pp. 101–12.

Johnson P.C. (1980). The myogenic response. In *Handbook of Physiology: circulation section 2, the cardiovascular system* vol. 2 (Bohr D.F., Somlyo A.T., Sparks H.V., eds). Baltimore: Williams and Wilkins, p. 409.

Kessek R.G., Kardon R.H. (1979). *Tissues and Organs: a text of scanning electron microscopy*. San Francisco: Freeman, p. 175.

Kvietys P.R. (1984). Microcirculation of the large intestine. In *The Physiology and Pharmacology of the Microcirculation* (Mortillaro N.A., ed.). Orlando: Academic, pp. 77–94.

Kvietys P.R., Granger D.N. (1982). Relationship between intestinal blood flow and oxygen uptake. *Am. J. Physiol.*, **242**, G202–8.

Lautt W.W. (1985). Mechanism and role of intrinsic regulation of hepatic arterial blood flow: hepatic arterial buffer response. *Am. J. Physiol.*, **249**, G549–56.

Lundgren O. (1967). Studies on blood flow distribution and countercurrent exchange in the small intestine. *Acta Physiol. Scand.*, **303**, 1.

Lundgren O., Haglund U. (1978). The pathophysiology of the intestinal countercurrent exchanges. *Life Sci.*, **23**, 1411.

Marston A., Bulkley R.G., Fiddain-Green R.G., Haglung U.H. (1989). *Splanchnic Ischaemia and Multiple Organ Failure*. London: Edward Arnold.

McAnena O.J., Moore F.A., Moore E.E. et al. (1991). Selective uptake of glutamine in the gastrointestinal tract: confirmation in a human study. *Br. J. Surg.*, **78**, 480–2.

McMichael J. (1937). The Oxygen Supply of the liver. *Q. J. Exp. Physio.*, **27**, 73–87.

McNeill J.R., Stark R.D., Greenway C.V. (1970). Intestinal vasoconstriction after hemorrhage: roles of vasopressin and angiotensin. *Am. J. Physiol.*, **219**, 1342–97.

McNeill J.R., Wilcox W.C., Pang C.C.Y. (1977). Vasopressin and angiotensin: reciprocal mechanisms controlling mesenteric conductance. *Am. J. Physiol.*, **232**, H260–6.

Meakins J.L., Marshall J.C. (1989). The gut as the motor of multiple system organ failure. In *Splanchnic Ischaemia and Multiple Organ Failure* (Marston A., Bulkley G.B., Fiddian-Green R.G., Haglund U.H., eds). London: Edward Arnold, p. 339.

Mersereau W.A., Hinchey E.J. (1973). Effect of gastric acidity on gastric ulceration induced by hemorrhage in the rat, utilizing a gastric chamber technique. *Gastroenterology*, **64**, 1130–5.

Peters J.H., Reilly P.M., Merine D.S. and Bulkley G.B. (1991). Vascular insufficiency. In *Textbook of Gastroenterology* (Yamada T. ed.). Philadelphia: J.B. Lippincott, p. 2213.

Porter J.M., Sussman M.S., Bulkley G.B. (1989). Splanchnic vasospasm in circulatory shock. In *Splanchnic Ischemia and Multiple Organ Failure* (Marston A., Bulkley G.B., Fiddian-Green R.G., Haglund U.H., eds). London: Edward Arnold, p. 74.

Ratych R.E., Chuknyiska R.S., Bulkley G.B. (1987). The primary localization of free radical generation after anoxia/reoxygenation in isolated endothelial cells. *Surgery*, **102**, 122–31.

Redfors S., Hallback D.A., Haglund U. et al. (1984). Blood flow distribution, villous tissue osmolality and fluid and electrolyte transport in the cat small intestine during regional hypotension. *Acta Physiol. Scand.*, **121**, 193–209.

Reilly P.M., Peters J.H., Merine D.S., Bulkley G.B. (1991a). Mesenteric vascular insufficiency. In *Atlas of Gastroenterology* (Powell D.W., ed.). Philadelphia: J.B. Lippincott.

Reilly P.M., Toung T.J.K., Miyachi M. et al. (1991b). The Fundamental Hemodynamic Mechanism of Pancreatic Ischemia in Cardiogenic Shock. Presented at Pancreas Club, AGA Meeting.

Reilly P.M., MacGowan S., Miyachi M. et al. (1992). Mesenteric vasoconstriction in cardiogenic shock in pigs. *Gastroenterology*, **102**, 1968–79.

Rothe C.F. (1983). Reflex control of veins and vascular capacitance. *Physiol. Rev.*, **63**, 1281–342.

Said S.I. (1983). Vasoactive peptides: state of the art review. Hypertension, **5**, (suppl. 1), I17–26.

Shepherd A.P. (1978). Intestinal O_2 consumption and 86-Rb extraction during arterial hypoxia. *Am. J. Physiol.*, **234**, E248–51.

Shepherd A.P., Granger D.N. (eds) (1984). *Physiology of the Splanchnic Circulation*. New York: Raven, p. 38.

Silen W., Merhav A., Simson J.N.L. (1981). The pathophysiology of stress ulcer disease. *World J. Surg.*, **5**, 165–74.

Swan K.G., Barton R.W., Reynolds D.G. (1971). Mesenteric hemodynanics during endotoxemia in the baboon. *Gastroenterology*, **61**, 872–6.

Taylor K.M., Bain W.H., Russell M. et al. (1979). Peripheral vascular resistance and angiotensin II levels during pulsatile and non-pulsatile cardiopulmonary bypass. *Thorax*, **34**, 594–8.

Vickers S.V., Bailey R.W., Bulkley G.B. (1989). Ischaemic hepatitis. In *Splanchnic Ischaemia and Multiple Organ Failure* (Marston A., Bulkley G.B., Fiddian-Green R.G., Heglund U.H., eds). London: Edward Arnold, p. 264.

Warshaw A., O'Hara P. (1978). Susceptibility of the pancreas to ischemic injury in shock. *Ann. Surg.*, **188**, 197–201.

Wells C.L., Maddaus M.A., Simmons R.L. (1987). The role of the macrophage in the translocation of intestinal bacteria. *Arch. Surg.*, **122**, 48–53.

Ambrose N.S., Johnson M., Burdon D.W., Keighley M.R. (1984). Incidence of pathogenic bacteria from mesenteric lymph nodes and ileal serosa during Crohn's disease surgery. *Br. J. Surg.*, **71**, 623–5.

Ziegler E.J., Fisher C.J. Jr, Sprung C.L. et al. (1991). Treatment of gram-negative bacteremia and septic shock with HA-A1 human monoclonal antibody against endotoxin. A randomized, double-blind, placebo-controlled trial. *New Engl. J. Med.*, **324**, 429–36.

Zinner M.J., Zuidema G.S., Smith P.L. et al. (1981). The prevention of upper gastrointestinal tract bleeding in patients in an intensive care unit. *Surg. Gynecol. Obstet.*, **153**, 214–20.

43. Biochemical Consequences of Lung Injury

Y. S. Bakhle

INTRODUCTION

This chapter is concerned with the biochemical consequences of lung injury rather than its morphological or physiological effects. However, only certain aspects of lung biochemistry and only certain forms of injury will be discussed. The biochemical systems discussed are those involved in the synthesis and catabolism of mediators, either circulating or locally acting endogenous substances utilized in cell to cell communication. The discussion also includes those exogenous, xenobiotic substances, usually drugs, that are substrates for binding or metabolism in lung. This grouping of pharmacologically relevant biochemical reactions in lung has been called the pharmacokinetic function of lung (Bakhle and Vane, 1974).

The lung injuries are also restricted to biochemical, rather than physical, trauma but cover a variety of inhaled or circulating injurious agents usually recognized by the physical damage they cause – oedema, endothelial or epithelial cell damage – and whose action is postulated to have a biochemical component as a precursor of the physical damage. Many of the experimental forms of lung injury have been developed in order to reproduce the high permeability oedema associated with several types of the clinically defined adult respiratory distress syndrome (ARDS), a condition which still has a mortality in excess of 50%, even in highly developed systems of medicine. However, it is likely that more attention will be paid in the future to the modelling and the clinical effects of inhaled environmental pollutants.

Injury to the lung can be characterized by clear and well-established effects on the respiratory function of this tissue, and failure to exchange gases adequately between inspired air and blood is often the final outcome of such injury. In many instances a concomitant of gas exchange failure is pulmonary oedema derived from increased microvascular permeability. Since the major permeability barrier in the microvasculature lies at the endothelium, high permeability oedema has been conceptually linked to endothelial cell dysfunction. Apart from maintaining the normal, low permeability of the microvasculature to high molecular weight solutes in blood, the endothelial cell is now recognized as the locus of many other important functions and properties (Ryan, 1986; Petty and Pearson, 1989). These include a wide range of biochemical proper-

ties – inactivation and synthesis of circulating vasoactive hormones, along with secretion of cytokines, eicosanoids, endothelium-derived relaxing factor (EDRF), endothelin and proteins such as von Willebrand Factor (vWF) and tissue plasminogen activator (TPA).

It is postulated that the loss of the physical structures that limit permeability at the endothelial layer is accompanied, and perhaps preceded, by loss of some of the endothelium's biochemical properties, many of which are associated with the cell membrane. These metabolic changes may be directly involved in the causal chain between injury and oedema as mediators or amplifiers of the injury process; for instance, through the generation of leucocyte chemoattractant molecules. The metabolic changes may also represent a response to the injury in an attempt to limit, break or inhibit the process leading to oedema. Lastly the metabolic change may be an epiphenomenon, an indicator of endothelial 'ill health', unconnected to the direct causal chain between injury and oedema, but providing a measurable side-effect of the injury process.

In any set of conditions, attempts to correlate physical changes (permeability, compliance, morphology) and biochemical changes would be valuable. If such correlations were shown to exist, they would suggest either new points of therapeutic attack or new biochemical indices of lung injury that could be used predictively, both outcomes of considerable clinical benefit. A search for these correlations has led to the many experimental and human studies of the pulmonary metabolism of pharmacologically active agents in lung injury states. A necessary background to a discussion of the metabolism in injury states is a brief description of the relevant metabolic reactions in normal lungs.

METABOLIC AND PHARMACOKINETIC FUNCTIONS OF NORMAL LUNG

The metabolism of blood-borne, biologically active, endogenous substrates during their passage through the pulmonary circulation alters their biological activity (Table 43.1). Because of this effect, the term 'pharmacokinetic' has been used to describe this property of lung (Bakhle and Vane, 1974). Development in this research area started over 25 years ago, with Vane and his colleagues publishing a series of papers clearly demonstrating the pulmonary metabolism of several different substrates, monoamines, peptides and prostaglandins (Vane, 1969). These initial findings have been extended and confirmed by several groups of workers and later work has been summarized in a series of reviews over the years (Bakhle and Vane, 1974; Gillis and Pitt, 1982; Junod, 1985; Gillis, 1986; Bakhle, 1990). Most of the experimental effort has

TABLE 43.1

ALTERATION OF THE BIOLOGICAL ACTIVITY OF ENDOGENOUS SUBSTRATES ON PASSAGE THROUGH THE PULMONARY CIRCULATION

Substrate	Effect of pulmonary transit on activity		
	Activation	Inactivation	No change
Biogenic amines		5-HT Noradrenaline Phenylethylamine	Dopamine Adrenaline Tyramine Histamine
Peptides	Angiotensin I	Bradykinin Enkephalin Atrial natriuretic peptide	Angiotensin II Oxytocin Vasopressin
Eicosanoids	Arachidonic acid	Prostaglandins D$_2$, E$_2$ and F$_{2\alpha}$	Prostacyclin (PGI$_2$)
Adenine derivatives		ATP, ADP, AMP Adenosine	
Steroids	Cortisone	Progesterone	

Note: This table summarizes the work of many authors which have been discussed in greater detail in previous reviews (Bakhle and Vane, 1974; Gillis and Pitt, 1982; Junod, 1985; Bakhle and Ferreira, 1985; Bend *et al.*, 1985; Gillis, 1986).

been concerned with the fate of endogenous substrates in order to assess the physiological function of this metabolic property of lung and later, its relevance to pathological conditions. The fate of *exogenous* xenobiotic compounds in lung is an important facet of the pharmacokinetic function of lung and has yielded results of physiological and clinical significance. However, there are important differences between the mechanisms involved and the two classes of substrate will be discussed separately.

Endogenous substrates

In Table 43.1, the fate of endogenous substrates is summarized using results from many authors and from both animal and human studies (Bakhle and Vane, 1974; Gillis and Pitt, 1982; Bakhle and Ferreira, 1985; Bend *et al.*, 1985; Junod, 1985; Gillis, 1986). Although a wide range of substrates is metabolized in lung (Table 43.1), they share some features of their fate in the pulmonary circulation which are essential to the understanding of this pulmonary function. First, the pharmacokinetic effect is *metabolic*, i.e. a biochemical transformation is the basis of the altered activity. This is in contrast to the fate of xenobiotic substrates (see later). It also means that *appearance* of metabolites, which are not retained in the lung, can be used as an assay, rather than disappearance of substrate. Furthermore, these transformations occur in conscious human subjects and within the physiological range of concentrations (Gillis *et al.*, 1979; Sole *et al.*, 1979). If high concentrations are used, selectivity of metabolism may be lost and sites and modes of metabolism

disclosed which are not relevant to low, physiological concentrations of substrate.

Two other features arise from the structure of the lungs. First, the entire cardiac output passes through the pulmonary circulation and blood from the lung passes very rapidly to the periphery. Thus these metabolic operations are carried out on the whole of the blood volume and the metabolic products are distributed almost immediately to the periphery to exert their effects there. Thus the lung can control the *pharmacodynamic* effects of vaso-active hormones on peripheral tissues by changes in their pharmacokinetics in the pulmonary circulation. In the present context, this possibility could link lung injury to the failure of other organs. Second, the respiratory function of the lungs brings the external environment (in terms of inspired air) into continuous and close contact with the epithelium of the airways and the cells of the alveolar capillaries, providing a means whereby external factors may alter internal biochemistry with pharmacodynamic consequences. Again this is relevant to lung injury; an injurious agent introduced via the airways could thus have an effect on the vascular endothelium as well as the airway epithelium.

Finally, the outcome of the pharmacokinetic process depends on the substrate and, as shown in Table 43.1, can result in activation, inactivation or no change. The process of activation entails the metabolic *product* being more biologically active than the *substrate* entering the pulmonary circulation and is well exemplified by the conversion of the inactive decapeptide, angiotensin (AI), to the highly potent octapeptide, AII. A more frequently observed fate is inactivation and is most clearly seen with 5-hydroxytryptamine (5-HT) and with prostaglandin E_2 (PGE$_2$) and PGF$_{2\alpha}$, all of which suffer extensive inactivation (>90%) on a single transit of the pulmonary circulation. However, the third category in this table – no change – is conceptually the most important because it demonstrates the selectivity of these metabolic functions in lung. For instance, the liver will inactivate prostaglandins and 5-HT entering via the portal circulation but it will not differentiate, as does the lung, between PGE$_2$ and PGI$_2$ or between noradrenaline, adrenaline and dopamine (Dusting et al., 1978; Youdim et al., 1980). This selectivity of the lung's metabolic functions led Vane (1969) to propose the idea of local and circulating hormones; the former, such as bradykinin, 5-HT and PGE$_2$, being largely inactivated in the pulmonary circulation and thus not able to reach the systemic arterial beds and the latter, such as histamine, adrenaline and vasopressin, passing freely through the pulmonary circulation and able to circulate to the periphery. This physiologically important property of selectivity in lung metabolism also has pathological significance. For instance, oedema formation induced by histamine is strongly potentiated by low concentrations of PGE$_2$ (Williams and Peck, 1977). It is possible to envisage situations in which both agents could be present in venous blood but the arterial blood would contain only histamine, as the PGE$_2$ had been removed by the lung. If, by injury, the lung's ability to remove PGE$_2$ were lost or decreased, then this mixture of histamine and PGE$_2$ could circulate to the peripheral vasculature and bring about increased permeability and oedema.

Sites of metabolism

The lung is said to comprise 40 different types of cell, many of which must be highly active metabolically – secretory cells, ciliated cells, mast cells, etc. However, as far as the metabolic functions operating on blood-borne substrates are concerned, the most relevant type is the endothelial cell of the pulmonary circulation. For many years, these cells were not considered to be metabolically interesting or even particularly active, but over the last 25 years evidence has been accumulating that they possess and exhibit a number of metabolic properties highly relevant to vasomotor control (Ryan, 1986; Petty and Pearson, 1989), such as conversion of AI to AII, inactivation of bradykinin, enkephalin and 5-HT, and synthesis of PGI$_2$ and endothelin. The metabolic functions of whole perfused lung are frequently taken as expressions of the activities of the pulmonary endothelium, and for many of these functions that would seem to be a justifiable assumption. The number of endothelial cells and their proximity to the blood-borne substrate strengthens the correlation between the properties of the endothelial cells and the phenomena observed in the pulmonary circulation in vivo or in perfused lungs.

Reference has already been made to the constant exposure of the lung to the external environment through ventilation and here the epithelial cell is the first to be encountered. The pharmacological biochemistry of the epithelial cell has been largely neglected during the vigorous analysis of endothelial cell function but some important new findings have emphasized the potential relevance of the epithelium to causation and repair of lung injury and these will be discussed later.

Mechanisms of selective metabolism

Some of the selectivity of the metabolic functions of lung may derive from the properties peculiar to the alveolar capillary endothelium, but there are at least two other more clearly defined mechanisms of selectivity which depend on the subcellular localization of the metabolic system involved.

First, some of the enzymes concerned are located on the outside of the endothelial cell membrane (ecto-enzymes), with free access to substrates in the extracellular or vascular space. For example, angiotensin converting enzyme (ACE) is found on the luminal surface of the endothelium in situ (Ryan, 1986), as are the ecto-nucleotidases, AMP-ase, ADP-ase and ATP-ase. For all these ecto-enzymes, the selectivity of metabolism must reflect the selectivity of the enzyme itself. This is certainly true of ACE, which will not hydrolyse peptides without a free carboxy terminal (Bakhle, 1974), and peptides with a C-terminal amide such as oxytocin and vasopressin pass freely through the pulmonary circulation (Bakhle and Vane, 1974). The free passage of AII also reflects the substrate specificity of ACE which will not hydrolyse certain peptide links involving proline (Bakhle, 1974).

Recently a different type of peptide inactivation has been shown in lung for the atrial natriuretic peptide (ANP). Radiolabelled ANP was rapidly removed on a single transit through rabbit lungs but it could then be recovered by displacement with un-labelled peptide (Turrin and Gillis, 1986). This unusual mode of inactivation is probably due to the presence of 'silent' receptors (binding sites which do not lead to effects) for ANP in lung (Needleman et al., 1989). However, in rat lung using 10-fold higher ANP concentrations there was some evidence of transformation of ANP by peptidase action into smaller fragments. This metabolism was a comparatively slow process with a 50% clearance time of 10 minutes (Numan et al., 1990). The relevance of these results to the rapid, first-pass binding demonstrated earlier is not obvious. However, as ANP can relax vascular smooth muscle and increase microvascular permeability (Needleman et al., 1989; Zimmerman et al., 1990), the clearance of ANP by lungs using either mechanism could have important consequences for peripheral microcirculations including the bronchial vascular bed.

The other relevant enzymes are within the cell and are consequently separated from their substrates in the blood by the cell membrane. Metabolism of the substrates such as 5-HT, noradrenaline, PGE_2 and adenosine comprises two distinct processes, uptake across the cell membrane and, subsequently, interaction with the intracellular enzyme. For the catecholamines, the uptake process is rate-limiting and is the source of the observed specificity (Bakhle and Vane, 1974; Gillis and Pitt, 1982; Junod, 1985). Pulmonary monoamine oxidase will metabolize noradrenaline, dopamine and adrenaline equally well *in vitro*, with a K_m between 300 and $400 \mu M$ (Bakhle and Youdim, 1979), whereas in whole lung only noradrenaline is metabolized, with a K_m of about $1 \mu M$ (Gillis and Pitt, 1982). Uptake is not rate limiting with PGE_2 or $PGF_{2\alpha}$ but the prostaglandin uptake system will not accept PGI_2 as a substrate, although the intracellular enzyme prostaglandin dehydrogenase (PGDH) hydrolyses PGI_2 faster than PGE_2 *in vitro* (Bakhle and Ferreira, 1985). Here, again, it is the specificity of the uptake system that determines the selectivity of the overall metabolism. This discrepancy between the enzymic content and the functions expressed in the organized tissue is frequently observed in lung and is also important in the pharmacokinetics of exogenous, xenobiotic drugs (see later).

Endocrine functions of lung

Apart from its pharmacokinetic modulation of circulating endogenous substrates, the lung also has the potential for a pseudo-endocrine function by virtue of its central position in the circulation. The release of von Willebrand Factor and tissue plasminogen activator from endothelium into the pulmonary blood could be considered an endocrine function (Petty and Pearson, 1989; Wiedemann et al., 1990). The endocrine function will also be expressed by the overflow into the pulmonary circulation of a mediator formed by lung tissue for intrapulmonary purposes. Such overflow is more likely in pathological situations. For instance, the release of eicosanoids and histamine from lung during immunological challenge (Bakhle and Ferreira, 1985) and of eicosanoids in acute injury states (endotoxin, embolism) (Brigham and Meyrick, 1986; Izumi and Bakhle, 1989; Malik and Johnson, 1989), into the systemic circulation, could add to the general cardiovascular derangements in these conditions. The generation of cytokines from the pulmonary endothelial cells (Mantovani and Dejana, 1989) could be regarded as being designed for local effect. However because the entire blood volume passes through the pulmonary circulation, cytokines in the pulmonary blood would be able to affect leucocytes and other cells in the periphery as well as those in the pulmonary circulation.

There are some other candidates for 'pulmonary vasoactive hormone' status as endothelial cells have been identified as the source of three more mediators, platelet activating factor (PAF), endothelium-derived relaxing factor (EDRF) and endothelin.

The phospholipid, PAF, has a wide spectrum of mostly pro-inflammatory activities (McManus and Deavers, 1989; Martin *et al.*, 1994). PAF is not structurally related to the lipid mediators derived from arachidonic acid (the eicosanoids), although the synthesis of PAF and of the eicosanoids are both inhibited by corticosteroids. The most important sources of PAF are leucocytes and platelets but cultured endothelial cells will release PAF on stimulation with a number of inflammatory mediators (Camussi *et al.*, 1987).

The vasodilator activity called EDRF (Furchgott and Zawadzki, 1980) has been identified as a comparatively simple molecule, nitric oxide (NO) (Moncada *et al.*, 1991) or a thiol derivative of NO (Ignarro, 1990). The EDRF is released from endothelial cells in culture or *in situ* by a number of stimuli, including histamine, bradykinin, ATP and acetylcholine. Although its vasodilator action *in vivo* depends on its diffusion abluminally to the underlying smooth muscle, NO can also be secreted into the lumen and exert potent anti-aggregatory effects on platelets (Moncada *et al.*, 1991) or be transferred downstream in the blood. Using blood-free perfusion media, NO was shown to be 'exported' from perfused isolated heart (Kelm and Schrader, 1990). However, export of NO from the large mass of endothelial cells in the pulmonary circulation was less easily demonstrated although there is evidence for EDRF/NO generation from the behaviour of activated platelets and neutrophils within the pulmonary circulation (May *et al.*, 1991) and the vasomotor responses of isolated lungs and strips of pulmonary artery (Chand and Altura, 1981; Crawley *et al.*, 1990; Rodman *et al.*, 1990). Now with highly sensitive chemiluminescence methods, NO in lung perfusate can be detected (Ishizaki *et al.*, 1995), as can NO in exhaled gas from healthy adults and patients (Borland *et al.*, 1993; Persson *et al.*, 1994).

Inhibition of NO synthesis by analogues of the natural precursor, L-arginine, has disclosed a continued basal release of NO in the systemic arterial beds in experimental animals (Ignarro, 1990; Moncada *et al.*, 1991) and man (Vallance *et al.*, 1989), implying a vasodilator 'tone' under normal physiological conditions. However, in the pulmonary bed, the presence of NO has been most convincingly inferred only during hypoxia (Brashers *et al.*, 1988; Mazmanian *et al.*, 1989; Archer *et al.*, 1990; Liu *et al.*, 1991). Furthermore, releasers of NO (ACh, bradykinin), NO itself and scavengers of NO (methylene blue) all were without effect on pulmonary perfusion pressures under normoxic conditions (Mazmanian *et al.*, 1989; Archer *et al.*, 1990). There are many other possible functions, immunological, neurophysiological and endocrine, attributed to NO and some may be demonstrable in lung (Jorens *et al.*, 1993; Quinn *et al.*, 1995). Its role in lung injury will be discussed later.

Endothelin is a peptide secreted by endothelial cells and originally described as a vasoconstrictor in the systemic arterial circulation (Yanagisawa *et al.*, 1988). Other properties include release of EDRF and eicosanoids from perfused tissues, bronchoconstriction and mitogenesis of vascular smooth muscle (Yanagisawa and Masaki, 1989). Endothelin release is stimulated by other vasoconstrictors, by thrombin, by hypoxia or by endotoxin (Morel *et al.*, 1989; Sugiura *et al.*, 1989; Yanagisawa and Masaki, 1989). Endothelin is vasoconstrictor in the pulmonary vascular bed (Brink *et al.*, 1991) and at the same time inactivated in this circulation (De Nucci *et al.*, 1988; Stewart *et al.*, 1991). Increased plasma levels of endothelin have been associated with pulmonary hypertension (Stewart *et al.*, 1991). The arteriovenous concentration ratio of immunoreactive endothelin in normal subjects was 0.5 (compatible with the 50% inactivation reported in rat isolated lung (De Nucci *et al.*, 1988)), but in patients with secondary or primary pulmonary hypertension (PPH) the ratio was 1.0 or 2.2 respectively, implying in the first instance loss of the inactivation function, and in the second net synthesis of endothelin by the lung. The initial hypothesis was that pulmonary hypertension was accompanied by endothelial damage and since endothelial cells synthesize endothelin, a *reduced* output of this peptide would have been predicted. However, endothelin was increased in endothelial cells from patients with PPH (Giaid *et al.*, 1993). Apart from a vasoconstrictor effect, this peptide is also mitogenic for smooth muscle cells (Yanagisawa and Masaki, 1989) and could thus mediate the morphological changes in the pulmonary vasculature typical of this condition. Plasma levels of this peptide could become a valuable marker for pulmonary hypertension. The relevance of endothelin to other lung disease states is still unclear (Levin, 1995).

Physiological control of lung metabolism

The physiological relevance of the metabolic function of lung is emphasized by its response to a variety of physiological control systems (Bakhle, 1990). This function changes during perinatal growth and later development. In female rats, lung metabolism of monoamines, arachidonate and prostaglandins, but not that of ADP were affected by the oestrous cycle. Experimental diabetes mellitus altered prostaglandin synthesis and ADP and adenosine metabolism but 5-HT metabolism was unchanged. A particularly significant finding is the species variation in lung metabolism between experimental animals and man. One such variation

for ADP degradation in isolated lungs from four species is illustrated in Figure 43.1, and demonstrates clearly that the level of 5'-nucleotidase (AMP-ase) varies markedly between species, although all exhibited a high level of ADP-ase activity. Whatever the significance of these differences for the physiology of each species might be, the practical importance of this work is that, in terms of *these* substrates, guinea-pig lung is the best analogue of human lung. This conclusion contrasts sharply with the finding that PG synthesis in guinea-pig lung is very different from that in human lung and that rat lung is a much closer analogue for this function (Bakhle and Ferreira, 1985). Knowledge of such species selective alterations in metabolism is essential to the good design and valid interpretation of animal models of human disorders.

It is clear that the metabolic function of lung is an important mechanism, under physiological control, for the manipulation of the arterial concentration of many potent endogenous vasoactive agents circulating in blood. There are also significant pharmacokinetic effects on xenobiotic substrates, involving processes of lesser specificity but detectable at therapeutic or subtherapeutic concentrations, in animals and man.

Exogenous substrates

The fate of exogenous xenobiotic substrates, usually drugs, in lung is markedly different from that of endogenous substrates discussed above, in three aspects. First, the immediate pharmacokinetic effect of passage through the pulmonary circulation is the reversible binding, without metabolism, of the exogenous substrate. The sites of this binding are not clearly defined. Some sites must be on the endothelium, as several drugs (tricyclic antidepressants) will interfere with the uptake systems for noradrenaline and 5-HT (Bakhle and Vane, 1974; Gillis and Pitt, 1982; Junod, 1985) located in these cells, but some must be elsewhere to account for the drug–drug interactions discussed below. Another probable location is the epithelial cell where some compounds can cause phospholipidosis (Bend *et al.*, 1985; Dunn and Glassroth, 1989). The lack of metabolism of blood-borne xenobiotic substrates is not due to the absence of enzymes, as lung tissue contains enough appropriate drug metabolizing enzymes – demethylases, mixed function oxidases, hydrolases – to handle the substrates that are bound (Bend *et al.*, 1985). There must be some restriction of access to the enzymes to explain this discrepancy. For instance, the relevant enzymes may be concentrated in the airway epithelial cells whereas the binding sites may be close to the pulmonary vasculature.

Second, the binding process has low specificity. The essential requirements, based on studies with

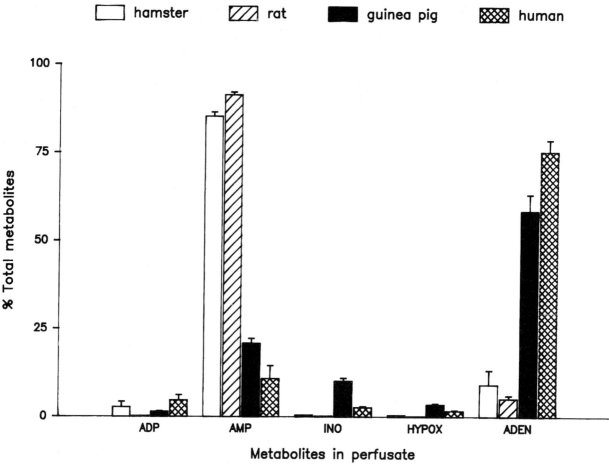

Figure 43.1 Species variation in metabolism of ADP by perfused lung. Whole lungs from hamsters, rats and guinea-pigs and samples of human lung were perfused via the pulmonary vessels with Krebs solution and the effluent perfusate collected after a single passage through the lung. Samples of the perfusate were analysed by thin layer chromatography with ADP, AMP, inosine (INO), hypoxanthine (HYPOX) and adenosine (ADEN) as markers. Following the administration of ^{14}C – ADP (10 nmoles) into the pulmonary circulation, there were two major metabolites, AMP and adenosine. For rat and hamster lungs, AMP was almost the sole metabolite (>80%) whereas guinea-pig and human lung exhibited further metabolism to adenosine with relatively little AMP (<20%). These results show that for this substrate (ADP), guinea-pig clearly provides the better analogue of human lung. (Results from Chelliah and Bakhle, 1983.)

local anaesthetics, β-adrenoceptor blocking drugs and analgesics, appear to be that the substrate is basic (pK_a >8.0) and lipophilic (Post *et al.*, 1979; Hemsworth and Street, 1981; Bend *et al.*, 1985; Roerig *et al.*, 1994). This wide range of substrates also explains the interactions between pharmacologically widely different drugs which nevertheless have enough physicochemical similarity to compete with each other. Thus local anaesthetics compete with and displace tricyclic antidepressants (Post *et al.*, 1979), the antidepressants with chlorpromazine (Bend *et al.*, 1985) and β-adrenoceptor antagonists with analgesics like fentanyl (Roerig *et al.*, 1994).

The third important difference in the fate of exogenous substrates is concerned with the airways. Entry into the lung via the airways is much

more common for drug molecules than for endogenous substrates and the cells encountered first in this method are epithelial rather than endothelial. Airway epithelium can also provide a physical barrier to drugs delivered to the airways in animals and man (Jeppsson *et al.*, 1991; Schmekel *et al.*, 1991; Sparrow and Mitchell, 1991). At least three important modes of lung injury, aspiration of gastric contents and inhalation of smoke or toxic vapours are likely to have their initial effects on the epithelium. Thus, assessing the health of the epithelium and its response to injury are essential components of studies of lung injury.

Important insights into the pharmacological biochemistry of the alveolar epithelial cells have also come from the extensive work on paraquat poisoning (Smith, 1985). The toxicity of this herbicide is primarily due to the destruction of Type I and Type II epithelial cells and their replacement by fibrotic tissue. These cells take up the herbicide by a transport system now known to have the endogenous polyamines (spermine, spermidine and putrescine) as its natural substrates (Smith, 1985; Nemery et al., 1987). Further studies of the epithelial uptake systems disclosed an uptake of cystamine (Lewis et al., 1989), which was rapidly metabolized to the sulphonic acid derivative taurine, which is itself taken up by epithelial cells (Banks et al., 1989; Lewis et al., 1990). The precise significance of these physiological epithelial uptake systems is not yet known. However, if we link the effects of the polyamines on cell growth (Heby, 1981) with the anti-oxidant effects of taurine (Banks et al., 1989; Lewis et al., 1990), it is possible that these epithelial uptake systems are a part of the normal protection and repair mechanisms of the alveolar epithelium.

EFFECTS OF LUNG INJURY ON THE PHARMACOKINETIC FUNCTION OF LUNG

How far are these metabolic and binding functions altered by lung injury and what can we hope to gain from such correlations? An answer to the first question will be provided by the review of different models given below but the second question will be attempted later.

Many of the models of lung injury in which the pharmacokinetic function has been assessed are designed to reproduce features of ARDS. However, there are a significant number representing other types of injury such as hyperoxia, pulmonary hypertension and environmental pollution. The greater awareness of atmospheric pollution will probably lead to an increased emphasis on the biochemical results of the chronic inhalation of 'urban' or 'industrial' air. It is not feasible to review every model or every study and a selection of injury models with measurable biochemical effects is summarized in the text below. The models have been divided, for convenience and without any mechanistic significance, into those where the injury is delivered via the airway and those delivered via the circulation.

Inhaled injury

Hyperoxia
Exposure to hyperoxic environments induces lung injury in which endothelial damage is an early and major feature (Crapo, 1989) and oxygen-induced lung injury in humans still presents real clinical problems (Klein, 1990). In a number of studies (Gillis and Catravas, 1982; Gillis and Pitt, 1982; Bakhle and Ferreira, 1985; De Nucci et al., 1986), lungs from animals exposed to hyperoxia showed decreased metabolism of several substrates in vivo

and in isolation, at a time when morphological signs of damage were not yet visible. In one study where several substrates were used (Toivonen et al., 1981), the earliest change appeared in PGE_2 metabolism even though this substrate is not metabolized by endothelial cells (Ody et al., 1979). The marked susceptibility of PGE_2 metabolism may reflect the susceptibility of the enzyme involved (PGDH) more than that of the cells in which it is located. By contrast, another endothelium-dependent function, vasodilatation induced by ACh (via its release of EDRF), was unaffected in rat lungs even with morphological evidence of hyperoxic endothelial damage (Feddersen et al., 1986).

Hypoxia
Local hypoxia and hypoxaemia may be present as a consequence of many injury states as the circulation or respiratory functions fail but acute hypoxia in an otherwise normal lung has been studied separately. The first reported metabolic effect – reduced conversion of angiotensin I to angiotensin II, an apparent inhibition of ACE – has now been explained as a haemodynamic effect consequent on hypoxic vasoconstriction (Gillis and Catravas, 1982). Two other metabolic effects are stimulated in acute hypoxia, synthesis of vasodilator prostaglandins and of EDRF. Inhibitors of prostaglandin synthesis (Weir et al., 1976) and of EDRF's effects (methylene blue, hydroquinone; Brashers et al., 1988; Mazmanian et al., 1989; Archer et al., 1990) or of NO synthesis (L-NMMA; Liu et al., 1991) potentiated hypoxic vasoconstriction. These findings and the increased output of PGI_2 from endothelial cell cultures exposed to hypoxia (Hamasaki et al., 1982) are compatible with an increased output of endogenous vasodilators during acute hypoxia, suggesting a physiological response antagonistic to the injury stimulus. However in chronic hypoxia (chronic obstructive lung disease) release of NO by acetylcholine or ADP, from pulmonary arterial rings was decreased (Dinh Xuan et al., 1993).

Tobacco smoke
Inhalation of tobacco smoke (active or passive) is probably the most common and chronic insult to the lung. However, smoking has cardiovascular as well as pulmonary sequelae and the effects of tobacco smoke on the metabolism of endogenous vasoactive substrates have been assessed in order to provide a link between smoking and cardiovascular disease. Isolated lungs from normal animals were ventilated with cigarette smoke and showed a decrease in metabolism of 5-HT and prostaglandins, with correlations to the tar content of the cigarette (Karhi et al., 1982; Matintalo et al., 1983). This was an acute effect of cigarette smoke as lungs from rats exposed in vivo for 10 days to smoke but not ventilated with smoke at the time of assay did not show these changes (Bakhle et al., 1979).

Decreased GSH levels in rat or rabbit isolated lungs following ventilation with cigarette smoke (Joshi *et al.*, 1988) could be linked to the earlier finding that *N*-acetylcysteine (NAC) which can restore depleted GSH levels (Berggren *et al.*, 1984) also protected against the toxic effects of cigarette smoke (Kobayashi *et al.*, 1990). In man a mixture of acute and chronic effects were observed, as an acute decrease in PGI$_2$ associated with smoking was observed only in habitual smokers not in non-smokers, suggesting that there was some long-lasting effect of smoking (Nadler *et al.*, 1983). Smoking also affects trans-epithelial transfer of a variety of substrates, including β-adrenoceptor agonists (Barrowcliffe and Jones, 1987; Schmekel *et al.*, 1991).

A major problem in interpreting results from these experimental studies is the relevance of the model chosen. What is the true model of 25 years of cigarette smoke inhalation? Is there a chronic effect on the endothelium? Such an effect would seem to be necessary to produce the chronic effects on the cardiovascular system. Can endothelial cell cultures treated with extracts of cigarette smoke (Holden *et al.*, 1989) yield results relevant to the human condition? This type of experiment is comparatively cheap and easy to perform and would lend itself to screening procedures aimed at identifying the active components of smoke. It is very clear that cigarette smoke in the airways can alter the biochemistry of the pulmonary circulation towards circulating endogenous substrates but the nature of the causal link between this alteration and cardiovascular disease induced by cigarette smoking is still unclear.

Atmospheric pollutants

The highly reactive atmospheric pollutants have generally been considered to attack the epithelium of the airways (Bils and Christie, 1978) and ozone is known to cause respiratory problems, including bronchial hyper-responsiveness, in normal human subjects (Ying *et al.*, 1990). Metabolism of arachidonate in rat isolated lung was affected by acute ventilation with high concentrations of ozone (Dutta *et al.*, 1990). Chronic exposure of rats *in vivo* to ozone also affected metabolism associated with pulmonary endothelium (Gross *et al.*, 1991) and these effects were reversed after 14 days in clean air. Furthermore, pre-exposure to lower levels of ozone followed by a higher concentration abolished the effect on metabolism, suggesting that some degree of tolerance could be induced. In none of these chronic exposure conditions was there any ultrastructural damage to endothelium. While it is difficult to relate the experimental findings directly to man at present, there is a clear need for more studies with ozone to clarify the relevance of these results.

Nitrogen dioxide is another oxidizing atmospheric pollutant and exposure of rats to a range of concentrations decreased the formation of PGI$_2$ in isolated lungs (Kobayashi, 1983; Kobayashi *et al.*, 1983) and also the catabolism of PGE$_2$ (Chaudhari *et al.*, 1979). However, more recently, no changes in metabolism *in vivo* could be measured in spite of an increase in permeability, respiratory changes and focal oedema following exposure of dogs to nitrogen dioxide (Man *et al.*, 1990). One of the test substrates was PGE$_1$ whose metabolism is known to be sensitive to oxidative injury (hyperoxia, free radicals) and these results contrast with the earlier findings of Chaudhari *et al.* (1979). The discrepancy between the two sets of results may derive from the use of indocyanine green as an intravascular marker in the later report. This dye has been shown to inhibit PGE$_2$ metabolism in perfused lung (Bakhle, 1981) and *in vivo* (Pitt *et al.*, 1983) and the possibility of artefactual interactions between dye marker and substrate might explain the unexpected results.

With the present and probably increasing levels of interest in environmental pollution, studies with inhaled atmospheric pollutants will be highly relevant to public health (Last *et al.*, 1994).

Volatile halogenated compounds

These divide clearly into two types; those used therapeutically as volatile anaesthetics and not normally considered as injurious agents and those more likely to be encountered as atmospheric pollutants in their industrial use as solvents, degreasing agents and cleaning fluids. However their grouping together emphasizes that effects on lung metabolism could be a general property of volatile, highly lipophilic compounds and thus distributed beyond those few compounds that have been tested so far.

The reports that halogenated anaesthetics interact with EDRF (Blaise *et al.*, 1987, 1994; Muldoon *et al.*, 1988; Stone and Johns, 1989) has consequences well beyond the pulmonary circulation, since the peripheral vasculature appears in man to have a vasodilator tone dependent on synthesis and release of EDRF (Vallance *et al.*, 1989; Moncada *et al.*, 1991). Another unrelated effect of halothane, its ability to increase the binding of propranolol to lung *in vivo* (Pang *et al.*, 1981), raises two important questions. First, what happens when the anaesthetic is discontinued and the excess propranolol is washed out of the lung? Will there be a rapid efflux, creating an arterial 'bolus' of drug, with pharmacodynamic consequences for instance on cardiac tissue? The second question is how widely is this potentiated binding found? Are other drugs bound by lung (fentanyl, meperidine, lignocaine; Jorfeldt *et al.*, 1983; Taeger *et al.*, 1988; Roerig *et al.*, 1994) equally susceptible? Both questions have real clinical meaning and deserve serious clinical assessment. The early experimental work showing decreased 5-HT and noradrenaline uptake in isolated lungs and *in vivo* after a variety of inhaled anaesthetics (Bakhle, 1990) was not confirmed by later studies in man (Gillis *et al.*, 1979; Dargent *et al.*, 1985b). However in view of the clinical implications of such interactions and of the improved methods of assay now available, a re-assessment of the interactions between commonly used general anaesthetics and the removal of monoamines or PGE_2 in human lung *in vivo* would be valuable.

The effects of the halogenated solvents (Hede *et al.*, 1985), although not striking in terms of their potency, are an indication that the toxicities of these and analogous compounds are not restricted to the liver. Indeed with the ability of the lung to affect the content of the blood circulating to the liver (as well as elsewhere), there is a possibility that some change in lung metabolism contributes to the more apparent hepatic damage.

Other forms of inhaled injury

At least two other forms of injury, acid aspiration and smoke inhalation, will have their initial gross effects on the epithelium. However both also cause pulmonary oedema (Jones *et al.*, 1978; Herndon and Traber, 1990), implying damage to the endothelium, and either can develop into clinically recognizable ARDS (Matthay, 1990; Pruitt *et al.*, 1990). The metabolic consequences of acid aspiration have not been studied, efforts being concentrated on the increased alveolar-capillary permeability (Jones *et al.*, 1978) and treatment of the injury. Exogenous VIP, a neuropeptide normally present in lung, prevented acid-induced pulmonary oedema in rats and this action was attributed to a VIP-induced increase in cyclic AMP levels which had fallen after the acid treatment (Foda *et al.*, 1988).

Smoke inhalation leading to pulmonary oedema and ARDS is already a major cause of death after fire in public places or private homes (Herndon and Traber, 1990) and an occupational hazard for some (Hansen, 1990). Protection is offered by xanthine oxidase inhibitors, protease inhibitors and prostacyclin analogues (Ahn *et al.*, 1990; Niehaus *et al.*, 1990; Witten *et al.*, 1990) and by inhibitors of leukotriene synthesis (Hales *et al.*, 1995). Another factor contributing to smoke injury is NO (Ischiropoulos *et al.*, 1994) and this variety of agents suggests further analysis of this type of lung injury is needed to clarify their mechanisms of action.

Circulating injury

Most of the forms of lung injury discussed below will induce primarily endothelial cell damage and emphasis has therefore been placed on those substrates that are metabolized by the endothelium. These injuries may appear at first sight to be an unrelated collection of models and a similar diversity of cause is one of the problems in the analysis of ARDS. However many of the experimental models and clinical forms involve oxygen-derived free radicals, either generated directly or via activated leucocytes, and this common feature is discussed later. The first two types of lung injury to be considered are essentially two forms of iatrogenic injury, cardiopulmonary bypass and ischaemic injury in transplant lungs.

Cardiopulmonary bypass

In the early years of this technique, post-perfusion syndrome and other descriptions of lung injury following cardiopulmonary bypass (CPB) were important side-effects of the procedure. In the first report of metabolic dysfunction, endothelial cell damage following CPB was suggested by the decreased removal of 5-HT and noradrenaline in patients exposed to CPB for more than 1 hour (mean duration 109 minutes) (Gillis *et al.*, 1972). In 1979, techniques had improved and with shorter CPB duration (mean 60 minutes), these effects were no longer present (Gillis *et al.*, 1979). Later still in 1985, longer periods of CPB (median duration 88 minutes) were also without effect on 5HT uptake in lung (Dargent *et al.*, 1985b). Another substrate affected by CPB was PGE_1 in patients (Hammond *et al.*, 1977), and in dogs (Pitt *et al.*, 1982) where time-related decreases were recorded. This last finding is relevant to the decreased PGE_2 metabolism in ANTU and endotoxin-injured lungs (Bakhle, 1982; Izumi and Bakhle, 1988) and to the use of PGE_1 as a marker for ARDS-induced damage in patients (Gillis *et al.*, 1986; Cox *et al.*, 1988). The severity and incidence of post-CPB lung injury has clearly diminished over the last 20 years, but it still causes concern (Kirklin, 1991; Treasure, 1994) and generates experimental analysis (Bando *et al.*, 1990; Gu *et al.*, 1991).

Ischaemia-reperfusion injury

This type of injury following thrombosis is a familiar concept with regard to the coronary circulation but another type of ischaemia-reperfusion injury is that occurring during the transplantation of organs. With the growing use of heart-and-lung transplants (Smyth *et al.*, 1991), there has been a concomitant growth of research on this form of lung injury. Although xanthine oxidase inhibitors are of some benefit in isolated reperfused lungs (Lynch *et al.*, 1988; Horgan *et al.*, 1989; Adkins and Taylor, 1990), this benefit was not seen *in vivo* (Bishop *et al.*, 1987). Another consequence of reperfusion is cytokine release (Serrick *et al.*, 1994) and prevention of such release may underlie the reversal of reperfusion injury by phosphodiesterase inhibitors (Endres, 1993; Barnard *et al.*, 1994). A more pragmatic approach is to improve preservation solutions to prevent ischaemic injury in the donated lung (Mulvin *et al.*, 1990). Clearly more work will be needed at either level to minimize this type of ischaemia-reperfusion injury.

α-Naphthylthiourea

This thiourea derivative is fairly selective for endothelial cells and damage to these cells has been well correlated with the progress of the oedema (Cunningham and Hurley, 1972; Meyrick et al., 1972). The mode of action of α-naphthylthiourea (ANTU) is not completely elucidated but it appears to involve oxygen derived free radicals, as free radical scavengers inhibit the oedema caused by this agent (Fox et al., 1983; Heffner and Repine, 1989). In this model both 5-HT removal and prostaglandin catabolism and synthesis were affected (Block and Schoen, 1981; Bakhle, 1982; Pankhania and Bakhle, 1985). However, the earliest change in lungs isolated after treatment of rats with ANTU in vivo was in adenosine uptake and occurred well before any sign of oedema; the uptake returned to normal over the same time as the oedema resolved (Bakhle and Grantham, 1987). Synthesis of PGI_2 was increased relatively late following ANTU, at about the same time as the oedema developed in this model, and was interpreted as a protective response to the injury (Pankhania and Bakhle, 1985).

Bleomycin

Lung toxicity of this antineoplastic agent also involves oxygen radicals and is usually associated with an interstitial pneumonitis leading to alveolar fibrosis with clear damage to epithelial cells. However, in the early stages endothelial injury is expressed as pulmonary oedema and neutrophil accumulation and this endothelial damage was more readily obtained with intratracheal administration (Hay et al., 1991). In this model, before changes in hydroxyproline levels (a marker for collagen metabolism) or lung morphology were detectable, metabolism of substrates typically handled by the endothelial cells was decreased (Gillis and Catravas, 1982; Lazo et al., 1986), compatible with an initial attack on the endothelium. It is interesting that after bleomycin (Chandler et al., 1985) and after ANTU (Bakhle, 1982), decreases in PGE_2 metabolism were noted; cultured endothelial cells do not metabolize PGE_2 (Ody et al., 1979) and the decreased metabolism seen in the lung could be due to the sensitivity of the rate-limiting enzyme, PGDH, to the oxidizing species produced in both models.

Free radical generating mixtures

A mixture of xanthine oxidase with hypoxanthine as substrate is a method of generating oxygen derived free radicals in situ. Perfusion of isolated lungs with such a mixture damages the endothelium and leads to decreased clearance of monoamines (Cook et al., 1982; Steinberg et al., 1982); an alternative but equivalent mixture (glucose oxidase and glucose) was equally effective in reducing lung uptake of 5-HT in vivo in dogs (Vigneswaran et al.,

1989). This injury also increased output of prostanoids from rat isolated lung (Berisha et al., 1990). Here both the physical injury (oedema, perfusion pressure and protein leakage) and the biochemical effect (increased prostanoid synthesis) were prevented by infusions of VIP but it was not clear whether the prostanoids were mediators of, or a response to, the cell injury.

Epithelial cell toxins

Two agents, paraquat and the insecticide-related toxin O,S,S-trimethyl phosphorodithioate, have been used to damage specifically epithelial cells, with subsequent analysis of metabolism. The selectivity of these agents for the epithelium has been confirmed by histology (Smith, 1985; Nemery et al., 1987). In these models, the uptake of polyamines associated with the epithelium was also decreased. These are important findings as they correlate the biochemical well-being with the physical integrity of the epithelium and provide a means of probing the epithelium's biochemical status. However, there are practical problems which need to be overcome before the full potential of these findings can be realized. One is that relatively little polyamine is taken up on a single transit through a perfused isolated lung (about 0.3%) compared with the endothelial substrates (40–90% uptake). Epithelial uptake is assayed using lung slices with exposure times of 15–60 minutes. It would clearly be better to develop a substrate and assay method that could be used in vivo and preferably non-destructively. For instance, it may be possible to give the substrate via the airway to increase the proportion taken up on a single pass. Other substrates for epithelial uptake which could serve as markers of epithelial health are cystamine (Lewis et al., 1989) or taurine (Banks et al., 1989; Lewis et al., 1990).

Endotoxin

The high prevalence of sepsis as a precursor to ARDS has been the driving force behind the many models of lung injury involving experimental septicaemia, injection of live bacteria or endotoxin. Most have used endotoxin and this agent has been accepted as providing a useful model for ARDS (Brigham and Meyrick, 1986; Welbourn and Young, 1992). One of the long established effects of endotoxin on lung metabolism is increased output of prostaglandins and many of endotoxin's effects were reduced by decreasing prostaglandin synthesis using cyclo-oxygenase inhibitors (Hubbard and Janssen, 1988; Davies et al., 1989; Said and Foda, 1989; Goldstein and Luce, 1990).

The beneficial effects of corticosteroids in animal models of endotoxin shock could reasonably be attributed to inhibition of the synthesis of eicosanoids, as a consequence of increased output of lipocortin (Flower, 1984). However, there are reports of unchanged or increased prostaglandin output after steroids in animals and man (Reines *et al.*, 1985; Chang *et al.*, 1989). In isolated lungs from rats, PGI_2 output was markedly decreased after treatment *in vivo* with endotoxin and methylprednisolone given 30 minutes after endotoxin prevented this fall in output (Izumi and Bakhle, 1989). In dogs, plasma levels of PGI_2 after endotoxin and steroid were higher than after endotoxin alone (Hales *et al.*, 1986). The mechanism of this increase is unknown, but since PGI_2 reduces activation of leucocytes and oedema formation when given intravenously (Rampart and Williams, 1986), such a change in prostaglandin production would clearly be beneficial in endotoxin-induced lung injury. An increase in PGI_2 would also imply protection of the endothelial cells, which produce this prostanoid, against direct or indirect (by marginated leucocytes) damage by endotoxin (Brigham and Meyrick, 1986).

There is an unexplained contrast between the widespread efficacy of corticosteroid treatment of animal models of endotoxin shock and lung injury and the generally poor results in ARDS patients (Goldstein and Luce, 1990). To some extent this must reflect the timing of the steroid treatment in the two groups. In the animal models, treatment is given either before or very soon after the endotoxin; in one series (Izumi and Bakhle, 1989), steroid was given before, at the same time, or after the endotoxin and it was noted that pretreatment was most effective. However, in the ARDS patient, treatment only follows the recognition of ARDS by a set of criteria based essentially on physical damage to the microvasculature, i.e. on changes in blood gases, compliance and radiographic appearance (Rocker *et al.*, 1989; Matthay, 1990). Thus the injury has been initiated and may still be continuing for many hours before steroids are given. A great improvement in the efficacy of steroids or any other drugs might be expected if treatment could be started much earlier, well before the physical signs have appeared. A biochemical early warning of the physical damage would allow the identification of those patients likely to progress to ARDS as presently defined, at a time when the physical signs of damage were not yet apparent. The early diagnosis of 'pre-ARDS' would also allow early treatment with greater chances of success.

One possible marker is exhaled NO; the output of this gas was markedly increased 2–3 hours after endotoxin was given intravenously to rats (Stewart *et al.*, 1995). As NO is exhaled by normal subjects (Borland *et al.*, 1993; Quinn *et al.*, 1995), this finding could be applied to patients at risk of ARDS as a non-invasive procedure. The source of the increased NO could be either leucocytes accumulating in lung or the lung tissue itself, as the inducible NO synthase was increased strikingly in bronchial epithelial cells by endotoxin or inflammatory cytokines (Robbins *et al.*, 1994; Gutierrez *et al.*, 1995).

Endotoxin also affects the catabolic function of lung. Endotoxin given to rats *in vivo* markedly decreased PGE_2 inactivation in isolated lung, this change preceding the onset of lung oedema and returning to normal as the oedema resolved (Grantham *et al.*, 1988; Izumi and Bakhle, 1988). Furthermore, methylprednisolone given after endotoxin prevented the oedema and the metabolic change (Izumi and Bakhle, 1988), as illustrated in

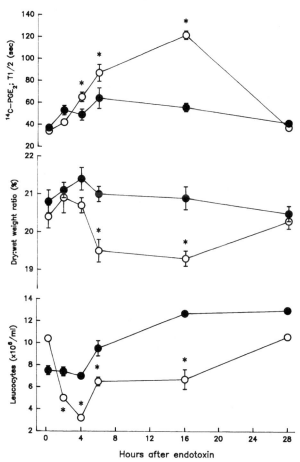

Figure 43.2 Effects of methylprednisolone (MP) on responses to endotoxin (Etx) in rats (Etx only, $-\bigcirc-$; Etx + MP, $-\bullet-$). The peripheral leucocyte count fell rapidly after Etx (3.5 mg/kg; IP) with a minimum at 4 hours. Lung oedema was detectable as decreased lung dry : wet weight ratios later, at 6 and 16 hours after Etx. The biochemical variable ($T_{\frac{1}{2}}$ for PGE_2) changed soon after Etx. At 4 hours it was almost twice the normal value (zero time) and increased to a maximum at 16 hours but returned to normal by 28 hours with both the other variables. Injection of MP (30 mg/kg SC, 30 minutes after Etx) either totally (oedema) or very markedly (leucocytes and $T_{\frac{1}{2}}$) reversed the changes due to Etx. These results demonstrate the value of the $T_{\frac{1}{2}}$ measurement as an early indicator of lung oedema and its response to treatment that prevented the lung injury. *$P < 0.05$. vs control (zero time) values, shown for Etx only, for clarity; $n > 6$. (Results from Izumi and Bakhle, 1988, 1989.)

Figure 43.2. In these experiments, the rapid fall in peripheral leucocytes was followed by a fall in dry : wet lung weight ratio, indicative of pulmonary oedema. The increase in $T_{\frac{1}{2}}$ for labelled PGE_2 reflecting decreased metabolism, was also rapid and preceded the oedema, although both variables returned to normal by 28 hours after endotoxin. Treatment with methylprednisolone, 30 minutes after endotoxin, totally reversed the oedema and severely attenuated the leucopenia. The metabolism of PGE_2 as measured by its $T_{\frac{1}{2}}$ value, responded equally well to treatment with the steroid.

However, endotoxin treatment *in vivo* did not affect the uptake of adenosine by rat isolated lung (Grantham *et al.*, 1988), even though this uptake was susceptible to ANTU-induced endothelial cell damage (Grantham and Bakhle, 1988). This differential effect of endotoxin on lung metabolism suggests that it is not merely disruption of or physical damage to the endothelium, which is present equally after either ANTU or endotoxin, but some particular consequence of endotoxin that causes a decrease in prostaglandin catabolism, such as the sensitivity of PGDH to oxidation and the generation of free radicals by either injurious agent.

Following the demonstration that endotoxin releases tumour necrosis factor (TNF) at an early stage in its action (Tracey *et al.*, 1986), several workers have shown that many of the effects of endotoxin *in vivo* can be mimicked by TNF (Stephens *et al.*, 1988; Ferrari-Baliviera *et al.*, 1989; Johnson *et al.*, 1989; Tracey and Lowry, 1990) and that antibodies to TNF prevent endotoxin shock (Tracey and Lowry, 1990). However, the effects of TNF on lung metabolism of endogenous substrates are largely unknown. Increased output of TxB_2 and other prostanoids has been reported from lungs *in vivo* and in isolation (Johnson *et al.*, 1989; Hocking *et al.*, 1990) and other consequences of TNF administration in man and in animals were decreased by cyclo-oxygenase inhibition (Michie *et al.*, 1988; Okusawa *et al.*, 1988; Kettelhut *et al.*, 1989; Simpson and Casey, 1989). Other important aspects of TNF's action on the metabolic function of lung remain to be systematically investigated.

Patients with adult respiratory distress syndrome

The theoretical and experimental predictions and findings from a number of experimental models have been extended to a limited series of patients with ARDS, using as endogenous test substrates 5-HT and PGE_1. In two separate studies, 5-HT removal was lower than in control patients (Morel *et al.*, 1985; Gillis *et al.*, 1986). In one group the severity of the ARDS and, where multiple assays were performed, worsening of the clinical signs was associated with a further decrease in 5-HT removal (Morel *et al.*, 1985). In both studies, values of 5-HT removal below 80% (the normal values

were 89–97%) were correlated with a fatal outcome.

Another substrate, PGE_1, was studied also in two separate groups of ARDS patients. Gillis *et al.* found decreased removal with low tracer doses of PGE_1 in their patients (Gillis *et al.*, 1986). This was confirmed in the second group who were receiving pharmacologically effective infusions of PGE_1 as a treatment for ARDS (Cox *et al.*, 1988). The second group also showed correlations between the severity of ARDS and the reduction in PGE_1 removal. These studies support the general prediction made from experimental work that clinical ARDS would be associated with a loss of the metabolic function of lung and that there is a qualitative correlation between severity of clinical signs, i.e., physical damage, and the extent of the metabolic dysfunction. Given the normal variability of man relative to inbred laboratory animal species, it is not surprising that there was a considerable variability in the absolute level of the dysfunction and a better correlation would be obtained with serial determinations in each patient.

The *predictive* value of the metabolic assay was only partially assessed in these studies. Fewer patients were placed in the 'at-risk' category, i.e. not yet with the clinical signs of ARDS; one out of two with lower PGE_1 removal (Cox *et al.*, 1988) but none of the at-risk patients with low 5-HT removal (Morel *et al.*, 1985) developed ARDS. These findings are difficult to assess fairly; it is possible that knowledge of the deficient 5-HT removal led to more active nursing and monitoring of those patients without obvious intent and with PGE_1, the numbers are too small for comment. Nevertheless, more predictive studies ought to be encouraged because it is in the at-risk patient that a biochemical early warning will have the greatest effect on treatment and on outcome.

Exogenous substrates

Exogenous, xenobiotic substrates have also been used in assessment of experimental lung injury states or different lung pathologies in man. The most frequently used substrate is propranolol and its first-pass uptake was decreased in lung injury induced by the phorbol esters (Merker and Gillis, 1988) and in shock lung models (Pang *et al.*, 1982a). Reduction of the vascular bed available for perfusion by ligation or occlusion also decreased uptake of propranolol, as did experimental atelectasis (Pang *et al.*, 1982a; Dargent *et al.*, 1985a; Merker and Gillis, 1988). These results were interpreted as showing changes in the total area perfused rather than the characteristics of the binding sites. In patients, a similar interpretation was placed on the diminished uptake of propranolol in emphysema, postoperative atelectasis and ARDS (Pang *et al.*, 1982b; Dargent *et al.*, 1985b; Morel *et al.*, 1985). Where a comparison could be made between 5-HT and propranolol as biochemical markers, the authors concluded that 5-HT was a better measure of metabolic quality, whereas propranolol appeared to reflect the perfused area available to the substrate (Dargent *et al.*, 1985b; Morel *et al.*, 1985).

If this were the correct interpretation, then the *increased* binding of propranolol caused by halothane *in vivo* (Pang *et al.*, 1981) could be due to an increase in perfused area consequent on the relaxation of pulmonary vascular smooth muscle by the anaesthetic. However, propranolol binding was also increased by lignocaine in isolated perfused lung (Dollery and Junod, 1976) where the pulmonary vasculature would be fully dilated. Another interpretation would therefore be that the lipid-soluble anaesthetic molecules cause reversible modification of the cell structures used as binding sites for propranolol; this effect might be comparable to the effects of anaesthetics on neuronal membranes.

Another exogenous substrate that may be useful to measure perfused area is an iodobenzylpropane diamine (HIPDM) (Slosman *et al.*, 1987; Shih *et al.*, 1988). This molecule can be labelled with γ-emitting radioisotopes of iodine, enabling the uptake or loss of radioactivity from lung to be measured by external detectors. Like the basic drugs, binding of this amine was open to competition by other basic drugs of dissimilar structure, but HIPDM was nevertheless very strongly bound to lung (Abrams *et al.*, 1987; Slosman *et al.*, 1987). Two studies have shown a decreased rate of loss from the lungs of smokers *in vivo* (Pistolesi *et al.*, 1988; Liu *et al.*, 1994) and use of this marker in other situations has been summarized (Miniati *et al.*, 1992).

The advantages of the γ-emitting radioisotopes of iodine have encouraged the study of other iodinated substrates, like *N*-isopropyl-iodo-amphetamine (IMP; Touya *et al.*, 1986) and the more useful iodoguanidines (Slosman *et al.*, 1988a). Lung uptake of one of these iodoguanidines, MIBG, was inhibited by cocaine, imipramine and noradrenaline (Slosman *et al.*, 1988a) as expected for a substrate for noradrenaline uptake in lung. However, uptake of MIBG was also inhibited by 5-HT (Slosman *et al.*, 1988a) which does not interfere with noradrenaline uptake (Alabaster, 1977; Gillis and Pitt, 1982) and by iodoamphetamine (Slosman *et al.*, 1989b) and labetalol (Khafagi *et al.*, 1989), both basic drugs. Clearly uptake of MIBG in lung involves at least two mechanisms. Another derivative, AIBG (Shulkin *et al.*, 1986), exhibited a lower single-pass uptake in lung but was said to have less non-specific binding (Weng *et al.*, 1990).

Uptake of MIBG was decreased by a reduction in vascular area by ligation of blood vessels, yielding a linear relationship between vascular surface and uptake (Slosman *et al.*, 1989). However MIBG uptake was also reduced in a model of minimal endothelial damage induced by intraperitoneal injections of bleomycin (Slosman *et al.*, 1990), but

this reduction was slight (20%) though significant. Two of the guanidines, MIBG and AIBG, were studied in the presence of an organo-gold antineoplastic agent with suspected pneumotoxicity (Weng *et al.*, 1990). Although the initial response of isolated lung to the organo-gold compound was vasoconstriction, when the perfusion pressure had returned to normal both MIBG and AIBG uptake were decreased, the latter by about 60%. Uptake of noradrenaline was not measured nor were any histological results provided.

These iodoamines offer considerable practical advantages in the measurement of lung pharmacokinetics but there has to be some doubt as to the relevance of these measurements to the crucial variable – the biochemical health of the endothelial cell. However the results obtained so far deserve further analysis in terms of the effects of established models of endothelial and epithelial injury on the uptake or loss of the iodoamines from lung.

CONCLUSIONS

At least three benefits of the correlation of physical lung injury and its biochemical precursors or consequences were proposed earlier in this chapter. The first benefit to be gained from a correlation of biochemistry and injury was the identification of mediators of the injury. This would lead to rational treatment by inhibition of their production or antagonism of their action. Such treatment would inhibit the development or, ideally, prevent the initiation of the injury process. A second benefit would derive from a better knowledge of the normal protection and repair mechanisms, the development of procedures to support and enhance those mechanisms and thus to limit the duration or intensity of the injury. The third gain would be a biochemical index of injury that could be used to give an early warning of the physical damage to come and thus allow treatment earlier than is possible at present. It is now appropriate to assess how far those benefits have been realized and, if possible, to identify areas of likely advance or trends of research effort.

Mediators of lung injury

A single group of chemical mediators essential to lung injury still remain to be identified. However there is strong evidence that the lipid mediators, eicosanoids (prostaglandins and leukotrienes) and PAF, play important roles in endotoxin-derived injury models (Brigham and Meyrick, 1986; Feuerstein and Hallenbeck, 1987; McManus and Deavers, 1989; Goldstein and Luce, 1990; Rinaldo and Christman, 1990). There was clear benefit in experimental injury from the use of cyclooxygenase inhibitors, especially ibuprofen, of corticosteroids (inhibitors of eicosanoid and PAF formation) and of antagonists of PAF. It is nevertheless significant that corticosteroids are no longer recommended as treatment for ARDS and neither ibuprofen nor PAF antagonists have yet supplanted them (Goldstein and Luce, 1990), although this may change as a result of a large-scale clinical trial (Dhainaut *et al.*, 1994).

A newer set of potential mediators are the cytokines (Rinaldo and Christman, 1990; Tracey and Lowry, 1990; Moldawer, 1994). Apart from the clear link between endotoxin and TNF, two other cytokines, IL-1 and IL-2, induced lung oedema in experimental models (Fairman *et al.*, 1987; Glauser *et al.*, 1988; Okusawa *et al.*, 1988; Klausner *et al.*, 1989; Rabinovici *et al.*, 1994) and, as a side-effect of anticancer therapies, in man (Lotze *et al.*, 1986). Another cytokine, IL-8, showed contractor activity on lung tissue susceptible to inhibition by indomethacin, implying the stimulation of prostaglandin synthesis (Burrows *et al.*, 1989). Several cytokines have leucocyte chemoattractant properties and the ability to enhance secretion of other cytokines or enzymes from those cells. Endothelial cells will both release and respond to a variety of cytokines (Mantovani and Dejana, 1989). Neither the complete range of cytokine activities nor their interrelationships have been fully explored (Movat *et al.*, 1987; Okusawa *et al.*, 1988; Moldawer, 1994) and therefore their place in the process of lung injury is still being assessed (Serrick *et al.*, 1994; Christman *et al.*, 1995; Shenkar and Abraham, 1995). Potent and selective antagonists and antibodies to these proteins or to their receptors will provide essential tools in this study (Suffredini, 1994; Bauer *et al.*, 1995; Bone *et al.*, 1995). The involvement of protein tyrosine kinase in models of inflammatory cytokine action (Novogrodsky *et al.*, 1994; Akarasereenont *et al.*, 1995) suggests that tyrosine kinase inhibitors may provide another route to the control of endotoxin's effects in lung.

There is now much evidence to support the involvement of leucocytes in the initiation of lung injury (Hogg, 1987; Rinaldo and Christman, 1990; Welbourn and Young, 1992), even though they are not obligatory for lung injury (Laufe *et al.*, 1986; Maunder *et al.*, 1986). However, in the majority of cases, leucocytes are present and functional and it is valid to accept these cells as important factors in most instances. These cells are the source of oxygen-derived free radicals implicated in the causation of injury in a variety of models, in culture, in perfused lung and *in vivo*; the same cells also are sources of proteases with deleterious actions on the microvasculature (Eisenberg *et al.*, 1990). It is therefore logical to seek to prevent the activation of leucocytes in order to prevent generation of free radicals and the secretion of proteases.

One method of 'deactivating' leucocytes is with prostacyclin or PGE$_1$. These two prostanoids will decrease the margination of leucocytes, the subsequent secretion of enzymes and generation of oxygen derived free radicals (Weissmann *et al.*, 1980; Fantone *et al.*, 1984; Jones and Hurley, 1984). *In vivo*, increased microvascular permeability dependent on leucocytes was markedly decreased by prostacyclin and PGE$_1$ analogues (Rampart and Williams, 1986) and elevated PGI$_2$ levels may protect against ARDS (Slotman *et al.*, 1985). The beneficial effects of corticosteroids in endotoxin-induced lung injury may be related to their ability to increase PGI$_2$ production (Hales *et al.*, 1986; Izumi and Bakhle, 1989) rather than to inhibition of prostanoid synthesis. Compounds that increase PGI$_2$ production have not been a major interest of pharmacological research, but such activity has been ascribed to a few compounds of varied structure – nafazatrom, suloctidil and Ph CL28A (Carreras *et al.*, 1980; Bakhle and Pankhania, 1987a,b; Pankhania and Bakhle, 1990). One of these, nafazatrom, decreased the damage due to cardiac ischaemia-reperfusion in dogs *in vivo*, a system in which leucocytes are involved (Coker and Parratt, 1984). Assessment of these compounds in lung injury *in vivo* would be helpful in an evaluation of the importance of these prostanoids as endogenous controllers of leucocyte activity.

The efficacy of pentoxifylline in experimental lung injury may also reflect deactivation of leucocytes (Ishizaka *et al.*, 1988; Welsh *et al.*, 1988; Lilly *et al.*, 1989). Pentoxifylline increases intracellular cAMP through inhibition of phosphodiesterase and prevents TNF and lysosomal enzyme release (Endres *et al.*, 1991; Sullivan *et al.*, 1991). Another chemically dissimilar agent with protective effects against a variety of lung injuries is the neuropeptide, VIP (Said and Foda, 1989; Pakbaz *et al.*, 1994). This peptide prevented injury and the increased output of prostanoids in isolated lungs induced by xanthine oxidase/xanthine mixtures (Berisha *et al.*, 1990) or paraquat (Berisha *et al.*, 1990; Pakbaz *et al.*, 1993). Inhibition of leukotriene synthesis in lung by VIP was linked to its stimulation of adenyl cyclase (DiMarzo *et al.*, 1989). VIP is normally present in lung and its release from perfused lung was markedly increased on injury (Berisha *et al.*, 1990).

It is therefore possible that both VIP and PGI$_2$ may be released from lung during injury as physiological antagonists to the harmful effects of marginated, activated leucocytes. Furthermore, deactivation of leucocytes may provide a point of therapeutic attack common to many clinically important lung injuries and this deactivation in turn may depend on increases in leucocyte cAMP (Torphy *et al.*, 1994) as the crucial biochemical event.

Repair processes in lung injury

There is much evidence for an increased formation of oxygen-derived free radicals in many forms of lung injury (Heffner and Repine, 1989). Restoration of the normal condition and recovery from the injury depends on a decrease in those free radicals by increased scavenging or decreased generation. Free radical scavengers are beneficial in a number of injury models (Heffner and Repine, 1989) but the application of compounds such as dimethylthiourea (Wong *et al.*, 1985; Gross *et al.*, 1989) and DMSO (Fox *et al.*, 1983) to clinical practice is unlikely.

Free iron is a catalyst for the generation of one of the more reactive oxidizing species, the hydroxyl free radical (Halliwell and Gutteridge, 1985). Potentiation of bleomycin toxicity by increased levels of iron (Hay *et al.*, 1991) and conversely inhibition of toxicity by depletion of whole body iron (Chandler *et al.*, 1988) strengthens the case for free iron as an important component in lung injury. Chelation of iron by desferrioxamine has been of benefit in culture and *in vivo* against a range of insults – ozone, phorbol esters, hyperoxia (Heffner and Repine, 1989), burn-induced lung injury (Demling and LaLonde, 1990) and paraquat (van der Wal *et al.*, 1992). There is certainly enough experimental data to encourage the study of chelating agents such as desferrioxamine or newer iron chelators (van der Wal *et al.*, 1992) in animal models of ARDS and, by extension, to patients with lung injury.

The contribution of NO, the other major free radical species produced in lung injury states, as a mediator of that injury is not easy to assess (Royall *et al.*, 1995). Although inhibition of NO synthase corrects many of the cardiovascular defects of septic shock (Thiemermann, 1994), there is still active discussion on the place of NO synthase inhibitors in patients with septic shock (Petros *et al.*, 1994; Quinn *et al.*, 1995). Experimental septic shock increased output of exhaled NO and in human lung tissue nitrotyrosine was increased in ARDS-like states (Haddad *et al.*, 1994; Kooy *et al.*, 1995); both findings indicative of increased NO synthesis. Nevertheless, direct local application by inhalation of exogenous NO has also been beneficial in ARDS (Benzing and Geiger, 1994; Fierobe *et al.*, 1995; Quinn *et al.*, 1995). It may be that a combination of systemic inhibition of NO synthase with local, inhaled NO will be the most beneficial mode of treatment.

Three likely candidates for clinical evaluation as antioxidants in lung injury are the sulphydryl compounds, NAC, cystamine and taurine. The latter two compounds are taken up avidly by epithelial cells (Banks *et al.*, 1989; Lewis *et al.*, 1989, 1990) and their protective effects might therefore be concentrated on these cells. Taurine decreased bleomycin-induced damage in hamster lung (Wang *et al.*, 1989) and injury induced by ozone or cyclophosphamide in rats (Schuller-Levis *et al.*, 1994; Venkatesan and Chandrakasan, 1994). Protection of epithelium may be an important feature as it is often the replacement of damaged epithelial cells with fibrotic tissue that is the irreversible step in lung injury.

These compounds could act either by supporting the endogenous free radical neutralizing systems or by direct reaction with the radicals. The cysteine-containing tripeptide glutathione (GSH) is an essential component of the cell's endogenous antioxidant capacity, as a substrate for GSH peroxidase and other enzymes as well as a direct scavenger of free radicals (Reed, 1990). Experimentally depleted GSH was restored by administration of NAC (Berggren *et al.*, 1984; Butterworth *et al.*, 1993) and oral NAC increased the concentration of GSH in plasma two-fold and in bronchoalveolar lavage fluid almost three-fold in patients (Bridgeman *et al.*, 1991). Lung injury from endotoxin, ANTU and hyperoxia was prevented by NAC given parenterally or orally (Bernard *et al.*, 1984; Bakhle and Stuart, 1988; Wagner *et al.*, 1989). The depletion of lung GSH by ANTU and the prevention of both

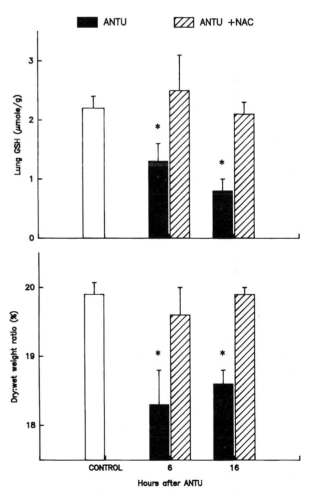

Figure 43.3 Prevention by oral *N* – acetylcysteine (NAC) of lung injury due to α-naphthylthiourea (ANTU) in rats. A single IP injection of ANTU (6 mg/kg) caused lung oedema (decreased lung dry : wet weight ratio) and depleted pulmonary tissue levels of glutathione (GSH). These changes were totally prevented by treatment with NAC (6% in drinking water, w/v) for 16 hours before ANTU injection. *$P < 0.05$ vs control; *n* = 3–6 rats per group. (J. J. Pankhania and Y. S. Bakhle, unpublished.)

oedema and GSH depletion by oral NAC is illustrated in Figure 43.3 (J.J. Pankhania and Y.S. Bakhle (1990), unpublished experiments). Here, a single injection of ANTU given to rats induced pulmonary oedema, shown by the fall in dry : wet lung weight ratio at 6 and 16 hours after ANTU. At the same times, lung GSH levels were reduced to about half normal values. Pretreatment with NAC (6% w/v in drinking water) overnight prevented the oedema and the fall in lung GSH at either 6 or 16 hours after ANTU. These results would support the general correlation between lung injury and a low level of endogenous antioxidants. Another potentially beneficial effect of NAC would be to increase nitrosothiols in lung; these compounds act as donors of NO and their formation may also prevent the conversion of inhaled NO to peroxynitrite (Kooy et al., 1995) or NO_2 (Gaston et al., 1994), both highly toxic to cells.

As a possible treatment for ARDS, NAC has practical advantages; its human pharmacokinetics are already known (Borgstrom et al., 1986) and it is available in oral, injectable and aerosol forms. The last could provide a means of giving large doses to the lung without having to expose the rest of the body to the same level of NAC. This selectivity has already been demonstrated in sheep where GSH in alveolar fluid but not in plasma was increased seven-fold after aerosol administration (Buhl et al., 1990). Furthermore, in models where epithelial damage is present or likely aerosols could carry antioxidants directly to the site of injury. It may be feasible to administer NAC by bronchoalveolar lavage in patients.

Biochemical index of lung injury

The search for a clinically feasible, biochemical index of lung injury has been the driving force for many of the studies of lung metabolic function. An essential feature of such an index is that it should change *before* physical injury is perceptible but otherwise should parallel the intensity and duration of the physical injury. The physical signs of injury would be increased vascular permeability (lung oedema), decreased lung compliance, changes in blood gases or radiological changes, which at present guide the diagnosis and treatment of lung injury (Rocker et al., 1989; Matthay, 1990; Demling, 1995). However attempts are being made to correlate endotoxin or cytokine levels in plasma with severity of illness indices as a guide to therapy (Barriere and Lowry, 1995).

One crucial consideration is the interpretation of change in the metabolic functions of lung – is it a change in 'quality' or 'quantity' (Toivonen et al., 1988; Dawson et al., 1989; Pitt and Lister, 1989)? For practical purposes, 'quality' equates with the biochemical well-being of the cells concerned, the efficiency of the uptake systems for the various substrates and the state of the enzymes required for their metabolism. Most workers in this field would agree that this 'quality' is the essential variable which is postulated to correlate with the other systems involved in the expression of injury. 'Quantity' approximates to the number of cells that have access and the duration of access, to the substrate. Exclusion of parts of the vascular bed or changes in blood flow rate and thus in transit time are clearly important determinants of the overall metabolism or binding of a substrate. This represents a haemodynamic variable and would only indirectly be a measure of metabolic status if, for instance, the metabolism concerned a vasoconstrictor substance.

In biochemical terms, the 'quality' variable is comparable to K_m and 'quantity' to V_{max} for the process studied. Although experimental methods to yield results independent of flow rate and heterogeneity of perfusion have been successfully devised and used (Dawson et al., 1989), in a clinical setting, concentrations of endogenous substrates well below the K_m values of the systems have to be used to avoid pharmacodynamic effects. At these concentrations, the kinetic analysis does not provide K_m and V_{max} values separately, but the ratio $A_{max} : K_m$ instead (A_{max} is V_{max} corrected for the amount of enzyme available and hence for the area perfused). A method of measuring this value under clinical conditions has been developed and is fully described elsewhere (Toivonen et al., 1988). These two methods essentially give the same answers from the same experimental conditions, particularly in terms of identifying the contribution of changes in haemodynamics or V_{max} to the overall result (Myers and Pitt, 1988; Catravas et al., 1990; Orfanos et al., 1994).

The substrate for the index has to be either pharmacologically beneficial or inert, as the patients in which they might be used would already be in cardiovascular difficulties. This consideration has led to the introduction of synthetic peptides such as BPAP, a tripeptide analogue of angiotensin I, to be used as a substrate for ACE assays *in vivo* (Ryan, 1983; Catravas et al., 1990). The tripeptide is pharmacologically inert, as are its metabolites, and BPAP has been used in assessments of experimental lung injury (McCormick et al., 1987; Riggs et al., 1988; Chen and Catravas, 1992). Other pharmacologically inert substrates that have been used are the non-metabolized xenobiotic compounds labelled with radioisotopes of iodine. Two of those already discussed, HIPDM (Pistolesi et al., 1988) and IMP (Touya et al., 1986), are clearly analogues of the xenobiotic amines (such as propranolol or amphetamine) and thus probably are better suited to measurement of vascular surface (quantity). The third type, the iodoguanidines MIBG or AIBG (Slosman et al., 1988b), are closer to endogenous substrates although they are not metabolized and retain some features of the exogenous substrate uptake systems. Clearly these xenobiotic substrates have not been fully characterized and it is not yet possible to assess their usefulness but they do offer enough advantages to merit further study.

The biochemical assay itself ought to be simple, avoiding if possible the time-consuming and labour-intensive extraction and separation of substrate and product in blood. It is here that the exogenous substrates have their advantage; they are not metabolized and a single assay of radioactivity in blood samples, if ^{14}C- or ^3H-labelled substrates are used, would suffice. The external counting possible with some radioisotopes of iodine confers an additional advantage. However the exogenous compounds are *non-metabolized* substrates and thus less likely to yield information on the metabolic state of the lung.

A compromise is offered by the experimentally successful method of assessing the wash-out of total radioactivity derived from radiolabelled PGE$_2$ (Bakhle, 1982). The $T_{1/2}$ value (time taken for 50% of the administered radioactivity to efflux from isolated lung) has shown a good correlation with metabolic changes for PGE$_2$ (and adenosine) following injury with ANTU (Bakhle, 1982; Izumi and Bakhle, 1988) or endotoxin (Grantham *et al.*, 1988; Izumi and Bakhle, 1988). The $T_{1/2}$ value for PGE$_2$ was increased by endotoxin injury and this occurred before pulmonary oedema developed but normalized as the oedema resolved (Grantham *et al.*, 1988; Izumi and Bakhle, 1988). Extension of this method to a clinical situation would mean that a simple total radioactivity measurement of arterial blood samples collected for about 30 seconds after the injection of a bolus of labelled PGE$_2$ should give a reliable indication of the biochemical state of the lung. The decreased metabolism of PGE$_2$ (or PGE$_1$) in experimental lung injury has already been substantiated in patients with established ARDS (Gillis *et al.*, 1986; Cox *et al.*, 1988). The fact that this variable ($T_{1/2}$) changes soon after endotoxin (Grantham *et al.*, 1988; Izumi and Bakhle, 1988) strengthens the possibility that it could provide a feasible and simple biochemical index of early lung injury.

A protein derived from endothelial cells and secreted into the blood, von Willebrand Factor (Factor VIII related antigen), has also been assessed as a predictor or indicator of lung injury (Wiedemann *et al.*, 1990). Although vWF was raised in experimental injury and in patients with sepsis, there are problems of specificity and rapidity of assay (Wiedemann *et al.*, 1990) that still have to be overcome.

SUMMARY

There is no doubt that lung injury alters the pharmacokinetic function of lung exhibited towards endogenous or exogenous substrates.

Analysis of these biochemical consequences of injury has strengthened the central position of oxygen-derived free radicals as agents of injury. This has directed attention to ways of preventing their generation – by deactivating leucocytes, for instance – or by increasing their neutralization, by supporting endogenous antioxidant mechanisms. The variety of drugs that have shown promise in experimental and clinical conditions may indeed all bring about a decrease in free radicals as a common feature. At least this would be a unifying hypothesis capable of test.

The hopes for an early warning, biochemical index of lung injury are still unfulfilled but the concept is still valid. The practical problems inherent in the development of a successful clinical test – how to achieve simplicity, speed and specificity, all simultaneously – are surmountable because the clinical rewards are high. Finally, in these efforts to analyse the mechanisms and solve the problems of lung injury, we have discovered more about the lung and the functions and the interactions of its 40 cell types. That in itself is a worthwhile achievement.

Acknowledgements

The support of the MRC and the Wellcome Trust for much of the work carried out in the author's laboratory is gratefully acknowledged.

REFERENCES

Abrams D.N., Man S.F., Noujaim A.A. (1987). Evaluation of the lung uptake of iodine-131 HIPDM by the single-pass multiple indicator dilution technique in a rabbit model. *J. Nucl. Med.*, **28**, 487–94.

Adkins W.K., Taylor A.E. (1990). Role of xanthine oxidase and neutrophils in ischemia-reperfusion injury in rabbit lung. *J. Appl. Physiol.*, **69**, 2012–18.

Ahn, S.Y., Sugi K., Talke P. et al. (1990). Effects of allopurinol on smoke inhalation in the ovine model. *J. Appl. Physiol.*, **68**, 228–34.

Akarasereenont P., Bakhle Y.S., Thiemermann C. et al. (1995). Cytokine-mediated induction of cyclo-oxygenase-2 by activation of tyrosine kinase in bovine aortic endothelial cells activated by bacterial lipopolysaccharide. *Br. J. Pharmacol.*, **115**, 401–8.

Alabaster V.A. (1977). Inactivation of endogenous amines in the lungs. In *Metabolic Functions of the Lungs* (Bakhle Y.S., Vane J.R., eds). New York: Marcel Dekker, pp. 3–31.

Archer S.L., Rist K., Nelson D.P. et al. (1990). Comparison of the hemodynamic effects of nitric oxide and endothelium-dependent vasodilators in intact lungs. *J. Appl. Physiol.*, **68**, 735–47.

Bakhle Y.S. (1974). Converting enzyme *in vitro*; measurement and properties. In *Angiotensin; handbook of experimental pharmacology*, Vol. 37 (Page I.H., Bumpus R.M., eds). Berlin: Springer-Verlag, pp. 41–80.

Bakhle Y.S. (1981). Inhibition by clinically used dyes of prostaglandin inactivation in rat and human lung. *Br. J. Pharmacol.*, **72**, 715–22.

Bakhle Y.S. (1982). Decreased inactivation of prostaglandin E_2 in isolated lungs from rats with α-naphthylthiourea induced pulmonary oedema. *Biochem. Pharmacol.*, **31**, 3395–401.

Bakhle Y.S. (1990). Pharmacokinetic and metabolic properties of lung. *Br. J. Anaesthesia*, **65**, 79–93.

Bakhle Y.S., Ferreira S.H. (1985). Lung metabolism of eicosanoids; prostaglandins, prostacyclin, thromboxane and leukotrienes. In *Handbook of Physiology; section 3, Respiratory System*; vol. 1, *circulatory and non-respiratory functions* (Fishman A.P., Fisher A.B., eds). Bethesda, MD: American Physiological Society, pp. 365–86.

Bakhle Y.S., Grantham C.J. (1987). Effects of pulmonary oedema on pharmacokinetics of adenosine in rat isolated lungs. *Br. J. Pharmacol.*, **91**, 849–56.

Bakhle Y.S., Pankhania J.J. (1987a). Drug effects on output of prostacyclin from isolated lungs. *Biochem. Pharmacol.*, **36**, 3540–3.

Bakhle Y.S., Pankhania J.J. (1987b). Inhibitors of prostaglandin dehydrogenase (Ph CL 28A and Ph CK 61A) increase output of prostaglandins from rat lung. *Br. J. Pharmacol.*, **92**, 189–96.

Bakhle Y.S., Stuart E.F. (1988). Oral N-acetylcysteine (NAC) prevents lung injury induced by α-naphthylthiourea in rats. *Br. J. Pharmacol.*, **95**, 768P.

Bakhle Y.S., Vane J.R. (1974). Pharmacokinetic function of the pulmonary circulation. *Physiol. Rev.*, **54**, 1007–45.

Bakhle Y.S., Youdim M.B.H. (1979). The metabolism of 5-hydroxytryptamine and β-phenylethylamine in perfused rat lung and *in vitro*. *Br. J. Pharmacol.*, **65**, 147–54.

Bakhle Y.S., Hartiala J., Toivonen H. (1979). Effects of cigarette smoke on the metabolism of vasoactive hormones in rat isolated lungs. *Br. J. Pharmacol.*, **65**, 495–500.

Bando K., Pillai R., Cameron D.E. et al. (1990). Leukocyte depletion ameliorates free radical-mediated lung injury after cardiopulmonary bypass. *J. Thorac. Cardiovasc. Surg.*, **99**, 873–7.

Banks M.A., Martin W.G., Pailes W.H. et al. (1989). Taurine uptake by isolated alveolar macrophages and type II cells. *J. Appl. Physiol.*, **66**, 1079–86.

Barnard J.W., Seibert A.F., Prasad V.R. et al. (1994). Reversal of pulmonary capillary ischemia-reperfusion injury by rolipram, a cAMP phosphodiesterase inhibitor. *J. Appl. Physiol.*, **77**, 774–81.

Barriere S.L., Lowry S.F. (1995). An overview of mortality risk prediction in sepsis. *Crit. Care Med.*, **23**, 376–93.

Barrowcliffe M.P., Jones J.G. (1987). Solute permeability of the alveolar–capilliary barrier. *Thorax*, **42**, 1–10.

Bauer C., Marzi I., Bauer M. et al. (1995). Interleukin-1 receptor antagonist attenuates leukocyte–endothelial interactions in the liver after hemorrhagic shock in the rat. *Crit. Care Med.*, **23**, 1099–105.

Bend J.R., Serabjit-Singh C.T., Philpot R.M. (1985). The pulmonary uptake accumulation and metabolism of xenobiotics. *Annu. Rev. Pharmacol. Toxicol.*, **25**, 97–125.

Benzing A., Geiger K. (1994). Inhaled nitric oxide lowers pulmonary capillary pressure and changes longitudinal distribution of pulmonary vascular resistance in patients with acute lung injury. *Acta Anaesthesiol. Scand.*, **38**, 640–5.

Berggren M., Dawson J., Moldeus P. (1984). Glutathione biosynthesis in the isolated perfused rat lung: utilization of extracellular glutathione. *FEBS Lett.*, **176**, 189–92.

Berisha H., Foda H., Sakakibara H. et al. (1990). Vasoactive intestinal peptide prevents lung injury due to xanthine/xanthine oxidase. *Am. J. Physiol.*, **259**, L151–5.

Bernard G., Lucht W., Niedermeyer M. et al. (1984). Effect of N-acetylcysteine on the pulmonary response to endotoxin in awake sheep and upon *in vitro* granulocyte function. *J. Clin. Invest.*, **73**, 1772–84.

Bils R.F., Christie B.R. (1978). The experimental pathology of oxidants and air pollutant inhalation. *Int. Rev. Exp. Pathol.*, **15**, 443–72.

Bishop M.J., Chi E.Y., Cheney F.W. Jr (1987). Lung reperfusion in dogs causes bilateral lung injury. *J. Appl. Physiol.*, **63**, 942–50.

Blaise G.A., Sill J.C., Nugent M. et al. (1987). Isoflurane causes endothelium-dependent inhibition of contractile responses of canine coronary arteries. *Anesthesiology*, **67**, 513–17.

Blaise G.A., To Q., Parent M. et al. (1994). Does halothane interfere with the release, action or stability of endothelium-derived relaxing factor/nitric oxide? *Anesthesiology*, **80**, 417–26.

Block E.R., Schoen F.J. (1981). Effect of α-naphthylthiourea on uptake of 5-hydroxytryptamine from the pulmonary circulation. *Am. Rev. Resp. Dis.*, **123**, 69–73.

Bone R.C., Balk R.A., Fein A.M. et al. (1995). A second large controlled clinical study of E5, a monoclonal antibody to endotoxin; results of a prospective, multicenter, randomized, controlled trial. *Crit. Care Med.*, **23**, 994–1006.

Borgstrom L., Kagedal B., Paulsen O. (1986). Pharmacokinetics of N-acetylcysteine in man. *Eur. J. Pharmacol.*, **31**, 217–22.

Borland C., Cox Y., Higgenbottam T.W. (1993). Measurement of exhaled nitric oxide in man. *Thorax*, **48**, 1160–2.

Brashers V.L., Peach M.J., Rose C.E. Jr (1988). Augmentation of hypoxic pulmonary vasoconstriction in the isolated perfused rat lung by *in vitro* antagonists of endothelium-dependent relaxation. *J. Clin. Invest.*, **82**, 1495–502.

Bridgeman M.M.E., Marsden M., MacNee W. et al. (1991). Cysteine and glutathione concentrations in plasma and bronchoalveloar lavage fluid after treatment with N-acetylcysteine. *Thorax*, **46**, 39–42.

Brigham K.L., Meyrick B. (1986). Endotoxin and lung injury. *Am. Rev. Resp. Dis.*, **133**, 913–27.

Brink C., Gillard V., Roubert P. et al. (1991). Effects and specific binding sites of endothelin in human lung preparations. *Pulmon. Pharmacol.*, **4**, 54–9.

Buhl R., Vogelmeier C., Critenden M. et al. (1990). Augmentation of glutathione in the fluid lining the epithelium of the lower respiratory tract by directly administering glutathione aerosol. *Proc. Nat. Acad. Sci.*, **87**, 4063–7.

Burrows L.J., Piper P.J., Lindley I. et al. (1989). Human recombinant neutrophil activating factor/interleukin 8 is a spasmogen of airway smooth muscle *in vitro*. *Br. J. Pharmacol.*, **98**, 789P.

Butterworth M., Upshall D.G., Hobbs M. et al. (1993). Elevation of cysteine and replenishment of glutathione in rat lung slices by cysteine isopropyl ester and other cysteine precursors. *Biochem. Pharmacol.*, **45**, 1769–74.

Camussi G., Bussolini F., Salvidio G. et al. (1987). Tumor necrosis factor/cachectin stimulates peritoneal macrophages, polymorphonuclear neutrophils and vascular endothelium to synthesize and release platelet activating factor. *J. Exp. Med.*, **166**, 1390–404

Carreras L.O., Chamone D.A.F., Klerckx P. et al. (1980). Decreased vascular prostacyclin (PGI$_2$) in diabetic rats. Stimulation of PGI$_2$ release in normal and diabetic rats by the antithrombotic compound BAY g 6575. *Thromb. Res.*, **19**, 663–70.

Catravas J.D., Ryan J.W., Chung A.Y. et al. (1990). Inhibition of endothelial-bound angiotensin converting enzyme, *in vivo*. *Br. J. Pharmacol.*, **101**, 121–7.

Chand N., Altura B.M. (1981). Acetylcholine and bradykinin relax intra-pulmonary arteries by acting on endothelial cells; role in lung vascular disease. *Science*, **213**, 1376–9.

Chandler D.B., Jackson R.M., Briggs A.D. et al. (1985). The effect of bleomycin on lung metabolism of prostaglandin E$_2$ in hamsters. *Prostaglandins Leukotrienes Med.*, **19**, 139–51.

Chandler D.B., Barton J.C., Briggs D.D. et al. (1988). Effect of iron deficiency on bleomycin-induced lung fibrosis in the hamster. *Am. Rev. Resp. Dis.*, **137**, 85–9.

Chang S.-W., Westcott J.Y., Pickett W.C. et al. (1989). Endotoxin-induced lung injury in rats: role of eicosanoids. *J. Appl. Physiol.*, **66**, 2407–18.

Chaudhari A., Sivarajah K., Warwick R. et al. (1979). Inhibition of pulmonary prostaglandin metabolism by exposure of animals to oxygen or nitrogen dioxide. *Biochem. J.*, **184**, 51–7.

Chelliah R., Bakhle Y.S. (1983). The fate of adenosine nucleotides in the pulmonary circulation of isolated lung. *Q. J. Exp. Physiol.*, **68**, 289–300.

Chen X., Catravas J.D. (1993). Neutrophil-mediated endothelial angiotensin converting enzyme dysfunction; role of oxygen-derived free radicals. *Am. J. Physiol.*, **265**, L243–9.

Christman J.W., Holden E.P., Blackwell T.S. (1995). Strategies for blocking the systemic effects of cytokines in the sepsis syndrome. *Crit. Care Med.*, **23**, 955–63.

Coker S.J., Parratt J.R. (1984). The effects of nafazatrom on arrhythmias and prostanoid release during coronary artery occlusion and reperfusion in anaesthetized greyhounds. *J. Molec. Cellular Cardiol.*, **16**, 43–52.

Cook D.R., Howell R.E., Gillis C.N. (1982). Xanthine oxidase-induced lung injury inhibits removal of 5-hydroxytryptamine from the pulmonary circulation. *Anesth. Analg.*, **61**, 666–70.

Cox J.W., Andreadis N.A., Bone R.C. et al. (1988). Pulmonary extraction and pharmacokinetics of prostaglandin E$_1$ during continuous intravenous infusion in patients with adult respiratory distress syndrome. *Am. Rev. Resp. Dis.*, **137**, 5–12.

Crapo J.D. (1989). Morphological changes in oxygen toxicity. *Annu. Rev. Physiol.*, **48**, 721–31.

Crawley D.E., Liu S.F., Evans T.W. et al. (1990). Inhibitory role of endothelium-derived relaxing factor in rat and human pulmonary arteries. *Br. J. Pharmacol.*, **101**, 166–70.

Cunningham A.L., Hurley J.V. (1972). Alpha-naphthylthiourea-induced pulmonary oedema in the rat: a topographical and electron microscope study. *J. Pathol.*, **106**, 25–35.

Dargent F., Gardaz J-P., Morel P. et al. (1985a). Effects of atelectasis and vascular occlusion on the simultaneous measurement of serotonin and propranolol pulmonary extraction in dogs. *Clin. Sci.*, **69**, 279–86.

Dargent F., Neidhart P., Bachmann M. et al. (1985b). Simultaneous measurement of serotonin and propranolol pulmonary extraction in patients after extracorporeal circulation and surgery. *Am. Rev. Resp. Dis.*, **131**, 242–5.

Davies E.A., Albert A.J., Devine M.J. et al. (1989). Ibuprofen plus prostaglandin E$_1$ in a septic porcine model of adult respiratory distress syndrome. *J. Trauma*, **29**, 284–91.

Dawson C.A., Roerig D.L., Linehan J.H. (1989). Evaluation of endothelial injury in human lung. *Clin. Chest Med.*, **10**, 13–24.

Demling R.H. (1995). The modern version of Adult Respiratory Distress Syndrome. *Annu. Rev. Med.*, **46**, 193–202.

Demling R.H., LaLonde C. (1990). Identification and modifications of the pulmonary and systemic inflammatory and biochemical changes caused by a skin burn. *J. Trauma*, **30**, S57–62.

De Nucci G., Astbury P., Read N. et al. (1986). Release of eicosanoids from isolated lungs of guinea pigs exposed to pure oxygen; effect of dexamethasone. *Eur. J. Pharmacol.*, **126**, 11–20.

De Nucci G., Thomas R., d'Orleans-Juste P. et al. (1988). Pressor effects of endothelin are limited by its removal in the pulmonary circulation and by the release of prostacyclin and endothelium derived relaxing factor. *Proc. Natl. Acad. Sci. USA*, **85**, 9797–800.

Dhainaut J-F.A., Tenaillon A., Le Tulzo Y. et al. (1994). Platelet-activating factor receptor antagonist BN 52021 in the treatment of severe sepsis; a randomized, double-blind, placebo controlled, multicenter clinical trial. *Crit. Care Med.*, **22**, 1720–8.

DiMarzo V., Tippins J.R., Morris H.R. (1989). The role of cyclic AMP in the inhibition of leukotriene biosynthesis by neuropeptides. *Eur. J. Pharmacol.*, **162**, 115–21.

Dinh-Xuan A.T., Pepke-Zaba J., Butt A.Y. et al (1993). Impairment of pulmonary-artery endothelium-dependent relaxation in chronic obstructive lung disease is not due to dysfunction of endothelial cell membrane receptors nor to L-arginine deficiency. *Br. J. Pharmacol.*, **109**, 587–91.

Dollery C.T., Junod A.F. (1976). Concentration of (+/−) propranolol in isolated perfused lungs of rat. *Br. J. Pharmacol.*, **57**, 67–71.

Dunn N., Glassroth J. (1989). Pulmonary complications of amiodarone toxicity. *Prog. Cardiovasc. Dis.*, **31**, 447–53.

Dusting G.J., Moncada S., Vane J.R. (1978). Recirculation of prostacyclin (PGI$_2$) in the dog. *Br. J. Pharmacol.*, **64**, 315–20.

Dutta S., Chatterjee M., Teknos T.N. et al. (1990). A study of ozone-induced edema in the isolated rat lung in relation to arachidonic acid metabolism, mixed-function oxidases and angiotensin converting enzyme activities. *Pulmonary Pharmacol.*, **3**, 65–72.

Eisenberg S.P., Evans R.J., Arend W.P. et al. (1990). Primary structure and functional expression from complementary DNA of a human interleukin-1 receptor antagonist. *Nature*, **343**, 341–6.

Endres S. (1993). Messengers and mediators: interactions among lipids, eicosanoids and cytokines. *Am. J. Clin. Nutr.*, **57**, (suppl. 5), 798S–800S.

Endres S., Fulle H.J., Sinha B. et al. (1991). Cyclic nucleotides differentially regulate the synthesis of tumor necrosis factor-alpha and interleukin-1 beta by human mononuclear cells. *Immunology*, **72**, 56–60.

Fairman R.P., Glauser F.L., Merchant R.E. et al. (1987) Increase of rat pulmonary microvascular permeability to albumin by recombinant interleukin-2. *Cancer Res.*, **47**, 3528–32.

Fantone J.C., Marasco W.A., Elgas L.J. et al. (1984). Stimulus specificity of prostaglandin inhibition of rabbit poylmorphonuclear leukocyte lysosomal enzyme release and superoxide anion production. *Am. J. Pathol.*, **115**, 9–16.

Feddersen C.O., McMurtry I.F., Henson P. et al. (1986). Acetylcholine-induced pulmonary vasodilation in lung vascular injury. *Am. Rev. Resp. Dis.*, **133**, 197–204.

Ferrari-Baliviera E., Mealy K., Smith R.J. et al. (1989). Tumor necrosis factor induces adult respiratory distress syndrome in rats. *Arch. Surg.*, **124**, 1400–5.

Fierobe L., Brunet F., Dhainaut J.F. et al. (1995). Effect of inhaled nitric oxide on right ventricular function in adult respiratory distress syndrome. *Am. J. Resp. Crit. Care Med.*, **151**, 1414–19.

Flower R.J. (1984). Macrocortin and the anti-phospholipase proteins. *Adv. Inflammation Res.*, **8**, 1–34.

Foda H.D., Iwanaga T., Liu L-W. et al. (1988). Vasoactive intestinal peptide protects against HCl-induced pulmonary edema in rats. *Ann. N.Y. Acad. Sci.*, **527**, 633–6.

Fox R.B., Harada R.N., Tate R.M. et al. (1983). Prevention of thiourea-induced pulmonary oedema by hydroxyl-radical scavengers. *J. Appl. Physiol.*, **55**, 1456–9.

Furchgott R.F., Zawadzki J.V. (1980). The obligatory role of endothelial cells in the relaxation of arterial smooth muscle by acetylcholine. *Nature*, **288**, 373–6.

Gaston B., Reilly J., Fackler J. et al. (1994). Endogenous bronchdilator *S*-nitrosothiols in human airways. In *The Biology of Nitric Oxide; physiological and clinical aspects* (Moncada S., Feelisch M., Busse R., Higgs, E.A., eds). London: Portland Press, pp. 444–6.

Giaid A., Yanagisawa M., Langleben D. et al. (1993). Expression of endothelin-1 in the lungs of patients with pulmonary hypertension. *New Engl. J. Med.*, **328**, 1732–9.

Gillis C.N. (1986). Pharmacological aspects of metabolic processes in the pulmonary microcirculation. *Annu. Rev. Pharmacol. Toxicol.*, **26**, 183–200.

Gillis C.N., Catravas J.D. (1982). Altered removal of vasoactive substances in the injured lung; detection of lung microvascular injury. *Ann. N.Y. Acad. Sci.*, **384**, 458–74.

Gillis C.N., Pitt B.R. (1982). The fate of circulating amines within the pulmonary circulation. *Annu. Rev. Physiol.*, **44**, 269–81.

Gillis C.N., Greene N.M., Cronau L.H. et al. (1972). Pulmonary extraction of 5-hydroxytryptamine and norepinephrine before and after cardiopulmonary bypass in man. *Circ. Res.*, **30**, 666–74.

Gillis C.N., Cronau L.H., Mendel S. et al. (1979). Indicator dilution measurement of 5-hydroxytryptamine clearance by human lung. *J. Appl. Physiol.*, **46**, 1178–83.

Gillis C.N., Pitt B.R., Wiedemann H.P. et al. (1986). Depressed prostaglandin E_1 and 5-hydroxytryptamine removal in patients with adult respiratory distress syndrome. *Am. Rev. Resp. Dis.*, **134**, 739–44.

Glauser F.L., Deblois G.G., Bechard D.E. et al. (1988). Cardiopulmonary effects of recombinant interleukin-2 infusion in sheep. *J. Appl. Physiol.*, **64**, 1030–7.

Goldstein G., Luce J.M. (1990). Pharmacologic treatment of the adult respiratory distress syndrome. *Clin. Chest Med.*, **11**, 773–87.

Grantham C.J., Bakhle Y.S. (1988). Effects of acute lung injury on metabolism of adenine nucleotides in rat perfused lung. *Br. J. Pharmacol.*, **94**, 1029–36.

Grantham C.J., Izumi T., Lewis D.H. et al. (1988). Effects of endotoxin-induced lung injury on the pharmacokinetics of prostaglandin E_2 and adenosine in rat isolated lung. *Circ. Shock*, **26**, 157–67.

Gross K.B., White H.J., Sargent N.E. (1991). The effect of ozone inhalation on metabolic functioning of vascular endothelium and on ventilatory function. *Toxicol. Appl. Pharmacol.*, **109**, 336–51.

Gross M.A., Viders D.E., Brown J.M. et al. (1989). Local skin burn causes systemic (lung and kidney) endothelial cell injury reflected by increased circulating and decreased tissue factor VIII-related antigen. *Surgery*, **106**, 310–16.

Gu Y.J., Wang Y.S., Chiang B.Y. et al. (1991). Membrane oxygenator prevents lung reperfusion injury in canine cardiopulmonary bypass. *Ann. Thorac. Surg.*, **51**, 573–8.

Gutierrez H.H., Pitt B.R., Schwarz M. et al. (1995). Pulmonary alveolar epithelial inducible NO synthase gene expression: regulation by inflammatory mediators. *Am. J. Physiol.*, **268**, L501–8.

Haddad I.Y., Pataki G., Hu P. et al. (1994). Quantitation of nitrotyrosine levels in lung sections of patients and animals with acute lung injury. *J. Clin. Invest.*, **94**, 2407–13.

Hales C.A., Musto S., Hutchinson W.G. et al. (1995). BW-755C diminishes smoke-induced pulmonary edema. *J. Appl. Physiol.*, **78**, 64–9.

Hales C.A., Brandstetter R.D., Neely C.F. et al. (1986). Methylprednisolone on circulating eicosanoids and vasomotor tone after endotoxin. *J. Appl. Physiol.*, **61**, 185–91.

Halliwell B., Gutteridge J.M.C. (1985). *Free Radicals in Biology and Medicine*. New York: Oxford University Press.

Hamasaki Y., Tai H-H., Said S.I. (1982). Hypoxia stimulates prostacyclin generation by dog lung *in vitro*. *Prostaglandins Leukotrienes Med.*, **8**, 311–16.

Hammond G.L., Cronau L.H., Whittaker D. et al. (1977). Fate of prostaglandins E_1 and A_1 in the human pulmonary circulation. *Surgery*, **81**, 716–22.

Hansen E.S. (1990). A cohort study on the mortality of firefighters. *Br. J. Indus. Med.*, **47**, 805–9.

Hay J., Shahzeidi S., Laurent G. (1991). Mechanisms of bleomycin-induced lung damage. *Arch. Toxicol.*, **65**, 81–94.

Heby O. (1981). Role of polyamines in the control of cell proliferation and differentiation. *Differentiation*, **19**, 1–20.

Hede A.R., Andersson L., Post C. (1985). Effect of a homologous series of halogenated methanes on pulmonary uptake of 5-hydroxytryptamine in isolated perfused rat lung. *Acta Pharmacol. Toxol.*, **57**, 291–6.

Heffner J.E., Repine J.E. (1989). Pulmonary strategies of antioxidant defense. *Am. Rev. Resp. Dis.*, **140**, 531–54.

Hemsworth B.A., Street J.A. (1981). Characteristics of $(+/-)[^{14}C]$ oxoprenolol and $(+/-)[^{14}C]$propranolol incorporation by rat lung slices. *Br. J. Pharmacol.*, **73**, 119–27.

Herndon D.N., Traber D.L. (1990). Pulmonary circulation and burns and trauma. *J. Trauma*, **30**, S41–4.

Hocking D.C., Phillips P.G., Ferro T.J. et al. (1990). Mechanisms of pulmonary edema induced by tumor necrosis factor-alpha. *Circ. Res.*, **67**, 68–77.

Hogg J.C. (1987). Neutrophil kinetics and lung injury. *Physiol. Rev.*, **67**, 1249–95.

Holden W.E., Maier J.M., Malinow M.R. (1989). Cigarette smoke extract increases albumin flux across pulmonary endothelium *in vitro*. *J. Appl. Physiol.*, **66**, 443–9.

Horgan M.J., Lum H., Malik A.B. (1989). Pulmonary edema after pulmonary artery occlusion and reperfusion. *Am. Rev. Resp. Dis.*, **140**, 1421–8.

Hubbard J.D., Janssen H.F. (1988). Increased microvascular permeability in canine endotoxic shock: protective effects of ibuprofen. *Circ. Shock*, **26**, 169–83.

Ignarro L.J. (1990). Biosynthesis and metabolism of endothelium-derived nitric oxide. *Annu. Rev. Pharmacol. Toxicol.*, **30**, 535–60.

Ischiropoulos H., Mendiguren I., Fisher D. et al. (1994). Role of neutrophils and nitric oxide in lung alveolar injury from smoke inhalation. *Am. J. Resp. Crit. Care Med.*, **150**, 337–41.

Ishizaka A., Wu Z., Stephens K.E. (1988). Attenuation of acute lung injury in septic guinea pigs by pentoxifylline. *Am. Rev. Resp. Dis.*, **138**, 376–82.

Ishizaki T., Shigemori K., Yamamura Y. et al. (1995). Increased nitric oxide biosynthesis in leukotoxin, 9,10-epoxy-12-octadecenoate injured lung. *Biochem. Biophys. Res. Commun.*, **210**, 133–7.

Izumi T., Bakhle Y.S. (1988). Modification by steroids of pulmonary oedema and prostaglandin E_2 pharmacokinetics induced by endotoxin in rats. *Br. J. Pharmacol.*, **93**, 955–63.

Izumi T., Bakhle Y.S. (1989). Output of prostanoids from rat lung following endotoxin and its modification by methylprednisolone. *Circ. Shock*, **28**, 9–21.

Jeppsson A-B., Sundler F., Luts A. et al. (1991). Hydrogen peroxide-induced epithelial damage increases terbutaline transport in guinea-pig tracheal wall: implications for drug delivery. *Pulmonary Pharmacol.*, **4**, 73–9.

Johnson J., Meyrick B., Jesmok G. *et al.* (1989). Human recombinant tumor necrosis factor alpha infusion mimics endotoxemia in awake sheep. *J. Appl. Physiol.*, **66**, 1448–54.

Jones G., Hurley J.V. (1984). The effect of prostacyclin on the adhesion of leukocytes to injured vascular endothelium. *J. Pathol.*, **142**, 51–9.

Jones G.J., Berry M., Hulands G.H. et al. (1978). The time course and degree of change in alveolar-capillary membrane permeability induced by aspiration of hydrochloric acid and hypotonic saline. *Am. Rev. Resp. Dis.*, **118**, 1007–13.

Jorens P.G., Vermeire P.A., Herman A.G. (1993). L-Arginine-dependent nitric oxide synthase: a new metabolic pathway in the lung and airways. *Eur. Resp. J.*, **6**, 258–66.

Jorfeldt L., Lewis D.H., Lofstrom J.B. et al. (1983). Lung uptake of lidocaine in man as influenced by anaesthesia, mepivacaine infusion or lung insufficiency. *Acta Anaesthesiol. Scand.*, **27**, 5–9.

Joshi U.M., Kodavanti P.R., Mehendale H.M. (1988). Glutathione metabolism and utilization of external thiols by cigarette smoke-challenged, isolated rat and rabbit lungs. *Toxicol. Appl. Pharmacol.*, **96**, 324–35.

Junod A.F. (1985). 5-Hydroxytryptamine and other amines in the lungs. In *Handbook of Physiology; section 3*, vol. 1 (Fishman A.P., Fisher A.B., eds). Bethseda, MD: American Physiological Society, pp. 337–50.

Karhi T., Rantala A., Toivonen H. (1982). Pulmonary inactivation of 5-hydroxytryptamine is decreased during cigarette smoke ventilation of rat isolated lung. *Br. J. Pharmacol.*, **77**, 245–8.

Kelm M., Schrader J. (1990). Control of coronary vascular tone by nitric oxide. *Circ. Res.*, **66**, 1561–75.

Kettelhut I.C., Fiers W., Goldberg A.L. (1989). The toxic effects of tumor necrosis factor *in vivo* and their prevention by cyclo-oxygenase inhibitors. *Proc. Natl. Acad. Sci.*, **84**, 4273–7.

Khafagi F.A., Shapiro B., Fig L.M. et al. (1989). Labetalol reduces iodine-131 MIBG uptake by pheochromocytoma and normal tissues. *J. Nucl. Med.*, **30**, 481–9.

Kirklin J.K. (1991). Prospects for understanding and eliminating the deleterious effects of cardiopulmonary bypass. *Ann. Thorac. Surg.*, **51**, 529–31.

Klausner J.M., Paterson I.S., Morel N.M.L. et al. (1989). Role of thromboxane in interleukin 2-induced lung injury in sheep. *Cancer Res.*, **49**, 3542–9.

Klein J. (1990). Normobaric pulmonary oxygen toxicity. *Anesth. Analg.*, **70**, 195–207.

Kobayashi T. (1983). Effect of ozone exposure on prostacyclin synthesis in lung. *Prostaglandins*, **26**, 1021–7.

Kobayashi T., Morita I., Murota S. (1983). Effects of nitrogen dioxide exposure of prostacyclin synthesis in lung and thromboxane A_2 synthesis in platelets in rats. *Prostaglandins*, **26**, 303.

Kobayashi T., Ganzuka M., Taniguchi K. et al. (1990). Lung lavage and surfactant replacement for hydrochloric acid aspiration in rabbits. *Acta Anaesthesiol. Scand.*, **34**, 216–21.

Kooy N.W., Royall J.A., Ye Y.Z. (1995). Evidence for *in vivo* peroxynitrite production in human acute lung injury. *Am. J. Resp. Crit. Care Med.*, **151**, 1250–4.

Last J.A., Sun W.M., Witschi H. (1994). Ozone, NO, and NO_2: oxidant air pollutants and more. *Environ. Health Perspect.*, **102**, (suppl. 10), 179–84.

Laufe M.D., Simon R.H., Flint A. (1986). Adult respiratory distress syndrome in neutropenic patients. *Am. J. Med.*, **80**, 1022–6.

Lazo J.S., Lynch T.J., McCallister J. (1986). Bleomycin-inhibition of angiotensin converting enzyme activity from serum, lungs and cultured pulmonary endothelial cells. *Am. Rev. Resp. Dis.*, **134**, 73–8.

Levin E.R. (1995). Endothelins. *New Engl. J. Med.*, **333**, 356–63.

Lewis C.P.L., Haschek W.M., Wyatt I. et al. (1989). The accumulation of cystamine and its metabolism to taurine in rat lung slices. *Biochem. Pharmacol.*, **38**, 481–8.

Lewis C.P.L., Cohen G.M., Smith L.L. (1990). The identification and characterisation of an uptake system for taurine into rat lung slices. *Biochem. Pharmacol.*, **39**, 431–7.

Lilly C.M., Sandhu J.S., Ishizaka, A. et al. (1989). Pentoxifylline prevents tumor necrosis factor-induced lung injury. *Am. Rev. Resp. Dis.*, **139**, 1361–8.

Liu S.F., Crawley D.E., Barnes P.J. et al. (1991). Endothelium-derived relaxing factor inhibits hypoxic pulmonary vasoconstriction in rats. *Am. Rev. Resp. Dis.*, **143**, 32–7.

Liu C.T., Wang D.L., Oliaro A. et al. (1994). Prolonged lung retention of ^{131}I-HIPDM in smokers. *Panminerva Med.*, **36**, 128–30.

Lotze M.T., Matory Y.L., Rayner A.A. et al. (1986). Clinical effects and toxicity of interleukin-2 in patients with cancer. *Cancer*, **58**, 2764–72.

Lynch M.J., Grum C.M., Gallagher K.P. et al. (1988). Xanthine oxidase inhibition attenuates ischemic-reperfusion lung injury. *J. Surg. Res.*, **44**, 538–44.

Maggart M., Stewart S. (1987). The mechanisms and management of noncardiogenic pulmonary edema following cardiopulmonary bypass. *Ann. Thorac. Surg.*, **43**, 231–6.

Malik A.B., Johnson A. (1989). Role of humoral mediators in the pulmonary vascular response to pulmonary embolism. In *Pulmonary Vascular Physiology and Pathophysiology* (Weir E.K., Reeves J.T., eds). New York: Marcel Dekker, pp. 445–68.

Man S.F.P., Williams D.J., Amy R.A. et al. (1990). Sequential changes in canine pulmonary epithelial and endothelial cell functions after nitrogen dioxide. *Am. Rev. Resp. Dis.*, **142**, 199–205.

Mantovani A., Dejana E. (1989). Cytokines as communication signals between leukocytes and endothelial cells. *Immunol. Today*, **10**, 370–5.

Martin T., Losa J.E., Garcia-Salgado M.J. et al. (1994). The role of platelet activating factor (PAF) in interstitial lung disease. *J. Investig. Allergol. Clin. Immunol.*, **4**, 149–57.

Matintalo M., Kuusisto T., Mannisto J. et al. (1983). The metabolism of PGE_2 is decreased by high- and medium-tar but not by low-tar cigarette smoke in isolated rat lungs. *Acta Pharmacol. Toxocol.*, **52**, 230–3.

Matthay M.A. (1990). The adult respiratory distress syndrome: definition and prognosis. *Clin. Chest Med.*, **11**, 575–80.

Maunder R.J., Hackman R.C., Riff E. et al. (1986). Occurrence of the adult respiratory distress syndrome in neutropenic patients. *Am. Rev. Resp. Dis.*, **133**, 313–16.

May G.R., Crook P., Moore P.K. et al. (1991). The role of nitric oxide as an endogenous regulator of platelet and neutrophil activation within the pulmonary circulation of the rabbit. *Br. J. Pharmacol.*, **102**, 759–63.

Mazmanian G.-M., Baudet B., Brink C. et al. (1989). Methylene blue potentiates vascular reactivity in isolated rat lungs. *J. Appl. Physiol.*, **66**, 1040–5.

McCormick J.R., Chrzanowski R., Andreani J. et al. (1987). Early pulmonary endothelial enzyme dysfunction after phorbol ester in conscious rabbits. *J. Appl. Physiol.*, **63**, 1972–8.

McManus L.M., Deavers S.I. (1989). Platelet activating factor in pulmonary pathobiology. *Clin. Chest Med.*, **10**, 107–18.

Merker M.P., Gillis C.N. (1988). Propranolol and serotonin removal in lung injury. *J. Appl. Physiol.*, **65**, 2579–84.

Meyrick B., Miller J., Reid L. (1972). Pulmonary oedema induced by ANTU, or by high or low oxygen concentrations in the rat – an electron microscope study. *Br. J. Exp. Pathol.*, **53**, 347–58.

Michie H.R., Manogue K.R., Spriggs D.R. et al. (1988) Detection of circulating tumor necrosis factor after endotoxin administration. *New Engl. J. Med.*, **318**, 1481–6.

Miniati M., Cocci F., Faci A. et al. (1992). Evaluation of non-respiratory function of the human lung by HIPDM lung scanning. *Clin. Physiol.*, **12**, 303–11.

Moldawer L.L. (1994). Biology of proinflammatory cytokines and their antagonists. *Crit. Care Med.*, **22**, S3–7.

Moncada S., Palmer R.M.J., Higgs E.A. (1991). Nitric oxide: physiology, pathophysiology and pharmacology. *Pharmacol. Rev.*, **43**, 109–42.

Morel D.R., Lacroix J.S., Hemsen A. et al. (1989). Increased plasma and pulmonary lymph levels of endothelin during endotoxin shock. *Eur. J. Pharmacol.*, **167**, 427–8.

Morel P., Dargent F., Bachmann M. et al. (1985). Pulmonary extraction of serotonin and propranolol in patients with adult respiratory distress syndrome. *Am. Rev. Resp. Dis.*, **132**, 479–84.

Movat H.Z., Burrowes C.E., Cybulski M.I. et al. (1987). Acute inflammation and a Schwartzman-like reaction induced by interleukin 1 and tumor necrosis factor: synergistic action of the cytokines in the induction of inflammatory and microvascular injury. *Am. J. Pathol.*, **129**, 463–76.

Muldoon S.M., Hart J.L., Bowen K.L. et al. (1988). Attenuation of endothelium-mediated vasodilation by halothane. *Anesthesiology*, **68**, 31–7.

Mulvin D., Jones K., Howard R. et al. (1990). The effect of prostacyclin as a constituent of a preservation solution in protecting lungs from ischaemic injury because of its vasodilatory properties. *Transplantation*, **49**, 828–30.

Myers C.L., Pitt B.R. (1988). Selective effect of phorbol ester on kinetics of serotonin removal and ACE activity of in situ perfused rabbit lungs. *J. Appl. Physiol.*, **65**, 377–84.

Nadler J.L., Velasco J.S., Horton R. (1983). Cigarette smoking inhibits prostacyclin formation. *Lancet*, **1**, 1248–50.

Needleman P., Blaine E.H., Greenwald J.E. et al. (1989). The biochemical pharmacology of atrial peptides. *Annu. Rev. Pharmacol. Toxicol.*, **29**, 23–54.

Nemery B., Smith L.L., Aldridge W.N. (1987). Putrescine and 5-hydroxytryptamine accumulation in rat lung slices; cellular localization and responses to cell specific injury. *Toxicol. Appl. Pharmacol.*, **91**, 107–20.

Niehaus G.D., Kimura R., Traber L.D. et al. (1990). Administration of a synthetic antiprotease reduces smoke-induced lung injury. *J. Appl. Physiol.*, **69**, 694–9.

Novogrodsky A., Vanichkin A., Patya M. et al. (1994). Prevention of lipopolysaccharide-induced lethal toxicity by tyrosine kinase inhibitors. *Science*, **264**, 1319–22.

Numan N.A., Gillespie M.N., Altiere R.J. (1990). Pulmonary clearance of atrial natriuretic peptides. *Pulmonary Pharmacol.*, **3**, 25–8.

Ody C., Dieterle Y., Wand I. et al. (1979). PGA_1 and $PGF_{2\alpha}$ metabolism by pig pulmonary endothelium, smooth muscle and fibroblasts. *J. Appl. Physiol.*, **46**, 211–16.

Okusawa S., Gelfand J.A., Ikejima T. et al. (1988). Interleukin 1 induces a shock-like state in rabbits. *J. Clin. Invest.*, **81**, 1162–72.

Orfanos S.E., Chen X., Ryan J.W. et al. (1994). Assay of pulmonary microvascular endothelial angiotensin converting enzyme *in vivo*; comparison of three probes. *Toxicol. Appl. Pharmacol.*, **124**, 99–111.

Pakbaz H., Foda H.D., Berisha H. et al. (1993). Paraquat-induced lung injury; prevention by vasoactive intestinal peptide and related peptide helodermin. *Am. J. Physiol.*, **265**, L369–73.

Pakbaz H., Berisha H., Sharaf H. et al. (1994). VIP enhances and nitric oxide synthase inhibitor reduces survival of rat lungs perfused *ex vivo*. *Ann. NY. Acad. Sci.*, **723**, 426–8.

Pang J.A., Blackburn J.P., Butland R.J.A. et al. (1982a). Propranolol uptake by dog lung; effect of pulmonary artery occlusion and shock lung. *J. Appl. Physiol.*, **52**, 393–402.

Pang J.A., Williams T.R., Blackburn J.P. et al. (1981). First pass lung uptake of propranolol enhanced in anaesthetized dogs. *Br. J. Anaesthesia*, **53**, 601–4.

Pang J.A., Butland R.J.A., Brooks N. et al. (1982b). Impaired lung uptake of propranolol in human pulmonary emphysema. *Am. Rev. Resp. Dis.*, **125**, 194–8.

Pankhania J.J., Bakhle Y.S. (1985). Effect of pulmonary oedema induced by α-naphthylthiourea on synthesis of cyclo-oxygenase products in rat isolated lungs. *Prostaglandins*, **30**, 37–50.

Pankhania J.J., Bakhle Y.S. (1990). Treatment *in vivo* with PhCL28A alters prostaglandin E$_2$, prostacyclin and leukotriene C$_4$ metabolism in rat isolated lungs. *Pulmonary Pharmacol.*, **3**, 73–7.

Persson M.G., Zetterstrom O., Argenius V. et al. (1994). Single-breath oxide measurements in asthmatic patients and smokers. *Lancet*, **343**, 133–5.

Petros A., Lamb G., Leone A. et al. (1994). Effects of a nitric oxide synthase inhibitor in humans with septic shock. *Cardiovasc. Res.*, **28**, 34–9.

Petty R.G., Pearson J.D. (1989). Endothelium – the axis of vascular health and disease. *J. R. Coll. Physicians*, **23**, 92–102.

Pistolesi M., Miniati M., Petruzelli S. et al. (1988). Pulmonary retention of iodobenzyl propanediamine in humans; effect of cigarette smoking. *Am. Rev. Resp. Dis.*, **138**, 1429–33.

Pitt B.R., Lister G. (1989). Interpretation of metabolic function of the lung. Influence of perfusion, kinetics, and injury. *Clin. Chest Med.*, **10**, 1–12.

Pitt B.R., Hammond G.L., Gillis C.N. (1982). Depressed pulmonary removal of (^{3}H) prostaglandin E$_1$ after prolonged cardiopulmonary bypass. *J. Appl. Physiol.*, **52**, 887–92.

Pitt B.R., Forder J.R., Gillis C.N. (1983). Drug induced impairment of pulmonary ^{3}H-prostaglandin E$_1$ removal *in vivo*. *J. Pharmacol. Exp. Ther.*, **227**, 531–7.

Post C., Andersson R.G.G., Ryrfeldt A. et al. (1979). Physico-chemical modifications of lidocaine uptake in rat lung tissue. *Acta Pharmacol. Toxol.*, **44**, 103–9.

Pruitt B.A., Cioffi W.G., Shimazu T. et al. (1990). Evaluation and management of patients with inhalation injury. *J. Trauma*, **30**, S63–8.

Quinn A.C., Petros A.J., Vallance P. (1995). Nitric oxide: an endogenous gas. *Br. J. Anaesthesia*, **74**, 443–51.

Rabinovici R., Sofronski M.D., Borboroglu P. et al. (1994). Interleukin-2-induced lung injury; the role of complement. *Circ. Res.*, **74**, 329–35.

Rampart M., Williams T.J. (1986). Polymorphonuclear leukocyte-dependent plasma leakage in rabbit skin is enhanced or inhibited by prostacyclin, depending on the route of administration. *Am. J. Pathol.*, **124**, 66–73.

Reed D.J. (1990). Glutathione: toxicological implications. *Annu. Rev. Pharmacol. Toxicol.*, **30**, 603–31.

Reines H.D., Halushka P.V., Cook J.A. et al. (1985). Lack of effect of glucocorticoids upon plasma thromboxane in patients in a state of shock. *Surg. Gynecol. Obstet.*, **160**, 320–2.

Riggs D., Havill A.M., Pitt B.R. et al. (1988). Pulmonary angiotensin converting enzyme kinetics after lung injury in the rabbit. *J. Appl. Physiol.*, **64**, 2508–16.

Rinaldo J.E., Christman J.W. (1990). Mechanisms and mediators of the adult respiratory distress syndrome. *Clin. Chest Med.*, **11**, 621–32.

Robbins R.A., Barnes P.J., Springall D.R. et al. (1994). Expression of inducible nitric oxide synthase in human bronchial epithelial cells. *Biochem. Biophys. Res. Commun.*, **203**, 209–18.

Rocker G.M., Pearson D., Wiseman M.S. et al. (1989). Diagnostic criteria for adult respiratory distress syndrome; time for reappraisal. *Lancet*, **1**, 120–3.

Rodman D.M., Yamaguchi T., Hasunuma K. et al. (1990). Effects of hypoxia on endothelium-dependent relaxation of rat pulmonary artery. *Am. J. Physiol.*, **258**, 207–14.

Roerig D.L., Ahlf S.B., Dawson C.A. et al. (1994). First pass uptake in the human lung of drugs used during anesthesia. *Adv. Pharmacol.*, **31**, 531–49.

Royall J.A., Kooy N.W., Beckman J.S. (1995). Nitric oxide-related oxidants in acute lung injury. *New Horizons*, **3**, 113–22.

Ryan J.W. (1983). Assay of peptidase and protease enzymes *in vivo*. *Biochem. Pharmacol.*, **32**, 2127–37.

Ryan U.S. (1986). Metabolic activity of pulmonary endothelium. *Annu. Rev. Physiol.*, **48**, 268–77.

Said S.I., Foda H.D. (1989). Pharmacologic modulation of lung injury. *Am. Rev. Res. Dis.*, **139**, 1553–64.

Schmekel B., Borgstrom L., Wollmer P. (1991). Difference in pulmonary absorption of inhaled terbutaline in healthy smokers and non-smokers. *Thorax*, **46**, 225–8.

Schuller-Levis G., Quinn M.R., Wright C. et al. (1994). Taurine protects against oxidant-induced lung injury; possible mechanism(s) of action. *Adv. Exp. Med. Biol.*, **359**, 331–9.

Serrick C., Adoumie R., Giaid A. et al. (1994). The early release of interleukin-2, tumor necrosis factor-alpha and interferon-gamma after ischaemia-reperfusion injury in the lung allograft. *Transplantation*, **58**, 1158–62.

Shenkar R., Abraham E. (1995). Effects of treatment with the 21-aminosteroid U7438F on pulmonary cytokine expression following hemorrhage and resuscitation. *Crit. Care Medi.*, **23**, 132–9.

Shih W.J., Coupal J.J., Dillon M.L. et al. (1988). Application of I-123 HIPDM as a lung imaging agent. *Eur. J. Nucl. Med.*, **14**, 21–4.

Shulkin B.L., Shapiro B., Tobes M.C. et al. (1986). Iodine-123–4-amino-3-iodobenzylguanidine, a new sympathoadrenal imaging agent: comparison with iodine-123 metaiodobenzylguanidine. *J. Nucl. Med.*, **27**, 1138–42.

Simpson S.Q., Casey L.C. (1989). Role of tumor necrosis factor in sepsis and acute lung injury. *Crit. Care Clin.*, **5**, 27–47.

Slosman D.O., Brill A.B., Polla B.S. et al. (1987). Evaluation of (iodine-125)-*N, N, N'*-trimethyl-(2-hydroxy-3-methyl-5-iodobenzyl)-1,3-propane diamine lung uptake using an isolated lung model. *J. Nucl. Med.*, **28**, 203–8.

Slosman D.O., Davidson D., Brill A.B. et al. (1988a).^{131}I-metaiodobenzylguanidine uptake in the isolated rat lung: a potential marker of endothelial cell function. *Eur. J. Nucl. Med.*, **13**, 543–7.

Slosman D.O., Morel D.R., Alderson P.O. (1988b). A new imaging approach to quantitative evaluation of pulmonary vascular endothelial metabolism. *J. Thorac. Imaging*, **3**, 49–52.

Slosman D.O., Donath A., Alderson P.O. (1989). ^{131}I-meta-iodobenzylguanidine and 125I-iodoamphetamine. Parameters of lung endothelial cell function and pulmonary vascular area. *Eur. J. Nucl. Med.*, **15**, 207–10.

Slosman D.O., Polla B.S., Donath A. (1990). ^{123}I-MIBG pulmonary removal: a biochemical marker of minimal lung endothelial cell lesions. *Eur. J. Nucl. Med.*, **16**, 633–7.

Slotman G.J., Burchard K.W., Gann, D.S. (1985). Thromboxane and prostacyclin in clinical acute respiratory failure. *J. Surg. Res.*, **39**, 1–7.

Smith L.L. (1985). Paraquat toxicity. *Philos. Trans. R. Soc. (Lond.) B*, **311**, 647–57.

Smyth R.L., Higenbottam T., Scott J. et al. (1991). The current state of lung transplantation for cystic fibrosis. *Thorax*, **46**, 213–16.

Sole M.J., Drobac M., Schwarz L. et al. (1979). The extraction of circulating catecholamines by the lungs in normal man and in patients with pulmonary hypertension. *Circulation*, **60**, 160–3.

Sparrow M.P., Mitchell H.W. (1991). Modulation by the epithelium of the extent of bronchial narrowing produced by substances perfused through the lumen. *Br. J. Pharmacol.*, **103**, 1160–4.

Steinberg H., Greenwald R.A., Sciubba J. et al. (1982). The effect of oxygen derived free radicals on pulmonary endothelial cell function in the isolated perfused rat lung. *Exp. Lung Res.*, **3**, 163–73.

Stephens K.E., Akitoshi I., Larrick J.W. et al. (1988). Tumor necrosis factor causes increased pulmonary permeability and edema. *Am. Rev. Resp. Dis.*, **137**, 1364–70.

Stewart D.J., Levy R.D., Cernacek P. et al. (1991). Increased plasma endothelin-1 in pulmonary hypertension: marker or mediator of disease? *Ann. Intern. Med.*, **114**, 464–9.

Stewart T.E., Valenza F., Ribeiro S.P. et al. (1995). Increased nitric oxide in exhaled gas as an early marker of lung inflammation in a model of sepsis. *Am. J. Resp. Crit. Care Med.*, **151**, 713–18.

Stone D.J., Johns R.A. (1989). Endothelium-dependent effects of halothane, enflurane and isoflurane on isolated rat aortic vascular rings. *Anesthesiology*, **71**, 126–32.

Suffredini A.F. (1994). Current prospects for the treatment of clinical sepsis. *Crit. Care Med.*, **22**, S12–18.

Sugiura M., Inagami T., Valentina K. (1989). Endotoxin stimulates endothelin-release *in vivo* and *in vitro* as determined by radioimmunoassay. *Biochem. Biophys. Res. Communi.*, **161**, 1220–7.

Sullivan G.W., Carper H.T., Novick W.J. (1991). Inhibition of the inflammatory action of IL-1 and TNF on neutrophil function by pentoxifylline. *Infections Immunol.*, **56**, 1722–9.

Taeger K., Weninger E., Schmelzer F. et al. (1988). Pulmonary kinetics of fentanyl and alfentanil in surgical patients. *Br. J. Anaesthesia*, **61**, 425–34.

Thiemermann C. (1994). The role of the L-arginine: nitric oxide pathway in circulatory shock. *Adv.-Pharmacol.*, **28**, 45–79.

Toivonen H., Hartiala J., Bakhle Y.S. (1981). Effects of high oxygen tension on the metabolism of vasoactive hormones in isolated perfused rat lung. *Acta Physiol. Scand.*, **111**, 185–92.

Toivonen H., Makari N., Catravas J.D. (1988). Monitoring of pulmonary endothelial enzyme function; an animal model for a simplified clinically applicable procedure. *Anesthesiology*, **68**, 44–62.

Torphy T.J., Barnette M.S., Hay D.W. et al. (1994). Phosphodiesterase IV inhibitors as therapy for eosinophil-induced lung injury in asthma. *Environ. Health Perspect.*, **102**, (suppl. 10), 79–84.

Touya J.J., Rahimian J., Corbus H.F. et al. (1986). The lung as a metabolic organ. *Semin. Nucl. Med.*, **16**, 296–305.

Tracey K.J., Lowry S.F. (1990). The role of cytokine mediators in septic shock. *Adv. Surg.*, **23**, 21–56.

Tracey K.J., Beutler B., Lowry S.F. et al. (1986). Shock and tissue injury induced by recombinant human cachectin. *Science*, **234**, 470–4.

Treasure T. (1994). A surgeon's view of adult respiratory distress syndrome. *Br. J. Hosp. Med.*, **52**, 108–14.

Turrin M., Gillis C.N. (1986). Removal of atrial natriuretic factor by perfused rabbit lungs in situ. *Biochemi. Biophy. Res. Commun.*, **140**, 868–73.

Vallance P., Collier J., Moncada S. (1989). Effects of endothelium-derived nitric oxide on peripheral arteriolar tone in man. *Lancet*, **ii**, 997–1000.

Vane J.R. (1969). The release and fate of vasoactive hormones in the circulation. *Br. J. Pharmacol.*, **35**, 209–42.

van der Wal N.A., Smith L.L., van Oirschot J.F. et al. (1992). Effect of iron chelators on paraquat toxicity in rats and alveolar type II cells. *Am. Rev. Resp. Dis.*, **145**, 180–6.

Venkatesan N., Chandrakasan G. (1994). *In vivo* administration of taurine and niacin modulate cyclophosphamide-induced lung injury. *Eur. J. Pharmacol.*, **292**, 75–80.

Vigneswaran W.T., Stanbrook H.S., Doctor R. et al. (1989). 5-Hydroxytryptamine uptake in oxygen radical-mediated acute lung injury. *Am. Rev. Resp. Dis.*, **139**, 382–6.

Wagner P.D., Mathieu-Costello O., Bebout D.E. et al. (1989). Protection against pulmonary O_2 toxicity by N-acetylcysteine. *Eur. Resp. J.*, **2**, 116–26.

Wang Q.J., Giri S.N., Hyde D.M. et al. (1989). Effect of taurine on bleomycin-induced lung fibrosis in hamsters. *Proc. Soc. Exp. Bio. Med.*, **190**, 330–8.

Weir E.K., McMurtry I.F., Tucker A. et al. (1976). Prostaglandin synthetase inhibitors do not decrease hypoxic vasoconstriction. *J. Appl. Physiol.*, **41**, 714–18.

Weissmann G., Smolen J.E., Korchak H. (1980). Prostaglandins and inflammation; receptor/cyclase coupling as an explanation of why PGEs and PGI_2 inhibit functions of inflammatory cells. In *Advances in Prostaglandin and Thromboxane Research* (Samuelsson B., Ramwell P.W., Paoletti R., eds). New York: Raven, pp. 1637–53.

Welbourn C.R.B., Young Y. (1992). Endotoxin, septic shock and acute lung injury; neutrophils, macrophages and inflammatory mediators. *Br. J. Surg.*, **79**, 998–1103.

Welsh C.H., Lien D., Worthen G.S. (1988). Pentoxifylline decrease endotoxin-induced neutrophil sequestration and extravascular protein accumulation in the dog. *Am. Rev. Resp. Dis.*, **138**, 1106–14.

Weng W., Lazo J.O., Gillis C.N. et al. (1990). Disposition of radioidinated benzylguanidines in perfused rabbit lung; pharmacokinetics and effect of an organo-gold complexed antineoplastic agent. *J. Pharmacol. Exp. Ther.*, **255**, 59–65.

Wiedemann H.P., Matthay M.A., Gillis C.N. (1990). Pulmonary endothelial cell injury and altered lung metabolic function. *Clin. Chest Medi.*, **11**, 723–36.

Williams T.J., Peck M.J. (1977). Role of prostaglandin-mediated vasodilatation in inflammation. *Nature*, **270**, 530–2.

Witten M.L., Grad R., Quan S.F. et al. (1990). Piriprost pretreatment attenuates the smoke-induced increase in ^{99m}Tc-DTPA lung clearance. *Exp. Lung Res.*, **16**, 339–53.

Wong C., Fox R., Demling R.H. (1985). Effect of hydroxyl radical scavenging on endotoxin-induced lung injury. *Surgery*, **97**, 300–7.

Yanagisawa M., Masaki T. (1989). Endothelin, a novel endothelium-derived peptide. *Biochem. Pharmacol.*, **38**, 1877–83.

Yanagisawa M., Kurihara H., Kimura S. et al. (1988). A novel potent vasoconstrictor peptide produced by vascular endothelial cells. *Nature*, **332**, 411–15.

Ying R.L., Gross K.B., Terzo T.S. et al. (1990). Indomethacin does not inhibit the ozone-induced increase in bronchial responsiveness in human subjects. *Am. Rev. Resp. Dis.*, **142**, 817–21.

Youdim M.B.H., Bakhle Y.S., Ben-Harari R.R. (1980). Inactivation of monoamines by the lung. In *Metabolic Activities of the Lung (Ciba Foundation Symposium 78)* (Porter R., Whelan J., eds). Amsterdam: North Holland, pp. 105–28.

Zimmerman R.S., Trippodo N.C., MacPhee A.A. et al. (1990). High-dose atrial natriuretic factor enhances albumin escape from the systemic but not the pulmonary circulation. *Circ. Res.*, **67**, 461–8.

44. The Pulmonary Circulation and Trauma

G. Schlag and H. Redl

INTRODUCTION

The pulmonary vessels play a decisive role in the response to trauma. Two pathomechanisms are involved: either direct trauma, such as lung contusion, aspiration or inhalation injury, or indirect trauma, i.e. due to release of tissue-damaging mediators. A combination of both mechanisms is possible (e.g. thoracic trauma in association with traumatic shock and/or polytrauma).

Due to the physiological role of the lung, pulmonary involvement is highly relevant for the post-traumatic course, and also because of the associated high mortality (> 50%).

Morphologically, the most important part of the lung is the alveolar septum where gas exchange takes place. This is also where early pathomorphological changes occur. In indirect damage the capillaries are primarily involved, while the alveolar space is not affected. In direct damage both the alveolar space and the capillaries are involved. Morphological evidence provides information about mediator effects at the cellular level, for example, as well as about the resulting development of interstitial lung oedema secondary to a permeability increase.

This chapter will mainly deal with the stages of development of failure in the lung as a response to trauma and discuss both the morphology and pathomechanisms leading to post-traumatic lung failure.

MORPHOLOGICAL CHANGES OF THE LUNG DURING THE POST-TRAUMATIC COURSE

Morphological alterations are seen within hours from the onset of shock and subsequently give rise to the formation of the organ in shock.

Lung in shock (Figure 44.1)

In the lung, the morphological substrate of shock is always related to leukostasis (sequestration of polymorphonuclear neutrophils (PMN)), confirmed in man (Schlag and Redl, 1972, 1980, 1985, 1988, 1991a; Schlag et al., 1976) and in three other species (Redl et al., 1978; Pretorius et al., 1987; Schlag and Redl, 1987).

PMN are seen within 1 hour from the onset of shock. Leukostasis could be confirmed experimentally during shock (low-flow syndrome) by way of

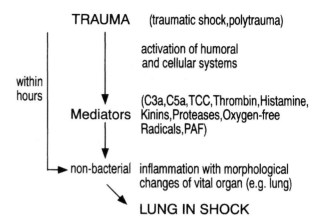

Figure 44.1 Reactions leading to the development of lung in shock.

[111]-Indium oxide labelled PMN. Leukostasis was highly significant when compared to control levels ($P < 0.001$). Autopsies in polytraumatized patients without direct lung damage (contusion, aspiration) and the use of a special esterase staining method for morphometric evaluation of PMN revealed significant leukostasis in all lobes of the lung as compared to deceased patients without trauma. Only patients who died within 48 hours after trauma were selected (Dinges et al., 1984) (Table 44.1). Leukostasis of the lung can be considered to be the morphological hallmark of traumatic shock (Figure 44.2) (Ratliff et al., 1971; Connell et al., 1975; Teplitz, 1976).

Endothelial swelling (Figure 44.3) is a further morphological symptom of the 'lung in shock' and is very common early in shock in the capillaries of the alveolar septa. Endothelial junctions are unaffected. Teplitz (1976) reported that endothelial cells lost their pinocytotic vesicles within a few hours after traumatic shock. This loss of pinocytotic vesicles is probably apparent rather than real, due to the presence of intracellular oedema. The number of vesicles is reduced in relation to the larger endothelial volume (Marquart and Caesar, 1970).

TABLE 44.1

LEUCOSTASIS AFTER POLYTRAUMA IN PATIENTS: QUANTITATIVE EVALUATION USING MORPHOMETRIC TECHNIQUES AFTER ESTERASE STAINING OF POLYMORPHONUCLEAR LEUCOCYTES IN HISTOLOGICAL SECTIONS (UNPAIRED T-TEST). (DATA FROM REDL ET AL., 1987)

Control	Polytrauma
2.4 ± 0.9	8 ± 2.3
$n = 6$	$n = 6$
	$p < 0.001$

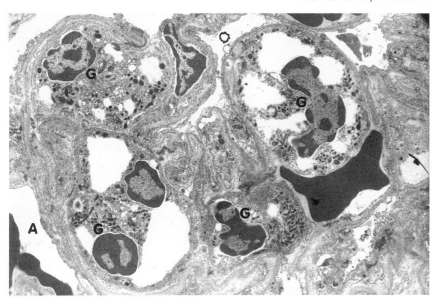

Figure 44.2 Leukostasis in the lung after hypovolaemic traumatic shock. A = alveoli; G = granulocyte.

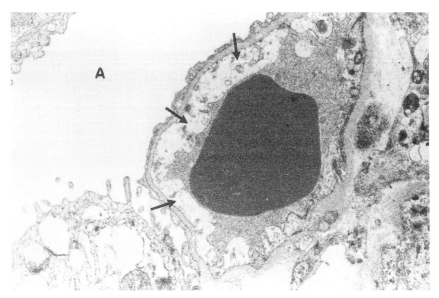

Figure 44.3 Endothelial swelling (arrows) in a human lung biopsy. A = alveoli. (Reproduced from Schlag and Redl, 1989, with permission.)

Mitochondria, endoplasmic reticulum and ribosomes were found to be drastically reduced in human lung biopsy specimens at 1 hour after injury. Endothelial cells revealed evidence of focal necrosis (Figure 44.4). Endothelial cell swelling persisted for several days after injury and led to bulbous evaginations into the vascular lumen.

In addition to evidence from human lung, endothelial damage to the capillaries is also demonstrated in a hypovolaemic-traumatic shock model in baboons, where endothelial bleb formation is found (Figure 44.5). Bulla formation results from endothelial shedding.

Endothelial cell damage constitutes the basis for permeability oedema extending into the interstitium. Perivascular oedema in the area of the alveolar septa marks incipient interstitial oedema, which can be observed within 1 hour of traumatic shock (Figure 44.6) and increases after several hours. This may explain why no disturbance of gas exchange is seen during the first hours after trauma, except in the case of direct lung injury (e.g. contusion). With lung contusion the prevalent morphological events are interstitial and alveolar haemorrhage secondary to damage of pulmonary capillaries. This haemorrhagic exudate further

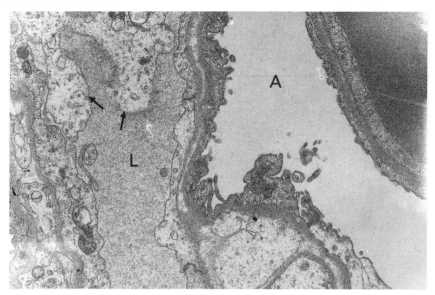

Figure 44.4 Massive swelling of endothelium with necrosis (arrows). Capillary lumen (L) and alveolus (A) in human biopsy specimen. (Reproduced from Schlag and Redl, 1985, with permission.)

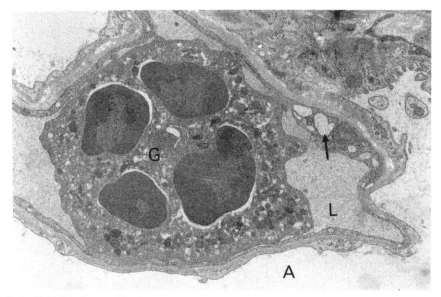

Figure 44.5 Endothelial bleb formation (arrow) in post-traumatic lung of baboon. A = alveoli; G = granulocyte; L = capillary lumen. (Reproduced from Schlag and Redl, 1988, with permission.)

affects the alveoli by inactivating surfactant. In addition, there is a rapid sequestration of PMN into the capillaries, which results in a localized inflammatory process quite similar to the indirect damage also caused by PMN. Contusion of the lung, as an expression of direct lung injury, results in early hypoxaemia, which is not seen during the early phase of indirect lung injury.

Immediately after trauma fat emboli often appear to occlude the capillary lumen completely (Figure 44.7). In lung biopsies performed in polytraumatized patients there was frequent evidence of fat in

the alveolar capillaries. It is thought that fat plays no major role, except for its mechanical properties such as blockade of the capillaries. Bosch *et al.* (1989) found intracellular fat in 91% of 80 autopsied polytraumatized patients, mostly in the macrophages, within 9 hours after trauma. In a series of lung biopsies performed 24 hours after trauma, fat was moved in the alveolar space and in the alveolar macrophages.

These acute morphological symptoms of the 'lung in shock' are mostly reversible with timely and adequate management.

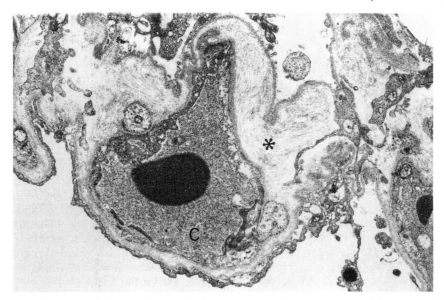

Figure 44.6 Interstitial oedema (asterisk) around alveolar capillaries (C). Patient biopsy specimen obtained 1 day after trauma. (Reproduced from Schlag and Redl, 1985, with permission.)

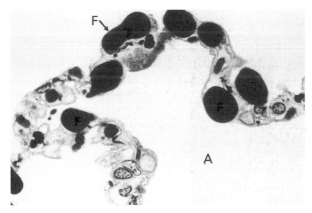

Figure 44.7 Fat-globuli (F) are blocking lung capillaries in a polytraumatized patients. A = alveoli. (Reproduced from Schlag *et al.*, 1977, with permission.)

However, with progressing pathomorphology, the cellular damage increases, perivascular oedema spreads and involves the alveolar space. As a consequence, the lung in early failure (also referred to as 'fat embolism syndrome' or 'shock lung syndrome') may occur.

Early failure of the lung

Early failure of the lung may develop within 24–72 hours after trauma, depending on whether direct lung injury is present. In this case there may be a rapid spread of the haemorrhage and interstitial oedema with very early impairment of lung function as an expression of organ failure.

Marked interstitial oedema (Figure 44.8) is caused by increased permeability of microvascular

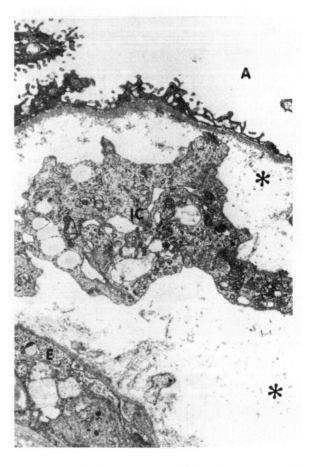

Figure 44.8 Fulminant interstitial oedema (asterisk) with several interstitial cells (IC), swollen endothelium (E) but normal epithelium around alveoli (A). Human biopsy specimen. (Reproduced from Schlag and Redl, 1985, with permission.)

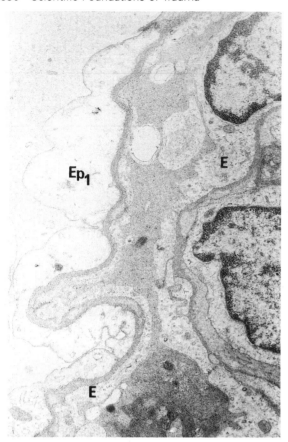

Figure 44.9 Oedematous swelling of capillary endothelium (E) and type I pneumocytes (Ep₁) in a human lung 24 hours after severe injury. (Reproduced from Schlag and Redl, 1985, with permission.)

walls. As the condition progresses and interstitial oedema becomes more prominent, alveolar epithelial cells tend to become oedematous if no direct lung injury is involved (Figure 44.9). In the areas of denuded alveolar cells type I interstitial oedema can lead to direct fluid leak into the alveolar space. This may explain the passage of intravascularly formed fibrin monomers into the alveolar space (Figure 44.10). As these fibrin monomers are polymerized, hyaline membranes develop in the alveolar spaces. Often a concomitant accumulation of PMN, erythrocytes and fat globules is seen in the alveolar space. Macrophages in the alveolar space frequently show pronounced vacuolization with large digestive vacuoles in the ultrastructure, suggesting macrophage overload. Clearing the alveolar space requires phagocytosis and digestion of the protein-rich and partly lipid-containing exudate, as well as of the fibrin deposits.

PMN migration may be seen at a very early stage ('lung in shock'), where specific adherence molecules may be expressed both by activated PMN and by stimulated endothelial cells. PMN adherence is the prerequisite for PMN migration through the capillary endothelium into the interstitial space and from there to the alveolar space.

An obvious symptom of PMN activation is degranulation (Figure 44.11), which is demonstrated by evidence of free granules intravascularly on electron microscopy (Figure 44.12), as well as in the interstitium.

At a very early stage the organism tries to compensate for the loss of surfactant type II by increasing the release of lamellar bodies from

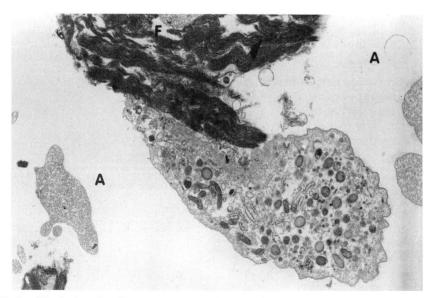

Figure 44.10 Fibrin (F) during hyaline membrane formation in a human lung with ARDS. A = alveoli. (Reproduced from Schlag and Redl, 1988, with permission.)

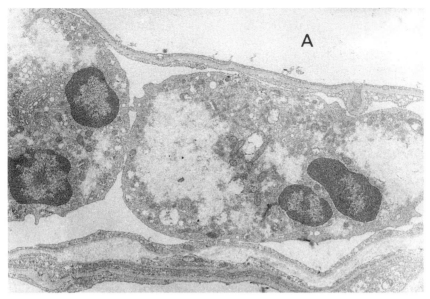

Figure 44.11 Partially degranulated granulocytes in a human lung after polytrauma. A = alveoli. (Reproduced from Schlag and Redl, 1980, with permission.)

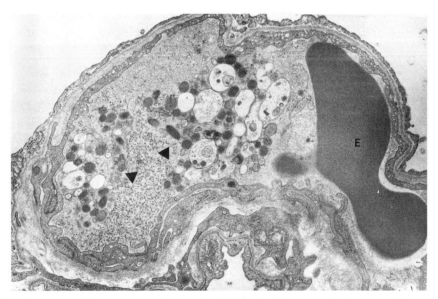

Figure 44.12 Free lysosomal-like granules (arrowheads) in the lumen of a lung capillary. E = erythrocytes. (Reproduced from Schlag and Redl, 1980, with permission.)

alveolar epithelial cells (responsible for surfactant production) (Figure 44.13). The type II alveolar epithelial cells only retain clear vacuoles near the surface.

This is followed by the spread of oedema into the interstitial and intra-alveolar space. PMNs accumulate in the intra-alveolar space, which leads to a change in the macrophage/PMN ratio in favour of the PMNs (i.e. up to 50% increase in PMN levels within the first 2 days vs a decrease of the macrophage count). Intracapillary fibrin deposits are not found at this early stage (Schlag *et al.*, 1976; Lium *et al.*, 1982).

Late failure of the lung

The transition between the stage of early organ failure in the lung and the onset of typical adult respiratory distress syndrome (ARDS) (late organ failure) extends over several days, with a peak commonly seen at the end of the first and the beginning of the second post-traumatic week. In this stage, the exudative phase of post-traumatic ARDS prevails. Gradually the proliferative stage develops and may often terminate as severe fibrosis.

Fibrosis may occur very early in the development of late organ failure; it first affects the interstitial

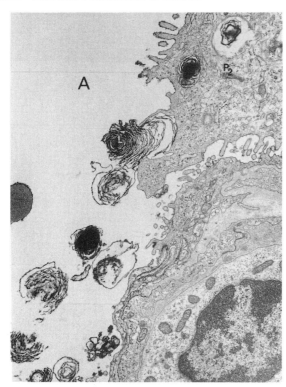

Figure 44.13 Numerous pneumocytes type II (P_2) have released lamellar bodies, which are also seen freely in the alveolar space (A). (Reproduced from Schlag *et al.*, 1976, with permission.)

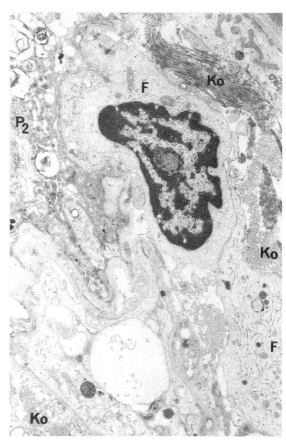

Figure 44.14 Nineteen days after multiple injuries leading to post-traumatic ARDS, a large number of fibrocytes (F), irregularly distributed collagen clusters (Ko) and high contrast elastic substances are seen in the interstitium. Patient biopsy specimen taken 19 days after traumatic injury. P_2 = pneumocytes type II. (Reproduced from Schlag and Redl, 1985, with permission.)

area and later on the intra-alveolar space. These alterations are largely irreversible. In rare instances the fibrotic processes may recede (Mittermayer *et al.*, 1978, 1979; Hassenstein *et al.*, 1980) and isolated scars remain. As a result a complete structural and functional recovery is not possible.

The collagen content of the interstitium increases (Lamy *et al.*, 1976; Zapol *et al.*, 1979) (Figure 44.14). Interstitial fibrosis is frequently associated with intra-alveolar fibrosis, which leads to severe impairment of gas exchange.

During the repair phase of the lung damage the restoration of denuded type I alveolar epithelial cells occurs via type II cells. These cells (pneumocytes) possess a mitotic potential; the rate of mitosis may be increased secondary to interstitial trauma. Also, type II cells show hyperplasia (Thal *et al.*, 1972; Redl and Schlag, 1980) (Figure 44.15). This hyperplasia may be explained by the urgent need for surfactant formation. On scanning electron microscopy the hyperplastic type II alveolar epithelial cells are seen as a nidal accumulation of cells abundantly covered with microvilli. Metaplasia of these cells in type I alveolar epithelial cells requires a certain amount of time, and epithelial defects associated with ARDS are very clearly seen. Hyperplasia of the type II cells develops within days.

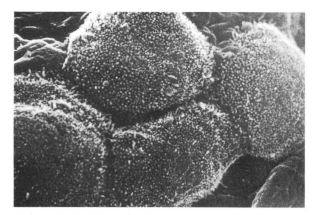

Figure 44.15 Hyperplasia of type II pneumocytes in the scanning electron microscope. (Reproduced from Redl and Schlag, 1980, with permission.)

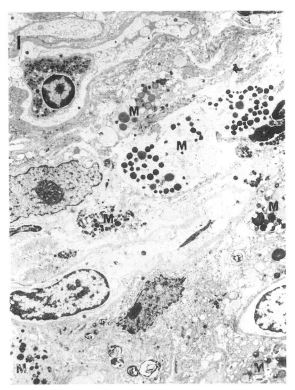

Figure 44.16 Partially oedematous fibrotic interstitial space (I) with numerous mast cells (M) in different stages of degranulation in a human lung 3 weeks after trauma. (Reproduced from Schlag *et al.*, 1980.)

Mast cells are also involved in the pulmonary alterations after shock, especially in the late phase. Elevated levels of these cells, very often showing partial degranulation, may be encountered in association with an already manifest fibrosis in the interstitium (Kawanami *et al.*, 1979) (Figure 44.16). A striking finding in lung biopsies is the heterogeneous pattern of the mast cell granulae, which are normally arranged in a snail-like pattern.

PATHOMECHANISMS AND CLINICAL IMPLICATIONS

Trauma-related activation of humoral systems secondary to lung damage

Complement system

Soft tissue trauma causes complement activation via the alternative pathway and subsequent activation of C3. C3 activation gives rise to the formation of C3b which increases conversion of C5 to C5a, a potent activator of PMN. C3a and C5a are involved in the increase in capillary permeability via PMN/endothelial interaction. C5a leads to PMN sequestration in the lung and liver, which may cause peripheral neutropenia (Ratliff *et al.*, 1971; Gallin, 1976; Hammerschmidt *et al.*, 1978).

Complement activation occurs very early in shock. The complement system induces lung damage due to interaction with other humoral systems (Pottemeyer *et al.*, 1986; Slotman *et al.*, 1986; Kongsgaard *et al.*, 1989) and activation of PMN. There is debate as to whether C3a and C5a are (Duchateau *et al.*, 1984; Langlois *et al.*, 1989; Zilow *et al.*, 1990; Roumen *et al.*, 1995) or are not (Maunder *et al.*, 1984; Weinberg *et al.*, 1989) specific predictors of the development of post-traumatic ARDS. The primary task of complement activation appears to be the development of an inflammatory response characterized by chemotaxis, opsonization and phagocytosis (Kunkel *et al.*, 1981; Bengtson and Haljamäe, 1988–89).

Zilow *et al.* (1990) showed increased C3a levels in the first 6 hours post-trauma, which were related to the subsequent development of ARDS. The C3a/C3 ratio served to identify patients prone to develop ARDS (Zilow *et al.*, 1990). In these patients, C5a could not be determined due to its very short half-life and very rapid binding to PMN. The reports by Zilow *et al.* (1990, 1991) confirm the importance of the complement system and its activation in acute trauma, especially with regard to damage of the pulmonary circulation.

Lung damage secondary to complement activation (anaphylatoxins) is best explained by the action of PMN and platelets. This complement effect together with PMN sequestration essentially accounts for the non-infectious inflammation of the lung, which constitutes the basis for the 'lung in shock'.

Polytrauma and thoracic injury increase C3d and terminal complement complex (C5b-9) levels (Fosse *et al.*, 1987). Presumably, this is caused by hypoperfusion resulting in hypoxic cell injury in the hypovolaemic phase. A further source of complement activation is tissue damage (trauma, ischaemia), as demonstrated for example by Heideman (1979) following the infusion of homogenized autologous muscle tissue.

Coagulation system

As a result of tissue trauma (muscle, fat) and fracture of long bones, tissue thromboplastin enters the bloodstream, whereupon the coagulation system is activated via factor X to Xa. There is also an activation via the contact system, which involves Hageman factor (factor XII), prekallikrein, factor XI and high-molecular-weight kininogen (HMWK).

The humoral systems, i.e. the complement, coagulation, fibrinolytic and kallikrein–kinin systems, are interrelated. Thus any activation of the complement system may in turn activate other humoral systems.

The local inflammatory reaction caused by trauma may be disseminated into the systemic circulation and thereby lead to the release of various mediators. Thrombin as a temporary end

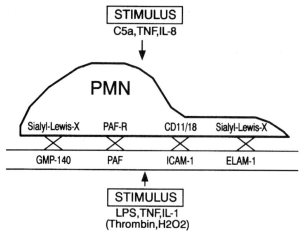

Figure 44.17 Stimuli and adherence molecules of PMN and endothelium responsible for leucocyte adherence.

product of the activated coagulation cascade plays a decisive role. As a result, fibrin formation may lead to an obstruction of the microvasculature in various organs (Risberg *et al.*, 1986). In the pulmonary circulation fibrin appears to be quite irrelevant during shock, as the fibrinolytic activity of the lung is very intense.

Thrombin and histamine are thought to be involved in stimulating the endothelial cells to provoke P-selectin (GMP-140) expression, an adherence molecule for PMN (Geng *et al.*, 1990).

Both humans and animals show very rapid sequestration of PMN in the lung. This is followed by immediate endothelial cell damage, prevalently caused by activated PMN and release of various mediators. This, however, requires very rapid adherence of PMN to the endothelial cells (GMP-140 induced adherence may occur within minutes) (Figures 44.17, 44.18).

Thrombin increases pulmonary vascular permeability for proteins to a certain extent. The increase in endothelial permeability may be due to an increase in interendothelial pore diameter or to gap formation (Taylor *et al.*, 1981; Johnson *et al.*, 1983; Lo *et al.*, 1985; Malik, 1986).

Fibrinolysis and the kallikrein–kinin system

Risberg *et al.* (1986) noted mild to moderate activation of the fibrinolytic system in polytraumatized patients on admission to hospital, although there was a decrease in antiplasmin complexes and fibrin degradation products over the subsequent days.

The initial activation of the fibrinolytic system may explain the absence of intravascular fibrin deposits in lung biopsies taken immediately after trauma. It is only on the second or third days after injury that fibrin deposits may be seen in the alveolar space, while intravascular fibrin deposits are only seen later. No definitive information is available on whether this is related to activation of the endothelium (endotoxin, cytokines) or the associated expression of tissue factor (TF) by type I alveolar cells (Idell *et al.*, 1992).

The inherent anticoagulative effect of the endothelial cells (EC; e.g. thrombomodulin) has shifted in favour of a prevalence of the coagulative properties, e.g. TF and plasminogen activator inhibitor (PAI-1).

Trauma also activates the contact system as part of the coagulation mechanism. As a result of this

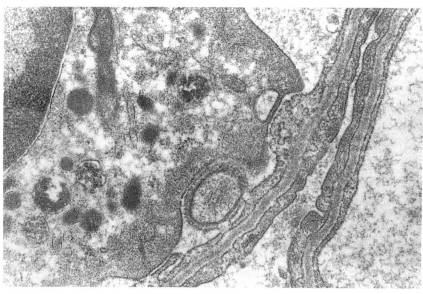

Figure 44.18 Contact between neutrophils and endothelial cells in lung capillaries. (Reproduced from Schlag and Redl, 1980, with permission.)

activation, factor XIIa triggers the kinin-forming pathway (Haberland, 1977). In shock, activation of factor XII may be due to local trauma and result in the formation of kallikrein, which in turn may interact with the activation of the humoral systems (complement, coagulation and fibrinolytic system).

As a representative of the kinins, bradykinin, among other effects, has the capacity to stimulate the contractile system of the EC. This may produce gap formation of the EC in the pulmonary capillary system and eventually interstitial oedema (Godin *et al.*, 1983). The bradykinin-induced increase in vascular permeability can play a role in the development of early perivascular oedema in the alveolar septa of the lung.

Trauma-related activation of cellular systems secondary to lung damage

Platelet activation

Thrombin generated within the coagulation cascade activates platelets and triggers the release of adenosine diphosphate (ADP) as well as platelet aggregation. Platelet aggregation may also occur directly at the site of injury due to exposed collagen.

Platelets may directly affect the lung by releasing thromboxane and serotonin, two potent mediators with a strong action on the vascular and bronchiolar tone of the lung.

Platelet involvement in trauma is expressed through their interaction with PMN. PMN aggregation is enhanced (Redl *et al.*, 1983), the cytotoxicity of PMN versus endothelial cells is elevated (Boogaerts *et al.*, 1982), and again platelets are activated by the platelet-activating factor (PAF) released by the activated PMN.

Phagocytes (PMN, monocytes, macrophages)

Leukostasis of the lung constitutes the substrate for the lung in early failure as the consequence of non-bacterial inflammation.

Reasons for leukostasis Essentially, leukostasis is the net effect of three different events, detailed below.

1. Reduction of blood flow during the 'low flow syndrome' in traumatic shock as demonstrated by Martin *et al.* (1982) The balance between PMN endothelial adhesive forces and haemodynamic dispersal forces is of major importance (Mayrovitz *et al.*, 1977). As the shear forces decrease, margination and adhesion of the leucocytes to the endothelium occurs almost exclusively in the postcapillary venules (House and Lipowsky, 1987). Adherence mainly depends on an increase in adhesive forces in contrast to diminished shear stresses. In a polytrauma model leukostasis

could not be significantly reduced (Redl *et al.*, 1984), probably due to adhesion phenomena, despite an increase in cardiac output during reinfusion and normalization of blood flow.

2. Activation of leucocytes (PMN) Among the different leucocyte populations granulocytes or PMN are the fastest-reacting cells within the body's inflammatory response mechanism and therefore the focus of the endothelial cell/leucocyte interaction. In traumatic shock activation of PMN mainly occurs via complement split products (C3a, C5a). PMN activation may be demonstrated both morphologically (ultrastructural) and biochemically via measurement of neutrophil elastase as the PMN-elastase-α_1-proteinase inhibitor complex (Neumann *et al.*, 1983; Neumann and Jochum, 1984). A positive correlation between trauma severity and plasma elastase levels has been demonstrated in patients (Nuytinck *et al.*, 1986) (Figure 44.19).

In a baboon traumatic shock model a significant increase in plasma elastase levels have been noted both at the end of the shock period and after retransfusion (Pretorius *et al.*, 1987). Early PMN activation caused by traumatic shock is evident both in humans and baboons, and represents a highly effective mediator stimulus for tissue damage, which is independent of any infectious component and may occur very soon after trauma.

Anaphylatoxins (C3a, C5a) stimulate neutrophils to perform the respiratory burst reaction with the formation of reactive oxygen species and the release of cytotoxic proteases. These complement products also induce an upregulation of neutrophil adherence molecules, especially of CD11b/CD18 (MAC-1) (Harlan *et al.*, 1985), which is both an important complement receptor (CR3) involved in phagocytosis and a ligand of the endothelial adherence

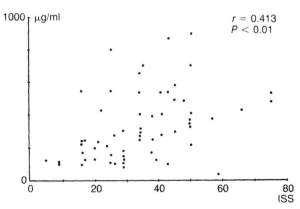

Elastase at admission (µg/ml)

Figure 44.19 Relationship between plasma granulocyte elastase and injury severity (ISS) in polytraumatized patients. (Reproduced from Nuytinck *et al.*, 1986, with permission.)

molecule intercellular adhesion molecule (ICAM-1).

The endothelial cell, especially in the lung, is a major target in shock and thus represents the substrate for generalized tissue damage.

3. Endothelial effects Activation of the endothelial cells (EC), e.g. via cytokines, requires a certain amount of time for expression of the adherence molecules endothelial leukocyte adhesion molecule (ELAM-1) and ICAM-1.

In the acute shock stage, analogous to the local inflammatory process, there is an EC response, which can be differentiated into endothelial stimulation (fast; protein synthesis-independent response) and endothelial activation (slower; protein synthesis-dependent response). The endothelial stimulation occurs in response to mediators such as thrombin, histamine, complement components and oxygen radicals. The molecules involved in endothelial stimulation are P-selectin and PAF on the endothelial level, and Sialyl-Lewis-X and PAF receptors as their PMN counterparts.

Recent investigations have shown that P-selectin also inhibits several aspects of neutrophil function, for example the production of superoxide anion (O_2^-) (Wong *et al.*, 1991). P-selectin interacts with neutrophils by a lectin-like mechanism. As soon as P-selectin is expressed it rapidly and reversibly binds to its receptors on leucocytes (Moore *et al.*, 1991).

PMN adherence to EC is also mediated by surface expression of the receptor CD11b/CD18 on PMN.

Post-traumatic ARDS patients (Simms and D'Amico, 1991) observed increased levels of CD11b/CD18 receptors on the PMN cell surface; the oxidative burst was upregulated. CD11b/CD18 expression is mainly relevant for PMN adherence in the pulmonary circulation, especially during sepsis (via tumour necrosis factor, TNF), and plays only a minor role in the acute traumatic setting. If TNF release or production has already occurred during traumatic shock, this could rapidly cause receptor expression at the PMN and thus also account for neutropenia.

In traumatic shock the EC are involved in PMN adherence, synthesis of mediators such as eicosanoids and PAF, as well as lipid peroxidation; the EC damage contributes to the permeability increase, which leads to perivascular oedema and later to interstitial oedema of the lung.

During this primary damage of the pulmonary circulation in shock a second factor, i.e. tissue damage induced by reinfusion, plays a major part with regard to the permeability increase. During the 'low flow syndrome' there may be severe hypoperfusion of all lobes of the lung, and especially in areas of zone I according to West (1978). Ischaemia may develop due to elevated alveolar

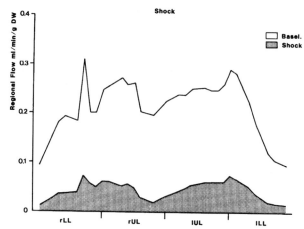

Figure 44.20 Flow distribution in canine lung during baseline and hypovolaemic shock measured by microspheres. rLL = Right lower lung; rUL = right upper lung; lUL = left upper lung; lLL = left lower lung.

pressure (Figure 44.20). Xanthine oxidase seems not to play a major role in the formation of reactive oxygen species. According to Gurtner *et al.* (1988), reactive oxygen species in the lung develop in relation to the respiratory chain or by cytochrome P-450 during reperfusion.

The prerequisite for EC damage by activated PMN is their adherence to the EC. An increased adherence in turn probably represents a precondition for the release of tissue-damaging mediators by PMN and for PMN migration and extravasation.

The assumption that EC have not yet been stimulated at an early stage of shock was also suggested by the fact that expression of the endothelial leucocyte adhesion molecule 1 (ELAM-1) was not confirmed by immunohistochemistry, while in animals (baboon) exposed to septic shock there was widespread expression of ELAM-1 in various organ systems (Table 44.2). At this very early stage we may assume that translocation of bacteria/endotoxin via the gut, which eventually triggers cytokine release and thus favours EC activation, has not yet taken place.

ELAM-1 expression is commonly detectable after 3–6 hours. During this period we were able to demonstrate incipient extravasation of PMN into the interstitium of the lung by way of electron-microscopic sections. Degranulation of PMN in the lung capillaries, a morphological proof of PMN activation, may be detected very early.

Oxygen products that appear in the initial stage (i.e. up to 4 hours) mainly account for damage of the EC, while proteases appear to play a minor role in the early phase of injury (Varani *et al.*, 1989).

PMN extravasation (migration) may occur either via the junctions of the EC or via the EC directly (Figure 44.21). In the interstitium of the lung there

TABLE 44.2

IMMUNOHISTOCHEMICAL LOCALIZATION OF ELAM-1 IN SEPTIC
AND TRAUMATIC SHOCK. (FROM REDL *ET AL.*, 1991)

	Septic shock		Traumatic shock	
	No. examined	Average score	No. examined	Average score
Lung	6	2.2+	13	0.03+
Liver	5	3.0+	12	0.16+
Kidney	3	2.7+	9	0.80+
Skin	2	3.0+	2	0.50+

The average score denotes average level of ELAM-1 expression, on a scale of 0 ± (0.5) 1, 2 and 3 + in the group examined.

may be further degranulation and thus release of mediators (protease, collagenase). At this point in time it is unclear if the PMNs play a role in the fibrogenetic process. More likely, there is a platelet–fibroblast interaction with the release of the platelet-derived growth factor (PDGF) via activation of intrapulmonary platelets (Heffner *et al.*, 1987). It is known that interstitial fibrosis in the lung may occur very early (within a week) (Hassenstein *et al.*, 1980; Auler *et al.*, 1986). Interstitial fibrosis is frequently associated with intra-alveolar fibrosis, which commonly becomes manifest in the second week after trauma and is responsible for the impairment of gas exchange.

Tissue fibrosis is often associated with a high morbidity (interstitial lung disorders). In the presence of lung fibrosis, the mononuclear cell/fibroblast interaction appears to be of decisive importance. This gives rise to the formation of a complex cytokine network, with inflammatory cells regulating fibroblast function.

Elias *et al.* (1990) have investigated the regulative potential of interleukin-1 (IL-1), TNF, interferon-gamma (IFN-γ) and IL-6. This mechanism controls fibroblast proliferation and collagen production. There is also a feedback mechanism from fibroblasts to regulate local inflammatory events. Fibroblasts additionally produce cytokines such as IL-1 and IL-6. Cytokine production in the tissue partly depends on the migration of mononuclear cells into the interstitium.

Further in the course of events associated with indirect lung damage (1–3 days after trauma), the alveolar space is also affected. Before this, the events are predominantly due to non-bacterial inflammation. The invasion of the alveolar space by PMN in the first 2–3 days can be explained by a chemotactic gradient. Parsons *et al.* (1985) have investigated the lavage fluid of lungs affected by ARDS and have noted marked accumulation of PMN as well as two chemotactic factors. Alveolar macrophages produce chemotactic factors for PMN, such as leukotriene B4 (LTB4), IL-8 and other peptides. The activation of macrophages commonly occurs in the later course of events, i.e. when infection (bacteramia, endotoxaemia) becomes manifest.

Joka *et al.* (1990) have encountered complement split products (C3a) in the lavage fluid of patients without direct lung damage already within the first hours post trauma. These complement split products may be released secondary to activation of macrophages, in the same way as other substances that may rapidly transport neutrophils into the alveolar space and/or into the interstitium of the

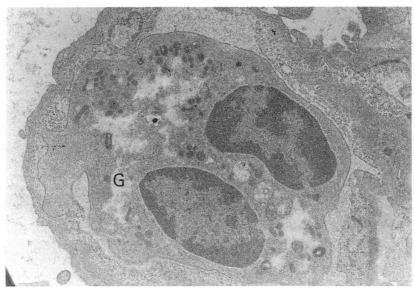

Figure 44.21 Granulocyte (G) leaving a lung capillary. (Reproduced from Schlag and Redl, 1991b, with permission.)

lung via the chemotactic route. Activation of macrophages immediately after trauma could be related to hypoxic periods during trauma.

As already discussed, the permeability increase is due to endothelial damage as well as to other factors that are unknown in the acute shock stage (leukotrienes, PAF, anaphylatoxins, fibrin, platelets, etc.). In animal experiments perivascular oedema was very frequently observed, the endothelial damage being quite moderate compared to humans.

Interstitial oedema may spread quite rapidly, especially in the presence of direct lung trauma (contusion). A major symptom in this situation is post-traumatic hypoxaemia. As a result of oedema and haemorrhage, the functional residual capacity (FRC) decreases, which in turn decreases the closing volume and blocks the terminal airways in association with a peripheral collapse of the alveoli.

The subsequent ventilation/perfusion disturbances (V/Q) may be caused by hypoventilation and by surfactant loss in the alveolar region as a consequence of flooding with blood and fibrin together with massive atelectasis. This in turn gives rise to additional V/Q disturbances and thus creates the substrate for hypoxaemia, which characterizes the clinical picture of severe lung contusion.

Sturm *et al.* (1986, 1991) investigated a group of severely injured patients with an Injury Severity Score (ISS) of 34 ± 7 and examined lung function and permeability very early after trauma (i.e. 12–48 hours). In the first 48 hours no major impairment of lung function was seen, and the situation only deteriorated after 48–72 hours (oxygenation quotient, dynamic compliance, alveolar–arterial oxygen difference, shunt fraction).

During the first 48 hours the extravascular lung water (EVLW) was stable but then started to increase. The extravasation of labelled albumin was determined scintigraphically and showed an elevation already within 24 hours after trauma. This finding clearly correlates with electron micrographic studies in humans and baboons.

The delayed EVLW increase can be explained by a lag time between the onset of increased permeability and its detection (Sturm, 1991). This steady increase of EVLW from 48 hours onwards indicates the development of the lung in early failure and involvement of the extravascular space (oedema fluid, fibrin deposits, cellular components). In the case of direct lung injury the distribution of interstitial oedema accompanied by haemorrhage is much faster. Also, the combination of contusion and traumatic shock may rapidly transform the 'organ in shock' into the 'early organ failure lung'. In this case, direct trauma is aggravated by the generalized non-bacterial inflammation.

Lung contusion may lead to bacterial infection of the lung, which may seriously impair the clearance function especially in the post-traumatic course and result in pneumonia. Indirect lung damage due to leukostasis and the release of tissue-damaging mediators creates a pathogenetic substrate for further damage. Regel *et al.* (1988) found that in their patients collective lung contusion was associated with a high incidence (59%) of subsequent ARDS.

The stage of early organ failure in the lung is a place of least resistance for infection. The infection may either be pre-existent, acquired (e.g. wound infection, peritonitis, nosocomial infection) or may occur in association with generalized endotoxaemia or bacteraemia via gut translocation.

The gut as an 'organ in shock' is increasingly gaining momentum as a potential pathomechanism of multiorgan failure (see Chapter 42). Bacterial translocation secondary to gut damage or even without evident histological damage caused by traumatic shock (perfusion/reperfusion damage) is a potential source of post-traumatic organ failure and especially of typical ARDS (late/or septic organ failure lung).

At this point a different mechanism leads to further lung damage, including the pulmonary circulation, due to the release of toxic mediators. Endotoxin – the most important trigger for activation processes of humoral and cellular systems – is a key pathomechanism of this late organ failure.

Septic challenge and the development of late failure in the lung (ARDS)

Endotoxin (lipopolysaccharide – LPS) has a direct effect on PMN, monocytes/macrophages (MO/MA) and EC, which results in the release of additional toxic mediators. It has recently become clear that the deleterious effects of endotoxin are caused via activation of cells by secondary mediators from humoral and cellular sources (Figure 44.22). Endotoxin may also act indirectly by increasing the binding capacity of different blood cells (PMN, lymphocytes, MO) to EC, and may thus induce EC damage.

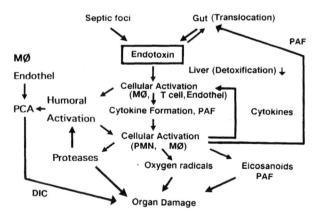

Figure 44.22 The central role of endotoxin in the stimulation of cells leading to organ failure. PCA = procoagulant activity; PAF = platelet activating factor. (Reproduced from Schlag and Redl, 1990, with permission.)

IL-1, which is released by EC after exposure to LPS, has a similar effect on bacterial adherence as LPS itself, which is necessary for bacteria to be able to penetrate the cell barrier. The binding of bacteria to EC is an active process requiring protein synthesis (Thomas *et al.*, 1988). LPS as a mediator and activator of different target cells is common in the plasma of critically ill patients. The morphological substrate of the organ failure syndrome is often disseminated intravascular coagulation (DIC). Low LPS concentrations may directly modulate endothelial cell haemostatic properties in the absence of other cell types. LPS may promote *de novo* synthesis and expression of procoagulant activity (TF).

The results of induced coagulation are fibrin deposits in direct contact with the EC, which have their own potential to damage EC. In animal endotoxaemia these fibrin deposits can be demonstrated in the pulmonary circulation, especially in the alveolar capillaries.

LPS stimulates the EC to produce eicosanoid derivatives, e.g. thromboxane 2 (TBX2) (Bahrami *et al.*, 1989), which is a potent vasoconstrictor of the pulmonary circulation and may contribute to pulmonary hypertension in ARDS.

Blood monocytes are transformed into long-lived tissue macrophages (MO/MA), which are easily susceptible to LPS stimulation. Macrophages have a major impact on the late organ failure due to the release of different cytokines (IL-1, TNF-α, IL-6, IL-8), proteinases, free oxygen radicals and phospholipid-derived products (thromboxane, leukotriene, prostaglandin E2 (PGE$_2$), PAF).

While cytokines are not necessarily cytotoxic by themselves, organ damage together with permeability changes may be mediated by their indirect effects on EC. The activated EC may trigger cytokine synthesis, expression of adhesive molecules like ELAM-1 (Bevilacqua *et al.*, 1987; Leeuwenberg *et al.*, 1989), ICAM-1, production of IL-1 resulting in biosynthesis and cell surface expression of tissue factor (TF) as well as PAF synthesis.

At present the most important cellular mediator of the organ-damaging effect of LPS is thought to be TNF (Beutler and Cerami, 1986; Tracey *et al.*, 1986), which is secreted by MO/MA in response to LPS.

Phospholipase A$_2$ (PLA$_2$), which is also released by activation of macrophages via a cascade system, may also have an important role. The major inducers of PLA$_2$ are the cytokines IL-1 and TNF. PLA$_2$ is produced by platelets, synovial fibroblasts, glomerular mesangial cells, vascular smooth muscle cells and various other tissue types (Pruzanski and Vadas, 1991). Sepsis is associated with a drastic increase in PLA$_2$ in the plasma. PLA$_2$ may especially cause lung injury via an inflammatory response (sequestration of PMN, impaired gas exchange, etc). A correlation of serum PLA$_2$ levels and an increased risk of ARDS has been reported (Vadas, 1984; Kellermann *et al.*, 1989; Koeniger *et al.*, 1989).

Numerous mediators combine to induce organ damage of the lung during sepsis, partly via an indirect and partly via a direct route. Primary damage of the cell during the 'organ in shock' and the lung in early failure is mainly due to activated PMN, toxic mediators such as proteinases (elastase, cathepsin), reactive oxygen species, cationic proteins and eicosanoids (e.g. leukotriene), all associated with non-bacterial inflammation.

During hypoxic damage, endotoxaemia and bacteraemia there is release of numerous toxic tissue-damaging mediators, with endotoxin as the most important primary mediator. These mediators (cytokines, proteinases, reactive oxygen species, PAF, eicosanoids, etc) are released through the direct and indirect action of endotoxin. Damage of the EC is decisive for further microcirculatory impairment, thus creating the substrate for organ damage, which in turn results in late or septic organ failure that is clinically evident at the end of the first and at the beginning of the second week after trauma.

REFERENCES

Auler J.O.C. Jr, Calheiros D.F., Brentani M.M. et al. (1986). Adult respiratory distress syndrome: evidence of early fibrogenesis and absence of glucocorticoid receptors. *Eur. J. Res. Dis.* **69**, 261–9.

Bahrami S., Redl H., Thurnher M. et al. (1989). Effects of PAF-antagonists in endotoxin shock – ovine and rat experiments. In *Second Vienna Shock Forum* (Schlag G., Redl H., eds). *Prog. Clin. Biol. Res.*, **308**, 931–6.

Bengtson A., Haljamäe H. (1988–89). Complement activation and organ function in critically ill surgical patients. *Acute Care*, **14–15**, 111–37.

Beutler B., Cerami A. (1986). Cachectin and tumor necrosis factor as two sides of the same biological coin. *Nature*, **320**, 584–8.

Bevilacqua M.P., Pober J.S., Mendrick D.L. et al. (1987). Identification of an inducible endothelial-leukocyte adhesion molecule. *Proc. Nat Acad. Sci. USA*, **84**, 9238–42.

Boogaerts M.A., Yamada O., Jacob J.S. et al. (1982). Enhancement of granulocyte endothelial cell adherence and granulocyte induced cytotoxicity by platelet release products. *Proc. Nat Acad. Sci. USA*, **79**, 7019–23.

Bosch U., Reisser S., Regel G. et al. (1989). Pulmonary fat embolism – an epiphenomenon of shock or a proper mediator mechanism? In *Second Vienna Shock Forum* (Schlag G., Redl, H., eds). *Prog. Clin. Biol. Res.*, **308**, 701–6.

Connell R.S., Swank R.L., Webb M.C. (1975). The development of pulmonary ultrastructural lesions during hemorrhagic shock. *J. Trauma*, **15**, 116–29.

Dinges H.P., Redl H., Schlag G. (1984). Quantitative estimation of granulocyte in the lung after polytrauma – dog and human autopsy data. *Eur. Surg. Res.*, **16**, 100–1.

Duchateau J., Haas M., Schreyen H. et al. (1984). Complement activation in patients at risk of developing the adult respiratory distress syndrome. *Am. Rev. Res. Dis.*, **130**, 1058–64.

Elias J.A., Freundlich B., Kern J.A. et al. (1990). Cytokine networks in the regulation of inflammation and fibrosis in the lung. *Chest*, **97**, 1439–45.

Fosse E., Mollnes T.E., Aasen A.O. et al. (1987). Complement activation following multiple injuries. *Acta Chir. Scand.*, **153**, 325–30.

Gallin J.I. (1976). The role of chemotaxis in the inflammatory immune response of the lung. In *Immunologic and Infectious Reactions in the Lung* (Kirkpatrick C.H., Reynolds H.Y., eds). New York: Marcel Dekker, pp. 161–79.

Geng J.G., Bevilacqua M.P., Moore K.L. et al. (1990). Rapid neutrophil adhesion to activated endothelium mediated by GMP-140. *Nature*, **343**, 757–60.

Godin D.V., Wright J.M., Tuchek J.M. et al. (1983). Plasma lysosomal enzymes in experimental and clinical endotoxemia. *Clin. Invest. Med.*, **6**, 319–25.

Gurtner G.H., Traystman R.J., Toung T.J.K. (1988). Letter to the editor. *J. Appl. Physiol.*, **64**, 1757.

Haberland G.L. (1977). Proteolytische Systeme, Steuerungseinheiten im Organismus. *Abhand. Mathematisch Naturwissenschaft. Klasse Akad. Wissenschaft.*, **2**, 1–20.

Hammerschmidt D.E., Craddock P.R., McCullogh J. et al. (1978). Complement activation and pulmonary leucostasis during nylon fiber filtration leucopheresis. *Blood*, **51**, 721–30.

Harlan J.M., Killes P.D., Snecal F. et al. (1985). The role of neutrophil membrane glycoprotein GP-150 in neutrophil adherence to endothelium *in vitro*. *Blood*, **66**, 167–78.

Hassenstein J., Riede U.N., Mittermayer C. et al. (1980). Zur Frage der Reversibilität der schockinduzierten Lungenfibrose. *Anaesth. Intensiv-ther. Notfallmed.*, **15**, 340–9.

Heffner J.E., Sahn S.A., Repine J.E. (1987). The role of platelets in the adult respiratory distress syndrome. Culprits or bystanders. *Am. Rev. Resp. Dis.*, **135**, 482–92.

Heideman, M. (1979) Complement activation *in vitro* induced by endotoxin and injured tissue. *J. Surg. Res.*, **26**, 670–5.

House S.D., Lipowsky H.H. (1987). Leukocyte-endothelium adhesion: microhemodynamics in mesentery of the cat. *Microvasc. Res.*, **34**, 363–79.

Idell S., James K.K., Coalson J.J. (1992). Fibrinolytic activity in bronchoalveolar lavage of baboons with diffuse alveolar damage: trends in two forms of lung injury. *Crit. Care Med.*, **20**, 1431–40.

Johnson A., Tahamont M.V., Malik A.B. (1983). Thrombin-induced lung vascular injury: role of fibrinogen and fibrinolysis. *Am. Rev. Resp. Dis.*, **128**, 38–44.

Joka T., Obertacke U., Sturm J.A. et al. (1990). Starreaktionen des traumatischen Schocks: Zelluläre Reaktionen. *Hefte Unfallheilkund.*, **212**, 45–53.

Kawanami O., Ferrans V.J., Fulmer J.D. et al. (1979). Ultrastructure of pulmonary mast cells in patients with fibrotic lung disorders. *Lab. Invest.*, **40**, 717–34.

Kellermann W., Frentzel-Beyme R., Welte M. et al. (1989). Phospholipase A in acute lung injury after trauma and sepsis: its relation to the inflammatory mediators PMN-elastase, C3a, and neopterin. *Klin. Wochenschr.*, **67**, 190–5.

Koeniger R., Hoffmann G.E., Schmid T.O. (1989). Serum activities of phospholipase A in acute posttraumatic pulmonary insufficiency. *Klin. Wochenschr.*, **67**, 212–16.

Kongsgaard U.E., Smith-Erichsen N., Geiran O. et al.

(1989). Different activation patterns in the plasma kallikreinkinin and complement systems during coronary bypass surgery. *Acta Anaesthesiol. Scand.*, **33**, 343–7.

Kunkel S.L., Fantone J.C., Ward P.A. (1981). Complement-mediated inflammatory reactions. *Pathobiol. Annu.*, **11**, 127–54.

Lamy M., Fallat R.J., Koeniger E. et al. (1976). Pathologic features and mechanisms of hypoxemia in adult respiratory distress syndrome. *Am. Rev. Resp. Dis.*, **114**, 267–84.

Langlois P.F., Gawryl M.S., Zeller J. et al. (1989). Accentuated complement activation in patient plasma during the adult respiratory distress syndrome: a potential mechanism for pulmonary inflammation. *Heart Lung*, **18**, 71–84.

Leeuwenberg J.F.M., Jeunhomme T.M.M.A., Buurman W.A. (1989). Induction of an activation antigen on human endothelial cells *in vitro*. *Eur. J. Immunol.*, **19**, 715–20.

Lium B., Aasen A.O., Saugstad O.D. et al. (1982). Experimental post-traumatic lung insufficiency in dogs. *Acta Pathol. Microbiol. Immunol. Scand. A*, **90**, 113–23.

Lo S.K., Perlman M.B., Niehaus G.D. et al. (1985). Thrombin-induced alterations in lung fluid balance in awake sheep. *J. of Appl. Physiol.*, **58**, 1421–7.

Malik A.B. (1986). Thrombin-induced endothelial injury. *Semin. Thromb. Hemost.*, **12**, 184–96.

Marquart K.-H., Caesar R. (1970). Quantitative Untersuchung über die sogenannten Pinocytosebläschen im Capillarendothel. *Virchows Arch. (Cell Pathol.)*, **6**, 220–33.

Martin B.A., Wright J.L., Thommasen H. et al. (1982). Effect of pulmonary blood flow on the exchange between the circulating and marginating pool of polymorpho-nuclear leukocytes in dog lungs. *J. Clin. Invest.*, **69**, 1277–85.

Maunder R.J., Harlan J.M., Talucci R.C. et al. (1984). Measurement of C3a and C5a in high-risk patients does not predict ARDS. *Am. Rev. Resp. Dis.*, **129**, A104.

Mayrovitz H., Wiedeman M., Tuma R. (1977). Factors influencing leukocyte adherence in microvessels. *Thromb. Haemost.*, **38**, 823–30.

Mittermayer C., Hassenstein J., Riede U.N. (1978). Is shock-induced lung fibrosis reversible? *Pathol. Res. Pract.*, **162**, 73–87.

Mittermayer C., Riede U.N., McEwan J.R. (1979). Pathologisch-anatomische Untersuchungen der Schocklunge. II. Spätschäden und Irreversibilität. In *Akutes progressives Lungenversagen* (Mayrhofer-Kramme O., Schlag G., Stoeckel H., eds). *Intensivmed. Notfallmed. Anästhesiol.*, **16**, 163–70.

Moore K.L., Varki A., McEver R.P. (1991). GMP-140 binds to a glycoprotein receptor on human neutrophils: evidence of a lectin-like-interaction. *J. Cell Biol.*, **112**, 491–9.

Neumann S., Jochum M. (1984). Elastase-alpha 1-proteinase inhibitor complex. In *Methods of Enzymatic Analysis* (Bergmeyer H.V., Bergmeyer J., Graßlc M., eds). Weinheim Chemie, pp. 184–98.

Neumann S., Hennrich N., Gunzer G. et al. (1983). Enzyme linked immunoassay for complexes of human granulocyte elastase with alpha 1-proteinase inhibitor in plasma. In *Progress in Clinical Enzymology II* (Goldberg D.M., Werner M., eds). New York: Masson, pp. 293–8.

Nuytinck J.K.S., Goris R.J.A., Redl H. et al. (1986). Posttraumatic complications and inflammatory mediators. *Arch. Surg.*, **121**, 886–90.

Parsons P.E., Fowler A.A., Hyers T.M. et al. (1985). Chemotactic activity in bronchoalveolar lavage fluid from patients with adult respiratory distress syndrome. *Am. Rev. Resp. Dis.*, **132**, 490–3.

Pottemeyer E., Vassar M.J., Holcroft J.W. (1986). Coagulation, inflammation and response to injury. *Crit. Care. Clin.*, **2**, 683–702.

Pretorius J.P., Schlag G., Redl H. et al. (1987). The 'lung in shock' as a result of hypovolemic-traumatic shock in baboons. *J. Trauma*, **27**, 1344–53.

Pruzanski W., Vadas P. (1991). Phospholipase A$_2$ – a mediator between proximal and distal effectors of inflammation. *Immunol. Today*, **12**, 143–6.

Ratliff N.B., Wilson J.W., Mikat E. et al. (1971). The lung in hemorrhagic shock. IV. The role of the polymorphonuclear leukocyte. *Am. J. Pathol.*, **65**, 325–34.

Redl H., Schlag G. (1980). Morphologische Untersuchungen der Lunge im Schock. *Anaesthesiol. Intensivmed.*, **125**, 19–26.

Redl H., Schlag G., Grisold W. et al. (1978). Early morphological changes of the lung in shock demonstrated in the light (LM), transmission electron (TEM) and Scanning Electron Microscopes (SEM). *Scanning Electron Microsc.*, **11**, 555–61.

Redl H., Hammerschmidt D.E., Schlag G. (1983). Augmentation by platelets of granulocyte aggregation in response to chemotaxines: studies utilizing an improved cell preparation technique. *Blood*, **61**, 125–31.

Redl H., Schlag G., Hammerschmidt D.E. (1984). Quantitative assessment of leukostasis in experimental hypovolemic-traumatic shock. *Acta Chir. Scand.*, **150**, 113–17.

Redl H., Dinges H.P., Schlag G. (1987). Quantitative estimation of leukostasis in the posttraumatic lung – canine and human autopsy data. In *First Vienna Shock Forum – Part A: Pathophysiological Role of Mediators and Mediator Inhibitors in Shock* (Schlag G., Redl H., eds). *Prog. Clin. Biol. Res.*, **236A**, 43–53.

Redl H., Dinges H.P., Buurman W.A. et al. (1991). Expression of endothelial leukocyte adhesion molecule-1 in septic but not traumatic/hypovolemic shock in the baboon. *Am. J. Pathol.*, **139**, 461–6.

Regel G., Sturm J.A., Friedl H.P. et al. (1988). Die Bedeutung der Lungenkontusion für die Letalität nach Polytrauma. Möglichkeiten der therapeutischen Beeinflussung. *Chirurg*, **59**, 771–6.

Risberg B., Medegard A., Heideman M. et al. (1986). Early activation of humoral proteolytic systems in patients with multiple trauma. *Crit. Care. Med.*, **14**, 917–25.

Risberg B., Andreasson S., Eriksson E. (1991). Disseminated intravascular coagulation. *Acta Anaesthesiol. Scand.*, **35**, (Suppl. 95), 60–71.

Roumen R.M.H., Redl H., Schlag G. et al. (1995). Inflammatory mediators in relation to the development of multiple organ failure in patients after severe blunt trauma. *Crit. Care Med.*, **23**, 474–80.

Schlag G., Redl H. (1980). Die Leukostase in der Lunge beim hypovolämisch-traumatischen Schock. *Anaesthesist*, **29**, 606–12.

Schlag G., Redl H. (1985). Morphology of the human lung after traumatic injury. In *Acute Respiratory Failure* (Zapol W.M., Falke K.J., eds). New York: Marcel Dekker, pp. 161–83.

Schlag G., Redl H. (1987). Oxygen radicals in hypovolemic-traumatic shock. In *Oxygen Free Radicals in Shock, International Workshop Florence 1985* (Novelli G.P., Ursini F., eds). Basel: Karger, pp. 94–108.

Schlag G., Redl H. (1988). The morphology of the adult respiratory distress syndrome. In *Shock and the Adult Respiratory Distress Syndrome* (Kox W., Bihari D., eds). Berlin: Springer, pp. 21–31.

Schlag G., Redl H. (1989). Lung in shock – posttraumatic lung failure (organ failure) – MOFS. In *Second Vienna Shock Forum* (Schlag G., Redl H., eds). *Prog. Clin. Biol. Res.*, **308**, 3–16.

Schlag G., Redl H. (1990). Effects of sepsis on the lung. In *The Open Packing – Laparostomy – in Pancreatitis and Peritonitis* (Waclawiczek H-W., Boeckl O., Pauser G., eds). Berlin: Springer, pp. 13–25.

Schlag G., Redl H. (1991a). Pathology of the acute posttraumatic lung failure. In *Thoracic Surgery: surgical management of chest injuries* (Webb W.R. and Besson A. eds) *International Trends in General Thoracic Surgery*, vol.7 (Webb W.R., Besson A., eds). St Louis: Mosby Year, pp. 49–54.

Schlag G., Redl H. (1991b). Acute lung injury following shock and major trauma. In *Immune Conference of Trauma, Shock and Sepsis – 1991* (Faist E., Ninnemann J.L., Green D.R., eds). Berlin: Springer.

Schlag G., Regel H. (1972). Lungenbiopsien bei hypovolämisch-traumatischem Schock. *Medizin. Welt.*, **23**, 1755–8.

Schlag G., Voigt W.H., Schnells G. et al. (1976). Die Ultrastruktur der menschlichen Lunge im Schock. *Anaesthesist*, **25**, 512–21.

Schlag G., Redl H., Glatzl A. (1977). Morphologische Veränderungen der Lunge im hypovolämisch-traumatischen Schock. *Unfallheilkunde*, **80**, 481–8.

Schlag G., Voigt W.H., Redl H., Glatzl A. (1980). Vergleichende Morphologie des posttraumatischen Lungenversagens. *Anaesth. Intensivther. Notfallmed.*, **15**, 315–39.

Simms H.H., d'Amico R.D. (1991). Increased PMN CD 11b/CD18 expression following post-traumatic ARDS. *J. Surg. Res.*, **50**, 362–7.

Slotman G.J., Burchard K.W., Williams J.J. et al. (1986). Interaction of prostaglandins, activated complement, and granulocytes in clinical sepsis and hypotension. *Surgery*, **99**, 744–51.

Sturm J.A. (1991). *Adult Respiratory Distress Syndrome – an aspect of multiple organ failure*. Berlin: Springer.

Sturm J.A., Wisner D.H., Oestern H.-J. et al. (1986). Increased lung capillary permeability after trauma: a prospective clinical study. *J. Trauma*, **26**, 409–18.

Taylor A.E., Parker J.C., Granger D.N. et al. (1981). Assessment of capillary permeability using lymphatic protein flux: estimation of the osmotic reflection coefficient. In *The Microcirculation* (Taylor A.E., ed.). New York: Academic, pp. 19–32.

Teplitz C. (1976). The core pathobiology and integrated medical science of adult acute respiratory insufficiency. *Surg. Clin. North Am.*, **56**, 1091–131.

Thal A.P., Brown E.B., Hermeck A.S. et al. (1972). *Shock – a physiologic basis for treatment*. Chicago: Year Book Medical.

Thomas P.D., Hampson F.W., Hunninghake G.W. (1988). Bacterial adherence to human endothelial cells. *J. Appl. Physiol.*, **65**, 1372–6.

Tracey K.J., Beutler B., Lowrey S.F. et al. (1986). Shock and tissue injury induced by recombinant human cachectin. *Science*, **234**, 470–4.

Vadas P. (1984). Elevated plasma phospholipase A_2 levels: correlation with the hemodynamic and pulmonary changes in gram-negative shock. *J. Lab. Clin. Med.*, **104**, 873–81.

Varani J., Ginsburg I., Schuger L. et al. (1989). Endothelial cell killing by neutrophils. Synergistic interaction of oxygen products and proteases. *Am. J. Pathol.*, **135**, 435–8.

Weinberg P.F., Matthay M.A., Webster R.O. et al. (1984). Biologically active products of complement and acute lung injury in patients with the sepsis syndrome. *Am. Rev. Resp. Dis.*, **130**, 791–6.

West J.B. (1978). *Ventilation/Blood Flow and Gas Exchange*, 3rd edn. Oxford: Blackwell Scientific Publications.

Wong C.S., Gamble J.R., Skinner M.P. et al. (1991). Adhesion protein GMP 140 inhibits superoxide anion release by human neutrophils. *Proc. Nat. Acad. Sci. USA*, **88**, 2397–401.

Zapol W.M., Trelstad R.L., Coffey J.W. et al. (1979). Pulmonary fibrosis in severe acute respiratory failure. *Am. Rev. Resp. Dis.*, **119**, 547–54.

Zilow G., Rother U., Kirschfink M. (1991). Adult respiratory distress syndrome and complement: significance of C3a in diagnosis and prognosis. In *Adult Respiratory Distress Syndrome – an aspect of multiple organ failure* (Sturm J.A., ed.). Berlin: Springer, pp. 59–74.

Zilow G., Sturm J.A., Rother U. et al. (1990). Complement activation and the prognostic value of C3a in patients at risk of adult respiratory distress syndrome. *Clin. Exp. Immunol.*, **79**, 151–7.

45 The Response of the Endocrine System to Injury

R. N. Barton and D. S. Gann

Alterations in endocrine activity form an essential part of the response to trauma. Broadly speaking, two phases of change can be identified, which roughly correspond to Cuthbertson's (1942) periods of ebb and flow. Initially injury provokes secretion of many hormones, which are usually referred to as stress hormones as they also respond to other forms of insult to the body. These hormones have clear circulatory and metabolic effects which can be seen as essential components of the body's attempts to maintain an adequate supply of fuel and oxygen to vital organs. The duration of these endocrine changes depends upon both the hormone and the severity of the injury. On average it corresponds fairly well to the 24–48 hours that Cuthbertson assigned to the ebb phase. The subsequent flow phase is also accompanied by changes in hormone concentration, but these tend to be different from those seen shortly after injury. The function of these later responses is by no means clear and they may not necessarily play a major role in the metabolic changes characteristic of the flow phase. After severe injury, or any injury with complications such as sepsis or delayed surgery, the flow-phase changes may be superimposed on persistent or reactivated elements of the ebb-phase response to give a picture of some complexity.

The early release of stress hormones is largely a response of the CNS to a variety of stimuli elicited by injury. Given that the primary function of the response is to preserve the energy supply to vital organs, one might expect fluid loss to be the most powerful stimulus, and recent evidence suggests that this is so (Bereiter et al., 1982). The signal elicited by fluid loss will depend upon its degree; if this is moderate the input from low-pressure baroreceptors in the right and left atria (reflecting changes in blood volume) will be diminished, while if the fluid loss is sufficient to reduce blood pressure the input from high-pressure baroreceptors in the carotid sinus will also decrease. Other stimuli undoubtedly contribute to the neuroendocrine response to injury to varying degrees, depending on its nature. Arterial chemoreceptors (described in Chapter 40) which respond to a fall in oxygen tension will be activated if fluid loss is sufficient to cause hypoxia or if direct chest or lung damage impairs oxygenation of the blood. Nociceptive afferents, again dealt with in detail in Chapter 38, are also a potent stimulus after injury

and do not necessarily involve conscious perception of pain as responses are seen in patients undergoing elective surgery under general anaesthesia. However, in the conscious patient, psychological factors such as fear and anxiety are also likely to contribute to the responses. None of these stimuli may be present after head injury, and yet this provokes neuroendocrine changes comparable to those after peripheral injuries. The mechanism is not known, although there is evidence that a raised intracranial pressure exacerbates the response (Feibel et al., 1983). An exception to this picture is the patient with direct damage to the hypothalamus or pituitary. This usually causes death but if the patient survives there may be impaired function of either the posterior pituitary (causing diabetes insipidus) or the anterior pituitary or both (Edwards and Clark, 1986).

The endocrine changes most characteristic of the flow phase are an increase in insulin secretion and decreased activity of the hypothalamo-pituitary-thyroid and hypothalamo-pituitary-gonadal systems. The time-course of these changes makes it unlikely that they are due to stimuli such as fluid loss and in fact there is evidence that they are not purely neuroendocrine responses. The increase in insulin secretion is unlikely to be central in origin while the decreases in thyroid and gonadal function are complex, involving disturbances at both central and peripheral levels. At present the cause of these delayed responses is unclear and it is unlikely to be the same for each of them.

In this chapter we first discuss the catecholamines and the hormones of the endocrine pancreas. These hormones are linked both with regard to their secretion, since the sympathoadrenal system has an important influence on the endocrine pancreas, and because they affect the same metabolic processes. We then describe the effects of injury on the hypothalamo-pituitary-adrenal (HPA) axis, with particular emphasis on the relevant neural pathways and neurotransmitters which have been much better studied than those of any other neuroendocrine system. We go on to consider, first the changes in other anterior pituitary hormones and the hormones of their peripheral target glands and then the effects of injury on hormones affecting the kidney, which have multiple control mechanisms, both central and peripheral. Finally, we discuss the role of hormones in the cardiovascular, metabolic, renal and immunological responses to injury.

CATECHOLAMINES AND PANCREATIC HORMONES

Catecholamines

Strictly only the catecholamines secreted by the adrenal medulla are hormones and therefore within the province of this chapter. However, the effects of circulating catecholamines are so difficult to distinguish from those of noradrenaline released locally by sympathetic nerve terminals in tissues that the sympathoadrenal system must be considered as a whole. The most important circulating catecholamine is adrenaline, produced by the adrenal medulla. Its release is accompanied by that of enkephalins, which are also stored in the chromaffin granules (Viveros *et al.*, 1985); the reason for this is uncertain, but these peptides may contribute to the opioid effects described in Chapter 38. A variable proportion of the circulating noradrenaline originates from the adrenal medulla, the remainder coming from postganglionic nerve endings. Plasma noradrenaline is sometimes taken as a general index of sympathetic activity but its interpretation is fraught with difficulties arising from variable local reuptake of noradrenaline and so forth (Hjemdahl, 1993). Studies in cats have shown that plasma noradrenaline is poorly correlated with adrenal noradrenaline output, and the same is true even for adrenaline (Bereiter *et al.*, 1986).

The activity of the sympathoadrenal system appears to be controlled by a discrete group of neurones in the rostral ventrolateral medulla. These receive projections from the nucleus of the tractus solitarius which acts as the primary relay station for afferent neural input from the baroreceptors. There are also connexions with higher centres such as the limbic system and hypothalamus. In ways that are not understood, different stimuli lead to tissue-specific activation of the sympathoadrenal system. This applies not only to local innervation of the different vascular beds but also to the adrenal medulla. Goldstein (1987) has pointed out that stresses large enough to pose a threat to life consistently produce an increase in circulating adrenaline, whereas sympathetic neural activity, as assessed either directly or by the plasma noradrenaline concentration, shows variable changes. There is increasing interest in the links between the sympathoadrenal and hypothalamo-pituitary-adrenal systems. Central administration of corticotrophin-releasing factor (CRF; see 'Hypothalamo-pituitary-adrenal axis' below) causes a pattern of selective stimulation of the sympathetic outflow similar to that in some types of stress and a CRF antagonist prevents the increases in circulating catecholamines caused by some stimuli (e.g. haemorrhage) but not others (e.g. interleukin-1; Fisher and Brown, 1991; Owens and Nemeroff, 1991). The ability of one small haemorrhage to potentiate the adrenal medullary response to another the following day (Lilly *et al.*, 1986) is also reminiscent of the behaviour of the adrenal cortex.

In practice, injury in man causes rather similar changes in plasma adrenaline and noradrenaline (reviewed by Barton, 1987), although there is no correlation between them. Both the magnitude and the duration of the increases in concentration depend upon the severity of injury. Thus, after elective surgery the changes are small and a rise in noradrenaline is not always seen; one study showed that the adrenaline response to hysterectomy was suppressed by epidural analgesia. In patients with uncomplicated accidental injury the catecholamine concentrations measured shortly after the injury increase exponentially with the Injury Severity Score and fall to normal levels over the next 2 days or so. After severe burns plasma noradrenaline is raised for around 10 days and a lowering of metabolic rate by β-adrenergic blockade has been observed even later. The concentrations of both catecholamines are very high in patients with shock after injury.

Insulin and glucagon

Secretion of insulin and glucagon is influenced by many of the same stimuli, including glucose, amino acids, fatty acids, the parasympathetic (vagus) and sympathetic nervous systems and circulating catecholamines (Miller, 1981; Shafrir *et al.*, 1987; see Figure 45.1). Some of their effects on the two hormones are in the same direction (notably for amino acids and vagal stimulation, both stimulatory) whereas others (especially glucose) have opposite effects. Regulation is extremely complex because glucagon stimulates insulin secretion while γ-aminobutyric acid from the pancreatic B cells inhibits glucagon secretion (Rorsman *et al.*, 1991). In addition, somatostatin (whose release is controlled

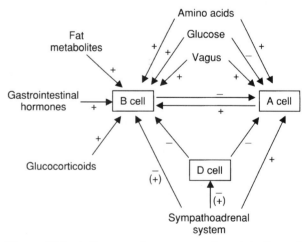

Figure 45.1 Influence of some neural, metabolic and endocrine factors on cells of the endocrine pancreas. + and – refer to stimulation and inhibition of the secretion of hormones, respectively glucagon, insulin and somatostatin for A, B and D cells. The interactions between the cells are mediated by these hormone products. The effects of the sympathoadrenal system are complex (and may differ between its neural and humoral components) and those likely to predominate after injury are shown here.

by many of the same factors) inhibits the secretion of both hormones (Shafrir *et al.*, 1987). The interactions between insulin, glucagon and somatostatin are paracrine, i.e. taking place locally within the pancreatic islets, and Samols and Stagner (1990) have recently questioned whether somatostatin actually influences insulin or glucagon secretion *in vivo* on the grounds that blood flow is in the wrong direction. Gastrointestinal hormones also have a major influence on insulin secretion.

Because of the overriding importance of glucose as a stimulus, the changes in plasma insulin must be considered in relation to those in plasma glucose. On this basis there is a tendency for a biphasic change in insulin (reviewed by Barton, 1987); the gain of the response to glucose is decreased in the ebb phase and increased in the flow phase. Shortly after most types of injury in man there is little change in the absolute plasma insulin concentration, but an increase might be expected because of the tendency of plasma glucose to rise. This is especially obvious after severe accidental injury, when the concentration of insulin tends to be lower and that of glucose higher than in patients with less severe injuries. A lowering of the sensitivity of insulin secretion to glucose has been confirmed by intravenous glucose-tolerance tests after burns and elective surgery. Animal experiments using adrenal medullectomy and α-adrenergic blockade show that this inhibition is due to circulating adrenaline, acting via α receptors in the pancreas (Cerchio *et al.*, 1973; Vigaš *et al.*, 1973), and in surgical patients the insulin response to glucose is negatively correlated with plasma adrenaline (Halter and Pflug, 1980). This is consistent with the consensus that, although catecholamines may have both stimulatory and inhibitory effects on insulin secretion, mediated respectively by β_2 and α_2 receptors, at high concentrations the inhibitory α_2 effect predominates (Miller, 1981). A high sympathetic nerve tone also inhibits insulin secretion, possibly through neurotransmitters such as galanin rather than catecholamines (Dunning and Taborsky, 1988), but the part played by this in inhibiting insulin secretion after injury is unclear.

During the flow phase after injury, the opposite change is seen. By a week after most types of injury plasma insulin is above normal, and it may stay high for another 2 weeks or so (reviewed by Barton, 1987). This cannot be explained by hyperglycaemia which is less prevalent than at short times after injury, and several studies have shown that the insulin response to glucose is enhanced in patients at this stage after elective surgery or burns. The mechanism has not been explored thoroughly. The concentrations of many amino acids are above normal but it has not been established whether they are sufficiently high to cause the observed increase in insulin. It is not yet possible to assess the relevance of reports that under suitable conditions cytokines such as interleukin 1 (IL-1) can stimulate insulin secretion (Kennedy and Jones, 1991).

Plasma glucagon rises after most types of injury, but the size and time-course of the effect vary between studies (Barton, 1987). Most workers have found a delay before the increase in glucagon concentration starts, but once it has taken place it persists for several days. This response is often attributed to sympathoadrenal stimulation. A number of studies have shown that adrenaline stimulates pancreatic glucagon secretion through a β receptor (Miller, 1981); there is also evidence for stimulation by splanchnic nervous input, but the identity of the receptors is unclear and it has again been suggested that galanin, rather than noradrenaline, is the neurotransmitter concerned (Dunning and Taborsky, 1988). There certainly appears to be a difference in time-course between the changes in plasma catecholamines and those in glucagon although the relationship between them has apparently not been studied in detail. Whether this discrepancy could be explained by non-noradrenergic sympathetic stimulation or whether some other stimulus such as amino acids is responsible is not known.

HYPOTHALAMO-PITUITARY-ADRENAL AXIS

Neural pathways and neurotransmitters

The area that constitutes the hypothalamic part of the HPA axis is the paraventricular nucleus (PVN). The signals called forth by injury are conveyed to the PVN mostly by neuronal means (Figure 45.2). It is known that a number of centres in the brain stem are important staging posts in the passage of this information (Lilly and Gann, 1992). One is the nucleus of the tractus solitarius (NTS) in the medulla. This receives tonic inhibitory input from the baroreceptors via the vagus nerve (and, in the case of the high-pressure baroreceptors, the sinus branch of the glossopharyngeal nerve) and stimulatory input from the arterial chemoreceptors. The NTS has direct connexions with the PVN, but part of the traffic between them is via the ventrolateral medulla. This contains nuclei that integrate the responses to noxious stimuli since it also receives input from the various types of nociceptors sensitive to tissue damage. This information ascends in the anterolateral quadrant of the spinal cord via the so-called spinothalamic tract, but the fibres are not those of the classical pain pathway (Stoner, 1986). The ventrolateral medulla also coordinates the sympathoadrenal response to injury. There are further important centres in the dorsal rostral pons (Carlson and Gann, 1991), which contains the locus coeruleus, locus subcoeruleus, parabrachial nucleus and dorsal raphe nuclei and receives projections from the NTS and ventrolateral medulla.

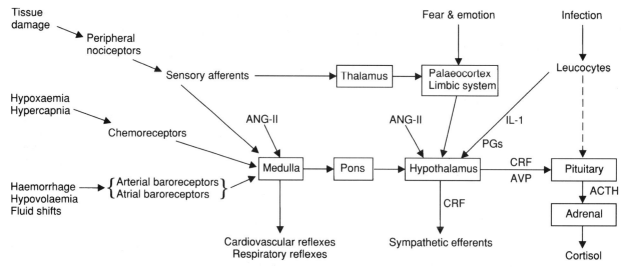

Figure 45.2 Schematic diagram of the hypothalamic-pituitary-adrenal system showing major afferent inputs, neural pathways and sites for modulation and for interaction. ANG-II = angiotensin II; PGs = prostaglandins; CRF = corticotrophin-releasing factor; AVP = arginine vasopressin; ACTH = adrenocorticotrophic hormone. (Reproduced from Lilly and Gann, 1992, with permission.)

The identity of the pathways by which these centres relay information to the PVN is not certain (Lilly and Gann, 1992). Most are noradrenergic and the medial forebrain bundle and the periventricular system appear to be important routes. Adrenergic pathways from the medulla and serotoninergic pathways from the raphe nuclei of the pons and midbrain may also play a role. Additional serotoninergic pathways reach the PVN indirectly via the suprachiasmatic nucleus of the hypothalamus. After experimental injury there is strong biochemical evidence for activation of noradrenergic but not serotoninergic pathways (Stoner, 1986). Physiological studies suggest at least three separate pathways conveying baroreceptor input to the hypothalamus, two stimulatory and one inhibitory (Lilly and Gann, 1992). There is evidence that the locus coeruleus or nearby areas is essential but the pathways cannot easily be related to anatomically defined tracts. In addition to this information arising initially from baroreceptors, chemoreceptors and nociceptors, the PVN also receives input from higher centres via the limbic system, especially the amygdala and septal area (Lilly and Gann, 1992). Some of this input reaches the PVN directly via the stria terminalis.

A great deal of work (reviewed by Assenmacher *et al.*, 1987; Jones and Gillham, 1988; Plotsky *et al.*, 1989) has been done on the neurotransmitters that, through the hypophysiotrophic hormones, influence ACTH secretion. There seems general agreement that acetylcholine and 5-hydroxytryptamine are excitatory neurotransmitters and that γ-aminobutyric acid (GABA) is inhibitory. To what extent changes in acetylcholine and GABA are responsible for the stimulation seen after injury is uncertain

since the anatomy and function of the cholinergic and GABAergic neurones to the hypothalamus are not understood; the latter are mostly short interneurones. Although catecholaminergic neurones are thought to be the only ones with direct synapses on CRF-secreting cells (Assenmacher *et al.*, 1987), their role in ACTH secretion is controversial. An earlier review (Weiner and Ganong, 1978) concluded that these neurones are mainly inhibitory, but the consensus is now against this (Assenmacher *et al.*, 1987; Plotsky *et al.*, 1989). Recent evidence indicates that noradrenergic neurones are primarily excitatory, acting mainly through α_1 receptors and possibly also through β receptors, although there are also inhibitory presynaptic α_2 receptors in the PVN and locus coeruleus (Carlson and Gann, 1992).

Stimulation by cytokines

Several members of the inflammatory cytokine family stimulate the HPA axis when administered either peripherally or centrally (Bateman *et al.*, 1989; Imura *et al.*, 1991; Kennedy and Jones, 1991; Lilly and Gann, 1992). This is thought to be largely independent of the pathways described above, although, especially at higher concentrations of cytokines, baroreceptors or nociceptors may be involved and activation of noradrenergic projections to the hypothalamus has been observed (Dunn, 1993). Most studies have been done with interleukin 1 (IL-1), although IL-6 has similar but less potent effects. IL-1 may act in a number of brain areas, including the hypothalamic paraventricular nucleus (see below). However, whether IL-1 administered peripherally can reach these sites is uncertain since it is unlikely to cross the blood–brain barrier. One possibility is that its primary action is at circumventricular organs where the barrier is defective, for example the organum vasculosum laminae terminalis or, as suggested by Rivier (1993), the median eminence. There is much evidence that the effects of IL-1 on the HPA axis are mediated by prostaglandins; whether these act in an autocrine or paracrine way is unknown. Both IL-1 and IL-6 have been reported to stimulate the HPA axis at the pituitary and adrenal as well as the hypothalamic level (Imura *et al.*, 1991; Kennedy and Jones, 1991), but, at least in the case of IL-1, it is doubtful whether these additional effects are physiologically relevant (Lilly and Gann, 1992; Dunn, 1993).

Except when sepsis supervenes, the contribution of cytokines to the HPA response to injury is uncertain. The circulating concentration of IL-1 is usually very low in the plasma of trauma patients. However, elective surgery (Cruickshank *et al.*, 1990), burns (Nijsten *et al.*, 1991) and accidental injury (Svoboda *et al.*, 1994) usually cause an increase in the concentration of IL-6. This occurs too slowly to initiate the HPA response but could play a part in potentiating it. Perhaps most interestingly, cytokines can be synthesized by glial and possibly neural cells within the brain and thus could contribute to the HPA response to head injury (see Chapter 9).

Hypothalamic releasing factors

The hypothalamus controls ACTH secretion largely through the tuberoinfundibular neurones which secrete the 41-residue corticotrophin-releasing factor (CRF) and vasopressin into the primary plexus of the median eminence where they are taken up by the capillaries of the portal system and transported to the anterior pituitary (Whitnall, 1993). These tuberoinfundibular neurones arise mainly from the parvicellular part of the PVN. It is likely that vasopressin from the magnocellular neurones of the supraoptic- and paraventricular-hypophyseal tracts also enters the portal capillaries; there are several possible mechanisms (Antoni, 1993), although these are controversial (Whitnall, 1993). In addition, there is evidence for the involvement of other stimulatory factors such as oxytocin and adrenaline (Plotsky, 1987) and of unknown release-inhibiting factors (Engler *et al.*, 1994).

There is evidence that full stress responses require the presence of both peptides, but the exact role that each plays is not clear. Changes in their secretion by the parvicellular neurones are not reflected in their concentrations in the systemic circulation. Most circulating CRF is derived from peripheral sources (Owens and Nemeroff, 1991), although pulses of plasma CRF corresponding to those of ACTH have been detected during major surgery (Calogero *et al.*, 1992). It has been proposed that under some conditions CRF acts in an essentially permissive manner; CRF has to be present for an ACTH response to occur, but the size of the response depends mainly on the quantity of vasopressin secreted (Plotsky, 1987). However, it is now clear that such notions are oversimplified and that the relative roles of the two peptides depend on many factors, including the type and duration of the stimulus and the species of animal used (Antoni, 1993; Whitnall, 1993). In the rat, there are two populations of parvicellular neurones, some containing CRF alone and some both CRF and AVP; during chronic stress the former appear to be converted to the latter (Tilders *et al.*, 1993).

An interesting recent development in connexion with these hypothalamic peptides is the discovery of a stimulus-specific role of nitric oxide (NO) in HPA activation. An inhibitor of NO synthase, L-NAME, potentiated the effects of IL-1β and endotoxin but attenuated the effects of mild electric shock on plasma ACTH and cortisol (Rivier, 1994; Rivier and Shen, 1994). L-NAME also potentiated stimulation by vasopressin but not CRF. However, not all these actions may have been due to inhibition of NO synthase since some could be counteracted by giving arginine, the substrate for the enzyme, whereas others could not.

Feedback inhibition

It is well known that the HPA axis is subject to feedback inhibition by corticosteroids; that is to say, if exogenous steroids are administered, secretion of ACTH decreases, whereas if endogenous corticosteroids are removed, for example by adrenalectomy, it increases. This feedback inhibition is complex. In gross terms it can be divided into fast, intermediate and slow feedback (Keller-Wood and Dallman, 1984; Jones and Gillham, 1988). Fast feedback occurs within minutes and is a function of the rate of rise of the corticosteroid concentration, whereas intermediate and slow feedback have time-scales of the order of a few hours and a few days respectively and depend on the actual concentrations (integrated over the appropriate time-period) of the corticosteroid. While fast feedback cannot be mediated by classical glucocorticoid actions involving changes in DNA transcription, intermediate and slow feedback probably are. There is currently interest in the possibility that feedback inhibition is mediated by lipocortin-1 (Buckingham *et al.*, 1994), which was thought to be responsible for the anti-inflammatory effects of glucocorticoids, although there is increasing evidence against this (Barnes and Adcock, 1993).

There are two types of corticosteroid receptor in the brain, Type I or mineralocorticoid receptors and Type II or glucocorticoid receptors. Both have a high affinity for all glucocorticoids, but Type I receptors have an especially high affinity for corticosterone and aldosterone (McEwen *et al.*, 1986; de Kloet, 1991). Type I receptors in the body can be divided into corticosterone-preferring and aldosterone-preferring. However, the distinction is thought to be due not to inherent differences in binding characteristics but to the relative concentrations of the two steroids at the receptor site. The predominant steroid, corticosterone, is oxidised to 11-dehydrocorticosterone by 11β-hydroxysteroid dehydrogenase whose activity is high in the vicinity of aldosterone-preferring receptors (de Kloet, 1991; Albiston *et al.*, 1994). Most Type I receptors in the brain are corticosterone-preferring. Their density is greatest in the hippocampus and septal area, whereas Type II receptors are fairly evenly distributed throughout the brain.

At one time it was thought that the hypothalamus was the main site of central feedback inhibition, but recently there has been much interest in the role of the hippocampus. Because Type I receptors have a higher affinity for corticosterone than Type II receptors, the hippocampus may play a particularly important role in feedback inhibition at very low concentrations of endogenous glucocorticoids. (The extensive use of the rat for this work accounts for the emphasis on corticosterone rather than cortisol, and there may well be species differences in the function of the two types of receptor.) However, when the body responds to stress the Type I receptors are likely to begin by being nearly saturated, whereas occupation of the Type II receptors will increase progressively with the corticosteroid concentration. Thus, modulation of the response by feedback inhibition probably involves the Type II receptors (Dallman *et al.*, 1987), which are present, *inter alia*, in the PVN; the role of the hippocampus appears to be limited (de Kloet, 1991; Jacobson and Sapolsky, 1991).

The role of feedback inhibition in limiting the response to injury is difficult to study and not fully understood. Many years ago Dallman and Yates (1968) showed that the responses to the component stimuli vary in their susceptibility to suppression by exogenous glucocorticoids. Thus haemorrhage or laparotomy with intestinal traction produces a response less attenuated by dexamethasone than a hind-limb scald, laparotomy alone or a period of hypoxia (Dallman and Yates, 1968). Keller-Wood and Dallman (1984) have pointed out that these differences are not merely a function of the 'strength' of the stimulus as assessed by its ability to raise plasma ACTH in the absence of dexamethasone. However, the relevance of these observations to the role of endogenous corticosteroids is uncertain, since there is evidence that short-term inhibition by dexamethasone is exerted mainly at the pituitary level, whereas endogenous steroids act at central sites (Miller *et al.*, 1992). Moreover, experiments in rats show that, with repeated or

chronic stress, feedback inhibition by corticosterone is counterbalanced by facilitation, which takes place by an unknown mechanism (Dallman *et al.*, 1992). Facilitation has also been observed with repeat of a small haemorrhage after 24 hours in dogs (Lilly *et al.*, 1992). Inhibition and facilitation with successive stimuli has also been observed at the level of adrenocortical sensitivity to ACTH (Jones and Gillham, 1988).

Stimulation independent of pituitary

Injury may stimulate the adrenal cortex by a number of mechanisms that act independently of or additionally to pituitary ACTH secretion. One route is through cells involved in the inflammatory and immunological responses to injury. The possibility of direct stimulation by cytokines is mentioned above. In addition, stimuli such as endotoxin and Newcastle disease virus, and also CRF and vasopressin, induce lymphocytes to express the gene for the ACTH precursor, pro-opiomelanocortin (POMC; Blalock, 1989). However, doubt has been cast on the significance of these effects because the POMC is not always processed to bioactive ACTH and because the output of peptides is low (Bateman *et al.*, 1989).

Another potentially important extrapituitary factor is the splanchnic nerve supply to the adrenal cortex, as shown by experiments involving stimulation or sectioning of these nerves (Charlton, 1990). However, there is disagreement over the mechanism of their stimulatory effect. Some studies suggest that they are secondary to an increase in adrenal blood flow (Breslow, 1992), which may stimulate corticosteroid synthesis by increasing the ACTH presentation rate or by mechanisms independent of ACTH (Charlton, 1990). However, other studies show that the effects of nerve stimulation on blood flow are minor (Breslow, 1992). Such stimulation releases a large number of peptides such as CRF and ACTH from the adrenal and these could, in principle, be responsible.

It is also possible that cortisol production is influenced by a recently identified family of peptides, the corticostatins, defensins or cryptdins, that are synthesized by peripheral tissues and attenuate the stimulatory effect of ACTH on cortisol secretion (Tominaga *et al.*, 1992). The most potent of these, CS-1 or NP3A, is found in neutrophils, lung and various other tissues. The role of these peptides after trauma is not known but there are claims that the concentration of CS-1 is increased in patients with peritonitis but not after haemorrhage (Tominaga *et al.*, 1992).

Effects of human trauma

In man, the rise in plasma cortisol after injury (reviewed by Barton, 1987) is one of its best-documented consequences. With minor and moderate injuries plasma cortisol tends to increase with the severity of injury. When the injury is severe, a levelling off of the response would be expected when the maximal capacity of the adrenal cortex to secrete cortisol is reached. In practice, a number of studies have shown that in severely injured patients plasma cortisol is less than maximal and in fact tends to fall as the severity of injury increases. However, the duration of the increase in plasma cortisol shows a better relationship with injury severity, normal levels being regained, on average, soonest after elective surgery and latest after severe burns, accidental injury (with a response lasting a few days) being intermediate. In patients dying after injury, very high cortisol concentrations may be seen before death. Elderly patients show a cortisol response that is prolonged inappropriately to the severity of their injury (Barton, 1996). In contrast, failure of plasma cortisol to respond to elective surgery in patients with rheumatoid arthritis has been reported (Chikanza et al., 1992).

There seems little doubt that at short times after injury a centrally driven increase in ACTH is responsible for the rise in cortisol. Plasma ACTH is raised and although in most studies it is poorly correlated with plasma cortisol this can probably be explained by its episodic release (Calogero et al., 1992). In severely injured patients the lower than expected cortisol concentrations could be due to impaired adrenal perfusion. At later times after injury the role of ACTH is by no means so certain; several studies (e.g. Naito et al., 1991; Doncaster et al., 1993) have shown that concentrations of ACTH are lower than expected from those of cortisol. These are not the first such observations: dissociations between cortisol and ACTH concentrations have been recorded during normal episodic secretion and after many forms of stress such as experimental haemorrhage (Charlton, 1990). Some of these discrepancies may be artefacts since the exquisite sensitivity of the adrenal cortex, combined with the pulsatile nature of ACTH secretion, makes it inherently difficult to detect changes in ACTH appropriate to moderate increases in plasma cortisol. These problems are compounded if the ACTH assay is insufficiently specific so that there is a high background immunoreactivity (Engeland et al., 1989). However, Naito et al. (1991) have convincingly demonstrated increased adrenal sensitivity to ACTH 2 days after major elective surgery, suggesting upregulation of ACTH receptors or the operation of extrapituitary factors such as cytokines or nerve stimulation.

The plasma concentration of cortisol may not always reflect its secretion rate after trauma. There are claims of an increased metabolic clearance rate at short times after elective surgery, which could be due to reduced concentrations of binding proteins (Barton, 1987). Another factor influencing cortisol clearance is interconversion with cortisone. It has long been known that surgery decreases both the ratio between cortisone and cortisol metabolites in the urine (Gold et al., 1958) and the ratio between plasma cortisone and cortisol (Srivastava et al., 1973). However, it is not known whether conversion of cortisol to cortisone is impaired or the reverse process enhanced; the kidney and liver respectively are major sites for these reactions (Walker et al., 1992). This question is of interest since the enzyme responsible, 11β-hydroxysteroid dehydrogenase, is now known to exist in two forms with quite different cofactors, substrate affinities, reversibilities and tissue distributions, one of which controls access to Type I receptors (Albiston et al., 1994). The decreased cortisone:cortisol ratio is not specific to trauma or even stress since it can be reproduced by administration of ACTH (Gold et al., 1958; Srivastava et al., 1973). Trauma also causes a decrease in adrenal androgen production, at least in relation to cortisol if not always in absolute terms (Parker, 1991). This occurs in other forms of stress but cannot be reproduced by ACTH; its mechanism is unknown.

OTHER ANTERIOR-PITUITARY SYSTEMS

Growth hormone and insulin-like growth factors

Growth hormone (GH) exhibits several unusual features. Its hypothalamic release-inhibiting hormone, somatostatin, plays a major role in its regulation and was in fact discovered before its releasing hormone. Unlike other hormones, GH shows qualitatively different changes after stress in different species; in particular, its concentration increases in man (Barton, 1987) but decreases in the rat (Barton, 1977) so that control mechanisms discovered in this species may not necessarily be relevant. Some of the effects of GH are mediated by proteins known as somatomedins or insulin-like growth factors, of which the major one is IGF-I.

The relative roles of GH-releasing hormone (GHRH) and somatostatin in the control of normal GH secretion, which occurs episodically, is not fully understood. Studies with antibodies in the rat suggest that somatostatin exerts a tonic inhibitory influence on GH secretion, while GHRH is responsible for its pulsatility (Müller, 1987). It is very likely that this difference in roles is achieved by differences in neural input to the relevant cells but the details are not yet clear. Both peptides occur in several regions of the hypothalamus, but the cell bodies of neurones secreting somatostatin are predominantly in the periventricular nucleus whilst those secreting GHRH are in the arcuate and ventromedial nuclei (Müller, 1987; Casanueva, 1992). In man, α-adrenergic and cholinergic agonists tend to stimulate GH release and β-adrenergic agonists to inhibit it; the role of dopaminergic, serotoninergic and GABAergic pathways is less clear (Müller, 1987; Casanueva, 1992). The relative roles of GHRH and somatostatin are more difficult to study in man but there is evidence that a decrease in somatostatin tone is at least partly responsible for normal pulses of secretion (Thorner *et al.*, 1990), which occur mainly at night. Feedback inhibition of GH secretion may occur at both the hypothalamic and pituitary levels and may involve both GH itself and IGF-I (Müller, 1987; Casanueva, 1992).

Both GH (Herington *et al.*, 1991) and IGF-I (Sara and Hall, 1990) bind to plasma proteins, and this is thought to be of particular significance for IGF-I. The great majority is bound to the 150 kD protein IGFBP-3. The control of this binding and its implications for bioactivity are not understood but the complex is thought to represent the body's main storage compartment for IGF-I. In contrast, the 25-kDa protein IGFBP-1, which binds a smaller quantity, shows a clear pattern of regulation: its concentration increases under conditions of carbohydrate storage and low insulin concentrations, putatively conferring protection against the insulin-like effects of IGF-I. Circulating IGF-I appears to be derived mainly from the liver and may play an endocrine role, but IGF-I is also produced locally in tissues in response to GH (Daughaday and Rotwein, 1989; Sara and Hall, 1990).

In man, plasma GH rises rapidly after accidental injury and elective surgery (reviewed by Barton, 1987); although a number of studies have shown no change in patients with burns, an early rise may have been missed because measurements did not start until 2 days or more after injury, by which time GH had returned to somewhere near its normal levels after other types of injury. Plasma somatomedin activity did not follow the GH concentration. Measurements by bioassay showed a rapid fall in activity after injury, with a gradual return to normal levels; in patients succumbing to severe burns somatomedin activity was low throughout. It was not correlated with plasma GH but one study showed a strong correlation with plasma insulin. Recently IGF-I concentrations have been measured in surgical patients by radioimmunoassay. After cholecystectomy plasma IGF-I either rose or remained unchanged, depending upon whether it was extracted before assay (Davenport *et al.*, 1992), whereas in patients critically ill after major surgery plasma IGF-I fell (Davies *et al.*, 1991). In both groups there was proteolytic degradation of IGFBP-3. The effect of these changes on IGF-I availability to tissues is uncertain. The critically ill patients had raised IGFBP-1 concentrations which were greatly decreased by parenteral feeding (Ross *et al.*, 1991).

Prolactin

Prolactin is also unusual in that its secretion is regulated primarily by tonic inhibition, which is lessened when prolactin secretion increases (Ben-Jonathan *et al.*, 1989). The most important inhibitory factor is dopamine, which is secreted by neurones with cell bodies in the arcuate and periventricular nuclei of the hypothalamus and passes down their axons in the tuberoinfundibular tract in the same way as polypeptide hypophysiotrophic hormones. Other inhibitory factors are found in hypothalamic extracts but their role is uncertain. Various forms of stress, including haemorrhage (Carlson *et al.*, 1990), increase plasma prolactin. There is evidence that this is not due to reduced dopamine secretion, and the existence of a prolactin-releasing factor has been postulated. A large number of candidates have been suggested, of which the best known is thyrotrophin-releasing hormone (TRH). However, its physiological role is uncertain and stimulation by vasoactive intestinal peptide, angiotensin II or peptides associated with the posterior lobe of the pituitary may be more important (Ben-Jonathan *et al.*, 1989). Most studies of prolactin secretion have used suckling rather than stress as a stimulus and the mechanism of the response may well vary between the two.

In man, the available evidence suggests that plasma prolactin usually rises shortly after injury, although most of the work has been done in patients undergoing elective surgery or suffering from thoracic trauma (Barton 1987; Delitala *et al.*, 1987). The interest in the latter arises from reports of galactorrhoea in patients with chest-wall injuries, suggesting that such patients have a particularly large prolactin response owing to stimulation of specific receptors in the areolar area. The response to injury is transient and although some authors have reported persistently raised prolactin concentrations after severe burns others have not (Barton, 1987).

Thyroid hormones

At first sight the control of thyroid-hormone secretion is similar to that of cortisol secretion: the stimulus is a pituitary hormone, thyroid-stimulating hormone (TSH), whose production is, in turn, controlled by secretion of a hypothalamic releasing hormone (TRH) by cells of the PVN into the hypophyseal portal system (Reichlin, 1985). Moreover, the system is subject to feedback inhibition by the thyroid hormones. However, there are differences between the two systems. Feedback inhibition is thought to lie mainly at the pituitary level; although there is evidence that thyroid hormones also act in the hypothalamus, causing the secretion of somatostatin and/or dopamine which inhibit the release of TSH, the role of this feedback inhibition at the hypothalamic level is not clear (Reichlin, 1985). Another difference is that stress does not stimulate the hypothalamo-pituitary-thyroid axis, and feedback inhibition is not overridden by central stimuli as it is for the HPA axis. Injury in fact tends to reduce the concentrations of thyroid hormones, and the main pituitary abnormality is that this usually fails to raise the concentration of TSH, or its response to exogenous TRH, as might be expected (Zaloga and Chernow, 1985; Barton, 1987).

The fall in thyroid-hormone concentration after injury is due largely to changes in the behaviour of peripheral tissues (Zaloga and Chernow, 1985; Barton, 1987). Thyroxine (T_4), the form secreted by the thyroid gland, is converted to the much more active triiodothyronine (T_3) peripherally, and this 5-deiodination is inhibited after injury, resulting in a decreased T_3 concentration. At the same time 5-deiodination to reverse T_3 is enhanced. There is also a tendency for plasma T_4 to fall, but this is pronounced only if the patient becomes critically ill. Both thyroid hormones bind strongly to thyroxine-binding globulin (TBG) in plasma, and it is the free hormones that are active. Normally a fall in plasma T_4 leads to a rise in the number of unoccupied binding sites on TBG, as measured by the T_3-resin-uptake test. However, after injury there is an increased T_3-resin-uptake index, and this suggests that binding of T_4 to TBG is inhibited. Consequently there may be no fall in the free T_4 concentration. It is, however, clear that free T_3, and thus the overall thyroid-hormone activity, in plasma is decreased. The changes may persist for several weeks and the reason why hypothyroidism is not observed clinically is not clear. Similar changes are seen in many forms of illness and have been described as the 'euthyroid sick syndrome'.

The mechanism of these effects of injury on thyroid function is not known. Corticosteroids can reproduce some of the changes, such as inhibited conversion of T_4 to T_3 and reduced TSH secretion (Utiger, 1986), but there is evidence against their involvement at least after elective surgery (Zaloga and Chernow, 1985). Starvation also produces a picture rather similar to that after trauma (although the subject may become clinically hypothyroid) (Utiger, 1986), but whether the transient decrease in food intake in most trauma patients would be sufficient to cause the marked changes observed is not known. Attempts to answer this question in experimental animals have been inconclusive because it has proved difficult to reproduce the effects of surgery in man (Hintze et al., 1991). It is possible that the only abnormalities are peripheral, and that the failure to observe a compensatory increase in TSH secretion is due to the lack of a fall in plasma free T_4, since both the pituitary and the hypothalamus can convert T_4 to T_3 (Utiger, 1986). Cytokines tend to inhibit the hypothalamo-pituitary-thyroid system but their role in the 'euthyroid sick syndrome' is unclear. The effects are mainly at the level of the hypothalamus and thyroid rather than on thyroid-hormone binding and metabolism and have mostly been demonstrated with IL-1 and

TNF (Imura et al., 1991), neither of which usually shows a sustained rise in plasma concentration.

Gonadal steroids

In men the hypothalamo-pituitary-testicular axis is regulated in an analogous way to the HPA axis and the hypothalamo-pituitary-thyroid axis, with the added complexity of two pituitary gonadotrophins, luteinizing hormone (LH) and follicle-stimulating hormone (FSH) (Reichlin, 1985). There is a common hypothalamic releasing factor, gonadotrophin-releasing hormone (GnRH), but feedback inhibition, which occurs at least partially at the pituitary level, is different for the two gonadotrophins, FSH secretion being inhibited by the polypeptide inhibin from the germinal cells of the testis as well as directly by testosterone. In women the picture is of course made much more complex by the menstrual cycle, but these complexities need not be considered in detail since little is known of the effects of trauma on female reproductive hormones. In part this reflects the relatively few premenopausal women succumbing to trauma.

Many studies have been done on reproductive hormones after trauma in men but a clear picture has not emerged (Barton, 1987). The only consistent finding, which resembles the effect of many forms of non-endocrine illness, is a fall in plasma testosterone, which can last for a considerable period, depending on the severity of injury. Most studies show no change in the concentration of sex-steroid binding globulin, so that the concentration of free, biologically active testosterone is also low, presumably accounting for the loss of libido after injury. Decreased concentrations of LH and FSH have been found, but the pattern varies between the two hormones and between studies, and the decrease, if any, in gonadotrophin concentrations does not correspond to that in testosterone. Injection of GnRH in patients with burns produced gonadotrophin responses that reflected the basal gonadotrophin concentrations, which were normal or decreased. This contrasts with patients with head injuries, in whom basal gonadotrophin concentrations were low but the response to GnRH was exaggerated (Clark et al., 1988). The few studies in premenopausal women show a fall in plasma oestrogens after injury; gonadotrophin concentrations may or may not fall, and in patients with head injury the response to GnRH is increased (Barton, 1987).

The results, at least in men, thus present a complex picture. The most striking finding would appear to be an impaired sensitivity of testosterone secretion to gonadotrophins in the testis. However, it has recently been claimed that this is secondary to abnormalities in hypothalamic GnRH release (Semple et al., 1987). The pulsatility of LH release was decreased after burns so that although its mean immunoreactivity did not change its bioactivity was reduced; that this could explain the low testosterone concentration was supported by a normal response to human chorionic gonadotrophin. Whatever the reason for the fall in testosterone, gonadotrophin concentrations fail to rise in consequence; this defect may evidently lie at the pituitary level or centrally, depending on the type of injury. In animal experiments, central inhibition of gonadotrophin secretion by stress has been attributed to CRF-41 (Owens and Nemeroff, 1991). In addition to these mechanisms, corticosteroids may play a role by inhibiting both LH secretion and its steroidogenic effect on the testis (Baxter and Tyrrell, 1986). IL-1 also has inhibitory effects at both the hypothalamic and the testicular level (Imura et al., 1991).

HORMONES AFFECTING THE KIDNEY

Vasopressin and oxytocin

The vasopressin and oxytocin in the circulation are largely derived from the magnocellular portions of the supraoptic and paraventricular nuclei of the hypothalamus (Zimmerman, 1983). The hormones pass down neural tracts into the posterior pituitary where they are released into its extensive capillary network. Although vasopressin, and perhaps oxytocin, synthesized by the parvicellular portions of these nuclei plays a major role in the control of ACTH secretion, it probably contributes little to the concentration in the general circulation. Much is known about the control of vasopressin secretion (Robertson, 1986). It is extremely sensitive to plasma osmolality (or, more precisely, to the concentration of certain solutes, especially those that do not readily enter cells), normal values for osmolality causing tonic vasopressin release. Hypovolaemia and hypotension, acting respectively through the low- and high-pressure baroreceptors, stimulate vasopressin secretion; the threshold is relatively high (at least 5% blood loss in the case of hypovolaemia), but once it has been exceeded, very high vasopressin concentrations can be achieved. Vasopressin secretion is still sensitive to changes in osmolality but the threshold and slope of the relationship are altered. Other important stimuli are pain, nausea, emotional stress and possibly hypoxia; at least the first two can again override the effects of the prevailing osmolality. Glucocorticoids inhibit vasopressin secretion by magnocellular neurones; for example, ACTH administration decreases the vasopressin response to haemorrhage in dogs, suggesting that the increase after trauma could to a certain extent depend on the size of the HPA response (Raff, 1987). The main stimulus to oxytocin secretion is suckling; much less is known about stimuli that might be relevant after injury.

Plasma vasopressin rises after injury of all types (Barton, 1987); after accidental injury the response increases with the severity of the injury (Anderson et al., 1989). The changes are not related to plasma osmolality and are clearly due to other stimuli. The most detailed studies have been done after elective surgery, where visceral traction is a particularly potent stimulus (Le Quesne et al., 1985). The rate at which plasma vasopressin returns to normal probably depends both on the severity of the injury and on plasma osmolality (Barton, 1987). The response can be transient after elective surgery. At the other extreme, vasopressin concentrations may continue to be higher than expected from the plasma sodium concentration for several weeks after severe burns, leading to trauma being included among the causes of the syndrome of inappropriate antidiuretic hormone secretion ('inappropriate' only in an osmotic context) (Robertson, 1986). An exception to this picture of raised vasopressin concentrations is the syndrome of traumatic diabetes insipidus, which occurs after head injury if there is sufficient tissue destruction or oedema in the hypothalamo-pituitary area (Edwards and Clark, 1986). Little is known about the oxytocin response to trauma. There is one report of a rise in oxytocin similar in size and duration to that in vasopressin shortly after elective surgery (Nussey et al., 1988), which would appear to conflict with the accepted idea that stress inhibits milk let-down in nursing mothers.

Renin-angiotensin system

The renin-angiotensin system is the name given to a proteolytic cascade with both endocrine functions and a role in vascular regulation in the kidney (Hackenthal et al., 1990). Renin is an aspartyl protease secreted by the juxtaglomerular apparatus, which comprises specialized cells in the afferent arterioles just before they enter the glomeruli of the kidney. Renin cleaves a circulating α_2-globulin, renin substrate or angiotensinogen, which is synthesized mainly in the liver, to the decapeptide angiotensin I. This in turn is cleaved to the active octapeptide angiotensin II by angiotensin-converting enzyme, which has a high activity in several tissues, notably the lungs, and is not thought to be rate-limiting although it can become so if inhibited pharmacologically.

The control of renin secretion is complex and three main mechanisms have been identified (Mitchell and Navar, 1989; Hackenthal et al., 1990), all of which could come into play after injury. First, activity in the renal nerves, which will be stimulated if hypovolaemia or hypotension is sensed by baroreceptors in the atria or carotid arteries, causes release of renin through a β_1-adrenergic mechanism. Second, the juxtaglomerular cells themselves act as baroreceptors; a decrease in the stretch of the arteriolar walls will directly stimulate renin production, although this mechanism requires a considerable fall in renal perfusion pressure because the arterioles proximal to the juxtaglomerular cells have the ability to autoregulate blood flow. Third, renin secretion is controlled by the flux of sodium chloride through the distal tubule. One ion, probably chloride, is sensed by specialized cells in an area of the tubule known as the macula densa, which lies close to the afferent arteriole of the same nephron and passes a signal (possibly decreased secretion of adenosine) to the adjacent juxtaglomerular cells. The role of the macula densa has been controversial but most evidence shows that the effect of chloride is inhibitory and that renin does not mediate the autoregulation of glomerular filtration (tubuloglomerular feedback). Clearly this mechanism may modulate the effects of stimuli such as hypovolaemia and hypotension on the renin–angiotensin system. Another potent feedback inhibitory mechanism is direct inhibition of renin secretion by angiotensin II.

Few studies have been done on the renin–angiotensin response to injury in man and the findings are divergent (Barton, 1987). In patients undergoing elective surgery, the reported response has varied from non-existent to large and prolonged. The reasons for these differences are not clear, but the response is enhanced in patients under epidural analgesia, probably owing to a greater fall in blood pressure. There are a few reports of plasma renin activity after burns and although raised values have been found their magnitude and time-course varies.

Aldosterone

Aldosterone secretion from the adrenal cortex is subject to regulation by three main stimuli (Baxter and Tyrrell, 1986; Carey and Sen, 1986). The first is angiotensin II; a heptapeptide metabolite, angiotensin III, is equipotent but its circulating concentration is normally much lower. The second factor is ACTH, which, although a potent stimulus, has only a transient effect, in contrast to angiotensin II. The third factor is the circulating K^+ concentration, to which the zona glomerulosa is very sensitive over the physiological range. Several additional factors may stimulate aldosterone secretion. One is hyponatraemia, but the required fall in plasma Na^+ (10–20 mM) is larger than is likely to occur physiologically. Experiments with administration of dopamine and its antagonists suggest tonic inhibition of aldosterone secretion by dopamine, attenuation of which may play a role in the aldosterone response to standing (Carey and Sen, 1986). However, the origin of this dopamine is unknown. Another inhibitor of aldosterone secretion, both under basal conditions and in response to various secretagogues, is atrial natriuretic peptide

(Kenyon and Jardine, 1989; Brenner *et al.*, 1990). Finally, there are reports of a glycoprotein aldosterone-stimulating factor in urine, which may be of pituitary origin and implicated in the pathogenesis of idiopathic hyperaldosteronism.

Angiotensin II and ACTH are thought to be the main stimuli to aldosterone secretion after injury but their relative contributions may vary greatly (Barton, 1987). A rise in plasma aldosterone has been observed in all the studies reported in patients with burns or after elective surgery (there appear to be few data after non-thermal accidental injury), irrespective of whether plasma renin activity increased. In those in whom it did not, ACTH is likely to have been the initial stimulus; however, in those showing a prolonged rise in plasma aldosterone – for example, if sodium intake was low – angiotensin II is likely to have perpetuated the response (Le Quesne *et al.*, 1985).

Atrial natriuretic peptide

Atrial natriuretic peptide (ANP) is a recently discovered hormone, which, like renin (whose secretion it inhibits), lies outside the control of the pituitary (Kenyon and Jardine, 1989; Brenner *et al.*, 1990). Most stimuli to its secretion, such as expansion of plasma volume and immersion of the body in water, probably act through atrial distension, and although there is evidence for stimulation by hormones such as glucocorticoids, adrenaline and vasopressin, this may be mediated, at least in part, by their haemodynamic effects. The few reports of the effects of trauma and hypovolaemia are consistent with this picture. Plasma ANP has usually been found to decrease after experimental haemorrhage (Carlson *et al.*, 1989) and did not change after elective cholecystectomy (Kidd *et al.*, 1987).

EFFECTS OF HORMONES AFTER INJURY

Cardiovascular effects

The effects of trauma on the control of the cardiovascular system are reviewed in Chapter 40. The picture shortly after injury is dominated by the sympathetic innervation of vascular smooth muscle, which has complex effects dependent on many factors (variations in discharge between vascular beds, density of different receptors, nature of initial stimulus, etc.) and is outside the scope of this review. Circulating adrenaline could also influence vasomotor tone directly, either by contributing to α_1-adrenergic vasoconstriction or by causing vasodilatation in vessels with a high density of β_2 receptors, for which noradrenaline has a lower affinity. However, these direct actions are likely to be complicated by indirect effects mediated by prejunctional receptors (Langer and Arbilla, 1990). Binding of adrenaline to these receptors will excite

(β_2) or inhibit (α_2) the secretion of noradrenaline by sympathetic nerve endings. Both vasopressin (acting through V1 receptors) and angiotensin II could enhance vasoconstriction after trauma, again either directly or by prejunctional effects. Vasopressin can reach a sufficiently high concentration after accidental injury; whether the same is true of angiotensin II, despite its great potency, is not known. Both of these hormones may have additional actions on the cardiovascular system at a central level via the area postrema of the medulla.

Precapillary vasoconstriction causes a fall in capillary hydrostatic pressure which leads to movement of fluids from the interstitial compartment into the circulation and thus helps to restore plasma volume. Completion of this process requires restitution of plasma protein and there is evidence that this too depends on hormones; glucocorticoids, glucagon and an unidentified pituitary hormone have all been implicated (Drucker *et al.*, 1981). Although vasomotor effects may contribute (Walker and Williams, 1992), the primary action of these hormones is to increase the extracellular concentration of solutes poorly permeable into cells, so that fluid is withdrawn from them osmotically. However, the identity of the major solute varies; under some circumstances it appears to be glucose (see below), whereas under other conditions glucose contributes only slightly to the rise in plasma osmolality.

Metabolic effects

Carbohydrate metabolism

Trauma causes characteristic changes in carbohydrate metabolism, described fully by Barton *et al.* (1990) and in Chapter 47. In the liver, glycogen is broken down, gluconeogenesis is stimulated from both new sources (amino acids, glycerol) and precursors derived from glycolysis (lactate, pyruvate) and suppression of glucose production by insulin is reduced. In insulin-sensitive peripheral tissues, uptake and oxidation of glucose are inhibited (peripheral insulin resistance) and glycogen breakdown in muscle is increased. These changes are not simultaneous; glycogenolysis is essentially an early ebb-phase event, although it may be delayed in humans undergoing elective surgery, while gluconeogenesis accompanies the increased net protein breakdown of the flow phase. In man, insulin resistance is best documented in the flow phase, but it probably starts in the ebb phase as it does in experimental animals. The result of all these changes is to cause hyperglycaemia, which is almost invariably seen after severe injury in man, although not always after moderate injuries; at later times it tends to be offset by a rise in plasma insulin, as mentioned above.

The early glycogen breakdown has a predominantly endocrine basis (Barton, 1985). Several hormones are capable of stimulating liver glycogen breakdown, including glucagon, adrenaline, vasopressin, angiotensin II and oxytocin. In the rat, in which fluid loss rather than nociception appears to be the glycogenolytic stimulus, adrenaline is not involved, but there is evidence for a role of glucagon. In man, this may well be reversed; hepatic glycogenolysis is much more sensitive to adrenaline than in the rat, and the lack of an immediate rise in glucagon in many studies makes its participation less likely. Vasopressin may well play a part but involvement of angiotensin II and oxcytocin is uncertain. Muscle glycogen breakdown after injury is mainly attributable to adrenaline. A direct effect of hypoxia may contribute to glycogen breakdown in both tissues after very severe injuries.

The role of hormones in stimulating gluconeogenesis after trauma is less certain. An increased rate of gluconeogenesis requires an adequate supply of precursors and this itself may partially have an endocrine basis as discussed below. However, hepatic extraction of these substrates is increased, owing at least in part to a rise in hepatic blood flow, the mechanism of which is uncertain. Cortisol, glucagon and adrenaline are capable of inducing key enzymes and thereby increasing gluconeogenic capacity. There is evidence for a role of glucagon after major burns (see Chapter 47), but after less severe injuries the concentrations of these hormones are not always still raised in the flow phase (Frayn, 1986). The same applies to peripheral insulin resistance after injury. In theory, glucocorticoids, adrenaline and growth hormone could all be involved, and the effects of injury can to some extent be reproduced by infusion of catecholamines, glucagon and cortisol. Glucocorticoids and adrenaline are very likely to cause the striking insulin resistance observed shortly after injury in the rat and plasma cortisol is inversely correlated with insulin sensitivity in patients during the first 48 hours after elective surgery (Brandi *et al.*, 1990). However, later on the concentrations of these hormones are usually lower than during triple-hormone infusions.

Fat metabolism

The most consistent effect of trauma on lipid metabolism is to cause lipolysis in adipose tissue (Barton, 1985; Barton *et al.*, 1990; see Chapter 47). This occurs in both the ebb and flow phases and is accompanied by an increase in the contribution of fat to oxygen consumption. In principle a number of hormones could be responsible for fat mobilization after injury, including adrenaline, growth hormone, glucagon and ACTH. The role of most of these hormones has not been tested, but the use of adrenergic blockers has consistently demonstrated the importance of the sympathoadrenal system after severe burns. However, adrenal medullectomy does not block the early lipolytic response to experimental injury in the rat, suggesting that sympathetic innervation of adipose tissue is more important than circulating adrenaline, in keeping with their accepted roles in fat mobilization. In patients with accidental injuries of moderate severity, the increase in plasma catecholamines wanes rapidly but the sympathoadrenal system might still contribute to lipolysis during the flow phase if selective sympathetic stimulation of adipose tissue were to persist. The flow phase is usually accompanied by reduced food intake, but the mechanism of fat mobilization after injury appears to be different from that in starvation, during which the concentration of insulin, a potent inhibitor of lipolysis, decreases.

This picture of sympathetically driven fat mobilization after injury is complicated by many factors, in particular a failure of the plasma non-esterified-fatty-acid (NEFA) concentration to increase as much as expected in both the ebb and flow phases (Barton, 1985; Barton *et al.*, 1990). Usually this would imply an increased rate of NEFA re-esterification within adipose tissue and a number of mechanisms may be responsible (see Figure 45.3). During the ebb phase there is experimental evidence for vasoconstriction in adipose tissue due to α_1-adrenergic stimuli and possibly also vasopressin. Such vasoconstriction has a proportionately greater effect on the release of NEFA than of glycerol because albumin is required for NEFA

transport. The rate of re-esterification is limited by the supply of glycerol 3-phosphate derived from glucose, which may be increased by a change in redox state (due, for example, to lactate), although decreased glucose uptake by adipose tissue resulting from insulin resistance would be expected to reduce this effect. The relative importance of these mechanisms depends on the model used and after injury in man it is difficult to distinguish between them. During the flow phase there is again evidence for increased re-esterification of NEFA within adipose tissue, but, more importantly, the metabolic clearance rate of plasma NEFA is raised so that their turnover rate is higher than expected from their concentration. A similar discrepancy has been reported for glycerol and triglyceride but the mechanisms are not known. In addition, experiments with labelled NEFA show that considerable quantities of the fat oxidized do not mix with the plasma NEFA pool.

In the liver, the major fates of NEFA are esterification to triglycerides (very-low-density lipoproteins, VLDL) and oxidation to ketone bodies. Both processes are controlled by hormones, glucagon increasing the proportion of NEFA converted to ketone bodies at the expense of VLDL and insulin doing the opposite. There is also some evidence for an anti-ketogenic effect of catecholamines at the hepatic level. It is often stated that ketogenesis is inhibited after injury and during sepsis. While this has been demonstrated in experimental sepsis and shown to be due to insulin, the evidence in man is not so convincing since many studies have failed to take proper account of the NEFA supply (Barton *et al.*, 1990). A recent thorough study in septic patients showed that ketone-body production was unaffected in the basal state but might or might not be lower than in control subjects when the NEFA supply was increased, depending on their antecedent nutrition; when ketogenesis was decreased, insulin did not appear to be responsible (Beylot *et al.*, 1989). The production of VLDL probably rises in the flow phase since, although their concentration is often not much higher than normal, their clearance is enhanced.

Protein metabolism

The well-known protein-catabolic effect of injury (reviewed by Barton *et al.*, 1990) may reflect either a decrease in the rate of protein synthesis or an increase in the rate of protein breakdown (see Chapter 48). The former is most often seen after elective surgery and may be mainly due to decreased food intake, whereas the latter occurs when injury is severe and is due to the trauma itself. Most recent work on the causation of these changes has been aimed at assessing factors such as cytokines and cyclo-oxygenase products and interest in hormones has been focused on the administration of exogenous hormones, especially GH

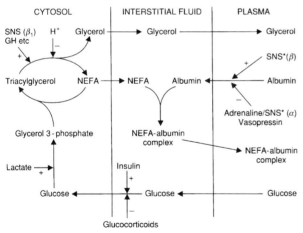

Figure 45.3 Factors influencing release of free fatty acids from adipose tissue in the ebb phase after injury. Not all the effects may be physiologically significant, and they may vary between species. SNS = sympathetic nervous system. *Neuronally released noradrenaline may cause vasoconstriction and increased microvascular permeability; these will have opposite effects on the availability of albumin for the removal of FFA. (Reproduced from Barton *et al.*, 1990, with permission.)

and IGF-1. Nevertheless, endogenous hormones, particularly glucocorticoids, could in principle contribute to the changes seen. Glucocorticoids are well known to cause net protein catabolism, with inhibition of protein synthesis and, less consistently, stimulation of protein breakdown (Sugden and Fuller, 1991). Many years ago the role of glucocorticoids after injury was dismissed as 'permissive' since adrenalectomy with constant steroid replacement did not prevent the increase in nitrogen excretion after long-bone fracture in the rat. In recent years this theory has implicitly been challenged with the attempts to reproduce the effects of injury by the 'triple-hormone infusion' described above. Although this causes an increase in nitrogen excretion, its relevance is again doubtful because plasma cortisol is higher than is usual during the flow phase (Frayn, 1986).

Recent animal experiments have addressed this question more directly. Matsusue and Walser (1992) studied wound healing 8 days after small-bowel transection and anastomosis in adrenalectomized rats maintained on different doses of corticosterone. Wound strength increased with the plasma corticosterone concentration up to a value approximating to its normal daily mean and then decreased as the concentration rose further. A similar concentration dependence for weight gain and other glucocorticoid actions has been attributed to opposing effects (respectively stimulatory and inhibitory) of occupation of Type I and Type II receptors (Devenport et al., 1989). Although these findings are not necessarily extrapolable to the general protein breakdown that follows injury, a role for Type II receptors has been demonstrated with the specific antagonist RU38486. This attenuated the stimulatory effect of experimental sepsis on protein breakdown but not its inhibitory effect on protein synthesis (Hall-Angerås et al., 1991). RU38486 also prevented the increase in both plasma urea and urea synthetic capacity in rats subjected to laparotomy and nephrectomy (Heindorff et al., 1991). Although these experiments were completed within 24 hours of inducing sepsis or injury, they suggest that glucocorticoids may well play a role in at least the early part of the protein-catabolic response.

Hormones may also play a part in the acute-phase response to trauma, but it is likely to be only a minor one (Fleck et al., 1985; Sehgal et al., 1989). This phenomenon, seen also in inflammation, infection and cancer, is characterized by increases in the concentrations of many plasma proteins (notably C-reactive protein and serum amyloid A in man, α_2-macroglobulin and α_1-acid glycoprotein in the rat; also fibrinogen, α_1-antitrypsin, caeruloplasmin and haptoglobin) and decreases in others (especially albumin, retinol-binding protein and transferrin). It is due in part to changes in the rates of synthesis of the relevant proteins in the liver, on

which trauma has a mostly anabolic effect, in contrast to muscle. There is strong evidence that these hepatic changes are mainly due to a direct action of IL-6 on hepatocytes. The hormones most likely to be involved are the corticosteroids, which have been reported to potentiate the effects of IL-6, but this seems to be very dependent on the preparation used.

Renal effects

Renal function after injury

The most prominent effect of injury on renal function is to cause sodium and water retention. The most complete descriptions are in patients undergoing elective surgery (Wynn, 1960; Clark, 1986). During and shortly after operation, urine output falls and a subnormal volume of hypertonic urine is excreted. However, the urine is not maximally concentrated and if sodium ion is given, only about half is excreted. Thereafter urine volume increases, but not as much as would be expected so that there is still positive water balance. The sodium balance depends upon the amount of sodium given, usually in parenteral fluids at this stage. If little sodium is administered, sodium excretion is also low so that the urine is hypotonic with respect to plasma; however, it is never maximally diluted. If saline is given, sodium excretion increases somewhat and the urine may well be hypertonic. However, less is excreted than given, so that the sodium balance is positive. After a few days these changes are reversed; there is a diuresis and sodium excretion rises, causing a net loss of sodium since intake (by now oral) is usually subnormal.

If injury is severe, variations in this pattern can sometimes be seen (Lucas, 1976, 1982; Davies, 1982). Marked hypotension may be associated with profound oliguria which in severe cases can progress to acute renal failure. Although urine output may not fall further, its concentration greatly decreases. Paradoxically, polyuria may be seen in patients who develop hyperdynamic sepsis after injury or even, in the early postoperative period, in severely injured patients who are not septic. This does not reflect restoration of fluid homoeostasis and may be superseded by oliguria.

Mechanism of urine formation

Before considering possible reasons for these changes, a brief discussion of the mechanism of urine formation (Burg, 1986; Klahr, 1988, Bankir et al., 1989) is appropriate. This is not completely understood and is usually described in terms of the function of the long-looped juxtamedullary nephrons. Although these compose only some 15% of the total, they play a disproportionate role in controlling sodium and water excretion. The kidney has a blood flow out of proportion to its size. Some of the plasma (around 20% under normal conditions) undergoes filtration in the glomerulus and enters the proximal tubule. There sodium ion is actively transported out of the protein-free ultra-filtrate and, owing to the high permeability of the nephron cells to water, is accompanied by an equivalent volume of water. The effluent from the proximal tubule is consequently approximately isotonic with the ultrafiltrate and normally has about 40% of its flow rate. It enters the thin descending limb of the loop of Henle which carries out little or no active transport but is fairly permeable to sodium; it is highly permeable to water but almost impermeable to urea. From the inner regions of the medulla the luminal fluid is returned towards the cortex first by the thin and then by the thick ascending limb of the loop of Henle. Neither is permeable to water. The thin limb does not perform active transport but is very permeable to sodium and moderately so to urea whereas the thick limb actively pumps sodium ion out of the nephron. The result of these character-istics is that an osmotic gradient composed mainly of sodium chloride and urea forms between the interstitial fluid of the cortex and that of the medulla, water is transported out of the descending limb of the loop so that its contents become hypertonic at the tip and sodium is transported out of the ascending limb so that the fluid emerging from the loop is very dilute. (In fact, computer models based on these characteristics cannot account fully for the concentrating ability of the kidney and additional mechanisms may be involved; for example, active transport of sodium into the descending loop of Henle.) The blood supply to the loop, in the form of the vasa recta, also has a counter-current arrangement so that the corticomedullary osmotic gradient is not dis-sipated.

The effluent from the loop of Henle enters the distal convoluted tubule and connecting tubule, both of which have little permeability to water but are capable of actively transporting sodium out of the tubular fluid. Their role in urine formation is not exactly understood, but it is likely to become even more hypotonic. The connecting tubule mer-ges into the collecting duct in which final regulation of the volume and composition of the urine takes place; the events in the more proximal parts of the nephron can be regarded as setting the scene for this. The collecting duct is divided functionally into three sections. The first, in the cortex, is again able to transport sodium ion out of the urine, but this capacity can now be increased by aldosterone. All three sections are almost impermeable to water unless vasopressin is present, when large quantities can be reabsorbed because of the high osmolality of the medullary interstitium; there is some evidence that aldosterone has a permissive effect on this response and that ANP decreases it. In addition, vasopressin increases the permeability of the third

section of the collecting duct, in the inner medulla, to urea.

Role of hormones

It is commonly believed that aldosterone is respon-sible for postoperative sodium retention and vaso-pressin, secreted in response to non-osmotic stimuli (the so-called 'syndrome of inappropriate anti-diuretic hormone secretion'), for the retention of water over the first day or two after surgery (Clark, 1986). However, not all the evidence is in support. Postoperative sodium retention persists after the aldosterone concentration has returned to normal and is not increased by adrenalectomy or spir-onolactone (Le Quesne et al., 1985; Clark, 1986). Likewise, during the first few hours after elective surgery there was little relationship between urine output and the plasma vasopressin concentration; a concentrated urine was frequently observed with-out a rise in vasopressin, while on some occasions there was positive free-water clearance in the presence of raised vasopressin concentrations (Le Quesne et al., 1985). Clearly, while it is likely that aldosterone and vasopressin do play a role after more severe injury when the rises in their concen-trations are larger and more persistent, they do not explain the renal response to elective surgery. Sodium retention is perhaps the greater mystery since it may be responsible for fluid retention beyond 2 days or so after surgery; for unknown reasons, fluid retention only persists if the patient is maintained on a high sodium intake (Clark, 1986).

In a series of carefully controlled experiments on experimental animals and patients, Wright and Gann (1965) concluded that postoperative sodium retention was due to increased reabsorption in the proximal and not the distal nephron. Part of the evidence was that the defect in urine-concentrating ability, which is part of the clinical picture, was still seen when mineralocorticoid and vasopressin con-centrations were high, implying a fall in medullary osmolality. Two interconnected hormone systems are known to stimulate sodium reabsorption in the proximal tubule: the renin–angiotensin system and the sympathoadrenal system. Both angiotensin II and noradrenaline have been postulated to cause preferential vasoconstriction of the efferent arter-iole, increasing the filtration fraction and thus protein concentration, oncotic pressure and water-absorbing capacity in the peritubular capillaries. Recent reviewers consider this mechanism may be oversimplified since both substances also cause preglomerular vasoconstriction (Kopp and DiBona, 1986; Mitchell and Navar, 1989); this applies partic-ularly to noradrenaline, and the evidence that angiotensin II increases the filtration fraction is not disputed. Besides their vasomotor effects, both angiotensin II and noradrenaline stimulate prox-imal tubular sodium transport directly, the effect of noradrenaline being mediated by α_1-adrenoceptors.

In addition, angiotensin II alters the sensitivity of tubuloglomerular feedback so that a decrease in flux of sodium chloride in the distal nephron does not cause a compensatory rise in glomerular filtration rate.

The effects of noradrenaline on proximal tubule function have mostly been described in experiments using renal nerve stimulation (either direct or elicited reflexly) and any such effects after trauma are much more likely to be due to renal nerve activity than to circulating catecholamines. Similarly, if angiotensin II plays a role the lack of consistent change in plasma renin activity suggests that it too is likely to be generated locally within the kidney. Excessive vasoconstriction by the sympathoadrenal and renin–angiotensin systems (exacerbated, after crush injury, by products of ischaemia such as myoglobin) is likely to be implicated in oliguria progressing to renal failure in patients with very severe injury or sepsis. The reason why some patients, such as those with hyperdynamic sepsis, exhibit polyuria is uncertain and various explanations have been proposed (Lucas, 1976, 1982). The mechanisms by which hormones might influence renal function after injury are summarized in Figure 45.4.

Consequences of renal changes

As implied by the description given earlier, the effects of post-trauma salt and water retention depend on the management of the patient. If sodium-poor fluids such as 5% glucose are given the consequence is hyponatraemia. In some patients, particularly those with severe injuries, this may be exacerbated by extrarenal events (Goldberg, 1981). Loss of sodium can occur into fluid sequestered at the site of injury, across burned surfaces or into cells as a result of hypoxic damage to membranes, causing increased permeability or impaired sodium pumping (Flear, 1970). Various groups may be at particular risk of post-trauma hyponatraemia. A large survey of postoperative patients concluded that it was almost invariable after renal transplant surgery, fairly frequent (about 20%) in patients undergoing cardiovascular or abdominal surgery and rare after other procedures, including orthopaedic surgery (Chung et al., 1986). In none was the hyponatraemia severe enough to cause obvious neurological abnormalities. However, recent data indicate a high prevalence in elderly patients after orthopaedic surgery (M.A. Horan, personal communication). Another study, in contrast, showed that premenopausal women were most susceptible to postoperative hyponatraemia, which was severe enough to cause seizures and respiratory arrest (Arieff, 1986). It is likely that these disparate reports reflect variations in fluid management in the centres concerned.

Immunological effects

It is well known that both trauma (see Chapter 49) and treatment with hormones, especially corticosteroids, are capable of depressing the body's defence mechanisms, including non-specific phagocytosis and the immune system. However, few

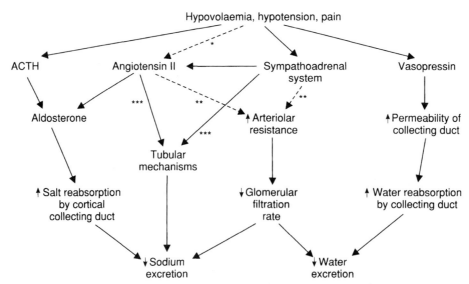

Figure 45.4 Endocrine mechanisms potentially able to cause sodium and fluid retention after injury. Many intermediate steps and possible interactions are omitted, e.g. tubuloglomerular feedback and other intrarenal feedback cycles involving local generation of angiotensin II and prostaglandin E_2, changes in the corticomedullary osmotic gradient, etc. The mechanisms shown do not always seem to apply in practice, as explained in the text. * Only likely to apply in marked hypotension. ** Applies to large rises in concentration or activity. *** Applies to smaller rises in concentration.

experiments have been directed specifically at evaluating the role of endogenous hormones in the changes in phagocytic and immunological function after injury. Usually the best one can do is to compare the nature and time-course of the changes seen after injury and after administration of a particular hormone, but even this is beset by difficulties. On the one hand, interest in host defence after injury has been focused on clinical problems such as septic shock or infection of burned skin. The patients studied have therefore tended to be those most at risk, in whom hormonally mediated events may be overshadowed by the effects of factors such as malnutrition and hypoxia. The same is true of animal models used to mimic such patients. On the other hand, most studies on the effects of corticosteroids on defence mechanisms have used large doses of synthetic glucocorticoids and in many experiments *in vitro* the concentrations of these steroids have been even higher than those found *in vivo*.

Polymorphonuclear leucocytes

Trauma, at least in the form of burn injury, leads to an increased number of circulating polymorphonuclear leucocytes (PMNs). However, the response is variable and the increase may be preceded or followed by neutropenia (Davies, 1982; Felix and Davis, 1986). Moreover, the PMNs may be less effective in defence against infection. The function of PMNs is usually divided into three components: chemotaxis to the site of the stimulus, phagocytosis of bacteria (which have been coated with opsonins) and intracellular killing of the phagocytosed bacteria. There is evidence for impairment of all three functions after severe injury, but chemotaxis and intracellular killing are affected more consistently than phagocytosis (Davies, 1982; Felix and Davis, 1986; see Chapter 49).

Both corticosteroids and adrenaline (acting through β receptors) are capable of causing neutrophilia (Calvano, 1986; Butterfield and Gleich, 1989). Both hormones decrease the adherence of PMNs to endothelium and thus mobilize the marginated pool; corticosteroids may potentiate the effects of adrenaline by inducing β-adrenergic receptors and preventing desensitization with prolonged stimulation (Calvano, 1986). Corticosteroids also cause release of PMNs from the bone-marrow storage compartment (Calvano, 1986) and decrease egress of cells from the circulation (Butterfield and Gleich, 1989). Corticosteroids are capable of impairing all three PMN functions but the evidence is contradictory. Studies of chemotaxis have mostly used very high concentrations of glucocorticoids and, although phagocytosis and bacterial killing have been studied in PMNs from corticosteroid-treated patients, the results have usually been negative, despite evidence for impairment of metabolic processes (such as superoxide ion formation)

necessary for bacterial killing (Butterfield and Gleich, 1989). Such observations suggest that corticosteroids are not responsible for the impairment in PMN function after severe injury, although they may well play a part in the accompanying neutrophilia (Calvano, 1986).

Mononuclear phagocytes

The mononuclear phagocytes (monocytes and macrophages) have a wide variety of roles in defences against infection and the effects of injury are likewise complex. The number of peripheral blood monocytes may increase after injury (Antonacci, 1986; Wood *et al.*, 1988). Impairment of phagocytosis by the reticuloendothelial system develops rapidly and persists for a period that depends on the severity of injury (Davies, 1982; Altura, 1986). The degree and characteristics of the change seem to vary between tissues (Davies, 1982) but circulating monocytes are among the cells affected (Calvano, 1986). The ratio of facilitatory to inhibitory monocytes decreases and associated with this is impairment of antigen presentation and processing (Miller-Graziano *et al.*, 1989). Another, related function of mononuclear phagocytes is to produce cytokines. The regulation of cytokine production is very complex because of many potential feedback loops, involving stimulatory and inhibitory (via prostaglandin E_2) effects of different cytokines on each other's production not only in monocytes but also in endothelial cells, fibroblasts, etc. The increased number of inhibitory monocytes would be expected to increase the production of tumour-necrosis factor (TNF) (Miller-Graziano *et al.*, 1989), but the cytokine whose plasma concentration increases most consistently is IL-6 (see 'Hypothalamo-pituitary-adrenal axis' above). Monocytes from severely injured patients may show decreased production of plasminogen activator and increased thromboplastin synthesis (Miller *et al.*, 1982).

The effects of glucocorticoids on mononuclear phagocytes are nearly all inhibitory. The number of monocytes in the peripheral circulation is reduced (Cupps and Fauci, 1982; Guyre and Munck, 1989). Maturation of monocytes to tissue macrophages is also inhibited (Guyre and Munck, 1989). At least some experiments show inhibition of monocyte chemotaxis but the effects of glucocorticoids on bacterial killing seem rather variable and lengthy exposure to the steroids is required. Glucocorticoids have inhibitory effects on antigen presentation by mononuclear phagocytes and on the production of IL-1, TNF, plasminogen activator and prostaglandins, but many of these actions have only been demonstrated *in vitro* and have yet to be confirmed *in vivo* (Bateman *et al.*, 1989; Guyre and Munck, 1989). It is clear that the effects of glucocorticoids differ in many respects from those of injury, although the possibility of their involvement in some of the changes in monocyte function after trauma cannot be ruled out. The effects of trauma on reticuloendothelial cell phagocytosis have been attributed to impairment of microcirculation and the hormones likely to play a role in it are those with vasoconstrictive properties (Altura, 1986).

Lymphocytes

The best-described immunological changes after trauma are those in T-lymphocyte function. There is a rapid loss of circulating T cells after moderate to severe injury and the number remains low for 24–48 hours (Davies, 1982; Wood et al., 1988). This represents a change in T-helper cells; the number of T-suppressor cells does not fall and after very severe injury may actually rise. Corticosteroids similarly cause a selective depletion of T-helper cells which in man (a 'steroid-resistant' species) is due to redistribution rather than lysis (Cupps and Fauci, 1982; Calvano, 1986; Wood et al., 1988). This similarity and the compatible time-course of the changes in T-cell numbers with those in plasma cortisol suggest a causal relationship, although direct verification is lacking. Unlike cortisol, adrenaline causes a transient increase in peripheral lymphocyte count although it too decreases the T-helper : suppressor cell ratio (Calvano, 1986).

There has been much interest in the function of T-lymphocytes after trauma, arising from the claim that impaired skin reactivity to recall antigens predicts the occurrence of septic complications after injury (Christou, 1986; see Chapter 49). There are reports that lymphocyte proliferation in response to non-specific mitogens is decreased after injury (Davies, 1982; Antonacci, 1986; Wood et al., 1988). The depression is related to the severity of injury and, if present at all, is usually small and transient; some studies have even shown enhancement, and persistent impairment of lymphocyte transformation is associated with fatal sepsis (Davies, 1982; Wood et al., 1988). There are also reports of decreased lymphocyte transformation in response to antigens (Wood et al., 1988). The changes in T-lymphocyte responses are delayed and occur after the number of circulating cells has returned to normal (Wood et al., 1988).

It is well known that corticosteroids cause decreases in the proliferative responses to both non-specific mitogens and antigens (Cupps and Fauci, 1982; Calvano, 1986; Wood et al., 1988). Catecholamines, acting through β-receptors, have also been reported to suppress T-cell responses to mitogens (Wood et al., 1988), and insulin resistance could conceivably have the same effect since insulin is mitogenic for lymphocytes once they have been stimulated by another mitogen, when they begin to express insulin receptors (Snow, 1985; Calvano, 1986). However, doubt has been cast on the role of hormones in causing impaired T-lymphocyte function after injury, largely because this response is not correlated, as regards either its magnitude or its time-course, with that in cortisol or other hormones (Wood et al., 1988). It has also been claimed that, with the exception of the autologous mixed lymphocyte reaction, the cortisol concentrations required are too high (Calvano, 1986). A preferred explanation is that an immunosuppressive factor, which is polypeptide or protein in nature, circulates after injury (Davies, 1982; Calvano, 1986; Wood et al., 1988). It is also likely that impairments of lymphocyte function are partly secondary to those in mononuclear phagocytes with their associated changes in cytokine production.

The changes in humoral immunity after injury are not so well defined. The number of circulating B lymphocytes may rise or fall, depending upon the severity of the injury (Davies, 1982; Wood et al., 1988). Patients with severe injury may show a decrease in the concentration of circulating immunoglobulins, particularly IgG (Davies, 1982; Wood et al., 1988). However, this is usually attributed to loss in the wound and there is little evidence for changes in immunoglobulin production by lymphocytes in vitro. Likewise, studies on the production of specific antibodies after injury have not given consistent results (Antonacci, 1986; Wood et al., 1988). The effects of corticosteroids on B-cell numbers and function are similarly not striking. The number of B cells in the circulation tends to fall but not as much as the number of T lymphocytes, while contradictory effects of corticosteroids on B-cell responses have been reported (Cupps and Fauci, 1982; Wood et al., 1988).

Glucocorticoids and inflammation

In 1984, Munck et al. proposed that the function of the adrenocortical response to stress was to counteract other responses and prevent them from developing to the point of causing harm, for example by causing autoimmunity by exposure to damaged tissues. Such a role would explain why glucocorticoid concentrations are invariably raised in stress, which is a mystery if their effects are merely permissive (see 'Protein metabolism' above). The hypothesis was focused particularly on the inflammatory and immunological systems but was also applied (rather less convincingly) to other aspects of the response to injury. In support of it, Munck et al. (1984) pointed out that the anti-inflammatory effects of glucocorticoids are mediated by the same receptors and have the same steroid specificity as other glucocorticoid effects, so that the distinction between physiological and pharmacological actions is artificial. Subsequent studies in experimental animals have confirmed that abolition of endogenous glucocorticoid effects, either by adrenalectomy or by treatment with RU38486, enhances the inflammatory responses to agents such as carrageenan (Laue et al., 1989). It is therefore probable that all the immunological sequelae of injury are influenced to some extent by glucocorticoids even though these do not appear to be primarily responsible for the impairment of defence mechanisms. It is worth noting that the changes most likely to be due directly to glucocorticoids, those in circulating neutrophil and lymphocyte numbers, may not conform to the hypothesis of Munck *et al.* (1984), since they occur rapidly and presumably represent a stage in the initial activation of defence mechanisms rather than their subsequent suppression.

Munck *et al.* (1984) were particularly interested in the inhibitory effects of glucocorticoids on cytokine production, part of a regulatory cycle involving also stimulation of the HPA axis by cytokines (see 'Hypothalamo-pituitary-adrenal axis' above). It is now clear that this cycle is even more complex than at first envisaged (Bateman *et al.*, 1989; Blalock, 1989). Glucocorticoids may also induce cytokine receptors, resulting in a biphasic dose-response curve, with first an increase and then a decrease in the concentration of cytokine-receptor complexes as the steroid concentration rises. The first phase has been postulated as a general explanation for the permissive effects of low glucocorticoid concentrations (Munck and Náraj-Fejes-Tóth, 1992); however, this does not take into account the possible contribution of Type I corticosteroid receptors (see Protein metabolism). Another interaction is between activated glucocorticoid receptors and AP-1, a major transcription factor for cytokines. Binding of these two proteins appears to cause loss of activity of both (Barnes and Adcock, 1993; Truss and Beato, 1993), so that not only may glucocorticoids antagonize the effects of cytokines at the transcriptional level but the presence of large quantities of cytokines could lead to general resistance to the effects of glucocorticoids. Many other interactions between transcription factors are being discovered, and their possible application to trauma is likely to be a question of great interest in the future.

REFERENCES

Albiston A.L., Obeyesekere V.R., Smith R.E., Krozowski, Z.S. (1994). Cloning and tissue distribution of the human 11β-hydroxysteroid dehydrogenase type 2 enzyme. *Molec. Cell. Endocrinol.,* **105**, R11–17.

Altura B.M. (1986). Endothelial and reticuloendothelial cell function: roles in injury and low-flow states. In *The Scientific Basis for the Care of the Critically Ill* (Little R.A., Frayn K.N., eds). Manchester: Manchester University Press, pp. 259–74.

Anderson I.D., Forsling M.L., Little R.A., Pyman J.A. (1989). Acute injury is a potent stimulus for vasopressin release in man. *J. Physiol.,* **416**, 28P.

Antonacci A.C. (1986). Immune dysfunction and immunomodulation following trauma. In *Advances in Host Defense Mechanisms*, Vol 6. *Host Defenses in Trauma And Surgery* (Davis J.M., Shires G.T., eds). New York: Raven, pp. 81–109.

Antoni F.A. (1993). Vasopressinergic control of pituitary adrenocorticotropin secretion comes of age. *Frontiers Neuroendocrinol.,* **14**, 76–122.

Arieff A.I. (1986). Hyponatremia, convulsions, respiratory arrest, and permanent brain damage after elective surgery in healthy women. *New Engl. J. Med.,* **314**, 1529–35.

Assenmacher I., Szafarczyk A., Alonso G., Ixart G., Barbanel G. (1987). Physiology of neural pathways affecting CRH secretion. *Ann.. NY Acad. Sci.,* **512**, 149–61.

Bankir L., Bouby N., Trinh-Trang-Tan M.-M. (1989). The role of the kidney in the maintenance of water balance. *Baillière's Clin. Endocrinol. Metab.,* **3**, 249–311.

Barnes P.J., Adcock I. (1993). Anti-inflammatory actions of steroids: molecular mechanisms. *Trends Pharmacol. Sci.,* **14**, 436–41.

Barton R.N. (1977). Effect of limb ischaemia and scalding on the concentrations of growth hormone and corticosterone in rat plasma. *J. Endocrinol.,* **73**, 347–53.

Barton R.N. (1985). Neuroendocrine mobilization of body fuels after injury. *Bri. Med, Bull.,* **41**, 218–25.

Barton R.N. (1987). The neuroendocrinology of physical injury. *Baillière's Clin. Endocrinol. Metab.,* **1**, 355–74.

Barton R.N. (1996). Endocrine responses to trauma in old age. In *Injury in the Aging* (Horan M.A., Little R.A., eds). Cambridge: Cambridge University Press (in press).

Barton R.N., Frayn, K.N., Little, R.A. (1990). Trauma, burns and surgery. In *The Metabolic and Molecular Basis of Acquired Disease*, Vol 1 (Cohen R.D., Lewis B., Alberti K.G.M.M., Denman A.M., eds). London: Baillière Tindall, pp. 684–717.

Bateman A., Singh A., Kral T., Solomon S. (1989). The immune hypothalamic-pituitary-adrenal axis. *Endocrine Rev.,* **10**, 92–112.

Baxter J.D., Tyrrell J.B. (1986). The adrenal cortex. In *Endocrinology and Metabolism*, 2nd edn (Felig P., Baxter J.D., Broadus A.E., Frohman L.A., eds). New York: McGraw-Hill, pp. 511–650.

Ben-Jonathan N., Arbogast L.A., Hyde J.F. (1989). Neuroendocrine regulation of prolactin release. *Prog. Neurobiol.,* **33**, 399–447.

Bereiter D.A., Plotsky P.M., Gann D.S. (1982). Tooth pulp stimulation potentiates the adrenocorticotropin response to hemorrhage in cats. *Endocrinology,* **111**, 1127–32.

Bereiter D.A., Engeland W.C., Gann D.S. (1986). Peripheral venous catecholamines versus adrenal secretory rates after brain stem stimulation in cats. *Am. J. Physiol.,* **251**, E14–20.

Beylot M., Guiraud M., Grau G., Bouletreau P. (1989). Regulation of ketone body flux in septic patients. *Am. J. Physiol.,* **257**, E665–74.

Blalock J.E. (1989). A molecular basis for bidirectional communication between the immune and neuroendocrine systems. *Physiol. Rev.,* **69**, 1–32.

Brandi L.S., Frediani M., Oleggini M., Mosca F., Cerri M., Boni C., Pecori N., Buzzigoli G., Ferrannini E. (1990). Insulin resistance after surgery: normalization by insulin treatment. *Clin. Sci.,* **79**, 443–50.

Brenner B.M., Ballermann B.J., Gunning M.E., Zeidel M.L. (1990). Diverse biological actions of atrial natriuretic peptide. *Physiol. Rev.,* **70**, 665–99.

Breslow M.J. (1992). Regulation of adrenal medullary and cortical blood flow. *Am. J. Physiol.,* **262**, H1317–30.

Buckingham J.C., Loxley H.D., Taylor A.D., Flower R.J. (1994). Cytokines, glucocorticoids and neuroendocrine function. *Pharmacol. Res.*, **30**, 35–42.

Burg M.B. (1986). Renal handling of sodium, chloride, water, amino acids and glucose. In *The Kidney*, 3rd edn (Brenner B.M., Rector F.C. Jr., eds). Philadelphia: Saunders, pp. 145–75.

Butterfield J.H., Gleich G.J. (1989). Anti-inflammatory effects of glucocorticoids on eosinophils and neutrophils. In *Anti-inflammatory Steroid Action* (Schleimer R.P., Claman H.N., Oronsky A., eds). San Diego: Academic Press, pp. 151–98.

Calogero A.E., Norton J.A., Sheppard B.C., Listwak S.J., Cromack D.T., Wall R., Jensen R.T., Chrousos G.P. (1992). Pulsatile activation of the hypothalamic-pituitary-adrenal axis during major surgery. *Metabolism*, **41**, 839–45.

Calvano S.E. (1986). Hormonal mediation of immune dysfunction following thermal and traumatic injury. In *Advances in Host Defense Mechanisms* Vol. 6. *Host Defenses in Trauma and Surgery* (Davis J.M., Shires G.T., eds). New York: Raven, pp. 111–42.

Carey R.M., Sen S. (1986). Recent progress in the control of aldosterone secretion. *Recent Prog. Hormone Res.*, **42**, 251–89.

Carlson D.E., Gann D.S. (1991). Response of plasma adrenocorticotropin to injections of L-glutamate or norepinephrine in the dorsal rostral pons of cats. *Endocrinology*, **128**, 3021–31.

Carlson D.E., Gann D.S. (1992). α-Adrenergic input in the locus coeruleus modulates plasma adrenocorticotropin in cats. *Endocrinology*, **130**, 2795–803.

Carlson D.E., De Maria E.J., Campbell R.W., Chrostek C., Graeber C.T., Gann D.S. (1989). Atrial peptide release after hemorrhage in unanesthetized swine. *Am. J. Physiol.*, **256**, R915–21.

Carlson D.E., Klemcke H.G., Gann D.S. (1990). Response of prolactin to hemorrhage is similar to that of adrenocorticotropin in swine. *Am. J. Physiol.*, **258**, R645–9.

Casanueva F.F. (1992). Physiology of growth hormone secretion and action. *Endocrinol. Metab. Clin. North Am.*, **21**, 483–517.

Cerchio G.M., Persico P.A., Jeffay H. (1973). Inhibition of insulin release during hypovolemic shock. *Metabolism*, **22**, 1449–58.

Charlton B.G. (1990). Adrenal cortical innervation and glucocorticoid secretion. *J. Endocrinol.*, **126**, 5–8.

Chikanza I.C., Petrou P., Kingsley G., Chrousos G., Panayi G.S. (1992). Defective hypothalamic response to immune and inflammatory stimuli in patients with rheumatoid arthritis. *Arthr. Rheum.*, **35**, 1281–8.

Christou N.V. (1986). Delayed hypersensitivity in the surgical patient. In *Advances in Host Defense Mechanisms*, Vol. 6. *Host Defenses in Trauma and Surgery* (Davis J.M., Shires G.T., eds). New York: Raven, pp. 143–68.

Chung H.-M., Kluge R., Schrier R.W., Anderson R.J. (1986). Postoperative hyponatremia. A prospective study. *Arch. Intern. Med.*, **146**, 333–6.

Clark R.G. (1986). Postoperative water and sodium metabolism. In *The Scientific Basis for the Care of the Critically Ill* (Little R.A., Frayn K.N., eds). Manchester: Manchester University Press, pp. 231–44.

Clark J.D.A., Raggatt P.R., Edwards O.M. (1988). Hypothalamic hypogonadism following major head injury. *Clin. Endocrinol.*, **29**, 153–65.

Cruickshank A.M., Fraser W.D., Burns H.J.G., van Damme J., Shenkin A. (1990). Response of serum interleukin-6 in patients undergoing elective surgery of varying severity. *Clin. Sci.*, **79**, 161–5.

Cupps T.R., Fauci A.S. (1982). Corticosteroid-mediated immunoregulation in man. *Immunol. Rev.*, **65**, 133–55.

Cuthbertson D.P. (1942). Post-shock metabolic response. *Lancet*, **i**, 433–7.

Dallman M.F., Yates F.E. (1968). Anatomical and functional mapping of central neural input and feedback pathways of the adrenocortical system. *Mem. Soc. Endocrinol.*, **17**, 39–72.

Dallman M.F., Akana S.F., Cascio C.S., Darlington D.N., Jacobson L., Levin N. (1987). Regulation of ACTH secretion: variations on a theme of B. *Recent Prog. Hormone Res.*, **43**, 113–67.

Dallman M.F., Akana S.F., Scribner K.A., Bradbury M.J., Walker C.-D., Strack A.M., Cascio C.S. (1992). Stress, feedback and facilitation in the hypothalamo-pituitary-adrenal axis. *J. Neuroendocrinol.*, **4**, 517–26.

Daughaday W.H., Rotwein P. (1989). Insulin-like growth factors I and II. Peptide, messenger ribonucleic acid and gene structures, serum, and tissue concentrations. *Endocrine Rev.*, **10**, 68–91.

Davenport M.L., Isley W.L., Pucilowska J.B., Pemberton L.B., Lyman B., Underwood L.E., Clemmons D.R. (1992). Insulin-like growth factor-binding protein-3 proteolysis is induced after elective surgery. *J. Clin. Endocrinol. Metab.*, **75**, 590–5.

Davies J.W.L. (1982). *Physiological Responses to Burning Injury*. London: Academic.

Davies S.C., Wass J.A.H., Ross R.J.M. et al. (1991). The induction of a specific protease for insulin-like growth factor binding protein-3 in the circulation during severe illness. *J. Endocrinol.*, **130**, 469–73.

de Kloet E.R. (1991). Brain corticosteroid receptor balance and homeostatic control. *Frontiers Neuroendocrinol.*, **12**, 95–164.

Delitala P., Tomasi P., Virdis R. (1987). Prolactin, growth hormone and thyrotropin-thyroid hormone secretion during stress states in man. *Baillière's Clin. Endocrinol. Metab.*, **1**, 391–414.

Devenport L., Knehans A., Sundstrom A., Thomas T. (1989). Corticosterone's dual metabolic actions. *Life Sci.*, **45**, 1389–96.

Doncaster H.D., Barton R.N., Horan M.A., Roberts N.A. (1993). Factors influencing cortisol-adrenocorticotrophin relationships in elderly women with upper femur fracture. *J. Trauma*, **34**, 49–55.

Drucker W.R., Chadwick C.D.J., Gann D.S. (1981). Transcapillary refill in hemorrhage and shock. *Arch. Surg.*, **116**, 1344–53.

Dunn A.J. (1993). Role of cytokines in infection-induced stress. *Ann. NY Acad. Sci.*, **697**, 189–202.

Dunning B.E., Taborsky G.J. Jr (1988). Galanin-sympathetic neurotransmitter in the endocrine pancreas? *Diabetes*, **37**, 1157–62.

Edwards O.M., Clark J.D.A. (1986). Post-traumatic hypopituitarism. Six cases and a review of the literature. *Medicine*, **65**, 281–90.

Engeland W.C., Miller P., Gann D.S. (1989). Dissociation between changes in plasma bioactive and immunoreactive adrenocorticotropin after hemorrhage in awake dogs. *Endocrinology*, **124**, 2978–85.

Engler D., Liu J.-P., Clarke I.J., Funder J.W. (1994). Corticotropin-release inhibitory factor. Evidence for dual stimulatory and inhibitory regulation over adrenocorticotropin secretion and biosynthesis. *Trends Endocrinol. Metab.*, **5**, 272–83.

Feibel J., Kelly M., Lee L, Woolf P. (1983). Loss of adrenocortical suppression after acute brain injury: role of increased intracranial pressure and brain stem function. *J. Clin. Endocrinol. Metab.*, **57**, 1245–50.

Felix J.C., Davis J.M. (1986). Neutrophil function in thermally injured patients. In *Advances in Host Defense Mechanisms*, Vol. 6. *Host Defenses in Trauma and Surgery* (Davis J.M., Shires G.T., eds). New York: Raven, pp. 63–79.

Fisher L.A., Brown M.R. (1991). Central regulation of stress responses: regulation of the autonomic nervous system and visceral function by corticotrophin releasing factor-41. *Baillière's Clin. Endocrinol. Metab.*, **5**, 35–50.

Flear C.T.G. (1970). Electrolyte and body water changes after trauma. *J. Clin. Path., 23 Suppl. (R. Coll. Pathologists)*, **4**, 16–31.

Fleck A., Colley C.M., Myers M.A. (1985). Liver export proteins and trauma. *Brit. Med. Bull.*, **41**, 265–73.

Frayn K.N. (1986). Hormonal control of metabolism in trauma and sepsis. *Clin. Endocrinol.*, **24**, 577–99.

Gold N.I., Singleton E., Macfarlane D.A., Moore F.D. (1958). Quantitative determination of the urinary cortisol metabolites, 'tetrahydro F,' 'allotetrahydro F' and 'tetrahydro E': effects of adrenocorticotropin and complex trauma in the human. *J. Clin. Invest.*, **37**, 813–23.

Goldberg M. (l98l). Hyponatremia. *Med. Clin. North Am.*, **65**, 251–69.

Goldstein D.S. (1987). Stress-induced activation of the sympathetic nervous system. *Baillière's Clin. Endocrinol. Metab.*, **1**, 253–78.

Guyre P.M., Munck A. (1989). Glucocorticoid actions on monocytes and macrophages. In *Anti-inflammatory Steroid Action* (Schleimer R.P., Claman H.N., Oronsky A., eds). San Diego: Academic Press, pp. 199–225.

Hackenthal E., Paul M., Ganten D., Taugner R. (1990). Morphology, physiology, and molecular biology of renin secretion. *Physiol. Rev.*, **70**, 1067–116.

Hall-Angerås M., Angerås U., Zamir O., Hasselgren P.-O., Fischer, J.E. (1991). Effect of the glucocorticoid receptor antagonist RU38486 on muscle protein breakdown in sepsis. *Surgery,* **109**, 468–73.

Halter J.B., Pflug A.E. (1980). Relationship of impaired insulin secretion during surgical stress to anesthesia and catecholamine release. *J. Clin. Endocrinol. Metab.*, **51**, 1093–8.

Heindorff H., Almdal T.P., Vilstrup H. (1991). Blockade of glucocorticoid receptors prevents the increase in urea synthesis after hysterectomy in rats. *Eur. J. Clin. Invest.*, **21**, 625–30.

Herington A.C., Ymer S.I., Tiong, T.S. (1991). Does the serum binding protein for growth hormone have a functional role? *Acta Endocrinol.*, **124**, (Suppl. 2), 14–20.

Hintze G., Braverman L.E., Ingbar, S.H. (1991). The effect of surgical stress on the *in vitro* metabolism of thyroxine by rat liver, kidney, and brain. *Endocrinology,* **128**, 146–52.

Hjemdahl P. (1993). Plasma catecholamines – analytical challenges and physiological limitations. *Baillière's Clin. Endocrinol. Metab.*, **7**, 307–53.

Imura H., Fukata J., Mori T. (1991). Cytokines and endocrine function: an interaction between the immune and neuroendocrine systems. *Clin. Endocrinol.*, **35**, 107–15.

Jacobson L., Sapolsky R. (1991). The role of the hippocampus in feedback regulation of the hypothalamic-pituitary-adrenal axis. *Endocrine Rev.*, **12**, 118–34.

Jones M.T., Gillham, B. (1988). Factors involved in the regulation of adrenocorticotropic hormone/β-lipotropic hormone. *Physiol. Rev.*, **68**, 743–818.

Keller-Wood M.E., Dallman M.F. (1984). Corticosteroid inhibition of ACTH secretion. *Endocrine Rev.*, **5**, 1–24.

Kennedy R.L., Jones, T.H. (1991). Cytokines in endocrinology: their roles in health and disease. *J. Endocrinol.*, **129**, 167–78.

Kenyon C.J., Jardine A.G. (1989). Atrial natriuretic peptide: water and electrolyte homeostasis. *Baillière's Clin. Endocrinol. Metab.*, **3**, 431–50.

Kidd J.E., Gilchrist N.L., Utley R.J. et al. (1987). Effect of opiate, general anaesthesia and surgery on plasma atrial natriuretic peptide levels in man. *Clin Exp. Pharmacol. Physiol.*, **14**, 755–60.

Klahr S. (1988). Structure and function of the kidneys. In *Cecil Textbook of Medicine*, 18th edn (Wyngaarden J.B., Smith L.H. Jr, eds). Philadelphia: Saunders, pp. 508–20.

Kopp U.C., Di Bona G.F. (1986). Catecholamines and neurosympathetic control of renal function. In *Kidney Hormones*, Volume III (Fisher J.W., ed). London: Academic, pp. 621–60.

Langer S.Z., Arbilla S. (1990). Presynaptic receptors on peripheral noradrenergic neurons. *Ann. NY Acad. Sci.*, **604**, 7–16.

Laue L., Kawai S., Udelsman R., Chrousos G.P. et al. (1989). Glucocorticoid antagonists: pharmacological attributes of a prototype antiglucocorticoid (RU486). In *Anti-inflammatory Steroid Action. Basic and Clinical Aspects* (Schleimer R.P., Claman H.N., Oronsky A., eds). San Diego: Academic, pp. 303–29.

Le Quesne L.P., Cochrane J.P.S., Fieldman N.R. (1985). Fluid and electrolyte disturbances after trauma: the role of pituitary and adrenocortical hormones. *Bri. Med. Bull.*, **41**, 212–17.

Lilly M.P., Gann D.S. (1992). The hypothalamic-pituitary-adrenal-immune axis: a critical assessment. *Arch. Surg.*, **127**, 1463–74.

Lilly M.P., Engeland W.C., Gann D.S. (1982). Adrenal response to repeated hemorrhage: implications for studies of trauma. *J. Trauma*, **22**, 809–14.

Lilly M.P., Engeland W.C., Gann D.S. (1986). Adrenal medullary responses to repeated hemorrhage in the conscious dog. *Am. J. Physiol.*, **251**, R1193–9.

Lucas C.E. (1976). The renal response to acute injury and sepsis. *Surg. Clin. North Am.*, **56**, 953–75.

Lucas C.E. (1982). Renal considerations in the injured patient. *Surg. Clin. North Am.*, **62**, 133–48.

Matsusue S., Walser M. (1992). Healing of intestinal anastomoses in adrenalectomized rats given corticosterone. *Am J. Physiol.*, **263**, R164–8.

McEwen B.S., de Kloet E.R., Rostene W. (1986). Adrenal steroid receptors and actions in the nervous system. *Physiol. Rev.*, **66**, 1121–88.

Miller R.E. (1981). Pancreatic neuroendocrinology: peripheral neural mechanisms in the regulation of the islets of Langerhans. *Endocrine Rev.*, **2**, 471–94.

Miller S.E., Miller C.L., Trunkey D.D. (1982). The immune consequences of trauma. *Surg. Clin. North Am.*, **62**, 167–81.

Miller A.H., Spencer R.L., Pulera M., Kang S., McEwen B.S., Stein M. (1992). Adrenal steroid receptor activation in rat brain and pituitary following dexamethasone: implications for the dexamethasone suppression test. *Biol. Psychiatry*, **32**, 850–69.

Miller-Graziano C.L., Szabo G., Takayama T., Wu J. (1989). Alterations of monocyte function following major injury. In *Immune Consequences of Trauma, Shock, and Sepsis* (Faist E., Ninnemann J., Green D., eds). Berlin: Springer-Verlag, pp. 95–108.

Mitchell K.D., Navar L.G. (1989). The renin-angiotensin-aldosterone system in volume control. *Baillière's Clin. Endocrinol. Metab.*, **3**, 393–430.

Müller E.E. (1987). Neural control of somatotropic function. *Physiological Rev.*, **67**, 962–1053.

Munck A., Náraj-Fejes-Tóth A. (1992). The ups and downs of glucocorticoid physiology. Permissive and suppressive effects revisited. *Molec. Cell. Endocrinol.*, **90**, C1–4.

Munck A., Guyre P.M., Holbrook, N.J. (1984). Physiological functions of glucocorticoids in stress and their relation to pharmacological actions. *Endocrine Rev.*, **5**, 25–44.

Naito Y., Fukata J., Tamai S., Seo N., Nakai Y., Mori K., Imura H. (1991). Biphasic changes in hypothalamo-pituitary-adrenal function during the early recovery period after major abdominal surgery. *J. Clin. Endocrinol. Metab.*, **73**, 111–17.

Nijsten M.W.N., Hack C.E., Helle M., ten Duis H.J., Klasen H.J., Aarden L.A. (1991). Interleukin-6 and its relation to the humoral immune response and clinical parameters in burned patients. *Surgery*, **109**, 761–7.

Nussey S.S., Page S.R., Ang V.T.Y., Jenkins J.S. (1988). The response of plasma oxytocin to surgical stress. *Clin. Endocrinol.*, **28**, 277–82.

Owens M.J., Nemeroff C.B. (1991). Physiology and pharmacology of corticotropin-releasing factor. *Pharmacol. Rev.*, **43**, 425–73.

Parker L.N. (1991). Control of adrenal androgen secretion. *Endocrinol. Metab. Clin. North Am.*, **20**, 401–21.

Plotsky P.M. (1987). Regulation of hypophysiotropic factors mediating ACTH secretion. *Ann. NY Acad. Sci.*, **512**, 205–17.

Plotsky P.M., Cunningham E.T. Jr, Widmaier E.P. (1989). Catecholaminergic modulation of corticotropin-releasing factor and adrenocorticotropin secretion. *Endocrine Rev.*, **10**, 437–58.

Raff H. (1987). Glucocorticoid inhibition of neurohypophysial vasopressin secretion. *Am. J. Physiol.*, **252**, R635–44.

Reichlin S. (1985). Neuroendocrinology. In *Williams Textbook of Endocrinology*, 7th edn (Wilson J.D., Foster D.W., eds). Philadelphia: W.B. Saunders, pp. 492–567.

Rivier C. (1993). Effect of peripheral and central cytokines on the hypothalamic-pituitary-adrenal axis of the rat. *Ann. NY Acad. Sci.*, **697**, 97–105.

Rivier C. (1994). Endogenous nitric oxide participates in the activation of the hypothalamic-pituitary-adrenal axis by noxious stimuli. *Endocrine J.*, **2**, 367–73.

Rivier C., Shen G.H. (1994). In the rat, endogenous nitric oxide modulates the response of the hypothalamic-pituitary-adrenal axis to interleukin-1β, vasopressin, and oxytocin. *J. Neurosci.*, **14**, 1985–93.

Robertson G.S. (1986). Posterior pituitary. In *Endocrinology and Metabolism*, 2nd edn (Felig P., Baxter J.D., Broadus A.E., Frohman L.A., eds). New York: McGraw-Hill, pp. 338–85.

Rorsman P., Ashcroft F.M., Berggren P.-O. (1991). Regulation of glucagon release from pancreatic A-cells. *Biochem. Pharmacol.*, **41**, 1783–90.

Ross R.J.M., Miell J.P., Holly J.M.P., Maheshwari H., Norman M., Abdulla A.F., Buchanan C.R. (1991). Levels of GH binding activity, IGFBP-1, insulin, blood glucose and cortisol in intensive care patients. *Clin. Endocrinol.*, **35**, 361–7.

Samols E., Stagner J.I. (1990). Islet somatostatin – microvascular, paracrine, and pulsatile regulation. *Metabolism*, **39**, (Suppl. 2), 55–60.

Sara V.R., Hall K. (1990). Insulin-like growth factors and their binding proteins. *Physiol. Rev.*, **70**, 591–614.

Sehgal P.B., Grieninger G., Tosato G. (eds) (1989). Regulation of the Acute Phase and Immune Responses: Interleukin-6. *Ann. NY Acad. Sci.*, **557**.

Semple C.G., Robertson W.R., Mitchell R. et al. (1987). Mechanisms leading to hypogonadism in men with burns injuries. *Bri. Med. J.*, **295**, 403–7.

Shafrir E., Bergman M., Felig P. (1987). The endocrine pancreas: diabetes mellitus. In *Endocrinology and Metabolism*, 2nd edn (Felig P., Baxter J.D., Broadus A.E., Frohman L.A., eds). New York: McGraw-Hill, pp. 1043–178.

Snow E.C. (1985) Insulin and growth hormone function as minor growth factors that potentiate lymphocyte activation. *J. Immunol.*, **135**, 776s–8s.

Srivastava L.S., Werk E.E. Jr, Thrasher K. et al. (1973). Plasma cortisone concentration as measured by radioimmunoassay. *J. Clin. Endocrinol. Metab.*, **36**, 937–43.

Stoner H.B. (1986). A role for the central nervous system in the responses to trauma. In *The Scientific Basis for the Care of the Critically Ill* (Little R.A., Frayn K.N., eds). Manchester: Manchester University Press, pp. 217–29.

Sugden P.H., Fuller S.J. (1991). Regulation of protein turnover in skeletal and cardiac muscle. *Biochem. J.*, **273**, 21–37.

Svoboda P., Kantorová I., Ochmann J. (1994). Dynamics of interleukin 1, 2, and 6 and tumor necrosis factor alpha in multiple trauma patients. *J. Trauma*, **36**, 336–40.

Thorner M.O., Vance M.L., Hartman M.L. et al. (1990). Physiological role of somatostatin on growth hormone regulation in humans. *Metabolism*, **39**. (Suppl. 2), 40–2.

Tilders F.J.H., Schmidt E.D., de Goeij D.C.E. (1993). Phenotypic plasticity of CRF neurons during stress. *Ann. NY Acad. Sci.*, **697**, 39–52.

Tominaga T., Fukata J., Hayashi Y. et al. (1992). Distribution and characterization of immunoreactive corticostatin in the hypothalamic-pituitary-adrenal axis. *Endocrinology*, **130**, 1593–8.

Truss M., Beato M. (1993). Steroid hormone receptors: interaction with deoxyribonucleic acid and transcription factors. *Endocrine Rev.*, **14**, 459–79.

Utiger R.D. (1986). The thyroid: physiology, hyperthyroidism, hypothyroidism, and the painful thyroid. In *Endocrinology and Metabolism*, 2nd edn (Felig P., Baxter J.D., Broadus A.E., Frohman L.A., eds). New York: McGraw-Hill, pp. 389–472.

Vigaš M., Németh Š., Jurčovičová J. (1973). The mechanism of trauma-induced inhibition of insulin release. *Hormone Meta Res.*, **5**, 322–4.

Viveros O.H., Unsworth C.D., Diliberto E.J. Jr (1985). Enkephalins in adrenal medulla and sympathetic nerves: storage, secretion, and synthesis. *Fed. Proc.*, **44**, 2851–5.

Walker B.R., Williams B.C. (1992). Corticosteroids and vascular tone: mapping the messenger maze. *Clin. Sci.*, **82**, 597–605.

Walker B.R., Campbell J.C., Fraser R., Stewart P.M., Edwards C.R.W. (1992). Mineralocorticoid excess and inhibition of 11β-hydroxysteroid dehydrogenase in patients with ectopic ACTH syndrome. *Clin. Endocrinol.*, **37**, 483–92.

Weiner R.I., Ganong W.F. (1978). Role of brain monoamines and histamine in regulation of anterior pituitary secretion. *Physiol. Rev.*, **58**, 905–76.

Whitnall M.H. (1993). Regulation of the hypothalamic corticotropin-releasing hormone neurosecretory system. *Prog. Neurobiol.*, **40**, 573–629.

Wood J.J., Rodrick M.L., McIrvine A.J., Mannick J.A. (1988). Lymphocyte abnormalities associated with impaired immunological defense. In *Trauma, Sepsis, and Shock. The Physiological Basis of Therapy* (Clowes G.H.A., Jr, ed.). New York: Marcel Dekker, pp. 371–421.

Wright H.K., Gann D.S. (1965). A defect in urinary concentrating ability during postoperative antidiuresis. *Surg., Gynecol. Obstet.*, **121**, 47–50.

Wynn V. (1960). Some problems of water metabolism following surgery. In *The Biochemical Response to Injury* (Stoner H.B., Threlfall C.J., eds). Oxford: Blackwell, pp. 291–309.

Zaloga G.P., Chernow, B. (1985). Thyroid function in acute illness. In *Endocrine Aspects of Acute Illness* (Geelhoed G.W., Chernow B., eds). New York: Churchill Livingstone, pp. 67–96.

Zimmerman E.A. (1983). Oxytocin, vasopressin, and neurophysins. In *Brain Peptides* (Krieger D.T., Brownstein M.J., Martin J.B., eds). New York: John Wiley, pp. 597–611.

SECTION 9
BIOCHEMICAL RESPONSES TO INJURY

46. Effects of Injury on Metabolic Rate

N. J. Rothwell

INTRODUCTION

The importance of changes in metabolic rate on the outcome of patients suffering trauma is not always apparent, probably because its effects are indirect and may occur after the very early phase, it is not routinely measured in clinical conditions, and perhaps also because awareness of nutritional problems in general is a rather recent phenomenon in hospital medicine.

Low metabolic rates, which may be associated with acute and severe illness, can lead to problems in maintaining body temperature and are often indicative of poor oxygen perfusion and/or multiple organ failure (Kinney, 1974; Long, 1977; Stoner, 1986; Little, 1988; Adolf and Eckart, 1990). In contrast high metabolic rates can, if not compensated by increased heat loss, produce fever which may offer some benefits in fighting infection, but is particularly detrimental when associated with neural damage such as that resulting from head injury or stroke or when tissue oxygen availability is limited. Sustained increases in metabolic rate impose additional energy demands on the patient resulting in depletion of body energy stores, i.e. cachexia. This latter phenomenon often occurs in the presence of low energy intakes, thus exacerbating the condition.

CHANGES IN METABOLIC RATE AFTER INJURY

Cuthbertson (1930, 1932) first described in detail the metabolic responses to injury, and defined two phases: He suggested that the early, or 'ebb' phase is characterized by a fall in metabolic rate, followed by a later, sustained 'flow phase' when metabolic rate is elevated above normal. However some controversy now exists over this characterization which is not always apparent after injury, particularly in man (Little *et al.*, 1981; Little and Stoner, 1981; Edwards *et al.*, 1988; Little, 1988). Several animal models of injury, for example, hind limb ischaemia and scald injury, do result in an early fall in metabolic rate and body temperature (ebb phase) which has been ascribed to inhibition of the central control of metabolic rate, and a subsequent rise in metabolic rate (Little, 1988,

1991). However a number of other rodent models of injury, such as turpentine-induced intramuscular abscess (Cooper and Rothwell, 1991) or cerebral ischaemia (O'Shaughnessy *et al.*, 1989), produce only a rise in metabolic rate which is apparent within 6 hours after injury. Similarly studies on patients have usually failed to reveal changes in metabolic rate consistent with an ebb and flow phase (for reviews see Little, 1988, 1991). Variable metabolic rates (i.e. decreases, no change or increases) have been reported in several studies in humans (Carli and Aber, 1987; Edwards *et al.*, 1988; Little, 1988), although the general consensus appears to be that metabolic rate is increased after injury, with low metabolic rates usually occurring in critically and terminally ill patients. The magnitude of the response to injury is dependent on many factors including the type and severity of injury. In reviewing the data on metabolic responses to injury, Little and Stoner (1981) and Long (1977) indicated that, in general, burn injury elicited the greatest increases in metabolic rate followed by multiple trauma and head injury.

Possible reasons for the apparent absence of an 'ebb phase' or early fall in metabolic rate in clinical studies may be that measurements have not been made early enough, and resuscitation is now initiated very rapidly. Recent data obtained by Childs (personal communication) indicates that in young children, metabolic rate increases shortly after thermal injury, and this effect does not appear to be directly related to the size of the burn, although in adult patients burn size does correlate with the magnitude of the metabolic response.

Several comprehensive reviews have discussed the magnitude, time-course and implications of changes in metabolic rate after injury (Long, 1977; Stoner, 1986; Little, 1988, 1991). The major purpose of this chapter is to consider the mechanisms responsible for those changes in metabolic rate, with particular emphasis on the central controls. However, because of the complex and varied terminology and definitions which exist in this field, these will first be considered briefly.

METABOLIC RATE – TERMINOLOGY AND DEFINITIONS

Metabolic rate is used synonymously with terms such as heat production and energy expenditure and can be divided into a number of components, such as basal metabolic rate, energy costs of physical activity, feeding, growth and reproduction, etc. However these distinctions are dependent on the conditions of measurement and can therefore be somewhat arbitrary. Increases in metabolic rate above 'normal' have been variously termed, nonshivering thermogenesis, diet-induced thermogenesis, luxusconsumption, adaptive or regulatory thermogenesis or hypermetabolism, depending on the stimulus and on the scientific background of the investigator. Changes in metabolic rate in response to cold or hyperphagia which participate in the regulation of body temperature and energy balance appear to be appropriate physiological responses. In contrast, increases in metabolic rate associated with injury or illness are not known to form part of a regulatory response (although future studies may reveal that this is the case), so that the most widely used term 'hypermetabolism' seems suitable. This literally means increased metabolism but immediately raises the important question of what is normal? Values for injured patients are usually compared to 'average' published values (mainly based on the Harris–Benedict equation (Harris and Benedict, 1919) for normal individuals of similar age and size. However, the comparison with an injured patient who is resting, if not sedated or paralysed, often has a very low food intake and may be subjected to a variety of treatments which could alter metabolic rate is clearly problematical. Large increases in metabolic rate are clearly discernible in some patients, but small changes in either direction must be treated with caution particularly when measurements are performed over relatively short periods of time in dynamic situations and in patients with marked changes in body composition. For these and other technical and ethical reasons most of the research into mechanisms of heat production, particularly the central control, has focused on animal studies. While these also have limitations, the results are usually more easily interpreted and in some cases have been applied successfully to clinical conditions.

PERIPHERAL MECHANISMS OF HYPERMETABOLISM

Increases in heat production in mammals must result from either increases in ATP utilization or a reduced efficiency of ATP synthesis – uncoupling of oxidative phosphorylation. Even if we exclude changes in muscular contraction, there are a number of pathways which will result in increased rates of ATP utilization (e.g. ion pumping, synthesis of fat, carbohydrate or protein, muscular contraction, 'futile cycles'). However, only one example of physiologically controlled uncoupling of oxidative phosphorylation has been demonstrated in vertebrates, that which occurs in brown adipose tissue (BAT). Increased rates of turnover of metabolic pathways such as protein synthesis and degradation or triglyceride synthesis/breakdown or cycling within pathways (e.g. 'substrate cycles' in glycolysis) will result in ATP utilization but with no net change in substrate concentration. It has been suggested that such pathways could contribute to diet-induced and non-shivering thermogenesis (Newsholme and Crabtree, 1976), although their quantitative importance is uncertain. Wolfe (1990) has also reported significant increases in the rates of triglyceride and glycolytic cycling in burn-injured patients, which appear to be under the control of the sympathetic nervous system. Calculations based on these measurements indicated that such cycles could contribute (15%) to the hypermetabolic response to burn injury. Rennie et al. (1990) have concluded from in vivo studies in patients and animals that protein turnover is usually unaltered or reduced after injury and is unlikely to be a major cause of hypermetabolism.

Increased heat production in BAT is the major effector of non-shivering (NST) and diet-induced thermogenesis (DIT) in small animals (Rothwell and Stock, 1984b, 1986a,b), although its importance and activity in large mammals, including man, is unknown. Thermogenesis in BAT is controlled by the sympathetic nervous system and dependent on interaction of noradrenaline with an atypical 'β_3 adrenoreceptor' on brown adipocytes (Arch et al., 1984). Uncoupling of oxidative phosphorylation in this tissue is due to the presence of a unique proton conductance pathway which allows dissipation of the protein gradient generated by mitochondrial respiration without obligatory synthesis of ATP (Nicholls and Locke, 1983). The activity of this pathway is dependent on the presence of a 32-kDa protein (uncoupling protein), and can be assessed in vitro from the binding of guanosine diphosphate (GDP) to isolated mitochondria. A close correlation has been observed between BAT activity and metabolic rates in a number of animal models of injury or inflammation, including cerebral ischaemia (O'Shaughnessy et al., 1990), endotoxin injection (Arnold et al., 1989), scald injury (Rothwell et al., 1990), intramuscular abscess in the rat (Cooper and Rothwell, 1991) and legionella infection in the guinea-pig (Cooper et al., 1989). In each case, the hypermetabolism and BAT activity are dependent on the sympathetic nervous system, and in endotoxin-treated rats the contribution of BAT to the rise in metabolic rate has been quantified from the measurements of blood flow (Jepson et al., 1987). The mass and activity of brown fat is inversely proportional to body size and is therefore very much smaller in humans than in laboratory rodents. Nevertheless, active BAT has been demonstrated in humans up to 80 years of age (Lean et al., 1986) and marked increases have been observed in activity of the tissue in children exhibiting cancer cachexia (Bianchi et al., 1989) or hypermetabolic responses to burn injury (Bruce et al., 1990). In adult (45–50 years) patients with severe sepsis high activity has also been observed in perianal adipose tissue (J. Bruce, K.E. Cooper and N.J. Rothwell, unpublished data).

The peripheral effector mechanisms of hypermetabolism are not fully understood, but their dependence on the sympathetic nervous system is more widely accepted (Wilmore *et al.*, 1976; Aulick and Wilmore, 1983; Landsberg and Young, 1983; Acheson, 1990). This can provide a focus for studies into the central mechanisms of hypermetabolism and indicates common features with diet-induced and non-shivering thermogenesis.

AREAS OF THE BRAIN CONTROLLING THERMOGENESIS

The major area of the brain which controls autonomic functions, particularly feeding behaviour and thermoregulation, is the hypothalamus, and it has been the focus for studies on thermogenesis. A close association between the ventromedial hypothalamus (VMH) and the regulation of body weight or energy balance was first demonstrated almost 40 years ago, when destruction of the ventromedial nucleus was shown to result in hyperphagia and obesity. The VMH has subsequently been referred to as a 'satiety' centre, acting inversely with the lateral hypothalamus (LH; known as the hunger centre) to control food intake (Stellar, 1954). However, obesity will develop in response to VMH lesions in the absence of hyperphagia, indicating that energy expenditure is simultaneously reduced (Han, 1965).

Shimazu and Takahashi (1980) suggested that the VMH might directly affect metabolism of BAT, since lipogenesis in the tissue was increased by electrical stimulation of this, but not other hypothalamic regions in the rat. Perkins *et al.* (1981) then reported marked increases in thermogenesis (assessed from changes in temperature) of brown fat in response to VMH stimulation, which were dependent on the sympathetic nervous system. Several groups have now confirmed the involvement of the VMH in the control of BAT thermogenesis. VMH stimulation raises brown fat temperature in conscious and anaesthetized animals and also causes marked increases in noradrenaline turnover (approximately three-fold; Saito *et al.*, 1989), and blood flow (almost 50-fold; Iwai *et al.*, 1987) to BAT, and 40% increases in resting oxygen consumption (Atrens *et al.*, 1985). Holt *et al.* (1987) reported that genetically obese Zucker rats exhibited normal temperature responses of brown fat following electrical stimulation of the VMH. Freeman and Wellman (1987) claimed that BAT was unresponsive to VMH stimulation in normal rats, but observed increases in temperature, following stimulation of other hypothalamic sites. However, closer study of their findings indicates that positive responses were elicited from the lateral region of the VMH (Freeman and Wellman, 1987), the same area that Perkins *et al.* (1981) found to be most sensitive. The VMH has also been implicated in the control of fever and responses to cytokines. Kuriyama *et al.* (1990) have demonstrated that interleukin-1β increased the firing rate of glucose-

sensitive neurones in the VMH. Many effects of VMH lesions, which were previously ascribed to destruction of the nucleus, have now been associated with disruption of the ventral noradrenergic bundle (VNAB) which passes through the lateral region of the VMH.

Inhibition of thermogenesis by surgical or chemical ablation of the VMH has been inferred from increases in the efficiency of weight gain (Han, 1965), reductions in the acute thermogenic responses to food (Carlisle *et al.*, 1988), in noradrenaline turnover and thermogenic activity of brown fat (Seydoux *et al.*, 1981; Hogan *et al.*, 1982), all of which will contribute to the development of obesity. It is difficult to distinguish the influence on thermogenesis of the VMH from that of the ventral noradrenergic bundle (VNAB). Sahakian *et al.* (1983) have shown that depletion of noradrenaline in or around the VNAB stimulates food intake and weight gain but inhibits BAT activity in the rat.

There is some doubt over whether the VMH is involved in the control of NST as well as DIT, and this may again relate to differential effects of the nucleus and of noradrenergic fibres. Hogan *et al.* (1982) reported impaired DIT, but no deficiency of NST in VMH-lesioned rats, whereas Imai-Matsumura *et al.* (1984) demonstrated that injection of lidocaine into the VMH prevented the increase in BAT temperature in response to cooling of the preoptic area in conscious rats.

The VNAB runs along the base of the brain and projects to the paraventricular (PVN) and dorsomedial nuclei (DMN), and the preoptic region of the hypothalamus and all of these areas have been implicated in the control of thermogenesis. The preoptic and anterior areas of the hypothalamus have been studied in some detail because of their general involvement in temperature regulation; both can apparently activate a variety of peripheral mechanisms of heat production and conservation. The PVN has been more specifically associated with dietary responses and its destruction results in obesity that shares some common features with the VMH syndrome, although PVN-induced obesity is generally more modest (Leibowitz *et al.*, 1984; Weingarten *et al.*, 1985; Leibowitz, 1986).

Many of the brain areas which activate BAT (Table 46.1) have already been associated with the control of thermogenesis or closely related functions. For example, the suprachiasmatic nucleus is thought to be responsible for diurnal variations in body temperature, while the supraoptic nucleus is involved in arousal from hibernation.

Investigations into the involvement of extra-hypothalamic areas in the control of thermogenesis are somewhat limited. Activation of thermogenesis in responses to conditioning (e.g. at the time of darkness) in laboratory rats and the sight and smell of food (Rothwell and Stock, 1981, 1986a,b; Rothwell, 1989b) suggests that there is some cortical

TABLE 46.1
EFFECTS OF ELECTRICAL STIMULATIONS ON BROWN ADIPOSE
TISSUE (BAT) TEMPERATURE

Brain area	BAT temperature*	Reference
VMH	+++	1,2
VMH	+	3
PVN	++	3,4
POAH	++	2,3,4
SCN	+	4
SON	+	2
SON	–	4
PH	–	4
PMV	–	3,4
DPM	–	4
DMN	–	2,4
PAG	–	4
ARH	–	3
Raphe	–	4
VTN	–	3
LH	–	2

VMH = ventromedial hypothalamus; PVN = paraventricular nucleus; POAH = preoptic anterior hypothalamus; SCN = suprachiasmatic nucleus; SON = supraoptic nucleus; PH = posterior hypothalamus; PMV = ventral premammillary nucleus; DPM = dorsal premammillary nucleus; PAG = periaqueductal grey; ARH = arcuate nucleus; VTN = ventromedial tegmental nucleus; LH = lateral hypothalamus.

* + = Rise in temperature; – = fall in temperature or no response.

1 = Perkins et al., 1981; 2 = Holt et al., 1987; 3 = Freeman and Wellman, 1987; 4 = R. LeFeuvre, N. J. Rothwell and M. J. Stock, unpublished results.

influence on thermogenesis, presumably via the hypothalamus.

Stereotaxic knife cuts or suction decerebration in the cat or the rat have indicated the presence of a tonic inhibitory centre in the upper pontine region. High-level decerebration in the prepontine region produces dramatic increases in body temperature (3–4°C) in several species (Bignall et al., 1975; Rothwell et al., 1983). In the rat, this is associated with dramatic increases in metabolic rate (Rothwell et al., 1983) which are dependent on the sympathetic nervous system. In contrast, premammillary transections prevent or inhibit these responses, indicating the presence of a tonic inhibitory system located somewhere between the lower mid-brain and upper pons which controls sympathetic outflow (Benzi et al., 1988; Rothwell et al., 1983).

Several pieces of evidence have implicated central noradrenergic pathways in the control of thermogenesis. The study of Sahakian et al. (1983) quoted earlier demonstrated that chemical destruction of noradrenergic pathways in the region of the VNAB resulted in inhibition of BAT activity and obesity. Conversely, Shimazu et al. (1986) have observed dramatic increases in body-weight gain in

rats in which noradrenaline was continuously infused into the VMH over several weeks. Although no direct measurements of food intake or thermogenesis were included in this study, a reduction in BAT activity was assumed from the increase in triglyceride turnover (Shimazu et al., 1986). After 12 weeks, food intake was increased by 67% in infused rats, but they were already 66% heavier by this time. The same group of workers found no changes in body weight in response to noradrenaline infusion into the PVN or the lateral hypothalamus, and only modest obesity in response to adrenaline infusion into the VMH. These apparently conflicting findings of Sahakian et al. (1983) and Shimazu et al. (1986) may represent subtle but crucial differences in the site of infusion and the location and type of receptors affected by experimental manipulation. For example, micro-injection of noradrenaline into the PVN can elicit feeding via an α-adrenoreceptor mechanism (Leibowitz, 1986), whereas activation of β-adrenoreceptors on the lateral hypothalamus may inhibit feeding (Grossman, 1962). It is likely that the control of thermogenesis is also dependent on both the site and on receptor subtype. There are some data indicating the involvement of central noradrenergic pathways, particularly the VNAB, in the metabolic responses to peripheral injury (Little, 1988). Changes in noradrenaline concentration or turnover, and particularly the ratio of activities of noradrenergic : serotonergic pathways within the hypothalamus, are considered of primary importance in the regulation of body temperature. These effects have been studied mainly within the preoptic region, but once again conflicting results have been obtained which are highly species dependent.

NUTRIENTS

Nutrient availability can exert direct effects on brain metabolism and neuronal function (Anderson, 1979; Fernstrom, 1986; Williamson, 1987; Rothwell and Stock, 1988a). There is also some evidence, although largely indirect, to suggest that specific nutrients may act as afferent signals causing selective activation of thermogenesis; for example, the work of Oomura (1976) has demonstrated potent effects of several endogenous sugar acids on feeding behaviour in the rat, and our preliminary data (unpublished) indicate that these may also stimulate metabolic rate. Davies et al. (1981) reported marked suppression of body weight in rats infused intracerebroventricularly with various nutrients, although food intake remained virtually unaltered.

Several amino acids can affect food intake by a central action and might therefore exert reciprocal effects on thermogenesis. For example, tryptophan, a precursor for 5-hydroxytryptophan (5-HT) inhibits food intake and the ratio of tryptophan to other large neutral amino acid is stimulated by insulin and by consumption of low protein diets (Leathwood, 1987), both of which increase thermogenesis. Although direct effects of these amino acids on metabolic rate have not been demonstrated, results of feeding studies provide a strong incentive for further research.

AMINERGIC PATHWAYS

Most of the evidence to support a role for noradrenergic mechanisms in CNS control of metabolism arises directly from studies on body-weight regulation. Sahakian *et al.* (1983) demonstrated that chemical destruction of noradrenergic pathways in the region of the VNAB resulted in inhibition of BAT activity and obesity. In contrast, Shimazu *et al.* (1986) reported rapid weight gains in rats following infusion of noradrenaline into the VMH of rats over several weeks, but found no changes in body weight in response to noradrenaline infusion into the PVN or the lateral hypothalamus, and only modest obesity in response to adrenaline infusion into the VMH. More recently, Siviy *et al.* (1989) found that infusion of noradrenaline into the PVN inhibited energy expenditure in the rat probably via an α_2-adrenoreceptor. These apparently conflicting findings may represent subtle but crucial differences in the site of infusion and the location and type of receptors affected by experimental manipulation. For example, microinjection of noradrenaline into the PVN can elicit feeding via an α-adrenoreceptor mechanism (Leibowitz, 1986), whereas activation of β-adrenoreceptors on the lateral hypothalamus may inhibit feeding (Grossman, 1962). It is likely that the control of thermogenesis is also dependent on both the site of action and receptor subtype.

Data on the actions of serotonergic pathways on thermogenesis are more consistent. Central or peripheral injections of 5-HT, serotonergic agonists or releasing agents such as D-fenfluramine stimulate metabolic rate and BAT thermogenesis by increasing sympathetic outflow (Rothwell and Stock, 1987b; LeFeuvre *et al.*, 1991). Chemical depletion of 5-HT pathways by injection of parachlorophenylalanine (PCPA) inhibits BAT activity (Fuller *et al.*, 1987) and causes hyperphagia and obesity in the rat (Breisch *et al.*, 1976). However, central injection of the slightly more selective neurotoxic agent 5,7-dihydroxytryptamine (5,7-DHT), in combination with desipramine to protect noradrenergic pathways, fails to induce obesity, but greatly enhances the thermogenic effects of D-fenfluramine, presumably because of increased receptor density or enhanced receptor sensitivity (LeFeuvre, 1990). The varied effects of PCPA and 5,7-DHT are probably due to selective destruction of 5-HT pathways in different brain regions. Some serotonergic pathways within the Raphe nucleus are not destroyed by 5,7-DHT and these are probably involved in the control of feeding and body weight (Coscina and Magder, 1984). Recently we have found that the thermogenic and anorectic effects of 5-HT or 5-HT releasing agents in the rat are dependent on central actions of corticotrophin releasing factor (CRF) since they are markedly attenuated by central injection of neutralizing anti-CRF antibody (LeFeuvre *et al.*, 1991).

There are relatively few studies on dopaminergic or cholinergic pathways and thermogenesis, although Shimazu *et al.* (1986) observed no changes in body weight after chronic infusions of acetylcholine into the hypothalamus.

AMINO ACIDS

Increasing brain γ-amino-n-butyric acid (GABA) concentrations by peripheral administration of GABA transaminase inhibitors inhibits the development of genetic obesity (Coscina and Nobrega, 1984) and stimulates thermogenesis (Horton *et al.*, 1988a). The use of selective GABA agonists and antagonists, injected centrally (into the VMH or third ventricle), has shown that activation of $GABA_B$ receptors, for example by baclofen, causes very large increases in thermogenesis (Addae *et al.*, 1986), whereas activation of the $GABA_A$ receptor inhibits metabolic rate and BAT activity (Horton *et al.*, 1988b). Several other amino acids could modify brain function and metabolic rate indirectly as they act as precursors for neurotransmitters (see above). Excitatory amino acids (e.g. glutamate and aspartate), however, act directly to influence CNS function and are released in response to local brain injury. Injection of excitatory amino acids stimulates brown fat thermogenesis in the rat (Amir, 1990). A physiological role of these transmitters has not been identified but they are strong candidates as mediators of hypermetabolic responses to brain injury and cerebral ischaemia (Choi and Rothman, 1990).

PEPTIDES AND THE CENTRAL CONTROL OF THERMOGENESIS

There is indirect evidence to implicate many peptides in the control of metabolic rate. Several peptides have been identified which elicit dose-dependent increases in metabolic rate in conscious animals when injected into the third ventricle of the brain, and in most cases these have been associated with increased BAT activity (LeFeuvre, 1990; Rothwell, 1989b, 1990b). Particularly notable is the fact that most of these peptides have been demonstrated to exert reciprocal effects on appetite and thermogenesis (Morley, 1987), although the physiological importance of endogenous peptides in appetite control or thermogenesis has not been elucidated.

One of the major peptide hormones implicated in the central control of energy balance is insulin (for reviews see Baskin *et al.*, 1987; Figlewicz *et al.*, 1987; Rothwell and Stock, 1988a) which when injected peripherally in high doses may cause obesity, but within physiological concentrations could have CNS actions to inhibit food intake and stimulate thermogenesis. Central infusion of insulin inhibits weight gain in the rat, and cerebroventricular injections enhance the thermogenic actions of glucose (for review see Rothwell and Stock, 1988a).

Thyrotropin releasing factor (TRH) or its chemical analogues are potent stimulators of metabolic rate in the rat (Griffiths *et al.*, 1988), and TRH has been suggested as an activator of the increased thermogenesis associated with arousal from hibernation and a mediator of neural thermoregulation and fever (Metcalfe, 1974; Lin, 1982). Lin *et al.* (1989) have recently reported a strong correlation between fever, thermogenesis and hypothalamic TRH concentrations in rats in response to pyrogenic agents. From these data the authors suggested that TRH mediates fever and interacts with serotonin and prostaglandins.

Another hypothalamic releasing factor with potent thermogenic actions is corticotrophin-releasing factor (CRF), which is now emerging as an important factor in the central control of energy balance and in the metabolic responses to stress, infection and injury (for review see Rothwell, 1990a).

CORTICOTROPHIN-RELEASING FACTOR

CRF is synthesized mainly in the paraventricular nucleus of the hypothalamus, although many other sites of synthesis within the CNS and the periphery have been identified (Gillies and Grossman, 1985; Emeric-Sauval, 1986). The most notable function of CRF is in the control of the synthesis and release of ACTH and other proopiomelanocortin (POMC)-derived peptides. However, CRF can also exert actions within the CNS which appear to be independent of the pituitary, and thus functions as a neurotransmitter or neuromodulator. The effects of CRF on thermogenesis, food intake and the sympathetic nervous system are included in this category.

The involvement of CRF in the control of energy balance was first implied from studies on the effects of adrenalectomy in genetically obese rodents (York, 1987, 1989). Briefly, adrenalectomy was found to almost completely normalize the defective energy balance of genetically obese and ageing rats and mice by both suppressing food intake and stimulating metabolic rate and brown fat activity (Yukimura *et al.*, 1978; Holt and York, 1982; Marchington *et al.*, 1983, 1986; Rothwell and Stock, 1984a, 1988b). These effects are inhibited by replacement of the animals with corticosterone or dexametha-

sone and, in the case of obese animals, only very low doses of replacement are required (Holt and York, 1982; King and Smith, 1985). Hypophysectomy exerts similar effects on energy balance (Rothwell and Stock, 1985; Holt *et al.*, 1988), leading to the suggestion that reduced synthesis, release or actions of CRF might be partially responsible for the impaired energy balance regulation and thermogenesis in obese mutants (Rothwell and Stock, 1985; York, 1989).

Central injection of CRF does indeed cause dose-dependent increases in metabolic rate, BAT blood flow and thermogenic activity which are prevented by inhibition of the sympathetic nervous system (LeFeuvre *et al.*, 1987). Brown (1982) first reported increased sympathetic outflow in response to CRF but in spite of an extensive study failed to identify its site of action within the brain. Genetically obese rats and mice can respond normally to injection of CRF (Carnie *et al.*, 1988), although preliminary reports have indicated reduced concentrations of CRF in specific hypothalamic nuclei (Moore and Routh, 1988), and these mutants may be unable to synthesize and/or release CRF in response to other stimuli (see later). Intracerebroventricular infusion of CRF in lean or obese animals inhibits body-weight gain and stimulates BAT and, like adrenalectomy, these effects appear greater in the obese mutants (Arase *et al.*, 1988; Rohner-Jeanrenaud *et al.*, 1988).

The actions of CRF on pituitary ACTH release are modified by glucocorticoid status but this is not the case for the thermogenic effects of CRF, which are almost identical in adrenalectomized animals or those treated with high doses of dexamethasone (for review see Rothwell, 1990b). However, glucocorticoids probably influence thermogenesis by inhibiting CRF synthesis. Peripheral or central administration of the glucocorticoid antagonist RU-486 stimulates thermogenesis and this effect is reversed by pretreatment of the animals with a CRF receptor antagonist (Hardwick *et al.*, 1989). The dissociation between the thermogenic and pituitary effects of CRF is supported by discrepancies in the relative potencies of CRF-like peptides from other species. Sauvagine is a very potent thermogenic agent when administered centrally in the rat but is much less effective in eliciting ACTH release (LeFeuvre *et al.*, 1989). Furthermore, the thermogenic effects of CRF are not modified by pretreatment of animals with a monoclonal antibody to ACTH (Rothwell *et al.*, 1991).

CRF could also mediate in the effects discussed earlier of serotonergic agonists on thermogenesis. 5-HT causes release of CRF both *in vivo* and *in vitro* (Gibbs and Vale, 1983; Calogero *et al.*, 1989), and results of our studies in conscious rats indicate that thermogenic responses to 5-HT and its precursors are attenuated by inhibition of CRF release or action (LeFeuvre *et al.*, 1991).

In addition to its effects on food intake, CRF has many other central actions, for example on behaviour, sleep, peripheral glucose metabolism and immune function (for review see Rothwell, 1990b). CRF could thus be of considerable importance in the central control of these processes in response to stress, injury or illness and this possibility has been enhanced by recent reports that CRF also mediates central effects of immune signals, most notably interleukin 1 (see below).

CYTOKINES

Bacterial, viral or parasitic infections are potent activators of thermogenesis usually resulting in fever (Cooper, 1987; Dinarello et al., 1988; Kluger, 1989). Peripheral release of a substance known originally as 'endogenous pyrogen' from macrophages was shown to induce fever and this was subsequently indentified as the cytokine interleukin 1 (IL-1; Blatteis, 1988; Dinarello et al., 1988; Kluger, 1989, 1990; Sternberg, 1989; Rothwell, 1991). Recombinant preparations of the two forms of IL 1 (IL-1α and β) have allowed detailed studies in experimental animals. IL-1 induces fever and activation of thermogenesis when injected peripherally or directly into the cerebroventricular space of rats, mice and rabbits (Dascombe et al., 1989a; Kluger, 1989), and these effects are dependent on the same peripheral effectors as the thermogenic responses to cold and diet – sympathetic activation of BAT (Rothwell, 1990d). Interestingly, genetically obese rodents (fatty Zucker rat and obese ob/ob mice) which show defective dietary activation of thermogenesis, also exhibit impaired responses to IL-1 (Dascombe et al., 1989b). The main site of action for IL-1 appears to be within the brain, since very low doses are required to induce fever compared to peripheral injection (ng range, Dascombe et al., 1989a) and central injection of antibody raised to IL-1β inhibits endotoxin-induced fever and hypermetabolism in the rat (Rothwell et al., 1989). However, the means by which IL-1 gains access to hypothalamic sites of action is unknown. Several studies have concluded that IL-1 is unable to cross the blood–brain barrier (Dinarello et al., 1988), while a recent report suggests that there is quite rapid transport of IL-1α into the brain (Banks et al., 1990). Another problem encountered in studies on IL-1 and fever has been the difficulty in detecting significant increases in circulating IL-1 in animals or humans during the development of fever in response to exogenous pyrogen or burn injury (Childs et al., 1989; Horan et al., 1989; Kluger, 1990; Rothwell, 1991). However dramatic increases in circulating concentrations of another pyrogenic cytokine, IL-6 (Busbridge et al., 1989a; LeMay et al., 1990), have been observed in response to infection, pyrogens, injury and even psychological stress (Childs et al., 1989; Horan et al., 1989, Kluger, 1989; Rothwell et al., 1989; LeMay et al., 1990). Since IL-1 is a potent releaser of IL-6, the latter may be a more important circulating pyrogen. Nevertheless, the involvement of IL-1 in fever and hypermetabolism is supported by the finding that administration of antibodies to IL-1β or to the IL-1 receptor attenuate the acute and chronic metabolic responses to endotoxin (Kluger, 1989; Long et al., 1989; Rothwell et al., 1989) or turpentine abscess (Gershenwald et al., 1990). It has now been demonstrated that central injection of IL-6 Ab attenuates endotoxin-induced fever in the rat, indicating that, like IL-1, it is also involved in the central control of fever (Rothwell et al., 1991b).

Tumour necrosis factor (TNF)α has been proposed as a mediator of cancer cachexia and was originally termed 'cachectin' because it induces wasting (Beutler and Cerami, 1986). TNF also causes activation of thermogenesis when injected centrally or peripherally into rodents (Rothwell, 1988), but the doses required are rather higher than for other cytokines, questioning its physiological importance. TNFα has, however, been strongly implicated in the control of fever (Dinarello et al., 1988; Nagai et al., 1988), although a recent report has suggested that administration of TNF antibody enhances fever in the rat (Long et al., 1990).

Interest in the central actions of cytokines has recently widened considerably with the realization that they exert important effects on neuroendocrine systems, forming a bidirectional communication between immune and endocrine systems (Besedovsky et al., 1985, 1986; Blalock, 1989; Buzzetti et al., 1989; see Chapter 45).

Berkenbosch et al. (1987) and Sapolsky et al. (1987) both reported that activation of the pituitary adrenal system by IL-1 involves hypothalamic release of CRF and pointed out that this may explain many of the endocrine responses to infection and injury. In particular, increases in glucocorticoid concentrations form an important feedback mechanism by subsequently inhibiting the metabolic and inflammatory effects of infection (Besedovsky et al., 1985, 1986). It has now also been demonstrated that the central effects of IL-1β on fever and thermogenesis are also dependent on CRF, since they are inhibited by treatment of animals with a CRF receptor antagonist (αhelical CRF 9–41), or monoclonal or polyclonal antibodies to CRF (Busbridge et al., 1989b; Rothwell, 1989a). The central effects of IL-6 and IL-8 are also dependent on CRF release, although the actions of IL-1α and TNFα are independent of CRF (Rothwell 1990d, 1991). Uehara et al. (1987) have reported differential effects of IL-1α and IL-1β on ACTH release in the rat and we have observed that, although genetically obese mutants fail to show significant thermogenic responses to IL-1β (Busbridge et al., 1990), they can respond normally to IL-1α (N.J. Busbridge et al., 1989b). This observation supports the suggestion that obese mutants cannot synthesize or release CRF in response to thermogenic stimuli such as IL-1β and strongly questions the dogma that IL-1α and IL-1β act on the same receptor (Dower *et al.*, 1986).

Although IL-1 appears unable to cross the blood–brain barrier, it could be synthesized within the central nervous system (Koenig, 1991; Rothwell, 1991). IL-1β has been identified by immunocytochemistry in several areas of the brain and a high density was observed in hypothalamic regions associated with CRF (Breder *et al.*, 1988). Messenger RNA for IL-1β has also been reported in the CNS and receptors have been identified in many brain areas (Farrar *et al.*, 1987; Haour *et al.*, 1990; Koenig, 1991).

Il-1β appears to be of greater importance in the control of fever and thermogenesis than IL-1α, since antibody to the β form but not to IL-1α inhibits these responses to endotoxin in the rat (Kluger, 1990; Rothwell *et al.*, 1990). It thus seems likely that IL-1β synthesized within the brain causes release of CRF, which then exerts a variety of metabolic and hormonal effects. It has also been reported that the inhibitory effects of IL-1 on food intake are dependent on CRF release (Uehara *et al.*, 1989). Thus inhibition of CRF release or action could be of benefit in the clinical management of cachexia. The site of action of cytokines is not known precisely, although *in vitro* effects on hypothalamic slice preparations have been reported (Tsagakaris *et al.*, 1989). Autoradiographic studies have identified IL-1 binding sites corresponding to the characteristics of Type I IL-1 receptor in the dentate gyrus and choroid plexus, but no binding was found in the hypothalmus (Haour *et al.*, 1990). However, we have now demonstrated that central effects of IL-1β on fever and thermogenesis in the rat are prevented by injection of an antibody to the Type II IL-1 receptor, indicating that this receptor is involved in some CNS actions of IL-1 (Lukeshi *et al.*, 1993).

EICOSANOIDS

Fever and the central effects of cytokines are generally mediated by eicosanoids, and inhibited by cyclo-oxygenase inhibitors. Prostaglandin E_2 (PGE_2) is generally thought to be the main mediator of fever, and therefore of the hypermetabolic responses to pyrogens (Dascombe, 1985). However a number of eicosanoids stimulate fever and thermogenesis, and in the rat $PGF_2\alpha$ is slightly more effective (Morimoto *et al.*, 1988). Bernadini *et al.* (1989) have reported that several arachidonic acid metabolites induce release of CRF from hypothalami *in vitro*. $PGF_2\alpha$ and thrombaxane A_2 (TXA_2) were both potent releasers of CRF, while PGE_2 was ineffective or inhibitory. Interestingly the thermogenic effects of $PGF_2\alpha$ but not PGE_2 *in vivo* are dependent on CRF (Rothwell, 1990c), which would strongly suggest that $PGF_2\alpha$ or TXA_2 rather than

PGE_2 mediate the effects of those cytokines which depend on CRF release for their action (i.e. IL-1β and IL-6).

Glucocorticoids are potent inhibitors of the inflammatory, pyrogenic and metabolic responses to injury and also inhibit diet-induced thermogenesis by central actions (York, 1989). These effects could be mediated by inhibition of either eicosanoid or CRF synthesis within the CNS. The antiinflammatory actions of steroids have been ascribed to inhibition of phospholipase A_2 activity, thus causing suppression of eicosanoid synthesis, and are thought to depend on the release of second mediators known as lipocortins (Flower, 1988). These proteins are synthesized in many tissues and have diverse actions on intracellular calcium, phospholipid binding and can act as substrates for receptor phosphorylation. Lipocortin-1 has been identified in the CNS (Smillie *et al.*, 1989; Strijbos *et al.*, 1991) and central injection of recombinant fragment of lipocortin-1 suppresses the thermogenic effects of cytokines in the rat (Carey *et al.*, 1990). Conversely, administration of antibody to lipocortin-1 enhances such responses, particularly in animals with impaired thermogenesis (Carey *et al.*, 1990). Thus lipocortin may act as an endogenous modulator of the metabolic responses to injury, but the factors controlling its synthesis and action are largely unknown.

SUMMARY AND CONCLUSIONS

Considerable advances have been made in our understanding of the mechanisms of hypermetabolism and particularly of the CNS control within the last few years. This has been due in large part to the availability of recombinant cytokines, of sensitive assays for cytokines and neuropeptides and to the realization that the brain forms an important component of the response to injury. Many aspects of the acute-phase response are under CNS control; the most widely recognized of these parameters are sleep, food intake, behaviour and hypothalamic-pituitary-adrenal function. However, results indicate that responses previously associated entirely with the peripheral immune system, such as antibody production, natural killer activity and IL-1-induced IL-6 release are also dependent on CNS mechanisms.

In spite of these important advances many questions remain to be answered. The most obvious are: what are the afferent signals, if these are cytokines, how do they gain access to the CNS and where is their site of synthesis, which CNS mechanisms are involved in the control of fever, thermogenesis and other acute-phase responses and, equally importantly, which parts of control can be dissociated, what are the peripheral effectors of hypermetabolism in man, how are hypermetabolic responses controlled and can they be modified pharmacologically? Perhaps one of the most fundamental questions relates to the biological value of hypermetabolism. The survival value of fever has been argued by Kluger (1989) and similar arguments can be used to support the value of increases in metabolic rate (Banet, 1981). However in some cases, for example when neuronal or ischaemic damage has occurred or when prolonged increases in metabolic rate lead to cachexia, hypermetabolism is clearly disadvantageous. It is important for us to distinguish these effects, as current research suggests that means of intervention and modification of metabolic rate in injured patients are likely to be available in the not too distant future.

REFERENCES

Acheson K.J. (1990). Sympathetic nervous system in the regulation of thermogenesis. In *Hormones and Nutrition in Obesity and Cachexia* (Muller M.J., ed.). Berlin: Springer, pp. 40–6.

Addae J.I., Rothwell N.J., Stock M.J., Stone T.W. (1986). Activation of brown fat thermogenesis in rats by baclofen. *Neuropharmacology,* **25**, 627–31.

Adolf M., Eckart J. (1990). Importance of indirect calorimetry for the nutrition of intensive care patients. In *Hormones and Nutrition in Obesity and Cachexia* (Muller M.J. et al., eds). Berlin: Springer, pp. 139–62.

Amir S. (1990). Intraventromedial injection of glutamate stimulates BAT thermogenesis. *Brain Res.,* **571**, 341–4.

Anderson G.H. (1979). Control of protein and energy intake: role of plasma amino acids and brain transmitters. *Can. J. Physiol. Pharmacol.,* **57**, 1043–57.

Arase K., York D.A., Shimazu H. et al. (1988). Effects of corticotropin releasing factor on food intake and brown adipose tissue thermogenesis in rats. *Am. J. Physiol.,* **255**, E255–9.

Arch J.R.S., Ainsworth A.T., Cawthorne M.A. et al. (1984). Atypical ß-adrenoreceptor on brown adipocytes: target for antiobesity drugs. *Nature,* **309**, 163–5.

Arnold J., Little R.A., Rothwell N.J. (1989). Energy balance and brown adipose tissue thermogenesis during chronic endotoxaemia in the rat. *J. Appl. Physiol.,* **66**, 1970–5.

Atrens D.M., Sinden J.D., Penicaud L. et al. (1985). Hypothalamic modulation of energy expenditure. *Physiol. Behav.,* **35**, 15–20.

Aulick L.H., Wilmore D.W. (1983). Hypermetabolism in trauma. In *Mammalian Thermogenesis* (Girardier L., Stock M.J., eds). London: Chapman Hall, pp. 259–304.

Banet M. (1981). Fever and survival in the rat – metabolic versus temperature response. *Experientia.,* **37**, 1302–4.

Banks W.A., Kastin A.J., Durham D.A. (1990). Bidirectional transport of interleukin-1 alpha across the blood brain barrier. *Brain Res. Bull.,* **23**, 439–42.

Baskin D.G., Porte D., Guest K., Dorsa D.M. (1987). Insulin in the brain. *Am. Rev. Physiol.,* **49**, 335–47.

Benzi R.H., Shibata M., Seydoux J., Girardier L. (1988). Prepontine knife cut induced hyperthermia in the rat. *Pflügers Archiv.,* **411**, 593–9.

Berkenbosch F., Van Oers J., Del Rey A. et al. (1987). Corticotropin releasing factor producing neurones in the rat – activation by interleukin 1β. *Science,* **238**, 524–8.

Bernadini R., Chiorenza A., Calogero A.E. et al. (1989). Arachidonic acid metabolites modulate rat hypothalamic corticotropin-releasing hormone secretion *in vitro. Neuroendocrinology,* **50**, 708–15.

Besedovsky H., del Rey A., Sorkin E. (1985). Immunological neuroendocrine feedback circuits. In *Neural Modulation of Immunity* (Guillemin R. et al., eds). New York: Raven, pp. 165–77.

Besedovsky H., del Rey A., Sorkin E., Dinarello C.A. (1986). Immunoregulatory feedback between interleukin-1 and glucocorticoid hormones. *Science,* **233**, 652–4.

Beutler B., Cerami A. (1986). Cachectin and tumour necrosis factor as two sides of the same biological coin. *Nature,* **320**, 584–8.

Bianchi A., Bruce J., Cooper A.L. et al. (1989). Increased brown adipose tissue activity in children with malignant diseases. *Horm. Metab. Res.,* **21**, 640–2.

Bignall K.E., Heggenness F.W., Palmer J.E. (1975). Effect of neonatal decerebration on thermogenesis during starvation and cold exposure in the rat. *Exp. Neurol.,* **40**, 174–88.

Blalock J.E. (1989). A molecular basis for bidirectional communication between the immune and neuroendocrine systems. *Physiol. Rev.,* **69**, 1–31.

Blatteis C.M. (1988). Neural mechanisms in the pyrogenic and acute phase responses to interleukin-1. *Int. J. Neurosci.,* **38**, 223–32.

Breder C.D., Dinarello C.A., Saper C.B. (1988). Interleukin-1, immunoreactive innervation of human hypothalamus. *Science,* **240**, 321–4.

Breisch S.T., Zemlan F.P., Hoebel B.G. (1976). Hyperphagic obesity following serotonergic depletion by intraventricular p-chlorophenylanine. *Science,* **192**, 382–4.

Brown M. (1982). Corticotropin releasing factor: central nervous system sites of action. *Brain Res.,* **399**, 10–14.

Bruce J., Childs C.C., Cooper A.L., Rothwell N.J. (1990). Brown adipose tissue activity in children in relation to disease status. *Proc. Nutr. Soc.,* **49**, 189A.

Busbridge N.J., Dascombe M.J., Hopkins S.J., Rothwell N.J. (1989a). Acute central effects of interleukin-6 on body temperature, thermogenesis and food intake in the rat. *Proc. Nutr. Soc.,* **48**, 48A.

Busbridge N.J., Dascombe M.J., Tilders F.J.A. et al. (1989b). Central activation of thermogenesis and fever by interleukin-1β and interleukin-1α involves different mechanisms. *Biochem. Biophys. Res. Commun.,* **162**, 591–6.

Busbridge N.J., Carnie J.A., Dascombe M.J. et al. (1990). Adrenalectomy reverses the impaired pyrogenic responses to interleukin 1β in obese Zucker rats. *Int. J. Obesity,* **14**, 809–19.

Buzzetti R., McLaughlin L., Scavo D., Rees L.H. (1989). A critical assessments of the interaction between the immune system and the hypothalamus-pituitary-adrenal axis. *J. Endocrinol.,* **20**, 183–7.

Calogero A.E., Bernadini R., Margioris A.N. et al. (1989). Effects of serotonergic agonists and antagonists on CRH secretion by explanted hypothalami. *Peptides,* **10**, 189–200.

Carey F., Forder R., Edge M.D. et al. (1990). Lipocortin 1 fragment modifies the pyrogenic actions of cytokines in the rat. *Am. J. Physiol.,* **259**, R266–9.

Carli F., Aber V.R. (1987). Thermogenesis after major electrosurgical procedures. *For. J. Surg.,* **74**, 1041–5.

Carlisle H.J., Rothwell N.J., Stock M.J. (1988). Thermic responses to food in rats with lesions of the ventromedial hypothalamus. *Proc. Nutr. Soc.*, **47**, 24A.

Carnie J.A., LeFeuvre R.A., Linton E.A. et al. (1988). Thermogenic effect of CRF in genetically obese Zucker rats. *Proc. Nutr. Soc.*, **47**, 165A.

Childs C., Ratcliffe R.J., Holt I., Hopkins S.J. (1989). Relationships between interleukin 1, interleukin 6 and pyrexia in burned children. *Cytokine*, **1**, 36.

Choi D.W., Rothman S.M. (1990). The role of glutamate neurotoxicity in hypoxic ischaemic neuronal death. *Annu. Rev. Neurosci.*, **13**, 171–82.

Cooper A.L., Rothwell N.J. (1991). Mechanisms of early and late hypermetabolism and fever after localised tissue injury in rats. *Am. J. Physiol.*, **261**, E698–705.

Cooper A.L., Fitzgeorge R.B., Baskerville A. et al. (1989). Bacterial infection (*Legionella pneumophilia*) stimulates fever, metabolic rate and brown adipose tissue activity in the guinea pig. *Life Sci.*, **45**, 843–7.

Cooper K.E. (1987). The neurobiology of fever: thoughts on recent developments. *Annu. Rev. Neurosci.*, **10**, 297–394.

Coscina D.V., Nobrega J.N. (1984). Anorectic potency of inhibiting GABA transaminase in brain: studies of hypothalamic dietary and genetic obesities. *Int. J. Obesity*, **8**, 181–200.

Coscina D.V., Magder R.J. (1984). Effects of serotonin depleting and brain lesions on the defence of hypothalamic obesity. *Physiol. Behav.*, **33**, 575–9.

Cuthbertson D.P. (1930). The disturbance of metabolism produced by bony injury, with notes in certain abnormal conditions of bone. *Biochem. J.*, **24**, 1244–63.

Cuthbertson D.P. (1932). Observations in the disturbance of metabolism produced by injury to the limbs. *Q. J. Med.*, **25**, 223–46.

Dascombe M.J. (1985). The pharmacology of fever. *Rev. Infect. Dis.*, **6**, 51–95.

Dascombe M.J., Rothwell N.J., Sagay B.O., Stock M.J. (1989a). Pyrogenic and thermogenic effects of interleukin 1β in the rat. *Am. J. Physiol.*, **256**, E7–11.

Dascombe M.J., Hardwick A., LeFeuvre R.A., Rothwell N.J. (1989b). Impaired effects of interleukin 1β in fever, thermogenesis and brown fat in genetically obese rats. *Int. J. Obesity*, **13**, 367–74.

Davies J.D., Wirtschaffer D., Askin K. E., Brief D. (1981). Sustained intracerebroventricular infusion of brain fuels reduces body weight and food intake of rats. *Science*, **212**, 81–2.

Dinarello C.A., Cannon J.G., and Wolfe S.M. (1988). New concepts on the pathogenesis of fever. *Rev. Infect. Dis.*, **10**, 168–87.

Dower S.K., Kronheim S.R., Hopp T.P. et al. (1986). The cell surface receptors for interleukin-1α and interleukin-1β are identical. *Nature*, **324**, 266–8.

Edwards J.D., Redmond A.D., Nightingale P., Wilkins R.G. (1988). Oxygen consumption following trauma: re-appraisal in severely injured patients requiring medical ventilation. *Br. J. Surg.*, **75**, 690–2.

Emeric-Sauval E. (1986). CRF: a review. *Psychoneuroendocrinology*, **11**, 277–94.

Farrar W.L., Kilian P.C., Ruff M.R. et al. (1987). Visualization and characterization of interleukin 1 receptors in brain. *J. Immunol.*, **139**, 459–63.

Fernstrom J.D. (1986). Acute and chronic effects of protein and carbohydrate ingestion on brain tryptophan levels and serotonin synthesis. *Nutr. Rev. Suppl.*, **5**, 25–36.

Figlewicz D.P., Lacour F., Sipols A. et al. (1987). Gastroenteropancreatic peptides and the central nervous system. *Ann. Rev. Physiol.*, **49**, 383–95.

Flower R.J. (1988). Lipocortin and the mechanisms of action of the glucocorticoids. *Br. J. Pharmacol.*, **65**, 987–1015.

Freeman P.H., Wellman P.J. (1987). Brown adipose tissue thermogenesis induced by low level electrical stimulation of the hypothalamus in rats. *Brain Res. Bull.*, **18**, 7–11.

Fuller M.J., Stirling D.M., Dunnett S. et al. (1987). Decreased brown adipose tissue thermogenic activity following a reduction in brain serotonin by intraventricular p-chlorophenylalanine. *Biosci. Rep.*, **7**, 121–7.

Gershenwald J.E., Fong Y., Chizzonite R. et al. (1990). Interleukin-1 receptor blockage attenuates the host inflammatory response. *Proc. Nat Acad. Sci.*, **87**, 4966–70.

Gibbs D.M., Vale W. (1983). Effect of the serotonin uptake inhibitor fluoxetine on corticotropin releasing factor and vasopressin secretion into hypophysial portal blood. *Brain Res.*, **280**, 176–9.

Gillies G., Grossman A. (1985). The CRF's and their control: chemistry, physiology and clinical implications. *Clin. Endocrinol. Metab.*, **14**, 821–45.

Griffiths E.C., Rothwell N.J., Stock M.J. (1988). Thermogenic effects of thyrotropin releasing hormone and its analogues in the rat. *Experientia*, **44**, 41–2.

Grossman S.P. (1962). Direct adrenergic and cholinergic stimulation of hypothalamic mechanisms. *Am. J. Physiol.*, **303**, 782–882.

Han P.W. (1965). Hypothalamic obesity in rats without hyperphagia. *Trans. NY Acad. Sci.*, **30**, 229–43.

Haour F.G., Ban E.M., Milon G.M. et al. (1990) Brain interleukin-1 receptors: characterisation and modulation after lipopolysaccharide injection. *Prog. Neurol. Endocrinol. Immunol.*, **3**, 196–204.

Hardwick A.J., Linton E.A., Rothwell N.J. (1989). Thermogenic effects of the antiglucocorticoid RU436 in the rat: involvement of corticotropin releasing factor and sympathetic activation of brown adipose tissue. *Endocrinology*, **124**, 1684–8.

Harris J.A., Benedict F.G. (1919). *A Biometric Study of Basal Metabolism in Man*. Carnegie Institute of Washington, Washington DC: Publ. No. 297.

Hogan S., Coscina D.V., Himms-Hagen J. (1982). Brown adipose tissue of rats with obesity inducing ventromedial hypothalamic lesions. *Am. J. Physiol.*, **243**, E334–8.

Holt S., York D.A. (1982). The effect of adrenalectomy on GDP binding to brown adipose tissue mitochondria of obese rats. *Biochem. J.*, **208**, 819–22.

Holt S., Wheal H., York D.A. (1987). Hypothalamic control of BAT in Zucker lean and obese rats; effects of electrical stimulation of the VMH and other hypothalamic nuclei. *Brain Res.*, **405**, 227–33.

Holt S., Rothwell N.J., Stock M.J., York D.A. (1988). Effect of hypophysectomy on energy balance and brown fat activity in obese Zucker rats. *Am. J. Physiol.*, **254**, E162–6.

Horan M.A., Gibbons L., Hopkins S.J. et al. Changes in plasma interleukin 6 during experimentally induced fever in normal humans. *Cytokine*, **1**, 138.

Horton R.W., Rothwell N.J., Stock M.J. (1988a). Chronic inhibition of GABA transaminase results in activation of thermogenesis and brown fat in the rat. *Gen. Pharmacol.*, **19**, 403–6.

Horton R.W., LeFeuvre R.A., Rothwell N.J., Stock M.J. (1988b). Opposing effects of activation of central GABAA and GABAB receptors on brown fat thermogenesis in the rat. *Neuropharmacology*, **27**, 363–6.

Imai-Matsumura K., Matsumura K., Nakayama T. (1984). Involvement of the ventromedial hypothalamus in brown adipose tissue thermogenesis induced by preoptic cooling in rats. *Jap. J. Physiol.*, **34**, 939–43.

Iwai M., Hell N.S., Shimazu T. (1987). Effects of VMH stimulation on blood flow of BAT in rats. *Pflügers Archiv.*, **410**, 44–7.

Jepson M.M., Cox M., Bates P.C. et al. (1987). Regional blood flow and skeletal muscle energy status in endotoxemic rats. *Am. J. Physiol.*, **252**, E581–7.

King B.M., Smith R.L. (1985). Hypothalamic obesity after hypophysectomy or adrenalectomy: dependence on corticosterone. *Am. J. Physiol.*, **249**, 522–6.

Kinney J.M. (1974). Energy requirements in injury and sepsis. *Acta Anaesthesiol. Acad.*, **55**, 15–20.

Kluger M.J. (1989). Body temperature changes during inflammation: their mediation and nutritional significance. *Proc. Nutr. Soc.*, **48**, 337–45.

Kluger M.J. (1990). Fever: role of pyrogens and cryogens. *Physiol. Rev.*, **71**, 93–127.

Koenig J.T. (1991). Presence of cytokines in the hypothalamic-pituatary axis. *Prog. Neurol. Endocrinol. Immunol.*, **4**, 143–53.

Kuriyama K., Hori T., Mori T., Nakashima, T. (1990). Actions of interferon α and interleukin-1β on the glucose responsive neurons in the ventromedial hypothalamus. *Brain Res. Bull.*, **24**, 803–10.

Landsberg L., Young J.B. (1983). Autonomic regulation of thermogenesis. In *Mammalian Thermogenesis* (Girardier L., Stock M.J., eds). London: Chapman & Hall, pp. 99–140.

Lean M.E.J., James W.P.T., Jennings G., Trayhurn P. (1986). Brown adipose tissue uncoupling protein content in human infants, children and adults. *Clin. Sci.*, **71**, 291–7.

Leathwood P.D. (1987). Tryptophan availability and serotonin synthesis. *Proc. Nutr. Soc.*, **46**, 143–56.

LeFeuvre R.A. (1990). The Hypothalamic Control of Thermogenesis. PhD Thesis, University of London.

LeFeuvre R.A., Rothwell N.J., Stock M.J. (1987). Activation of brown fat thermogenesis in response to central injection of CRF in the rat. *Neuropharmacology*, **26**, 1217–21.

LeFeuvre R.A., Rothwell N.J., White A. (1989). Comparison of the thermogenic effects of CRF, sauvagine and urotensin 1 in the rat. *Horm. Metab. Res.*, **21**, 525–6.

LeFeuvre R.A., Aisenthal L., Rothwell N.J. (1991). Involvement of corticotrophin releasing factor (CRF) in the thermogenic and anorexic actions of serotonin (5HT) and related compounds. *Brain Res.*, **555**, 245–50.

Leibowitz S.F. (1986). Brain monoamines and peptides: role in the control of eating behaviour. *Fed. Proc.*, **45**, 1396–403.

Leibowitz S.F., Roland C.R., Hor L., Squillari V. (1984). Noradrenergic feeding via the paraventricular nucleus is dependent upon circulating corticosterone. *Physiol. Behav.*, **32**, 857–64.

LeMay L.G., Vander A., Kluger M. (1990). The effects of psychological stress and anaesthesia on plasma inter-leukin 6 (IL-6) activity in rat. *Cytokine*, **1**, 123.

Lin M.T. (1982). Metabolic respiratory, vasomotor and body temperature responses to TRH, angiotensin II, substance P, neurotensin, somatostatin, LH-RH, beta endorphin, oxytone and vasopressin in the rat. *Adv. Biosci.*, **38**, 229–51.

Lin M.T., Wang P.S., Chuang J. et al. (1989). Cold stress on a pyrogenic substrate deviates tryptophan releasing hormone levels in rat hypothalamus and induces thermogenic reactions. *Neuroendocrinology*, **50**, 177–81.

Little R.A. (1988). Metabolic rate and thermoregulation after injury. In *Recent Advances in Critical Care Medicine*, Vol. 3 (Ledingham I., eds). London: Churchill, pp. 159–72.

Little R.A. (1991). Metabolic rate and its control after accidental injury. In *Proceedings of the Biological Council Symposium: Obesity and cachexia* (Rothwell N.J., Stock M.J., eds). Chichester: Wiley, pp. 197–208.

Little R.A., Stoner H.B. (1981). Body temperature after accidental injury. *Br. J. Surg.*, **68**, 221–4.

Little R.A., Stoner H.B., Frayn K.N. (1981). Substrate oxidation shortly after accidental injury in man. *Clin. Sci.*, **61**, 789–91.

Long C.L. (1977). Energy balance and carbohydrate metabolism in infection and sepsis. *Am. J. Clin. Nutr.*, **30**, 301–10.

Long N., LeMay L.G., Otterness I. et al. (1989). The roles of IL-1α and β TNF and IL-6 in LPS fever in the rat. In The physiological and pathological effects of cytokines. *Prog. Leukocyte Biol*, **10**, 313–18.

Long N.C., Kunkel S.L., Vander A.J., Kluger M.J. (1990). Antiserum against tumour necrosis factor enhances lipopolysaccharide fever in rats. *Am. J. Physiol.*, **258**, R332–7.

Luheshi G., Hopkins S.J., LeFeuvre R.A., Deascombe M.J., Ghiara P., Rothwell N.J. (1993). Importance of brain type-II receptors in fever and thermogenesis in the rat. *Am. J. Physiol.*, **265**, E585–E591.

Marchington D., Rothwell N.J., Stock M.J., York D.A. (1983). Energy balance diet-induced thermogenesis and brown adipose tissue in lean and obese (fa/fa) Zucker rats after adrenalectomy. *J.Nutr.*, **113**, 1395–402.

Marchington D., Rothwell N.J., Stock M.J., York D.A. (1986). Thermogenesis and sympathetic activity in BAT of overfed rats after adrenalectomy. *Am. J. Physiol.*, **250**, E362–6.

Metcalfe G. (1974). TRH: a possible mediator of thermoregulation. *Nature*, **252**, 310–11.

Morimoto A., Murakami N., Watanabe T. (1988). Is the central arachidonic acid cascade system involved in the development of acute phase response in rabbits? *J. Physiol.*, **397**, 281–9.

Moore B.J., Routh V.H. (1988). Corticotropin releasing factor (CRF) levels are altered in the brain of the genetically obese fatty Zucker rat. *Fed. Proc.*, **22**, 5386.

Morley J.E. (1987). Neuropeptide regulation of appetite and weight. *Endocrine Rev.*, **8**, 256–87.

Nagai M., Saigusa T., Shimada Y. et al. (1988). Antibody to tumour necrosis factor (TNF) reduces endotoxin fever. *Experientia*, **44**, 606.

Newsholme E., Crabtree B. (1976). Substrate cycles in metabolic regulation and in heat generation. *Biochem. Soc. Symp.*, **41**, 61–109.

Nicholls D.G., Locke R. (1983). Thermogenic mechanism in brown fat. *Physiol. Rev.*, **64**, 1–64.

Oomura Y. (1976). Significance of glucose, insulin and free fatty acid in the hypothalamic and satiety neurones. In *Hunger: basic mechanisms and diurnal implications* (Novin D., Wyrwicka W., Bray G., eds). New York: Raven, pp. 145–57.

O'Shaughnessy C.T., Rothwell N.J., Shrewsbury-Gee J. (1990). Sympathetically mediated hypermetabolic response to cerebral ischaemia in the rat. *Can. J. Physiol. Pharmacol.*, **68**, 1334–7.

Perkins M.N., Rothwell N.J., Stock M.J., Stone T.W. (1981). Activation of brown adipose tissue thermogenesis by the ventromedial hypothalamus. *Nature*, **89**, 401–2.

Rennie M.J., Bennett W., Connacher A. et al. (1990). Physiological and pathophysiological regulation of human muscle protein turnover. In *Hormones and Activities in Obesity and Cachexia* (Muller M.J., eds.). Berlin: Springer, pp. 107–22.

Rohner-Jeanrenaud F., Walker C., Greco Perotto R., Jeanrenaud B. (1988). Chronic intracerebroventricular administration of corticotropin releasing factor (CRF) to genetically obese fa/fa rats arrests the further increase of their body weight. In *Obesity in Europe '88: Proceedings of the European Congress on Obesity* (Bjorntorp P., Rossner S.J., eds). London: Libbey, pp. 253–8.

Rothwell N.J. (1988). Central effects of TNFα in the rat. *Biosci. Rep.*, **8**, 345–52.

Rothwell N.J. (1989a). CRF is involved in the pyrogenic and thermogenic effects of interleukin 1β in the rat. *Am. J. Physiol.*, **256**, E111–15.

Rothwell N.J. (1989b). Central control of thermogenesis. *Proc. Nutr. Soc.*, **48**, 241–50.

Rothwell N.J. (1990a). Thermogenesis in obesity and cachexia. In *Endocrinology and Metabolism – hormones and nutrition in obesity and cachexia* (Muller M., ed.). Heidelberg: Springer, pp. 77–85.

Rothwell N.J. (1990b). Central effects of CRF on metabolism and energy balance. *Neurosci. Biobehav. Rev.*, **14**, 263–71.

Rothwell N.J. (1990c). Central activation of thermogenesis by prostaglandins, dependence on CRF. *Horm. Metab. Res.*, **22**, 616–18.

Rothwell N.J. (1990d). Mechanisms of the pyrogenic effects of cytokines. *Eur. Cytokine Network*, **1**, 211–13.

Rothwell N.J. (1991). Functions and mechanisms of interleukin-1 in the brain. *Trends Pharm. S.*, **12**, 430–6.

Rothwell N.J., Stock M.J. (1981). *Obesity and Leanness – basic aspects*. London: J. Libbey.

Rothwell N.J., Stock M.J. (1984a). Sympathetic and adrenocorticoid influences on diet-induced thermogenesis and brown fat activity in the rat. *Comp. Biochem. Physiol.*, **79A**, 575–9A.

Rothwell N.J., Stock M.J. (1984b). Brown adipose tissue. *Rec. Adv. Physiol.*, **10**, 349–85.

Rothwell N.J., Stock M.J. (1985). Thermogenesis and BAT activity in hypophysectomized rats with and without corticotropin replacement. *Am. J. Physiol.*, **249**, E333–30.

Rothwell N.J., Stock M.J. (1986a). Brown adipose tissue and diet-induced thermogenesis. In *Brown Adipose Tissue* (Trayhurn P., Nicholls D.G., eds). London: Arnold, pp. 269–98.

Rothwell N.J., Stock M.J. (1986b). Whither brown fat? *Biosci. Rep.*, **6**, 3–18.

Rothwell N.J., Stock M.J. (1986c). Possible involvement of prostaglandins in diet-induced thermogenesis of cafeteria fed rats. *Proc. Nutr. Soc.*, **45**, 111A.

Rothwell N.J., Stock M.J. (1987a). Influence of carbohydrate and fat intake on diet-induced thermogenesis and brown fat activity in rats fed low protein diets. *J. Nutr.*, **117**, 1721–6.

Rothwell N.J., Stock M.J. (1987b). Effects of diet and fenfluramine on thermogenesis on the rat: possible involvement of serotonergic mechanisms in the rat. *Int. J. Obesity*, **11**, 319–24.

Rothwell N.J., Stock M.J. (1988a). Insulin and thermogenesis. *Int. J. Obesity*, **1**, 93–102.

Rothwell N.J., Stock M.J. (1988b). Influence of adrenalectomy on age-related changes in energy balance thermogenesis and brown fat activity in the rat. *Comp. Biochem. Physiol.*, **89A**, 265–9.

Rothwell N.J., Stock M.J., Thexton A.J. (1983). Decerebration activates thermogenesis in the rat. *J. Physiol.*, **342**, 15–22.

Rothwell N.J., Busbridge N.J., Humphray H., Hissey P. (1989). Central actions of interleukin-1β on fever and thermogenesis. *Cytokine*, **1**, 153.

Rothwell N.J., Rose J.G., Little R.A. (1990). Brown adipose tissue activity after scald injury in the rat. *Circ. Shock*, **33**, 33 6.

Rothwell N.J., Hardwick A.J., LeFeuvre R.A. et al. (1991). Central actions of CRF on thermogenesis are mediated by proopio melanocortin products. *Brain Res.*, **541**, 89–92.

Rothwell N.J., Busbridge N.J., LeFeuvre R.A. et al. (1991b). Interleukin-6 is a centrally acting endogenous pyrogen in the rat. *Can. J. Physiol. Pharmacol.*, **69**, 1465–9.

Sahakian B.J., Trayhurn P., Wallace M. et al. (1983). Increased weight gain and reduced activity in brown adipose tissue produced by depletion of hypothalamic noradrenaline. *Neurosci. Lett.*, **39**, 321–6.

Saito M., Minokoshi Y., Shimanin R. (1989). Accelerated norepinephrine turnover in peripheral tissues after ventromedial hypothalamic stimulation in rats. *Brain Res.*, **481**, 298–303.

Sapolsky R.M., Rivier C., Yamamoto G. et al. (1987). Interleukin 1 stimulates the secretion of hypothalamic corticotropin releasing factor. *Science*, **238**, 522–4.

Seydoux J., Rohner-Jeanrenaud F., Assimacopoulos-Jeannet F. et al. (1981). Functional disconnection of brown adipose tissue in hypothalamic obesity in rats. *Pflügers Archiv.*, **390**, 1–4.

Shimazu T., Takahashi A. (1980). Stimulation of hypothalamic nuclei has differential effects on lipid synthesis in brown and white adipose tissue. *Nature*, **284**, 62–4.

Shimazu T., Noma M., Saito M. (1986). Chronic infusion of norepinephrine into the VMH induces obesity in rats. *Brain Res.*, **369**, 215–23.

Siviy S.M., Kritikos A., Atrens D.M., Shepherd A. (1989). Effects of norepinephrine infusion in the paraventricular hypothalamus on energy expenditure in the rat. *Brain Res.*, **487**, 79–88.

Smillie F., Boulton C., Peers S., Flower R.J. (1989). Distribution of lipocortins I, II and V in tissues of the rat, mouse and guinea pig. *Br. J. Pharmacol.*, **97**, P90.

Stellar E. (1954). The physiology of motivation. *Psychol. Rev.*, **61**, 522.

Sternberg E.M. (1989). Monokines, lymphokines and the brain. In *The Year in Immunology* (Cruse J.M., Lewis R.E., eds). Basel: Karger, pp. 205–17.

Stoner H.B. (1986). Metabolism after trauma and in sepsis. *Circ. Shock*, **19**, 75–87.

Strijbos P.J.C.M., Tilders F.J.H., Carey F. et al. (1991). Localisation of immunoreactive lipocortin-1 in the brain and the pituitary gland of the rat: effects of adrenalectomy, dexamethanne and colchicine treatment. *Brain Res.*, **553**, 249–60.

Tsagakaris S., Gillies G., Rees L.H. et al. (1989). Interleukin 1 directly stimulates the release of corticotrophin releasing factor from rat hypothalamus. *Neuroendocrinology*, **49**, 98–101.

Uehara A., Gottschall P.E., Dahl R.R., Arimura A. (1987). Stimulation of ACTH release by human interleukin-1 beta but not by interleukin-1 alpha in conscious freely moving rats. *Biochem. Biophys. Res. Commun.*, **146**, 1286–90.

Uehara A., Sekuya C., Takasagi Y. et al. (1989). Anorexia induced by interleukin 1: involvement of corticotropin releasing factor. *Am. J. Physiol.*, **257**, R613–17.

Weingarten H.P., Chang P., McDonald T.J. (1985). Comparison of the metabolic and behavioural disturbances following PVN and VMH lesions. *Brain Res. Bull.*, **14**, 551–9.

Williamson D.H. (1987). Brain substrates and the effect of nutrition. *Proc. Nutr. Soc.*, **46**, 81–7.

Wilmore D.W., Long J.M., Mason A.D. et al. (1976). Catecholamines: mediator of the hypermetabolic response to thermal injury. *Ann. Surg.*, **870**, 653–70.

Wolfe R.R. (1990). Physiological significance of substrate cycling in humans. In *Hormones and Nutrition in Obesity and Cachexia* (Muller M.J., ed.). Berlin: Springer, pp. 59–68.

York D.A. (1987). Neural activity in hypothalamic and genetic obesity. *Proc. Nutr. Soc.*, **46**, 105–17.

York D.A. (1989). Corticosteroid inhibition of thermogenesis in obese animals. *Proc. Nutr. Soc.*, **48**, 231–5.

Yukimura Y., Bray G.A., Wolfsen A.R. (1978). Some effects of adrenalectomy in the fatty rat. *Endocrinology*, **103**, 1924–8.

47. Substrate Metabolism in Injury

R. R. Wolfe

Three aspects of metabolic regulation are fundamental to the determination of substrate oxidation: (1) the requirement for energy production; (2) the availability of energy substrates; (3) the intracellular capacity for substrate oxidation. This chapter will focus on regulation of the availability of endogenous substrates, and their intracellular oxidation. The predominant endogenous substrates are glucose, which is produced in the liver and released into the blood, and free fatty acids, which are released into the circulation from fat cells by the process of lipolysis. Factors regulating alterations in glucose production and lipolysis in critical illness will be discussed, and related to observed effects on substrate oxidation.

GLUCOSE PRODUCTION

The organ normally responsible for glucose production is the liver, and in some circumstances the kidney can also contribute. In the production of glucose from either glycogen or gluconeogenesis from non-glucose precursors, glucose-6-phosphate (G-6-P) formation is the penultimate step. G-6-P is trapped inside the cell because it cannot pass through the membrane into the plasma. The formation and release of plasma glucose is dependent on the presence of the enzyme glucose-6-phosphatase to catalyse the conversion of G-6-P to glucose, and this enzyme can be found in significant quantities only in the liver and the kidneys. Thus, although glycogen can be produced and stored in rather large amounts in the muscle, the G-6-P resulting from the breakdown of muscle glycogen can only supply the precursor for glycolysis in that tissue, and cannot contribute to the maintenance of the plasma glucose concentration. Glucose production in the liver is derived from either stored glycogen or gluconeogenesis from non-glucose precursors.

GLYCOGEN METABOLISM

Following the ingestion of a high-carbohydrate meal, a significant portion of the absorbed glucose ends up as glycogen in the liver. However, recent evidence indicates that most of this glycogen is not derived from glucose taken up in the liver. Rather, most of ingested or infused glucose is taken up peripherally (Katz *et al.*, 1983) and metabolized to actate (Wolfe and Burke, 1978) or, to a lesser extent,

to alanine (Wolfe *et al.*, 1986). These molecules are transported back to the liver, where they are taken up and converted into glycogen (Newgard *et al.*, 1983). When glucose absorption or infusion stops and the blood glucose level drops, a hormonal response is triggered that stimulates the breakdown of glycogen and the release of glucose into the bloodstream. Glucagon is probably the most potent stimulus of glycogen breakdown in this circumstance. In fact, stimulation of hepatic glycogenolysis is one of the most sensitive and reproducible metabolic effects of a hormone on any tissue (Cahill, 1988). Other hormones that stimulate glycogenolysis are adrenaline, noradrenaline, vasopressin and angiotensin II. In the first few hours after a meal (or cessation of a glucose infusion), glycogenolysis can account for as much as 50% of the total glucose production, but by 24 hours of fasting most of the liver glycogen is depleted (Felig *et al.*, 1975). If the hormones that stimulate glycogenolysis are elevated above normal (as is the case with glucagon in stress), glycogen is depleted more rapidly.

GLUCONEOGENESIS

Gluconeogenesis refers to the formation of new glucose from non-carbohydrate precursors. Gluconeogenesis is a complex reaction sequence of many intermediate steps; it involves some reactions of glycolysis in reverse and some additional reactions that overcome the energy barriers, preventing a direct reversal of glycolysis. A variety of substrates can serve as gluconeogenic precursors, but under most circumstances lactate is the most important.

Since most lactate is derived from plasma glucose via glycolysis, the resynthesis of glucose from lactate is a cyclic reaction, originally described by Cori (1931), and is commonly called the Cori cycle. Resynthesis of glucose from lactate in the liver is an important route of lactate disposal, for although other tissues can also dispose of lactate, animals with surgical hepatectomies develop lactic acidosis (Cahill, 1988). For example, when the ability of a tissue to completely catabolize substrates to carbon dioxide and water is limited because of a lack of sufficient oxygen, the Cori cycle maintains a supply of fuel (glucose) that can provide a certain amount of energy anaerobically. The 'net' glucose formation does not increase via the Cori cycle, and in that sense it may be considered a waste of energy, since energy is required to resynthesize the glucose from lactate. However, the energy to resynthesize the glucose comes from fat oxidation in the liver (Exton, 1975), so that the Cori cycle results in an energy transfer from adipose tissue to muscle, with glucose and lactate serving as the 'currency' in situations in which the muscle is unable to fully rely on fat oxidation. The resting rate of Cori cycle activity in normal man has been determined to account for approximately 10–15% of the total glucose production in fasting (Wolfe *et al.*, 1979a; Cahill, 1988).

Glycerol is potentially an excellent gluconeogenic substrate, in that it enters the gluconeogenic pathway closer to glucose than any other substrate. The extent to which glycerol is converted to glucose is primarily a function of its availability, since the conversion of glycerol to glucose is the major route by which glycerol is cleared from the blood. Glycerol contributes only about 3% of the total glucose produced during a short fast in a normal, lean subject. When there is stimulation of fat mobilization, such as during a long fast (Bortz *et al.*, 1972) or sepsis (Wolfe, 1986), glycerol can contribute as much as 20% of the total glucose production.

Alanine and glutamine account for 50–60% of the total amino acids released from muscle. In non-acidotic conditions, little glutamine is taken up by the kidney; rather, it is taken up by the mucosal cells of the small intestine and converted to alanine (Windmueller and Spaeth, 1975). Thus, alanine is the major amino acid precursor for gluconeogenesis. Alanine is released from muscle in far greater quantities than present in muscle protein, but its origin is controversial. It has been suggested that pyruvate resulting from the glycolytic catabolism of glucose is transaminated and the resulting alanine is released into the bloodstream, where it travels to the liver for reincorporation into glucose (Felig, 1973). According to this proposal, alanine functions in a metabolic cycle analogous to the Cori cycle in that no new 'net' glucose is produced. The nitrogen required for the transamination of pyruvate is derived from the amino acids that are oxidized by muscle, including the branched-chain amino acids valine, leucine and isoleucine, as well as aspartate and glutamate. The role of this process has been proposed to be the transfer of ammonia from muscle to liver in the non-toxic form of alanine.

There are different potential sites of control of gluconeogenesis, most of which involve the rate of pyruvate production in the liver. Gluconeogenesis is only one of a variety of potential fates for pyruvate, including the tricarboxylic aid cycle (for ATP generation) or fatty acid synthesis. Although various factors are known to affect the rate of gluconeogenesis *in vitro*, the most important factors *in vivo* are the hormones glucagon, epinephrine and cortisol, which stimulate gluconeogenesis; insulin, which inhibits gluconeogenesis; and the plasma glucose level itself. An elevated plasma glucose concentration, independent of any change in hormonal levels, inhibits hepatic glucose production (Wolfe *et al.*, 1986).

GLUCOSE PRODUCTION IN CRITICAL ILLNESS

Glucose production is elevated in almost all critically ill patients (Figure 47.1) (Wolfe *et al.*, 1979b; Shaw *et al.*, 1985; Shaw and Wolfe, 1986a,b, 1987). Studies have particularly focused on the response in burn patients, because their relatively stable (yet critical) condition allows reproducible experimental conditions. From our experience in a wide variety of critical illnesses, however, it seems likely that the regulation of glucose production is similar in most patients. Gluconeogenesis, particularly from alanine (Wilmore *et al.*, 1980), is elevated, and glycogenolysis is also stimulated subsequent to carbohydrate intake. The increased rate of gluconeogenesis from amino acids renders those amino acids unavailable for reincorporation into body protein. Rather, the nitrogen is excreted, primarily in urea, therefore contributing to the progressive depletion of body protein stores.

Relationship between muscle amino acid release and gluconeogenesis

The rate of protein breakdown in critical illness is increased when compared to the rate in normal individuals fed comparable levels of protein and calories (Wolfe *et al.*, 1983). This results in an increased efflux of amino acids from the muscle, including gluconeogenic amino acids. Alanine in particular is released at an increased rate (Newsholme, 1976) and seems to be a systemic response to injury, since the release was found to be elevated not only from the burned legs, but also from the unburned legs of patients with burns elsewhere (Newsholme, 1976). The increased alanine released into the plasma is cleared in the liver and converted to glucose at an increased rate. It has been proposed that the rate of glucose production is directly influenced by the availability of alanine (Blackburn *et al.*, 1977). However, when alanine was infused into normal volunteers, contrary to the proposed theory, increased alanine delivery to the liver did

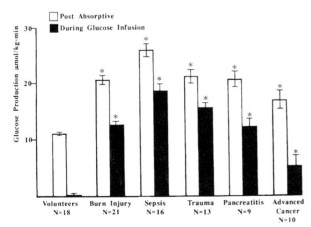

Figure 47.1 Glucose production in critically ill patients.

not stimulate the total rate of glucose production (Wolfe *et al.*, 1985a). In contrast, infusing glucose increased alanine release from muscle, indicating that pyruvate availability is rate limiting for the peripheral formation of alanine. Thus, the increase in total glucose production in critical illness cannot be attributed to an increased rate of alanine delivery to the liver. Rather, the high rate of glucose production and thus glucose uptake (see below) drives the rate of peripheral release of alanine. This general notion is further supported by the fact that plasma amino acid concentrations, including gluconeogenic amino acids, are generally below normal in burn patients. It is unclear how low concentrations of amino acids could be the driving force for gluconeogenesis in the liver. Thus, it can be concluded that factors directly stimulating glucose production at the liver are more important than changes in peripheral metabolism in dictating the rate of glucose production.

Responsiveness of glucose production to glucose and insulin

Plasma insulin levels are usually normal or elevated in burn patients (Wolfe *et al.*, 1979b). The fact that the basal rate of glucose production is elevated, despite a normal or elevated plasma insulin level, can be defined as hepatic insulin resistance, since normally the elevated insulin concentration would lower the rate of glucose production. Furthermore, the plasma glucose concentration is also frequently increased, which would normally directly inhibit glucose production (Wolfe *et al.*, 1986). When glucose is infused into patients, glucose production is suppressed to some extent, but at all glucose infusion rates tested, the residual endogenous glucose production is higher than would be expected in normal volunteers (Wolfe *et al.*, 1979a) because of this hepatic 'insulin' and 'glucose' resistance.

The failure of glucose production to respond to altered substrate delivery, and the sustained glucose production in the face of elevated insulin and glucose levels, argue for a potent hepatic stimulation of glucose production in critically ill patients. Studies in burn patients indicate this stimulation is hormonal.

The best way to determine if a hormone is exerting an effect is to lower pharmacologically that hormone concentration acutely, or block its action, and observe the response in order to deduce the pre-blockade action of the hormone. When this approach is used to study the role of the catecholamines by giving adrenergic blocking agents, the stimulation of glucose production in burn injury cannot be explained by increased catecholamine activity. In fact, when adrenergic blockade was administered to burned guinea-pigs, glucose production increased, as opposed to the expected decrease had pre-existent catecholamine activity been stimulating glucose

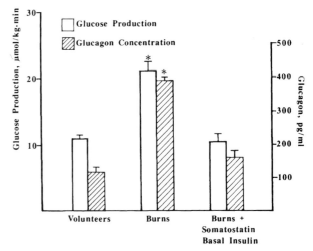

Figure 47.2 Relationship between glucagon and glucose production in patients with severe burns.

production (Durkot and Wolfe, 1981). This unexpected increase in glucose production was subsequently explained on the basis of the blockade effect on fatty acid metabolism (Wolfe and Shaw, 1984). When the changes in fatty acid levels after blockade were eliminated by lipid infusion, it became evident that adrenergic blockade had no effect on glucose production in the basal state.

In contrast to the situation with the catecholamines, blocking glucagon secretion has a pronounced effect on glucose production in burn patients (Jahoor *et al.*, 1986). Patients were infused with somatostatin, which inhibits the secretion of glucagon and insulin, and insulin was replaced in order to maintain the pre-existent basal concentration. When glucagon was lowered to the normal concentration, glucose production fell and remained depressed through the infusion (Figure 47.2) (Jahoor *et al.*, 1986). This study proves the role of an elevated concentration of glucagon as the pre-eminent stimulator of glucose production in burn patients.

The role of cortisol and other hormones as simulators of glucose production in burn injury has not been assessed in the same manner as glucagon and the catecholamines. The results of hormone infusion experiments, however, indicate that cortisol may play an important role (Blackburn *et al.*, 1977), probably via enhancing and prolonging the effectiveness of glucagon.

REGULATION OF LIPOLYSIS

In normal man, lipids constitute more than 80% of the stored fuel reserve. Additionally, fat stores, along with very small carbohydrate stores, can be almost completely depleted without detriment to the individual. Conversely, the use of protein reserves is limited, since even moderate depletion can adversely affect an organism exposed to stress

(Blackburn *et al.*, 1977). Consequently, when an individual must rely on endogenous fuel supplies for energy, lipids are physiologically the most desirable source. Most tissues, including heart and skeletal muscle (Neely *et al.*, 1972; Hochachka *et al.*, 1977), can readily use fatty acids as substrates for energy metabolism. The use of fatty acids by these tissues preserves the limited carbohydrate stores for use by central nervous tissue and red blood cells. Additionally, the brain can partially adapt to use of ketone bodies (β-hydroxybutyrate and acetoacetate) as an energy substrate. Thus, in the postabsorptive state in man, fat may supply approximately 50–60% of the energy. If food deprivation continues for several days, adaptive mechanisms occur whereby a greater percentage of energy is derived from fat, consequently body nitrogen is spared as a consequence (Cahill, 1970). The extent to which an animal is able to tolerate starvation appears to be related to its ability to rely on fat as an energy source. For example, the dog adapts to starvation poorly, in that a proportionate increase in energy derived from fat is evident only after several days of fasting. As a result, the dog may become physiologically compromised within 4–5 days of starvation because of protein depletion. In contrast, the hibernating bear withstands food deprivation throughout the winter by utilizing endogenous fat to such an extent that its lean body mass is preserved (Nelson *et al.*, 1975). Thus, it seems reasonable that a theoretically optimal 'stress' response would involve the mobilization and utilization of fat. The pattern of hormonal response generally associated with varieties of stress – increased adrenaline, cortisol and glucagon levels and low insulin levels, as well as increased sympathetic nervous system activity – would be expected to favour the mobilization of lipid from storage depots. However, other factors may be simultaneously operative that would tend to suppress the mobilization or utilization of fat. For example, elevations in the lactate concentration resulting from the stimulation of muscle glycolysis (another catecholamine effect) stimulates re-esterification within the adipose cell (Fredholm, 1971), meaning that even though lipolysis may be stimulated, the amount of fatty acids released into the plasma may not reflect that stimulation. A decrease in pH inhibits lipolysis (Fredholm, 1971) and hyperglycaemia may inhibit lipolysis directly (Schulman *et al.*, 1980) and stimulate re-esterification by leading to an increased rate of formation of α-glycerophosphate, which forms the backbone to which fatty acids attach to form triacylglycerols. In addition, adequate blood flow through fat is necessary for an increased lipolytic rate to be reflected by enhanced fatty acid mobilization (Kovach *et al.*, 1970). Since sympathetic stimulation decreases fat blood flow, this is another potential impediment to the mobilization of fat in injury and sepsis. In summary, although the generalized 'stress response' would seem to favour the

mobilization of fat from adipose tissues to the readily usable form of plasma free fatty acids (FFAs), many factors interact to determine if that response actually occurs.

Given all of these potentially interacting variables, it is interesting that in any form of stress a stimulation of lipolysis and concomitant release of fatty acids into plasma is a fundamental metabolic response (Figure 47.3). The principal mediator of this response is increased adrenergic activity (Wolfe *et al.*, 1987a,b), as beta adrenergic blockade in patients will acutely reduce the rate of release of FFA to the normal range. However, there is a tachyphylaxis to the repetitive administration of beta-blockade, such that chronic blockade in patients does not diminish FFA concentrations (Hernden *et al.*, 1988). There are consequently other factors in patients that can also stimulate lipolysis if adrenergic activity wanes, or is blocked.

FFA are released at a rate well in excess of the requirement of tissues for FFA as an energy substrate. In severely burned patients, over 70% of released fatty acids are not oxidized, but rather re-esterified into triglyceride (TG). Since the rate of release of fatty acids is markedly elevated, the total rate of re-esterification is also greatly elevated in patients. The major site of clearance and re-esterification of plasma FFA is the liver; the major determinant of TG synthesis is the rate of delivery of FFA to the liver. Under normal conditions, even a high rate of hepatic fatty acid uptake can be accommodated by a proportionate synthesis of TG and secretion into the plasma as VLDL-TG. This plasma TG is returned to the adipose tissue for storage, thereby forming a cycle between TG and FFA (Figure 47.4) (Wolfe *et al.*, 1985b). However, in critically ill patients, there may be a limit to the amount of TG that can be exported from the liver, perhaps reflecting impaired Apo B protein synthesis, which is necessary for the formation of the VLDL-

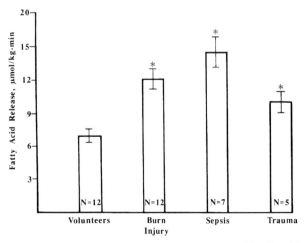

Figure 47.3 Release of fatty acid in critically ill patients.

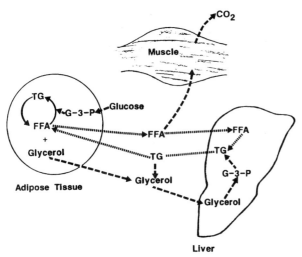

Figure 47.4 Relationship between fatty acid release and triglyceride production.

TG prior to secretion. In this case, fat will accumulate in the liver, even in the absence of a significant amount of hepatic fatty acid synthesis. This response could possibly be antagonized by a large dose of glucose that would stimulate hepatic fatty acid synthesis. On the other hand, insulin and glucose suppress the peripheral mobilization of FFA, and thus the delivery of FFA to the liver. In septic dogs, we found the suppressive effect of hyperinsulinae-mia on FFA release to actually result in a decrease in hepatic TG production, even though glucose uptake was markedly greater than in the basal state (Wolfe *et al.*, 1985b). The clinical observation that the amount of fat in the liver in seriously ill patients is directly related to the severity of illness, and unrelated to the nature of the nutritional support (Wolfe *et al.*, 1988), is predicted from the physiological basis of the production of hepatic TG.

SUBSTRATE OXIDATION IN CRITICAL ILLNESS

Measurement by indirect calorimetry

Several factors are important in determining the relative ability to oxidize substrates, not the least of which is the methodology chosen to assess the response. Indirect calorimetry has long been the principle approach, yet both technical and theoretical limitations may cause problems in patients. The potential technical problem may arise when attempting to measure oxygen consumption (V_{O_2}) in patients receiving oxygen via a ventilator, because it is difficult to obtain a well-mixed sample of the inspired air for accurate oxygen concentration measurement. This can be overcome technically. Perhaps more substantive, theoretical problems arise in patients due to uncertainties regarding the contribution of protein metabolism to the observed respiratory quotient (RQ, V_{O_2} divided by V_{CO_2}),

which is the cornerstone of the calculation of substrate oxidation rates (Frayn, 1983). It is classically assumed that 6.04 litres of O_2 are consumed for each gram of urinary nitrogen, based on the elemental composition of beef muscle protein. However, depending on the amino acid proportion in the protein mixture, the use of the general factor of 6.04 litres O_2/g urinary nitrogen will result in substantial error since the O_2 to urinary nitrogen value can range from 2.2 litres O_2/g N for arginine to 16.01 litres O_2/g N for phenylalanine. An error in the factor between +12% and –39% of the true value can be incurred if the general factors are used, since the O_2 to urinary nitrogen value for the major dietary proteins and artificial amino acid mixtures range from 5.34 to 9.88 litres O_2/g urinary nitrogen (Livesey and Elia, 1988). Another problem of potential importance is that when nitrogen is excreted in urea, one carbon is lost from the bicarbonate pool with each molecule of urea, but of course this does not occur with ammonia. Consequently, the physiological RQ of protein oxidation (R_p) will depend on the proportion of nitrogen excreted as NH_3, creatinine, or urea. Thus, when nitrogen is eliminated in creatinine, urea or ammonia, the R_p is 0.823, 0.826 and 0.95, respectively (Kleibu, 1975). The higher RQ of ammonia stems from the fact that all the CO_2 from oxidation comes out in the breath as opposed to some of the CO_2 coming out in urea or creatinine if they are the end products containing the nitrogen. A normal distribution of nitrogen among urea, creatinine, and ammonia is around 90:5:5. However, in special circumstances (acidosis; starvation; diabetes; under conditions of impaired urea synthesis such as severe liver injury, hepatectomy, decreased hepatic blood flow, and so forth) the contribution of ammonia may considerably increase. From the difference in R_p it can be calculated that R_p increases by 0.00127 for each 1% increase in the proportion of nitrogen excreted as ammonia. A combination of errors in R_p and O_2 urinary nitrogen can produce significant errors in the rates of fuel utilization. The following example is from Livesey and Elia (1988). Two patients in nitrogen balance, with identical energy expenditures (2930 kcal/day) and $R_p = 0.85$, receive 14 g N as either Amin-Aid or Aminofusin (commercially available amino acid mixtures):

	Amino acid oxidation (kcal/day)	R_p	Fat oxidation (kcal/day)
Amin-Aid	9.88 × 4.65 × 14 = 643	0.889	636
Aminofusin	5.48 × 4.65 × 14 = 359	0.853	989
Δ (AA-AF)	−44%		+55%

This large potential error does not cover possible errors for a change in the distribution of urea, creatinine and ammonia in the urine, which may also be substantial. Thus, classical indirect calorimetry as applied to critically ill patients receiving nutritional support is subject to considerable error when computing absolute rates of carbohydrate and fat oxidation.

GLUCOSE UTILIZATION

The glucose concentration in the blood is normally regulated within narrow limits, but the rate of glucose uptake and oxidation can vary greatly. Following a high carbohydrate meal, or during a high dose glucose infusion, glucose is the major fuel for the body; after several hours of fasting, only about 25% of total carbon dioxide production is from glucose oxidation (Wolfe *et al.*, 1979a). Certain tissues, most notably the brain and erythrocytes, depend on glucose for energy and have a relatively constant rate of glucose uptake under most conditions. An exception to this occurs in prolonged starvation, when the brain adapts to the use of ketones (acetoacetate and beta-hydroxybutyrate) for energy, but this is a special situation that is not relevant to the day-to-day regulation of glucose utilization when nutrition is available. Therefore, even though the brain and erythrocytes may account for more than 50% of the glucose uptake during fasting, they probably do not play an important role in the observed fluctuations in the rate of glucose oxidation in different physiological and pathological states. The liver can play a role in the disposition of a glucose load (Felig and Wahren, 1971), but since most of this glucose uptake is not oxidized, the liver is not a site where the rate of glucose oxidation varies much either. The muscle mass, on the other hand, exerts a profound influence on an individual's overall rate of glucose utilization. Since muscle constitutes approximately 40% of the body mass, any change in the rate of glucose uptake by muscle will significantly affect the overall rate of glucose uptake by the individual. In the resting postabsorptive state, it is debatable whether the muscle takes up any glucose at all (Andres *et al.*, 1956), but in the individual with hyperglycaemia or one who is exercising, the rate of glucose utilization by the muscle can increase several fold. Because of the important role of changes in muscle glucose metabolism in the overall energy metabolism, considerable attention has been focused on regulating glucose utilization by the muscle.

The rate of glucose entry into the muscle cell is a rate-limiting step of glucose metabolism. Glucose is rapidly phosphorylated to G-6-P once inside the cell, so the intracellular glucose concentration is lower than the extracellular concentration, and glucose moves down its concentration gradient into the cell. Glucose diffusion is facilitated by a carrier-transport system that, when combined with glucose, renders the glucose sufficiently lipid soluble to move through the cell membrane. No energy is expended in this process, so it is considered a passive (as opposed to active) transport mechanism. The rate of glucose uptake increases in the muscle cell as the blood glucose level increases, and insulin increases the ability of the muscle cell to take up glucose. Insulin works on the surface of the cells by binding to specific receptors that then initiate its action (Cutarecasas, 1971).

In normal volunteers, the rate of muscle glucose uptake and utilization are influenced strongly by the physical state. Muscle glucose uptake and utilization increase significantly during exercise, and bed rest causes decreased forearm glucose uptake during glucose infusion (Lipman *et al.*, 1972). The latter response is only evident during glucose infusion, since in the resting state without glucose infusion the muscle takes up little glucose. The mechanism whereby exercise enhances glucose transport into muscle has not been elucidated, but it seems to involve an amplification of the normal stimulatory effect of insulin on glucose clearance (Koivisto *et al.*, 1980). The implications of the role of the physical state on glucose clearance is obvious in relation to critically ill patients, since such patients usually are recumbent and perform little exercise.

Whereas it is generally accepted that insulin regulates muscle glucose utilization by controlling the rate of glucose entry, there is an alternative explanation that was originally described as the 'glucose-fatty acid cycle' (Randle *et al.*, 1963). The cornerstone of the theory is that free fatty acid (FFA) inhibits glucose utilization. Since insulin inhibits lipolysis and thereby reduces the circulating levels of FFA in the plasma, a low level of insulin (e.g. during fasting) releases that inhibition and results in a high FFA level. The high FFA level in turn inhibits glucose utilization, and since the rate of glucose uptake is reduced, a given blood glucose concentration can be maintained at a reduced rate of glucose production.

Evidence supporting the role of the 'glucose-fatty acid cycle' in controlling glucose uptake is controversial. Some *in vitro* experiments have demonstrated an inhibitory effect of FFA on glucose oxidation (Rennie and Holloszy, 1977). In contrast, other experiments have failed to find an FFA effect on glucose utilization in the perfused rat hind limb (Goodman *et al.*, 1974). Evidence obtained *in vivo* regarding the glucose-fatty acid cycle is even more controversial. This controversy is a result of the close interactions between glucose, fatty acids and insulin, which make it impossible to alter only the pertinent variable without in some way affecting another. In any case, there does appear to be a close interrelationship between glucose and fatty acid metabolism, and although the exact details have not been clearly resolved, in a general sense, there is no doubt that their respective oxidation rates are inversely related.

Role of insulin

Insulin is the single most important hormone for controlling glucose metabolism. The burn patient has been described for many years as 'insulin resistant', implying that the altered glucose metabolism in such patients is in some way due to the failure of insulin to function properly as a metabolic regulator. To understand the concept of 'insulin resistance', it is first necessary to consider the normal function of insulin with regard to glucose metabolism.

Insulin serves to decrease the plasma glucose concentration by inhibiting the rate of hepatic glucose production, and also by stimulating glucose uptake in certain peripheral tissues. However, the threshold for the action of insulin on peripheral glucose uptake is higher than the threshold for the effect of insulin on hepatic glucose production. The concentration of insulin necessary to elicit one-half the maximal effect on either glucose production or peripheral glucose clearance has been determined by using the glucose-insulin clamp technique (De Fronzo *et al.*, 1979). Using this approach, insulin is increased to a prescribed concentration by infusion. The plasma glucose concentration is then measured at frequent intervals and enough glucose is infused to maintain the plasma glucose concentration at the same level as before the insulin infusion. This technique is called a 'euglycaemic clamp', and is useful in evaluating the effect of a change in plasma insulin concentration, independent of changes in the plasma glucose concentration. Using this approach, along with a tracer infusion of labelled glucose to measure the plasma glucose kinetics, it has been estimated that one-half the maximal suppressive effect of insulin on glucose production is elicited at a plasma concentration of 29 uU/ml, whereas one-half the maximal effect on glucose uptake is not achieved until there is an incremental increase of insulin concentration of 55 uU/ml (meaning a plasma concentration of about 65 mU/ml) (Rizza *et al.*, 1981). Other investigators have determined that the peripheral effect requires an even higher concentration of insulin (Kolterman *et al.*, 1979).

Not only is a high concentration of insulin required to elicit one-half the maximal effect on glucose clearance, very nearly that much insulin is needed to exert any peripheral effect at all. Zierler and Rabinowitz (1964) measured glucose uptake across the forearm, and then infused insulin into an artery supplying blood to the arm. They found that if the insulin concentration was increased to 30 uU/ml, there was no effect on glucose uptake, although effects on fat mobilization, potassium flux and amino acids were elicited. Thus, of all the known metabolic effects of insulin, its effect on the peripheral clearance of glucose is the least sensitive or responsive, yet it is this aspect of insulin action that

has received the most attention in relation to the response to stress.

The ability of insulin to stimulate glucose uptake peripherally is diminished with stress. This insulin resistance is evident after injury and during sepsis after a wide range of doses of insulin (Wolfe *et al.*, 1979b; Black *et al.*, 1982) and does not seem to be overcome, even at supraphysiological plasma insulin concentrations (Henderson *et al.*, 1991). A number of indirect lines of evidence have been used to deduce that an impaired ability to oxidize glucose is responsible for the peripheral insulin resistance in patients. For example, plasma lactate concentration is often high, particularly during glucose infusion, even with adequate tissue oxygenation. However, until recently a direct determination of the ability to oxidize pyruvate had not been made. Using stable isotope methodology, the intracellular pyruvate pool of severely burned patients was labelled to quantify both the total rate of production and oxidation of pyruvate. Results indicate that not only is there no impairment in pyruvate oxidation, but also the total rate of oxidation is significantly increased, both in the basal state and during glucose infusion (Figure 47.5) (Wolfe *et al.*, 1991). Thus, high lactate concentrations result in these patients simply from a mass-action effect secondary to a high rate of pyruvate production, and thus do not necessarily reflect any impairment in pyruvate oxidation.

The lack of a significant role of an impairment in glucose oxidation on the overall metabolic response in critically ill patients is further substantiated by the results of a recent experiment, in which the rate of glucose oxidation in septic patients was stimulated with dichloroacetate (DCA), a specific stimulator of pyruvate dehydrogenase. The experiment

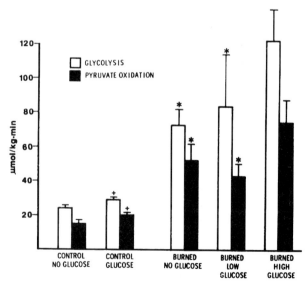

Figure 47.5 Effects of burn injury on pyruvate metabolism.

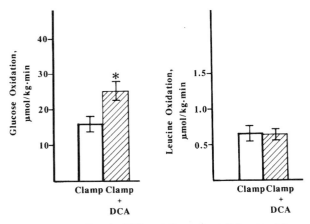

* **Significantly Different From Basal Value,** $P < .05$

Figure 47.6 Effect of stimulation of glucose oxidation in sepsis or burn injury on leucine oxidation.

was done under conditions in which the insulin and glucose concentrations were clamped experimentally at constant values. DCA significantly stimulated glucose oxidation in septic patients, as expected, but this had no effect on leucine oxidation (Figure 47.6) (Jahoor *et al.*, 1989). Leucine flux was also not affected, meaning that the alterations in amino acid oxidation and protein kinetics in patients is not directly related to the rate of glucose oxidation.

SUMMARY

The mix of endogenous substrates (glucose, fatty acids) oxidized for energy in critically ill patients is largely determined by their relative availability. In particular, the rate of glucose oxidation is directly related to the availability of plasma glucose, as there appears to be no impairment in its oxidation. The oxidation of fatty acids could be considered to make up the balance between energy requirement and availability of glucose. Fatty acids are released well in excess of their oxidation rate, meaning that in patients as much as 70% of FFA are re-esterified into triglyceride in the liver, potentially contributing to the development of fatty infiltration of the liver. The extent of re-esterification, as opposed to oxidation, is largely determined by the availability of glucose, in that an abundance of glucose will decrease FFA oxidation and stimulate re-esterification.

These observations with regard to the metabolism of endogenous substrates can generally be extrapolated to the metabolism of exogenous substrate given as nutritional support. Carbohydrate intake dictates the rate of glucose oxidation, and, by deduction, fat oxidation. Thus, when given at rates below caloric requirement in order to prevent fat synthesis, exogenous glucose is an optimal energy substrate. Whereas fat may be utilized to some

extent, if sufficient glucose is given simultaneously, the rate of fat oxidation is usually minimal.

Acknowledgements

Supported by a Grant from the Shriners Hospital and NIH Grant DK 33965.

REFERENCES

Andres R., Cader G., Zierler K.L. (1956). The quantitatively minor role of carbohydrate in oxidative metabolism by skeletal muscle in intact man in the basal state. Measurements of oxygen and glucose uptake and carbon dioxide and lactate production in the forearm. *J. Clin. Invest.*, **35**, 671.

Black P.R., Brooks D.C., Bessey P.Q. et al. (1982). Mechanisms of insulin resistance following injury. *Ann. Surg.*, **196**, 420–35.

Blackburn G.L., Maini B.S., Pierce E.C. (1977). Nutrition in the critically ill patient. *Anesthesiology*, **47**, 181–94.

Bortz W.M., Paul P., Haff A.G., Holmes W.L. (1972). Glycerol turnover and oxidation in man. *J. Clin. Invest.*, **51**, 1537–46.

Cahill G.F. Jr (1970). Starvation in man. *N. Engl. J. Med.*, **282**, 668–75.

Cahill G.F. Jr. (1988). Starvation: some biological aspects. In *Nutrition and Metabolism in Patient Care* (Kinney J.M., Jeejeebhoy K.N., Hill G.L., Owen O.E., eds). London: W.B. Saunders Company, pp. 193–204.

Cori C.F. (1931). Mammalian carbohydrate metabolism. *Physiol. Rev*, **11**, 143–285.

Cutarecasas P. (1971). Insulin-receptor interactions in adipose tissue cells: Direct measurement and properties. *Proc. Natl. Acad. Sci. USA*, **68**, 1264–8.

De Fronzo R.A., Tobin J.D., Andres R. (1979). Glucose clamp technique: a method for quantifying insulin secretion and resistance. *Am. J. Physiol.*, **237**, E214–23.

Durkot M.J., Wolfe R.R. (1981). Effects of adrenergic blockade on glucose kinetics in septic and burned guinea pigs. *Am. J. Physiol.*, **241**, R222–7.

Exton J.H. (1975). Gluconeogenesis. *Metabolism*, **21**, 945–90.

Felig P. (1973). The glucose-alanine cycle. *Metabolism*, **22**, 179.

Felig P., Wahren J. (1971). Influence of endogenous insulin secretion on splanchnic glucose and amino acid metabolism in man. *J. Clin. Invest.*, **59**, 1702–11.

Felig P., Wahren J., Hendler R. (1975). Influence of oral glucose ingestion on splanchnic glucose and gluconeogenic substrate metabolism in man. *Diabetes*, **24**, 468.

Frayn K. (1983). Calculation of substrate oxidation rates *in vivo* from gaseous exchange. *J. Appl. Physiol.*, **55**, 628–34.

Fredholm B.B. (1971). The effect of lactate in canine subcutaneous adipose tissue in situ. *Acta Physiol. Scand.*, **81**, 110–13.

Goodman M.N., Berger M., Ruderman, N.B. (1974). Glucose metabolism in rat skeletal muscle at rest. Effect of starvation, diabetes, ketone bodies, and free fatty acids. *Diabetes*, **23**, 881–8.

Henderson A.A., Frayn K.N., Galasko C.S.B., Little R.A. (1991). Dose–response relationships for the effects of insulin on glucose and fat metabolism in injured patients and control subjects. *Clin. Sci.*, **80**, 25–32.

Herndon D.N., Barrow R.E., Rutan T.C. et al. Effect of propranolol administration on hemodynamic and metabolic responses of burned pediatric patients. *Ann. Surg.*, **208**, 484–92.

Hochachka P.W., Neely J.R., Driedzic N.R. (1977). Integration of lipid utilization with Krebs cycle activity in muscle. *Fed. Proc.*, **36**, 2809–14.

Jahoor F., Herndon D.N., Wolfe R.R. (1986). Role of insulin and glucagon in the response of glucose and alanine kinetics in burn-injured patients. *J. Clin. Invest.*, **78**, 807–14.

Jahoor F., Shangraw R.E., Miyoshi H. et al. (1989). Role of insulin and glucose oxidation in mediating the protein catabolism of burns and sepsis. *Am. J. Physiol.*, **257**, E323–31.

Katz D., Glickman M.G., Rapoport S. (1983). Splanchnic and peripheral disposal of oral glucose in man. *Diabetes*, **32**, 675–9.

Kleibu M. (1975). *Fire of Life: an introduction to animal energetics*. New York: Kreigenic.

Koivisto V., Soman V., Nadel E. (1980). Exercise and insulin: studies on insulin binding, insulin mobilization and counter regulatory hormone secretion. *Fed. Proc.*, **39**, 1481–6.

Kolterman O., Sackow M., Olefsky J. (1979). The effects of acute and chronic starvation on insulin binding to isolate human adipocytes. *J. Clin. Endocrinol. Metab.*, **48**, 836–42.

Kovach A.G.B., Rosell S., Sandor P. (1970). Blood flow, oxygen consumption and free fatty acid release in subcutaneous adipose tissue during hemorrhagic shock in control and phenoxybenzamine-treated dogs. *Circ. Res.*, **26**, 733–48.

Lipman R.L., Raskin P., Love T. (1972). Glucose intolerance during decreased physical activity in man. *Diabetes*, **21**, 101–7.

Livesey G., Elia M. (1988). Estimation of energy expenditure, net carbohydrate utilization, and net fat oxidation and synthesis by indirect calorimetry: evaluation of errors with special reference to the detailed composition of fuels. *Am. J. Clin. Nutr.*, **47**, 608–28.

Neely J.R., Rovetto M.J., Oram J.R. (1972). Myocardial utilization of carbohydrate and lipids. *Prog. Cardiovasc. Res.*, **15**, 289–329.

Nelson R.A., Jones J.D., Wahner H.W. (1975). Nitrogen metabolism in bears: urea metabolism in summer starvation and in winter sleep and role of urinary bladder in water and nitrogen conservation. *Mayo Clin. Proc.*, **50**, 141–6.

Newgard C.B., Hirsch L.J., Foster D.W., McGarry J.D. (1983). Studies on the mechanism by which exogenous glucose is converted into liver glycogen in the rat. *J. Biol. Chem.*, **258**, 8046–52.

Newsholme E.A. (1976). Carbohydrate metabolism *in vivo*, regulation of blood glucose level. *Clin. Endocrinol. Metab.*, **5**, 543–78.

Randle P.J., Garland P.B., Hales C.N., Newsholme E.A. (1963). The glucose and fatty acids cycle. Its role in insulin sensitivity and the metabolic disturbance of diabetes mellitus. *Lancet*, **i**, 785–9.

Rennie M.J., Holloszy J.O. (1977). Inhibition of glucose uptake and glycogenolysis by availability of oleate in well-oxygenated perfused skeletal muscle. *Biochem. J.*, **168**, 161.

Rizza R.A., Mandarino I.J., Gerich J.E. (1981). Dose–response characteristics for effects of insulin or production and utilization of glucose in man. *Am. J. Physiol.*, **240**, E638–9.

Schulman G.I., Williams P.E., Liljenquist J.E., Cherrington A.D. (1980). Effect of hyperglycemia independent of changes in insulin or glucagon on lipolysis in the conscious dog. *Metabolism*, **29**, 317–20.

Shaw J.H., Wolfe R.R. (1986a). Determinations of glucose turnover and oxidation in normal volunteers and septic patients using stable and radio-isotopes: the response to glucose infusion and total parenteral feeding. *Aust. NZ J. Surg.*, **56**, 785–91.

Shaw J.H.F., Wolfe R.R. (1986b). Glucose, fatty acid, and urea kinetics in patients with severe pancreatitis. The response to substrate infusion and total parenteral nutrition. *Ann. Surg.*, **204**, 665–72.

Shaw J.H.F., Wolfe R.R. (1987). Glucose and urea kinetics in patients with early and advanced gastrointestinal cancer: the response to glucose infusion, parenteral feeding, and surgical resection. *Surgery*, **101**, 181–91.

Shaw J.H.F., Klein S., Wolfe R.R. (1985). Assessment of alanine, urea, and glucose interrelationships in normal subjects and in patients with sepsis with stable isotopic tracers. *Surgery*, **97**, 557–67.

Wilmore D.W., Goodwin C.W., Aulick L.H. (1980). Effect of injury and infection on visceral metabolism and circulation. *Ann. Surg.*, **192**, 491–582.

Windmueller H.G., Spaeth A.E. (1975). Intestinal metabolism of glutamine and glutamate from the lumen as compared to glutamine from blood. *Arch. Biochem. Biophys.*, **171**, 662–77.

Wolfe B.M., Walker B.K., Shaul D.B. et al. (1988). Effect of total parenteral nutrition on hepatic histology. *Arch. Surg.*, **123**, 1084–90.

Wolfe R.R. (1986). Substrate kinetics in sepsis. In *The Scientific Basis for the Care of the Critically Ill* (Frayn K.N., Little R.A., eds). Manchester: Manchester University Press, pp. 123–51.

Wolfe R.R., Burke J.F. (1978). Effect of glucose infusion on glucose and lactate metabolism in normal and burned guinea pigs. *J. Trauma*, **18**, 800–5.

Wolfe R.R., Shaw J.H. (1984). Inhibitory effect of plasma free fatty acids on glucose production in the conscious dog. *Am. J. Physiol.*, **246**, E181–6.

Wolfe R.R., Allsop J.R., Burke J.F. (1979a). Glucose metabolism in man: responses to intravenous glucose infusion. *Metabolism*, **28**, 210–20.

Wolfe R.R., Durkot M.J., Allsop J.R., Burke J.F. (1979b). Glucose metabolism in severely burned patients. *Metabolism*, **28**, 1031–9.

Wolfe R.R., Goodenough R.D., Burke J.F., Wolfe M.H. (1983). Response of protein and urea kinetics in burn patients to different levels of protein intake. *Ann. Surg.*, **197**, 163–71.

Wolfe R.R., Jahoor F., Herndon D.N., Wolfe M.H. (1985a). The glucose alanine cycle: origin of control. *J. Parenter. Enter. Nutr.*, **9**, 107 (abstr.).

Wolfe R.R., Shaw J.H., Durkot M.J. (1985b). Effect of sepsis on VLDL kinetics: responses in basal state and during glucose infusion. *Am. J. Physiol.*, **248**, E732–40.

Wolfe R.R., Shaw J.H., Jahoor F. et al. (1986). Response to glucose infusion in humans: role of changes in insulin concentration. *Am. J. Physiol.*, **250**, E306–11.

Wolfe R.R., Herndon D.N., Peters E.J. et al. (1987a). Regulation of lipolysis in severely burned children. *Ann. Surg.*, **206**, 214–21.

Wolfe R.R., Herndon D.N., Jahoor F. et al. (1987b). Effect

of severe burn injury on substrate cycling by glucose and fatty acids. *N. Engl. J. Med.*, **317**, 403–8.

Wolfe R.R., Jahoor F., Herndon D.N., Miyoshi H. (1991). Isotopic evaluation of the metabolism of pyruvate and related substrates in normal adult volunteers and severely burned children: effect of dichloroacetate and glucose infusion. *Surgery,* **110**, 54–67.

Zierler K.L., Rabinowitz D. (1964). Effect of very small concentrations of insulin on forearm metabolism. Persistence of its action on potassium and free fatty acids without its effect on glucose. *J. Clin. Invest.*, **43**, 950–6.

48. Protein Metabolism in Injury

P. J. Garlick and
J. Wernerman

INTRODUCTION

One of the first to recognize the central role of protein metabolism in life was von Liebig in 1842, who stated that 'the amount of tissue metamorphosis in a given time may be measured by the quantity of nitrogen in the urine'. Following this, his pupil Voit described nitrogen balance as a method for studying protein metabolism (Bischoff and Voit, 1860), but it was Cuthbertson in the 1930s who used the nitrogen balance technique to establish the basis of our current knowledge of the metabolic response to trauma (reviewed by Cuthbertson, 1976). He showed that there was an increase in total urinary nitrogen excretion after fractures, and that the amount excreted was proportional to the magnitude of the trauma and to the muscle mass of the individual (Cuthbertson, 1930). Cuthbertson also concluded that the urinary nitrogen loss was derived largely from skeletal muscle and showed that nutrition would not cause these patients to regain nitrogen equilibrium (Cuthbertson, 1931). Later he defined the 'ebb' and 'flow' phases of the response (Cuthbertson, 1942). The 'ebb' is the immediate response, characterized by circulatory instability and a depression in metabolic processes. The 'flow' phase takes longer to develop and persists for much longer. It is associated with the lysis and repair of injured tissue and is the period when energy expenditure is elevated and the disturbances in body protein metabolism which are the subject of this chapter occur.

For many years the management of protein metabolism after trauma was connected to the problems of surgical starvation or semistarvation (Moore, 1959). The obvious disadvantage of not being able to eat was, of course, a major problem for these patients. Intravenous nutrition was clearly needed, but the inadequacy of being able to give only energy substrate (i.e. glucose) was soon recognized, leading to experiments with amino acids in parenteral nutrition. The pioneer work was done by Elman in the 1930s using protein hydrolysates (Elman, 1939), but it was not until the 1950s that crystalline amino acids became available.

Progress beyond this point has to a large extent been delayed by the lack of appropriate techniques for investigating the physiology and pathophysiology of protein metabolism. New therapeutic possibilities have also failed to be evaluated fully because of this deficiency. This chapter, therefore, whilst describing our present knowledge of the response of protein metabolism to trauma, emphasizes what is actually known and what is only hypothesized. The techniques that are presently in use are described in some detail, because knowledge of the assumptions, strengths and weaknesses of each method is often necessary to fully comprehend the results presented in this field. Finally, our knowledge on the mechanisms of the changes following trauma are described, leading to a discussion of current therapies and how effectively these modify the responses of protein metabolism to trauma.

The substantial loss of body protein after trauma leads to wasting and loss of function, particularly in the skeletal musculature. However, because the body contains no stores of protein equivalent to the stores of glycogen and fat, all of the depletion of body nitrogen represents the loss of functional proteins and enzymes. The penalty for this is that with prolonged trauma or sepsis this deficit itself contributes to morbidity and mortality. The benefit, presumably, is that the amino acids released by proteolysis are available to support the defence mechanisms. Thus there is a redistribution of nutrient resources, in the (presumed) absence of their availability from the diet.

Knowledge of the mechanisms of these responses has been sought by a number of routes. Because of the difficulty of performing the necessary studies in traumatized patients, such studies have frequently been supported by measurements in experimental animals and animal tissues *in vitro*. Interpretation of these data requires caution and careful consideration of the relevance of the particular animal model chosen to mimic human trauma. For the same reasons, many measurements have been made in elective surgical patients. The interindividual variability and the level of control by the experimenter in these studies are better than is possible after severe trauma, but the results must also be interpreted with some caution, as the response is much attenuated and of shorter duration. Despite these limitations, however, a body of biochemical and metabolic knowledge has been gained which has resulted in continuing improvements in treatment over the last few decades. For example, the values for urinary nitrogen losses after surgery published a decade or two ago would now be considered excessive (Table 48.1). None the less, with prolonged illness there is still a steady loss of body protein, and research continues in an effort to find how treatments, such as total parenteral nutrition (TPN), can minimize this. However, the potential dangers of this strategy must also be fully understood. Any treatment which limits protein mobilization might also interfere with the activation of the defence systems, and hence might be detrimental rather than beneficial. For this reason metabolic

690

TABLE 48.1
NITROGEN LOSSES AFTER VARIOUS TYPES OF TRAUMA.
(ADAPTED FROM RANDALL, 1970)

Peak daily nitrogen loss after operations		Cumulated nitrogen loss during 10 days following catabolic illness	
Minor surgery	4 g	Minor operation	25 g
Appendectomy	5 g	Major operation	50 g
Cholecystectomy	10 g	Simple fracture	115 g
Vagotonomy and pyloroplasty	15 g	Peritonitis	135 g
		Multiple injury	150 g
Peritonitis and fistula	16 g	Major burn	170 g
Ruptured aneurysm	22 g		
Severe trauma, sepsis	27 g		
Ulcerative colitis, fever	35 g		

evidence, for example for the attenuation of nitrogen loss, might not be adequate. As will be seen below, for practical reasons the majority of studies of therapy have been metabolic or biochemical, but clinical evaluation of outcome must be the final assessment.

BODY PROTEIN LOSSES

Nitrogen balance

The observation that the urinary N excretion is increased in trauma, in the absence of any increase in dietary nitrogen intake, is evidence that body protein is being lost. This conclusion can be made because the bulk of both dietary and body N is contained in protein, which comprises some 15–20% of lean body mass. The nitrogen balance technique, which was first introduced 150 years ago, therefore requires that the nitrogen content of all inputs and outputs of the body be measured, allowing the difference, or balance, to be equated with the loss or gain of body protein, by the equation:

protein loss (grammes) = N loss (grammes) × 6.25

The outputs from the body are generally in the form of urinary, faecal and integumental (skin, hair and sweat) nitrogen, but in trauma victims there may be additional outputs via blood, other fluid and wound losses. Similarly, inputs are from the diet (either intravenous or oral) and from any other nitrogen-containing substances that may be given, such as blood and albumin. Much has been written about the difficulties and precision of this approach, but if measurements are made over a long enough

period to allow for day to day variations and the intake of nutrients is maintained constant, quite consistent data can be obtained.

It is common to assume that the non-urinary losses of N are small and constant in magnitude, so in many studies their measurement is neglected. It is also quite common practice to measure the urinary urea rather than the total urinary N, on the assumption that urea forms a constant proportion of total N. This has been pointed out by Kinney (1983) to be inappropriate. Although urea is the major component of urinary N in healthy subjects, contributing about 85%, compared with 5% for creatinine, 3% for ammonia and 1.5% for uric acid, in a large group of hypercatabolic patients the amount of urea varied widely, from 60 to 90% of total N.

The net loss of nitrogen varies both with the severity of the trauma and with the time period after the initial insult. The time-course of negative N balance depends on the type of trauma (Figure 48.1), but typically reaches a peak during the early part of the 'flow' phase and then gradually declines, before becoming positive during convalescence. Table 48.1 shows the peak daily loss and the cumulated N loss for a range of catabolic conditions. These illustrative values are given for comparison only: as they were derived from studies performed some 20 years ago, the equivalent values with more modern surgical techniques would almost certainly be lower. It is clear that the greater the extent of the injury, the greater the N loss, and that the occurrence of sepsis or other complications also aggravates the losses. When routes of loss other than the urine contribute substantially, this also enhances the overall effect. Thus, major burns, with the desquamation of large areas of damaged tissue and secretions of plasma through the wounds, in addition to a very high urinary loss, top the list.

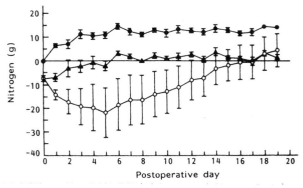

Figure 48.1 The daily and cumulative nitrogen balances in patients over 20 days following cholecystectomy. Patients were allowed free access to normal food. Values are presented as mean ± SEM. (Reproduced from Petersson et al., 1990, with permission.)

From the cumulated losses given in Table 48.1 it is possible to estimate the total loss of lean tissue. In the case of major burns this amounts to almost 6 kg, but even with a minor operation there may be almost 1 kg of loss over 10 days. It is therefore evident that prolonged illness, which might result in a substantial cumulative loss of N even when the daily N loss is moderate, will result in a serious depletion of the lean tissues of the body.

Changes in body composition

After trauma the loss of protein and fat is qualitatively similar to the pattern seen during starvation (Figure 48.2(a); see also 'Effects of altered nutrient intake' below). The pattern of loss of lean tissue from the various organs is, however, different (Figure 48.2(b)). Most of the loss of lean tissue after surgery is from skeletal muscle, while gut, blood proteins and liver are well preserved. This characteristic depletion of muscle was one of the early findings of Cuthbertson (1931, 1976), who noted the high sulphur to nitrogen ratio in the urine and equated this to a loss from a tissue, such as muscle, with a high sulphur content. Muscle wasting and weakness are also apparent clinically.

A notable exception to the generally catabolic response is the increase in the concentrations of certain proteins in the blood – the so-called acute-phase proteins. The most pronounced increase occurs for C-reactive protein, but each has its own characteristic time-course and pattern of response to trauma (Table 48.2). The role of some of the acute-phase proteins, such as fibrinogen, after injury is clearly apparent, and although they do not all have such obvious functions, it is generally assumed that they serve a protective function, which is beneficial to survival. The relative conservation of liver, which is the site of synthesis of acute-phase proteins, is therefore consistent with this. However, it is not true that all liver-derived plasma proteins increase after trauma: there are decreases in the plasma concentrations of albumin, transferrin, retinol-binding protein and pre-albumin (Table 48.2). These changes are discussed further in 'Circulating proteins' below.

Thus, although the overall response to trauma is body protein loss, this is accompanied by a redistribution of the available resources to support survival and recovery. The loss of muscle protein can then be seen as a penalty paid by the body for the benefits of preserving its defences, i.e. the acute-phase proteins and the immune system, and supplying substrates for repair of damaged tissues.

THE DYNAMICS OF PROTEIN METABOLISM

Whole-body protein turnover

Basic principles

Nitrogen balance and body composition techniques give information on the net loss of body protein, but give no insight into its mechanism. It has been recognized since the work of Schoenheimer in the 1940s that the body proteins are in a dynamic state, being continuously degraded and resynthesized from free amino acids. This process is known as protein turnover and involves every single protein

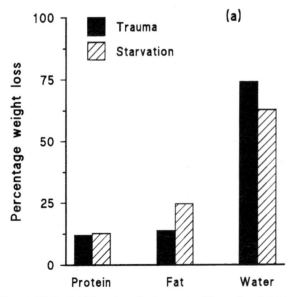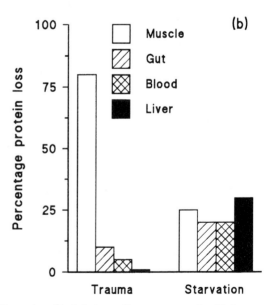

Figure 48.2 (a) The chemical composition of weight loss after 3 weeks of total starvation compared with trauma without nutritional support, illustrating the similarity of total body protein loss in the two conditions. (b) The contribution of individual organs to protein loss, showing substantial differences between starvation and trauma. (Adapted from Kinney, 1978.)

Table 48.2
ACUTE-PHASE PROTEINS CLASSIFIED ACCORDING TO THEIR USUAL CHANGE IN CONCENTRATION. (ADAPTED FROM KUSHNER AND MACKIEWICZ, 1987)

Approx 50% increase	Approx 2- to 4-fold increase	Up to 1000-fold increase	Decrease
Caeruloplasmin	α_1 acid glycoprotein	C-reactive protein	Albumin
Complement components	α_1 proteinase inhibitor	Serum amyloid A	Transferrin
	α_1 anti-chymotrypsin		α_2HS-glycoprotein
	Haptoglobin		
	Fibrinogen		

in each tissue, each protein being turned over at its own characteristic rate. This allows the body to continuously repair damaged components. It also facilitates a rapid response to changes in circumstances (e.g. dietary intake, trauma) that might require a redirection of available nutrients to bring about a redistribution of body proteins. Thus, some proteins, such as those in skeletal muscle, might need to be rapidly mobilized to free amino acids, to supply the substrates for gluconeogenesis and the synthesis of new proteins as part of the host defence.

The healthy adult human turns over about 300 g of protein each day: thus comparatively small changes in the rates of synthesis or degradation can bring about quite rapid losses or gains in protein content. For example, a fall of only 10% in the rate of protein synthesis without any change in degradation would cause a loss of body protein of 30 g/day (i.e. almost 200 g/day of lean tissue loss). The same argument applies to the proteins of each individual tissue or organ, and also to individual proteins, so a fall in the synthesis rate in one organ can rapidly supply the substrate for increased synthesis at another site.

Protein synthesis and degradation take place through separate processes and are able to be regulated independently. It is also important to recognize that an increase in protein degradation can have exactly the same net effect as a decrease in synthesis. Thus the same loss of protein of 30 g/day can be brought about by several distinct mechanisms: a decrease in synthesis; an increase in degradation; a combination of these two; increases in both synthesis and degradation (but with the change in degradation being the larger), or by decreases in both processes (but with a larger change in synthesis). In all cases the protein loss is a reflection simply of the difference between synthesis and degradation. However, when investigating the effects of physiological and pathological factors on protein metabolism, it is important to distinguish the various different possible mechanisms for an observed change in protein balance. For example, an increase in protein synthesis would

have different implications for energy conservation than a decrease in protein degradation, because protein synthesis has a substantial requirement for energy in the form of ATP (Waterlow et al., 1978a).

A variety of isotopic labelling techniques have been used to study rates of whole-body protein metabolism after trauma. Before considering the results of these studies, however, a brief description of the principles of the methods will be given, together with their validity and limitations, as an understanding of these might be crucial to the interpretation of experimental results. Detailed descriptions can be found elsewhere (Waterlow et al., 1978a; Garlick, 1980; Halliday and Rennie, 1982; Wolfe, 1984; Bier, 1991).

Measurement of whole-body protein turnover
Methods have been developed for measuring whole-body protein turnover rates with a variety of different isotopes. The early work of Schoenheimer and Rittenberg (for details see Waterlow et al., 1978a) was based on the stable isotope, ^{15}N, but more recent studies have also used ^{14}C or [3]H (radioactive) or ^{13}C or [2]H (stable). In general the principles are the same with all isotopes, and involve measurements of isotopic enrichment in one or more body compartments (e.g. plasma, urine) following administration of an isotopically labelled amino acid or protein. The data are then analysed by means of a metabolic model, which is a simplified representation of the major pathways and pools of either total N or of that particular amino acid in the body. The model shown in Figure 48.3 is the simplest and most commonly used, although more complex models have sometimes been employed. In this model there are two compartments comprising the free amino acid (or 'metabolic') pool and the pool of protein-bound amino acids. Protein synthesis (S) and degradation (D) are represented by the arrows between these two pools. There are additional pathways of entry to the free amino acid pool from dietary intake and de novo synthesis, and exit by oxidation (O) to CO_2 and urinary end products, and by conversion to

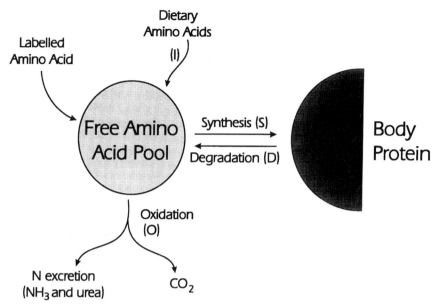

Figure 48.3 Simplified illustration of whole-body protein metabolism. This two-pool model is frequently used to calculate rates of whole-body protein turnover from data obtained by labelling with carbon-13 or nitrogen-15 labelled amino acids. For details, see text.

other metabolites. For the purposes of the analysis *de novo* synthesis and conversion to other metabolites are usually regarded as negligible.

Analysis of the model assumes that the free amino acid pool remains in balance, so that total entry and total exit are equal. Hence:

$$I + D = O + S = Q \qquad (48.1)$$

Q, the total turnover rate of the free amino acid pool, is known as the flux rate. Alternative terms for Q are entry, appearance (R_a), disposal rate (R_d) or irreversible loss (Shipley and Clark, 1972). The procedure is to estimate Q from the isotopic data, and then to calculate S and D from equation (48.1), knowing O and I.

The method for determining Q varies somewhat, depending on the isotopic label used and its method of administration. The simplest example is when [1–^{14}C]leucine is given as a constant infusion. This label was chosen because leucine is essential (i.e. no intake except from the diet) and has no metabolic pathways except to CO_2 (James *et al.*, 1974, 1976). During the first few hours of infusion, and more rapidly if a bolus (or prime) dose of label is given initially, the specific radioactivity of leucine in the blood reaches a constant (plateau) value (A), which is used to calculate the flux:

$$Q = i / A \qquad (48.2)$$

where i is the rate of infusion of isotope. In the subsequent calculation of protein synthesis and degradation from Q by equation (48.1), the value of I is the dietary leucine intake and O is the rate of leucine oxidation. The oxidation rate can be esti-

mated separately from the rate of production of $^{14}CO_2$ in the breath.

In recent years there has been an increasing use of the stable isotope ^{13}C: the calculations are the same (with isotopic enrichment in atom % excess substituted for specific radioactivity), except that the amount of leucine infused as [1–^{13}C]leucine must be allowed for in the formulae, as it cannot be given at a low enough rate to be regarded as a true tracer.

The assumptions of this approach are that the free amino acid pool is in a steady state and that the pool of leucine is homogeneous and represented by the blood. The former can usually be achieved in volunteers, but might be difficult in traumatized patients. The latter is certainly not true, in that the metabolic pool is highly compartmented, so that the plasma leucine is not the direct precursor of either protein synthesis or leucine oxidation, which occur within tissues. This gives rise to values of protein turnover that are underestimates. The metabolite of leucine, α-ketoisocaproate (KIC), might give more accurate values for turnover rates, but this cannot completely overcome the problem, since it can only represent the isotopic enrichment at the site of its own synthesis from leucine, most of which is thought to occur in skeletal muscle (Matthews *et al.*, 1982). It is also assumed that the production of breath $^{13}CO_2$ quantitatively represents leucine oxidation, but fixation of $^{13}CO_2$ into other compounds and difficulties with CO_2 collection in traumatized patients introduce some uncertainty. Moreover, for a plateau in plasma enrichment to be maintained, the isotope that has been incorporated into protein must not be returned (recycled) to the metabolic pool. The resulting rise in the plateau would cause artifactually low rates of turnover. This factor limits the time period over which infusions can be made to less than 12 hours in adults (Schwenk *et al.*, 1985; Melville *et al.*, 1989).

The advantages of the primed infusion of labelled leucine are that the measurement can be made in a reasonably short period (about 4 hours) and is repeatable if non-radioactive amino acids are used. It is thus the method of choice when precision is required in a highly controlled environment, such that a steady state, a continuous dietary intake of known composition and amount, and continuous respiratory gas analysis can be achieved. Thus a dedicated laboratory or metabolic ward is advisable, if not obligatory.

When measurements are to be made in free living subjects, with little interference with their normal life and relatively few invasive procedures, the techniques using ^{15}N are more suitable. ^{15}N has most commonly been given in the form of $[^{15}N]$glycine as a continuous infusion, either orally or intravenously (Waterlow *et al.*, 1978a,b). There are three major differences from carbon labelling. First, the label is assumed to be transferred metabolically to other amino acids, so that the derived rates of turnover are in the units of grams of nitrogen. Secondly, measurements of ^{15}N are not made directly on the metabolic pool, but on an end product of nitrogen metabolism in the urine (urea or ammonia), which is assumed to be derived directly from the metabolic pool and therefore has the same isotopic enrichment. Thirdly, the rate of amino acid oxidation is not derived from the isotopic data, but instead is assumed to be represented by the rate of total N excretion in the urine. In other respects the calculations and assumptions are the same. Both the N and C labelling techniques can be modified so that the label can be given as a single dose, but the method of calculation is similar and the assumptions are identical (Waterlow *et al.*, 1978a,b; Fern *et al.*, 1981).

The assumption of a homogeneous metabolic pool is clearly an over-simplification with ^{15}N, since the two urinary end products, urea and ammonia, give different rates of turnover (Fern *et al.*, 1981). Moreover, different rates are obtained with both end products when the label is given orally as opposed to intravenously (Fern *et al.*, 1981). Urea is made in the liver and ammonia in the kidney, so the enrichments of these two products are representative of the different metabolism of nitrogen in the two organs. This difficulty can be partially overcome by a method in which the values from the two end products are combined, allowing consistent data to be obtained with intravenous and oral isotope administration (Fern *et al.*, 1985a). It is also necessary to assume that of the amino acids

labelled by $[^{15}N]$glycine, the relative proportions entering protein synthesis will be the same as those entering urinary end products. The implications of this assumption are very difficult to assess in any particular experimental situation, which has led some workers to use proteins uniformly labelled with ^{15}N (Fern and Garlick, 1983; Wutzke *et al.*, 1983).

The disadvantages of ^{15}N methods are firstly that the metabolism of N from glycine is less well understood than that of the C from leucine, so the sources of error are less easy to recognize. Secondly, the time taken to reach plateau enrichment of urea is very lengthy because of the delaying effect of the body urea pool, so that infusions of 48–72 hours have been commonly performed (Picou and Taylor-Roberts, 1969). With such chronic infusions the rates of turnover obtained must be significantly modified by isotope recycling. To minimize the time period, priming with $[^{15}N]$glycine has been used to achieve plateau in ammonia within a few hours (Jeevanandam *et al.*, 1985; Jackson *et al.*, 1987). In addition, a more rapid plateau in urea could be obtained by priming with $[^{15}N]$urea. However, short periods of measurement are more easily achieved when the isotope is given as a single dose, rather than a constant infusion (Waterlow *et al.*, 1978a,b). Because it is then possible to estimate the amount of label that has been delayed in the body urea pool, without waiting for it to be excreted, the method can conveniently be used in volunteers or patients with measurement periods as short as 9 hours (Fern *et al.*, 1981).

Simultaneous comparisons of carbon and nitrogen labelling have shown that in general the two approaches give similar values for whole-body protein synthesis in healthy adult man of about 200–300 g protein per day (Garlick and Fern, 1985). Moreover, in subjects given diets with altered protein and energy content, the effect of the change on protein synthesis and degradation has been shown to be the same when measured with $[^{15}N]$glycine or $[1-^{14}C]$leucine. The choice of which method is used is likely to be determined by what is practical in a given set of volunteers or patients: can they be restrained in a respiration chamber, can blood or urine be sampled, what analytical facilities are available for isotope measurements? When attention is paid to the requirements and limitations of each of the methods, there is reason to suppose that either can give reproducible results. However, the inhomogeneity of the free amino acid pool and the resulting inability to estimate the isotopic enrichment of the free amino acid at the site of whole-body synthesis remains a major problem, which affects the interpretation of all methods. In the future, it is expected that techniques for non-invasive measurements in specific tissues and organs will continue to be developed and that these will provide more detailed and accurate information. However, despite the limitations of the whole-body measurements, there are situations where they are the only option, because they are relatively non-invasive.

Changes in whole-body turnover rates after trauma

The use of the term 'Catabolic response to injury' led in the past to the supposition that the loss of body protein after injury or trauma was the result of an increase in protein degradation (catabolism). Studies of whole-body protein turnover have shown, however, that the true mechanism of this response is more complex (see reviews by Clague, 1981; Gelfand et al., 1983; Waterlow, 1984; Burns, 1988; Wolfe et al., 1989). Early measurements with isotopes (O'Keefe et al., 1974; Crane et al., 1977) showed that after surgery involving minor to moderate trauma, there was a decrease in protein synthesis, with no change in degradation (Figure 48.4). Later work with more severe trauma seemed to be inconsistent with this, showing in some cases that there was indeed an increase in protein degradation, sometimes also accompanied by an increase in synthesis (Long et al., 1977; Kien et al., 1978; Birkhahn et al., 1980; Figure 48.4). Thus, the loss of body protein resulted from a larger increase in degradation than synthesis. Such increases in whole-body synthesis and degradation seem to be characteristic of a wide range of pathological states. These include, in addition to major skeletal injury (Birkhahn et al., 1980, 1981), other highly catabolic conditions such as sepsis (Long et al., 1977) and burns (Jahoor et al., 1988), as well as with elective surgery (Carli et al., 1990). A similar response occurs with infections (Tomkins et al., 1983): indeed, increases in turnover rates have also been demonstrated in volunteers made pyrexic by cholera/TAB vaccination, despite the fact that they remained in N balance (Garlick et al., 1980a). Cancer is also frequently associated with elevated protein synthesis and degradation, particularly when at an advanced stage with metastases or with aggressive tumours (Fearon et al., 1988; Melville et al., 1990), but not with less advanced disease (Glass et al., 1983). Stimulation of whole-body turnover rates has also been demonstrated in animals with bacteraemia (Pomposelli et al., 1985) and injury (Sakamoto et al., 1983).

Although the reason for this increase in turnover is not known, it is sufficiently widely reported that it is unlikely not to be real. Similar data have been obtained with a range of techniques, using isotopes of carbon and nitrogen, so it is unlikely that the apparent discrepancies result from methodological artefacts (Birkhahn et al., 1980, 1981). However, difficulties of interpretation have arisen because of differences in experimental protocols in different laboratories. The majority of studies have made a measurement at a single point in time after the initial trauma, and have compared this with values from healthy controls or the same patients before injury (i.e. for elective surgery). However, it is to be expected that the metabolic response will change over time, as the patient passes through the ebb, flow, convalescent and recovery phases. Data from burned children suggest that accelerated protein degradation persists from the time of injury throughout convalescence, with the peak occurring during the flow phase (Wolfe et al., 1989).

A further variable is the state of nutrition at the time the measurements were made. With early studies on elective surgical patients (O'Keefe et al., 1974; Crane et al., 1977), they were fed during the presurgery measurement, but received only dextrose or had a reduced oral intake postsurgery. There was an apparent fall in the rate of protein synthesis (Figure 48.4), but this was quite small, in fact smaller than the decrease in synthesis observed when healthy subjects changed from a normal diet to one containing only 500 Kcal/day of glucose (Garlick et al., 1980b). To explain this, Clague (1981) proposed the hypothesis illustrated in Figure 48.5 in which protein turnover rates are altered independ-

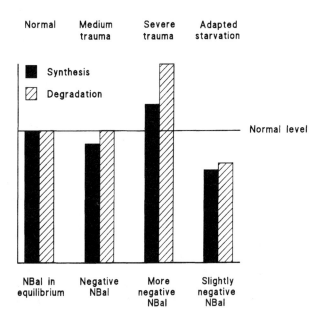

Figure 48.4 Illustration of different ways in which whole-body rates of protein synthesis and degradation contribute to protein loss after trauma and during starvation. In all cases the protein loss occurs because synthesis is lower than degradation. However, with moderate surgical trauma involving a reduction in dietary intake a depression in synthesis with little change in degradation has been observed (e.g. O'Keefe et al., 1974), whereas with severe trauma in intravenously fed patients increases in both synthesis and degradation are seen (e.g. Birkhahn et al., 1980, 1981). Conversely, in starvation both synthesis and degradation are depressed.

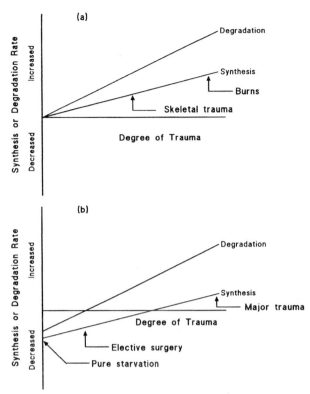

Figure 48.5 Modification of the apparent responses of protein synthesis and degradation to trauma by concurrent starvation. The graphs illustrate the increases in both synthesis and degradation with increasing severity of trauma: the higher gradient for degradation over synthesis results in higher rates of protein loss with more severe trauma. (a) Traumatized patients and controls fed normally during measurements. At zero degree of trauma, synthesis and degradation are equal and subjects are in protein balance. All levels of trauma cause an elevation of both synthesis and degradation and negative protein balance. (b) Patients fed for control measurements but starved after trauma. At zero trauma, both synthesis and degradation are depressed and protein balance is negative. At all levels of trauma the rate of protein loss is higher than in (a), but only with the most severe trauma is synthesis elevated in comparison with fed controls. Adapted from Claque (1981).

ently by the degree of trauma and by the level of dietary intake. When patients are given the same intake during control and post-trauma measurements, protein synthesis and degradation both increase with increasing degree of trauma, but the lines diverge, resulting in greater losses of body protein with more severe trauma. This is illustrated in Figure 48.5(a) and is in agreement with experimental data from studies when healthy (control) and traumatized patients were fed the same amounts of diet (Birkhahn *et al.*, 1981). When the nutritional intake is reduced postoperatively, as frequently occurs in hospital patients, the effect of the low dietary intake is to reduce rates of protein turnover (see 'Effects of altered nutrient intake' below), and hence to shift the lines for both synthesis and degradation downwards (Figure 48.5(b). Under these circumstances, the effect of relatively minor trauma is to lower protein synthesis, with little or no effect on degradation, as observed by O'Keefe *et al.* (1974). Only when the degree of trauma is great, do the increases in turnover rates due to trauma predominate. In general, the experimental data fit this hypothesis, which is therefore able to explain why the majority of the studies described above showed elevations in turnover rates while some of the earlier measurements did not.

Protein turnover in individual tissues

Measurements of whole-body protein turnover are able to explain protein losses and gains in terms of alterations in synthesis or degradation, but give no indication of the site of these changes. Moreover, the complexity of amino acid metabolism in the whole body causes difficulties with interpretation. These methods have been used widely because they are practical in a clinical environment. However, more detailed information can be obtained if measurements are made on individual tissues. Because these techniques are invasive, relatively little work has been done on human tissue protein turnover until recently, and most of the existing knowledge has been gained from work in experimental animals, with measurements made either *in vivo* or on isolated tissue samples *in vitro*.

Measurement of tissue protein turnover rates *in vivo*.

As with protein turnover in the whole body, methods for individual tissues and proteins generally rely on isotopic labelling (for reviews see Waterlow *et al.*, 1978a; Zak *et al.*, 1979; Garlick, 1980; Garlick *et al.*, 1991a, 1994). For measurement of protein synthesis, the incorporation of the isotope into the protein under study is measured, which requires a sample of the tissue. In addition, it is necessary to know the isotopic enrichment or specific radioactivity of the free amino acid precursor. It is this latter requirement that has created much difficulty and controversy, and this is illustrated in Figure 48.6. As the isotopic label is generally given by injection into the circulation, its enrichment in the plasma tends to be higher than in the free amino acid pools of the tissues. Moreover, as Figure 48.6 shows, the direct precursor for protein synthesis is the tRNA, which appears to be synthesized from a small subcompartment of the tissue free pool. As a consequence, the enrichment of the precursor is likely to be different from that of either the plasma or tissue free amino acids. This problem has had a significant bearing on the

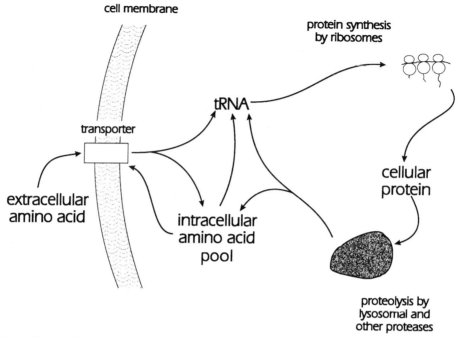

cell membrane

protein synthesis
by ribosomes

tRNA

transporter

cellular
protein

extracellular
amino acid

intracellular
amino acid
pool

proteolysis by
lysosomal and
other proteases

Figure 48.6 The cellular origin of amino acids destined for protein synthesis. The isotopic enrichment of the tRNA during isotopic labelling experiments depends on relative charging from each of three possible sources: (i) direct from the membrane transporter at an enrichment similar to that in the plasma; (ii) from the mixed intracellular pool, with a lower enrichment than that in the plasma; (iii) directly recycled from proteolysis, with zero enrichment. If (i) predominates, the enrichment of aminoacyl tRNA will be higher than that of the intracellular pool; if (iii) predominates, the aminoacyl tRNA enrichment will be lower than the intracellular pool. In practice, the relative proportions of these three pathways are likely to vary in different metabolic and nutritional states.

development of methods, because direct measurement of tRNA enrichment is not suited to routine studies.

One commonly used method is to give the tracer amino acid (e.g. leucine labelled with ^{13}C, ^{14}C or ^{3}H) by continuous intravenous infusion for a few hours, and to assess the incorporation of isotope into protein at the end. The average enrichment of the free amino acid pool during the incorporation period can then be readily assessed, because a plateau value is quickly attained and can be evaluated from a single measurement taken at the time of tissue sampling. This method was used widely for studies in experimental animals with radioactive amino acids in the 1960s and 1970s (Waterlow and Stephen, 1968; Garlick, 1969; Waterlow et al., 1978a) and more recently with stable isotopes in human tissues (Halliday and McKeran, 1975; Stein et al., 1978; Rennie et al., 1982; Halliday et al., 1988). Generally the free amino acid enrichment in the tissue was taken as the precursor, because protein synthesis is an intracellular process. Difficulties in interpretation have, however, been encountered with some tissues, because the tissue and plasma free amino acid enrichments differed appreciably (e.g. up to four-fold in liver and gut; McNurlan et al., 1979), making the choice of which to use as precursor crucial.

To avoid this problem a technique was developed whereby the labelled amino acid was given as a very large, non-tracer dose, which raises the free amino acid concentration in the blood and tissues by several fold. This results in very rapid equilibration of the free amino acid in all compartments to similar isotopic enrichments, so that either plasma or tissue free amino acids can be used for the precursor measurement. This approach has been very widely adopted for measurements of protein synthesis in cultured cells (Ballard, 1982; McNurlan and Clemens, 1985), tissues in vitro (Mortimore et al., 1972; Watkins and Rannels, 1980) and in tissues of animals in vivo (Henshaw et al., 1971; Scornik, 1974; McNurlan et al., 1979; Garlick et al., 1980c) using radioactively labelled amino acids. Recently it has also been used with stable isotopes in human volunteers and patients, when the large dose of amino acid given (e.g. 4 g of [1-^{13}C] leucine or 3 g phenylalanine in an adult) has not proved harmful (Garlick et al., 1989; McNurlan et al., 1994). Table 48.3 shows rates of protein synthesis in a range of human tissues obtained by this method. For comparison, values for tissues of growing rats are also given, showing that rat tissues turnover some 10 times faster than those of the human.

Although the constant infusion and flooding methods do not always produce the same values,

TABLE 48.3
PROTEIN SYNTHESIS RATE (%/DAY) OF DIFFERENT TISSUES IN
ADULT HUMANS AND GROWING RATS

	Human	Rat
Skeletal muscle	1–2	13
Heart	5	17
Liver	23	87
Large intestine	10	62
Lymphocytes	8	–
Albumin	7	30
Tumour tissue		
Colon	23	–
Breast	11	–

Rates are expressed as the percentage of the tissue protein (for albumin, the percentage of the intravascular pool) synthesized per day (%/day). Human data are from Garlick *et al.* (1991a) and rat data from Garlick (1980).

they have both contributed substantially to our knowledge of the regulation of protein synthesis *in vivo*, both in animals and latterly in humans. In addition to these methods there is one semi-quantitative index of protein synthesis rate which does not use isotopes. If a small sample of tissue such as muscle can be obtained, the ribosomes can be isolated from it by sucrose gradient centrifugation and the degree of polyribosome aggregation can be assessed. When ribosomes are actively engaged in protein synthesis, they travel along the strands of messenger RNA, which are usually long enough to accommodate several ribosomes simultaneously (polyribosomes). The total number of polyribosomes in the tissue is therefore an index of the rate of protein synthesis (Munro, 1970a; Wernerman *et al.*, 1986a,b). Data are usually expressed as the total concentration of ribosomes and the proportion of these that are aggregated into polyribosomes, both these values in human muscle being sensitive to nutritional state and trauma (see below).

Protein degradation has proved far more difficult to measure than synthesis with any degree of confidence (Waterlow *et al.*, 1978a; Garlick, 1980). Prelabelling by injection of a labelled amino acid, followed by observation of the decay of label in tissue protein, has been used in the past, but suffers from serious problems of recycling of the label released by degradation into new protein synthesis, thus giving artefactually low rates. Although this can be avoided in some cases by use of non-reutilizable labels (McFarlane, 1963; Millward, 1970), with mixed tissue proteins there are additional problems because the decay of label does not follow the simple exponential (first order) kinetics needed to derive degradation rates. Instead, multi-exponential decay curves are observed (Garlick *et al.*, 1976). This technique is therefore limited to the

study of the degradation of single proteins in experimental animals.

A commonly used alternative to direct measurement of degradation is to measure the rate of synthesis and the rate of growth of tissue protein and to calculate degradation from the expression: growth rate = synthesis rate – degradation rate. This has proved very valuable for measurements in small animals (Turner and Garlick, 1974; Garlick *et al.*, 1975; Millward *et al.*, 1976), when the growth rate can be obtained by measurements on tissues removed at death, although the level of precision that can be obtained is rather low. This method is obviously not practical for studies in man, but a similar approach which uses the uptake or release of an amino acid from an organ or limb has been used for human measurements (see 'Interorgan fluxes' below).

In the case of the myofibrillar proteins of muscle, there is an alternative procedure which does not use isotopes. The amino acid, 3-methylhistidine, is present only in actin and myosin, and is produced by modification of specific histidine residues after synthesis of the protein. Following degradation of these proteins, the 3-methylhistidine is not reincorporated, but is excreted quantitatively in the urine. Thus, the rate of excretion of this amino acid in the urine has been widely used as a convenient and non-invasive method for assessing the rate of myofibrillar protein degradation, which has particular value for clinical studies in man (Munro and Young, 1981). There are certain drawbacks, such as the contribution of 3-methylhistidine from non-muscle tissues (Rennie and Millward, 1983) and the methylhistidine derived from the diet (Sjölin *et al.*, 1987), which have received considerable emphasis in the last few years. However, more recent data (see below) suggest that this method is no more imprecise than other techniques for evaluating protein metabolism at the whole-body level, and this technique provides a valuable addition to the isotopic methods described above.

Measurements on isolated tissues *in vitro*
As an alternative to measurement of protein turnover rates *in vivo*, many researchers have chosen to remove tissues from experimental animals and to incubate or perfuse them *in vitro*. This has a dual advantage that measurements can be made more precisely, since the system under study is less complex, and the environment of the tissue can be rigidly controlled. Thus, the responses of the tissue to potential controlling factors, such as hormone or substrate levels, can be investigated without complications arising from secondary changes in other factors that would occur in the intact animal.

It is very important to recognize the differences of interpretation between *in vitro* and *in vivo* studies. When measurements are made *in vivo*, one observes the overall change brought about by a particular treatment of the whole animal or person. This change might, however, be mediated by a variety of hormonal and other factors, whose individual contributions might be difficult to assess with certainty *in vivo*. The strength of the *in vitro* experiment is that it enables potential regulatory factors to be studied independently, and mechanisms to be deduced. It is not, however, the best approach for assessing the overall response *in vivo*, since the tissue will not only be reflecting the situation in the live animal, but also the hormone and substrate concentrations in the incubation medium. The *in vivo* and *in vitro* approaches are therefore best regarded as complementary, one to reflect the *in vivo* changes, the other to analyse possible mechanisms.

The main drawback of *in vitro* systems is their viability. This is not so much of a problem with perfusion of whole organs or limbs, when the circulation can be kept intact. However, with tissue slices and other preparations involving cutting of the sample, protein synthesis may proceed at only a fraction of the *in vivo* rate (Seider *et al.*, 1980). Even with intact tissues, such as the small leg muscles of rodents (soleus and extensor digitorum longus), which are frequently used in metabolic studies, the rates of protein synthesis are much lower than those *in vivo* and degradation much higher (Goldspink *et al.*, 1983). Only the very smallest of muscles can be used in this way, since oxygen transport through the tissue becomes limiting, resulting in the development of hypoxic cores (Maltin and Harris, 1985). Thus these preparations might not accurately reflect the *in vivo* metabolism of the muscle, as they are frequently in a highly stepped-down state.

Measurement of rates of protein synthesis and degradation *in vitro* is much more precise than *in vivo*. Synthesis is commonly measured by adding a labelled amino acid at a high concentration (flooding) and assessing the incorporation into protein (Mortimore *et al.*, 1972). The precursor specific radioactivity at the high concentration used can safely be assumed to equal that of the incubation or perfusion medium, which remains constant over several hours. Degradation can be measured simultaneously by measuring the net balance of an amino acid in the medium (e.g. phenylalanine or tyrosine which are not metabolized in muscle or valine in liver: thus degradation is the sum of synthesis plus amino acid release) (Mortimore *et al.*, 1972). Alternatively, many workers have added cycloheximide to the medium to inhibit synthesis, so that degradation is then equal to the net release of a non-metabolized amino acid (Fulks *et al.*, 1975; Jefferson *et al.*, 1977).

Changes in muscle protein turnover after trauma
Despite the *increase* in whole-body protein turnover after trauma, studies on surgical patients have

suggested that protein synthesis in skeletal muscle *decreases*. After surgery involving moderate trauma (cholecystectomy) there is a fall in the muscle content of ribosomes and in the proportion of these that are present as polysomes, which are qualitative indications of a decrease in synthesis (Wernerman *et al.*, 1986a,b). This effect was observed on the day following surgery, when the negative nitrogen balance was increasing and the muscle amino acid concentrations are deranged (see 'Free amino acid pools' below). In parallel with changes in the concentration of free amino acids in muscle (Vinnars *et al.*, 1990), the changes in polysomes become more pronounced on the third day after surgery and are still not restored to normal by the 30th day (Petersson *et al.*, 1990).

Direct measurements of protein synthesis in muscle of surgical patients by the flooding dose method have confirmed that a decrease of about 50% occurs on the third day (Essén *et al.*, 1992a). However, this fall is extremely rapid: rates of synthesis were already reduced by 30% compared with preoperative levels by 2–3 hours after the first incision (Essén *et al.*, 1992b). By contrast, the changes in critically ill patients are more complex, involving depressed protein synthesis in some but elevations in others (Essén *et al.*, 1996).

Our knowledge of the changes in protein degradation in human muscle have been derived almost entirely from measurements of the excretion of 3-methylhistidine in the urine. A large number of studies have shown an increase in the excretion of 3-methylhistidine with a range of types of trauma. For example, patients admitted for elective surgery or volunteers with experimentally induced infection show a peak in methylhistidine excretion at about 2–4 days post-trauma and a subsequent decline (Wannemacher *et al.*, 1975; Williamson *et al.*, 1977; Carli *et al.*, 1990). Higher rates of methylhistidine excretion are observed in the more traumatized patients, and it has been shown that those patients who have not adapted to the utilization of ketone bodies display higher rates of methylhistidine and total nitrogen excretion (Williamson *et al.*, 1977).

The origin of the additional 3-methylhistidine after trauma has, however, been controversial. Experiments in patients undergoing abdominal surgery seemed to show an increase in urinary excretion of methylhistidine without any concomitant increase in its release from the leg (Rennie *et al.*, 1984). The suggestion was that the relatively small amounts of methylhistidine-containing proteins in the gastrointestinal tract had much faster rates of turnover than skeletal muscle proteins, and thus contributed a substantial proportion of whole-body methylhistidine production. In separate experiments in starved rats there was an immediate elevation in urinary methylhistidine, which coincided with an apparent rise in the degradation of smooth muscle in the gut, but an elevation in skeletal muscle breakdown did not occur until later (Emery et al., 1986). More recent work, however, has shown that the contribution of the gut is much smaller than was thought. It has been shown that neither patients nor rats display low rates of methylhistidine excretion after small bowel resection (Brenner et al., 1987; Long et al., 1988). Moreover, in a series of careful measurements of leg balance by Sjölin et al. (1989, 1990), the increase in methylhistidine excretion in infected and septic patients was shown to result from an increase in the release of the amino acid by skeletal muscle. In addition, release by the splanchnic area was shown to be small. The conclusion from this series of experiments was that increased methylhistidine excretion in trauma is indeed an indication of increased skeletal muscle proteolysis.

Because of the difficulty of performing experiments on human tissues, knowledge in this area has benefited substantially from experiments in animals. Measurements in vivo by either constant infusion or flooding dose of labelled amino acids have in many cases confirmed the changes in muscle synthesis seen in human studies. Thus, surgery (Lee et al., 1988a), sepsis (Hall-Angeras et al., 1991a), infection (Fern et al., 1985b), cancer (Pain et al., 1984) and experimental trauma induced by injection of endotoxin (Jepson et al., 1986) or turpentine (Ballmer et al., 1991) lead to a substantial reduction in the rate of protein synthesis in various skeletal muscles. With sepsis, it has been shown that the decrease in synthesis is associated with decrease in peptide chain initiation, resulting from a lower activity of initiation factor 2B (eIF-2B) activity (Vary et al., 1994). Also the inhibition by surgery was observed within the first 2–3 hours (Bakic et al., 1988), which is analogous to the changes occurring in human surgical patients (Essén et al., 1992b). By contrast, in other laboratories, bacteraemia (Pomposelli et al., 1985) and fracture of the femur (Stein et al., 1976) have been shown to elevate muscle synthesis. In addition, experimental burn injury was shown to stimulate protein synthesis in soleus muscle from both the burned and uninjured limbs (Shangraw and Turinsky, 1984). In plantaris muscle, however, the increase was only seen in the injured tissue.

Protein degradation in muscle of traumatized animals is more difficult to measure in vivo, but estimates derived from the rates of synthesis and growth have shown a substantial increase during endotoxaemia (Jepson et al., 1986) and after surgery (Lee et al., 1988b). In the latter case, however, degradation returned to normal by 4 days after surgery, when protein synthesis remained low: after more major trauma there was an inhibition of degradation at 4 days, possibly in order to recover lost tissue. The increase in protein breakdown after burn injury relates to a stimulation of several known proteolytic systems, including the lysosomal, calcium dependent and ubiquitin dependent pathways (Fang et al., 1995a), the latter being particularly important for degrading the contractile proteins. By contrast, sepsis-induced proteolysis does not appear to involve the lysosomal pathway (Tiaro et al., 1994).

Measurements on isolated muscles in vitro have also shown variations in response. For example, thermal injury has been shown to have a stimulatory (Shangraw and Turinsky, 1982), inhibitory (Frayn and Maycock, 1979; Fang et al., 1995b) or no effect (Odessey and Parr, 1982) on protein synthesis in incubated muscles in different laboratories. Degradation rates in the same studies were similarly variable, showing an increase (Odessey and Parr, 1982; Shangraw and Turinsky, 1982; Fang et al., 1995b) or no change (Frayn and Maycock, 1979). However, in muscles taken from animals with a variety of other types of trauma, reduced rates of synthesis and elevated rates of degradation have been demonstrated; for example, as a result of surgery (Lee et al., 1988b), sepsis (Hall-Angeras et al., 1991a; Breuillé et al., 1994) and endotoxaemia (Ash & Griffin, 1989).

Because of the wide range of muscle protein synthesis rates in critically ill patients (Essén et al., 1996), it is important to attempt to clarify whether the variable responses of muscle seen in animal models protein synthesis result from variations in the type or degree of the trauma studied, or possibly from some other aspect of the experimental protocols. Methodological differences do not appear to be responsible: both increases and decreases in synthesis have been observed with both constant infusion and flooding dose of labelled amino acids, and the stimulation brought about by bacteraemia was demonstrated by both techniques in the same laboratory (Pomposelli et al., 1985). Moreover, both the decreases due to surgery, sepsis and endotoxaemia and the increase due to thermal injury were apparent when measured in vivo or in vitro in the same laboratories (Shangraw and Turinsky, 1982, 1984; Lee et al., 1988a,b; Ash and Griffin, 1989; Hall-Angeras et al., 1991a,b). Thus, it appears that the variations in response result from differences in the experimental models studied. Food intake is certainly an important variable, because trauma usually results in a lower food intake. Thus, the inhibitory effect of septicaemia on protein synthesis was much less pronounced in fasted than in fed animals (Ash and Griffin, 1989), and the inhibition of synthesis by surgery was absent in fasted rats (Preedy et al., 1988). Since reduced food intake lowers muscle protein synthesis in the young animals that are generally used in these experiments, it is essential to equalize the intakes of traumatized and control animals by fasting, intravenous feeding or by 'pair feeding'. When pair feeding was done in experiments on infection (Fern *et al.*, 1985b) and surgery (Lee *et al.*, 1988a), rates of muscle synthesis in the traumatized animals were much lower than those in *ad libitum* fed controls, but the differences due to the trauma alone, as shown by comparison with the pair-fed animals, were much less pronounced.

Other variables include the site, type and degree of the trauma. Changes in protein synthesis after single leg scalding were different in the muscles from the injured and non-injured sides (Shangraw and Turinsky, 1984). Moreover, the large urinary output of methylhistidine after accidental injury in man might result in part from autolysis of the damaged tissue (Threlfall *et al.*, 1981). It has been suggested that creatine is also produced by the damaged tissue and its urinary excretion might be used as an indicator of the post-traumatic 'flow phase' (Threlfall *et al.*, 1984). Urinary creatine excretion is much elevated after musculoskeletal trauma and this increase correlates in both magnitude and duration with the Injury Severity Score (Threlfall *et al.*, 1984). In experimental ischaemia of the hind limb in rats the creatinuria was correlated with the duration of ischaemia and was shown to originate partly in the injured muscle and partly in non-injured muscle (Threlfall *et al.*, 1984).

The degree of trauma is difficult to evaluate in animal studies, but no differences are apparent between the studies with increases and those with decreases in protein synthesis. In a study designed to investigate the influence of the degree of trauma induced by surgery in rats, it was shown that more severe trauma resulted in increases in synthesis that were both greater and longer lasting, but the direction of change was not altered (Lee *et al.*, 1988a). Moreover, differences in response do not seem to depend on the presence of pyrexia. Small rodents, such as rats, might respond to trauma with either an increase (e.g. turpentine injection, Ballmer *et al.*, 1991) or a decrease (e.g. malaria infection, Fern *et al.*, 1985b) in body temperature, yet in both the examples cited, a decrease in muscle protein synthesis was observed. The reasons for these differences in response therefore remain to be elucidated.

In summary, the loss of muscle protein after surgery and most other types of stress appears to be a consequence of an elevation of protein degradation and an inhibition of synthesis. The fall in synthesis is particularly rapid and can persist for considerable periods of time. More work needs to be done, however, particularly in human patients, to discover how the changes relate to the type and degree of trauma.

Changes in liver protein turnover after trauma

As pointed out earlier, the mass of the liver after trauma is well preserved, and indeed, in animal models is even increased. The contributions of changes in protein synthesis and degradation to the increase in mass are not, however, well described. There have been a number of studies of changes in synthesis, but little on degradation, because of lack of adequate methods for measurement. Protein synthesis in the liver consists of two components: the synthesis of the endogenous structural and enzyme proteins of the tissue, and the synthesis of proteins that are subsequently secreted into the circulation (i.e. the plasma proteins, which will be discussed individually under 'Circulating proteins' below). The latter remain in the liver for only a short period (about half an hour) during processing before secretion into the plasma. Thus, techniques for measuring protein synthesis which take only a short period of time (i.e. less than the secretion time) measure the total liver synthesis, which includes both components. Methods involving incorporation of isotopic tracers for periods of several hours, by contrast, measure only the synthesis of endogenous protein, as the label incorporated into plasma proteins has by that time largely exited from the liver.

There have been very few studies of liver protein kinetics in human patients, because of the difficulty in making direct measurements. However, it has been demonstrated that the total rate of protein synthesis is elevated in patients with inflammatory bowel disease, but is unaltered in patients with early colorectal cancer (Heys *et al.*, 1992). In another study on colorectal cancer, in patients with advanced disease, however, the rate of synthesis of endogenous protein was depressed (Fearon *et al.*, 1991).

Studies in experimental animals *in vivo* have given a much clearer picture. With stress resulting from surgery (Preedy *et al.*, 1988), cancer (Pain *et al.*, 1984; Warren *et al.*, 1987), turpentine injection (Ballmer *et al.*, 1991), sepsis (Breuillé *et al.*, 1994; Vary and Kumball, 1992) and endotoxin injection (Jepson *et al.*, 1986; Ash and Griffin, 1989), elevations in the rate of total liver protein synthesis, measured with short periods of isotope incorporation, have been reported. With malaria infection, however, a decrease was observed (Fern *et al.*, 1985b). When increases are observed, they are more apparent when compared with controls fed the same amount of food, since the fall in food intake after trauma causes an opposing decrease in synthesis (Pain *et al.*, 1984; Preedy *et al.*, 1988). Although these rates include both endogenous and secreted proteins, the increase with trauma appears to represent an increase in the synthesis of the endogenous fraction, since elevated rates have also been demonstrated with much longer periods of isotope incorporation during bacteraemia (Pomposelli *et al.*, 1985), after burn injury (Shangraw and Turinsky, 1984) or fracture of the femur (Stein *et al.*, 1976). An elevation in the rate of protein degradation has also been reported (Shangraw and Turinsky, 1984). Although the liver contains a proportion of non-parenchymal cells, particularly the

Kupffer cells of the immune system, which might be expected to be altered by trauma, the stimulation in the turnover of hepatic proteins is not a consequence of this. Hepatocytes purified from the livers of tumour-bearing rats showed much higher rates of protein synthesis *in vitro* than those from control animals (Warren *et al.*, 1987).

Effects of trauma in other tissues
Although skeletal muscle and liver have been studied most extensively, there is evidence of changes in protein synthesis in a number of other tissues of experimental animals. Of particular interest are the heart and diaphragm muscles, which appear to respond differently from the skeletal muscles by showing an increase in synthesis at some times after injury (Preedy *et al.*, 1988), infection (Fern *et al.*, 1985b) or turpentine injection (Ballmer *et al.*, 1991). This might be a consequence of the increased work demand on these tissues as a result of hypermetabolism (Ballmer *et al.*, 1991). Similarly, stimulations of lung and spleen protein synthesis have also been demonstrated after surgery and during malaria infection (Fern *et al.*, 1985b; Preedy *et al.*, 1988). Protein synthesis in the small and large intestinal mucosa is also enhanced during sepsis, but in the gastric mucosa there is an inhibition (Higashiguchi *et al.*, 19944: Breuillé *et al.*, 1994). By contrast, decreases in synthesis have been reported for the mucosa and smooth muscle of the small intestine during malaria infection (Fern *et al.*, 1985b), with no change after surgery (Preedy *et al.*, 1988) or turpentine injection (Ballmer *et al.*, 1991). It appears, therefore, that the responses vary, depending on the tissue and the type of trauma. The data are consistent with a scenario in which rates of protein turnover respond in order to redistribute body proteins to meet the specific needs of particular situations. Thus, rates of synthesis in relatively non-essential or unused tissues (e.g. leg muscles, gut) decrease, while those in more essential tissues are maintained, or even elevated when an additional workload is called for (e.g. respiratory and cardiac muscles, lung, spleen). These changes should not therefore be seen as an undesirable consequence of the trauma, but instead as part of the body's defence mechanisms, specifically aimed at counteracting the pathological processes.

When considering the pattern of changes in protein turnover in the individual tissues, one particular point needs further clarification. We need to reconcile the observations of increases in synthesis in some tissues and decreases in others with the consistent increases in whole-body turnover rates that have been observed in states of trauma. The major decrease seems to be in skeletal muscle, which is believed to contribute about 25% of whole-body turnover in healthy adults (Halliday *et al.*, 1988). Therefore, it must be concluded that elevations in turnover occur in a number of other tissues, which

together more than compensate for the decrease in muscle. At present only liver has been shown consistently to have increased rates, but data are lacking for many other tissues, particularly for human patients. Moreover, the information on changes in the mass of individual tissues is not available for human studies, and this could be crucial if those tissues with rapid rates of turnover were to increase in mass in relation to muscle. It must also be appreciated that apparent inconsistencies might be methodological in origin. Rates of protein turnover in individual tissues are intrinsically more reliable than those for the whole body, because the whole body is more heterogeneous and the assumptions needed to make the measurements in separate tissues are fewer in number. However, in view of recent developments in techniques both for measuring protein synthesis in human tissues and for assessing organ size non-invasively, it seems likely that answers to these questions are not far away.

Circulating proteins

In the present context the most important circulating proteins are the 'acute-phase' proteins, which have been defined as those which increase in concentration by more than 25% after trauma or other inflammatory stimulus (Kushner, 1982). Also included are those proteins which decrease in concentration after trauma, the most notable being albumin, and these are sometimes known as 'negative acute-phase proteins'. The magnitude of the change in concentration varies considerably within the group (see Table 48.2), some increasing by only 25% and others by up to 1000-fold. Although a small amount of some of these proteins might be made in non-hepatic tissues (Kushner and Mackiewicz, 1987), they are largely synthesized by the parenchymal cells of the liver. Together they might contribute 30–50% of total liver protein synthesis, and thus probably account for the increase in liver protein synthesis seen after various forms of trauma (see 'Protein turnover in individual tissues' above).

After synthesis by the ribosome, the secretory proteins are retained within the cell for a fixed interval (typically about 30 minutes) while they are processed and packaged for secretion, before they appear in the circulation. As with cellular proteins, their concentrations are regulated by changes in either or both of synthesis (more correctly, secretion) and degradation, with an increase in synthesis being particularly prominent in those which increase markedly in concentration. However, a third process, that of distribution between the intra- and extravascular spaces, is also an important factor in controlling their concentrations. After secretion of the protein into the plasma the molecules can then leak through the capillary walls into the extravascular space. Thus, alterations in the 'transcapillary escape rate' can rapidly influence the concentration in the plasma.

Rates of both synthesis and degradation of plasma proteins have traditionally been determined by injecting the purified protein labelled with a radioactive isotope of iodine (^{131}I or ^{125}I), and then measuring the kinetics of loss of the label from the plasma or whole body over several days. A second method has been to label the plasma protein by injecting $NaH^{14}CO_3$ and measuring the incorporation into the specific protein and into urea (McFarlane, 1963). These techniques, which are described in detail by Bianchi *et al.* (1976), have been much used in the past, but are technically difficult, require long periods of measurement and use radioactive isotopes. More recently stable isotopes have been employed, by modifications of the constant infusion (Gersovitz *et al.*, 1986; Olufemi *et al.*, 1990) and flooding (Ballmer *et al.*, 1990) methods.

Useful general descriptions of the acute-phase proteins have been provided by Fleck *et al.* (1985), Fleck (1989) and Kushner and Mackiewicz (1987). The increases in concentration of the 'positive' acute-phase proteins occur after a delay period of about 8 hours (Figure 48.7). During this period there is often a fall in their concentrations, in parallel with the fall in concentration of the 'negative' acute-phase proteins (Fleck *et al.*, 1985). The main factor responsible for the increase is believed to be an increase in their synthesis, with changes in degradation being of minor significance (Kushner, 1982). This stimulation in synthesis has been shown to result from changes in gene expression. For a number of acute-phase proteins, an increase in the cytoplasmic concentration of their specific mRNA has been demonstrated. Usually this is brought about by a parallel increase in transcription, but in some instances the message may be stabilized (Kushner, 1982).

With the 'negative' acute-phase proteins the fall in concentration occurs very soon (within 4 hours) after the initial insult (Figure 48.7). Serum albumin is

a good example, which has been quite extensively studied. It is the most abundant protein of the plasma, comprising about 50% of total plasma proteins in the healthy subject, and its synthesis contributes about 10–15% of total liver protein synthesis in rats (Pain *et al.*, 1978). Its concentration is influenced by a number of other factors, in addition to the fall seen during an acute-phase response. Important among these are physiological factors such as dietary protein intake and whether the subject is standing or lying, and pathological conditions such as impaired liver function and loss through the kidney or intestine (Fleck *et al.*, 1985; Whicher and Spence, 1987; Fleck, 1989). For this reason its frequent use as a clinical marker of nutritional status is open to serious misinterpretation (Fleck *et al.*, 1985; Whicher and Spence, 1987; Klein, 1990).

Descriptions of the factors that control albumin concentration have been given previously (Fleck *et al.*, 1985; Whicher and Spence, 1987; Fleck, 1989; Klein, 1990). A fall in concentration occurs very rapidly after severe injury or inflammation, but might not be observed with less severe trauma. Despite the rise in liver protein synthesis during stress, albumin synthesis as a proportion of total liver synthesis declines during experimental inflammation, because of a fall in the amount of albumin mRNA (Moshage *et al.*, 1987; Ballmer *et al.*, 1995). Although there may be a decrease in albumin synthesis and an increase in degradation, these are insufficient to account for the rapidity of the change in concentration. This is caused by an increase in the vascular permeability, resulting in an increase in the transcapillary escape rate and net movement of albumin into the extravascular space. Changes in vascular permeability have the capacity to alter albumin concentration much more rapidly than changes in synthesis or degradation, because the transcapillary escape rate of albumin (about 100%/day) is about ten times faster than its synthesis and degradation (7%/day).

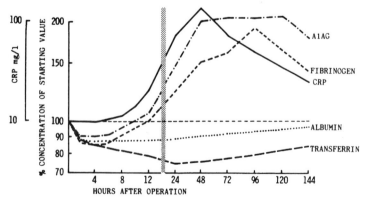

Figure 48.7 The time-course of change in acute-phase protein concentrations after surgical trauma. Percentage changes are shown on a logarithmic scale, except for C-reactive protein, which is given in mg/l. (Reproduced from Fleck *et al.*, 1985, with permission.)

Interorgan fluxes

In addition to the passage of amino acids into and out of protein, there is a continual flux between the tissues by way of the blood (for reviews see Felig, 1975; Wernerman and Vinnars, 1987). This is measured by sampling the arterial and venous blood across an organ or limb and measuring the arteriovenous difference in concentration. If the blood flow through the region under study is also measured, then it is possible to calculate the net uptake or loss of each of the amino acids.

In the fed state there is a flux of free amino acids passing nitrogen from the intestine to the liver. There is also a net uptake by the peripheral tissues, largely skeletal muscle (Wahren *et al.*, 1976). In the postabsorptive state this flux is reversed, with a net transport of amino acid nitrogen from the peripheral tissues to the splanchnic area, mainly the liver (Felig *et al.*, 1969; Felig and Wahren, 1971; Figure 48.8). Although the net loss from muscle in the postabsorptive state originates from muscle protein, the pattern of individual amino acids does not resemble that of muscle protein. The major part of the efflux consists of non-essential amino acids, in particular alanine and glutamine. Indeed, skeletal muscle actually produces glutamine constantly, irrespective of food intake, for export to the splanchnic area, particularly the intestinal mucosa and lymphoid tissue. Similarly, the peripheral tissues are also net producers of alanine, which is exported to the liver for gluconeogenesis. Another

amino acid which shows a constant pattern irrespective of food intake is glutamate, which is synthesized in the liver and exported to the peripheral tissues (Felig *et al.*, 1973).

The determinant of these patterns is the metabolism of the individual amino acids within the tissues. In the muscle many amino acids, in particular the branched chains, are transaminated to their keto acids, which are transported to the liver or oxidized completely within the muscle. The recipients of the nitrogen are intermediates of glucose metabolism, notably pyruvate and α-ketoglutarate, giving rise to alanine and glutamic acid. Deamination of some amino acids gives ammonia, which in combination with glutamate gives glutamine. Alanine and glutamine are therefore the main vehicles for transporting nitrogen from the periphery to the splanchnic area, where they are used for urea synthesis and gluconeogenesis or as energy substrates. The glucose is returned to the periphery, so these processes have been termed the glucose-alanine cycle and the glucose-glutamine cycle, which are analogous to the Cori cycle (Felig, 1981; Souba *et al.*, 1985).

Measurement of the fluxes of amino acids across tissues gives information about the net amino acid balance for that tissue, but the knowledge gained about protein metabolism is only qualitative in nature. There are, however, a few exceptions. The efflux of 3-methylhistidine is a good measure of the degradation of contractile proteins, since after release it is not reutilized for protein synthesis

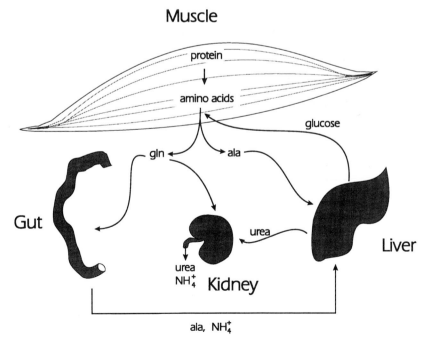

Figure 48.8   The passage of amino nitrogen, mainly in the form of glutamine and alanine, from the muscle to the splanchnic tissues during fasting. In trauma the net efflux of amino acids from muscle is increased three- to five-fold, but the proportions of the individual amino acids are unaltered. (Adapted from Souba *et al.*, 1985.)

(Sjölin *et al.*, 1989, 1990; see 'Protein turnover in individual tissues' above). Phenylalanine or tyrosine, by contrast, are reutilized for protein synthesis, so their efflux from peripheral tissues is widely used as an index of net (rather than total) protein degradation, as they are not metabolized peripherally. A third approach combines a constant infusion of a labelled amino acid with its tissue balance (Cheng *et al.*, 1985; Gelfand and Barrett, 1987). This enables separate values for rates of synthesis and degradation of tissue protein to be determined, and is potentially a very valuable method, because of the relative lack of techniques for assessing total protein degradation in individual tissues. An additional refinement of this approach, which requires the intracellular amino acid enrichment to be measured in a tissue biopsy, enables the inward and outward transport of the amino acid across the membrane to be evaluated (Biolo *et al.*, 1995).

The main difficulties with the balance technique are the accurate measurement of blood flow and the maintenance of an adequate steady state. If the free amino acid pool size is changing during the measurement period, then the flux will reflect the net balance of the total tissue amino acid, including the free pool, rather than the balance of protein. For example, the hourly efflux of phenylalanine from the forearm in the postabsorptive state is only about 20% of the total free phenylalanine pool in the muscle (Garlick *et al.*, 1991a). Thus a 10% per hour increase in the free pool size would appear as a halving of the rate of efflux, without there being any change in protein turnover rates. The method also assumes that the only source of influx and efflux is by free amino acids. However, over 24 hours it appears that the peripheral tissues are net exporters of free amino nitrogen (Elia and Livesey, 1983; Wernerman and Vinnars, 1987). This might be explained by the uptake of circulating peptides and plasma proteins and their degradation to free amino acids by peripheral tissues. This represents another route of transport of amino acids from the liver to the periphery, which cannot be measured because the concentration of plasma proteins is quite high in comparison to that of free amino acids. The calculation of net protein degradation would then be invalidated, but if the uptake of protein could be considered to be constant, the relative changes would be valid for comparative purposes. Additional sources of error apply when the technique is modified to include a labelled amino acid. These are outlined under 'Protein turnover in individual tissues' above, and mainly arise from the need to determine the true precursor enrichment, which affects the accuracy of the estimates of both synthesis and degradation. It must also be recognized that measurements across a limb include more than only muscle and that the contributions of skin and bone might not be negligible (Preedy and Garlick, 1981). However, despite the theoretical limitations of this approach, it is becoming widely accepted, both for understanding the physiology of interorgan amino acid fluxes, as a routine technique for assessing changes in protein or amino acid metabolism in experimental and clinical investigations.

In patients with trauma, burns or sepsis the efflux of alanine and other amino acids from peripheral tissues increases three- to five-fold (reviewed by Clowes *et al.*, 1980; Gelfand *et al.*, 1983). However, the proportions of the individual amino acids are the same as those found in normal postabsorptive subjects (Clowes *et al.*, 1980). This efflux reflects the net degradation of muscle protein characteristic of these states. In infected patients it has been shown that the efflux of 3-methylhistidine from the leg increases, showing that the protein loss results from an increase in proteolysis (Sjölin *et al.*, 1989, 1990). Furthermore, from the observed positive correlation between the release of methylhistidine by the leg and that of tyrosine and phenylalanine, it was deduced that protein synthesis was depressed during infection, and that with mild infection this was the dominant effect.

In concert with the increased efflux from peripheral tissues, there is an elevation in the rate of uptake of amino acids by the splanchnic bed (Wilmore *et al.*, 1979, 1980). The increased uptake of alanine by the liver complements the elevation in gluconeogenesis (Gelfand *et al.*, 1983), and there is also a doubling of the uptake of glutamine by the intestine (Souba and Wilmore, 1983). These findings support the conclusion that the breakdown of muscle protein supplies the precursors for oxidative metabolism in the splanchnic area and the tissues involved in the host defence.

Free amino acid pools

Alterations in protein turnover rates and in the fluxes between tissues result in changes in the concentrations of free amino acids in plasma and tissue water. The concentrations in the blood plasma are readily measured, yet despite considerable investigation, they have not proved very useful in understanding the response to trauma (Gelfand *et al.*, 1983; Harper, 1990). The total concentration is about 2.5 mmol/l, but there is a wide range (approx 100-fold) in concentration among individual amino acids. Glutamine and alanine predominate, but other non-essentials (e.g. glycine, serine) and some essentials (e.g. lysine, valine) also have comparatively high concentrations. The total concentration tends to increase slightly after trauma, with rises also in the branched chains, but most of the glucogenic amino acids fall. However, these changes are rather inconsistent, except for the pronounced rise in phenylalanine, perhaps because the levels are much influenced by a number of other physiological factors, such as feeding (Bergström *et al.*, 1990), and dietary composition (for review see Munro, 1970b).

The free amino acid concentrations in the intracellular water of the tissues are in general higher than in the plasma (for review see Fürst, 1983, 1985). The only tissue that is well characterized in man is skeletal muscle. Here the total concentration is ten-fold higher than in the plasma, and individual amino acids, such as glutamate (80-fold) and glutamine (30-fold), are even more concentrated (Bergström *et al.*, 1974). Glutamine is the most abundant intracellular amino acid in muscle, with a normal concentration of 20 mmol/l of intracellular water, and it constitutes more than 50% of the total intracellular amino acid pool (with the exception of taurine, which is not present in protein, but exists almost exclusively in the intracellular pool at very high concentration).

The pattern of intracellular amino acids in muscle is only marginally affected by food intake (Bergström *et al.*, 1990), but characteristic changes occur after trauma, with an increase in the essentials, especially the branched chains and aromatics, and a marked decrease in glutamine (Vinnars *et al.*, 1975; Figure 48.9). As a result of this loss of glutamine, there is also a pronounced depletion of total free amino acids in severe illness (Roth *et al.*, 1982). The decrease in muscle glutamine correlates with the fall in muscle protein synthesis in malnourished and endotoxin-treated animals (Jepson *et al.*, 1988) and in elective surgery patients (Wernerman *et al.*, 1986a,b). Hence, the level of glutamine is sometimes used as an index of muscle protein catabolism after trauma and of malnutrition in intensive care.

Similar changes in muscle free amino acids are seen after starvation, and also in semistarvation accompanied by bed-rest, as well as in malnutrition (Askanazi *et al.*, 1978, 1980). However, the depletion in muscle glutamine seen after starvation is rapidly restored on refeeding (Vinnars *et al.*, 1987). By contrast, provision of food or of intravenous nutrition not containing glutamine does not influence the changes seen after surgical trauma (Vinnars *et al.*, 1980; Hammarqvist *et al.*, 1989, 1990). Moreover, the changes occurring after trauma are normalized rather slowly: normal muscle concentrations of glutamine are not obtained until several weeks after elective surgery (Petersson *et al.*, 1992).

The intracellular pools of other tissues are less well characterized in comparison to muscle. For example, in the intestinal mucosa the non-essential amino acids are also relatively abundant, but glutamine is not dominant (Ollenschläger *et al.*, 1990) and the total amino acid concentration is only half that of muscle.

The concentration of tissue free amino acids are highly reproducible, as are, by contrast with plasma, the changes seen in response to catabolic states. Measurements of free amino acids have helped in understanding the changes in amino acid metabolism after trauma, whereas the glutamine level in muscle has given quantitative information about the effectiveness of nutritional therapy. Although these measurements give no direct information on the dynamics of protein and amino acid metabolism, and the sampling of muscle is an invasive procedure, the analysis is simple compared with techniques based on stable isotopes. Therefore, determination of amino acids is an important adjunct to the more complex techniques for assessing protein metabolism described earlier, and is particularly valuable for longitudinal studies in post-trauma patients.

MEDIATORS AND MODIFIERS OF THE METABOLIC RESPONSE

Effects of altered nutrient intake

The metabolic response to trauma bears some similarity to starvation, so it is important to ask how much it is mediated by a lack of food intake. Moreover, unless nutritional support is provided, starvation will exacerbate the response to trauma. The effects of nutrient intake on body protein metabolism have been reviewed extensively (Waterlow *et al.*, 1978a; Garlick, 1980; Young *et al.*, 1983a; Reeds and Garlick, 1984; Waterlow, 1984; McNurlan and Garlick, 1989; Garlick *et al.*, 1991b). The responses of whole-body, liver and muscle protein turnover to nutrition, in comparison with the effects of trauma, are summarized in Table 48.4.

Responses to nutrient intake can be conveniently separated into acute (postabsorptive) and chronic (adapted starvation) effects. In the postabsorptive state the body utilizes its stores of nutrients. Accordingly, the oxidation of amino acids continues, with loss of body protein and negative

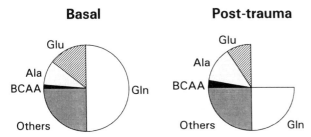

Figure 48.9 The effect of trauma on the intracellular pools of free amino acids in skeletal muscle. In healthy man the intracellular pool is dominated by glutamine (Gln), glutamate (Glu) and alanine (Ala). After trauma the total pool size is decreased by about 25%, mainly as a result of a 50% loss of glutamine, but glutamine, glutamate and alanine still dominate. By contrast, the concentrations of the branched-chain amino acids (BCAA) increase after trauma.

TABLE 48.4

SUMMARY OF RESPONSES OF PROTEIN SYNTHESIS (S) AND DEGRADATION (D) TO PHYSIOLOGICAL AND PATHOLOGICAL STIMULI

	Whole-body		Liver		Muscle	
	S	*D*	*S*	*D*	*S*	*D*
Pathological States						
Trauma	↑	↑	↑	↑	↓	↑
Anaesthetics – volatile	↓	↓ (?)	↓		→	
Anaesthetics – intravenous			→		→	
Immobility	↓	→			↓	→
Physiological States						
Fasting (acute)	→	↑	↓	↑	→ (?)	↑
Starvation (chronic)	↓	↓	↓		↓	↓
Activity/work					↑	↑
Hormones						
Insulin	→ (?)	↓	→	↓	→ (?)	↓
Corticosteroids		↑	↑ (?)	↑	↓	↑
Glucagon	→	↑	↓	↑	↓	
Adrenaline		↓			→	↓
Growth hormone			↑		↑	→
Cytokines						
IL-1	→	→	↑		↓	↑ (?)
IL-6			↑			
TNF	→	→	↑	↓	↓	↑

The arrows indicate the direction of change resulting from the particular physiological or pathological state or from an increase in the circulating level of the hormone. The information is taken from the literature on both human and animal studies. Question marks indicate where there is uncertainty regarding a response, but in no case should this table be read without reference to the relevant text.

nitrogen balance. Feeding then reverses these processes by replacing lost proteins. At the whole-body level, the switch from catabolism to anabolism is achieved by modulating the rate of protein degradation, with little change in the rate of protein synthesis (Melville *et al.*, 1989). At the tissue level, much of the protein lost during fasting is thought to originate from skeletal muscle, as shown by the limb efflux of amino nitrogen in the postabsorptive state, described in 'Interorgan fluxes' above. Animal studies suggest that other tissues, particularly liver and intestine, also contribute to the protein loss (Addis *et al.*, 1936). The mechanism of this protein loss from muscle is, however, controversial. In adult human volunteers there is disagreement about the response of muscle protein synthesis to fasting/feeding. Measurements by infusion of [1-^{13}C]leucine suggest that fasting inhibits synthesis (Halliday *et al.*, 1988). By contrast, both the flooding method (McNurlan *et al.*, 1992) and polyribosome analysis (Wernerman *et al.*, 1985) show little difference in synthesis between the fed and overnight fasted states, implying that degradation is the important site of regulation. This disagreement probably arises from the different assumptions on which the methods are based (see 'Protein turnover in individual tissues' above), and remains to be

resolved. The results from animal experiments are, however, informative. Young growing rats show a large and rapid decrease in muscle protein synthesis when food is withdrawn for a few hours, and this can be rapidly reversed by refeeding (Garlick *et al.*, 1983). Work on isolated muscles *in vitro* suggests that there is also a stimulation of protein degradation by fasting (Fulks *et al.*, 1975). By contrast, *in vivo* experiments in adult rats have shown quite different responses: muscle protein synthesis is resistant to fasting for short periods (Baillie and Garlick, 1992). These data suggest that responses to nutrients in growing animals might be qualitatively different from those in adults. This lends credibility to the results from adult man, described above, showing no change in muscle protein synthesis with fasting, and implies that changes in protein degradation might bring about the loss of muscle protein.

There are no studies of the effects of fasting or feeding on liver and intestine in humans, but animal experiments suggest that fasting results in a small fall in synthesis (McNurlan *et al.*, 1979, 1982). However, both *in vivo* and *in vitro* measurements show that the main cause of the loss of liver protein in the postabsorptive period is a large increase in degradation (Waterlow *et al.*, 1978a).

During longer-term starvation the priority is to restrict the loss of protein by minimizing the need for gluconeogenesis. Thus, over a period of a few days the brain begins to adapt by using ketone bodies as its main oxidative substrate in place of glucose, and there is a concomitant reduction in the oxidation of amino acids and urinary nitrogen excretion. Typically, the rate of N excretion is about 12 g/day in well-nourished subjects, and falls to only about 3 g/day in the fully starvation-adapted state (Cahill, 1970). Starvation in man is accompanied by a fall in whole-body protein synthesis and degradation relative to the post-absorptive values (Henson and Heber, 1983; Nair et al., 1983). There is also a small, but significant fall in protein synthesis in human skeletal muscle (Essén et al., 1992c). Muscle protein degradation, as assessed from the excretion of 3-methylhisti-dine, rises initially (Giesecke et al., 1989), but then falls progressively (Young et al., 1973). In starved rats there is a fall in protein synthesis in most tissues, particularly in skeletal muscle, where degradation may also be depressed (Garlick et al., 1975; Millward et al., 1976; McNurlan et al., 1982). This fall in both synthesis and degradation limits both the loss of protein and the expenditure of energy which would be needed to maintain these processes. Only during the terminal phase, when other supplies of energy have become exhausted, is there an increase in muscle protein degradation, resulting in a very rapid loss of protein (Millward et al., 1976).

It is clear from the above that many of the effects of trauma cannot be attributed to a lack of nutrient intake. The main contrasts between simple starvation and starvation after trauma are shown in Table 48.5. Although both trauma and starvation result in negative protein balance, their mechanism is different, both synthesis and degradation of whole-body protein increasing with trauma, but decreasing with starvation. Clague (1981) has suggested that trauma and starvation can have independent but additive effects, and has rationalized their interactions in the scheme presented earlier (Figure 48.5; see 'whole-body protein turnover' above).

The actions of trauma and starvation on individual tissues are also different. Starvation inhibits liver protein synthesis, but trauma stimulates, whilst in muscle they act similarly, both in general depressing protein synthesis. However, these effects are consistent with the overall responses of body protein, which involve a loss of protein from all tissues in starvation, compared with the redistribution of protein among the tissues in trauma.

TABLE 48.5
COMPARISON OF METABOLISM IN STARVATION AND TRAUMA. (ADAPTED FROM WRETLIND, 1985)

	Starvation	Starvation after trauma
Protein metabolism	Urinary nitrogen excretion decreases progressively as adaption to the starved state occurs. The decreasing contribution of skeletal muscle to gluconeogenesis spares muscle protein. Liver protein content is reduced early in the course of starvation	Prolonged increase of urinary nitrogen excretion. The contribution of muscle amino acids to gluconeogenesis is elevated. Liver protein levels are not reduced
Fat metabolism	Fat oxidation increases and eventually provides most of the energy needed. An adaptation of energy metabolism in muscle and brain to oxidation of ketone bodies occurs	A marked increase in fat oxidation in combination with an increase in circulating free fatty acid levels, while the ketone bodies show only a moderate elevation
Carbohydrate metabolism	Utilization of glucose in the tissues decreases	The oxidation of glucose in the tissues increases, as does glucose turnover
Hormonal changes	A slight increase in adrenaline, glucagon and growth hormone levels in the early phase of starvation. Insulin levels are low	Elevated levels of catecholamines, growth hormone, glucagon and corticosteroids. Insulin is also high, but is accompanied by insulin resistance
Energy expenditure	Resting energy expenditure decreases progressively during starvation	Resting energy expenditure increases by 10–20%: even higher values are seen after extensive burns
Effect of nutrition	The effect of dietary carbohydrate and fat on nitrogen balance is prompt	Only limited effect of dietary carbohydrate and fat on nitrogen balance

Responses to hormones

Current views on the responses of whole body, liver and muscle to the administration of various hormones are summarized in Table 48.5, which incorporates data obtained in both humans and animals. The most important hormones in relation to the response to trauma are outlined below.

Insulin

This is thought to be the main hormone governing the disposition of nutrients after feeding. However, although insulin is clearly anabolic, its effects on protein synthesis are not entirely clear. Data from growing rats are unequivocal, showing both an increase in synthesis and a decrease in degradation in muscle (Jefferson et al., 1977; Garlick et al., 1983; Pain et al., 1983), but in adult rats there is no increase in muscle synthesis (Baillie and Garlick, 1992). Also, the effect of insulin in the liver of animals is to depress proteolysis without any clear effect on synthesis (Mortimore and Mondon, 1970). Similarly in adult humans, insulin infusion depresses degradation in both the whole body and muscle, but synthesis is unaltered or even decreased (Gelfand and Barrett, 1987; Pacy et al., 1989; McNurlan et al., 1994). In an effort to explain this discrepancy between animal and human studies, it has been suggested that the primary effect of insulin is to inhibit protein degradation: as a result, the free amino acid levels fall, either preventing an increase in synthesis or causing a fall (Flakoll et al., 1989; Bennet et al., 1990). It is not yet clear, however, whether synthesis rises in the absence of this fall in amino acid availability, or whether protein synthesis in adult muscle is insensitive to insulin, as in the adult rat.

In trauma the concentration of insulin rises, but this is countered by the development of insulin resistance. However, it is not yet possible to say whether this resistance to insulin affects protein, as well as glucose metabolism, and insulin's role in the response of protein metabolism to trauma is therefore not known.

Stress hormones

Circulating levels of cortisol, catecholamines and glucagon rise after trauma, and collectively these are known as the 'stress hormones'. When infused together into human volunteers, they cause protein loss and bring about some of the responses typical of trauma, such as increased nitrogen and 3-methylhistidine excretion (Bessey et al., 1984; Gelfand et al., 1984) and alterations in muscle polyribosomes and free amino acid concentrations (Wernerman et al., 1989). However, there was no effect on whole-body protein turnover rates measured with [1-^{13}C]leucine (Gelfand et al., 1984). Muscle protein synthesis has been reported to be unaltered by stress hormone infusion in one study (McNurlan et al., 1996),

or increased, but with a greater increase in protein breakdown, in another (Gore et al., 1993). When the hormones have been studied separately, both cortisol and adrenaline had almost the same effect on muscle as all three (Wernerman et al., 1989), but had no effect on whole-body protein synthesis (Miles et al., 1984). No effect of adrenaline was seen on muscle protein synthesis, but protein degradation was inhibited, suggesting an anti-catabolic role for this hormone (Fryburg et al., 1995). The effect of cortisol alone on nitrogen excretion was delayed relative to the effect of the three hormones together (Gelfand et al., 1984) and an elevation of whole-body protein degradation has been demonstrated (Brillon et al., 1995). In animal studies, both corticosteroids and glucagon administration have been shown to depress muscle protein synthesis within a few hours (Garlick et al., 1987; Preedy and Garlick, 1985, 1988). The discrepancy between these studies could arise because in some the concentrations studied were different from those in traumatized patients. However, there remains an inconsistency with catecholamines, on which kinetic studies are few. In human muscle in vivo (Castellino et al., 1990; Fryburg et al., 1995) and in rat muscle in vitro (Garber et al., 1976) it has been shown to be anabolic, which contrasts with its inclusion among the 'stress hormones'.

It has not yet been shown that the changes induced by stress hormone infusion occur as rapidly as the fall in muscle protein synthesis due to injury, which has been detected within 2 hours of surgery (Essén et al., 1992b). Therefore, the exact role of the stress hormones in the response to trauma remains to be elucidated, as other mediators, such as the cytokines, are likely to be acting concurrently.

Cytokines

These products of activated macrophages are dealt with in more detail in Chapters 46 and 49. Both interleukin-1B (IL-1B) and tumour necrosis factor (TNF) reproduce the effects of trauma on muscle and liver protein synthesis when injected into growing rats (Charters and Grimble, 1989; Ballmer et al., 1991). Moreover, protein degradation is inhibited by TNF in liver and stimulated in muscle, and these effects are enhanced by simultaneous administration of IL-1 (Flores et al., 1989). However, whole-body rates of synthesis and degradation appear to be unaffected by these factors, either individually or in combination (Flores et al., 1989). In addition, IL-6 has been shown to stimulate the synthesis of acute-phase proteins by the liver (Ramadori et al., 1988). In addition, it has been shown that the catabolic response to sepsis or endotoxaemia is reduced when cytokines are inhibited by administration of TNF antiserum (Zamir et al., 1992), pentoxifilline (to inhibit TNF production Breuillé et al., 1993), or interleukin-1 receptor antagonist (Zamir *et al.*, 1994). The cytokines are therefore believed to play an important role in mediating the metabolic responses to trauma. However, as with the stress hormones, it is not yet certain whether they can act quickly enough to be responsible for the rapid effect of surgery on muscle protein synthesis. Moreover, their role in relation to each other and to the stress hormones requires clarification.

Anaesthesia

Traumatized patients usually receive some form of anaesthetic or sedative procedure, involving a range of agents, each of which might modify metabolism and hence contribute to the metabolic response to trauma. General anaesthesia is often a combination of sedation, pain relief and muscle relaxation, and these components should be considered separately. There is no evidence that sedation itself has any impact on amino acid or protein metabolism, except when given in very large doses (e.g. fentanyl; Giesecke *et al.*, 1988). Also there is no direct information on the effects of muscle relaxants. However, a number of studies have been performed on the volatile anaesthetic agents, which provide both analgesia and sedation. In both man and animals halothane has been reported to lower protein synthesis. In surgical patients given halothane plus fentanyl there was a reduction in both the synthesis and degradation of whole-body protein, but there was no change in leucine oxidation (Rennie and MacLennan, 1985). However, in dogs given halothane/nitrous oxide anaesthesia, there was a substantial increase in leucine oxidation, as a result of a decrease in whole-body protein synthesis (Horber *et al.*, 1988). Several studies have shown that halothane inhibits protein synthesis in various tissues studied *in vitro* and *in vivo*. Measurements in rats *in vivo* showed a pronounced inhibition in the liver and a smaller effect in lung, but skeletal and cardiac muscle were not affected (Heys *et al.*, 1989). However, these effects appear to be reversed rapidly when the halothane is removed (Rannels *et al.*, 1983; Ferguson *et al.*, 1991), suggesting that this agent will contribute little to the overall response to trauma.

There have been fewer studies of other anaesthetic agents. In surgical patients muscle protein synthesis was measured before and during a period of modified neurolept anaesthesia without surgery, and no change was detected (Essén *et al.*, 1992b). Studies of the other volatile gases have shown that enfluorane has a similar effect on rat liver to that of halothane, but isofluorane does not (Ferguson *et al.*, 1990). Measurements in rats have also shown that pentobarbitone inhibits protein synthesis in liver and lung, but a combination of fentanyl and midazolam only depressed synthesis in lung (Heys *et al.*, 1989). It is notable that none of these studies have demonstrated any effect in skeletal muscle, implying that the loss of muscle protein after trauma is not mediated by the anaesthetic procedures used.

Body temperature

The elevation of body temperature seen in connection with trauma coincides with the increase in energy expenditure (Wilmore *et al.*, 1976). A parallel increase in nitrogen excretion is also seen, but the independent contributions of the increases in temperature and energy expenditure to this protein loss are not yet clear. It has been shown that a period of hyperthermia in a hot room results in an increase in nitrogen excretion (Beisel *et al.*, 1968). Moreover, an increase of 11% in net protein degradation per °C rise in temperature was noted in rat muscles incubated at temperatures between 33 and 42°C. This resulted mainly from an increase in proteolysis, but there was also a rise in synthesis with temperature up to 39°C and a fall at higher temperatures (Baracos *et al.*, 1984). Thus, the hyperthermia might be expected to contribute to the changes in protein metabolism in trauma. However, it is unlikely that the increase either in temperature or energy expenditure is the primary reason for the protein loss, as this still occurs when there is little elevation in body temperature and no increase in energy expenditure (Shanbhogue *et al.*, 1987).

Low body temperature is also of significance, because this is often seen during surgical procedures under general anaesthesia. When a very low temperature occurs, such as in open heart surgery, there is a reduction in the magnitude of the protein catabolic response (Johnson *et al.*, 1986). However, a major difficulty, especially when extracorporeal circulation is used, is the very pronounced stress involved with heating to regain normal body temperature, which can reverse any potential benefit (Wong, 1983). Indeed, when the body temperature is maintained at its normal level during abdominal surgery, the metabolic response is attenuated (Carli *et al.*, 1989). With burns the problem of cooling is markedly aggravated because of evaporative losses from the burned area, resulting in stimulation of heat production (Wilmore *et al.*, 1976). Therefore, modern treatment of burns involves an ambient temperature of above 30°C. This markedly diminishes the nitrogen losses by reducing the degree of stress which would otherwise be involved in maintaining the body temperature (Liljedahl, 1980).

Immobility

Trauma is frequently accompanied by immobility, which might itself contribute to the loss of muscle protein. Early studies in human volunteers showed that immobilization of the lower half of the body in a plaster cast caused a substantial negative N balance (Schønheyder et al., 1954) resulting from a decrease in whole-body protein degradation, measured with [15N]glycine. The negative N balance took several days to develop, however. More recently, Stuart et al. (1990) have studied the effect of bed-rest on protein metabolism and have concluded that whole-body protein degradation was unaltered, but synthesis was decreased, resulting in negative protein balance. However, these changes could be prevented by increasing the intake of dietary protein.

Measurements during immobilization or tail suspension of rats have demonstrated that the muscle atrophy results mostly from a decrease in protein synthesis. Moreover, both the onset of this decrease and its reversal during recovery could be detected within 6 hours (Booth and Seider, 1979; Tucker et al., 1981).

It is therefore clear that immobility could contribute to the metabolic effects of trauma. However, it is not the main cause of protein loss or of the changes in protein turnover, because the negative N balance resulting from bed-rest is quite small (Stuart et al., 1990) and the changes in whole-body protein turnover are different from those after trauma (Table 48.4).

BENEFITS OF INTERVENTION

Nutritional support

Because a part of the body wasting in traumatized unfed patients results directly from the lack of nutrient intake, nutritional support is universally regarded as essential whenever the expected period of reduced intake exceeds a few days. However, the optimal route of nutrient administration, enterally or parenterally, is less clear cut. Whenever both routes are accessible, enteral feeding is considered to be superior. The documentation in man for this statement is, however, not very convincing. Disuse of the gastrointestinal tract has been shown to lead to mucosal atrophy and intestinal barrier damage in animals (Wilmore et al., 1988), but the clinical implications of this in man are still controversial. It is of course cheaper to eat food, and this avoids the risks associated with parenteral feeding, but in terms of nitrogen balance or whole-body protein economy, no clear-cut differences have been demonstrated when all other factors were comparable (McMahon, 1988). Rates of whole-body protein synthesis and degradation were higher in volunteers and patients fed intravenously compared with orally (Sim et al., 1979; Jeevanandam et al., 1987) even though there was no difference in balance. However, this might have resulted from changes in the distribution of the [15N]glycine tracer, as occurs when the tracer itself is given intravenously or

orally (Fern et al., 1981, see 'Measurement of whole-body protein turnover' above).

Healthy subjects are able to maintain nitrogen equilibrium while receiving a wide range of dietary protein intakes. Below about 50 g of protein intake per day, however, body protein is gradually lost. Changes in dietary protein intake require a period of time before a new equilibrium between intake and loss is achieved. During the adaptation period positive N balance in response to an increase in protein intake might occur for a substantial period of time. The protein gained during this period has been termed the 'labile protein reserve'. This has been discussed by Munro (1964) and is not thought to consist of a special storage protein, but instead might involve an expansion of the normal proteins of the body and thus comprise a 'functional' reserve. This might be of importance after trauma, when malnourished patients are known to suffer a higher morbidity and mortality than well-nourished patients (Studley, 1936; Lawson, 1965). However, during the post-trauma period they display less negative nitrogen balances (Kinney, 1977), presumably because their 'reserve' is already depleted.

Energy intake in healthy subjects also influences body protein equilibrium. As illustrated in Figure 48.10, intakes below that required to balance energy expenditure result in an appreciable negative nitrogen balance. There is also an interaction between energy and protein intake. At any particular energy intake, increasing the intake of protein will limit protein loss, but only up to a maximum, which is determined by the deficit in energy. Thus, deficiencies of either energy or protein in the diet will result in body protein loss, even in healthy subjects. In traumatized patients, maintenance, much less restoration, of lean body mass will not occur unless adequate protein and energy are given.

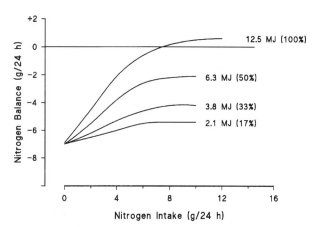

Figure 48.10 The relation between the nitrogen content of the diet and nitrogen balance at different levels (% of normal) of caloric intake in healthy subjects. (Adapted from Calloway and Spector, 1954.)

During the 1960s and 1970s the concept of hyperalimentation of severely ill patients was suggested (Dudrick *et al.*, 1968; Kaplan *et al.*, 1969). The basis of this was the elevated basal energy expenditure (BEE) seen in various patients with trauma, infection or burns. Today we know that with modern hospital care these patients have near to normal rates of BEE. Historically there have been two misinterpretations: the false concept that the BEE is also high in patients subjected to modern hospital care and also the idea that a non-malnourished patient would benefit from a 'positive energy balance'. This latter notion immediately leads to overfeeding as one of the major risks with parenteral nutrition today (Detsky, 1991). When the effect of nutrition is examined in terms of nitrogen balance, very little is gained by giving more calories than the actual requirement. The quality of any nitrogen retention is also disputable, since there are no indications that important body proteins can be saved in traumatized patients by giving calories above the actual EE. The composition of the energy given is, however, important. Both fat and carbohydrate should be given. If the energy is given only as glucose, a somewhat better nitrogen balance is sometimes seen (Henneberg *et al.*, 1985), but in parallel there is an inhibition of utilization of endogenous fat.

The total amount of nitrogen given to patients has also proved controversial to some extent, but nowadays there seems to be agreement worldwide that not more than 0.15 g nitrogen/kg body wt/24 h should be provided. The rationale for this recommendation rests largely upon the finding that larger amounts of nitrogen do not improve nitrogen balance after trauma (Larsson *et al.*, 1990; see Figure 48.11). On the contrary, more nitrogen will lead to oxidation of the amino acids with extra urea and heat production. The former may be handled by the patient with normal kidney function, but might necessitate dialysis treatment for some. Elevated heat production might also cause difficulty because of increased respiration and perhaps an elevated body temperature. The latter may be misinterpreted as an infection and hence be treated with antibiotics: these powerful drugs might have side-effects, especially on kidney function.

The composition of the amino acids given has been debated extensively during the last decade or so. Initially amino acid solutions for parenteral use were based on the concept that a balanced or nutritionally ideal mixture was required, similar to that for healthy subjects. However, because of evidence that supplements might be beneficial or because certain amino acids were generally omitted from the 'standard' mixtures, much research into specific amino acids has been performed. Moreover, intravenous feeding with a conventional mixture of amino acids does not appear to reverse the decrease in muscle protein synthesis following surgery (Essén *et al.*, 1992a; Tjader *et al.*, 1996; Figure 48.12).

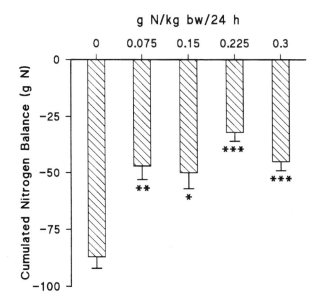

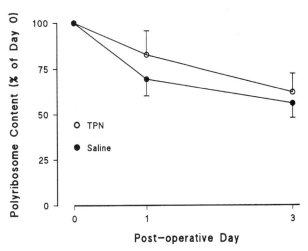

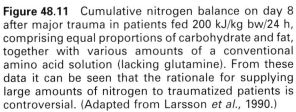

Figure 48.11 Cumulative nitrogen balance on day 8 after major trauma in patients fed 200 kJ/kg bw/24 h, comprising equal proportions of carbohydrate and fat, together with various amounts of a conventional amino acid solution (lacking glutamine). From these data it can be seen that the rationale for supplying large amounts of nitrogen to traumatized patients is controversial. (Adapted from Larsson *et al.*, 1990.)

Figure 48.12 The fall in muscle protein synthesis after elective surgery, as reflected by the changes in concentration of polyribosomes. This decrease is not influenced by postoperative total parenteral nutrition comprising 135 kJ/kg bw/24 h and 0.2 g nitrogen/kg bw/24 h. The amino acid solution was of a conventional type, lacking glutamine. (Data from Wernerman *et al.*, 1986b.)

Branched chain amino acids (BCAA)

Experiments on isolated animal muscles *in vitro* have shown that elevated concentrations of leucine, isoleucine and valine can inhibit protein loss by stimulating protein synthesis and inhibiting protein degradation (Buse and Reid, 1975; Fulks *et al.*, 1975; Li and Jefferson, 1978). However, despite some studies showing that supplements of leucine or BCAA in various groups of patients can improve nitrogen balance (see reviews by Adibi, 1980; Smith and Elia, 1983; Walser, 1984; Brennan *et al.*, 1986), attempts to demonstrate a clinical benefit have not been successful. Thus, Brennan *et al.* (1986), in a workshop sponsored by the American Society for Parenteral and Enteral Nutrition, concluded that as little major effect on outcome had yet been demonstrated, no widespread application of BCAA formulations could be endorsed. More recent studies have also shown no effect of BCAA supplements on nitrogen retention (e.g. Hammarqvist *et al.*, 1988; Vente *et al.*, 1991; Sandstedt *et al.*, 1992). A number of factors might explain the apparent discrepancies between the experimental and clinical studies. The *in vitro* work showing effects of BCAA was performed in muscle from growing animals and, as pointed out earlier, there appear to be differences in the responses of skeletal muscle to nutrients in growing versus adult animals. Li and Jefferson (1978) were unable to demonstrate an effect of BCAA on protein metabolism in perfused muscle from older animals. Also, the experiments *in vitro* inevitably involve muscle which is in negative protein balance, because of deteriorating viability. When experiments have been performed *in vivo*, effects of BCAA on muscle protein synthesis have not been detected (McNurlan *et al.*, 1982; Louard *et al.*, 1990). The role of BCAA in growing animals *in vivo* might be as part of the mechanism for stimulating protein synthesis after feeding, by enhancing insulin sensitivity (Garlick and Grant, 1988), but the evidence for a stimulation of synthesis by feeding in adults is controversial (see 'Mediators and modifiers of the metabolic response' above) and there is no indication that additional leucine would stimulate above the normal fed level. However, it is possible that additional leucine might be of benefit by stimulating insulin sensitivity when insulin levels are low or during insulin resistance. It has been noted that insulin can have a beneficial effect on nitrogen balance, but only in the most severely catabolic patients (Woolfson *et al.*, 1979). Moreover, the workshop on clinical uses of BCAA (Brennan *et al.*, 1986) concluded that positive benefits of BCAA on nitrogen metabolism had been shown only in the most severely ill patients.

Glutamine

This amino acid is not included in the conventional amino acid mixtures because of stability problems when in solution. Since it is classed as a dispensable amino acid, this has not until recently been considered to be a problem. However, the depletion of muscle glutamine concentration after trauma (see 'Circulating proteins' above and Vinnars *et al.*, 1975) and the correlation between low muscle glutamine and mortality (Roth *et al.*, 1982) have led to the provision of extra glutamine or glutamine analogues in experimental studies. These have been shown to result in an improvement in muscle protein metabolism as well as in whole-body nitrogen economy after trauma (Hammarqvist *et al.*, 1989; Stehle *et al.*, 1989; Vinnars *et al.*, 1990; Wernerman *et al.*, 1990). However, despite the demonstration of a correlation between protein synthesis rate and glutamine concentration in rat muscle (Jepson *et al.*, 1988), it has not proved possible to restore protein synthesis to normal by infusion of glutamine in traumatized or starved animals (Jepson and Millward, 1991; Khan *et al.*, 1991; Wusteman and Elia, 1991; Wusteman *et al.*, 1995), or by increasing the concentration of glutamine in the medium of muscle incubated *in vitro* (Fang *et al.*, 1995c). Even if protein synthesis rate and glutamine concentration are sometimes statistically correlated, there are several examples when they are not (Khan *et al.*, 1991).

As stated above (See 'Free amino acid pools' page 706), skeletal muscle is the major producer of glutamine, so it is natural that muscle glutamine depletion should be the first sign of the central role of glutamine in post-traumatic amino acid metabolism. Glutamine is continuously transported by the blood to the splanchnic area to be used as an oxidative fuel in the intestine. The major part of the carbons of glutamine reaching the intestine appear as CO_2, lactate or alanine in the portal blood (Windmueller and Spaeth, 1974), whereas the amino groups are metabolized to portal ammonia, to be cleared by the liver. The cells shown to be most likely to use glutamine as an oxidative fuel in the intestine are enterocytes and immunocompetent cells (Ardawi and Newsholme, 1984; Souba *et al.*, 1985). In support of this there is a large number of studies in animals showing better tolerance to burns, cortisol or cytostatic drugs (Souba *et al.*, 1990) when glutamine-supplemented TPN is provided. However, animals receiving ordinary food by the oral route show a similar tolerance to such stressful events. Moreover, the preference of immunocompetent cells for glutamine is exclusively documented by *in vitro* tests of lymphocyte proliferation, etc. (Newsholme *et al.*, 1985). Thus, the clinical documentation for a beneficial effect of glutamine supplementation of TPN in man is sparse. However, in bone marrow transplant patients, beneficial effects on nitrogen balance, the number of positive cultures, the need for blood transfusions and on hospital stay, have been reported (Ziegler *et al.*, 1992b).

The instability of glutamine in aqueous solutions may be overcome by manufacturing the amino acid solution immediately before use (Elia and Livesay, 1983) or by providing glutamine as dipeptides, which are stable in aqueous solutions, but are rapidly hydrolysed when infused intravenously (Albers et al., 1988). Another approach is to give the corresponding carbon skeleton of glutamine, alpha-ketoglutarate, which is also stable in aqueous solutions (Hammarqvist et al., 1990; Wernerman et al., 1990). In critically ill patients, alpha-ketoglutarate has been shown to maintain the free glutamine level in muscle (Petersson et al., 1992), while glutamine-containing dipeptides only show a marginal effect (Karner and Roth, 1990). However, the route of administration, dosage and tolerance are controversial issues. So far in man, only parenterally administered glutamine/alpha-ketoglutarate has been shown to have beneficial effects, and the efficacy of glutamine-enriched enteral formulae remains to be established. Most studies so far have used a higher content of glutamine than its proportion in naturally occurring proteins, but no dose–response relationship has been established. In contrast, a very high rate of glutamine supplementation to rats caused a depression of the muscle protein synthesis rate (Jepson and Millward, 1991). In general, however, intravenous glutamine or glutamine analogues have been well tolerated and are readily cleared from plasma. This is particularly well documented for the dipeptides (Albers et al., 1989). Amino acid solutions containing glutamine dipeptides are becoming available commercially, but the indications for the use of such products are still to be settled.

Arginine

This amino acid is classed as conditionally indispensable, as it can be synthesized by humans, but is required for optimal growth. It is a precursor of several compounds of metabolic significance, including polyamines, creatine and nitric oxide. Arginine has been reported to have a wide range of important effects, including the stimulation of secretion of several hormones, improvement of wound healing and inhibition of tumour implantation and growth. The latter two effects have been attributed to the ability of arginine supplements to enhance various aspects of the immune system. These biological effects of arginine have been reviewed in detail (Visek, 1986; Barbul, 1986, 1990a; Kirk and Barbul, 1990).

In traumatized animals, the involution of the thymus and reduced sensitivity of blood lymphocytes to stimulation by mitogens have been shown to be reversed by the provision of arginine supplements (Barbul et al., 1980a). Moreover, weight loss is reduced (Seifter et al., 1978) and nitrogen retention is improved (Barbul et al., 1981a). During sepsis in the rat the synthesis of acute-phase proteins and

histones are enhanced (León et al., 1991). In patients with surgical trauma of moderate severity the provision of 15 g/day of arginine parenterally substantially reduced nitrogen losses (Elsair et al., 1978), whereas in volunteers oral supplements of arginine (25 g/day) enhanced wound healing and stimulated the responses of lymphocytes to mitogens (Barbul et al, 1990; Daly et al., 1992).

The mechanism of the effects of arginine on recovery from trauma and on wound healing are not at present clear and several possibilities have been suggested (Barbul, 1986; Kirk and Barbul, 1990). The secretagogue effects could be responsible for increased secretion of several hormones, notably growth hormone. However, attempts to correlate the improved nitrogen retention following trauma with growth hormone levels in animals and humans were not successful, although increased IGF-1 after arginine supplementation has been observed (Barbul et al., 1984; Daly et al., 1988; Kirk et al., 1993). Arginine is also a precursor of proline, which is particularly abundant in the collagen synthesized by the healing wound, and for polyamines, which are involved in cell division. A relatively newly discovered pathway, by which arginine is converted to nitric oxide, has been shown to be involved in the activation of several components of the immune system (e.g. cytotoxicity of activated macrophages; Hibbs et al., 1988) and activation of lymphocytes (Kirk et al., 1990). Activation of the immune system by arginine supplements has been widely reported in both animals (Barbul et al., 1977, 1980b, 1988; Saito et al., 1987) and in man (Barbul et al., 1981b; Daly et al., 1988; Park et al., 1991), and macrophages and lymphocytes are recognized as important participants in wound repair (Barbul, 1990b). However, despite the present lack of definitive evidence for its mechanism of action, arginine-supplemented products are becoming available for enteral feeding of traumatized patients.

Other amino acids

Tyrosine and cysteine are not classically regarded as indispensable in man. However, because their only source is by synthesis from phenylalanine and methionine, which are indispensable, they rely on an adequate provision and conversion of these precursors. Moreover, neither tyrosine nor cysteine can be included in conventional amino acid solutions because tyrosine is insoluble and cysteine is unstable. Attempts are therefore being made to make derivatives of these two amino acids (e.g. dipeptides, N-acetyl derivatives), which can be included in intravenous feeds (Bässler, 1989).

Overall it is clear that nutrition of the traumatized patient is an important adjuvant therapy, especially in depleted and/or malnourished subjects. However, the limitations of nutritional support as a medical therapy must be recognized, as parenteral nutrition can never replace proper surgical and pharmacological treatment of the underlying pathology. The aim is to win time, in order to create the optimal conditions for the traumatized subject to recover and improve tolerance of other treatments, rather than to counteract and reverse the natural metabolic responses. With this aim one important goal of intravenous nutrition is to avoid producing any adverse effects, not only those related to caloric overfeeding, but also those related to protein metabolism.

Hormonal therapy

Growth factors

The ability of young individuals to maintain a positive nitrogen balance after surgery has led to the suggestion that growth hormone might have a beneficial effect on protein metabolism after trauma. Moreover, infusion of growth hormone into healthy humans stimulates muscle protein synthesis (Fryburg and Barrett, 1993). Many years ago it was shown that a pituitary extract spares body nitrogen when given to traumatized rats (Cuthbertson et al., 1941), and experiments in man have demonstrated that extracts of human growth hormone confer a beneficial effect on whole-body nitrogen economy after surgical trauma (Manson and Wilmore, 1986; Ward et al., 1987; Ponting et al., 1988) and after burns (Soroff et al., 1960; Liljedahl et al., 1961). More recently, the biosynthetic human growth hormone has shown similar effects (Ziegler et al., 1988; Jiang et al., 1989; Mjaaland et al., 1990; Hammarqvist et al., 1992). As an adjunct to parenteral nutrition in patients with gastrointestinal disease or to critically ill patients with burns or after trauma, biosynthetic human growth hormone enhances the efficiency of nutrient utilization and stimulated wound healing (Herndon et al., 1990; Ziegler et al., 1990, 1992a). It is thought that insulin-like growth factor-1 (IGF-1) plays a role in the anabolic response to growth hormone (Clemmons and Underwood, 1991), and IGF-1 acutely stimulates muscle protein synthesis in humans and animals (Fryburg 1994; Sandström et al., 1995; Jacob et al., 1996). IGF-1 is now being studied in its own right as a possible enhancer of protein retention after trauma. Currently, the role of IGF-1 binding proteins in the responses to growth hormone and IGF-1 and their regulation are being studied in relation to nutritional status.

The doses of growth hormone given are far in excess of those used for hormone replacement in growing children. However, with periods of treatment of up to 6 weeks, it seems to be well tolerated. Elevated levels of C-peptide and insulin have been observed and hypoglycaemia sometimes occurs, requiring extra glucose, so high doses of growth hormone cannot be recommended in diabetics. The positive effect on nitrogen economy may be explained by the protective effect of growth hormone on muscle after surgical trauma (Mjaaland et al., 1990; Lundeberg et al., 1991; Hammarqvist et al., 1992). Reports that muscle strength is maintained after surgery (Jiang et al., 1989), as well as an improved inspirational force in patients with chronic obstructive pulmonary disease (Clemmons and Underwood, 1991), also point towards skeletal muscle as an important site of action of growth hormone.

Biosynthetic growth hormone is now available in sufficient quantity to be used as an adjuvant to protein metabolism in various pathological states. However, many important questions remain to be answered before growth factors can be recommended for routine clinical practice.

Insulin

Because of the development of insulin resistance after trauma and the anabolic nature of insulin, additional insulin has been investigated as a possible promoter of nitrogen retention. In burned patients improvements in nitrogen balance were achieved by this means, but only in the most traumatized patients, with rates of nitrogen excretion in excess of 30 g/day (Woolfson et al., 1979). Similarly in highly traumatized patients following major operative resections, nitrogen excretion was diminished by insulin infusion and the efflux of amino acids from the forearm was reduced, implying an improved retention of protein in skeletal muscle (Inculet et al., 1986). However, no benefit of insulin infusion on nitrogen balance, 3-methylhistidine excretion or whole-body protein kinetics measured with [^{15}N]glycine could be detected in relatively unstressed patients (Powell-Tuck et al., 1984; Powell-Tuck and Glynn, 1985; Glynn et al., 1987). Improvements in body cell mass have been detected by body composition measurement with multiple isotopes. In a range of patients with different degrees of stress, the higher rates of recovery of cell mass resulting from insulin infusion correlated with the degree of malnutrition and inversely with the age of the patients (Shizgal and Posner, 1989). Thus in some patients, insulin could result in a doubling of the rate of recovery of body cell mass, but the corresponding improvement of nitrogen retention is less than 1 g/day, which is too small to be detected by the nitrogen balance technique.

Overall, it appears that there might be some benefit to be gained by insulin infusion in terms of nitrogen balance and lean tissue recovery, at least in those patients who are very highly traumatized or malnourished. There might also be some disadvantages, however. Adipose tissue deposition might result from insulin's stimulation of triglyceride synthesis (Jeejeebhoy et al., 1976) and the stimulation of glucose oxidation might cause increases in carbon dioxide production and oxygen consumption (Askanazi *et al.*, 1981), which can both be harmful to the stressed patient. At present, therefore, insulin infusion is not recommended for treatment of the trauma victim.

Pharmacological agents

Anabolic steroids

Anabolic steroids have long been known to increase muscle mass in farm animals and in healthy humans. They have also been used clinically in various conditions to improve lean tissue deposition and spare body protein. Retention of protein has been demonstrated as a positive nitrogen balance, at least in malnourished subjects (Tweedle *et al.*, 1973; Michelsen *et al.*, 1982). However, other investigators have failed to demonstrate such potentially beneficial effects (Lewis *et al.*, 1981; Yule *et al.*, 1981; Young *et al.*, 1983b). The effect has been suggested to be located in muscle tissue (Michelsen *et al.*, 1982), but the mechanistic basis for such an action is unknown. In patients with lung cancer, beneficial effects have been reported, not only on body weight, but also on survival (Chlebowski *et al.*, 1983). This is not necessarily related to an effect on protein metabolism, however, since steroids in general are known to have similar effects.

The use of anabolic steroids has recently diminished, possibly because of its misuse by athletes, which has made the manufacturers withdraw their products. Overall, the evidence in favour of anabolic steroids in the depleted post-traumatic state is not overwhelming, but on the other hand, the possible benefits have not been evaluated with modern quantitative techniques.

Non-steroidal anti-inflammatory drugs

There is evidence that some of the actions of the cytokines are mediated through the eicosanoids. Notably, the hyperthermic effect of IL-1 depends on the production of prostaglandin-E_2 from arachidonic acid in the cell membrane by the cyclo-oxygenase pathway (Dinarello and Wolff, 1982). An increase in PGE_2 is also involved in the stimulation of proteolysis in skeletal muscle by IL-1 (Rodeman and Goldberg, 1982). Non-steroidal anti-inflammatory drugs, which interfere with the synthesis of PGE_2 by inhibiting cyclo-oxygenase, have therefore been investigated as potential inhibitors of the stress response. In isolated muscles it was shown that indomethacin blocked the rise in both the PGE_2 concentration and proteolysis (Baracos *et al.*, 1983), whereas in septic rats, muscle wasting was reduced (Ruff and Secrist, 1984). Also, prostaglandin blockade with ibuprofen or diclofenac has been shown to minimize the metabolic abnormalities associated with experimental endotoxaemic shock in animals (Slotman *et al.*, 1985; Urbascheck *et al.*, 1985) and to diminish muscle protein loss seen in association

with experimental tumours (Strelkov *et al.*, 1989). By contrast, however, administration of fenbufen in endotoxaemic rats abolished the rise in body temperature, but failed to prevent the loss of body weight and muscle protein, as well as the fall in protein synthesis in muscle and the rise in liver (Jepson and Millward, 1989).

In critically ill patients few reports exist concerning the effects of NSAID on protein metabolism or the metabolic response to trauma. In severely ill surgical patients it has been shown that diclofenac administration decreases glucose turnover, but whole-body protein turnover was not affected (Shaw and Wolfe, 1988). However, indomethacin has been reported to decrease nitrogen loss by about 20% after elective gastrectomy (Asoh *et al.*, 1987). More work on NSAID needs to be done, but it should be recognized that not all of the effects of prostaglandin blockade are potentially beneficial. Prostaglandins, specifically $PGF_{2\alpha}$, have also been implicated in the increase in protein synthesis in isolated muscles induced by work, which can be blocked by NSAID (Smith *et al.*, 1983). Moreover, the stimulation of muscle protein synthesis in growing rats by insulin and by feeding can be inhibited by indomethacin (Reeds and Palmer, 1984; Reeds *et al.*, 1985; McNurlan *et al.*, 1987), although the effect on the response to feeding could not be reproduced in adult man (McNurlan *et al.*, 1987). Recovery from trauma requires that each of these responses should be operating correctly.

Adrenergic blockade

The role of catecholamines in the initiation of the metabolic response to trauma is still debated. It is controversial whether they induce the cytokine response via activation of macrophages, or whether the cytokines are the primary event which among other things causes a rise in catecholamine levels. However, as detailed in 'Responses to hormones' above, infusion of the stress hormones brings about many of the metabolic changes seen after trauma. Moreover, in volunteers the acute effect of stress hormones on muscle amino acid metabolism is inhibited by simultaneous administration of propranolol (Ejeson *et al.*, 1991). However, in dogs the urinary nitrogen loss following surgery was not affected by combined α- and β-blockade, despite a decrease in the efflux of amino acids from the hind limb (Hulton *et al.*, 1985). While there is a number of reports of the effects of α- or β-blockade on aspects of carbohydrate or fat metabolism in traumatized patients, there seems to be little on protein metabolism. Nitrogen economy is improved by β-blockade in thyrotoxicosis in man (Georges *et al.*, 1975) and in animal models of sepsis (Dickerson *et al.*, 1990). This effect is thought to be mediated through an attenuation of muscle protein degradation, as indicated by a reduction in 3-methylhistidine excretion (Dickerson *et al.*, 1990).

The use of pharmacological β-blockade in clinical practice is limited by its circulatory effects, which may be very hazardous to patients. In critically ill patients there are particular difficulties if the circulation is not stable. This is probably the main reason for the absence of controlled clinical trials of β-blockade in traumatized patients, despite its theoretical advantages. However, an alternative method for limiting the effects of catecholamines is an epidural blockade, which can give a total sympathetic block with certain types of surgery (see below).

Epidural anaesthesia

A complete nervous block attenuates the metabolic response to trauma. These effects have been reviewed by Kehlet (1990a,b, 1991). For example, epidural anaesthesia during and for 3 days after hip replacement surgery or hysterectomy completely restores the otherwise negative nitrogen balance to normal (Brandt et al., 1978; Kehlet et al., 1979). On the other hand, a spinal or epidural block given perioperatively, but discontinued postoperatively, does not influence the metabolic responses (Norlén et al., 1990). It appears, therefore, that once the response to trauma has been triggered by the afferent nervous stimuli from the site of injury, it will be irreversible. Similarly, the metabolic effects of major abdominal or upper abdominal surgery are not attenuated by preoperative epidural blockade (Vesterberg et al., 1982), presumably because it is not possible to prevent the afferent stimuli from reaching the brain.

This type of anaesthetic technique is known to alter the hormonal response to injury (Rutberg et al., 1984) and therefore its effects are thought to be attributable to an altered pattern of stress hormones. This explains the variable results described above, since in clinical practice it is very difficult to maintain an effective epidural block for several days after trauma, as a complete sympathetic block up to the level of T4 is needed to produce this effect. On the other hand, the pain relief obtained by using epidural or subarachnoid administration of local anaesthetics can be of great benefit to the patient, although no dramatic effects on nitrogen economy are seen.

CONCLUDING REMARKS

Management of traumatized patients is dominated by the need for repair of the damaged tissue, so our aim is to provide the best possible environment for the healing process. Repair and healing are closely related to protein metabolism and require optimal conditions for protein metabolism to be maintained. Hence, in order to provide the best possible care for the patient, knowledge of the underlying pathophysiological and physiological mechanisms controlling protein metabolism are mandatory. In parallel, reliable techniques are also needed for evaluating experimental therapies. This chapter has dealt with the present state of knowledge concerning the pathophysiology of protein metabolism in connection with trauma. In addition, available techniques have been discussed and commented on, to give the reader information on the methodological difficulties involved and how our present knowledge may be expanded. Finally, metabolic studies have also paved the way for a variety of suggested therapies, presented above in 'Benefits of intervention'.

To summarize the present position, excellent general care of the patient subjected to trauma stands out as the cornerstone of treatment. If the activations of mediators can be modified by early and adequate care, in terms of reduction of tissue damage, circulatory stability, pain control, good oxygenation, etc., the negative effects upon protein metabolism become less extensive. Following the initial phase of trauma, one goal of therapy should be to optimize the conditions for protein metabolism, especially in critical tissues. This is accomplished by adequate caloric and protein/amino acid support. Today, the emphasis is not to overfeed the patient, which is potentially hazardous. In biochemical terms, the aim is to achieve the most favourable whole-body economy, which is thought to involve the least possible tissue loss. In the future, this strategy may have to be re-evaluated, however, when better knowledge of protein metabolism in individual organs is established.

The obvious goal for the treatment of the traumatized patient is to keep mortality and morbidity as low as possible. However, when the type of therapy or level of metabolic care of the patient needs to be evaluated, such end-points are not very useful. Obviously the background to mortality and morbidity is multifactorial, and this calls for large groups of patients to be compared to allow for definite conclusions. Since only a very limited number of such studies can be performed, a large part of the development of new concepts for treatment must rely on biochemical measurements, which brings us back to the fundamental importance of our knowledge of the pathophysiology. Since biochemical measurements such as nitrogen balance or protein synthesis rate can be made with reasonable precision, the use of such indices depends entirely upon how studies are designed in relation to what questions are asked. This dualism between studies with clinical end-points and those with biochemical end-points is a necessity in the field of human protein metabolism. The conditions and limitations of this dualism provide the fascination that can be experienced when studying the relationship between protein metabolism and clinical outcome.

REFERENCES

Addis T., Poo L.J., Lew W. (1936). Protein loss from liver during a two day fast. *J. Biol. Chem.*, **115**, 117–18.

Adibi S.A. (1980). Roles of branched-chain amino acids in metabolic regulation. *J. Lab. Clin. Med.*, **95**, 475–84.

Albers S., Wernerman J., Stehle P. et al. (1988). Availability of amino acids supplied intravenously in healthy man as synthetic dipeptides. Pharmokinetic evaluation of L-alanyl-L-glutamine and L-glycyl-L-tyrosine. *Clin. Sci.*, **75**, 463–8.

Albers S., Wernerman J., Stehle P. et al. (1989). Availability of amino acids supplied by constant infusion of synthetic dipeptides in healthy man. *Clin. Sci.*, **76**, 643–8.

Ardawi M.S.M., Newsholme E.A. (1984). Glutamine metabolism in lymphoid tissues. In *Glutamine Metabolism in Mammalian Tissues* (Häussinger D., Sies H., eds). Berlin: Springer-Verlag, pp. 235–46.

Ash S.A., Griffin G.E. (1989). Effect of parenteral nutrition on protein turnover in endotoxaemic rats. *Clin. Sci.*, **76**, 659–66.

Askanazi J., Elwyn D.H., Kinney J.M. et al. (1978). Muscle and plasma amino acids after injury: the role of inactivity. *Ann. Surg.*, **188**, 797–803.

Askanazi J., Fürst P., Michelsen C.B. et al. (1980). Muscle and plasma amino acids after injury; hypocaloric glucose vs. amino acid infusion. *Ann. Surg.*, **191**, 465–572.

Askanazi J., Nordenshom J., Rosenbaum S.H. (1981). Nutrition of the patient with respiratory failure. *Anesthesiology*, **54**, 373–7.

Asoh T., Shirasaka C., Uchidia I., Tsuji H. (1987). Effects of indomethacin on endocrine responses and nitrogen loss after surgery. *Ann. Surg.*, **206**, 770–6.

Baillie A.G.S., Garlick P.J. (1992). Attenuated response of muscle protein synthesis to fasting and insulin in adult female rats. *Am. J. Physiol.*, **262**, E1–5.

Bakic V., MacFadyen B.V., Booth F.W. (1988). Effect of elective surgical procedures on tissue protein synthesis. *J. Surg. Res.*, **44**, 62–6.

Ballard F.J. (1982). Regulation of protein accumulation in cultured cells. *Biochem. J.*, **208**, 275–87.

Ballmer P.E., McNurlan M.A., Milne E. et al. (1990). Measurement of albumin synthesis in humans: a new approach employing stable isotopes. *Am. J. Physiol.*, **259**, E797–803.

Ballmer P.E., McNurlan M.A., Southorn B.G. et al. (1991). Effects of human recombinant interleukin-1β on protein synthesis in rat tissues compared with a classical acute-phase reaction induced by turpentine. *Biochem. J.*, **279**, 683–8.

Ballmer P.E., McNurlan M.A., Grant I. et al. (1985). Down-regulation of albumin synthesis in the rat by human recombinant interleukin-1β or turpentine and the response to nutrients. *J. Parenter. Enter. Nutr.*, **19**, 266–71.

Baracos V., Rodemann H.P., Dinarello C.A., Goldberg A.L. (1983). Stimulation of muscle protein degradation and prostaglandin E2 release by leukocytic pyrogen (interleukin 1). A mechanism for the increased degradation of muscle proteins during fever. *N. Engl. J. Med.*, **308**, 553–8.

Baracos V.E., Wilson E.J., Goldberg A.L. (1984). Effects of temperature on protein turnover in isolated rat skeletal muscle. *Am. J. Physiol.*, **246**, C125–30.

Barbul A. (1986). Arginine: Biochemistry, physiology, and therapeutic implications. *J. Parent. Enter. Nutr.*, **10**, 227–38.

Barbul A. (1990a). Arginine and immune function. *Nutrition*, **6**, S56–62.

Barbul A. (1990b). Immune aspects of wound repair. *Clin. Plast. Surg.*, **17**, 433–42.

Barbul A., Rettura G., Levenson S.M. (1977). Arginine: thymotrophic and wound healing promoting agent. *Surg. Forum*, **28**, 101–3.

Barbul A., Wasserkrug H.L., Seifter E. et al. (1980a). Immunostimulatory effects of arginine in normal and injured rats. *J. Surg. Res.*, **29-a**, 228–35.

Barbul A., Wasserkrug H.L., Sisto D.A., Efron G. (1980b). Thymic and immune stimulatory actions of arginine. *J. Parent. Enter. Nutr.*, **4-b**, 446–9.

Barbul A., Sisto D.A., Wasserkrug H.L. et al. (1981a). Metabolic and immune effects of arginine in postinjury hyperalimentation. *J. Trauma*, **21**, 970–4.

Barbul A., Wasserkrug H.L., Sisto D.A., Efron G. (1981b). Arginine stimulates lymphocyte immune response in healthy humans. *Surgery*, **902**, 244–51.

Barbul A., Wasserkrug H.L., Yoshimura N. et al. (1984). High arginine levels in intravenous hyperalimentation abrogate post-traumatic immune suppression. *J. Surg. Res.*, **36**, 620–4.

Barbul A., Sisto D.A., Wasserkrug H.L., Efron G. (1988). Arginine stimulates thymic immune functions and ameliorates the obesity and hyperglycaemia of genetically obese mice. *J. Parent. Enter. Nutr.*, **3**, 492–5.

Barbul A., Lazarou S.A., Efron D.T. et al. (1990). Arginine enhances wound healing and lymphocyte immune responses in humans. *Surgery*, **108**, 331–7.

Bässler K.H. (1989). Metabolic basis for inclusion of tyrosine and cysteine in amino acid solutions. In *Nutrition in Clinical Practice* (Hartig W., Dietze G., Weiner R., Fürst P., eds). Basel: Karger, pp. 46–55.

Beisel W.R., Goldman R.F., Joy R.J.T. (1968). Metabolic balance studies during induced hyperthermia in man. *J. Appl. Physiol.*, **24**, 1–10.

Bennet W.M., Connacher A.A., Scrimegeour C.M. et al. (1990). Euglycemic hyperinsulinemia augments amino acid uptake by human leg tissues during hyper-aminoacidemia. *Am. J. Physiol.*, **259**, E185–94.

Bergström J., Fürst P., Norée L-O., Vinnars E. (1974). Intracellular free amino acid concentration in human muscle tissue. *J. Appl. Physiol.*, **36**, 693–7.

Bergström J., Fürst P., Vinnars E. (1990). Effect of a test meal, without and with protein, on muscle and plasma free amino acids. *Clin. Sci.*, **79**, 331–7.

Bessey P.Q., Watters J.M., Aoki T.T., Wilmore D.W. (1984). Combined hormonal infusion simulates the metabolic response to injury. *Ann. Surg.*, **200**, 264–81.

Bianchi R., Mariani G., McFarlane A.S. (1976). *Plasma Protein Turnover*. London: MacMillan Press.

Bier D.M. (1991). Methodology for the study of metabolism: kinetic techniques. In *Principles of Perinatal and Neonatal Metabolism* (Cowett R.M., ed.). New York: Springer-Verlag, pp. 1–14.

Biolo G., Declan Fleming R.Y., Maggi S.P. et al. (1995). Transmembrane transport and intracellular kinetics of amino acids in human skeletal muscle. *Am. J. Physiol.*, **268**, E75–84.

Birkhahn R.H., Long C.L., Fitkin D. et al. (1980). Effects of major skeletal trauma on whole body protein turnover in man measured by L-[1, ¹⁴C]-leucine. *Surgery*, **88**,

294–300.

Birkhahn R.H., Long C.L., Fitkin D. et al. (1981). Whole-body protein metabolism due to trauma in man as estimated by L-[^{15}N]alanine. *Am. J. Physiol.*, **241**, E64–71.

Bischoff T.L.W., Voit C. (1860). *Die Gesetze der Ernährung des Fleischfressers.* Leipzig: Winter.

Booth F.W., Seider M.J. (1979). Early change in skeletal muscle protein synthesis after limb immobilization of rats. *J. Appl. Physiol.*, **47**, 974–7.

Brandt M.R., Fernandes A., Mordhorst R., Kehlet H. (1978). Epidural analgesia improves postoperative nitrogen balance. *Br. Med. J.*, **1**, 1106–8.

Brennan M.F., Cerra F., Daly J.M. et al. (1986). Branched chain amino acids in stress and injury. *J. Parent. Enter. Nutr.*, **10**, 446–52.

Brenner U., Herbertz L., Thul P. et al. (1987). The contribution of small gut to the 3-methylhistidine metabolism in the adult rat. *Metabolism*, **36**, 416–18.

Breuillé D., Farge M.C., Rosé F. et al. (1993). Pentoxifylline decreases body weight loss an muscle protein wasting characteristic of sepsis. *Am. J. Physiol.*, **265**, E660–6.

Breuillé D., Rose F., Arnal M. et al. (1994). Sepsis modifies the contribution of different organs to whole-body protein synthesis in rats. *Clin, Sci,.*, **86**, 663–9.

Brillon D.J., Zheng B., Campobell R.G., Matthews D.E. (1995). Effect of cortisol on energy expenditure and amino acid metabolism in humans. *Am. J. Physiol.*, **268**, E501–13.

Burns H.J.G. (1988). The metabolic and nutritional effects of injury and sepsis. In *Ballière's Clinical Gastroenterology*, vol. 2(4) (Burns H.J.G., eds). London: Ballière Tindall, pp. 849–67.

Buse M.J., Reid S.S. (1975). Leucine: a possible regulator of protein turnover in muscle. *J. Clin. Invest.*, **56**, 1250–61.

Cahill G.F. (1970). Starvation in man. *N. Engl. J. Med.*, **282**, 668–75.

Calloway D.H., Spector H. (1954). Nitrogen balance *as related to* caloric and protein intake *in* active young men. *Am. J. Clin. Nutr.*, **2**, 405–12.

Carli F., Emery P.W., Freemantle C.A.J. (1989). Effect of peroperative normothermia on postoperative protein metabolism in elderly patients undergoing hip arthroplasty. *Br. J. Anaesth.*, **63**, 276–82.

Carli F., Webster J., Ramachandra V. et al. (1990). Aspects of protein metabolism after elective surgery in patients receiving constant nutritional support. *Clin. Sci.*, **78**, 621–8.

Castellino P., Luzi L., del Prato S., DeFronzo R. (1990). Dissociation of the effects of epinephrine and insulin on glucose and protein metabolism. *Am. J. Physiol.*, **258**, E117–25.

Charters Y., Grimble R.F. (1989). Effect of recombinant human tumour necrosis factor α on protein synthesis in liver, skeletal muscle and skin of rats. *Biochem. J.*, **258**, 493–7.

Cheblowski R.T., Herrold J., Richardson B., Block J.B. (1983). Effects of Deca-Durabolin in patients with advanced non-small cell lung cancer. *Cancer Res.*, **31**, 95A.

Cheng K.N., Dworzak F., Ford G.C. et al. (1985). Direct determination of leucine metabolism and protein breakdown in humans using L-[1-^{13}C, ^{15}N]-leucine and the forearm model. *Eur. J. Clin. Invest.*, **15**, 349–54.

Clague M.B. (1981). Turnover in pathological states. In *Nitrogen Metabolism in Man* (Waterlow J.C., Stephen J.M.L., eds). London: Applied Science, pp. 525–39.

Clemmons D.R., Underwood L.E. (1991). Nutritional regulation of IGF-1 and IGF binding proteins. *Ann. Rev. Nutr.*, **11**, 393–412.

Clowes G.H.A., Randall H.T., Cha C-J. (1980). Amino acid and energy metabolism in septic and traumatized patients. *J. Parent. Enter. Nutr.*, **4**, 195–205.

Crane C.W., Picou D., Smith R., Waterlow J.C. (1977). Protein turnover in patients before and after elective orthopaedic operations. *Br. J. Surg.*, **64**, 129–33.

Cuthbertson D.P. (1930). The disturbance of metabolism produced by bony and non-bony injury, with notes on certain abnormal conditions of bone. *Biochem. J.*, **24**, 1244–63.

Cuthbertson D.P. (1931). The distribution of nitrogen and sulphur in the urine during conditions of increased catabolism. *Biochem. J.*, **25**, 236–44.

Cuthbertson D.P. (1942). Post-shock metabolic response. *Lancet*, **i**, 433–4.

Cuthbertson D.P. (1976). Surgical metabolism: historical and evolutionary aspects. In *Metabolism and the Response to Injury* (Wilkinson A.W., Cuthbertson D.P., eds). Bath: Pitman Medical, pp. 1–34.

Cuthbertson D.P., Shaw G.B., Young F.G. (1941). The anterior pituitary gland and protein metabolism. II The influence of anterior pituitary extract on the metabolic response to the rat to injury. *J. Endocrinol.*, **2**, 468–74.

Daly J.M., Reynolds J., Thom A. et al. (1988). Immune and metabolic effects of arginine in the surgical patient. *Ann. Surg.*, **208**, 512–22.

Daly J.M., Lieberman M.D., Goldfine J. et al. (1992). Enteral nutrition with supplemental arginine, RNA, and omega-3 fatty acids in patients after operation: Immunologic, metabolic, and clinical outcome. *Surgery*, **112**, 56–67.

Detsky A.S. (1991). Parenteral nutrition – is it helpful? *N. Engl. J. Med.*, **325**, 573–5.

Dickerson R.N., Fried R.C., Bailey P.M. et al. (1990). Effect of propranol on nitrogen and energy metabolism in sepsis. *J. Surg. Res.*, **48**, 38–41.

Dinarello C.A., Wolff S.M. (1982). Molecular basis of fever in humans. *Am. J. Med.*, **72**, 799–818.

Dudrick S.J., Wilmore D.W., Vars H.M., Rhoads J.E. (1968). Long-term total parenteral nutrition with growth, development, and positive nitrogen balance. *Surgery*, **64**, 134–42.

Ejeson B., Vinnars E., Wernerman J. (1991). Beta-blockade counteracts the changes in muscle free amino acids evoked by stress hormones. *Clin. Nutr.*, **10**, (Spec. Suppl. 2), 97.

Elia M., Livesey G. (1983). Effects of ingested steak and infused leucine on forelimb metabolism in man and the fate of the carbon skeletons and amino groups of branched-chain amino acids. *Clin. Sci.*, **64**, 517–26.

Elman R. (1939). Time factor in retention of nitrogen after intravenous injection of a mixture of amino acids. *Proc. Soc. Exp. Biol. Med.*, **40**, 484–7.

Elsair J., Poey J., Issad H. et al. (1978). Effect of arginine chlorhydrate on nitrogen balance during the three days following routine surgery. *Biomed. Express*, **29**, 312–17.

Emery P.W., Cotellessa L., Holness M. et al. (1986). Different patterns of protein turnover in skeletal and gastrointestinal smooth muscle and the production of N-methylhistidine during fasting in the rat. *Biosci. Rep.*, **6**, 143–53.

Essén P., McNurlan M.A., Wernerman J. et al. (1992b). Uncomplicated surgery, but not general anesthesia, decreases muscle protein synthesis. *Am. J. Physiol.*, **262**, E253–60.

Essén P., McNurlan M.A., Wernerman J. et al. (1992c). Short-term starvation decreases skeletal muscle protein synthesis rate in man. *Clin. Physiol.*, **12**, 287–99.

Essén P., McNurlan M.A., Sonnenfeld T., Milne E. et al. (1993). Muscle protein synthesis after operation – the effects of intravenous nutrition. *Eur. J. Surg.*, **159**, 195–200.

Essén P., McNurlan M.A., Gamrin L. et al. (1996). Tissue protein synthesis rates in critically ill patients. *Ann. Surg.*, (in press).

Fang C., Tiao G., James H. et al. (1995a). Burn injury stimulates multiple proteolytic pathways in skeletal muscle, including the ubiquitin-energy-dependent pathway. *J. Am. Coll. Surg.*, **180**, 161–70.

Fang C., James H.J., Ogle C. et al. (1995b). Influence of burn injury on protein metabolism in different types of skeletal muscle and the role of glucocorticoids. *J. Am. Coll. Surg.*, **180**, 33–42.

Fang C.H., James J.H., Fischer J.E., Hasselgren P.O. (1995c). Is muscle protein turnover regulated by intracellular glutamine during sepsis? *J. Parenter. Enter. Nutr.*, **19**, 279–85.

Fearon K.C.H., Hansell D.T., Preston T. et al. (1988). Influence of whole body protein turnover rate on resting energy expenditure in patients with cancer. *Cancer Res.*, **48**, 2590–5.

Fearon K.C., McMillan D.C., Preston T. et al. (1991). Elevated circulating interleukin-6 is associated with and acute-phase response but reduced fixed hepatic protein synthesis in patients with cancer. *Ann. Surg.*, **213**, 26–31.

Felig P. (1975). Amino acid metabolism in man. *Ann. Rev. Biochem.*, **44**, 933–55.

Felig P. (1981). Inter-organ amino acid exchange. In *Nitrogen Metabolism in Man* (Waterlow J.C., Stephen J.M.L. eds). London: Applied Science, pp. 45–61.

Felig P., Wahren J. (1971). Amino acid metabolism in exercising man. *J. Clin. Invest.*, **50**, 2703–14.

Felig P., Owen O.E., Wahren J., Cahill G.F. (1969). Amino acid metabolism during prolonged starvation. *J. Clin. Invest.*, **48**, 584–94.

Felig P., Wahren J., Räf L. (1973). Evidence of inter-organ amino-acid transport by blood cells in humans. *Proc. Natl. Acad. Sci.*, **70**, 1775–9.

Ferguson K., Heys S.D., Norton A.C. et al. (1990). Effect of volatile anaesthetic agents on liver protein synthesis. *Proc. Nutr. Soc.*, **49**, 182A.

Ferguson K., Baillie A.G.S., Norton A.C. et al. (1991). Time course effect of volatile anaesthetic agents on tissue protein synthesis. *Proc. Nutr. Soc.*, **50**, 167A.

Fern E.B., Garlick P.J. (1983). The rate of nitrogen metabolism in the whole body of man measured with (^{15}N) glycine and uniformly labelled (^{15}N) wheat. *Hum. Nutr. Clin. Nutr.*, **37C**, 91–107.

Fern E.B., Garlick P.J., McNurlan M.A., Waterlow J.C. (1981). The excretion of isotope in urea and ammonia for estimating protein turnover in man with [^{15}N]glycine. *Clin. Sci.*, **61**, 217–28.

Fern E.B., Garlick P.J., Waterlow J.C. (1985a). The concept of the single body pool of metabolic nitrogen in determining the rate of whole body nitrogen turnover. *Hum. Nutr. Clin. Nutr.*, **39C**, 85–99.

Fern E.B., McNurlan M.A., Garlick P.J. (1985b). Effect of malaria on rate of protein synthesis in individual tissues of rats. *Am. J. Physiol.*, **249**, E485–93.

Fischer J.E. (1991). A teleological view of sepsis. *Clin. Nutr.*, **10**, 1–9.

Flakoll P.J., Kulaylat M., Frexes-Steed M. et al. (1989). Amino acids augment insulin's suppression of whole body proteolysis. *Am. J. Physiol.*, **257**, E839–47.

Fleck A. (1989). Clinical and nutritional aspects of changes in acute-phase proteins during inflammation. *Proc. Nutr. Soc.*, **48**, 347–54.

Fleck A., Colley C.M., Myers M.A. (1985). Liver export proteins and trauma. *Br. Med. Bull.*, **41**, 265–73.

Flores E.A., Bistrian B.R., Pomposelli J.J. et al. (1989). Infusion of tumor necrosis factor/cachectin promotes muscle catabolism in the rat. A synergistic effect with interleukin 1. *J. Clin. Invest.*, **83**, 1614–22.

Frayn K.N., Maycock P.F. (1979). Regulation of protein metabolism by a physiological concentration of insulin in mouse soleus and extensor digitorum longus muscles. Effects of starvation and scald injury. *Biochem. J.*, **184**, 323–30.

Fryburg D.A. (1994). Insulin-like growth factor I exerts growth hormone- and insulin-like actions on human muscle protein metabolism. *Am. J. Physiol.*, **267**, E331–6.

Fryburg D.A., Barrett E.J. (1993). Growth hormone acutely stimulates skeletal muscle but not whole-body protein synthesis in humans. *Metabolism*, **42**, 1223–7.

Fryburg D.A., Gelfand R.A., Jahn L.A. et al. (1995). Effects of epinephrine on human muscle glucose and protein metabolism. *Am J. Physiol.*, **268**, E55–9.

Fulks R.M., Li J.B., Goldberg A.L. (1975). Effects of insulin, glucose, and amino acids on protein turnover in rat diaphragm. *J. Biol. Chem.*, **250**, 290–8.

Fürst P. (1983). Intracellular muscle free amino acids – their measurement and function. *Proc. Nutr. Soc.*, **42**, 451–62.

Fürst P. (1985). Regulation of intracellular metabolism of amino acids. In *Nutrition in Cancer and Trauma Sepsis. Proc. 6th Congress of ESPEN, Milan 1984* (Bozzetti F., Dionigi R., eds). Basel: Karger, pp. 21–53.

Garber A.J., Karl I.E., Kipnis D.M. (1976). Alanine and glutamine synthesis and release from skeletal muscle; β-adrenergic inhibition of amino acid release. *J. Biol. Chem.*, **251**, 851–7.

Garlick P.J. (1969). Turnover rate of muscle protein measured by constant intravenous infusion of ^{14}C-glycine. *Nature*, **223**, 61–2.

Garlick P.J. (1980). Protein turnover in the whole animal and specific tissues. In *Comprehensive Biochemistry* (Neuberger A., ed.). Amsterdam: Elsevier, pp. 77–210.

Garlick P.J., Fern E.B. (1985). Whole-body protein turnover: theoretical considerations. In *Substrate and Energy Metabolism in Man* (Garrow J.S., Halliday D., eds). London: John Libbey, pp. 7–15.

Garlick P.J., Grant I. (1988). Amino acid infusion increases the sensitivity of muscle protein synthesis *in vivo* to insulin: effect of branched-chain amino acids. *Biochem. J.*, **254**, 579–84.

Garlick P.J., Millward D.J., James W.P.T., Waterlow J.C., (1975). The effect of protein deprivation and starvation on the rate of protein synthesis in tissues of the rat. *Biochim. Biophys. Acta*, **414**, 71–84.

Garlick P.J., Waterlow J.C., Swick R.W. (1976). Measurement of protein turnover in rat liver: analysis of the complex curve for decay of label in a mixture of proteins. *Biochem. J.*, **156**, 657–63.

Garlick P.J., McNurlan M.A., Fern E.B. et al. (1980a). Stimulation of protein synthesis and breakdown by vaccination. *Br. Med. J.*, **281**, 263–4.

Garlick P.J., Clugston G.A., Waterlow J.C. (1980b). Influence of low-energy diets on whole-body protein turnover in obese subjects. *Am. J. Physiol.*, **238**, E235–44.

Garlick P.J., McNurlan M.A., Preedy V.R. (1980c). A rapid and convenient technique for measuring the rate of protein synthesis in tissues by injection of [³H]phenylalanine. *Biochem. J.*, **192**, 719–23.

Garlick P.J., Fern M., Preedy V.R. (1983). The effect of insulin infusion and food intake on muscle protein synthesis in postabsorptive rats. *Biochem. J.*, **210**, 669–76.

Garlick P.J., Grant I., Glennie R.T. (1987). Short term effects of corticosterone treatment on muscle protein synthesis in relation to the response to feeding. *Biochem. J.*, **248**, 439–42.

Garlick P.J., Wernerman J., McNurlan M.A. et al. (1989). Measurement of the rate of protein synthesis in muscle of postabsorptive young men by injection of a 'flooding dose' of [1-¹³]leucine. *Clin. Sci.*, **77**, 329–36.

Garlick P.J., Wernerman J., McNurlan M.A., Heys S.D. (1991a). Organ-specific measurements of protein turnover in man. *Proc. Nutr. Soc.*, **50**, 217–25.

Garlick P.J., McNurlan M.A., Ballmer P.E. (1991b). Influence of dietary protein intake on whole-body protein turnover in humans. *Diabetes Care*, **14**, 1189–98.

Garlick P.J., McNurlan M.A., Essén P., Wernerman J. (1994). Measurement of tissue protein synthesis rates, *in vivo*: a critical analysis of contrasting methods. *Am. J. Physiol.*, **266**, E287–97.

Gelfand R.A., Barrett E.J. (1987). Effect of physiologic hyperinsulinemia on skeletal muscle protein synthesis and breakdown in man. *J. Clin. Invest.*, **80**, 1–6.

Gelfand R.A., deFronzo R.A., Gusberg R. (1983). Metabolic alterations associated with major injury or infection. In *New Aspects of Clinical Nutrition* (Kleinberger G., Deutsch E.C., eds). Basel: Karger, pp. 221–39.

Gelfand R.A., Matthews D.E., Bier D.M., Sherwin R.S. (1984). Role of counterregulatory hormones in the catabolic response to stress. *J. Clin. Invest.*, **74**, 2238–48.

Georges L.P., Santangelo R.P., Mackin J.F., Canary J.J. (1975). Metabolic effects of propranolol in thyrotoxicosis. I. Nitrogen, calcium, and hydroxyproline. *Metabolism*, **24**, 11–21.

Gersovitz M., Munro H.N., Udall J., Young V.R. (1986). Albumin synthesis in young and elderly subjects using a new stable isotope. *Metabolism*, **29**, 1075–86.

Giesecke K., Hamberger B., Järnberg P.-O. et al. (1988). High- and low-dose fentanyl anaesthesia: hormonal and metabolic responses during cholecystectomy. *Br. J. Anaesth.*, **61**, 575–82.

Giesecke K., Magnusson I., Ahlberg M. et al. (1989). Protein and amino acid metabolism during early starvation as reflected by excretion of urea and methylhistidines. *Metabolism*, **38**, 1196–200.

Glass R.E., Fern E.B., Garlick P.J. (1983). Whole-body protein turnover before and after resection of colorectal tumours. *Clin. Sci.*, **64**, 101–8.

Glynn M.J., Metzner S., Halliday D., Powell-Tuck J. (1987). The effect of exogenous insulin on whole body protein metabolism during the total parenteral nutri-

tion (TPN) of critically ill intensive care patients. *Clin. Nutr.*, **6**, 45.

Goldspink D.F., Garlick P.J., McNurlan M.A. (1983). Protein turnover measured *in vivo* and *in vitro* in muscles undergoing compensatory growth and subsequent denervation atrophy. *Biochem. J.*, **210**, 89–98.

Gore D.C., Jahoor F., Wolfe R.R., Herndon D.N. (1993). Acute response of human muscle protein to catabolic hormones. *Ann. Surg.*, **218**, 679–84.

Hall-Angeras M., Angeras U., von Allmen D. et al. (1991a). Influence of sepsis in rats on muscle protein turnover *in vivo* and in tissue incubated under different *in vitro* conditions. *Metabolism*, **40**, 247–51.

Hall-Angeras M., Hasselgren P.-O., Dimlich R.V., Fischer J.E. (1991b). Myofibrillar proteinase, cathepsin B, and protein breakdown rates in skeletal muscle from septic rats. *Metabolism*, **40**, 302–6.

Halliday D., McKeran R.O. (1975). Measurement of muscle protein synthetic rate from serial muscle biopsies and total body protein turnover in man by continuous intravenous infusion of L-[α-¹⁵N]lysine. *Clin. Sci. Mol. Med.*, **49**, 581–90.

Halliday D., Rennie M.J. (1982). The use of stable isotopes for diagnosis and clinical research. *Clin. Sci.*, **63**, 485–96.

Halliday D., Pacy P.J., Cheng K.N. et al. (1988). Rate of protein synthesis in skeletal muscle of normal man and patients with muscular dystrophy; a reassessment. *Clin. Sci.*, **74**, 237–40.

Hammarqvist F., Wernerman J., von der Decken A. et al. (1988). The effects of branched chain amino-acids upon postoperative muscle protein synthesis and nitrogen balance. *Clin. Nutr.*, **7**, 171–5.

Hammarqvist F., Wernerman J., Ali R. et al. (1989). Addition of glutamine to total parenteral nutrition after elective abdominal surgery spares free glutamine in muscle, counteracts the fall in muscle protein synthesis, and improves nitrogen balance. *Ann. Surg.*, **209**, 455–61.

Hammarqvist F., Wernerman J., Ali R., Vinnars E. (1990). Effects of an amino acid solution enriched with either branched chain amino acids or ornithine-α-ketoglutarate on the postoperative intracellular amino acid concentration of skeletal muscle. *Br. J. Surg.*, **77**, 214–18.

Hammarqvist F., Strömberg C., von der Decken A. et al. (1992). Biosynthetic human growth hormone preserves both muscle protein synthesis and the decrease in muscle free glutamine and improves whole body nitrogen economy after operation. *Ann. Surg.*, **216**, 184–91.

Harper A. (1990). Physiological significance of changes in plasma amino acid concentrations. *Nutrition*, **6**, 494–5.

Henneberg S., Eklund A., Stjernström H. et al. (1985). Post-operative substrate utilisation and gas exchange using two different TPN-systems: glucose versus fat. *Clin. Nutr.*, **4**, 235–42.

Henshaw E.C., Hirsch C.A., Morton B.E., Hiatt H.H. (1971). Control of protein synthesis in mammalian tissues through changes in ribosomal activity. *J. Biol. Chem.*, **246**, 436–46.

Henson L.C., Heber D. (1983). Whole body protein breakdown rates and hormonal adaptation in fasted obese subjects. *J. Clin. Endocrinol. Metab.*, **57**, 316–19.

Herndon D.N., Barrow R.E., Kunkel K.R. et al. (1990).

Effects of recombinant human growth hormone on donor-site healing in severely burned children. *Ann. Surg.*, **212**, 424–31.

Heys S.D., Norton A.C., Dundas C.R. et al. (1989). Anaesthetic agents and their effect on tissue protein synthesis in the rat. *Clin. Sci.*, **77**, 651–5.

Heys S.D., Park K.G.M., McNurlan M.A. et al. (1992). Protein synthesis rates in colon and liver: stimulation by gastrointestinal pathologies. *Gut*, **33**, 976–81.

Hibbs J.B., Taintor R.R., Vavarin S., Rachlin E.M. (1988). Nitric oxide: a cytotoxic activated macrophage effector molecule. *Biochem. Biophys. Res. Commun.*, **157**, 87–94.

Higashiguchi T., Noguchi Y., O'Brien W. et al. (1994). Effect of sepsis on mucosal protein synthesis in different parts of the gastrointestinal tract in rats. *Clin. Sci.*, **87**, 207–11.

Horber F.F., Krayer S., Rehder K., Haymond M.W. (1988). Anesthesia with halothane and nitrous oxide alters protein and amino acid metabolism in dogs. *Anesthesiology*, **69**, 319–26.

Hulton N., Johnson D.J., Smith R.J., Wilmore D.W. (1985). Hormonal blockade modifies post-traumatic protein catabolism. *J. Surg. Res.*, **39**, 310–15.

Inculet R.I., Finley R.J., Duff J.H. et al. (1986). Insulin decreases muscle protein loss after operative trauma in man. *Surgery*, **99**, 752–8.

Jacob R., Hu X., Niederstock D. et al. (1996). IGF-I stimulation of muscle protein synthesis in the awake rate: permissive role of insulin and amino acids. *Am. J. Physiol.*, **270**, E60–6.

Jackson A.A., Persaud C., Badaloo V., deBenoist B. (1987). Whole-body protein turnover in man determined in three hours with oral or intravenous ^{15}N-glycine and enrichment in urinary ammonia. *Hum. Nutr. Clin. Nutr.*, **41C**, 263–76.

Jahoor F., Desai M., Herndon D.N., Wolfe, R.R. (1988). Dynamics of the protein metabolic response to burn injury. *Metabolism*, **37**, 330–7.

James W.P.T., Sender P.M., Garlick P.J., Waterlow J.C. (1974). The choice of label and measurement technique in tracer studies in man. In *Dynamic Studies with Radioisotopes in Medicine*, vol. 1. Vienna: IAEA, pp. 461–72.

James W.P.T., Garlick P.J., Sender P.M., Waterlow J.C. (1976). Studies of amino acid and protein metabolism in normal man with L-(U-^{14}C)tyrosine. *Clin. Sci. Mol. Med.*, **50**, 525–32.

Jeejeebhoy K.N., Anderson G.H., Nakhooda A.F. et al. (1976). Metabolic studies in total parenteral nutrition with lipid in man. Comparison with glucose. *J. Clin. Invest.*, **57**, 125–36.

Jeevanandam M., Brennan M.F., Horowitz G.D. et al. (1985). Tracer priming in human protein turnover studies with [^{15}N]glycine. *Biochem. Med.*, **34**, 214–25.

Jeevanandam M., Lowry S.F., Brennan M.F. (1987). Effect of the route of nutrient administration on whole-body protein kinetics in man. *Metabolism*, **36**, 968–73.

Jefferson L.S., Li J.B., Rannels S.R. (1977). Regulation by insulin of amino acid release and protein turnover in the perfused rat hemicorpus. *J. Biol. Chem.*, **252**, 1476–83.

Jepson M.M. and Millward D.J. (1989). Effect of the cyclo-oxygenase inhibitor fenbufen on muscle and liver protein metabolism, muscle glutamine and plasma insulin in endotoxaemic rats. *Clin. Sci.*, **77**, 13–20.

Jepson M.M., Millward D.J. (1991). Impact of glutamine infusions on muscle protein synthesis in fasted and endotoxin treated rats. *Clin. Nutr.*, **10**, (suppl.), 43–6.

Jepson M.M., Pell J.M., Bates P.C., Millward D.J. (1986). The effects of endotoxaemia on protein metabolism in skeletal muscle and liver of fed and fasted rats. *Biochem. J.*, **235**, 329–36.

Jepson M.M., Broadbent P., Bates P.C., Millward D.J. (1988). The relationship between skeletal muscle glutamine concentration and protein synthesis in rats. *Am. J. Physiol.*, **225**, E166–72.

Jiang Z.M., He G.Z., Zhang S.Y. et al. (1989). Low-dose growth hormone and hypocaloric nutrition attenuate the protein-catabolic response after major operation. *Ann. Surg.*, **210**, 513–24.

Johnson D.J., Brooks D.C., Pressler V.M. et al. (1986). Hypothermic anesthesia attenuates postoperative proteolysis. *Ann. Surg.*, **204**, 419–29.

Kaplan M.S., Mares A., Quintana P. et al. (1969). High caloric glucose-nitrogen infusions. Post-operative management of neoneatal infants. *Arch. Surg.*, **99**, 567–71.

Karner J., Roth E. (1990). Alanyl-glutamine infusions to patients with acute pancreatitis. *Clin. Nutr.*, **9**, 43–4.

Kehlet H. (1990a). Neural release mechanisms in the response to injury. In *Surgical Pathophysiology* (Aasen A.O., Risberg B., eds). London: Harwood Academic, pp. 77–90.

Kehlet H. (1990b). Effect of pain-relieving techniques on posttraumatic protein economy. *Beitr. Anaesth. Intens. Notfallmed.*, **32-b**, 15–19.

Kehlet H. (1991). Neurohumoral response to surgery and pain in man. In *Proceedings of the VIth World Congress on Pain* (Bond M.R., Charlton J.E., Woolf C.J., eds). Amsterdam: Elsevier Science, pp. 35–40.

Kehlet H., Brandt M.R., Prange-Hansen A., Alberti K.G.M.M. (1979). Effect of epidural analgesia on metabolic profiles during and after surgery. *Br. J. Surg.*, **66**, 543–6.

Khan K., Wusteman M., Elia M. (1991). The effect of severe dietary restriction on intramuscular glutamine concentrations and protein synthetic rate. *Clin. Nutr.*, **10**, 120–4.

Kien C.L., Young V.R., Rohrbaugh D.K., Burke J.F. (1978). Increased rates of whole body protein synthesis and breakdown in children recovering from burns. *Ann. Surg.*, **187**, 383–91.

Kinney J.M. (1977). The metabolic response to injury. In *Nutritional Aspects of Care in the Critically Ill* (Richards J.R., Kinney J.M., eds). Edinburgh: Churchill Livingstone, pp. 95–133.

Kinney J.M. (1978). The tissue composition of surgical weight loss. In *Advances in Parenteral Nutrition* (Johnston J.D.A., ed.). Lancaster, UK: Medical and Technical Press, pp. 511–20.

Kinney J.M. (1983). Amino acid support in the hypercatabolic patient. In *Amino Acids, Metabolism and Medical Applications* (Blackburn G.L., Grant J.P., Young V.R., eds). Boston: John Wright, PSG Inc., pp. 377–86.

Kirk S.J., Barbul A. (1990). Role of arginine in trauma, sepsis, and immunity. *J. Parent. Enter. Nutr.*, **14**, 226S–9S.

Kirk S.J., Regan M.C., Barbul A. (1990). Activated cloned murine T lymphocytes synthesis a molecule with the biochemical characteristics of nitric oxide. *Biochem. Biophys. Res. Commun.*, **173**, 660–5.

Kirk S.J., Hurson M., Regan M.C. et al. (1993). Arginine

stimulates wound healing and immune function on elderly human beings. *Surgery*, **114**, 155–60.

Klein S. (1990). The myth of serum albumin as a measure of nutritional status. *Gastroenterology*, **99**, 1845–51.

Kushner I. (1982). The phenomenon of the acute phase response. *Ann. N.Y. Acad. Sci.*, **389**, 39–48.

Kushner I., Mackiewicz A. (1987). Acute phase proteins as disease markers. *Dis. Markers*, **5**, 1–11.

Larsson J., Lennmarken C., Mårtensson J. et al. (1990). Nitrogen requirements in severely injured patients. *Br. J. Surg.*, **77**, 413–16.

Lawson L.J. (1965). Parenteral nutrition in surgery. *Br. J. Surg.*, **52**, 795–9.

Lee V.M., Hansen R.J., Wolfe B.M., Clifford A.J. (1988a). Muscle protein metabolism of rats in surgical trauma. *J. Parent. Enter. Nutr.*, **12**, 445–51.

Lee V.M., Wolfe B.M., Hansen R.J., Clifford A.J. (1988b). Postsurgical muscle protein turnover in perfused hindquarters of the rat. *J. Parent. Enter. Nutr.*, **12**, 452–6.

León P., Redmond H.P., Stein T.P. et al. (1991). Arginine supplementation improves histone and acute-phase protein synthesis during gram-negative sepsis in the rat. *J. Parent. Enter. Nutr.*, **15**, 503–8.

Lewis L., Dalm M., Kirkpatrick J.R. (1981). Anabolic steroid administration during nutritional support: a therapeutic controversy. *J. Parent. Enter. Nutr.*, **5**, 64–6.

Li J.B., Jefferson L.S. (1978). Influence of amino acid availability on protein turnover in perfused skeletal muscle. *Biochim. Biophys. Acta*, **544**, 351–9.

Liljedahl S-O. (1980). Treatment of the hypercatabolic state in burns. *Ann. Chir. Gynaecol.*, **69**, 191–6.

Liljedahl S-O., Gemzell C.A., Plantin L.O. (1961). Effect of human growth hormone in patients with severe burns. *Acta Chir. Scand.*, **122**, 1–14.

Long C.L., Jeevanandam M., Kim B.M., Kinney J.M. (1977). Whole body protein synthesis and catabolism in septic man. *Am. J. Clin. Nutr.*, **30**, 1340–4.

Long C.L., Dillard D.R., Bodzin J.H. et al. (1988). Validity of 3-methylhistidine excretion as an indicator of skeletal muscle protein breakdown in humans. *Metabolism*, **37**, 844–9.

Louard R.J., Barrett E.J., Gelfand R.A. (1990). Effect of infused branched-chain amino acids on muscle and whole-body amino acid metabolism in man. *Clin. Sci.*, **79**, 457–66.

Lundeberg S., Belfrage M., Wernerman J. et al. (1991). Growth hormone improves muscle protein metabolism and whole body nitrogen economy in man during a hyponitrogenous diet. *Metabolism*, **40**, 315–22.

Maltin C.A., Harris C.I. (1985). Morphological observations and rates of protein synthesis in rat muscles incubated *in vitro*. *Biochem. J.*, **232**, 927–30.

Manson J.M., Wilmore D.W. (1986). Positive nitrogen balance with human growth hormone and hypocaloric intravenous feeding. *Surgery*, **100**, 188–97.

Matthews D.E., Schwartz H.P., Young R.D. et al. (1982). Relationship of plasma leucine and α-ketoisocaproate during a L-[1-^{13}C]leucine infusion in man: a method for measuring human intracellular leucine tracer enrichment. *Metabolism*, **31**, 1105–12.

McFarlane A.S. (1963). Measurement of synthesis rates of liver-produced plasma proteins. *Biochem. J.*, **89**, 277–90.

McMahon M.J. (1988). Perioperative nutritional support. In *Ballière's Clinical Gastroenterology*, vol. 2(4) (Burns H.J.G., ed.). London: Ballière Tindall, pp. 751–63.

McNurlan M.A., Clemens M.J. (1985). Inhibition of cell proliferation by interferons. *Biochem. J.*, **237**, 871–6.

McNurlan M.A., Garlick P.J. (1989). Influence of nutrient intake on protein turnover. *Diabetes Metab. Rev.*, **5**, 165–89.

McNurlan M.A., Tomkins A.M., Garlick P.J. (1979). The effect of starvation on the rate of protein synthesis in rat liver and small intestine. *Biochem. J.*, **178**, 373–9.

McNurlan M.A., Fern E.B., Garlick P.J. (1982). Failure of leucine to stimulate protein synthesis *in vivo*. *Biochem. J.*, **204**, 831–8.

McNurlan M.A., McHardy K.C., Broom J. et al. (1987). The effect of indomethacin on the response of protein synthesis to feeding in rats and man. *Clin. Sci.*, **73**, 69–75.

McNurlan M.A., Essén P., Milne, E. et al. (1993). Temporal responses of protein synthesis in human skeletal muscle to feeding. *Br. J. Nutr.*, **69**, 117–26.

McNurlan M.A., Essén P., Thorell A. et al. (1994). Response of protein synthesis in human skeletal muscle to insulin: an investigation with L-[^{2}H$_5$]phenylalanine. *Am. J. Physiol.*, **267**, E102–8.

McNurlan M.A., Sandgren A., Hunter K. et al. (1996). Protein synthesis rates of skeletal muscle, lymphocytes, and albumin with stress hormone infusion in healthy man. *Metabolism*, in press.

Melville S., McNurlan M.A., McHardy K.C. et al. (1989). The role of degradation in the acute control of protein balance in adult man: failure of feeding to stimulate protein synthesis as assessed by L-[1-^{13}C]leucine infusion. *Metabolism*, **38**, 248–55.

Melville S., McNurlan M.A., Calder A.G., Garlick P.J. (1990). Increased protein turnover despite normal energy metabolism and response to feeding in patients with lung cancer. *Cancer Res.*, **50**, 1125–31.

Michelsen C.B., Askanazi J., Kinney J.M. et al. (1982). Effect of an anabolic steroid on nitrogen balance and amino acid patterns after total hip replacement. *J. Trauma*, **22**, 410–13.

Miles J.M., Nissen S.L., Gerich J.E., Haymond M.W. (1984). Effects of epinephrine infusion on leucine and alanine kinetics in humans. *Am. J. Physiol.*, **247**, E166–72.

Millward D.J. (1970). Protein turnover in skeletal muscle. I. The measurements of rates of synthesis and catabolism of skeletal muscle protein using ^{14}C-Na$_2$CO$_3$ to lable protein. *Clin. Sci.*, **39**, 577–90.

Millward D.J., Garlick P.J., Nnanyelugo D.O., Waterlow J.C. (1976). The relative importance of muscle protein synthesis and breakdown in the regulation of muscle mass. *Biochem. J.*, **156**, 185–8.

Mjaaland M., Unneberg K., Hotvedt R., Revhaug A. (1990). Growth hormone after gastrointestinal surgery: effect on skeletal muscle metabolism. *Clin. Nutr.*, **9**, (suppl.), O.43.

Moore F.D. (1959). *Metabolic Care of the Surgical Patient*. Philadelphia: W.B. Saunders.

Mortimore G.E., Mondon C.E. (1970). Inhibition by insulin of valine turnover in liver. *J. Biol. Chem.*, **245**, 2375–83.

Mortimore G.E., Woodside K.H., Henry J.E. (1972). Compartmentation of free valine and its relation to protein turnover in perfused rat liver. *J. Biol. Chem.*, **247**, 2776–84.

Moshage H.J., Janssen J.A.M., Franssen J.H. et al. (1987). Study of the molecular mechanism of decreased liver synthesis of albumin in inflammation. *J. Clin. Invest.*, **79**, 1635–41.

Munro H.N. (1964). General aspects of the regulation of protein metabolism by diet and hormones. In *Mammalian Protein Metabolism* (Munro H.N., Allison J.B., eds). New York: Academic, pp. 381–481.

Munro H.N. (1970a). Survey of general mechanisms. In *Mammalian Protein Metabolism*, vol. IV (Munro H.N., eds). New York: Academic, pp. 3–130.

Munro H.N. (1970b). Free amino acid pools and their role in regulation. In *Mammalian Protein Metabolism* (Munro H.N., ed). New York: Academic, pp. 299–386.

Munro H.N., Young V.R. (1981). Use of N$^\tau$-methylhistidine excretion as an *in vivo* measure of myofibrillar protein breakdown. In *Nitrogen Metabolism in Man* (Waterlow J.C., Stephen J.M.L., eds). London: Applied Science, pp. 495–508.

Nair K.S., Ford G.C., Halliday D., Garrow J.S. (1983). Effect of total starvation on protein synthesis in obese women. *Proc. Nutr. Soc.*, **42**, 135A.

Newsholme E.A., Crabtree B., Ardawi, M.S.M. (1985). Glutamine metabolism in lymphocytes: its biochemical, physiological and clinical importance. *Q. J. Exp. Physiol.*, **70**, 473–89.

Norlén H., Dimberg M., Allgén L-G., Vinnars E. (1990). Water and electrolytes in muscle tissue and free amino acids in muscle and plasma in connection with transurethral resection of the prostate. II Isotonic 2.2% glycine solution as an irrigating fluid. *Scand. J. Urol. Nephrol.*, **24**, 95–101.

O'Keefe S.J.D., Sender P.M., James W.P.T. (1974). 'Catabolic' loss of body nitrogen in response to surgery. *Lancet*, **ii**, 1035–7.

Odessey R., Parr B. (1982). Effect of insulin and leucine on protein turnover in rat soleus muscle after burn injury. *Metabolism*, **31**, 82–7.

Ollenschläger G., Langer K., Steffen H-M. et al. (1990). Intracellular free amino acid patterns in duodenal and colonic mucosa. *Clin. Chem.*, **36**, 378–81.

Olufemi O.S., Humes P., Whittaker P.G. et al. (1990). Albumin synthetic rate: comparison of arginine and alpha-ketoisocaproate precursor methods using stable isotope techniques. *Eur. J. Clin. Nutr.*, **44**, 351–61.

Pacy P.J., Nair K.S., Ford C., Halliday D. (1989). Failure of insulin infusion to stimulate fractional muscle protein synthesis in type 1 diabetic patients. *Diabetes*, **38**, 618–24.

Pain V.M., Clemens M.J., Garlick P.J. (1978). The effect of dietary protein deficiency on albumin synthesis and on the concentration of active albumin messenger RNA in rat liver. *Biochem. J.*, **172**, 129–35.

Pain V.M., Albertse E.C., Garlick P.J. (1983). Protein metabolism in skeletal muscle, diaphragm, and heart of diabetic rats. *Am. J. Physiol.*, **245**, E604–10.

Pain V.M., Randall D.P., Garlick P.J. (1984). Protein synthesis in liver and skeletal muscle of mice bearing an ascites tumor. *Cancer Res.*, **44**, 1054–7.

Park K.G.M., Hayes P.D., Garlick P.J. et al. (1991). Stimulation of lymphocyte natural cytotoxicity by L-arginine. *Lancet*, **337**, 645–6.

Petersson B., Wernerman J., Waller S.-O. et al. (1990). Elective abdominal surgery depresses muscle protein synthesis and increases subjective fatigue: effects lasting more than 30 days. *Br. J. Surg.*, **77**, 796–800.

Petersson B., Vinnars E., Waller S.-O., Wernerman J. (1992). Long-term changes in muscle free amino acid levels after elective abdominal surgery. *Br. J. Surg.*, **79**, 212–16.

Picou D., Taylor-Roberts T. (1969). The measurement of total protein synthesis and catabolism and nitrogen turnover in infants in different nutritional states and receiving different amounts of dietary protein. *Clin. Sci.*, **36**, 283–96.

Pomposelli J.J., Palombo J.D., Hamawy K.J. et al. (1985). Comparison of different techniques for estimating rates of protein synthesis *in vivo* in healthy and bacteraemic rats. *Biochem. J.*, **226**, 37–42.

Ponting G.A., Halliday D., Teale J.D., Sim A.J. (1988). Postoperative positive nitrogen balance with intravenous hyponutrition and growth hormone. *Lancet*, **i**, 438–40.

Powell-Tuck J., Glynn M.J. (1985). The effect of insulin infusion on whole body protein metabolism in patients with gastro-intestinal disease fed parenterally. *Hum. Nutr. Clin. Nutr.*, **39c**, 181–91.

Powell-Tuck J., Fern E.B., Garlick P.J., Waterlow J.C. (1984). The effect of surgical trauma and insulin on whole body protein turnover in parenterally fed undernourished patients. *Hum. Nutr. Clin. Nutr.*, **38c**, 11–22.

Preedy V.R., Garlick P.J. (1981). Rates of protein synthesis in skin and bone and their importance in the assessment of protein degradation in the perfused rat hemicorpus. *Biochem. J.*, **194**, 373–6.

Preedy V.R., Garlick P.J. (1985). The effect of glucagon administration on protein synthesis in skeletal muscles, heart and liver *in vivo*. *Biochem. J.*, **228**, 575–81.

Preedy V.R., Garlick P.J. (1988). Inhibition of protein synthesis by glucagon in different rat muscles and protein fractions *in vivo* and in perfused rat hemicorpus. *Biochem. J.*, **251**, 727–32.

Preedy V.R., Paska L., Sugden P.H. et al. (1988). The effects of surgical stress and short-term fasting on protein synthesis *in vivo* in diverse tissues of the mature rat. *Biochem. J.*, **250**, 179–88.

Ramadori G., van Damme J., Rieder H., Meyer zum Buschenfelde K.H. (1988). Interleukin 6, the third mediator of acute-phase reaction, modulates hepatic protein synthesis in human and mouse. Comparison with interleukin 1β and tumor necrosis factor-α. *Eur. J. Immunol.*, **18**, 1259–64.

Randall H.T. (1970). Indications for parenteral nutrition in postoperative catabolic states. In *Parenteral Nutrition* (Meng H.C., Law D.H., eds). Springfield, IL: Thomas, pp. 13–39.

Rannels D.E., Christopherson R., Watkins C.A. (1983). Reversible inhibition of protein synthesis in the lung by halothane. *Biochem. J.*, **210**, 379–87.

Reeds P.J., Garlick P.J. (1984). Nutrition, and protein turnover in man. In *Advances in Nutritional Research* (Draper H.H., ed.). New York: Plenum Press, pp. 93–138.

Reeds P.J., Palmer R.M. (1984). Changes in prostaglandin release associated with inhibition of muscle protein synthesis by dexamethasone. *Biochem. J.*, **219**, 953–7.

Reeds P.J., Hay S.M., Glennie R.T. et al. (1985). The effect of indomethacin on the stimulation of protein synthesis by insulin in young postabsorptive rats. *Biochem. J.*, **227**, 255–61.

Rennie M.J., MacLennan P. (1985). Protein turnover and amino acid oxidation: the effects of anaesthesia and surgery. In *Substrate and Energy Metabolism in Man*

(Garrow J.S., Halliday D., eds). London: John Libbey, pp. 213–21.

Rennie, M.J., Millward D.J. (1983). 3-Methylhistidine excretion and the urinary 3-methylhistidine/creatine ratio are poor indicators of skeletal muscle protein breakdown. *Clin. Sci.*, **65**, 217–25.

Rennie M.J., Edwards R.H.T., Halliday D. et al. (1982). Muscle protein synthesis measured by stable isotope techniques in man: the effects of feeding and fasting. *Clin. Sci.*, **63**, 519–23.

Rennie M.J., Bennegård, K., Edén E. et al. (1984). Urinary excretion and efflux from the leg of 3-methyhistidine before and after major surgical operation. *Metabolism*, **33**, 250–6.

Rodemann H.P., Goldberg A.L. (1982). Arachidonic acid, prostaglandin E2 and F2a influence rates on protein turnover in skeletal and cardiac muscle. *J. Biol. Chem.*, **257**, 1632–8.

Roth E., Funovics J., Mühlbacher F. et al. (1982). Metabolic disorders in severe abdominal sepsis: glutamine deficiency in skeletal muscle. *Clin. Nutr.*, **1**, 25–41.

Ruff R.L., Secrist D. (1984). Inhibitors of prostaglandin synthesis or cathepsin B prevent muscle wasting due to sepsis in the rat. *J. Clin. Invest.*, **73**, 1483–6.

Rutberg H., Håkansson E., Anderberg B. et al. (1984). Effects of the extradural administration of morphine, or bupivacaine, on the endocrine response to upper abdominal surgery. *Br. J. Anaesth.*, **56**, 223–33.

Saito H., Trocki O., Wang S., Alexander W. (1987). Metabolic and immune effects of dietary arginine suplementation after burn. *Arch. Surg.*, **12**, 784–9.

Sakamoto A., Moldawer L.L., Palombo J.D. et al. (1983). Alterations in tyrosine and protein kinetics produced by injury and branched chain amino acid administration in rats. *Clin. Sci.*, **64**, 321–31.

Sandstedt S., Jorfeldt L., Larsson J. (1992). Randomized, controlled study evaluating effects of branched chain amino acids and alpha-ketoisocaproate on protein metabolism after surgery. *Br. J. Surg.*, **79**, 217–20.

Schønheyder F., Heilskov N.S.C., Olesen K. (1954). Isotopic studies on the mechanism of negative nitrogen balance produced by immobilization. *Scand. J. Clin. Lab. Invest.*, **6**, 178–88.

Schwenk W.F., Tsalikian E., Beaufrere B., M.W. (1985). Recycling of an amino acid label with prolonged isotope infusion: implications for kinetic studies. *Am. J. Physiol.*, **248**, E482–7.

Scornik O. (1974). *in vivo* rate of translation by ribosomes of normal and regenerating liver. *J. Biol. Chem.*, **249**, 3876–83.

Seider M.J., Kapp R., Chen C-P., Booth F.W. (1980). The effects of cutting or of stretching skeletal muscle *in vitro* on the rates of protein synthesis and degradation. *Biochem. J.*, **188**, 247–54.

Seifter E., Rettura G., Barbul A., Levenson S.M. (1978). Arginine: an essential amino acid for injured rats. *Surgery*, **84**, 224–30.

Shanbhogue R.L.K., Bistrian B.R., Jenkins R.L. et al. (1987). Increased protein catabolism without hypermetabolism after human orthotopic liver transplantation. *Surgery*, **101**, 147–9.

Shangraw R.E., Turinsky J. (1982). Effect of disuse and thermal injury on protein turnover in skeletal muscle. *J. Surg. Res.*, **33**, 345–55.

Shangraw R.E., Turinsky J. (1984). Altered protein kinetics *in vivo* after single-limb burn injury. *Biochem. J.*, **223**,

Shaw J.H.F., Wolfe R.R. (1988). Metabolic intervention in surgical patients. *Ann. Surg.*, **207**, 274–82.

Shipley R.A., Clark R.E. (1972). *Tracer Methods for In Vivo Kinetics*. New York: Academic Press.

Shizgal H.M., Posner B. (1989). Insulin and the efficacy of total parenteral nutrition. *Am. J. Clin. Nutr.*, **50**, 1355–63.

Sim A.J.W., Wolfe B.M., Young V.R. et al. (1979). Glucose promotes whole-body protein synthesis from infused amino acids in fasting man. *Lancet*, **i**, 68–72.

Sjölin J., Hjort G., Friman G., Hambraeus L. (1987). Urinary excretion of 1-methylhistidine: a qualitative indicator of exogenous 3-methylhistidine and intake of meats from various sources. *Metabolism*, **36**, 1175–84.

Sjölin J., Stjernström H., Henneberg S. et al. (1989). Splanchnic and peripheral release of 3-methylhistidine in relation to its urinary excretion in human infection. *Metabolism*, **38**, 23–9.

Sjölin J., Stjernström H., Friman G. et al. (1990). Total and net muscle protein breakdown in infection determined by amino effluxes. *Am. J. Physiol.*, **258**, E856–63.

Slotman G.T., Burchard K.W., Williams J.A. et al. (1985). Interactions of prostaglandins, activated complement, and granulocytes in clinical sepsis and hypotension. *Circ. Shock*, **16**, 67.

Smith R., Elia M. (1983). Branched chain amino acids in stress and injury. *J. Parenter. Enter. Nutr.*, **10**, 446–52.

Smith R.H., Palmer R.M., Reeds P.J. (1983). Protein synthesis in isolated rabbit forelimb muscles. The possible role of metabolites in arachidonic acid in the response to intermittant stretching. *Biochem. J.*, **214**, 153–61.

Soroff H.S., Pearson E., Green N.L. (1960). The effect of growth hormone on nitrogen balance at various levels of intake in burned patients. *Surg. Gynecol. Obstet.*, **111**, 259–73.

Souba W.W., Wilmore D.W. (1983). Postoperative alteration of arteriovenous exchange of amino acids across the gastrointestinal tract. *Surgery*, **94**, 342–50.

Souba W.W., Smith R.J., Wilmore D.W. (1985). Glutamine metabolism by the intestinal tract. *J. Parenter. Enter. Nutr.*, **9**, 608–17.

Souba W.W., Klimberg S., Plumley D.A. et al. (1990). The role of glutamine in maintaining a healthy gut and supporting the metabolic response to injury and infection. *J. Surg. Res.*, **48**, 383–91.

Stehle P., Zanders J., Mertes N. et al. (1989). Effect of parenteral glutamine peptide supplements on muscle glutamine loss and nitrogen balance after major surgery. *Lancet*, **i**, 231–3.

Stein T.P., Oram-Smith J.C., Wallace H.W., Leskiw M.J. (1976). The effect of trauma on protein synthesis. *J. Surg. Res.*, **21**, 201–3.

Stein T.P., Mullen J.L., Oram-Smith J.C. et al. (1978). Relative rates of tumor, normal gut, liver and fibrinogen synthesis in man. *Am. J. Physiol.*, **234**, E648–52.

Strelkov A.B., Fields A.L.A., Baracos V.E. (1989). Effects of systemic inhibition of prostaglandin production on protein metabolism in tumor-bearing rats. *Am. J. Physiol.*, **257**, C261–9.

Stuart C.A., Shangraw R.E., Peters E.J., Wolfe R.R. (1990). Effect of dietary protein on bed-rest-related changes in whole-body-protein synthesis. *Am. J. Clin. Nutr.*, **52**, 509–14.

Studley H.O. (1936). Percentage weight loss. A basic

indicator of surgical risk in patients with peptic ulcer. *JAMA*, **106**, 458–60.

Threlfall C.J., Stoner H.B., Galasko C.S.B. (1981). Patterns in the excretion of muscle markers after trauma and orthopedic surgery. *J. Trauma*, **21**, 140–7.

Threlfall C.J., Maxwell A.R., Stoner H.B. (1984). Post-traumatic creatinuria. *J. Trauma*, **24**, 516–23.

Tiao G., Fagan J.M., Samuels N. et al. (1994). Sepsis stimulates nonlysosomal, energy-dependent proteolysis and increases ubiquitin mRNA levels in rat skeletal muscle. *J. Clin. Invest.*, **94**, 2255–64.

Tjäder I., Essén P., Thörne A. et al. (1996). Muscle protein synthesis rate decreases 24 hours after abdominal surgery irrespective of total parenteral nutrition. *J. Parenter. Enter. Nutr.*, **20**, 135–8.

Tomkins A.M., Garlick P.J., Scholfield W.N., Waterlow J.C. (1983). The combined effects of infection and malnutrition on protein metabolism in children. *Clin. Sci.*, **65**, 313–24.

Tucker K.R., Seider M.J., Booth F.W. (1981). Protein synthesis rates in atrophied gastrocnemius muscles after limb immobilization. *J. Appl. Physiol.*, **51**, 73–7.

Turner L.V., Garlick P.J. (1974). The effect of unilateral phrenicectomy on the rate of protein synthesis in rat diaphragm *in vivo*. *Biochim. Biophys. Acta*, **349**, 109–13.

Tweedle D., Walton C., Johnston I.D.A. (1973). The effect of anabolic steroid on post-operative nitrogen balance. *Br. J. Clin. Pract.*, **27**, 130–2.

Urbascheck R., Patscheke H., Stegmeier K., Urbaschek B. (1985). The effect of a thromboxane receptor blockade in endotoxic shock. *Circ. Shock*, **16**, 71.

Vary T.C., Kimball S.R. (1992). Regulation of hepatic protein synthesis in chronic inflammation and sepsis. *Am. J. Physiol.*, **262**, C445–52.

Vary T.C., Jurasinski C.V., Karinch A.M., Kimball S.R. (1994). Regulation of eukaryotic initiation factor-2 expression during sepsis. *Am. J. Physiol.*, **266**, E193–201.

Vente J.P., Soeters P.B., von Meyenfeldt M.F. et al. (1991). Prospective randomized double-blind trial of branched chain amino acid enriched versus standard parenteral nutrition solutions in traumatized and septic patients. *World J. Surg.*, **15**, 128–33.

Vesterberg K., Leander U., Fürst P., Vinnars E. (1982). Nitrogen sparing effect of Ornicetil[R] in trauma. II Muscle and plasma amino acids. *Clin. Nutr.*, **1**, (suppl.), 138.

Vinnars E., Bergström J., Fürst P. (1975). Influence of the postoperative state on the intracellular free amino acids in human tissue. *Ann. Surg.*, **182**, 665–71.

Vinnars E., Fürst P., Liljedahl S-O. et al. (1980). Effect of parenteral nutrition on intracellular free amino acid concentration. *J. Parenter. Enter. Nutr.*, **4**, 184–7.

Vinnars E., Bergström J., Fürst P. (1987). Effects of starvation on plasma and muscle amino acid concentrations in normal subjects. *Clin. Nutr.*, **6**, (suppl.), P.16.

Vinnars E., Hammarqvist F., von der Decken A., Wernerman J. (1990). Role of glutamine and its analogs in posttraumatic muscle protein and amino acid metabolism. *J. Parenter. Enter. Nutr.*, **14**, 125S–9S.

Visek W.J. (1986). Arginine needs, physiological state and usual diets. A reevaluation. *J. Nutr.*, **116**, 36–46.

Wahren J., Felig P., Hagenfeldt J. (1976). Effect of protein ingestion on splanchnic and leg metabolism in normal man and in patients with diabetes mellitus. *J. Clin.*

Invest., **57**, 987–99.

Walser M. (1984). Therapeutic aspects of branched-chain amino and keto acids. *Clin. Sci.*, **66**, 1–15.

Wannemacher R.W., Dinterman R.E., Pekarek R.S. et al. (1975). Urinary amino acid excretion during experimentally induced sandfly fever in man. *Am. J. Clin. Nutr.*, **28**, 110–18.

Ward H.C., Halliday D., Sim A.J.W. (1987). Protein and energy metabolism with biosynthetic human growth hormone after gastrointestinal surgery. *Ann. Surg.*, **206**, 56–61.

Warren R.S., Jeevanandam M., Brennan M.F. (1987). Comparison of hepatic protein synthesis *in vivo* versus *in vitro* in the tumor-bearing rat. *J. Surg. Res.*, **42**, 43–50.

Waterlow J.C. (1984). Protein turnover with special reference to man. *Q. J. Exp. Physiol.*, **69**, 409–38.

Waterlow J.C., Stephen J.M.L. (1968). The effect of a low protein diet on the turnover rates of serum, liver and muscle proteins in the rat measured by continuous infusion of L-[14C]lysine. *Clin. Sci.*, **35**, 287–305.

Waterlow J.C., Garlick P.J., Millward D.J. (1978a). *Protein Turnover in Mammalian Tissues and in the Whole Body*. Amsterdam: North Holland.

Waterlow J.C., Golden M.H.N., Garlick P.J. (1978b). Protein turnover in man measured with [15]N: comparison of end products and dose regimes. *Am. J. Physiol.*, **235**, E165–74.

Watkins C.A., Rannels D.E. (1980). Measurement of protein synthesis in rat lungs perfused *in situ*. *Biochem. J.*, **188**, 269–78.

Wernerman J., Vinnars E. (1987). The effect of trauma and surgery on interorgan fluxes of amino acids in man. *Clin. Sci.*, **73**, 129–33.

Wernerman J., von der Decken A., Vinnars E. (1985). The diurnal pattern of protein synthesis in human skeletal muscle. *Clin. Nutr.*, **4**, 203–5.

Wernerman J., von der Decken A., Vinnars E. (1986a). Protein synthesis after trauma as studied by muscle ribosome profiles. In *Clinical Nutrition and Metabolic Research. Proc. 7th Congress ESPEN, Munich 1985* (Dietze G., Grünert A., Kleinberger S., Wolfram G., eds). Basel: Karger, pp. 66–85.

Wernerman J., von der Decken A., Vinnars E. (1986b). Protein synthesis in skeletal muscle in relation to nitrogen balance after abdominal surgery: the effect of total parenteral nutrition. *J. Parenter. Enter. Nutr.*, **10**, 578–82.

Wernerman J., Botta D., Hammarqvist F. et al. (1989). Stress hormones given to healthy volunteers alter the concentration and configuration of ribosomes in skeletal muscle, reflecting changes in protein synthesis. *Clin. Sci.*, **77**, 611–16.

Wernerman J., Hammarqvist F., Vinnars E. (1990). Alpha-ketoglutarate and postoperative muscle catabolism. *Lancet*, **335**, 701–3.

Whicher J., Spence C. (1987). When is serum albumin worth measuring? *Ann. Clin. Biochem.*, **24**, 572–80.

Williamson D.H., Farrell R., Kerr A., Smith R. (1977). Muscle-protein catabolism after injury in man, as measured by urinary excretion of 3-methylhistidine. *Clin. Sci. Molec. Med.*, **52**, 527–33.

Wilmore D.W., Long J.M., Mason A.D., Pruitt B.A. (1976). Catecholamines as mediators of the metabolic response to thermal injury. In *Metabolism and the Response to Injury* (Wilkinson A.W., Cuthbertson D., eds). Bath:

Pitman Medical, pp. 287–99.

Wilmore D.W., Aulick H.L., Goodwin C.W. (1979). Glucose metabolism following severe injury. *Acta Chir. Scand. Suppl.*, **498**, 43–7.

Wilmore D.W., Goodwin C.W., Aulick H.L. et al. (1980). Effect of injury and infection on visceral metabolism and circulation. *Ann. Surg.*, **192**, 491–504.

Wilmore D.W., Smith R.J., O'Dwyer S.T. et al. (1988). The gut: a central organ after surgical stress. *Surgery*, **104**, 917–23.

Windmueller H.G., Spaeth A.E. (1974). Uptake and metabolism of plasma glutamine by the small intestine. *J. Biol. Chem.*, **249**, 5070–9.

Wolfe R.R. (1984). *Tracers in Metabolic Research. Radioisotope and stable isotope/mass spectrometry methods*. New York: Alan R. Liss.

Wolfe R.R., Jahoor F., Hartl W.H. (1989). Protein and amino acid metabolism after injury. *Diabetes Metab. Rev.*, **5**, 149–64.

Wong K.C. (1983). Physiology and pharmacology of hypothermia. *West. J. Med.*, **138**, 227–32.

Woolfson A.M.J., Heatley R.V., Allison S.P. (1979). Insulin to inhibit protein catabolism after injury. *N. Engl. J. Med.*, **300**, 14–17.

Wretlind A. (1985). *Allmän Näringslära Malnutrition, Svälttillstånd*. Stockholm: Kabi Witrum.

Wusteman M., Elia M. (1991). Effect of glutamine infusions on glutamine concentration and protein synthetic rate in rat muscle. *J. Parenter Enter Nutr.*, **15**, 521–5.

Wusteman M., Tate H., Elia M. (1995). The use of a constant infusion of [^{3}H]phenylalanine to measure the effects of glutamine infusions on muscle protein-synthesis in rats given turpentine. *Nutrition*, **11**, 27–31.

Wutzke K., Heine W., Drescher U. et al. (1983). ^{15}N-labelled yeast protein – a valid tracer for calculating whole-body protein parameters in infants: a comparison between ^{15}N-yeast protein and ^{15}N-glycine. *Hum. Nutr. Clin. Nutr.*, **37C**, 317–27.

Young V.R., Yang R.D., Meredith C. et al. (1983a). Modulation of amino acid metabolism by protein and energy intakes. In *Amino Acids, Metabolism and Medical Applications* (Blackburn G.L., Grant J.P., Young V.R., eds). Boston: John Wright, PSG Inc., pp. 13–28.

Young G.A., Yule A.G., Hill G.L. (1983b). Effects of an anabolic steroid on body composition in patients receiving intravenous nutrition. *J. Parenter. Enter. Nutr.*, **7**, 221–5.

Young V.R., Haverberg L.N., Bilmazes C., Munro H.N. (1973). Potential use of 3-methylhistidine excretion as an index of progressive reduction in muscle protein catabolism during starvation. *Metabolism*, **22**, 1429–36.

Yule A.G., Macfie J., Hill G.L. (1981). The effect of anabolic steroid on body composition in patients receiving intravenous nutrition. *Aust. NZ J. Surg.*, **51**, 280–4.

Zak R., Martin A.F., Blough R. (1979). Assessment of protein turnover by use of radioisotopic tracers. *Phys. Rev.*, **59**, 407–47.

Zamir O., Hasselgren P.O., Kunkel S.L. et al. (1992). Evidence that tumor necrosis factor participates in the regulation of muscle proteolysis during sepsis. *Arch Surg.*, **127**, 170–4.

Zamir O., O'Brien W., Thompson R. et al. (1994). Reduced muscle protein breakdown in septic rats following treatment with interleukin-1 receptor antagonist. *Int. J. Biochem.*, **26**, 943–50.

Ziegler T.R., Young L.S., Mason J.M., Wilmore D.W. (1988). Metabolic effects of recombinant human growth hormone in patients receiving parenteral nutrition. *Ann. Surg.*, **208**, 6–16.

Ziegler T.R., Young L.S., Ferrari-Baliviera E. et al. (1990). Use of human growth hormone combined with nutritional support in a critical care unit. *J. Parenter Enter Nutr.*, **12**, 574–81.

Ziegler T.R., Rombeau J.L., Young L.S. et al. (1992a). Recombinant human growth hormone enhances the metabolic efficacy of parenteral nutrition: a double-blind, randomized controlled study. *J. Clin. Endocrinol. Metab.*, **74**, 865–73.

Ziegler T.R., Young L.S., Benfell K. et al. (1992b). Clinical and metabolic efficacy of glutamine-supplemented parenteral nutrition after bone marrow transplantation: a randomized double-blind controlled study. *Ann. Intern. Med.*, **116**, 821–8.

Acknowledgement

The authors express their gratitude to Ann White for her skilful and valuable assistance during the preparation of this chapter.

49. Mechanisms of Infection
E. A. Deitch

In many ways, the history of trauma and infection is the history of surgery, since throughout the treatment of wounds and the prevention of infection have been major responsibilities of the surgeon. Today, as more complex and physiologically demanding operative and reoperative procedures are being performed on sicker and more severely injured patients, the importance of understanding the mechanisms of infection and the physiology of host antibacterial defence systems is of ever greater importance. This is especially true in the trauma victim, since injury not only predisposes to infection by promoting bacterial contamination of normally sterile tissues and spaces, but also induces the development of an immunocompromised state. In spite of the development of successive generations of new and improved antibiotics, infection and multiple organ failure remain the most common causes of late death in trauma patients. This fact is not surprising, since it appears to be ultimately of little importance which antibiotics are used or which organisms are causing the infection if the patient's intrinsic antibacterial defences cannot respond effectively.

Realization of the clinical limitations of antibiotics has led to a resurgence of interest in basic studies of the host's immune and inflammatory defence systems. This increased interest in host antibacterial defence mechanisms reflects the growing acceptance that our therapeutic manoeuvres must be directed not only toward the eradication of invading bacteria but also toward increasing the host's resistance to infection.

In order optimally to apply existing therapeutic options and successfully to utilize new therapeutic approaches directed at bolstering host defences, the surgeon must have a working knowledge of the immune and inflammatory host defence systems as well as understand how these systems are modulated by stress, trauma, surgery and current therapy. Additionally, since infection can be a cause as well as the result of impaired host defences, knowledge of the mechanisms of how infection disrupts normal host defence systems is also critical for patient care. It is further necessary to understand that the host defence systems, and especially the inflammatory response, are a two-edged sword. When they are properly controlled and regulated, they are effective in eliminating invading microorganisms and clearing tissue debris. However, unchecked or inadequately regulated, they may produce or potentiate the development of local or distant organ injury and failure. Thus, the goal of this chapter will be to review the normal biology of the host's antibacterial defence systems as well as the complex interrelationships between these defence systems, trauma, infection and the development of multiple organ failure.

HOST DEFENCE MECHANISMS

Conceptually, the immune system can be viewed as a system developed both to protect the host against infection with pathogenic microorganisms and to prevent the development and limit the spread of malignant tumours. Thus, infection represents a failure of the host's immune defences due either to impaired immune function, overwhelming bacterial challenge or a combination of these events.

Because a fundamental role of the immune system is the preservation of the body's integrity against invading microorganisms that threaten to disrupt the body's homoeostasis, the host has developed both local and systemic defence systems to protect against this threat. The systemic defences consist primarily of the non-specific inflammatory response and the specific immune system. The local defences consist of mechanical barriers such as the skin and the mucosa lining the gastrointestinal, respiratory and urinary tracts. The latter are frequently disrupted by trauma, leaving the further protection of the host to the systemic host defence systems. Familiar examples of traumatized patients with diminished local defences include patients who have sustained a severe thermal injury where the skin barrier has been destroyed and patients with blunt or penetrating abdominal trauma who have hollow viscus perforations with contamination of the peritoneal cavity by intestinal flora. Additionally, therapeutic manoeuvres, such as the use of indwelling venous, arterial or urinary catheters, which breach the body's local defences, may provide conduits for the systemic invasion of nosocomial surface organisms. However, trauma affects more than local defences. After a major injury many elements of the systemic host defence system become impaired. This combination of impaired local and systemic host defences plus bacterial contamination results in a high incidence of infection.

Antibacterial defence systems

The host's antibacterial defences follow the classification already outlined – local defences, such as the skin and mucous membranes, and systemic defences. The components of the local defence system function to prevent or limit colonization with potential pathogens in addition to providing mechanical barriers against tissue invasion by resident flora. Although the components of this local defence system vary from one anatomical region to another, they share common features. These include: (1) the presence of a mechanical barrier, such as the skin and mucous membranes; (2) physical defences, such as intestinal mucus or ciliary action in the lung; (3) local secretions that contain bactericidal agents such as lysozyme and secretory immunoglobulins; and (4) the normal microbial flora, which serves to prevent colonization by potential pathogens. The clinical importance of these local defences will be covered in greater detail in the section on specific infectious complications.

The systemic host defences are the non-specific inflammatory and the specific immune systems (Table 49.1). The first is the primary defence of the non-immune host to invading bacteria, since it is activated immediately after injury or upon bacterial invasion and does not require a previous exposure to the invading organism for activation. The initiation of an inflammatory response by invading bacteria or injury not only serves to limit the potential local and systemic spread of invading bacteria, but also signals to the host that the body's mechanical barriers have been breached, which in turn initiate a cascade of events which primes the host's systemic defences.

The major elements initially contributing to the local inflammatory response include vasoactive amines, plasma proteins, mast cells, tissue macrophages and systemically recruited neutrophils and monocytes (Solomkin and Simmons, 1983). The non-cellular components of the inflammatory response modify the local environment to limit the spread of invading bacteria, render the invading bacteria more susceptible to phagocytosis and recruit phagocytic cells to the inflammatory focus. The major non-cellular mediators involved in this phase of the inflammatory process are components of the coagulation and complement cascades plus

the vasoactive amines. Activation of the coagulation cascade at the inflammatory site creates a fibrin matrix that entraps microorganisms and limits their dissemination, while capillary thrombosis at the perimeter of the inflammatory process prevents the egress of microorganisms through the microcirculation. Once the tissue injury recognition phase has been initiated, activated complement components and other humoral factors amplify the local humoral response and recruit functional phagocytes from the systemic circulation. The locally recruited phagocytes then function in concert with locally and systemically generated humoral factors to eradicate the invading bacteria.

The neutrophil is the most important effector cell recruited into the wound by the inflammatory response. Its primary function is the detection, ingestion and destruction of organisms that have penetrated the local defences and invaded living tissue. Increased susceptibility to infection has been associated with defects in all of the steps of neutrophil function leading up to the ingestion and killing of invading bacteria. These are illustrated schematically in Figure 49.1 and include: adherence to the vascular endothelium at the site of the inflammatory response (margination), migration through the vascular wall to the site of bacterial invasion (chemotaxis) and the ingestion and intracellular killing of the bacteria. Each of these *in vivo* neutrophil functions can be measured *in vitro*. Thus,

TABLE 49.1

MAJOR COMPONENTS OF THE NON-SPECIFIC (INFLAMMATORY) AND SPECIFIC HOST DEFENCE SYSTEMS

System	Cellular	Humoral
Non-specific	Neutrophils Reticuloendothelial system Monocytes/ macrophages	Alternative complement system Fibronectin Coagulation/ fibrinolytic
Specific	B-Lymphocytes T-Lymphocytes Macrophages Plasma cells	Antibodies Lymphokines Monokines Classical complement system

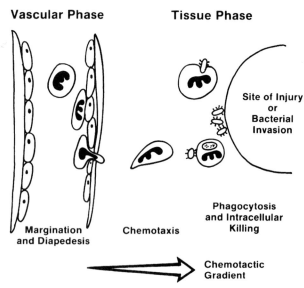

Vascular Phase   **Tissue Phase**

Site of Injury or Bacterial Invasion

Phagocytosis and Intracellular Killing

Margination and Diapedesis   **Chemotaxis**

Chemotactic Gradient

Figure 49.1 Locally generated chemotactic factors induce the recruitment of circulating neutrophils to a nidus of infection or an inflammatory focus. The circulating neutrophils sense these factors and respond by endothelial margination and subsequent diapedesis through the vascular wall. Once the neutrophils reach the extravascular space, they migrate along the chemotactic gradient phagocytosing and killing whatever bacteria they meet.

the classic signs of the inflammatory response (rubor, calor, tumour and dolor) can be seen to reflect the body's attempts to eradicate or limit the spread of bacteria that have breached the host's mechanical defences. The low incidence of wound infections complicating clean surgery or traumatic lacerations highlights the intrinsic effectiveness of this inflammatory defence system in eradicating contaminating bacteria.

The antibacterial action of the neutrophil is most effective against bacteria lodged in tissues or in areas where blood flow is slow (e.g. pulmonary circulation) or has stopped (e.g. site of inflammation or injury). Blood-borne organisms are not effectively cleared by circulating neutrophils, since the flow of blood is too rapid in the systemic vasculature to allow sufficient contact time between neutrophils and bacteria for phagocytosis to occur. Removal of circulating bacteria is primarily a function of the reticuloendothelial system (RES), which consists of the fixed macrophages of the liver, spleen and lymph nodes. The architecture of the RES is specifically developed for this function. The RES organs contain a complex meshwork of reticular fibres and collagenous proteins embedded in a mucopolysaccharide matrix with the phagocytic cells inhabiting the lattice. This special anatomical arrangement promotes intimate contact between phagocytic cells and circulating particulate and soluble debris, including bacteria. The intimate and prolonged contact between fixed phagocytic cells and circulating bacteria promotes the efficient phagocytosis and subsequent killing of microorganisms.

The non-specific humoral system assists the cellular system by coating invading bacteria with proteins that the phagocytes recognize through surface receptors. Such coating is termed 'opsonization' and the term 'opsonin' refers to a protein that when bound to an antigen (i.e. bacteria), increases the affinity of that antigen for the phagocytic cell. The major opsonin systems are composed of: proteins of the classical and alternative complement systems, fibronectin and antibody. Conceptually, opsonins can be viewed as links between the humoral and cellular elements of the non-specific and specific immune systems (Figure 49.2).

The specific immune system consists of macrophages, lymphocytes, plasma cells and their humoral products (Table 49.1). It is only recently, with the development of monoclonal antibodies, that the complex interactions between cellular subpopulations of the immune system have begun to be understood at the cellular level. In contrast to the phylogenetically more primitive inflammatory host-defence system, the specific immune system responds precisely to antigenic sites on the surfaces of invading bacteria to produce antigen-specific antibodies formed against the invading organism. The antibody molecule is structurally bifunctional,

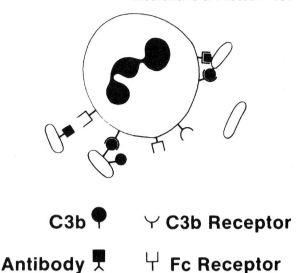

C3b

Antibody

Y C3b Receptor

Fc Receptor

Figure 49.2 The antibody and complement systems are the two major classes of bacterial opsonins. Both antibody and the C3b component of complement serve as bridges which facilitate bacterial phagocytosis by physically connecting the bacteria to the neutrophil. This process is mediated through specific receptors expressed on the surface of the neutrophil.

containing a constant region (Fc) that binds to the effector cell and a variable region (Fab2) that binds to the antigen. Antibodies serve as specific opsonins that increase the affinity of bacterial binding to neutrophils and fixed-tissue macrophages of the RES. In addition, antibody can directly activate the classical complement cascade by binding to the first component of complement (C1q). In this way, the specific and non-specific host-defence systems interact to defend the body against invading microorganisms.

For most antigens, including bacterial antigens, the initial step in the induction of humoral immunity (antibody production) is the presentation of the foreign antigen by macrophages or other antigen-presenting cells to helper thymus-derived lymphocytes (T cells). Activation of the helper T cells results in the liberation of soluble mediators (cytokines) that instruct B lymphocytes to proliferate and differentiate into antibody-producing plasma cells. Plasma cells can be viewed as antibody-producing factories, with each cell secreting more than 2000 identical antibody molecules per second throughout its several-day life-span. This highly complex antibody-producing system has many checks and balances. Although the exact mechanisms and pathways that regulate antibody production are not fully known, there is clear evidence that this process can be blocked or suppressed in a number of ways. For example, antibody production can be prevented by the failure of antigen to be presented to the helper T cell or by the activation of suppressor T cells or inhibitory macrophages.

Cell-mediated immunity includes a wide range of functions directly carried out by immune cells or their products, exclusive of antibody production. These include the activation of macrophages to become more effective phagocytes, the induction of null lymphocytes (killer [K] cells) that destroy antibody-coated target cells and the production of cytotoxic T cells (natural killer [NK] cells) that lyse foreign cells. The exact mechanisms controlling cell-mediated immunity are incompletely understood. However it appears that both macrophages and lymphocytes are composed of multiple subpopulations, some of which induce or augment the immune response while others suppress or down-regulate it (Paul, 1986).

Evidence that T lymphocytes develop into different subpopulations specialized for certain functions was first presented by Kisielow et al. in 1975. These investigators documented that post-thymic mouse lymphocytes capable of exerting either helper or suppressor functions could be identified by the presence of the cell surface antigens Thy1 and Ly. This work indicated that microscopically identical lymphocytes could be separated into functionally distinct subpopulations based on their surface antigenic phenotype. Today, by using commercially available monoclonal antibodies, helper T cells can be distinguished from suppressor T cells, and both can be differentiated from B cells, NK and K cells (Table 49.2). Although exceptions exist, it now appears that by determining the in vitro cell surface receptor expression of a cell, it is possible to predict its biological activity. For example, through studies which correlated cell surface receptor expression with functional assays, it appears that when suppressor T cells are preferentially activated, the immune response will be downregulated. In contrast, when helper T cells are activated, the immune response will be augmented. Under normal conditions, these mononuclear-cell populations maintain immunological homoeostasis through a complex and poorly understood series of feedback and regulatory loops. In contrast, in certain diseases or after injury these regulatory systems can fail. Thus, disruption of this immunological balance can lead to an uncontrolled inflammatory response at one extreme or to impaired resistance to infection at the other extreme.

To summarize, the non-specific host-defence system is the primary defence against invading bacteria in the non-immune host. The key components of this system are neutrophils (migrate to sites of inflammation and infection), the alternative complement system (primary opsonins for gram-negative bacteria when preformed antibodies are absent) and the RES (clears the circulation of blood-borne bacteria and particulate debris). The specific immune system contributes to the defence of the host by the production of specific antibody and by activating blood monocytes to release cytokines and to become more effective phagocytes. However, prior to the induction of specific immunity, a lag phase of 10–14 days for a primary immune response or 3–5 days for a secondary response must elapse. Thus, although the specific immune system can aid in the defence of the host against bacteria, its major role is in the eradication of intracellular pathogens, such as viruses, fungi or intracellular bacteria such as Listeria monocytogenes. Since these microorganisms are infrequent or late pathogens in the trauma victim, it appears that the non-specific host-defence system is of major clinical importance in the trauma victim.

Effect of trauma on non-specific and specific immunity

Although each of the components of the host-defence systems has been described above separately, they are generally activated simultaneously and function synergistically in vivo to prevent and control infection. Furthermore, many of the systems overlap and this immunological redundancy helps compensate for certain trauma-induced immune defects. Before the effects of trauma on the immune and inflammatory defences are described, it is important to state that the immune status of an individual patient can be significantly modified by non-trauma-related factors, such as the patient's age, nutritional state and premorbid physiological status.

It should come as no surprise that the risk of infection is increased in patients sustaining major thermal or mechanical injuries, since widespread defects in multiple aspects of the immune and inflammatory antibacterial host defences have been found in these patients (Table 49.3).

TABLE 49.2
PHENOTYPIC CHARACTERIZATION OF FUNCTIONALLY DISTINCT
LYMPHOCYTES

Lymphocyte population	Human	Murine
T cells	CDT3+, CDT11+	Thy 1+
T-helper/inducers	CDT4+, CDT8–	Lyt–1+
T-suppressor/cytotoxic	CDT4–, CDT8+	Lyt–2, 3+
NK (natural killer)	FcR+, Ig–	Fcr+, Ig–
K cells	FcR+, Ig–	FcR+, Ig–
B cells	FcR+, Ia+, Ig+	FcR+, Ia+, Ig+

Monoclonal antibodies of the CD series are used to identify human lymphocyte subpopulations, while the Thy(Ly) series are used to identify murine lymphocyte cell populations. FcR+ indicates that the surface receptor for the constant (Fc) region of the immunoglobulin molecule is present; Ig+, that the surface of the cell expresses immunoglobulin (Ig); Ig–, that immunoglobulin is not expressed on the cell surface, Ia+, that this Ia antigen is present on the surface of the cell.

TABLE 49.3

GENERAL TRENDS IN SYSTEMIC HOST DEFENCES AFTER THERMAL INJURY OR MECHANICAL TRAUMA OR DURING MALNUTRITION

		Burn patient		
	Trauma	Non-septic	Septic	Malnutrition
Cellular immunity				
Neutrophils				
Chemotaxis	D	D	D	D
Phagocytosis	N	N	N	D
Bacterial activity	N,D	N,D	D	D
Lymphocytes				
Endogenous (SBT)	–	I	I	–
Stimulated (PMA,MLR)	D	N,D	N,D	N,D
NK activity	N,D	N,D	D	N,D
Helper T cells	N,D	N,D	N,D	D
Suppressor T cells	N,I,D	N,I,D	N,I,D	D
Macrophages	D	D	D	D
Humoral immunity				
Complement	D > N	D > N	D	D
Fibronectin	D > N	D > N	D	D
Antibody	N	D > N	N	N,D

N = normal; I = increased; D = decreased; – = not done; > = changes to.

The relationship between the magnitude of the injury and the risk of infectious complications has been clearly documented in the burn patient, where the risk of infection is increased in patients with burns involving more than 40% of the body surface area. Furthermore, the ability of a patient to survive an infectious episode is inversely related to the size of the burn. A similar relationship has been demonstrated between the magnitude of mechanical trauma, as reflected in the Injury Severity Score, and the risk of infectious complications (Meakins *et al.*, 1978; Maderazo *et al.*, 1983). In fact, changes in certain aspects of both humoral and cellular immunity induced by both thermal and mechanical trauma correlate with the magnitude of the injury. This concept is most clearly illustrated in the burn victim where the magnitude of the injury is reflected in the percentage of the body burned (Deitch *et al.*, 1984) (Figure 49.3).

That trauma leads to an immunocompromised state is no longer controversial, but uncertainty still exists concerning which abnormalities are of prognostic importance. For many years, it has been known that patients sustaining major injuries develop multiple defects in their immune systems. These include alterations in immunoglobulin levels, changes in the concentrations and activities of components of both the classical and the alternative complement pathways, reduced circulating plasma fibronectin, depressed serum opsonic activity, and impairment of macrophage, lymphocyte and neutrophil functions, as well as reduced RES activity (Table 49.3). Although it is clear that injury is associated with multiple defects in the humoral and

cellular components of both the non-specific defence system and the specific immune system, no firm consensus has been reached on their prognostic and clinical significance.

This confusion is compounded by the fact that different laboratories employ different methods to measure specific immune parameters in patients treated with different clinical regimens. Perhaps of greater significance is the fact that in many studies, only one immunological variable is measured. In that immune defects do not occur in isolation, it is difficult to determine whether a particular abnormality is a primary event of clinical importance or is secondary to another, unmeasured, abnormality. The clinical profile on which many of the immunological predictors of sepsis and death have been based is schematically illustrated in Figure 49.4. It can be seen that the immunological parameter measured initially decreases postinjury and in patients who do not survive or become septic, remains depressed. In patients who survive, the immunological parameter ultimately returns to normal. Studies of this kind represent only associations and should not be interpreted as showing cause and effect relationships. *In vivo* the host-defence systems act synergistically to prevent and control infections. Consequently, clinically just because one specific host-defence parameter is decreased after trauma it does not mean that restoration of that specific parameter will necessarily reduce the risk of infection. This fact has been a major reason for the discouraging results to date with the use of various immune adjuvants. This problem of overinterpreting a specific immune

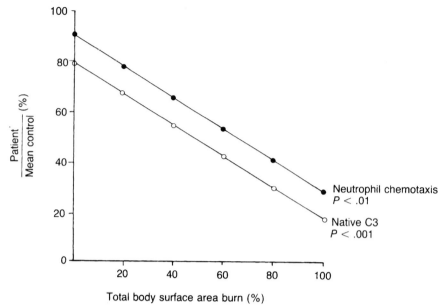

Figure 49.3 There is a direct relationship between the magnitude of the injury (burn size) and the magnitude of the decrease in several immunological variables. This concept is illustrated using neutrophil chemotaxis and native C3 serum levels as examples.

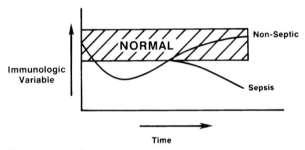

Figure 49.4 Schematic drawing illustrating the concept that many of the elements of the host's antibacterial defences (humoral and cellular) follow a biphasic course, in which they are initially depressed but return to normal as the patient recovers.

defect can best be avoided by measuring several aspects of immune function simultaneously.

Neutrophils

Abnormalities in neutrophil chemotaxis or microbicidal activity are frequently associated with recurrent bacterial infections of soft tissues and systemic sepsis in patients with congenital defects in neutrophil function. This observation has led many investigators to measure neutrophil function after trauma or burns. As illustrated in Figure 49.1, the sucessful eradication of invading bacteria requires several successive neutrophil responses, the failure of any of which could lead to an established infection. Decreased neutrophil chemotaxis frequently occurs after thermal injury or mechanical trauma and the magnitude of the initial impairment

in chemotaxis appears to be related directly to the magnitude of the injury. However, in spite of this relationship between impaired chemotaxis and trauma, there is conflicting evidence as to whether this chemotactic defect is prognostically important in identifying the patient at increased risk of becoming infected. Furthermore, Meakins *et al.* (1979) in a prospective trial using levamisole to reverse the *in vitro* chemotactic defect in surgical patients, were not able to demonstrate a decrease in the incidence of infection.

No consistent defect in neutrophil bacterial phagocytosis after burn or trauma has been documented and, in fact, several groups have found phagocytosis to be increased in trauma or burn victims. Of all the neutrophil functions measured, impaired neutrophil bactericidal activity appears to correlate best with an increased risk of infection (Table 49.3).

In spite of active investigations into the possible causes of abnormal neutrophil function after trauma or burns, the causes of neutrophil dysfunction remain speculative. There is controversy over whether they are due to humoral suppressive factors or circulating toxins, are cytokine mediated or are the result of cellular deactivation. The last is the term used to describe the phenomenon of *in vivo* activation of neutrophils leading to *in vitro* paralysis – cells, which have been activated in the body, become relatively or absolutely refractory to subsequent stimuli *in vitro*. Evidence in support of this theory consists of the association of signs of *in vivo* neutrophil activation in the face of decreased *in vitro* function (Figure 49.5). Regardless of the

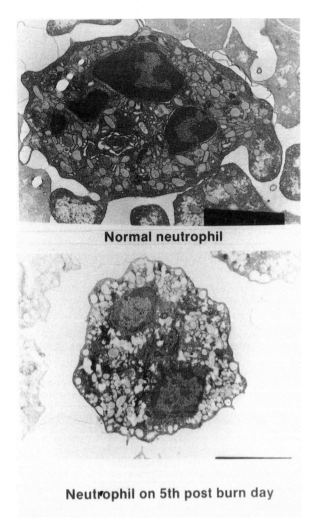

Normal neutrophil

Neutrophil on 5th post burn day

Figure 49.5 Electron micrograph of a normal neutrophil and a neutrophil from a non-infected burn patient. The neutrophil from the burn patient shows evidence of *in vivo* activation, which is manifest as degranulation and vacuole formation.

aetiology of abnormal neutrophil function after traumatic injury, the presence of impaired neutrophil function is associated with an increased risk of infection. Since the neutrophil is the primary cell involved in the eradication of bacteria that typically cause infection in these patients, to some extent, any or all of the defects in neutrophil function described above probably contribute to the increased risk of infection in the trauma victim.

Reticuloendothelial system

The RES clears circulating debris, such as aggregated protein, damaged cells and fibrin from the blood stream, in addition to removing blood-borne bacteria. Efficient RES phagocytosis requires the presence of humoral factors, which coat the particles to promote their recognition, attachment and ingestion by the fixed macrophages of the RES.

During the last decade, it has become apparent that normal serum levels of the opsonic protein, fibronectin, in addition to complement and antibody are necessary for optimal RES function. A large body of information now exists indicating that RES activity and plasma fibronectin levels are transiently depressed in trauma victims and that the magnitude of this initial decrease in plasma fibronectin levels is greater in non-survivors than survivors. Additionally, a secondary decrease in fibronectin levels during sepsis identifies the thermally or mechanically injured patient at increased risk of sepsis (Table 49.3).

The potential clinical importance of impaired RES function is highlighted by studies demonstrating that RES stimulants increase host resistance to trauma and infection, while RES depressants can convert a sublethal injury or infection into a lethal event. The clinical consequences of impaired RES activity and depressed fibronectin levels may extend to other organs. For example, after RES depression, the role of clearance of circulating debris and bacteria shifts from the liver to other organs, especially the lung. This RES blockade-induced increase in the pulmonary clearance of bacterial and non-bacterial particles is associated with the margination and sequestration of circulating neutrophils within the lung. In this way, RES blockade may ultimately result in pulmonary dysfunction due to the activation of neutrophils sequestered in the lungs. Thus, based on human and animal studies documenting that RES function is decreased and plasma fibronectin levels are depressed after burns or trauma, it appears that impaired RES activity may contribute to the development of infection or distant organ failure.

There are anecdotal reports of fibronectin repletion improving host resistance to infection and impaired organ function in injured or septic hypoopsonic patients. Although these are encouraging, prospective controlled clinical trials of fibronectin repletion have not verified the clinical efficacy of fibronectin replacement therapy (Mansberger *et al.*, 1989). Thus, currently there does not appear to be a role for fibronectin replacement therapy in the trauma victim.

Humoral defences

Although there is evidence that many humoral factors may be potentally important in the control of bacterial infections (Simmons and Howard, 1988), this discussion will concentrate on the two major classes of opsonins generally present in biological fluids, the heat-stable immunoglobulins and the heat-labile complement components. In the non-immune host, the alternative complement system is the major opsonin system, while in the immune host, with high levels of specific antibody, complement plays only an adjuvant role as a bacterial opsonin. Complement can be activated through one of two major pathways. The classical pathway is activated when bacterial antigens interact with specific antibodies and, therefore, requires an immune host. The alternative pathway can be activated by endotoxin, denatured serum proteins or damaged cells and, therefore, does not require an immune host. Consequently, the alternative pathway of complement activation acts as an immediate first line of defence after trauma.

Serum opsonic activity has been studied most extensively in patients with thermal injuries. These patients exhibit depressed serum opsonic activity for *Pseudomonas aeruginosa*, *Escherichia coli* and occasionally *Staphylococcus aureus*. However, impaired opsonic activity does not appear to be a reliable indicator of sepsis, since it has been observed during both septic and non-septic periods. When present, it appears to be related to the systemic activation and subsequent consumption of certain components of the alternative complement system. The defect in opsonic activity due to complement consumption is not limited to the thermally injured patient but also occurs after mechanical trauma and in patients with gram-negative bacterial infections. In addition to their systemic role as opsonins, these humoral factors are important locally. For example, complement components serve as local opsonins in tissues and one of the complement breakdown products, C5a, is a major chemoattractant for neutrophils. Although the complement system plays a major role in the control and eradication of invading bacteria, excessive activation of this system can damage the host. For example, persistent or recurrent episodes of complement activation are believed to contribute to the development of the adult respiratory distress syndrome (ARDS). That is, complement-induced neutrophil aggregation and activation may lead to the sequestration of activated neutrophils within the pulmonary vasculature where the activated neutrophils liberate oxidants and proteases that damage the endothelium.

Although serum immunoglobulin levels are transiently decreased after thermal or mechanical injury, they return to normal levels quickly and this early hypoimmunoglobulinaemia does not appear to be associated with increased susceptibility to infection. Thus, in general, serum immunoglobulin levels are not accurate indicators or predictors of sepsis or recovery in the trauma victim. Therefore, it is not entirely unexpected that clinical trials of prophylactic immune globulin therapy have not been clinically beneficial (Waymack *et al.*, 1989).

Specific immune system
Beginning with the observation that burn and trauma patients are frequently anergic and that burn victims have delayed rejection of skin allografts, many studies have been performed to evaluate cell-mediated immunity in the trauma victim. Its

importance as an antibacterial defence system in the trauma victim is unclear, since cell-mediated immunity is not critical in controlling acute bacterial infections with extracellular pathogens. Rather, cell-mediated immunity is more important in the defence against infections caused by slow-growing intracellular bacteria, fungi and viruses – infections not commonly seen after trauma (Howard, 1980). Furthermore, controversy exists over whether trauma causes impaired cell-mediated immunity and whether this results in an increased risk of infection.

This confusion can be clarified to some degree by classifying the studies into those that measured cell-mediated immunity by *in vivo* tests, such as the response to skin tests, and those that used *in vitro* measurement. The presence of skin test anergy after trauma is associated with an increased risk of sepsis. However, the skin test response is a complicated phenomenon requiring both lymphocyte activation and the subsequent recruitment of effector cells from the inflammatory host defence system to the skin test site. Over the past several years, Meakins *et al.*, (1979) have attempted to determine which elements of this response are abnormal in the anergic patient. Their results suggest that anergy is not primarily due to lymphocyte dysfunction, since these cells can be activated *in vitro*. Instead, anergy is the outcome of multiple factors, including impaired neutrophil function. In contrast to anergy, there is no consensus as to whether *in vitro* cell-mediated immunity is normal, increased or decreased. Furthermore, there is debate whether changes in cell-mediated immunity measured *in vitro* correlate prognostically with sepsis or death (Table 49.3). This failure of *in vitro* tests of cell-mediated immunity to correlate tightly with outcome is not unexpected, since a potential weakness of all standardized *in vitro* assays is the fact that the assays may not accurately reflect the complex interactions that are taking place *in vivo* (Xu *et al.*, 1988).

This controversy cannot be resolved until we have a better understanding of the mechanisms involved in the development of impaired cell-mediated immunity after trauma. Many putative causes of lymphocyte dysfunction have been proposed including: decreased helper T-cell activity, increased suppressor T-cell activity, increased inhibitory macrophage activity and the presence of circulating humoral suppressive substances or modulatory cytokines (Figure 49.6). Currently, it is not possible to say with certainty which of these alternatives occur at the cellular level. However, a clear understanding of the process at the cellular level will be critical for the development of rational therapeutic modalities to augment host defences.

Mediators of the immunocompromised state
That trauma can lead to depression of immunity is no longer a matter of debates although controversy

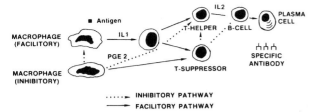

Figure 49.6 The major relationships between the various mononuclear cell subpopulations. Humoral factors (monokines and lymphokines) serve as the primary messengers that transmit information between the cell populations. Three of the best described messengers are interleukin 1 (IL1) produced by facilitatory macrophages, prostaglandin E_2 (PGE 2) produced by inhibitory macrophages, and interleukin-2 (IL2), produced by helper T cells.

and confusion still exist about the mechanisms by which trauma induces immunosuppression in an otherwise healthy individual. The hypothesis that has received the greatest attention is that trauma, hypotension, tissue injury or stress will induce, generate or liberate immunosuppressive factors that directly or indirectly downregulate or suppress the normal immune response. Some of the earliest work in this field was performed by Schoenenberger *et al.* (1975) who isolated a burn toxin from the serum and skin of severely burned patients. Since then, a wide variety of putative immunosuppressive factors have been obtained from the sera of victims of blunt or penetrating trauma. Clinical interpretation of these studies is limited by the inability of investigators to identify the origin of these factors. Recently, Ozkan and Hinneman (1985) have isolated and biochemically characterized a low-molecular-weight peptide from the sera of burn and trauma patients that suppresses both lymphocyte and neutrophil activity *in vitro* (e.g. Hoyt *et al.*, 1988). This suppressive active peptide has been termed 'SAP' and is composed of normal cellular or humoral factors that are modified or released into the circulation at the time of injury. However, further investigations of the relationship between the level of SAP, the incidence of infectious complications and the immune status of the host must be performed before any firm conclusions can be drawn about the clinical importance of SAP as a key factor in the development of an immunocompromised state after trauma. Other factors, such as prostaglandin E_2 (PGE$_2$), endotoxin, tumour necrosis factor (TNF), complement products, various interleukins, as well as others, have been implicated as potential mediators of the immunosuppressed state following trauma or stress. Further work is required to clarify the role of these factors as clinically significant mediators of immune suppression *in vivo*. In addition to these humoral mediators, there is evidence, albeit con-

flicting, that thermal and mechanical trauma can induce alterations in cellular immunity by affecting the balance of helper and suppressor T-cell activity in favour of increased suppression or decreased helper activity.

Studies attempting to determine why patients develop widespread changes in immune competence after thermal or mechanical trauma have largely neglected to explore the relationships between the stress state and immune dysfunction. This area may be important, since it appears that stress hormones and neurotransmitters such as the endogenous opiates, may represent an information channel between the immune, endocrine and central nervous systems (see also Chapter 45). In support of this concept is recent evidence indicating that immune homoeostasis may require not only the regulatory influence of immunocompetent cells but also effects from the central nervous system and a balanced endocrine environment (Adler, 1981). For example, adrenergic and corticosteroid receptors are present on both lymphocytes and neutrophils and these hormones have been implicated in modulating the various immune effector functions of these cells. In fact, lymphocytes contain receptors for many other hormones and mediators including insulin, growth hormone, acetylcholine and endorphins. Since both direct manipulation of the brain and chronic stress influence the immune response, it appears that potential brain messengers (hormones and endogenous opiates) can be recognized by immune cells and affect cellular function.

Another area which is receiving increasing attention is the effect of hypotension on the immune state. Based on recent studies, it appears that transient hypotension, even in the absence of any significant tissue trauma, will produce a marked depression in elements of both the specific and non-specific host-defence systems (Chaudry *et al.*, 1990). Whether the trauma-induced, immunosuppressed state is mediated by hormones, opiates, trauma-induced toxins, endotoxin, prostaglandins, cytokines, such as IL-1 or TNF, or other products, singly or in combination, must await further investigation.

Integrated hypothesis of infection: the burn wound as an example

From the previous discussion, it is clear that trauma causes profound changes in many aspects of the host-defence system. Although the absolute importance of each of these acquired immunological defects to host resistance to infection is not completely understood, it is reasonable to conclude that each component contributes to the host's overall immunological reserve in some fashion. Based on our studies of multiple components of the local and systemic host defence systems in thermally injured patients (Deitch *et al.*, 1985), the following hypo-

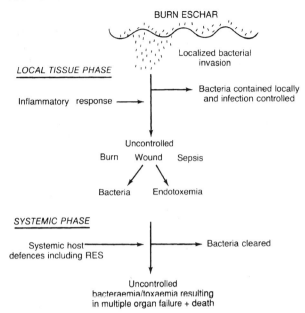

Figure 49.7 Schematic representation of burn wound sepsis. If the local tissue defences do not control the invading bacteria, systemic infection results.

thetical model is offered to explain the immunological basis of the increased susceptibility of the burn patient to life-threatening infections originating from the burn wound (Figure 49.7). This model is designed to illustrate the interdependence of various components of the host-defence systems in preventing and controlling infection and can also be conceptually applied to the mechanically injured patient, in whom the site of invading bacteria may be the lung, peritoneal cavity or soft tissue. It is based primarily on failure of the local defence barriers against bacteria due to injury of the skin plus failure of the non-specific, inflammatory defence system. However, dysfunction of the specific immune system may also be important, since one of its major roles is to amplify and focus the ability of the non-specific host-defence system towards the control of invading bacteria.

The combination of the destruction of the skin barrier to bacteria plus failure in the recruitment of neutrophils to the burn wound (impaired chemotaxis) and the decreased ability of burn blister fluid to opsonize bacteria allows organisms that colonize (contaminate) the burn wound to multiply and reach sufficient population densities to invade and propagate in viable tissues under the eschar. If the invading bacteria can be opsonized, phagocytosed and killed by local phagocytes in combination with the late-arriving neutrophils, the infection will be contained locally. However, if local bacterial control fails because of impaired neutrophil bactericidal activity, then the survivors may multiply and the infection extend further into contiguous viable

tissue. At some point, the numbers of bacteria in the tissue rises to the extent that they enter the systemic circulation. These blood-borne bacteria are initially cleared by the RES. Eventually, the continued bacteraemia from the uncontrolled local infection results in RES overload, which is generally reflected as a secondary decrease in plasma fibronectin levels. At this point, the clearance of circulating bacteria and immunologically generated humoral and cellular factors shifts from the liver to other organs, especially the lung. The net result of this process ultimately can lead to the development of haematogenous pneumonia as well as contribute to the development of pulmonary insufficiency and multiple organ failure.

This scheme highlights the concept that the increased susceptibility to infection is not likely to be due to a single, isolated defect in antibacterial defences, but instead is related to multiple abnormalities in several different host-defence systems.

HOST–MICROBE RELATIONSHIPS

The development of infection requires both a susceptible host and the presence of a bacterial pathogen. These infections are generally caused by organisms that are already colonizing the patient, some of which are hospital acquired. Since these infections tend to originate from microorganisms colonizing mucosal or skin surfaces at sites of thermal, mechanical or surgical trauma, knowledge of the normal microflora at various body sites as well as an understanding of the factors that alter it are important. For example, by knowing the characteristic microflora of different anatomical regions, it is possible to predict which microorganisms are most likely to cause an infection when a specific anatomical region is injured. This information is essential in selecting an appropriate empiric antibiotic regimen. Similarly, in the bacteraemic patient with a clinically occult focus of infection, knowledge of the normal microecology will help determine the potential portal of entry for that infecting organism. More information on the specific microflora of different anatomical regions and how they are modified in the trauma patient will be presented below in the section on specific infectious complications.

Microbial-induced modulation of host defences

In the previous section on the effects of trauma on host antibacterial defences, the contribution of trauma-induced immune suppression in the pathogenesis of infection was stressed. However, the presence of bacteria, and especially endotoxin, can have profound immunomodulatory effects on host-defence systems. That is, infection can be a cause as well as an effect of impaired host defences. Since it appears that the physiological effects of gram-negative bacterial sepsis appear to be primarily mediated directly or indirectly by endotoxin, an understanding of the biology of endotoxin-induced alterations in host-defence systems is clinically important.

Although the terms endotoxin and lipopolysaccharide are frequently used interchangeably, the two terms are not identical (see also Chapter 34). Endotoxin contains protein as well as the lipopolysaccharide moiety and consists of the following three regions: polysaccharide side-chains; a core lipopolysaccharide; and a lipid A component consisting of a glucosamine backbone to which are linked long-chain fatty acids. Since lipid A appears to be primarily responsible for the effects of endotoxin and its structure appears to be constant among the different genera of gram-negative bacilli, considerable effort has been directed towards producing antibodies against lipid A. This topic will be discussed in more detail later.

The concept that endotoxin mediates the pathophysiological changes associated with sepsis is based on extensive *in vivo* experimental studies. These documented that many of the effects observed when endotoxin is injected into experimental animals are similar to those observed in septic man. For example, both septic man and endotoxin-treated animals display fever, shock, disseminated intravascular coagulation and similar changes in intermediary metabolism. Endotoxin appears to exert the majority of its toxic effects indirectly by triggering the overproduction and release of endogenous factors by the host and endotoxic shock appears to be due to the activation of endogenous host systems and cells, especially the macrophage/monocyte system. In fact, the lethal effects of endotoxin appear to be the consequence of the fact that 'our arsenals for fighting off bacteria are so powerful and involve so many defence mechanisms, that we are in more danger from them than from the invaders' (Thomas, 1974).

Before discussing the effects of endotoxin on the immune system, it is important to realize that the exact *in vivo* effects of endotoxin depend on the route of administration, dose, timing and frequency of administration, the response measured and the experimental species tested. For example, multiple small doses of intravenously administered, but not intradermally injected, endotoxin will induce a state of endotoxin tolerance. Similarly, endotoxin can augment or suppress the host's ability to withstand a septic challenge: animals receiving sublethal doses of endotoxin are more resistant to bacterial challenge than control animals when tested 24–48 hours after receiving endotoxin. In contrast, endotoxin-treated animals are less resistant to the same bacterial challenge when tested shortly after receiving endotoxin. Lastly, it is important to remember that the response to endotoxin varies greatly between species: rodents are much more resistant to endotoxin

than man, while other species, such as the dog, show major differences in their haemodynamic response to endotoxin challenge. These caveats should be kept in mind when assessing the results of studies investigating the mechanisms of endotoxin-induced toxicity as well as the efficacy of potential therapeutic agents.

Haemodynamic, metabolic and immunological disturbances have all been documented after endotoxin challenge and endotoxic shock remains a clinically common cause of death. Endotoxin activates both the classical and alternative pathways of complement. The lipid A region can activate the classical pathway, in the absence of specific antibody, by directly binding to the first component (C1). Activation of the alternative pathway appears to be due to the polysaccharide moiety. Once activated, the anaphylatoxins C3a and C5a are produced, which have vasodilatory properties and may contribute to endotoxin shock. Furthermore, complement breakdown products may modulate neutrophil and lymphocyte activity, since these cells have been documented to have complement receptors. Clinical and experimental endotoxaemia is associated with diffuse microvascular thrombosis and activation of the coagulation system, which may take place directly by endotoxin-induced activation of Hageman factor (factor XII) or indirectly by endotoxin-stimulated secretion of tissue procoagulation factor by macrophages.

Arachidonic acid metabolites produced by endotoxin-activated macrophages also appear to play a role in endotoxin-mediated disease. This conclusion is based on the fact that endotoxin can elicit the production of prostaglandins and leukotrienes and that inhibitors or antagonists of these metabolites can modulate the physiological effects of endotoxin. Other macrophage products have been shown to be induced by endotoxin. These include interleukin 1 (IL-1), tumour necrosis factor (TNF), colony stimulating factors and interferon. Each of these, alone or in combination, can have profound effects on multiple homoeostatic systems including immune integrity. However, at this point in time, it is generally agreed that TNF is responsible for most of endotoxin's systemic effects, including the induction of endotoxin shock (Beutler and Cerami, 1987). Another potential mediator of endotoxin shock is platelet activating factor (PAF). PAF is produced by many cells, including macrophages, neutrophils, platelets and endothelial cells and its biological effects include increased vascular permeability, hypotension and death. Furthermore, endotoxin-induced hypotension is associated with detectable levels of plasma PAF and PAF antagonists reverse endotoxin-induced shock. Determination of the exact role of these endotoxin-induced mediators and cytokines in endotoxin shock is compounded by the fact that these mediators appear to interact synergistically.

In addition to endotoxin's direct effect on host-defence factors, many of the same mediators that potentiate endotoxin shock can also alter neutrophil, lymphocyte and macrophage function. Bacteria and endotoxin are among the most powerful stimulants of the immune system. In spite of endotoxin's deleterious effects, it should not be forgotten that, in most circumstances, the immune response to a bacterial or endotoxin challenge is beneficial. B cells are activated to produce antibodies, macrophages are activated to become more efficient phagocytes, neutrophils are released from the bone marrow, and the RES is primed to clear the circulation more efficiently of blood-borne bacteria and debris.

Endotoxin's effect on B-cell activation, in contrast to most antigens, is not T-cell dependent. Although endotoxin has no direct effect on T cells, it can modulate the T-cell response to other antigens that are T-cell dependent. In fact, endotoxin's modulating effects on T-cell proliferation and the host's immune response vary from complete suppression to immune enhancement and increased resistance to an infectious challenge. The ability of endotoxin to modulate T-cell activity appears to be mediated to a large extent by cytokines produced by activated macrophages. Depending upon which cytokines are produced by the activated macrophages, the immune response will be enhanced or suppressed. Endotoxin-mediated immune enhancement appears to be associated with the preferential production and secretion of IL-1 by activated macrophages, while suppression is associated with PGE_2 release. Thus, endotoxin appears to induce a stimulatory circuit that is associated with increased bactericidal activity and the secretion of IL-1, or a suppressive circuit associated with PGE_2 secretion. In the suppressive circuit, PGE_2 downregulates macrophage activity as well as other effector cells via a feedback suppression loop.

Thus, endotoxin has a wide range of immunological activities. On the one and positive hand, endotoxin stimulates B-cell proliferation, activates macrophages, primes the RES, induces granulocytosis, increases serum complement levels and promotes an inflammatory response. On the other and negative hand, depending on the dosage and timing of its administration, endotoxin can induce suppressor T-cell activity and PGE_2 secretion by macrophages, as well as decrease the resistance of experimental animals to an infectious challenge. Thus, endotoxin initiates a complex series of events leading to the production of numerous mediators many of which, such as IL-1, TNF, CSF, PGE_2 and the interferons, have their own immunomodulating effects. Therefore, in considering the effects of endotoxin on the immune response, it is important to keep in mind the fact that endotoxin, in addition to its direct effects on the immune system, also induces the production and release of numerous cytokines and inflammatory mediators, all of which induce their own cascade of effects.

INFECTIOUS COMPLICATIONS: PATHOPHYSIOLOGY AND THERAPY

General concepts

The development of infection requires both a susceptible host and the presence of a bacterial pathogen. Thus, only by paying attention to both the host and the pathogen will it be possible to reduce the incidence and consequences of infections in the immunocompromised trauma victim. That is, therapeutic manoeuvres must be directed not just towards the eradication of invading bacteria, but also at mechanisms to increase the host's resistance to infection. In this regard, there is no substitute for mature surgical judgement, early definitive surgery and good operative technique. For example, by debriding necrotic tissue, controlling bacterial contamination and preventing the development of postoperative seromas and haematomas, the surgeon not only removes the milieu in which bacteria multiply but also improves the delivery of host resistance factors, nutrients and oxygen to the sites of injury and inflammation. In addition, early definitive surgery and removal of necrotic tissue may bolster host defences by reducing the circulating levels of potential injury or inflammatory-induced suppressive factors, such as PGE_2, as well as by limiting the period of stress and thereby allowing the hormonal and metabolic state of the patient to return more rapidly to normal. Thus, early definitive surgery utilizing good operative technique plus the use of appropriate perioperative antibiotics and nutrition to bolster host defences are critically important in reducing the risk of infection. In consequence, immunomodulation begins in the emergency area by restoring intravascular volume and improving oxygen delivery to the tissues and continues in the operating room where the injuries are definitively treated and necrotic tissue is removed.

In addition to the direct effects of trauma on host resistance, other factors can also influence host defences, including anaesthetic agents, antibiotics and starvation. Over the past decade, the important relationship between nutrition, immunity and infection has been the focus of intensive investigation. In fact, most of the abnormalities of host defences that have been documented after thermal or mechanical trauma can also be induced by protein-calorie malnutrition (Alexander, 1986). For example, protein-calorie malnutrition causes atrophy of lymphoid tissue, decreases T- and B-cell function, depresses neutrophil bactericidal activity and is associated with decreased levels of components of both the classic and alternative complement pathways (Table 49.3). The clinical importance of aggressive nutritional support in improving host defences and decreasing infection and death has been clearly shown in a prospective study of burned children (Alexander, 1986) and similar results appear to hold in victims of blunt trauma (Border *et al.*, 1987). The immune enhancing effects of appropriate nutritional support cannot be overstated, since at the present time nutritional manipulation is the most practical and important means of non-operative immune modulation in the trauma victim.

Immunotherapy

Interest in immunotherapeutic approaches that prevent, correct or potentiate host defences against infectious agents has increased as our understanding of and ability to manipulate the immune response has increased. The use of agents to prevent infections has a long history, the most famous of these early studies being the use of cowpox as a vaccine by Jenner in 1798 to prevent the development of smallpox. Although active immunization with vaccines has been effective in preventing certain infections, such as tetanus, rabies and polio, the use of vaccines directed against common pathogens in the trauma victim, such as the enteric bacilli or pseudomonads, has been largely unsuccessful. The reason is the antigenic diversity of these microorganisms and the need for the host to be able to respond immunologically to the administered antigens. Likewise, based on the results of a controlled, double-blind, prospective study of the passive administration of intravenous gamma globulin to burn victims (Waymack *et al.*, 1989), nonspecific passive immunization also does not appear to be effective in preventing infection – clinical failure which was largely predictable. Although serum immunoglobulin levels are transiently decreased after thermal or mechanical injury, they return to normal quickly and the transient hypoimmunoglobulinaemic state has not been shown to be associated with an increased risk of infection. In that clinical studies have indicated that serum immunoglobulin levels are not accurate indicators or predictors of sepsis or recovery in the trauma victim, it is not surprising that clinical trials have not documented prophylactic immune globulin therapy to be of clinical benefit.

In contrast to these negative results, a prospective, randomized study employing an antibody made in humans to the mutant J5 strain of *E. coli* was found to reduce the mortality rate of patients with gram-negative sepsis (Ziegler *et al.*, 1982). Similar results have been obtained in burn patients, where the use of hyperimmune anti-*Pseudomonas* gamma globulin reduced the mortality from *Pseudomonas* infections (Jones *et al.*, 1973). Although these two clinical trials and subsequent experimental studies using anti-LPS antibodies are encouraging, the limited bacterial cross-reactivity of current hyperimmune antisera and specific polyclonal and monoclonal antibodies renders their clinical utility undefined. Thus, interest has focused on other modalities, such as the use of the immunologically active compounds, known as biological response modifiers.

Compounds altering immunological responses were formerly termed immunadjuvants, immunopotentiators or immunomodulators. These terms have been replaced by the more descriptive term 'biologic response modifier' (BRM). A partial list of these compounds and their mechanisms of action are outlined in Table 49.4. Since almost all of these compounds have multiple diverse immunological effects, they may function as stimulatory or suppressive agents, according to the exact immune function measured. This fact is not surprising since drugs that non-specifically stimulate macrophages or T cells can activate suppressive as well as helper circuits. Although these BRMs have all been documented to be effective in experimental models, the results of clinical studies have not been as encouraging. For example, although thymopentin (TP-5) was effective in reducing infectious mortality in animal studies, a controlled clinical trial of TP-5 in seriously burned patients failed to show any benefit (Waymack *et al.*, 1987). This was not completely surprising, since the primary effect of TP-5 is on cell-mediated immunity which is not critical in controlling acute bacterial infections.

TABLE 49.4
BIOLOGICAL RESPONSE MODIFIERS (BRM)

BRM*	Actions
Interleukin 1	T-cell activator
Interleukin 2	Augments T-cell proliferation and NK-cell cytoxicity
Interleukin 6	B-cell growth factor and hepatocyte stimulator
Interferons	Augment PMNs, macrophages, B and T cells
Colony-stimulating factors	Augment differentiation and function of PMNs and macrophages
Thymopentin	Stimulates T-cell proliferation and activates NK cells
Levamisole	Enhances PMN, macrophage and T-cell function
Glucan	Activates PMN, macrophage and T cells
C. parvum	Stimulates PMN, macrophage and T cells
Muramyl depeptide	Activates PMN, macrophage, B cell and NK cells

*This is only a partial list of BRMs and only selected major actions of each BMR are listed.

Since human and animal studies have documented a clear association, agents which enhance neutrophil and RES function are more likely to be effective in reducing the incidence of infection than agents whose primary effects are on cell-mediated immunity. In this regard, BRMs, such as the colony-stimulating factors or glucan, which increase macrophage and neutrophil bactericidal activity, appear to be potentially beneficial. Currently, human trials with these agents are in progress. Another option being investigated is the combined use of BRMs with antibiotics, the concept being that the BRM will function synergistically with the antibiotic by increasing the host's intrinsic antibacterial defence systems. The utility of this approach awaits clinical studies.

Since many of the lethal effects of gram-negative sepsis are due to endotoxin, interest in reducing the risk or biological consequences of systemic endotoxaemia is receiving increasing attention. In this regard, several different approaches have been taken to protect the host against endotoxaemia. These approaches include attempts to prevent or limit endotoxaemia as well as the use of drugs or antibodies, directly or indirectly, to neutralize the effects of endotoxin. Since endotoxin generally originates from the gut or from areas of localized infection, such as intra-abdominal abscesses or infected soft tissue, in order to prevent or limit endotoxaemia it is necessary to maintain intestinal barrier function and to prevent or treat infections. The judicious use of broad-spectrum antibiotics to reduce the risk of disruption of the normal gut flora, the use of enteral nutrition to prevent gut mucosal atrophy, and the avoidance of intestinal ischaemia appear to be critical elements in maintaining gut integrity. Prompt drainage of abscesses, early resection of necrotic tissue, optimal nutritional and physiological support and good infection control policies all play a role in the prevention or limitation of infectious complications. It is clear that the prevention of uncontrolled endotoxaemia is superior to attempts at its treatment.

In general, therapeutic manoeuvres to neutralize endotoxin have concentrated on the use of specific antisera, polyclonal and monoclonal antibodies, or drugs, such as polymixin B. All these therapeutic agents share one characteristic property: they bind directly to the endotoxin molecule and neutralize its biological activity. Recently, Munster *et al.* (1986) have evaluated the use of prophylactically administered polymyxin B to neutralize endotoxin and thereby reverse postburn immunosuppression. Although the results of this study are not conclusive, the concept is appealing. The use of specific agents to block or neutralize endotoxin-induced mediators from activated macrophages is in its infancy. However, this approach may be more widely used in the future. For example, it has been documented that inhibition of cyclo-oxygenase activity by ibuprofen

will attenuate the metabolic response to intravenous endotoxin in healthy human volunteers. Further work in this field is needed to determine if specific inhibitors or antibodies to endogenous mediators, such as TNF or PAF, will be clinically beneficial. The role of BRMs in the treatment of endotoxaemia is not clear, since experimentally BRMs, such as *C. Parvum*, that activate macrophages may predispose the host to endotoxic shock. Unfortunately, there is inadequate information available at present to reach any conclusions about the clinical efficacy of these potential agents in the treatment of endotoxaemia in humans.

Concepts in antibiotic use

Although a detailed review of the currently available antimicrobial agents and their spectrum of activity is beyond the scope of this chapter, no discussion of the mechanisms of infection would be complete without some discussion of the principles of antibiotic use as well as their limitations and liabilities. Antibiotics are two-edged swords. When used appropriately, they are effective in the prevention and treatment of certain infectious complications; however, they can also predispose to super-infections by inducing the emergence of antibiotic-resistant strains or by disrupting the host's indigenous (normal) microflora. The key to reducing the incidence of antibiotic-induced super-infections is to use the narrowest spectrum agents for the shortest time possible to achieve the desired clinical endpoint. In this regard, differentiating between prophylaxis and therapy is critical. However, this distinction can be difficult at times in the trauma victim where injury-induced bacterial contamination may have occurred. This point can best be illustrated in the patient undergoing laparotomy for blunt or penetrating trauma. Preoperatively, the patient receives antibiotics (generally a second generation cephalosporin, such as cefoxitin or cefotetan) which usually are stopped within 24 hours postoperatively if no or only mininimal bacterial contamination is found. However, if a major degree of contamination is present, such as from a colon injury, the antibiotics are generally continued for 3–5 days and in this situation they serve both prophylactic (wound) and therapeutic (peritoneum) roles.

A second principle that must be remembered is that antibiotics are only adjuvant agents in certain infections and that their effectiveness can be influenced by local factors. For example, certain antibiotics, such as the aminoglycosides, are inactivated by purulent material. Since many antibiotics as well as host phagocytic cells require oxygen for optimal activity, antibiotics play only an adjuvant role to drainage in the treatment of infections associated with a low oxygen tension such as abscesses. Likewise, antibiotics are secondary to surgical intervention in infections complicated by the presence of necrotic tissue or haematomas.

In seriously ill patients with suspected or diagnosed infections, antibiotic therapy must frequently be initiated empirically before the results of culture and sensitivity tests are available and, in some instances, even before samples can be obtained for culture. Which antibiotics should be used depends on the suspected site of infection and the organisms that commonly inhabit that location. However, antibiotic choice may have to be modified for patients likely to have an abnormal flora, such as patients who have received a previous course of antibiotics or patients who have become colonized with hospital-acquired pathogens. In these circumstances, antibiotic therapy is initiated with a single agent or combination of agents with the lowest possible toxicities, whose spectrum of activity is broad enough to cover all the suspected pathogens. This empirical therapy is modified as necessary based on the patient's clinical response and the results of bacterial culture and sensitivity tests. Since victims of major trauma are at increased risk of developing additional infections, it is mandatory that the antibiotics be stopped as soon as possible to limit the emergence of antibiotic-resistant bacteria and/or subsequent superinfections.

Even when these principles are followed, antibiotic-induced disruption of the indigenous microflora leading to colonization and subsequent superinfections with hospital-acquired pathogens may occur. In normal circumstances, modulation of the local environment by the indigenous microflora influences how many and which microorganisms can colonize that environment. This regulatory role of the indigenous microflora prevents non-indigenous microorganisms acquired from the external environment from establishing themselves as part of the normal microflora. This ability of the indigenous microflora to interfere with or antagonize the growth of exogenous bacteria and thereby prevent colonization, is referred to as 'colonization resistance'. Thus, the elimination of microorganisms responsible for colonization resistance by the use of prophylactic or therapeutic antibiotics promotes the colonization and multiplication of previously inhibited or newly acquired pathogens. In this way, antibiotics can predispose to superinfection with endogenous drug-resistant or hospital-acquired pathogens. Because of this risk and other side-effects, antibiotic therapy should be as specific as possible and antibiotics should not be used lightly.

Site-specific infections

To this point, the chapter has focused on clarifying the basic principles of immunobiology and discussing the relevance of bacterial and host factors to the development of infection. Little attention has been focused on the development of specific infectious complications, such as wound infections, nosocomial pneumonias or peritonitis. Each of these three infectious complications will be discussed individually for three reasons. First, they account for much of the infectious morbidity and mortality in the trauma victim. Second, their incidence or severity can be reduced by the clinician who understands the specific and unique factors that influence their development. Third, a discussion of the different factors that promote and prevent infection in these three different locations will help reinforce the specific concepts presented earlier in this chapter.

Wound infections

Nowhere else is the concept that clinical care can influence the incidence of infection better illustrated than in the surgical wound. As previously described, when bacteria breach the skin barrier, the humoral and cellular components of the non-specific inflammatory system are the major defence against the development of a wound infection with the neutrophil the primary effector cell. However, each neutrophil has a finite capacity to ingest and kill invading bacteria. Thus, the key to preventing a wound infection is to ensure that the number of bacteria present in the wound does not exceed the bactericidal capacity of the inflammatory response. Although, in any tissue, there will be a critical inoculum of bacteria that will cause an infection, as illustrated in Figure 49.8, this host–pathogen balance can be shifted in either direction. For example, the balance is shifted to favour the pathogen if factors important in host defences are reduced, such as oxygen delivery or tissue perfusion, or if bacterial growth is promoted, such as by the presence of necrotic tissue or haemoglobin.

Optimal tissue perfusion and oxygen delivery to the wound is critical in reducing the risk of a wound infection. For example, since the wound space is hypoxic with a Po_2 of 5–10 mmHg, and oxygen-mediated neutrophil bactericidal activity is reduced in low oxygen environments, especially when the Po_2 drops below 5 mmHg, it is possible to significantly augment neutrophil function and reduce the incidence of infection by increasing the inspired oxygen concentration above that of room air (Knighton et al., 1986). Maintaining an adequate intravascular volume to ensure tissue perfusion is also critical in preventing infection, since even small decreases in circulatory volume, which cause terminal capillaries at the wound–tissue interface to close, will increase the hypoxic zone and thereby potentiate bacterial growth. This concept is well illustrated by the clinical observations that ischaemia predisposes to infection of injured tissues and that fewer bacteria are required to cause an infection in patients who are in shock. Adequate removal of devitalized or injured tissue is also critical, since devitalized tissue acts as a foreign

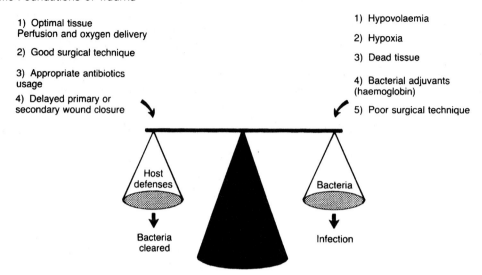

1) Optimal tissue
Perfusion and oxygen delivery

2) Good surgical technique

3) Appropriate antibiotics
usage

4) Delayed primary or
secondary wound closure

1) Hypovolaemia

2) Hypoxia

3) Dead tissue

4) Bacterial adjuvants
(haemoglobin)

5) Poor surgical technique

Host
defenses

Bacteria

Bacteria
cleared

Infection

Figure 49.8 Factors that shift the host–pathogen equation.

body and foreign bodies create an anoxic micro-environment that impairs the ability of the host to effectively clear invading or contaminating bacteria.

There are factors that influence the patient's ability to control a bacterial change over which the surgeon has no control, such as the magnitude of the injury, the immunosuppressive effects of the operative procedure or the patient's premorbid physiological status. However, the appropriate use of preoperative prophylactic antibiotics to bolster the host's antibacterial defences can frequently shift the host–pathogen equation in favour of the host. For these antibiotics to be fully effective, they must be administered parenterally in full doses prior to the operative procedure. Based on the classic and elegant studies of Burke (1961), it is now clear that prophylactic antibiotics must be present in the wound prior to bacterial challenge to be optimally effective. Nevertheless, in some circumstances, the bacterial inoculum will be clearly too high to be controlled by host defences even when augmented with antibiotics. Thus, in the situation of the heavily contaminated wound, consideration should be given to delayed primary wound closure or healing by secondary intention. By ensuring that the wound is not closed over a bacterial inoculum that would almost certainly cause an infection, the incidence and consequences of wound infection can be reduced.

Nosocomial pneumonia

Nosocomial pneumonias occur in less than 1% of all hospitalized patients. However, the incidence of this complication approaches 15% in the postoperative patient and exceeds 25% in the ICU patient, especially if mechanical ventilation is required. These postoperative or ICU pneumonias differ from community-acquired pneumonias in that many are polymicrobial and the majority are caused by *Staphylococcus aureus* or gram-negative bacteria, such as *Pseudomonas aeruginosa, Klebsiella* sp., *Escherichia coli, Enterobacter* sp. or *Proteus* sp. Since the mortality rate of gram-negative nosocomial pneumonia approaches or exceeds 50% in most reported series, and this infectious complication is relatively common after trauma, a thorough understanding of the pathophysiology of nosocomial pneumonias is of obvious clinical importance.

Although the pathogens causing pneumonia in these patients may reach the patient via contaminated ventilator circuits or via the hands of the hospital staff, in most instances, the most common mechanism is by the aspiration of bacteria colonizing the patient's oropharynx or stomach. In normal circumstances, the oropharynx is colonized with a mixed flora of aerobic plus facultative and strict anaerobic bacteria, while the trachea and distal respiratory tract are sterile. Although low numbers of gram-negative aerobic bacilli, *S. aureus*, or yeast may transiently be found in the oropharynx of the normal individual, these potential pathogens are prevented from reaching high numbers and permanently colonizing the oropharynx by the host's defence systems functioning in concert with the indigenous microflora. As outlined in Figure 49.9, oropharyngeal colonization with gram-negative bacilli and *S. aureus* commonly occurs within 24–96 hours of admission to the hospital and is the first step in the development of pneumonia.

The two most common factors associated with colonization of the oropharynx with potential pathogens are the use of antibiotics, which decrease colonization resistance of the oropharynx, and agents, such as antacids or H_2 blockers, which by

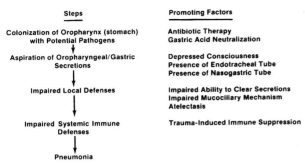

**Sequence of Events in
the Development of Nosocomial Pneumonia**

Steps	Promoting Factors
Colonization of Oropharynx (stomach) with Potential Pathogens	Antibiotic Therapy Gastric Acid Neutralization
Aspiration of Oropharyngeal/Gastric Secretions	Depressed Consciousness Presence of Endotracheal Tube Presence of Nasogastric Tube
Impaired Local Defenses	Impaired Ability to Clear Secretions Impaired Mucociliary Mechanism Atelectasis
Impaired Systemic Immune Defenses	Trauma-Induced Immune Suppression
Pneumonia	

Figure 49.9 The development of nosocomial pneumonia.

neutralizing gastric acidity promote bacterial colonization of the normally sterile stomach. Since the population level of bacteria colonizing the oropharynx is about 10^8 per ml, even a small degree of aspiration can lead to a large bacterial challenge. Thus, conditions that promote aspiration, such as a depressed level of consciousness (diminished gag reflex), or the presence of an endotracheal or nasogastric tube, increase the risk of the development of pneumonia. Once the lower respiratory tract has become colonized with aspirated organisms, impaired local defence mechanisms, especially the inability to cough and clear secretions, allow the aspirated organisms to multiply and potentially develop into a deep lung infection. This failure of the local defences is especially important in the pathogenesis of pulmonary infection in the trauma victim since, in these patients, multiple arms of the local and systemic inflammatory and immune defences are impaired.

Knowledge of the factors promoting or potentiating the development of nosocomial pneumonias is important, since this information serves as the basis for therapeutic options directed at preventing this complication. For example, knowledge that gastric bacterial colonization leads to oropharyngeal and trachea colonization and potentiates the development of pneumonia (especially in intubated patients) has led to a major change in stress ulcer prophylaxis (Driks *et al.*, 1987). In this regard, the use of sucralfate rather than antacids or H_2 blockers appears to reduce the incidence of pneumonia by preventing upper gastrointestinal bacterial overgrowth. Similarly, topical hypopharyngeal and oral antibiotics have been utilized to reduce the incidence of pneumonias in trauma victims by preventing or limiting oropharyngeal and upper gastrointestinal colonization with potential pathogens (Stoutenbeek *et al.*, 1987). Furthermore, since the development of pneumonia is potentiated by factors that promote pulmonary stasis and impair the clearance of secretions, manoeuvres that facilitate ambulation and encourage effective coughing are

critical in these patients. These range from good pulmonary toilet, early definitive surgery (including operative stabilization of fractures which allows earlier extubation and ambulation), and the avoidance of excessive sedation (prevents impairment of the cough reflex), to the provision of adequate analgesia in patients with abdominal or thoracic pain (promotes effective coughing). Maintenance of a good cough reflex cannot be stressed too forcefully, since it is one of the principal means by which the airways are cleared of foreign materials, excessive secretions and contaminating microorganisms.

Postoperative peritonitis

Principles of the management of penetrating or blunt trauma to the abdomen are discussed elsewhere in this text. Nevertheless, in spite of appropriate initial surgical therapy, postoperative intraabdominal infections remain a common cause of morbidity and mortality in the trauma victim.

In normal circumstances, the peritoneal cavity is relatively resistant to a bacterial challenge, since following bacterial contamination a series of events is initiated that will eradicate or localize and thereby minimize bacterial spread. The first step in this process is the initiation of a local inflammatory response, which is mediated by the release of histamine and other vasoactive factors by resident mesothelial cells. These stimulated mesothelial cells also release thromboplastin, which converts the fibrinogen present in the inflammatory exudate into fibrin, the net effect of which is the deposition of fibrinous exudates that serve to localize and trap the contaminating bacteria. Bacterial localization and trapping are further facilitated by the development of an adynamic ileus and the adherence of contiguous bowel and omentum to the sticky, fibrinous adhesions. As elsewhere in the body, the humoral factors produced during the inflammatory response serve to activate and attract phagocytic cells (initially resident macrophages and subsequently neutrophils) to the inflammatory focus. In addition, these humoral factors, especially components of the complement system, enhance bacterial opsonization and facilitate bacterial phagocytosis and intracellular killing by the recruited phagocytes.

In addition to the inflammatory response, the peritoneum protects itself against contaminating bacteria by mechanically clearing these bacteria. In contrast to fluids and solutes, which cross the peritoneal membrane, particulate material and bacteria are cleared exclusively through fenestrations that overlie lymphatic channels within the diaphragm. Based on experimental studies, it appears that bacterial clearance via the diaphragmatic lymphatics is a very rapid process, since within a few minutes of an intraperitoneal bacterial challenge, bacteria can be recovered from the thoracic duct and blood stream. In fact, it is this diaphragmatic clearance mechanism that seems to be the cause of bacteraemia in patients with intra-abdominal infections. Thus, the three major defence mechanisms involved in controlling or eradicating intraperitoneal bacteria are: (1) the mechanical clearance of bacteria by the diaphragmatic lymphatics; (2) the physical localization of the invading bacteria; and (3) the ingestion of bacteria by phagocytes.

The effectiveness of these peritoneal host defences in eradicating contaminating or residual bacteria in the absence of microbial adjuvants or the presence of a continuing source of bacterial seeding is well documented both clinically and experimentally. However, in the presence of factors that impair host defences or facilitate bacterial growth or virulence, the balance will be shifted in favour of infection. One of the best studied and most clinically relevant adjuvant agent which potentiates infection is haemoglobin. Although the exact mechanisms by which it potentiates infection remains to be defined, it appears to both promote bacterial growth and impair phagocyte function. Other substances, such as faeces or bile salts, as well as necrotic tissue, also seem to potentiate infection. In addition to these endogenous adjuvants, exogenous materials, such as drains, suture material or haemostatic agents potentiate infection by acting as foreign bodies. Thus, one major principle in the prevention or treatment of intra-abdominal sepsis is the removal of adjuvant substances from the peritoneal cavity that might interfere with normal host-defence mechanisms. In this regard, meticulous haemostasis, debridement of devitalized tissue, copious lavage to remove blood and other adjuvants, plus the avoidance of foreign bodies may help reduce the incidence of postoperative intra-abdominal infections.

Thus, although the peritoneal cavity is relatively resistant to a bacterial challenge, in the presence of adjuvant substances, such as fibrin or haemoglobin, bacteria can overcome normal host defences, and intra-abdominal infection results. To put the process of intra-abdominal sepsis into perspective, it is useful to view the various types of abdominal infections (peritonitis, phlegmon, abscess) as a continuum. This point is illustrated by considering what occurs when a colonic anastamosis leaks. First, the peritoneal host defences attempt to isolate the site of bacterial contamination from the rest of the peritoneal cavity. This is accomplished by the induction of a local inflammatory response with the resultant influx of neutrophils and the deposition of fibrin to trap the invading bacteria and to help seal the site of perforation. If the locally deposited fibrin, with the aid of the omentum and surrounding viscera, can wall off the colonic leak, a generalized peritonitis does not occur. Instead, a phlegmon or abscess develops, which generally requires debridement or drainage, although in some circum-

stances, local host defences in conjunction with antibiotics can lead to complete resolution of the inflammatory process. None the less, even in the best of circumstances, this inflammatory response results in the formation of adhesions, which may cause problems in the future.

THE GUT AS A RESERVOIR FOR SYSTEMIC INFECTIONS

Although the originating site or focus of infection can be identified in most patients, there is an increasing number of patients with bacteraemia in whom a source of infection is never found even at autopsy. For example, Goris *et al.* (1985) reported that no septic focus could be identified either clinically or at autopsy in more than 30% of their bacteraemic patients dying of sepsis and multiple organ failure. The fact that many of these bacteraemic patients are infected with bacteria that are normally found within the GI tract suggests that these infections may have originated there. The concept of the intestinal tract as a source or reservoir for bacterial infections is consistent with recent experimental studies by Deitch and Berg documenting that under certain conditions bacteria contained within the gut will cross the mucosal barrier to cause systemic infections, a process termed 'bacterial translocation' (Deitch, 1988).

Clinical evidence

Some of the earliest clinical studies documenting that bacteria and endotoxin from the gut may gain access to the systemic circulation were performed in the 1960s. However, the work was largely ignored and the concept that the gut can be a reservoir for portal or systemic bacteraemia or endotoxaemia fell into disfavour. Only to be resurrected by the results of epidemiological studies which showed that the reservoir of intestinal organisms was a clinically important source for bacteria and fungi which caused systemic infection in several immunocompromised patient populations including victims of trauma. This relationship between gut-associated microorganisms and systemic infection was based on surveillance cultures documenting that the bacterial serotypes causing infection were the same as those contained in the patient's stool samples. Once the gut was identified as a reservoir for bacteria causing systemic infections, several groups of investigators attempted to reduce the incidence of infection in these high-risk patients by prophylactic treatment with oral antibiotics.

The earliest clinical trials attempted to reduce the incidence of nosocomial infections in cancer patients receiving chemotherapy by sterilizing the gut with broad-spectrum oral antibiotics. This approach was not successful due to the emergence of antibiotic-resistant enteric bacteria. The realization that it is not possible to sterilize the gut, plus the fact that broad-spectrum antibiotics suppress not only potentially pathogenic microorganisms, such as enteric bacilli, but also the non-pathogenic strict anaerobes which may be protective, led to the development of a policy of selective antibiotic decontamination of the gut. This approach was based largely on the experimental work of van der Waaij, who documented that anaerobic intestinal microflora play a protective role in preventing intestinally based systemic infections and termed this 'colonization resistance' (van der Waaij *et al.*, 1971).

In most studies, the use of prophylactic oral antibiotics to selectively decontaminate the gut significantly reduced the incidence of lethal and non-lethal infections but their effect on overall survival was less consistent. For example, a recent prospective trial in trauma patients indicates that selective antibiotic decontamination of the gut in combination with topical hypopharyngeal antibiotics will reduce the incidence of primary bacter-aemias, respiratory tract, urinary tract and wound infections (Stoutenbeek *et al.*, 1987). However, the decreased incidence of systemic infections was not associated with an improvement in overall survival. Similar results were recently reported in two prospective randomized trials of selective gut decontamination involving a total of 420 ICU patients. Thus, gut decontamination is unlikely by itself to significantly improve survival.

Although clinical studies (Tancrede *et al.*, 1985; Border *et al.*, 1987; Stoutenbeek *et al.*, 1987; Deitch, 1988) have established that the gut can be a reservoir for systemic infections after trauma, there has been little information on the underlying mechanisms of how bacteria contained within the gut translocate across the mucosal barrier. Therefore, we and others have investigated the relationships between the GI tract microflora, host defences and injury to clarify the mechanisms by which bacteria contained with the GI tract translocate from the gut to cause systemic infections. Prior to presenting the results of these experimental studies, the major antibacterial defences of the gut will be reviewed.

Normal intestinal and hepatic antibacterial defences

The gut contains high concentrations of bacteria and endotoxin that must be excluded, in addition to nutrients that must be selectively absorbed. Therefore, the host has developed multiple defence mechanisms that function together to prevent intestinal bacteria and endotoxin from reaching systemic organs and tissues (Table 49.5). These include mechanical and immunological defences and the stabilizing influence of a normal intestinal microflora.

TABLE 49.5

INTESTINAL ANTIBACTERIAL AND ANTI-ENDOTOXIN HOST DEFENCES

Mechanical
  Intestinal peristalsis
  Mucous production
  Epithelial desquamation
  Epithelial barrier
Bacterial
  Colonization resistance
  Bacterial antagonism
Immunological
  Secretory immunoglobulins
  GALT system
Hepatobiliary
  Bile salts
  RES function
Other
  Gastric acidity

An initial step in the translocation of bacteria from the intestinal tract appears to be the adherence or close association of bacteria to the epithelial cell surface or to ulcerated areas of the intestinal mucosa. The mechanical defences of the intestine limit the ability of bacteria to reach or cross the epithelial mucosal barrier. For example, in the small intestine, normal peristalsis prevents the prolonged stasis of bacteria in close proximity to the intestinal mucosa and thereby reduces the chances that any individual bacterium will have adequate time to penetrate the mucous layer and attach to the epithelium. If the peristaltic clearing of bacteria is altered, either by mechanical obstruction or the development of an ileus, bacterial stasis occurs. In this circumstance, bacteria will have an increased opportunity to penetrate the mucous layer and adhere directly to the epithelial mucosa. Therefore, under normal conditions, the combination of peristaltic waves and the mucous layer serve to limit the direct attachment of bacteria to the intestinal mucosa.

Certain bacteria normally colonizing the gut, especially the obligate anaerobic bacteria, act synergistically with the host's mechanical defences to limit growth and epithelial attachment of potential pathogens (i.e. colonization resistance). The obligate anaerobes not only are the most numerous bacteria within the gut, but they appear to play an important role in colonization resistance, since they associate closely with the intestinal epithelium and are thought to form a barrier that limits the direct attachment of potential pathogens to the mucosa. This anaerobic bacterial barrier is lost when broad-spectrum antibiotics are administered since the obligate anaerobes are in general more sensitive to antibiotic suppression than the rest of the intestinal microflora.

The intestinal immune system, known as the gut-associated lymphoid tissue (GALT), consists of Peyer's patches, lymphoid follicles, lamina propria lymphocytes, intraepithelial lymphocytes and cells of the mesenteric lymph nodes. The gut lymphoid tissue contains the same full repertoire of lymphocytes and macrophage subsets as the systemic immune system. These intestinal lymphocyte subsets regulate the local immune response to soluble and particulate oral antigens, such as bacteria and endotoxin. The exact role of the immune system in preventing bacterial adherence and translocation is not clear, although it is generally accepted that secretory immunoglobulins (IgA and IgM) play a major role in the defence against mucosal invasion by bacteria. Secretory IgA is unique among the various classes of immunoglobulins in that it binds to bacteria but does not activate the effector arms of the immune system. In this way, secretory IgA can bind to bacteria and prevent their attachment to epithelial cells without creating a local inflammatory response, which might impair the normal absorptive processes of the gut.

Much less is known about intestinal anti-endotoxin defences than the antibacterial defences of the gut. The presence of bile within the intestinal tract appears to be a major factor responsible for preventing the escape of endotoxin from the gut. Bile salts appear to prevent portal endotoxaemia by binding directly to intraluminal endotoxin and forming detergent-like complexes which are poorly absorbed. Thus, conditions that decrease bile flow or increase intestinal permeability may lead to increased portal endotoxaemia. Although portal endotoxaemia may sporadically occur even in normal circumstances, systemic endotoxaemia does not follow unless the RES function of the liver has been impaired.

Experimental results: animal studies

In order to study the phenomenon of bacterial translocation, *in vivo* animal models have been developed. In these, the blood, peritoneal cavities and organs (mesenteric lymph node complex, liver, and spleen) were harvested and quantitatively cultured for translocating bacteria. The mesenteric lymph node complex (MLN) consists of an aggregated group of lymph nodes that drain most of the small intestine, caecum and proximal colon. Since the MLNs are normally sterile, the presence of bacteria in these nodes as well as other systemic organs is a sensitive marker of bacterial translocation.

Although bacterial translocation can be induced in a variety of animal models, it appears that at least one of three basic pathophysiological factors must be present for bacterial translocation to occur. These three promoting factors are: (1) disruption of the ecological balance of the intestinal microflora

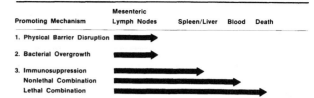

Figure 49.10 Diagram illustrating combined injuries interacting synergistically to promote systemic infection.

resulting in overgrowth with certain bacteria (especially, enteric bacilli); (2) impaired host immune defences; and (3) physical disruption or impairment of the gut mucosal barrier.

A second important concept that has evolved from these studies is that bacterial translocation is not an all or none phenomenon. Disruption or impairment of a single major intestinal defence system will consistently promote bacterial translocation to the mesenteric lymph node and occasionally to the liver or spleen; however, the bacteria do not usually multiply in the mesenteric lymph node or spread systemically. Instead, they are locally contained and eventually eradicated as the animal recovers. In conditions that more closely mimic the clinical situation, in which the animal receives several simultaneous or sequential insults, translocating bacteria not only reach the mesenteric lymph nodes but also invade systemic organs and the blood stream. In some of these combined injury models, the majority of the animals survive, although bacteria can be transiently cultured from their RES organs. In other models, death frequently occurs from the translocating bacteria. This concept is shown schematically in Figure 49.10 and has been reviewed by Deitch (1988). To more clearly illustrate the phenomenon of bacterial translocation, the results of some specific experiments will be presented.

Non-lethal burn injuries were chosen as the initial model to examine the relationship between trauma and bacterial translocation, since by altering the size of the burn injury, the effect of varying levels of trauma on gut barrier function could be assessed. In these initial experiments, bacterial translocation occurred only in rats receiving major (40% TBSA) burns, indicating that bacterial translocation does not occur routinely after trauma in otherwise healthy animals with a normal gut flora. However, when the gut flora was disrupted resulting in bacterial overgrowth with *E. coli* C25, the burned animals could not prevent the systemic spread of translocating bacteria as well as control uninjured animals whose gut flora were similarly disrupted (Table 49.6).

Because of the clinical association between hypotension, infection, and the development of multiple

TABLE 49.6

INCIDENCE (%) AND MAGNITUDE OF BACTERIAL TRANSLOCATION IN ANTIBIOTIC-DECONTAMINATED MICE AND RATS COLONIZED WITH *E. COLI* C25 SUBJECTED TO SHAM OR BURN INJURY

Group	MLN	Spleen	Liver	Blood	CFU/MLN*
Mice					
Sham burn	77%	3%	49%	0	5.3
30% burn	100%	60%	90%	25%	73 000
P values	NS	< 0.01	< 0.01	< 0.05	< 0.0001
Rats					
Sham burn	100%	11%	22%	0%	600
40% burn	100%	100%	100%	0%	142 000
P values	NS	< 0.01	< 0.01	NS	< 0.001

*Mean colony-forming units (CFU) of bacteria per mesenteric lymph node (MLN). NS = not significant.

organ failure, the effects of limited periods of haemorrhagic shock (30, 60 or 90 minutes at 30 mmHg) on intestinal barrier function were tested. Bacteria were translocated to the MLNs of all three groups of shocked rats, although the rats subjected to 90 minutes of shock had more mucosal damage and a higher incidence of translocating bacteria in their livers, spleens and blood streams than rats subjected to the shorter periods of shock. Haemorrhagic shock appeared to promote bacterial translocation by injuring the intestinal mucosa (Figure 49.11). In fact, the histological appearance of the ileal and caecal mucosa of the shocked rats was similar to that documented in humans experiencing periods of hypotension. The mechanisms of mucosal injury and bacterial translocation appeared to be mediated through a pathway involving xanthine oxidase-generated oxidants, since oxygen radical scavengers as well as drugs which prevented xanthine oxidase activation largely prevented mucosal injury and reduced the incidence of shock-induced bacterial translocation (Figure 49.11) (Deitch *et al.*, 1988). Although the mechanism primarily responsible for promoting bacterial translocation after 30 minutes of haemorrhagic shock appears to be a reperfusion injury related to xanthine oxidase activation, based on other experimental studies (Rush *et al.*, 1988), ischaemia-induced tissue hypoxia may be more important when gut hypoperfusion persists for longer periods.

The effect of endotoxaemia, alone and in combination with other insults, on bacterial translocation was also investigated, since endotoxaemia is relatively common after thermal or mechanical trauma,

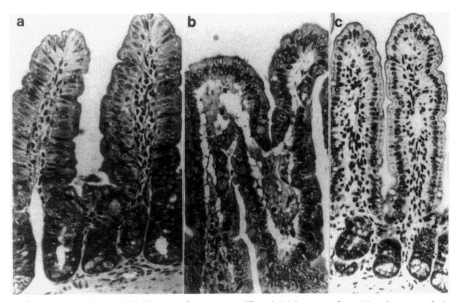

Figure 49.11 (a) Control rat ileum. (b) Ileum of a rat sacrificed 24 hours after 30 minutes of shock. The lamina propria is oedematous and the epithelial mucosa is being lifted off the lamina propria. (c) Ileum of a rat pretreated with an inactivator of xanthine oxidase. The villi and lamina propria appear normal. (× 260.)

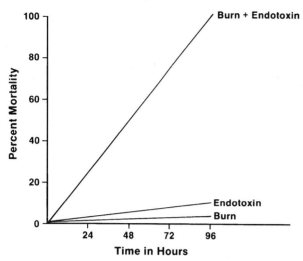

Figure 49.12 Mortality rates of mice receiving endotoxin plus burn was significantly greater than mice receiving endotoxin or burn only.

is associated with conditions leading to multiple systems organ failure, may increase intestinal permeability, and impair host defences. In mice with a normal gut flora, non-lethal doses of endotoxin consistently promote bacterial translocation to the MLN. However, the translocated bacteria remained localized and did not spread to other systemic organs, tissues or to the blood stream. In contrast, the same non-lethal dose of endotoxin caused systemic spread of translocating bacteria to the liver, spleen and blood stream of thermally injured mice. Furthermore, the mortality rate of mice receiving only endotoxin or only a thermal injury was less than 10%, while the combination of endotoxin plus a thermal injury increased the mortality rate to 100% (Figure 49.12). The results in protein-malnourished animals challenged with endotoxin were similar to those observed in the burned animals. Thus, it appears that the combination of endotoxin plus either a thermal injury or a protein-malnourished state results in a rapidly fatal septic syndrome that originates from bacteria inhabiting the gut. Furthermore, in a fashion similar to haemorrhagic shock, endotoxin appears to promote mucosal injury and bacterial translocation through an ischaemia-reperfusion injury mediated by xanthine oxidase-generated oxidants.

Because nutritional deficiencies are relatively common and may impair the normal antibacterial defences of the gut as well as predispose to infection, increasing attention has focused on the relationship between malnutrition and loss of intestinal barrier function. Currently it appears that parenteral alimentation or the enteral administration of certain elemental diets will lead to loss of intestinal barrier function and bacterial translocation (Deitch, 1990). Although the mechanisms by which these diets cause loss of barrier function have not been fully worked out, there appears to be some evidence that barrier function can be bolstered by the administration of glutamine or non-absorbable dietary fibres. Dietary fibre may be beneficial since it is important in maintaining the normal ecological balance of the gut microflora and bacterial fermentation end products of fibre are trophic for intestinal epithelial cells. Glutamine's protective role in maintaining intestinal barrier function (especially during stress states) may be related to the fact that it is the major fuel for enterocytes as well as immune effector cells, such as lymphocytes and macrophages.

There is also evidence that bacteria can translocate across the histologically intact mucosal barrier to invade abdominal abscesses or sterile abdominal inflammatory lesions. However, the mechanisms by which intestinal bacteria translocate to abdominal fluid collections has not been determined. In fact, the routes by which the translocating bacteria reach the MLN, liver, spleen and blood stream once the bacteria have breached the mucosal barrier and reached the lamina propria are not known with certainty, although it appears that these bacteria can leave the gut both via the portal blood and the mesenteric lymphatics.

Experimental results: human studies

Human data on bacterial translocation to the MLNs are extremely limited. We recently documented that MLNs obtained at laparotomy from patients undergoing elective surgery rarely contain bacteria (1 of 25 patients) (Deitch, 1989). In contrast, 10 of 17 (59%) patients operated on for simple intestinal obstruction had viable bacteria in their MLNs, although none had necrotic bowel and cultures of their peritoneal cavities were sterile. The result of this study was similar to that reported in patients with Crohn's disease in which 33% of the lymph nodes from the Crohn's patients contained bacteria, while only 5% of the patients without Crohn's disease had viable bacteria in their MLNs. Most recently, Moore *et al.* (1991) found that about one-third of trauma victims had bacteria in their MLNs at laparotomy, although their portal blood was sterile. Finally, based on clinical studies and an anecdotal report in which candida was recovered from the blood and urine of a volunteer who drank a large quantity of *Candida albicans*, it appears that candida also translocates from the gut in humans.

In addition to these studies, three clinical reports have appeared indicating that intestinal permeability is increased in patients during an infectious episode, shortly after a major thermal injury or in healthy volunteers receiving a single dose of endotoxin. Additionally, bacteria have been cultured from the blood of hypotensive victims of blunt trauma upon presentation to the emergency room. Thus, the limited direct clinical information that is available supports the concept that bacterial translocation does occur in humans.

Therapeutic options directed towards preventing bacterial translocation and bolstering intestinal barrier function are discussed in the next section on multiple organ failure.

MULTIPLE SYSTEMS ORGAN FAILURE

Recognition of the multiple organ failure syndrome (MOFS) as a distinct clinical entity is a relatively recent event dating from the mid-1970s (Baire, 1975). Since that time, multiple organ failure (MOF) has emerged as a common final pathway leading to death in a wide variety of patients including the trauma victim. The development of organ failure in this syndrome is unusual, since in MOF the organs that fail are not limited to or even necessarily involved in the original injury or infection. Instead, MOFS appears to be a stereotyped response to a major physiological insult, in which the sequence of organ failure follows a largely predictable course (Fry, 1988). Although MOFS has been the focus of extensive clinical and laboratory studies over the past decade, the exact mechanisms responsible for the development or perpetuation of this syndrome remain uncertain.

In evaluating any of the current hypotheses proposed to explain the development of MOF, several clinical observations must be considered. First, in most patients who develop MOFS, the organs that fail are not necessarily directly injured or involved in the primary disease process. Additionally, there is generally a lag period of days to weeks between the initial physiological insult and the clinical appearance of distant organ dysfunction. These two clinical observations strongly suggest that MOFS is a systemic process mediated by endogenous or exogenous circulating factor(s), whose effects are not clinically evident immediately after the initiating insult. These findings, plus the fact that patients appear clinically septic and many have untreated septic foci, prompted investigators in the late 1970s to propose that MOF was the external expression of a septic syndrome due to an occult septic focus (usually intra-abdominal).

Although it is clear that an untreated focus of infection is a common cause of MOF, as more patients underwent empirical exploration in search of occult intra-abdominal abscesses, it became clear that MOF could exist in the absence of an identifiable focus of infection. The fact that many patients dying of sepsis and MOF have enteric bacteraemias for which no septic focus can be identified clinically or at autopsy (Goris *et al.*, 1985) has led some investigators to postulate that the infections originated from the gut (Deitch, 1990). Gut barrier failure may also contribute to MOF in the subgroup of 'uninfected' patients with MOF who die with clinical features akin to those of sepsis. In these, gut barrier failure may contribute to the development of MOF by allowing endotoxin normally contained within the gut to reach the portal and systemic circulations where it helps to produce the septic process. Thus, gut-derived endotoxin may be the link between gut failure and MOF in the septic-appearing patient without microbiological evidence of infection. Therefore, although uncontrolled infection is the most common initiator of MOF, it appears that it can occur in the absence of an established focus of infection or even in the absence of microbiological evidence of infection.

One point deserving special emphasis is the physiological similarities between systemic infection (sepsis), MOF and a septic state in which there is no evidence of infection. The observation that patients displaying systemic signs of infection may not have underlying infections has led many investigators and clinicians to adopt the term 'septic state' to describe this syndrome. In fact, it is frequently impossible to clinically differentiate the patient with systemic infection from the patient who appears septic (septic state) but does not have microbiological evidence of systemic infection. All three states appear to share certain physiological similarities, such as altered intermediary metabolism, a hyperdynamic state and signs of systemic inflammation. Thus, it appears likely that the mediators responsible for the external expression of these three clinical syndromes are similar.

Although the exact cause of MOF is not known, certain associations appear clear. The development of MOF is most commonly associated with one or more of the following clinical conditions; infection (endotoxaemia), trauma with retained necrotic tissue or shock. All three of these clinical conditions are associated with distant organ injury and theoretically can initiate distant organ failure in a number of ways. They can impair gut barrier function resulting in systemic endotoxaemia or bacteraemia, generate or induce the release of endogenous mediators, promote reticuloendothelial system dysfunction, or disrupt oxygen delivery to the tissues. Although the

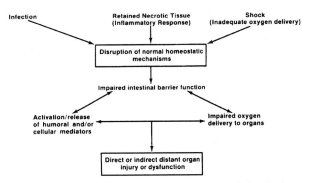

Figure 49.13 Diagram illustrating potential relationships between initiating events and effector systems in the pathogenesis of multiple organ failure.

author's own bias is that gut barrier failure, especially in conjunction with hepatic dysfunction, plays a key role in promoting or potentiating the development of MOF in many patients, it is likely that these and other mechanisms interact to produce organ failure. Figure 49.13 schematically outlines a simpled version of how this could occur.

First, there is an initiating clinical event that disrupts multiple normal homoeostatic mechanisms. These then interact to amplify or modulate each other. For example, during shock oxygen delivery to the gut is impaired resulting in increased intestinal permeability. Increased permeability of the gut subsequently results in luminal bacteria and endotoxin reaching the portal and systemic circulations, where they activate resident macrophages and circulating neutrophils, as well as multiple humoral plasma protein cascades. Products of these in turn may further impair oxygen deliver by their effects on the microcirculation, as well as potentiate the continued translocation of products from the gut by increasing the degree of intestinal permeability. A similar scenario may occur during infectious or inflammatory states where activation of endogenous inflammatory mediators may lead to changes in tissue oxygen delivery as well as impair intestinal barrier function. Therefore, it appears that under the right conditions, the cumulative disruption of multiple interacting systems may ultimately result in distant organ injury. A necessary corollary of this multifactorial hypothesis of MOF is that treatment must also be multimodal. Therefore, based on the current limited understanding of MOF, it is unlikely that any single therapeutic manoeuvre will be fully effective in treatment or prevention.

In the previous section of this chapter on bacterial translocation and gut barrier failure, clinical and experimental evidence supporting the concept that failure of intestinal barrier function promotes a 'septic state' was presented. This information plus knowledge that endotoxin exerts a profound effect on many other organ systems, including the lung, kidney and liver, as well as the immune and cardiovascular systems, supports the hypothesis that MOF may be directly or indirectly related to the uncontrolled escape of bacteria and/or endotoxin from the intestine.

Evidence for the gut–liver axis in multiple organ failure

There is increasing evidence that a clinically important relationship may exist between the state of intestinal barrier function and Kupffer cell activity. Since the hepatic reticuloendothelial system (Kupffer cells) appears to play a role in the clearance of translocating bacteria or endotoxin from the portal blood, impaired hepatic RES activity could potentiate the systemic effects of gut barrier failure by allowing gut-derived bacteria or

endotoxin to reach the systemic circulation. In addition, the presence of bacteria and endotoxin in the portal circulation would promote hepatic macrophages to secrete various factors, including cytokines, oxidants and proteases. These macrophage-derived products may directly injure or alter hepatocyte function and in concert with other soluble or cellular factors exacerbate the septic state and lead to impaired distant organ function. In this manner, the gut–liver axis may promote or potentiate the development or progression of MOF.

Clinically, the development of established MOF is preceded by a phase of persistent hypermetabolism which is usually associated with some degree of respiratory dysfunction. Progression of this syndrome is characterized first by a rising bilirubin and clinical evidence of liver dysfunction followed by a rising creatinine and progressive renal failure. The hypothesis that loss of intestinal barrier function and the escape of bacteria and endotoxin induce a hypermetabolic response is consistent with experimental observations that endotoxin infused through the portal vein will induce a hypermetabolic response and that immediate enteral feeding blunts the hypermetabolic response after thermal injury (Mochizuki et al., 1984). Since immediate enteral feeding also maintains gut mass and prevents the excessive secretion of catabolic hormones, a possible mechanism is that intestinal barrier function is maintained and translocation of bacteria or endotoxin into the portal or systemic circulations with consequent hypermetabolism prevented. Further studies are necessary to verify these findings and conclusions.

Thus, there is evidence to suggest that alterations in intestinal barrier function leading to excessive portal endotoxaemia or bacteraemia may contribute to hepatic dysfunction. Similarly, impaired hepatic dysfunction resulting in decreased bile flow and systemic endotoxaemia could additionally compromise intestinal barrier function leading to the further leak of bacteria and endotoxin from the gut. In this way dysfunction of various aspects of the gut–liver axis could initiate a vicious cycle of hepatic injury and bacterial (endotoxin) translocation. Furthermore, in circumstances where RES activity is impaired, spillover of intestinal and other antigens into the systemic circulation may occur. For example, portal and systemic endotoxaemia are relatively common in patients with obstructive jaundice, cirrhosis and acute or chronic liver disease. Additionally, Border et al. (1987) have documented in blunt trauma patients that the appearance of bacteraemia of gut origin occurs only after clinical evidence of liver dysfunction is apparent. In this fashion, impaired hepatic RES activity could potentiate the systemic effects of gut barrier failure by allowing gut-derived bacteria or endotoxin to reach the systemic circulation leading to the injury of other organs. In addition, the presence of bacteria and endotoxin in the portal circulation would promote hepatic macrophages to secrete various factors into the systemic circulation that may further exacerbate distant organ function.

In this chapter, no attempt has been made to discuss all the proposed mechanisms, potential mediators or effector systems involved in the pathogenesis of distant organ injury after failure of the gut–liver axis. Yet, it appears clear that the development or progression of MOF and distant organ injury represents the summation of many interacting factors and is not due to alterations in a single system. In cases where elements of the gut–liver axis have failed, endotoxin or bacteria appear to be the initial triggers that initiate the cascade of events leading to MOF. Once this has taken place, multiple systems are incorporated into the process including neutrophils, macrophages, platelets and their products, as well as products of the complement and coagulation cascades plus a host of other soluble factors. The products of these activated cellular and humoral systems, such as the cytokines, the third component of complement, and activated Hageman's factor in turn activate and recruit other potential effectors of organ injury.

Therapeutic concepts

Many, if not all, of the defences that prevent bacteria and endotoxin from escaping from the gut are impaired in trauma victims. These patients are frequently immunosuppressed and the antibiotic regimens they receive may disrupt the normal ecology of the gut microflora resulting in impaired colonization resistance and subsequent bacterial overgrowth with potential pathogens. Therapeutic regimens, such as prophylactic and therapeutic H_2 blockers or antacid therapy to alkalinize the stomach, may result in the colonization of the stomach with bacteria due to the increased survival of orally ingested bacteria. Hyperosmolar enteral or parenteral feedings may not only disrupt the normal bacterial ecology of the gut but also result in mucosal atrophy and altered intestinal mechanical defences. The hypoalbuminaemia and capillary leak syndrome that commonly occur in these patients can result in intestinal oedema, impaired jejunoileal peristalsis, intestinal stasis, bacterial overgrowth and altered intestinal permeability. These and other changes can easily be seen to theoretically promote the failure of the gut barrier to bacteria and endotoxin.

It is not surprising that attempts to control the gut flora by selective decontamination may not increase survival, since the patients enrolled in these studies are almost always immunosuppressed and their intestinal barrier function is impaired. In fact, based on the experimental work presented earlier, it appears that neither the maintenance of a normal gut flora nor selective decontamination of the gut will prevent gut-origin sepsis if the mucosal barrier is mechanically disrupted or the animal is severely immunocompromised. What this means clinically is that selective decontamination of the gut microflora is unlikely to be fully effective in patients with a damaged intestinal mucosa or profound immune suppression. More is required. Attention must be focused on ways to bolster the host's local and systemic antibacterial defence systems, so that bacteria translocating from the gut can be promptly killed. In addition, means of preventing, limiting or speeding the repair of the acquired intestinal mucosal injury that frequently occurs after shock, sepsis or trauma are required.

Progress being made in this area includes the use of specific nutrients (glutamine and dietary fibre), growth factors and trophic gut hormones, as well as early enteral feeding to prevent or limit gut atrophy or injury. Since the starved gut loses mucosal mass and villous height, and becomes more permeable to intraluminal bacteria and endotoxin, early enteral feeding may be important in maintaining gut mucosal integrity. Wilmore *et al.* (1988) have recently reviewed the concept that gut barrier failure may occur in critically ill patients due to the fact that current methods of parenteral nutrition do not support mucosal structure or function.

Whether maintenance of mucosal integrity and the preservation of the mucosal barrier to bacterial translocation and endotoxin will prevent sepsis of gut origin or the development or progression of MOF is unknown. Nor is it apparent whether the restoration of mucosal integrity and barrier function in the patient with MOF will result in improved survival. It is known that, in normal circumstances, the normal gut flora acts in concert with the mechanical and immunological defences of the host to directly and indirectly prevent intestinal colonization or overgrowth with potential pathogens. Although many factors may influence the gut flora, including intestinal motility, diet and antibiotics, attempts must be made to maintain the normal ecology of the patient's intestinal microflora. This consideration does not mean that appropriate antibiotics should not be used to treat established infections but it does highlight an additional potential risk of antibiotic therapy.

The classical studies of Border and coworkers have clearly established that a policy of early definitive surgery in trauma victims will improve survival by reducing the incidence of organ failure and sepsis associated with gut dysfunction (Border *et al.* 1987). To explain these observations, Border has proposed that a causal relationship exists between retained necrotic tissue, macrophage activation, gut barrier failure and the subsequent development of MOF. Thus, a policy of immediate definitive surgery to reduce the inflammatory response and the incidence or magnitude of gut failure may prevent the development of a vicious

TABLE 49.7
POTENTIAL THERAPEUTIC OPTIONS

Maintain normal gut microflora
1. Judicious use of systemic and oral antibiotics to maintain colonization resistance
2. Selective antibiotic decontamination with oral antibiotics
3. Maintain gastric acidity by using cytoprotective agents to prevent stress ulceration

Support gut barrier function
1. Early enteral feeding
2. Use of trophic hormones, such as growth hormone

Limit stress state
1. Early definitive surgery
2. Control systemic factors that may affect the gut
3. Prompt diagnosis and control of systemic infections
4. Optimize oxygen delivery to the tissues

Potential therapeutic agents
1. Antioxidants to prevent mucosal damage
2. Use of agents to neutralize or block endotoxin
3. Biological response modifiers to increase host resistance

cycle of gut failure and uncontrolled inflammation leading to more gut failure and further exacerbation of the inflammatory response.

Non-intestinal factors may also impair gut function and lead to gut-mediated distant organ dysfunction. Hypotension, haemodynamic instability or vasoactive agents that decrease intestinal perfusion may promote bacterial translocation or systemic endotoxaemia by increasing intestinal permeability. Systemic insults or drugs that decrease intestinal motility may be deleterious, because ileus is associated with bacterial overgrowth and loss of colonization resistance. Uncontrolled distant infections, such as pneumonias, or the presence of endotoxaemia may alter intestinal permeability and promote the translocation of intestinal bacteria or the escape of endotoxin from the gut. Thus, attention should be paid to systemic factors that may influence intestinal function, as well as factors that directly affect the gut. A summary of the potential clinical options available to prevent or treat gut barrier function is presented in Table 49.7.

SUMMARY AND CONCLUSIONS

The exact relationship of gut failure, bacterial translocation and endotoxaemia to clinical infection, the septic state or MOFS is not known with certainty. However, it is clear that gut failure and the translocation of intestinal bacteria/endotoxin to the portal or systemic circulation is part of the MOFS. Normal GI function is unquestionably altered in patients at risk of developing MOFS and many, if not all, of the defence mechanisms that normally contain bacteria or endotoxin within the intestinal tract are impaired in these patients. They are immunosuppressed and the antibiotic regimens they receive frequently disrupt the normal ecology of the gut microflora, resulting in impaired colonization resistance and intestinal overgrowth with potential pathogens. Gut failure can take many forms, including stress ulcers, ileus and intolerance to enteral feedings, all of which may weaken the gut mucosal barrier to luminal bacteria and endotoxin. Episodes of hypotension or decreased regional perfusion of intestinal segments may lead to gastric or intestinal erosions which could act as portals of entry for intestinal bacteria or endotoxin. Although these clinical studies do not establish a cause and effect relationship between gut failure, systemic sepsis or MOFS, experimental studies clearly document that trauma, impaired host antibacterial defences, shock, malnutrition, intestinal obstruction or disruption of the normal gut flora will promote gut barrier failure and bacterial translocation.

Furthermore, it appears reasonable to assume that in some circumstances gut barrier failure can become self-perpetuating. For example, the endotoxaemic or bacteraemic state can both lead to the further absorption of intestinal endotoxin or bacteria. Since endotoxaemia occurs in patients at risk of developing MOFS and experimentally endotoxin increases intestinal permeability, promotes bacterial translocation, and in combination with other nonlethal insults will induce the development of a lethal septic syndrome, it seems that endotoxaemia may be an important link between gut failure and MOFS. Additionally, it appears that the gut can fuel the septic process in endotoxaemic or bacteraemic patients, in that endotoxaemia or bacteraemia can induce gut barrier failure leading to the further absorption of intestinal endotoxin or bacteria.

Hepatic RES function may be especially important in determining whether translocating bacteria or endotoxin are neutralized or cause organ dysfunction. Not only are Kupffer cells important in preventing portal endotoxin from reaching the systemic circulation but also their state of activity and the mediators and products they liberate may modulate both hepatocyte and distant organ function. Thus, a clinically important relationship appears to exist between the state of the intestinal barrier, Kupffer cell function and distant organ dysfunction.

In putting the phenomena of gut failure and bacterial translocation into perspective, it is important to realize that neither is an all or none phenomenon. Although many of the factors associated with the care of the critically ill patient predispose to gut barrier failure, if the host's other defences are intact, the translocating bacteria are killed and their products, such as endotoxin, are cleared or inactivated. Thus, although disruption or impairment of a single major intestinal defence system consistently promotes bacterial translocation, the translocating bacteria are usually limited to the mesenteric lymph nodes and do not spread systemically. Instead, these translocating bacteria are locally contained and eventually eradicated as the animal or patient recovers. However, if the host's systemic defences are impaired, the translocating bacteria or endotoxin may spread systemically and induce or potentiate distant organ failure ultimately resulting in a lethal septic syndrome.

Thus, there is abundant clinical and extensive experimental evidence to support the hypothesis that gut failure may promote or potentiate the development or progression of MOFS. This is not to say that gut failure is the only cause of MOFS. Nor is failure of the gut–liver axis the only mechanism by which distant organ injury may occur in these patients. It is clear that, in many patients who develop MOFS, gut barrier failure is not the inciting cause. Rather it is the failure to diagnose and/or adequately treat septic foci in the lung, abdomen or elsewhere. None the less, there is a distinct group of patient who develop MOFS, in whom failure of the gut–liver axis is likely to be of aetiological importance.

REFERENCES

Adler R. (1981). *Psychoneuroimmunology*. Orlando: Academic.

Alexander J.W. (1986). Nutrition and infection: new perspectives for an old problem. *Arch. Surg.*, **121**, 966–72.

Ambrose N.S., Johnson M., Burdon D.W. et al. (1984). Incidence of pathogenic bacteria from mesenteric lymph nodes and ileal serosa during chronic disease surgery. *Br. J. Surg.*, **71**, 623–5.

Baue A.E. (1975). Multiple, progressive, or sequential systems failure: a syndrome of the 1970s. *Arch. Surg.*, **110**, 779–81.

Beutler B., Cerami A. (1987). The endogenous mediator of endotoxic shock. *Clin. Res.*, **35**, 192–7.

Border J.R., Hassett J., LaDuca J. et al. (1987). The gut origin septic states in blunt multiple trauma (ISS = 40) in the ICU. *Ann. Surg.*, **206**, 427–48.

Burke J.F. (1961). The effective period of preventive antibiotic action in experimental incisions and dermal lesions. *Surgery*, **50**, 161–8.

Chaudry I.H., Ayala A., Ertel W., Stephan R.N. (1990). Hemorrhage and resuscitation: immunological aspects. *Am. J. Physiol.*, **256**, R663–78.

Deitch E.A. (1988). Does the gut protect or injure patients in the ICU? In *Perspectives in Critical Care, vol. 1* (Cerra F., ed.). St Louis, MO: Quality Medical Publishing Inc., pp. 15–32.

Deitch E.A. (1989). Simple intestinal obstruction causes bacterial translocation in man. *Arch. Surg.*, **124**, 699–701.

Deitch E.A. (1990). Gut failure its role in the multiple organ failure syndrome. In *Multiple Organ Failure* (Deitch E.A., eds). New York: Thieme, pp. 40–59.

Deitch E.A., Gelder F., McDonald J.C. (1984). Sequential prospective analysis of the nonspecific host defense system after thermal injury. *Arch. Surg.*, **119**, 83–9.

Deitch E.A., Dobke M., Baxter C.R. (1985). Failure of local immunity: a predisposing cause of burn wound sepsis. *Arch. Surg.*, **120**, 78–84.

Deitch E.A., Bridges W., Baker J. et al. (1988). Hemorrhagic shock-induced bacterial translocation is reduced by xanthine oxidase inhibition or inactivation. *Surgery*, **104**, 191–8.

Driks M.R., Craven D.E., Celli B.R. et al. (1987). Nosocomial pneumonia in intubated patients given sucralfate as compared with antacids of histamine type 2 blockers: the role of gastric colonization. *N. Engl. J. Med.*, **317**, 1376–82.

Fry D.E. (1988). Multiple system organ failure. *Surg. Clin. North Am.*, **68**, 107–22.

Goris R.J., Beokhorst P.A., Nuytinck K.S. et al. (1985). Multiple organ failure: generalized autodestructive inflammation. *Arch. Surg.*, **120**, 1109–15.

Howard R.J. (1980). Host defense against infection. *Curr. Prob. Surg.*, **17**, 267–317.

Hoyt D.B., Ozkan A.N., Easter D., Pinney E. (1988). Isolation of an immunosuppressive trauma peptide and its relationship to fibronectin. *J. Trauma*, **28**, 907–13.

Jones C.E., Alexander J.W., Fisher M.W. (1973). Clinical evaluation of pseudomonas hyperimmune globulin. *J. Surg. Res.*, **14**, 87–96.

Kisielow P., Hirst J.A., Shiku H., Beverley P.C. et al. (1975). Ly antigens as markers for functionally distinct subpopulations of thymus-derived lymphocytes of the mouse. *Nature*, **253**, 219–20.

Knighton D.R., Halliday B., Hunt T.K. (1986). Oxygen as an antibiotic: a comparison of the effects of inspired oxygen concentration and antibiotic administration on *in vivo* bacterial clearance. *Arch. Surg.*, **121**, 191–5.

Maderazo E.G., Albano S.D., Woronick C.L. et al. (1983). Polymorphonuclear leukocyte migration abnormalities and their significance in seriously traumatized patients. *Ann. Surg.*, **198**, 736–42.

Mansberger A.R., Doran J.E., Treat R. et al. (1989). The influence of fibronectin administration on the incidence of sepsis and septic mortality in severely injured patients. *Ann. Surg.*, **210**, 297–307.

Meakins J.L., McLean A.P., Kelly R. et al. (1978). Delayed hypersensitivity and neutrophil chemotaxis: effect of trauma. *J. Trauma*, **18**, 240–7.

Meakins J.L., Christou N.V., Shizgal H.M. et al. (1979). Therapeutic approaches to anergy in surgical patients: surgery and levamisole. *Ann. Surg.*, **190**, 286–96.

Mochizuki H., Trocki O., Dominioni L. et al. (1984). Mechanism of prevention of postburn hypermetabolism and catabolism by early enteral feeding. *Ann. Surg.* **200**, 297–310.

Moore F.A., Moore E.E., Poggetti R. et al. (1991). Gut bacterial translocation via the portal vein: a clinical prospective with major torso trauma. *J. Trauma*, **31**, 629–38.

Munster A.M., Winchurch R.A., Thupari J.N., Ernst C.B. (1986). Reversal of postburn immunosuppression with low-dose polymyxin B. *J. Trauma*, **26**, 995–8.

Ozkan A.N., Hinnemann L. (1985). Suppression of in

vitro lymphocyte and neutrophil responses by a low molecular weight suppressor active peptide. *J. Clin. Immunol.*, **5**, 172–9.

Paul W.E. (1986). *Fundamental Immunology.* New York: Raven.

Rush B.F. Jr., Sori A.J., Murphy T.F. et al. (1988). Endotoxemia and bacteremia during hemorrhagic shock: the link between trauma and sepsis? *Ann. Surg.*, **207**, 549–54.

Schoeneberger G.H., Burkhardt F., Kalberer F. et al. (1975). Experimental evidence for a significant impairment of host defense for gram-negative organisms by a specific cutaneous toxin produced by severe burn injuries. *Surg. Gynecol. Obstet.*, **141**, 555–61.

Simmons R.L., Howard R.J. (eds) (1988). *Surgical infectious diseases*, 2nd edn. New York: Appleton-Century-Crofts.

Solomkin J.L., Simmons R.L. (1983). Cellular and subcellular mediators of acute inflammation. *Surg. Clin. North Am.*, **63**, 225–43.

Stoutenbeek C.P., Van Saene H.K.F., Miranda D.R. et al. (1987). The effect of oropharyngeal decontamination using topical nonabsorbable antibiotics on the incidence of nosocomial respiratory tract infections in multiple trauma patients. *J. Trauma*, **27**, 357–64.

Tancrede C.H., Andremont A.O. (1985) Bacterial translocation and gram-negative bacteremia in patients with hematological malignancies. *J. Infect. Dis.*, **152**, 99–103.

Thomas L. (1974). *The Lives of a Cell: notes of a biology watcher.* New York: Viking.

van der Waaij D., Berghuis-de Vries J.M., Lekkerkerk-van der Wees J.E.C. (1971). Colonization resistance of the digestive tract in conventional and antibiotic-treated mice. *J. Hyg. (Camb.)*, **69**, 405–11.

Waymack J.P., Jenkins M., Warden G.D. et al. (1987). A prospective study of thymopentin in severely burned patients. *Surg. Gynecol. Obstet.*, **164**, 423–30.

Waymack J.P., Jenkins M., Alexander J.W. et al. (1989). A prospective trial of prophylactic intravenous immune globulin for the prevention of infections in severely burned patients. *Burns*, **15**, 71–6.

Wilmore D.W., Smith R.J., O'Dwyer S.T. et al. (1988). The gut: a central organ after surgical stress. *Surgery*, **104**, 917–23.

Xu D., Deitch E.A., Sittig K. et al. (1988). *In vitro* cell mediated immunity after thermal injury is not impaired: density gradient purification of mononuclear cells is associated with spurious (artifactual) immunosuppression. *Ann. Surg.*, **208**, 768–75.

Ziegler E.J., McCutchan J.A., Fierer J. et al. (1982). Treatment of gram-negative bacteremia and shock with human antiserum to a mutant *Escherichia coli*. *N. Engl. J. Med.*, **307**, 1225–30.

Index

Coventry University

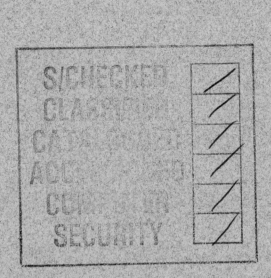